Mastering Refractive IOLs
The Art and Science

EDITOR

DAVID F. CHANG, MD

CLINICAL PROFESSOR, UNIVERSITY OF CALIFORNIA

SAN FRANCISCO, CALIFORNIA

ASSOCIATE EDITORS

STEVEN J. DELL, MD
DELL LASER CONSULTANTS
TEXAN EYE
AUSTIN, TEXAS

WARREN E. HILL, MD
EAST VALLEY OPHTHALMOLOGY
MESA, ARIZONA

RICHARD L. LINDSTROM, MD
MINNESOTA EYE CONSULTANTS
BLOOMINGTON, MINNESOTA

KEVIN L. WALTZ, OD, MD
EYE SURGEONS OF INDIANA
INDIANAPOLIS, INDIANA

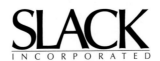

SLACK
INCORPORATED

*Delivering the best in health care information
and education worldwide*

www.slackbooks.com

ISBN: 978-1-55642-859-3

The procedures and practices described in this book should be implemented in a manner consistent with the professional standards set for the circumstances that apply in each specific situation. Every effort has been made to confirm the accuracy of the information presented and to correctly relate generally accepted practices. The authors, editor, and publisher cannot accept responsibility for errors or exclusions or for the outcome of the material presented herein. There is no expressed or implied warranty of this book or information imparted by it. Care has been taken to ensure that drug selection and dosages are in accordance with currently accepted/recommended practice. Due to continuing research, changes in government policy and regulations, and various effects of drug reactions and interactions, it is recommended that the reader carefully review all materials and literature provided for each drug, especially those that are new or not frequently used. Any review or mention of specific companies or products is not intended as an endorsement by the author or publisher.

SLACK Incorporated uses a review process to evaluate submitted material. Prior to publication, educators or clinicians provide important feedback on the content that we publish. We welcome feedback on this work.

Contact SLACK Incorporated for more information about other books in this field or about the availability of our books from distributors outside the United States.

Published by: SLACK Incorporated
                 6900 Grove Road
                 Thorofare, NJ 08086 USA
                 Telephone: 856-848-1000
                 Fax: 856-853-5991
                 www.slackbooks.com

Library of Congress Cataloging-in-Publication Data

Mastering refractive IOLs : the art and science / editor, David F. Chang.
       p. ; cm.
  Includes bibliographical references and index.
  ISBN 978-1-55642-859-3 (alk. paper)
  1. Intraocular lenses. I. Chang, David F., 1954-
  [DNLM: 1. Lens Implantation, Intraocular--methods. WW 358 M423 2008]
  RE988.M37 2008
  617.7'1--dc22

                        2008002676

Printed in the United States of America.

Last digit is print number: 10 9 8 7 6 5 4 3 2

Dedication

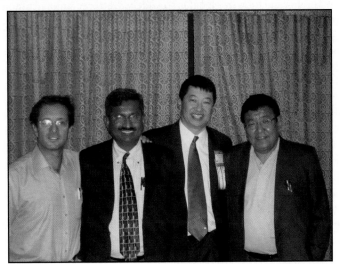

From l to r: Drs. Geoff Tabin, R. D. Ravindran, David F. Chang, and Sanduk Ruit.

This textbook highlights the latest advances in refractive IOL technology and surgery. No longer satisfied with simply treating cataracts, our efforts are now focused on reversing lens aging through the pseudophakic correction of presbyopia. Amidst such exciting advances, it is easy to forget that the greatest challenge in the field of cataract and IOL surgery continues to be the staggering and increasing backlog of cataract blindness in developing countries.

Modern phacoemulsification machines are expensive to purchase and maintain, incur relatively high disposable costs, and require extensive surgical training. Furthermore, for the more advanced and mature cataracts typical of underserved populations, performing phacoemulsification becomes more difficult and complication prone. What is needed is a high-volume, cost-effective, "low tech" procedure that can treat the most advanced of cataracts with a low complication rate in the shortest amount of time.

This very goal is being achieved in a handful of international programs that are providing a hopeful paradigm for overcoming cataract blindness worldwide. I have had the privilege of visiting and collaborating with doctors at both the Aravind Eye Hospital network in Southern India, and the Tilganga Eye Center in Kathmandu, Nepal. Observing first-hand how these 2 systems provide low-cost, high-volume and quality cataract surgery is an awe-inspiring experience for any visiting ophthalmologist.

Founded in 1976 by the legendary Dr. G. Venkataswamy, Aravind Eye Hospital has grown into a network of 5 regional eye hospitals providing high-level ophthalmic care to the poor population of Southern India. Private paying patients comprise approximately 30% of their patient base. This revenue funds the 70% of Aravind's services that are provided at no cost to the indigent via a financially self-sustaining program that receives minimal government reimbursement. In terms of cataract surgery, this means that of the approximately 200,000 procedures performed annually in the Aravind system, 70% are provided for free.

While private cataract patients at Aravind may pay anywhere from $200 to $300 to undergo phacoemulsification with foldable IOLs imported from the United States, the nonpaying cataract patients are treated for less than $15 per case, including the IOL. This is accomplished by performing a manual, sutureless, small incision extracapsular procedure with reusable equipment and supplies. Their IOL manufacturing facility, Aurolab, produces PMMA IOLs for less than $5 per lens. Following a retrobulbar block, the nucleus is expressed through a capsulorrhexis and a temporal, self-sealing 6.0- to 6.5-mm scleral pocket incision. Manual cortical cleanup precedes capsular bag implantation of a square edge PMMA IOL. The technique is commonly abbreviated as manual SICS (small incision cataract surgery).

While the procedure itself seems straightforward, it is the stunning speed, skill, and efficiency with which it is performed that must literally be seen to be believed. By alternating between 2 parallel operating room tables, a single surgeon is able to perform over 15 cases per hour by consistently completing sub-5-minute procedures on the densest of cataracts with no intervening turnover time. To ensure efficiency across different surgical teams, every aspect of the procedure is standardized, from preoperative patient and instrument preparation to the surgical steps themselves. Having been screened in outlying rural eye camps, as many as 300 to 400 cataract patients will be bused to a regional Aravind eye hospital where they will all undergo their surgery on one single day. After several days of in-house follow-up, they are transported back to their rural villages where a local postoperative visit and refraction are performed 1 month later by the Aravind staff.

Founded in 1994 by Dr. Sanduk Ruit, the Tilganga Eye Center is a shining example of an efficient eye care delivery system on a smaller scale. Dr. Ruit has developed his own variation of the manual, sutureless SICS. Our prospective randomized trial comparing phaco and manual, sutureless SICS in a camp population showed that the latter method produces excellent results at a fraction of the cost of phaco.[1] Tilganga Eye Center is also financially self-sustaining wherein private care subsidizes charity care. They also have their own IOL manufacturing facility, which, like that at Aravind, is able to supply low-cost IOLs to other developing countries. Because the rural population in Nepal is so widely scattered amongst mountain villages that are accessible only by foot, the Tilganga system strives to deliver portable cataract care by transporting the necessary staff and equipment to remote eye camps. Using a single portable operating table, the Tilganga surgeons can also perform more than 10 cataract surgeries per hour. As at Aravind, the high-volume, cost-effective Tilganga surgical techniques and protocols are standardized across their surgical teams. Since 1994 when Dr. Ruit and Dr. Geoff Tabin co-founded the Himalayan Cataract Project, Tilganga ophthalmologists and staff have provided mobile cataract surgical care and physician training in numerous developing countries across mountainous Asia.

Though of a different scale and serving different types of communities, Aravind and Tilganga are complimentary models of how best to address the world's backlog of cataract blindness. They demonstrate that the solution requires not only a cost-effective surgical technique, but also an entire system of efficient and financially self-sustaining cataract care delivery. Beyond the impressive productivity of these 2 institutions, equally important has been their mission to train surgical teams from other developing countries in their methods of cataract surgery. An efficient, high-volume system utilizing low cost, sub-5-minute procedures to tackle advanced cataracts with minimal complications is clearly the best way to leverage the scarcest and most precious asset of the system—the cataract surgeon.

I consider this work to be the most inspiring and impressive accomplishment in our field of cataract surgery and it is with great respect and admiration that I dedicate this textbook to my friends at the Aravind and Tilganga Eye Hospitals. They are the unsung but true heroes in our field, and as we struggle to meet the high refractive expectations of our premium IOL patients, we must remember and salute our colleagues in developing countries that are on the frontlines of the most important surgical battlefield.

Reference

1. Ruit S, Tabin G, Chang DF, et al. A prospective randomized clinical trial of phacoemulsification vs manual sutureless small incision extracapsular cataract surgery in Nepal. *Am J Ophthalmol.* 2007;143:32-38.

In addition to his Advanced Medical Optics, Alcon, and Visiogen consulting fees, Dr. Chang will also donate any royalties from this book to the Himalayan Cataract Project.

Contents

Acknowledgments

Compiling this textbook was a colossal venture and adventure that was completed in record time. I first approached SLACK Incorporated with the idea during the 2007 ASCRS meeting where, judging from attendance at symposia and instruction courses, interest in refractive IOLs was rising along a steep trajectory. The need for more physician-to-physician education on the subject was very obvious. However, whether it was a symposium, instruction course, booth presentation, or users meeting, there was always far too much material to cover in the available time. So many of the pearls I learned were beyond the realm of evidence-based medicine. Where could all of this information be found or collected? Recognizing the pressing and unmet need for a comprehensive textbook, we established the ambitious goal of completing this book in time for the 2008 ASCRS meeting—a 9-month publishing cycle.

My initial plan was to assemble a manual for transitioning to refractive IOLs. So many colleagues have yet to embark on this odyssey and the number of hurdles for the beginning refractive IOL surgeon is daunting. It soon became obvious, however, that the educational process is far more than a series of "transitioning" steps because there really is no endpoint. Regardless of our experience, we are all continually learning new insights and approaches in our quest to improve. What began as a modest beginner's manual therefore morphed into a comprehensive 236-chapter textbook on mastering the multidisciplinary and multidimensional skills necessary for success as a refractive IOL surgeon.

I am truly grateful to my 4 associate editors, Steven J. Dell, Warren E. Hill, Richard L. Lindstrom, and Kevin L. Waltz, each of whom is among the most influential innovators, opinion leaders, and educators in the refractive IOL field. Whether as authors, editors, or as a collective sounding board for selecting topics and authors, their influence and guidance is evident throughout the book. I have enjoyed creating a lasting testament to our collaboration and friendship.

I particularly want to thank the more than 200 authors who have written original chapters for this textbook. To possess the expertise that makes each of them an effective teacher means that they are all very busy clinicians. Writing and illustrating chapters during weekends under tight deadlines is a thankless job. I hope you readers appreciate the generosity of their time in sharing their personal experiences and lessons with you.

Finally, this was a project that put SLACK Incorporated's fine Book Division to the ultimate test. I am fortunate to have such an excellent working relationship with John Bond and Jennifer Briggs, who gave me the freedom and flexibility to steer this, our third textbook project, in the direction that I wanted. They are truly dedicated professionals who managed the entire process from pilot concept to final deadline. With the support of Managing Editor, Kimberly Shigo, Senior Project Editor, April Billick turned in another unbelievable job with the layout and the editing process. Managing so much material from so many authors under such tight deadlines is a testament to April's organizational skills and excellence as an editor. That I would even consider undertaking such an ambitious project is a measure of my respect and high regard for the SLACK Incorporated team.

Finally, writing on behalf of my 4 associate editors and our more than 200 coauthors, we would like to thank our families for allowing us to devote our precious time and energy toward compiling a resource that we hope will help all refractive IOL surgeons and their patients worldwide.

David F. Chang, MD

About the Editor

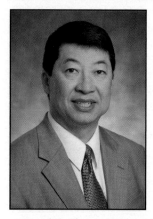

David F. Chang, MD is a Summa Cum Laude graduate of Harvard College and earned his MD at Harvard Medical School. He completed his ophthalmology residency at the University of California, San Francisco (UCSF) where he is now a clinical professor. Dr. Chang is Chairman of the American Academy of Ophthalmology (AAO) Annual Meeting Program Committee, having previously chaired the Cataract Program Subcommittee. He organized and was the program cochair for the first 7 AAO "Spotlight on Cataracts" Symposia. He is also on the program committees for the ASCRS Annual Meeting and the OSN Hawaiian Eye Meeting.

He has been selected to deliver the following named lectures: Transamerica Lecture (UCSF), Williams Lecture (UCSF), Wolfe Lecture (University of Iowa), DeVoe Lecture (Columbia-Harkness), Gettes Lecture (Wills Eye Hospital), Helen Keller Lecture (University of Alabama), Kayes Lecture (University of Washington, St. Louis), Thorpe Lecture (Pittsburgh Ophthalmology Society), Schutz Lecture (New York University Medical Center), Wallace-Evan Lecture (Casey Eye, Oregon), Proctor Lecture (UCSF/Proctor Foundation), and the keynote address at the Chinese American Ophthalmological Society's 20th anniversary meeting. He is a 3-time AAO Secretariat Award recipient (2003, 2006, 2007). He was the inaugural recipient of the UCSF Department of Ophthalmology's Distinguished Alumni Award (2005) and in 2006 became only the third ophthalmologist to ever receive the Charlotte Baer Award honoring the outstanding clinical faculty member at the UCSF Medical School. He was the third recipient of the Strampelli Medal from the Italian Ophthalmological Society (2007).

Dr. Chang is chairman of the AAO Practicing Ophthalmologists' Curriculum Panel for Cataract and Anterior Segment, which developed the American Board of Ophthalmology knowledge base for the MOC examination. He is also on the AAO Cataract Preferred Practice Pattern Panel and the AAO Revitalization Study Group. Dr. Chang is chair of the ASCRS Cataract Clinical Committee and is a member of the ASCRS Eye Surgery Education Council Presbyopia Task Force. He is on the Board of Directors for the Pan American Association of Ophthalmology. He is on the scientific advisory board for the UCSF Collaborative Vision Research Group, American Medical Optics, Allergan ATLAS, Calhoun Vision, Medennium, Peak Surgical, and Visiogen, and is the medical monitor for the Visiogen Synchrony accommodating IOL FDA monitored trial. He is cochief medical editor for *Cataract and Refractive Surgery Today* and developed the *CRSToday Virtual Textbook of Cataract Surgery*. He is the cataract editor for 2 online educational sites: the AAO's "Specialty Clinical Updates" and the *Ocular Surgery News'* "Ophthalmic Hyperguides." He is an associate editor for the 3rd edition of *Cataract Surgery* (Elsevier 2008, Roger F. Steinert, editor). He was the chief editor for *Curbside Consultation in Cataract Surgery* (SLACK Incorporated, 2007), the series editor for the 7 SLACK Incorporated Curbside Consultation in Ophthalmology textbooks, and the principal author of *Phaco Chop* (SLACK Incorporated, 2004), which was the first ophthalmic textbook with a paired DVD featuring instructional surgical video. Finally, his coauthored 2005 report on IFIS and tamsulosin is one of the 5 most cited papers from the *Journal of Cataract and Refractive Surgery* (Source: Editorial, *JCRS* 1/08).

About the Associate Editors

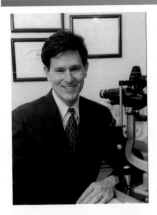

Steven J. Dell, MD is Medical Director of Dell Laser Consultants and Director of Refractive and Corneal Surgery at Texan Eye in Austin, Texas. He serves on the Refractive Surgery Clinical Committee of the American Society of Cataract and Refractive Surgery and is a popular lecturer at meetings worldwide. He is the inventor of several popular surgical instruments and medical devices. Dr. Dell serves on the editorial boards of *Ocular Surgery News, Cataract and Refractive Surgery Today, The Video Journal of Ophthalmology,* and *Cataract and Refractive Surgery Today—Europe.* Dr. Dell is a board-certified member of the American Board of Ophthalmology, a Fellow of the American Academy of Ophthalmology, and a member of the American Society of Cataract and Refractive Surgery. He works closely with a variety of ophthalmic companies in the development of new products and technologies and serves as a consultant to several major companies in the industry.

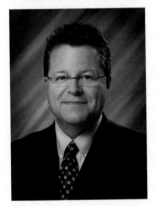

Warren E. Hill, MD has served as the Medical Director of East Valley Ophthalmology in Mesa, Arizona for the past 22 years, specializing in consultative ophthalmology, challenging anterior segment surgery and intraocular lens power calculations.

Dr. Hill received BS and BA undergraduate degrees at the University of Maryland, a Doctor of Medicine from the University of Arizona, and completed an ophthalmology residency at the University of Rochester, in Rochester, New York. Dr. Hill is also a member of the International Intra-Ocular Implant Club, a Fellow of the American College of Surgeons, the American Academy of Ophthalmology, the International College of Surgeons, and the American College of Eye Surgeons.

Dr. Hill has devoted much of his professional activities to the mathematics of intraocular lens power calculations in complex and unusual clinical situations. He is a consultant to industry in the field of intraocular lens mathematics, intraocular lens design, and optical coherence biometry. He has published many scientific articles, served as visiting professor for numerous grand rounds, and has delivered more than 200 presentations to ophthalmic societies in both the United States and internationally in 20 countries and on 6 continents.

Aside from his interest in ophthalmology, Dr. Hill is a multi-engine, instrument-rated commercial pilot.

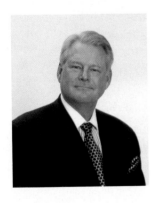

Richard L. Lindstrom, MD, founder and attending surgeon of Minnesota Eye Consultants and Adjunct Professor Emeritus at the University of Minnesota Department of Ophthalmology, is a board-certified ophthalmologist and internationally recognized leader in corneal, cataract, refractive, and laser surgery. He has been at the forefront of ophthalmology's evolutionary changes throughout his career, as a recognized researcher, teacher, inventor, writer, lecturer, and highly acclaimed physician and surgeon.

After graduating Magna Cum Laude from the College of Liberal Arts at the University of Minnesota, Dr. Lindstrom completed his doctorate degree in medicine in 1972. He conducted research, residency, and fellowship training in cornea at the University of Minnesota and affiliated hospitals and extended his anterior segment surgery fellowship training at Mary Shiels Hospital in Dallas and was a Heed Fellow in Glaucoma at University Hospital in Salt Lake City. In 1980, Dr. Lindstrom returned to the University of Minnesota, where he spent 10 years on the faculty of the Department of Ophthalmology, the last two as a full professor and the Harold G. Scheie Research Chair. He continues as Adjunct Professor Emeritus, Chairman of the Vision Foundation, and Associate Director of the Minnesota Lions Eye Bank at the University of Minnesota. He entered private practice in 1989 and has led the growth and expansion of Minnesota Eye Consultants, serving as managing partner for 15 years. He is also medical director of TLC Vision, Midwest Surgical Services, and Refractec. He is Chief Medical Editor of the USA and International editions of *Ocular Surgery News,* which reaches 82,000 ophthalmologists worldwide.

Dr. Lindstrom currently served as President (2007-2008) of the American Society of Cataract and Refractive Surgeons; he also serves on the Executive Committee and is the Chair of the Corporate Gifts Committee for the ASCRS Foundation. He has in the past served as the President of the International Society of Refractive Surgery, the International Intraocular Implant Club, and the International Refractive Surgery Club. He is the Global Education Liaison of the International Society of Refractive Surgery of the American Academy of Ophthalmology.

He is Chairman and CEO of Lindstrom Cleaning and Construction, a three-generation family business. He has endowed funds supporting the University of Minnesota Department of Ophthalmology, the Eye Bank Association of America, and the University of Minnesota Tennis Team.

Dr. Lindstrom holds over 30 patents in ophthalmology and has developed a number of solutions, intraocular lenses, and instruments that are used in clinical practices globally. He serves on the Board of Directors of AcuFocus, Inc, TLC Vision, Occulogix, Eyeonics, Refractec, the Minnesota Medical Foundation, and Inner City Tennis.

A frequent lecturer throughout the world on cornea, cataract, and refractive surgery, he has presented over 37 named lectures and keynote speeches before professional societies in the United States and abroad, most recently giving the Blumenthal Memorial lecture in Jerusalem, Israel, the Benedetto Strampelli Medal Lecture in Rome, Italy, and the Albrecht von Garefe-Vorlesung Innovator's Lecture in Nuremberg, Germany.

Dr. Lindstrom serves on a number of journal editorial boards, including *Journal of Cataract and Refractive Surgery, Journal of Refractive Surgery,* and *Ophthalmic Surgery.* He is the Honorary Editor-in-Chief of the US/Chinese *Journal of Ophthalmology.* He has coedited 7 books, published over 350 peer-reviewed journal articles, and 60 book chapters. His professional affiliations are extensive, including Liaison of the International Society of Refractive Surgery of the American Academy of Ophthalmology.

He is the recipient of numerous awards for distinguished service by national and international ophthalmology associations, including the LANS, Barraquer and the first lifetime achievement award from the International Society of Refractive Surgery in October 1995 and also was honoured with another lifetime achievement award in October 2002, the Binkhorst Lecture Award from the American Society of Cataract and Refractive Surgery, the Bausch and Lomb Lifetime Achievement Award, April 2005, and the Paton Award and NACT from the Eye Bank Association of America.

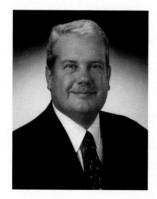

Kevin L. Waltz, OD, MD was a founding partner of Eye Surgeons of Indiana in Indianapolis in 1993. He has a long-standing interest in refractive surgery as one of the few doctors who was trained in both optometry and ophthalmology. He graduated from the Indiana University School of Optometry in 1981 and the Meharry Medical College in 1987. He completed a 2-year fellowship at the Southern College School of Optometry in 1983. He completed an internship at Vanderbilt University in 1988 and his residency in ophthalmology at the University of Florida in 1991. He completed a 1-year fellowship in ophthalmic plastic and reconstructive surgery in 1992. He was the first ophthalmologist in the world to receive the Array Multifocal IOL as a patient in 1998 and one of the first ophthalmologists in the world to implant the Array in refractive surgery patients. He coined the name PRELEX or presbyopic lens exchange to describe refractive lens surgery. He has taught other doctors from around the world how to successfully incorporate PRELEX into their practice. He first described accommodative arching of the Crystalens in 2004. He remains actively involved in the research and development of surgical eye care.

Contributing Authors

Richard L. Abbott, MD
Thomas W. Boyden Health Sciences Clinical Professor of Ophthalmology
Beckman Vision Center
University of California San Francisco
Research Associate
Francis I. Proctor Foundation
San Francisco, CA
Board Member
Chairman of Underwriting Committee
Ophthalmic Mutual Insurance Company
San Francisco, CA

Natalie A. Afshari, MD
Associate Professor of Ophthalmology
Cornea and Refractive Surgery
Duke University Eye Center
Duke University Medical Center
Durham, NC

Iqbal Ike K. Ahmed, MD
University of Toronto
Toronto, Ontario

Yachna Ahuja, MD
Case Western Reserve University
Cleveland, OH

Leonardo Akaishi, MD
Member of the Editorial Board of Oftalmologia em FOCO
Director of HOB
Brasilia Ophtalmologic Hospital

Alan B. Aker, MD
Medical Director, Aker-Kasten Eye Center
Boca Raton, FL

Avery Alexander, MD
Theda Clark Medical Center
Neenah, WI
Appleton Medical Center
Appleton WI

José F. Alfonso, MD, PhD
Instituto Ofthalmológico Fernández-Vega
Oviedo, Spain
Surgery Department, School of Medicine
University of Oviedo
Oviedo, Spain

Jorge L. Alió, MD, PhD
Department of Ophthalmology
Miguel Hernández University School of Medicine
VISSUM—Instituto Oftalmológico de Alicante
Department of Cornea and Refractive Surgery
Alicante, Spain

David Allen, BSc, FRCS, FRCOphth
Consultant Ophthalmologist, Sunderland Eye Infirmary
Sunderland, England

Noel Alpins, FRANZCO, FRCOphth, FACS
Associate Fellow
University of Melbourne
Victoria, Australia

Lisa Brothers Arbisser, MD
Eye Surgeons Associates, PC
Iowa and Illinois Quad Cities
Adjunct Associate Clinical Professor
University of Utah Moran Eye Center
Salt Lake City, UT

Pablo Artal, PhD
Laboratorio de Optica
Centro de Investigacion en Optica y Nanofisica (CiOyN)
Universidad de Murcia
Campus de Espinardo
Murcia, Spain

Kerry K. Assil, MD
CEO and Medical Director
Assil Eye Institute
Beverly Hills, CA

Federico Badala, MD
Fellow, CODET Aris Vision Institute
Toluco, Mexico

Jay Bansal, MD
Medical Director, LaserVue Eye Center
Santa Rosa, CA

Graham D. Barrett, MBBCh, FRANZCO, FRACS
Lions Eye Institute
Perth, Australia

George Beiko, BM, BCh, FRCS(C)
Assistant Prof, McMaster University
Hamilton, Ontario, Canada
Lecturere, University of Toronto
Toronto, Ontario, Canada

Roberto Bellucci, MD
Chief of the Hospital Ophthalmic Unit
Hospital and University of Verona
Verona, Italy

Joshua Ben-Nun, MD
Vitro-retinal specialist
NuLens Founder & CSO
Hertzliya-Pituach, Israel

Abdhish R. Bhavsar, MD
Director, Clinical Research, Retina Center, PA
Minneapolis, MN
Attending Surgeon, Phillips Eye Institute
Minneapolis, MN
Adjunct Associate Professor, University of Minnesota
Minneapolis, MN

Brian S. Boxer Wachler, MD
Boxer Wachler Vision Institute
Beverly Hills, CA

Rosa Braga-Mele, MD, MEd, FRCSC
Associate Professor, University of Toronto
Director of Cataract Unit, Mt. Sinai Hospital
Director of Clinical Research, Kensington Eye Institute
Toronto, Canada

Michael B. Brenner, MD, FICS
Clinical Adjunct Professor
Southern California College of Optometry
Surgical Director, Presbyopic Services
TLC Laser Eye Center
Torrance, CA

Frank A. Bucci, Jr, MD
Medical Director
Bucci Laser Vision Institute and Ambulatory Surgery Center
Wilkes Barre, PA

Carlos Buznego, MD
President and Anterior Segment Surgeon
Center for Excellence in Eye Care
Miami, FL
Voluntary Assistant Professor of Ophthalmology
Bascom Palmer Eye Institute
Miami, FL

Stephen Bylsma, MD
Assistant Clinical Instructor
Department of Ophthalmology
UCLA
Los Angeles, CA
Private Practice
Santa Maria, CA

Matthew C. Caldwell, MD
Cornea and Refractive Surgery Fellow
Duke University Eye Center
Durham, NC

Fabrizio I. Camesasca, MD
Department of Ophthalmology
Istituto Clinico Humanitas
Rozzano, Milano, Italy

Charles Campbell

Harvey Carter, MD
LSU Medical School
New Orleans, LA
Presbyterian Hospital of Dallas, North Dallas Surgicare
Dallas, TX

Jeffrey J. Caspar, MD
Associate Professor
Residency Program Director
University of California Davis Medical Center
Sacramento, CA

David Castillejos, MD
Chula Vista, CA

Timothy B. Cavanaugh, MD
President and Medical Director, Cavanaugh Eye Center and Laser Vision Center
Kansas City, KS
Director, Deer Creek Surgery Center
Kansas City, KS

Shiao Chang, PhD
V.P. Materials
Calhoun Vision
Pasadena, CA

William Jerry Chang, MD
Chief, Department of Ophthalmology
Kaiser Permanente Medical Group
Redwood City, CA

Geoff Charlton
President, ForSight Strategies
Olympia, WA

Arturo Chayet, MD
Director CODET Aris Vision Institute
Toluco, Mexico

William K. Christian, MD
Associate Cataract and Refractive Surgeon
Assil Eye Institute
Beverly Hills, CA

Y. Ralph Chu, MD
Founder and Medical Director, Chu Vision Institute, PA
Edina, MN
Adjunct Assistant Professor of Ophthalmology
University of Minnesota
Minneapolis, MN
Professor of Ophthalmology
University of Utah (Moran Eye Institute)
Salt Lake City, UT

John Ciccone
Director of Communications
American Society of Cataract and Refractive Surgery
Fairfax, VA

Robert J. Cionni, MD
Medical Director
Cincinnati Eye Institute
Cincinnati, OH
The Eye Institute of Utah
Salt Lake City, UT
Adjunct Professor of Ophthalmology
The University of Cincinnati
Cincinnati, OH
The John Moran Eye Center
The University of Utah
Salt Lake City, UT

Tom M. Coffman, MD
Clinical Assistant Professor
Nova Southeastern University
Ft. Lauderdale, FL
Private practice, Visual Health
Palms Springs, FL

D. Michael Colvard, MD, FACS
Associate Clinical Professor
Doheny Eye Institute
Keck School of Medicine
University of Southern California
Encino, CA

J. Andy Corley
Chairman and CEO
Eyeonics, Inc
Aliso Viejo, CA

Kay Coulson, MBA
President
Elective Medical Marketing
Boulder, CO

Alan S. Crandall, MD
Professor and Senior Vice Chair of Ophthalmology & Visual Sciences,
Director of Glaucoma and Cataract
John A. Moran Eye Center
University of Utah
Salt Lake City, Utah

William W. Culbertson, MD
Professor of Ophthalmology,
Bascom Palmer Eye Institute
University of Miami Miller School of Medicine
Miami, Florida

James A. Davies, MD, FACS
InnoVision EyeCare Centers
Medical Director, Surgical Eye Care Center/Ambulatory Surgical Center
Carlsbad, CA

Dan Davis, OD
Clinical Associate, Chu Vision Institute, PA
Edina, MN

Elizabeth A. Davis, MD, FACS
Adjunct Clinical Assistant Professor of Ophthalmology
University of Minnesota Department of Ophthalmology
Director, Minnesota Eye Laser and Surgery Center
Minnesota Eye Consultants
Minneapolis, MN

James A. Davison, MD, FACS
Wolfe Eye Clinic
Marshalltown, IA

James D. Dawes, MHA, CMPE, COE
Chief Administrative Officer, Center For Sight
Venice, FL

Sheraz M. Daya, MD, FACP, FACS, FRCS(Ed)
Centre for Sight
Corneoplastic Unit & Eye Bank
Queen Victoria Hospital
Sussex, United Kingdom

David J. Deitz, MPhil
McDonald Eye Associates
Fayetteville AR

Jim Denning, BS
CEO, Discover Vision Centers
Independence, MO

Kevin Denny, MD
Chief, Cataract and Anterior Segment Surgery
Department of Ophthalmology
California Pacific Medical Center
San Francisco, CA

Uday Devgan, MD, FACS
Maloney Vision Institute
Chief of Ophthalmology, Olive View—UCLA Medical Center
UCLA School of Medicine
Los Angeles, CA

Steven Dewey, MD
Private Practice
Colorado Springs, CO

H. Burkbard Dick, MD
Professor and Chairman, Director
Center for Vision Science
Ruhr University Eye Hospital
Bochum, Germany

John F. Doane, MD
Refractive Surgeon, Discover Vision Centers
Kansas City, MO
Associate Clinical Professor
University of Kansas Department of Ophthalmology
Lawrence, KS

Eric Donnenfeld, MD
Ophthalmic Consultants of Long Island
Long Island, NY
Trustee, Dartmouth Medical School
Hanover, NH

Paul Dougherty, MD
Clinical Instructor of Ophthalmology
Jules Stein Eye Institute
University of California, Los Angeles
Medical Director
Dougherty Laser Vision
Los Angeles and Camarillo, CA

Paul Ernest, MD
TLC Eyecare and Laser Center
Jackson, MI

Ahmad M. Fahmy, OD, FAAO
Attending Optometrist, Minnesota Eye Consultants
Minneapolis, MN

Luis E. Fernández de Castro, MD
Magill Research Center for Vision Correction
Storm Eye Institute
Medical University of South Carolina
Charleston, SC

Luis Fernández-Vega, MD, PhD
Instituto Ofthalmológico Fernández-Vega
Oviedo, Spain and
Surgery Department, School of Medicine,
University of Oviedo, Spain.

I. Howard Fine, MD
Clinical Professor
Oregon Health & Science University
Drs. Fine, Hoffman and Packer
Eugene, OR

William J. Fishkind, MD, FACS
Co-Director, Fishkind and Bakewell Eye Care and Surgery Center
Tucson, AZ
Clinical Professor of Ophthalmology
University of Utah
Salt Lake City, Utah
Clinical Instructor
University of Arizona
Tucson, AZ

Michael T. Furlong, MD
Medical Director, Furlong Vision Correction
San Jose, CA

Ron P. Gallemore, MD, PhD
Director and Founder
Retina Macula Institute
Torrance, CA
Assistant Clinical Professor
Jules Stein Eye Institute
UCLA School of Medicine
Los Angeles, CA

Andrea Galvis, MD
Department of Ophthalmology
Fundacion Clinica Valle del Lili
Cali, Colombia

William D. Gaskins, MD, FACS
Gaskins Eye Care and Surgery Center
Naples, FL

Johnny L. Gayton, MD
Eyesight Associates
Warner Robins, GA

Pietro Giardini, MD
Polivisus
Brescia, Italy

James P. Gills, MD
Clinical Professor of Ophthalmology
University of South Florida
Tampa, FL
Consulting Professor of Ophthalmology
Duke University
Durham, NC
St. Luke's Cataract and Laser Institute
Tarpon Springs, FL

Pit Gills, MD
St. Luke's Cataract and Laser Institute
Tarpon Springs, FL

Frank Jozef Goes, MD
GOES Eye Centre
Antwerp, Belgium

Harry B. Grabow, MD
Clinical Assistant Professor, University of South Florida
Tampa, FL
Medical Director, Sarasota Cataract & Laser Institute
Center for Advanced Eye Surgery
Sarasota, FL

Oscar Gris, MD
Cornea and Refractive Surgery Unit
Instituto de Microcirugía Ocular
Barcelona, Spain

Jose L. Güell, MD
Associate Professor of Ophthalmology
Autonoma University of Barcelona
Director of Cornea and refractive Surgery Unit
Instituto Microcirugia Ocular de Barcelona
Barcelona, Spain

D. Rex Hamilton, MD, MS, FACS
Director, UCLA Laser Refractive Center
Assistant Professor of Ophthalmology
Jules Stein Eye Institute
Los Angeles, CA

David R. Hardten, MD
Adjunct Associate Professor of Ophthalmology
University of Minnesota Department of Ophthalmology
Director of Refractive Surgery
Minnesota Eye Consultants
Minneapolis, MN

R. Lee Harman, MD, FACS
President/CEO
The Harman Eye Clinic
Arlington, WA
Co-Owner, LEGACY Strategic Consultant, LLC
Camano Island, WA

David Harmon
President and Executive Editor
Market Scope

Nicola Hauranieh, MD
Polivisus
Brescia, Italy

Weldon W. Haw, MD
Associate Clinical Professor of Ophthalmology
Cornea, Cataract, and Refractive Surgery
UCSD School of Medicine
La Jolla, CA

Bonnie An Henderson, MD
Assistant Clinical Professor, Harvard Medical School
Partner, Ophthalmic Consultants of Boston
Boston, MA

Jerry Tan Tiang Hin, MBBS, FRCS, FRCOphth
Jerry Tan Eye Surgery
Singapore

Kenneth J. Hoffer, MD, FACS
Clinical Professor of Ophthalmology
UCLA
Los Angeles, CA

Richard S. Hoffman, MD
Clinical Associate Professor
Oregon Health & Science University
Drs. Fine, Hoffman and Packer
Eugene, OR

Jack T. Holladay, MD, MSEE, FACS
Clinical Professor of Ophthalmology
Baylor College of Medicine
Houston, TX

Edward Holland, MD
Director, Cornea Services
Cincinnati Eye Institute
Professor of Ophthalmology
University of Cincinnati
Cincinnati, OH

Jeffrey D. Horn, MD
Medical Director, Vision For Life
Nashville, TN

John A. Hovanesian, MD
Refractive Surgeon, Harvard Eye Associates
Laguna Hills, CA
Clinical Instructor, UCLA Jules Stein Eye Institute
Los Angeles, CA

Suber S. Huang, MD, MBA
Philip F. and Elizabeth G. Searle—Suber S. Huang Professor
and Vice-Chairman
Director, Vitreoretinal Diseases and Surgery
Department of Ophthalmology
University Hospitals Case Medical Center
Cleveland, OH

Conall F. Hurley, MB, BCh, BAO, FRCSI
Director & Owner, The Ardfallen Eye Clinic
Cork, Ireland

Randolph T. Jackson, MD
Discover Vision Centers
Kansas City, MO

J. Michael Jumper, MD
Retina Service Chief
California Pacific Medical Center
West Coast Retina Medical Group
San Francisco, CA

Paul Kaufman, MD
University of Madison Wisconsin
Madison, WI

Hakan Kaymak, MD
Department of Ophthalmology
Knappschaft´s Hospital
Sulzbach, Germany

Robert M. Kershner, MD, MS, FACS
Clinical Professor of Ophthalmology
John A. Moran Eye Center
University of Utah School of Medicine
Salt Lake City, UT
IK HO Visiting Professor of Ophthalmology
Chinese University of Hong Kong
Adjunct Professor of Anatomy and Physiology
Palm Beach Community College
Palm Beach Gardens, FL

Guy M. Kezirian, MD, FACS
President, SurgiVision® Consultants, Inc.
Scottsdale, AZ

Terry Kim, MD
Associate Professor of Ophthalmology
Duke University School of Medicine
Director of Fellowship Programs
Associate Director
Cornea and Refractive Surgery
Duke University Eye Center
Durham, NC

Guy E. Knolle, MD, FACS
Knolle & Young Associates
Austin, TX

Michael C. Knorz, MD
Professor of Ophthalmology
Medical Faculty Mannheim of the University of Heidelberg
Heidelberg, Germany

Olga Konykhov, MD
Fellow in Corneal and Refractive Surgery
Pepose Vision Institute
St. Louis, MO

Marie Czenko Kuechel, MA
President, Czenko Kuechel Consulting
Suburban Chicago, IL

George D. Kymionis, MD, PhD
Cornea Research Fellow
Bascom Palmer Eye Institute
University of Miami Miller School of Medicine
Miami, Florida

Stephen S. Lane, MD
Adjunct Clinical Professor
University of Minnesota
Managing Partner, Associated Eye Care
Stillwater, MN

Michael Lawless, MD
Medical Director, Vision Group
Ophthalmic Surgeon, The Eye Institute
Sydney Australia

Yunhee Lee, MD
Assistant Professor of Clinical Ophthalmology
Bascom Palmer Eye Institute
University of Miami Miller School of Medicine
Miami, FL

Robert P. Lehmann, MD, FACS
Clinical Associate Professor of Ophthalmology
Baylor College of Medicine
Houston, TX
Private practice
Nacogdoches and Southlake, TX

John Lehr, OD
Regional Clinical Director/Advisor
TLC The Laser Eye Centers
Chicago, IL

Jess C. Lester, MD, FACS
Atlanta, GA

Richard A. Lewis, MD
Consultant in glaucoma and cataract
Private practice
Sacramento, CA

Brian Little, FRCS, FRCOphth, FHEA
Consultant Ophthalmologist
Honorary Senior Lecturer
Royal Free Hospital NHS Trust
London, United Kingdom

Dwayne Logan, MD
Atlantis Eyecare
Anaheim, CA

Angel López-Castro, MD
Laservision Eye Clinic
Madrid, Spain

Brian D. Lueth, MD
Physicians Eye Clinic
Everett, WA

Richard J. Mackool, MD
Director, The Mackool Eye Institute (Ambulatory Surgery Center)
Astoria, NY
Senior Attending Surgeon, New York Eye and Ear Infirmary
New York, NY

Richard J. Mackool, Jr, MD
The Mackool Eye Institute
Astoria, NY

Scott MacRae, MD
Departments of Ophthalmology and Biomechanical Engineering
University of Rochester
Rochester, NY

Shareef Mahdavi, BA
President, SM2 Strategic
Pleasanton, CA

Martin A. Mainster, PhD, MD, FRCOphth
Luther L. Fry Endowed Professor of Ophthalmology
University of Kansas School of Medicine
Kansas City, KS

Michael W. Malley, BA
President/Founder, CRM Group
Houston, TX

William F. Maloney, MD
Maloney Eye Center
Vista, CA

Edward E. Manche, MD
Director of Cornea and Refractive Surgery
Associate Professor of Ophthalmology
Stanford University School of Medicine
Stanford, CA

Felicidad Manero, MD
Cornea and Refractive Surgery Department
Instituto De Microcirugía Ocular De Barcelona (Imo)
Barcelona, Spain

Paul Mann, MD
Mann Eye Institute and Laser Center
Houston, TX

William Martin, MD
Assistant Professor and Section Chief for Ophthalmology
University of Toledo School of Medicine
Toledo, OH

Samuel Masket, MD
Clinical Professor , UCLA
Private Practice
Los Angeles, CA

W. Andrew Maxwell, MD, PhD
California Eye Institute
Fresno, CA

J. E. "Jay" McDonald II, MD
McDonald Eye Associates
Fayetteville AR

Marguerite B. McDonald, MD, FACS
Cornea/refractive/anterior segment specialist
Ophthalmic Consultants of Long Island
Lynbrook, NY
Adjunct Clinical Professor of Ophthalmology
Tulane University School of Medicine
New Orleans, LA
Clinical Professor of Ophthalmology
New York University (NYU)
Manhattan, NY
Staff physician
Manhattan Eye Ear and Throat Hospital
New York, NY
Staff physician
Island Eye Center
Carle Place, NY

Javier A. Gaytan Melicoff, MD
Cornea and Refractive Surgery Consultant
Angles Puebla Hospital, MOP Microcirugia Ocular De Puebl SC
Puebla, Mexico

Ulrich Mester, MD
Department of Ophthalmology
Knappschaft's Hospital
Sulzbach, Germany

Marc A. Michelson, MD
Alabama Eye & Cataract Center, PC
Birmingham, AL
Clinical Associate Professor of Ophthalmology
University of Alabama School of Medicine
Birmingham, AL

Kevin M. Miller, MD
Kolokotrones Professor of Clinical Ophthalmology
David Geffen School of Medicine at UCLA
Jules Stein Eye Institute
Los Angeles, CA

Rick Milne, MD
Private practice
President, The Eye Center
Columbia, SC

Robert A. Mittra, MD
Assistant Clinical Professor University of Minnesota,
VitreoRetinal Surgery, P.A.
Minneapolis, MN

Satish Modi, MD, FRCS(C), CPI
Assistant Clinical Professor of Ophthalmology
Albert Einstein College of Medicine
Bronx, NY
Seeta Eye Centers
Poughkeepsie, NY

Robert Montés-Micó, PhD
Optics Department, Faculty of Physics
University of Valencia, Spain

Merce Morral, MD
Cornea and Refractive Surgery Consultant.
Instituto De Microcirugía Ocular De Barcelona (Imo)
Barcelona, Spain.

Robert Morris, MRCP, FRCS, FRCOphth
Southampton Eye Unit
Southampton University Hospitals NHS Trust
Southampton, England

Con Moshegov, MD, FRANZCO, FRACS
Medical Director, Perfect Vision Eye Surgery
Sydney, Australia
Consultant, Concord Hospital
Sydney, Australia

Lana J. Nagy, BS
Departments of Ophthalmology and Biomechanical
Engineering
University of Rochester
Rochester, NY

Louis D. "Skip" Nichamin, MD
Medical Director
Laurel Eye Clinic
Brookville, PA

Lee T. Nordan, MD
Assistant Clinical Professor of Ophthalmology
Jules Stein Eye Institute
UCLA
Los Angeles, CA

Terrence P. O'Brien, MD
Professor of Ophthalmology
Bascom Palmer Eye Institute
University of Miami Miller School of Medicine
Palm Beach Gardens, FL

Thomas A. Oetting, MD
Clinical Professor
Residency Program Director
University of Iowa
Iowa City, IA

Roger V. Ohanesian, MD
Founding Partner, Harvard Eye Associates
Laguna Hills, CA
Associate Clinical Professor, UC-Irvine Department of
Ophthalmology
Irvine, CA

Randall J. Olson, MD
The John A. Moran Presidential Professor and Chair of
Ophthalmology
CEO, John A. Moran Eye Center
Department of Ophthalmology and Visual Sciences
Salt Lake City, UT

Robert H. Osher, MD
Medical Director Emeritus
Cincinnati Eye Institute
Professor of Ophthalmology
University of Cincinnati
Cincinnati, OH

Ivan L. Ossma, MD, MPH
Department of Ophthalmology
Fundacion Clinica Valle del Lili
Cali, Colombia
Clinical Professor
School of Medicine
Santander Industrial University
Bucaramanga, Colombia

Mark Packer, MD, FACS
Clinical Associate Professor
Oregon Health & Science University
Drs. Fine, Hoffman and Packer
Eugene, OR

Parag D. Parekh, MD, MPA
Minnesota Eye Consultants
Minneapolis, MN

Natalia Pelaez, MD
Cornea And Refractive Surgery Fellow
Universidad Autónoma De Barcelona
Instituto De Microcirugía Ocular De Barcelona (Imo),
Barcelona, Spain.

Jay S. Pepose, MD, PhD
Director, Pepose Vision Institute
Professor of Clinical Ophthalmology and Visual Sciences
Washington University School of Medicine
St. Louis, MO

Matteo Piovella, MD
Founder and Scientific Director
CMA, Centro Microchirurgia Ambulatoriale
Monza, Italy

John W. Potter, OD, FAAO
Vice President for Patient Services
TLC Laser Eye Centers
Dallas, TX

Thomas C. Prager, PhD, MPH
Vale Asche Russell Professor of Ophthalmology
Department of Ophthalmology and Visual Science
The University of Texas Medical School
Houston, TX

Louis Probst, MD
Medical Director, TLC The Laser Eye Centers
Chicago, IL

Mujtaba A. Qazi, MD
Pepose Vision Institute
Instructor of Clinical Ophthalmology and Visual Sciences
Washington University School of Medicine
St. Louis, MO

Sherman W. Reeves, MD, MPH
Corneal/Refractive Surgeon
Minnesota Eye Consultants, P.A.
Minneapolis, MN

Paul Rhee, OD
Calhoun Vision
Pasadena, CA

Allan M. Robbins, MD, FACS
Robbins Eye Associates
Assistant Clinical Professor at the University of Rochester
Rochester, NY

Kenneth J. Rosenthal, MD, FACS
Surgeon Director
Rosenthal Eye and Facial Plastic Surgery
Associate Professor of Ophthalmology
The John A. Moran Eye Center, University of Utah Medical School
Salt Lake City, UT
Assistant Clinical Professor of Ophthalmology
New York University Medical School
New York, NY

Sheri L. Rowen, MD, FACS
Director of Ophthalmology
Mercy Medical Center, Baltimore, MD
Clinical Assistant Professor
University of Maryland

Jonathan B. Rubenstein, MD
Rush Medical College
Chicago, IL

James J. Salz, MD
Clinical Professor of Ophthalmology
University of Southern California
Los Angeles, CA

Thomas W. Samuelson, MD
Minnesota Eye Consultants
Minneapolis, MN
Associate Clinical Professor of Ophthalmology
University of Minnesota
Minneapolis, MN

Helga P. Sandoval, MD, MSCR
Magill Research Center for Vision Correction
Storm Eye Institute
Medical University of South Carolina
Charleston, SC

Christian Sandstedt, PhD
Director Optics
Calhoun Vision
Pasadena, CA

John A. Scholl, MS
Vice President of Research & Development
PowerVision
Belmont, CA

Daniel M. Schwartz, MD
Shirley Reich Chair in Ophthalmology
Director Retina Service
University of California, San Francisco
San Francisco, CA

Jim Schwiegerling, PhD
Ophthalmology and Vision Sciences
University of Arizona
Tucson, AZ

Barry S. Seibel, MD
Clinical Assistant Professor of Ophthalmology
UCLA Medical School
Los Angeles, CA

Mohamed H. Shabayek, MD, PhD
Research Institute of Ophthalmology
Giza, Egypt

Alan Shiller, MD
Shiller Vision Center
Palestine and Waco, TX

Joel K. Shugar, MD, MSEE
Medical Director
Nature Coast EyeCare Institute
Perry, FL

Jack A. Singer, MD
Private Practice
Randolph, VT

Maite Sisquella, OPT
Instituto Microcirugia Ocular de Barcelona
Barcelona, Spain

Stephen G. Slade, MD, FACS
Slade & Baker Vision
Houston, TX

Michael E. Snyder, MD
Specialist in Cataract, Cornea, and Refractive Surgery
Cincinnati Eye Institute
Volunteer Assistant Professor of Ophthalmology
University of Cincinnati
Cincinnati, OH

Kerry D. Solomon, MD
Magill Research Center for Vision Correction
Storm Eye Institute
Medical University of South Carolina
Charleston, SC

Renée Solomon, MD
Private Practice
New York, NY

Michael Sopher
VP of Business Development, Eyemaginations, Inc
Towson, MD

Jason E. Stahl, MD
Cataract and Refractive Surgery
Durrie Vision
Overland Park, KS
Assistant Clinical Professor of Ophthalmology
Kansas University Medical Center
Kansas City, KS

George Stamatelatos, BSc Optom
Senior Optometrist
NewVision Clinics
Melbourne, Australia

Roger F. Steinert, MD
Professor of Ophthalmology
Professor of Biomedical Engineering
Vice Chair of Clinical Ophthalmology
University of California Irvine
Irvine, CA

Julian D. Stevens, MRCP, FRCS, FRCOphth
Consultant Ophthalmic Surgeon
Moorfields Eye Hospital
London, United Kingdom

Tracy Swartz, OD, MS, FAAO
Wang Vision Institute, Nashville, TN
Adjunct Faculty, Indiana University School of Optometry
Bloomington, IN

Audrey Talley-Rostov, MD
Northwest Eye Surgeons
Seattle, WA

Joshua Teichman, MD
University of Toronto
Toronto, Ontario

Richard Tipperman, MD
Associate Surgeon/Active Staff
Wills Eye Institute
Philadelphia, PA

William Trattler, MD
Director of Cornea
Center for Excellence in Eye Care
Miami, FL
Voluntary Assistant Professor of Ophthalmology
Bascom Palmer Eye Institute
Miami, FL

Patricia L. Turner, MD
Clinical Assistant Professor of Ophthalmology
University of Kansas School of Medicine
Kansas City, KS

Farrell Tyson, MD, FACS
Director, Cape Coral Eye Center
Cape Coral, FL

Carlos Vergés, MD, PhD
Professor and Head Department of Ophthalmology CIMA
Universidad Politécnica de Cataluña
Barcelona, Spain

Paolo Vinciguerra, MD
Chairman, Department of Ophthalmology
Istituto Clinico Humanitas
Rozzano, Milano, Italy

Vanee Virash, MD

Daniel Vos, MD
Wolfe Clinic
Ames, IA

David T. Vroman, MD
Magill Research Center for Vision Correction
Storm Eye Institute
Medical University of South Carolina
Charleston, SC

John A. Vukich, MD
Assistant Clinical Prof.
University of Wisconsin, Madison
School of Medicine
Director of the Davis Duehr Dean
Center for Refractive Surgery
Madison, WI

R. Bruce Wallace, III, MD, FACS
Clinical Professor of Ophthalmology
LSU Medical School
New Orleans, LA
Assistant Clinical Professor of Ophthalmology
Tulane Medical School
New Orleans, LA
Medical Director, Wallace Eye Surgery
Alexandria, LA

Ming Wang, MD, PhD
Medical Director of Refractive Surgery, Aier Eye Hospital System, PR China
Clinical associate professor of ophthalmology of University of Tennessee
Attending Surgeon, Saint Thomas Hospital
Director, Wang Vision Institute
Nashville, TN

Robert D. Watson
President, Patient Education Concepts, Inc
Houston, TX

Robert Jay Weinstock, MD
Director of Cataract and Refractive Surgery
The Eye Institute of West Florida
Associate Clinical Professor
University of South Florida
Tampa, FL

Darrell E. White, MD
President and CEO, Skyvision Centers
Westlake, OH

Jeffrey Whitman, MD
Key-Whitman Eye Center
Dallas, TX

Stephen Wiles, MD
Deligeorges & Wiles Eye Center
Kansas City, MO

John R. Wittpenn, MD
Associate Clinical Professor
Department of Ophthalmology
State University of New York at Stony Brook
Stony Brook, NY
Partner, Ophthalmic Consultants of Long Island
Stony Brook, NY

Michael Y. Wong, MD
Private Practice
Princeton, NJ
Clinical Instructor
Robert Wood Johnson Medical School
New Brunswick, NJ
Medical Director
Wills Eye Laser
Princeton, NJ

J. Trevor Woodhams, MD
Surgical Director, Woodhams Eye Clinic
Atlanta, GA

Helen Wu, MD
Tufts New England Eye Center
Boston, MA

Sandra Yeh, MD
Prairie Eye Center
Springfield, IL

Sonia H. Yoo, MD
Associate Professor of Clinical Ophthalmology
Bascom Palmer Eye Institute
University of Miami Miller School of Medicine
Miami, Florida

Geunyoung Yoon, PhD
Departments of Ophthalmology and Biomechanical Engineering
University of Rochester
Rochester, NY

Leonard Yuen, MD, MPH
Boxer Wachler Vision Institute
Beverly Hills, CA

Charles M. Zacks, MD
Chair, Ethics Committee, American Academy of Ophthalmology
Partner, Maine Eye Center
Portland, ME

Harvey Zalaznick, MD
Tenzel, Weiner, & Zalaznick, MDs, PA
Practice to Ophthalmology
Aventura, FL

Foreword

Ophthalmology is entering an exciting new era. The technology is rapidly changing, our boundaries are expanding, and today every cataract patient can expect to receive an intraocular lens that will not only replace their natural failing lens, but will, in the vast majority of cases, function safely, and at a better optical level, than the lens of a "normal" phakic individual of the same age.

The goal four or five decades ago was to restore useful vision after cataract removal without resorting to thick cataract spectacles; today we are able to provide clarity of vision unequaled even by the natural lens. The rapidly developing field of IOLs began with correction of basic power, then, aided by corneal surgery, astigmatism was conquered. Now a new frontier—presbyopia—has been targeted. In this monumental work, the editors and contributing authors, all active in clinical practice and research, have sought to bring the latest information to the reader. In *Mastering Refractive IOLs: the Art and Science*, Dr. David Chang and his coeditors, along with more than 200 contributors, have provided a comprehensive textbook on the art and science of refractive IOLs for the practicing ophthalmologist.

This new technology will continue to improve, and with it we share the joy, the excitement, and the sheer exhilaration of restoring sight to those who have never been able to see the world clearly. The premium IOL, the presbyopia-correcting IOL, offers a restoration of vision to pre-presbyopic levels with "better than ever" clarity.

Dr. Chang and his associate editors, Dr. Steven J. Dell, Dr. Warren E. Hill, Dr. Richard L. Lindstrom, and Dr. Kevin L. Waltz, present a comprehensive text, designed for surgeons wanting guidance from experts in making presbyopia-correcting IOLs part of their practice.

Covering everything from patient selection and education to management of complications, the text begins with the question, "Why Offer Premium IOLs?" In this section 16 authors share their experience and explain why they have transitioned from monofocal to premium presbyopia-correcting IOLs. Then other experts explain how to select the best IOL for patient needs.

Three things determine the outcome. 1) The patient potential (ie, the visual need and the health of the eye). 2) The technology, and 3) the skill and mind-set of the surgeon. The technology should be determined for the eye, not the eye for the technology. Premium IOLs are not "one size fits all." The lens should be chosen to meet the patient's needs and expectations.

It has been said that one who has a watch knows what time it is. If he has 2 watches, he is never sure. Optical characteristics of presbyopia-correcting lenses vary considerably, and the patient's visual needs factor significantly in the decision of which lens to offer each patient. Each of these lenses has a unique combination of advantages and disadvantages.

Patients are much more interested in the visual outcome than a particular technology, and so the surgeon needs to make decisions that will meet their needs without confusing them with choices that only a scientist can understand. They are more interested in what you tell them about how they will be able to see.

Preoperative education and counseling is critical for success with any presbyopic IOL. Some lessons are clear. One should never promise the patient that he will not need glasses again, but tell him that he will need glasses at least "some of the time." Then, if he does, you have prepared him and he is satisfied. But if he doesn't need them, you are his hero.

That we have no universally perfect solution increases the importance of careful patient selection. The premium IOL appropriately allows surgeons to differentiate between refractive surgical goals. Understanding the differences between the available presbyopia IOL designs permits the surgeon to individualize his approach, which for some patients may include mixing different lenses.

This is one of the most thoroughly referenced texts to be published on the science, and the art, of vision correction with IOLs. It is truly a classic. I encourage any serious practitioner of refractive eye surgery to read this book to gain solid instruction in the use of presbyopia-correcting IOLs.

Spencer P. Thornton, MD, FACS

Preface

Prior to 2004, the distinction between refractive and cataract surgeons was straightforward. Our procedures, reimbursement process, and patient populations were entirely different. All of this changed with the introduction of new presbyopia-correcting IOLs and the landmark Center for Medicare and Medicaid Services (CMS) ruling allowing patients to pay out of pocket for them. Suddenly a major segment of refractive surgery was intraocular, and nearly everyone needing cataract surgery was a potential refractive patient. The following editorial, "A Day to Remember," which I wrote for the June 2005 issue of *Cataract and Refractive Surgery Today*, recalls our initial sense at that time of just how much things were about to change.

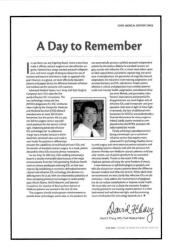

In case there was any lingering doubt, recent events have made it official: cataract surgeons are also refractive surgeons. Patients have always wanted spectacle independence, and we've sought all along to reduce the size of incisions and improve biometry in order to approach this goal. However, as a group, we never effectively educated patients and payers about the difference between refractive and medical care for someone with cataracts. AMO's Array and Staar's toric IOLs were the first purely refractive IOL innovations. The new technology intraocular lens (NTIOL) designation for ASC reimbursement made by CMS allowed manufacturers an extra $50 of reimbursement, but the patient did not pay, nor did the surgeon receive any additional premium for this service. In hindsight, implanting advanced refractive IOL technologies for no additional charge was a mistake, because it diminished their perceived value and made it even harder for patients to differentiate between the capabilities of multifocal and toric IOLs and the benefits of standard cataract surgery. As a result, patient demand for these IOLs became almost nonexistent.

For me, May 10, 2005 (my 25th wedding anniversary), became a doubly memorable date because of the major announcement from the CMS permitting Medicare beneficiaries to choose presbyopia-reducing IOLs at their own expense. By establishing an economic delineation between cataract and refractive IOL technology, this decision is a defining event for us all. With the newsworthy availability of three competing premium technologies to tackle presbyopia (Alcon's ReSTOR, AMO's ReZoom, and Eyeonics' Crystalens), the injustice of denying these options to Medicare patients was averted in the nick of time. That surgeons should receive greater reimbursement to provide these technologies seems clear, as the products do not automatically produce satisfied, spectacle-independent patients by themselves.

Relative to standard cataract surgery, success with refractive IOLs is much more reliant upon an ideal capsulorrhexis and pristine capsular bag, the avoidance of complications, the prevention of surgically induced astigmatism, the reduction of pre-existing astigmatism, and accurate biometry and IOL calculations. Proper patient selection is critical, and physicians must consider patients' ocular and macular health, astigmatism, contralateral refractive error, lifestyle, and personality traits. Patients' expectations and potential for disappointment are much higher with all refractive IOLs and increase pre- and postoperative chair time. In light of these higher demands, the lack of additional reimbursement for NTIOLs was undoubtedly a financial disincentive for many surgeons.

Indeed, hardly anyone noticed or complained when the NTIOL provision officially expired last month. Clearly, achieving a pseudo-accommodating emmetropic eye is a premium refractive service that requires more advanced IOL technology, flawless biometry and surgery, and more extensive patient evaluation and counseling.

Eyeonics blazed a trail with the premium IOL channel whereby non-Medicare cataract patients could pay a fair market, out-of-pocket premium for an uncovered refractive benefit. Thanks to the recent CMS ruling, Medicare patients will enjoy the same freedom of choice. It now behooves us ophthalmologists to properly and ethically educate our cataract patients about the difference between medical and refractive services. When asked what we recommend, we must clarify that refractive IOLs are discretionary—they address the inconvenience of eyeglasses but do not reduce complications or improve ocular health. We must take care not to abuse the economic freedom recently granted to our trusting cataract patients. It is their hard-earned and well-deserved right, and the promising future of refractive IOL technology depends on it.

Today, I think we would all agree that the CMS ruling and the new premium refractive IOLs have dramatically and permanently altered the clinical practice of every cataract and refractive surgeon. Ready or not, we are suddenly faced with the new challenge of educating patients about these multiple options, and then managing and meeting their expectations. Navigating these previously uncharted waters has been both interesting and intimidating, and we are still continually searching for better approaches.

Wouldn't it be wonderful if we could glean the collective wisdom of more than 200 experienced refractive IOL colleagues? This nontraditional textbook seeks to provide such a compendium of practical advice and pearls, reflecting the consensus, controversy, and diversity of our varied opinions, approaches, and practices. To provide as much balance as possible between differing preferences and philosophies, the products and the most important and controversial topics are addressed by multiple different authors.

Refractive IOLs have provided surgeons and patients with exciting new opportunities that also entail different risks and the increased potential for dissatisfaction. For this reason, we must all improve our surgical proficiency, our understanding of clinical optics, our communication skills, our clinical judgment, and our expertise in avoiding and managing complications. In short, we must all remain committed to mastering both the science and the art of refractive IOL surgery.

David F. Chang

SECTION I

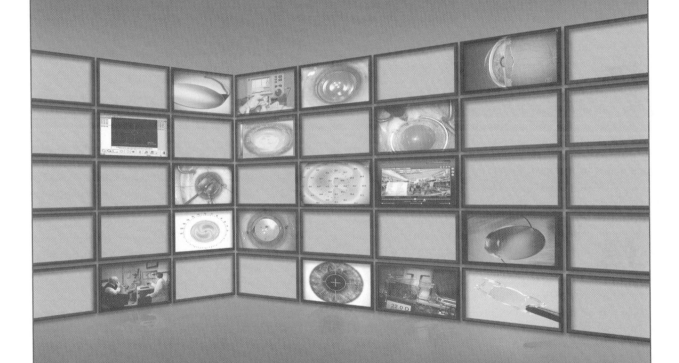

Why Offer
Premium IOLs?

THE BIRTH OF THE PREMIUM IOL CHANNEL

Jim Denning, BS

"The real winners in this whole process are the patients. Health care is not a God-given right, but purchasing a life-enhancing procedure with your own hard-earned money sure is."

The Premium Intraocular Lens (IOL) Channel has been more of a journey than a destination. For me it began at an American Academy of Ophthalmology meeting in 1999. Stephen Slade, MD gave a 3-minute talk about an accommodating IOL called the AT-45 from a company called C&C Vision (Aliso Viejo, CA). This was the same period in time when we actually thought if we complained loud enough that Medicare would stop cutting our fees. Dr. Slade made an opening comment that went something like "with all the bad news surrounding Medicare reimbursement I'm still going to talk about new technology for cataract patients." I thought, "what a great lens technology for all the baby boomers who were becoming presbyopic." I did not really have an initial interest in the AT-45 for cataract patients; my reasoning was that I assumed the manufacturer would get it approved as a new technology IOL (NTIOL). What that meant to me back in 1999 was the manufacturer makes a nice profit, the taxpayers pay for it, and the surgeons promote it as unpaid salesmen. At that instant I stored the C&C accommodating AT-45 lens in my brain database. I spoke with my partner, John Doane, MD, about Dr. Slade's talk and confirmed that we were talking about an accommodating IOL. He said he was way ahead of me and had already visited with the owners of the company to see if he could be involved with the Food and Drug Administration (FDA) phase II trials. The owners were Stuart Cumming, MD and Andy Corley, CEO. C&C Vision later changed its name to Eyeonics, Inc (Aliso Viejo, CA) and renamed the AT-45 the Crystalens.

We started the phase II trials of the AT-45 accommodating lens in the third quarter of 2000. John Doane, MD was the investigator. Alcon (Fort Worth, TX) started trials of its multifocal IOL—the ReSTOR—about the same time. The trial went well, and the ReSTOR multifocal IOL was eventually approved by the FDA in March 2005. The ReZoom multifo-

cal IOL by Advanced Medical Optics (Santa Ana, CA) would also be approved in March 2005. During the early years, I had many discussions with Andy Corley about his vision for marketing this IOL. To my surprise he had no intention of bringing it to market as a covered service. He planned to bring it to market as an uncovered device and have the patients pay out of pocket for it as well as the services required to achieve a refractive outcome. What a great concept. Finally, the surgeons and Ambulatory Surgery Centers (ASCs) could participate in the free market on a high-technology device. The free market would be huge as it included everyone over the age of 45. Ignorance is certainly bliss. We had no idea how difficult it would be for that concept to become a reality. There were a lot of bumps in the road. We hit every one of them. Eyeonics offered physician courses to educate surgeons on how to implant the accommodating IOL and to explain to them that the IOL could not be offered to Medicare patients. One of the first courses took place in Atlanta on October 4, 2003. Dr. Doane was one of the course directors. He arrived back home about 11:00 PM and called me on his way home from the Kansas City airport. He described the portion of the meeting where the panelists were trying to explain to the doctors that the IOL could not be used in cataract surgery on Medicare patients. The reason was the IOL sold for $825.00 and Medicare would not pay any extra for the IOL. The surgeons' reactions ranged from "the IOL is a God-given right to patients and Medicare must pay" to "I'm resigning from the Medicare program so I can use the IOL in cataract surgery to anyone willing to pay for it." He went on to tell me that the panelists were telling the surgeons it was ok to implant the presbyopia-correcting (Pr-C) IOL in any patient who had cataracts and commercial insurance. Since these patients had commercial insurance and not Medicare, they would automatically be charged out of pocket for the IOL. Hearing that, I bolted straight out of bed. In reality, the commercial insurance status was no different than Medicare. All commercial insurance companies had language in their (ASC) contracts that read "the facility fee shall be considered payment in full for professional fees, nursing care, tests, and implantable lenses." In other words, the IOL could not be used in Medicare or commercial patients for cataract surgery. Neither would pay extra for the Pr-C IOL. What we quickly found out was that both Medicare and the commercial insurance companies wanted to consider the Pr-C IOLs "covered" services, but neither wanted to pay extra for the IOL. This was a big bump in the road. We will discuss this more later.

The commercialization of the presbyopic IOLs centered around several large issues. The first issue was that Medicare, the big gorilla that controlled 80% of the cataract market, considered the presbyopic IOLs a standard covered service IOL. That meant the $150.00 it allows for an IOL would result in a loss of approximately $700.00 to the surgical facility. Since the AT-45 was considered a covered service, no additional services required to achieve a refractive outcome would have been paid by Medicare nor could they be passed on to the patient. The covered service rules prohibited that. The second issue was that commercial insurance, which controlled the remaining 20% of the cataract market, bundled any type of IOL implant inside their typical ASC contracts. They were not even paying any extra for a NTIOL. The third issue was that the pure refractive market could not support the roll out of the presbyopic IOL on its own. We had a great new lens technology, but we were locked out of the large cataract market from bureaucratic policies associated with Medicare and commercial managed care contracts that bundled all IOLs in the facility fee payment.

Eyeonics' CEO, Andy Corley, stood firm on his business plan to change the Medicare policy to allow the free market to set the price of the presbyopic IOL and all services required to achieve a refractive outcome. He could have caved in and taken the easy road with no bumps. This would have meant going for NTIOL status. It would have been successful in the short term. In the long term, he knew that this would have basically killed the advancement of presbyopic IOLs. His reasoning was simple. If the surgeons were not paid for their efforts to achieve a refractive outcome, the presbyopic IOLs would be just like any other standard IOL. We had plenty of those to choose from and certainly did not need another one on the shelf.

The Medicare solution ended up being mostly political. It was worked on everyday from 2000 through May 2005. We had countless meetings and discussions with members of Congress and with Medicare directors. Congressman Christopher Cox represented California, the home state of Eyeonics. Congressman Cox was a huge supporter of allowing Medicare patients access to the presbyopic IOLs. He believed that it should be a noncovered service from Medicare and that if patients wanted to spend their own money to reduce their dependency on reading glasses, then they should have that right. He was comfortable with this position since the traditional government-issue IOL produced excellent results and Medicare covered a pair of glasses to refine any refractive errors remaining after traditional cataract surgery. Congressman Dennis Moore represented Kansas. Dr. Doane did the investigative work for Eyeonics at Discover Vision Centers located in Kansas. Although Congressman Moore never took a position on the presbyopic IOL issue, his staff was instrumental in identifying key Medicare directors for us

to talk to about the proposed policy change. The commercial insurance companies virtually number in the hundreds, and this posed almost as big a hurdle as Medicare. We approached this by going to each commercial insurance company one by one. It was a long and tedious task. The game plan was to deal with medical directors that we personally knew at various commercial insurance companies. Once the medical directors understood that these IOLs addressed presbyopia, a noncovered service, and that we were not going to implant the IOL without compensation from the patient, they agreed to allow their members to pay out of pocket. The process began in Kansas City and we obtained written letters from the major insurers confirming presbyopic IOLs were noncovered and we could charge patients out of pocket for the IOL and extra services needed to achieve a desired refractive outcome. This grassroots effort was explained at every course Eyeonics gave over the years, and the other refractive IOL manufacturers adopted a similar approach. This approach was ultimately very successful in resolving the issue with commercial insurers.

Changing Medicare's policy proved to be more difficult. Even with Congressman Cox pressing Center for Medicare and Medicaid Services (CMS) officials to consider the policy change, it seemed we were making very little progress. One of the grassroots tactics we used was to have CMS constituents, the Medicare patients, participate in the process. After all it should be their choice to use a new technology device or not. We provided Medicare patients with the phone numbers of their representatives and they called high-level CMS directors directly in large enough numbers to be heard. One thing we learned early on was Medicare patients generally expect any health care service to be free and unlimited. This expectation is especially true of children of Medicare beneficiaries, who want unlimited health care services for their parents. More importantly, however, is that they will not tolerate being told they cannot have something even if they are willing to pay for it out of pocket. We freely distributed the CMS contact information to any practice who wanted it and gave it out at every Eyeonics course.

On September 7, 2004, Andy Corley hastily summoned several individuals for a meeting directly with CMS officials in Baltimore, MD. The meeting attendees included myself, along with Andy Corley, Bill Link, Steven Dell, MD, Jim Largent, Eyeonics' attorney Grant Bagley, and an entire room full of CMS department heads. The CMS officials were very gracious to us and were open to discussion, but there was still a great divide between our different agendas. Eyeonics wanted a policy in which the noncovered presbyopic function of the IOL would be considered a noncovered service. CMS wanted the IOL covered under the NTIOL reimbursement protocol. Dr. Dell and the Eyeonics team gave compelling arguments that the presbyopia-correcting function of the IOL and extra services to achieve a refractive outcome should be noncovered services.

It was very clear at the end of the meeting that Eyeonics was not going to bring the accommodating IOL to market as a covered service, nor were they going to reduce the price of the IOL. Andy later told us that CMS privately told him 2 important things immediately after the meeting ended. Number one was the CMS director said something to the effect that "We had all of the department heads in here today because we could not figure out a way to tell you no." Number two was "Please tell your users of the IOL to stop giving out the phone numbers of the CMS department heads. We already understand the issue." As soon as Andy told me this, I knew we had won the war.

A few days after returning to work, I received a call from Congressman Moore's office. His Chief of Staff had close ties with CMS officials and said that CMS would need a letter of support from either the American Academy of Ophthalmology (AAO) or the American Society of Cataract and Refractive Surgery (ASCRS) to ever consider a policy change that would make presbyopic IOLs a noncovered service. I sent that message up the flag pole and many others did the same. In February 2005, ASCRS issued a position statement that was sent to CMS, which in effect stated that "developments that are determined to be 'elective' should be available to every patient by offering an option to pay out-of-pocket over and above the basic 'essential' benefit." CMS adopted the principal concept of the ASCRS position statement.

On May 3, 2005 CMS issued Ruling No. 05-01. The historical policy was well written and made the following statement: "the presbyopia-correcting functionality of an IOL does not fall into the benefit category and is not covered. Any additional provider or physician services required to insert or monitor a patient receiving a Pr-C IOL are also not covered." A large new market was created on this day. Manufacturers have devoted enormous resources toward developing new Pr-C IOLs and techniques, and new premium channel IOLs will be brought through the development pipeline at a healthy pace.

Of all the awards and certificates I have received over the years, I have kept a personal note from Andy Corley framed in my office. It reads, "Dear Jim, Thank you for all your contributions to the CMS effort. I wanted to quit about ½ dozen times but you and Largent wouldn't let me. Of all the small victories we've had this is the most satisfying, with great respect, Andy."

I'm grateful that Dr. Doane called me late at night on October 4, 2003 to vent about the surgeon bedlam over patients not having access to accommodating IOLs. I doubt if I would have ever gotten involved had we not had that discussion. The real winners in this whole process are our patients. Health care is not a God-given right, but purchasing a life-enhancing procedure with your own hard-earned money sure is.

CHAPTER 2

REFRACTIVE IOLS—
ECONOMIC DEMOGRAPHICS

David Harmon

Multifocal and accommodating intraocular lenses (IOLs) offer significant opportunities to expand ophthalmic practice revenues, while providing patients with an expanded range of vision. However, these IOLs are not for everyone. Many cataract and refractive patients may not be good candidates for these new lenses for reasons that extend well beyond simple medical issues. In addition, not all cataract and refractive surgeons are prepared to successfully integrate these IOLs into their offered services.

Cataract patients account for the vast majority of all patients electing refractive IOLs today. Most patients with a vision-limiting cataract are good candidates for refractive IOLs. These patients are motivated to undergo cataract surgery to avoid further vision loss, and in most cases a portion of the cost of the surgery is covered by Medicare and/or private insurance. Surgeons responding to an April 2007 Market Scope survey reported that cataract patients account for approximately 97% of refractive IOL procedures. A subcategory of these patients, those with a cataract in one eye who undergo a refractive lens exchange in the other eye, make up approximately 1% of patients.

Some surgeons consider presbyopic patients with refractive errors good candidates for refractive IOLs. Surgeons responding to the Market Scope survey reported that these patients represented 2.3% of US IOL surgery patients (about 70,000 procedures, 38,000 patients per year). While this is a very small portion of the population of eligible patients, with improvements in technology and safety, many expect this number to increase dramatically.

Refractive IOLs carry premium charges for a host of reasons. These premium charges are designed to cover the additional cost of the IOL, additional preoperative counseling, additional preoperative exams, more postoperative counseling and testing, and increased enhancement rates. In the United States, multifocal and accommodating lenses cost $850 to $900, a significant premium over the $80 to $200 charged for conventional IOLs. Many surgeons report that preoperative counseling for refractive IOLs takes twice as long, with much

of this time spent explaining the compromises associated with these lenses and ensuring that patient expectations are in line with anticipated results.

Many practices employ different preoperative testing protocols for refractive IOL patients. Surgeons may perform tests—corneal topography, ocular coherence tomograph (OCT) imaging of the anterior chamber, and in some cases retinal scans—that are not typically used for patients undergoing cataract surgery with conventional IOLs. In many cases, refractive IOL patients also require more postoperative visits due to adaptation issues, and in some cases prolonged therapy may be necessary. Patients implanted with refractive IOLs often require enhancements in order to correct astigmatism, adjust for spherical errors, or introduce some myopia to improve near vision. Although enhancements are rare with conventional cataract surgery, surgeons responding to the Q1-2007 Market Scope survey reported an average enhancement rate of 9% for refractive IOLs.

Fortunately, many of these additional costs can be passed on through a premium charged directly to the patient that is separate from the reimbursement amount allowable by Medicare. In some cases, surgeons charge a global fee that includes the surgeon and the facility fees along with the cost of any required enhancements. Others charge a surgeon fee and leave the ambulatory surgery center (ASC) or hospital to collect the facility fee. Facility fees range from $650 to $1300, depending on the location and IOL purchase arrangements.

Market Scope surveyed US surgeons to determine average prices charged for these procedures during the first quarter of 2007. Although fees ranged widely for cataract patients implanted with presbyopia-correcting IOLs, an average premium charge of $1876 was reported by those surgeons charging a global fee, while the average premium charge was $1491 for those charging only for the surgeon portion. For patients without the benefit of Medicare coverage, reported global fees averaged $3959 and surgeon-only fees averaged $2586 (Table 1).

Premium charges for refractive IOLs are simply unaffordable for a large segment of the senior population. However,

Table 1

AVERAGE FEES FOR REFRACTIVE IOL SURGERY

Procedure	Surgeon-Only Fee	Global Fee
Premium for cataract with refractive IOL	$1491	$1876
RLE with refractive IOL	$2586	$3959

Table 2

PROSPECTS FOR REFRACTIVE IOLs

	Unlikely	Only Highly Motivated	Few Income Barriers
Annual income levels	>$35K	>$35K and <$75K	>$75K
55 to 64 years old	25.7%	34.9%	39.4%
65 to 74 years old	43.4%	35.7%	20.9%
75 years old or more	58.4%	30.5%	11.1%

income levels of patients opting for refractive IOLs vary widely, and income level is just one of several factors involved in a refractive IOL decision. Nonetheless, patient income levels remain a key predictor for which patients will elect the more expensive procedure.

Those with household incomes of below $35,000 per year from all sources are unlikely candidates for simple economic reasons, while those candidates with household incomes above $75,000 per year are generally in a financial position to elect the premium price procedure. The additional cost of refractive IOLs makes a significant dent in the budgets of those patients with income levels less than $75,000 but more than $35,000. Patients in this income category must be highly motivated to choose the procedure (Table 2).

Average income levels vary widely throughout the United States; however, in many cases higher income seniors are concentrated in some geographic areas, and lower income seniors in others. As an example, 2005 median household income in STAAR County, TX was $16,504, while it was $86,677 in Suffolk County, NY. A practice located in the former county would struggle to find patients able to afford the additional cost of a refractive IOL, while practices located in Suffolk County might find it worthwhile to offer this option to all cataract patients.

In addition, patients' lifestyles play an important role in the benefits of the presbyopia-correcting features of these IOLs. Cataract patients that view themselves as active and highly involved in visually demanding tasks are typically more motivated to spend the additional money to optimize vision in all distant ranges. Although an early retirement was a common goal for many of today's elderly, expectations have changed significantly among members of the baby boom generation. These individuals often look forward to a second career or pursuing other lifelong goals after retirement from a first career. Also, the rapidly changing technologies of cell phones, computers, and other devices have become an integral part of life and have raised visual demands.

Population demographics, including an aging baby boom generation and increasing life expectancy, will expand the

demand for refractive IOLs significantly during the next 2 decades. In 2006, the US population segment age 65 and older totaled approximately 37.3 million, but by 2016 this population segment is expected to include 47.8 million and by 2026 forecasts call for this number to reach 65.5 million (Figure 1).

Although the surgical techniques employed for refractive IOLs are the same basic techniques as those used in cataract surgery, surgeons' interactions with patients are remarkably different. Historically, cataract patients have been satisfied with a level of vision improvement still dependent upon multifocal glasses for correction of spherical error, astigmatism, and near vision. By contrast, refractive IOL patients expect good vision at all distance ranges without any correction. These expectations have been fueled by advances in vision correction such as laser in situ keratomileusis (LASIK), which has provided a remarkably successful option for younger patients. Also, a lack of understanding of eyesight, visually demanding lifestyles, and the premium prices charged for refractive IOLs have further raised patients' expectations. Much of the additional time requirements involved with refractive IOL implantations are associated with setting (or resetting) patient expectations and managing those expectations through the postoperative period.

Many cataract surgery practices are ill suited for the additional time required to educate patients, manage patient expectations, and handle the demanding sales process associated with refractive IOLs. Although the surgeon may be quite capable of performing the surgery, the practice may lack the marketing, counseling, and business skills necessary for selling a patient-pay procedure. Traditionally these business skills and resources have been found in practices focused on laser refractive surgery rather than in cataract practices where fees are paid by Medicare and patient expectations have been different. However, cataract patients are less likely to seek laser centers for cataract surgery. In addition, many laser refractive surgeons have focused on office-based laser surgery, electing not to offer IOL surgery.

Practices that offer both refractive and cataract surgery are better positioned to also provide refractive IOLs. These

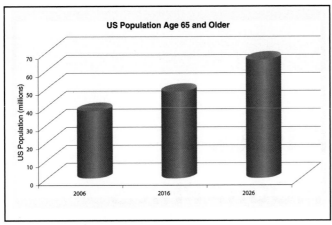

Figure 1. US population age 65 and older.

practices are well organized to market and sell patients on relatively expensive elective surgical procedures and to counsel patients regarding expectations. These surgeons also have the skill set required for IOL surgery and the refractive laser equipment and skills required for the enhancements that may be necessary.

Refractive IOLs offer significant opportunities to increase practice revenues. Changing demographics, including an expanding senior population segment, increasing visual demands, and changing lifestyles, are expected to fuel the market for these products. Nonetheless, not all patients are good economic candidates for the relatively expensive procedure. The potential for the refractive IOL market varies widely by geography, as well. Finally, marketing, counseling, and patient management skills are keys to the success of any refractive IOL practice.

CHAPTER 3

REFRACTIVE IOLs—
ECONOMIC DEMOGRAPHICS

Geoff Charlton

One of the cornerstones in business is the concept of the marketing mix, commonly referred to as the 4 Ps. Simply stated, the successful marketing of a product or service is derived from an optimal combination of product, price, place (distribution), and promotion. In theory, the intersection of a properly balanced marketing mix defines the target market.

In today's world of rapid technological advances, it often seems as if the presence of new technology alone is sufficient to drive market demand. The recent introduction of presbyopia-correcting IOLs (Pr-C IOLs) seems to refute this and the doctrine of the 4 Ps. Without the 2005 ruling by the Center for Medicare and Medicaid Services allowing ophthalmologists to recoup the additional costs associated with the insertion of the PC-IOL following cataract surgery, it is doubtful that a significant target market would exist at all.

In reality, the success of any new product or service may have more to do with the target market's influence on the marketing mix rather than the other way around. With this in mind, this chapter will examine the specific demographic, economic, and social trends in the United States that predispose one group in particular to embrace the benefits of PC-IOLs.

The Graying of America

We are entering an unprecedented time in our history as the first of 78 million baby boomers (those born between 1946 and 1964) reach age 65 in 2011, heralding the much anticipated "age wave" in the United States. While it is true that individuals from previous generations lived beyond age 65, it certainly was not as common as it is today and will be in the decades to come. In 1900, the average age at death in the United States was 47; the average current lifespan today is 77 years. In fact, US Census Bureau projections (Figure 1) indicate that in the not-too-distant future, Americans can expect a good 20 years or more life expectancy beyond age 65!

By 2030, nearly 71 million people will be age 65 and over (Figure 2), accounting for roughly 20% of the total US population. Clearly, the generation that dominated the American political, business, and cultural landscape during the last half of the 20th century will continue to do so during the first decades of the 21st century.

Baby boomers, unlike their predecessors, are not necessarily looking to retire or slow down when they reach age 65. As recently as just a decade ago, only 18% of men and 9% of women age 65 and older were still active in the workforce. In contrast, a recent study by the American Association of Retired Persons (AARP) found that 80% of baby boomers fully expect to continue working at least part time during their retirement years. This may be due in part to the shift away from agricultural and industrial occupations that predominated in the years prior to World War II. Presently, 60% of baby boomers are professional, managerial, or white-collar workers, and their collective skills and experience will still be in high demand in today's global business environment.

This desire to work may have as much to do with funding their eventual retirement as it does with staying busy—84% of baby boomers feel that their generation will need more money in retirement than their parents' generation in order to live comfortably. Uncertain about the future of Social Security and Medicare benefits, many boomers today are resigning themselves to extending their careers or even beginning new careers beyond the traditional retirement age. Faced with competition from younger colleagues and a desire to maintain a youthful appearance, many aging Americans will prefer options for vision correction that minimize or eliminate the need for glasses.

Maintaining 20/20 Vision in the Year 2020

An estimated 20.5 million Americans past age 40 have a cataract in either eye, but by 2020 that number is expected to increase to 30.1 million. Historically, cataract surgery volumes have consistently grown at an annual rate of about 3%

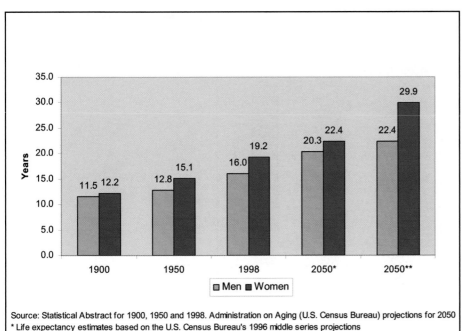

Figure 1. US life expectancy 1900 to 2050.

Source: Statistical Abstract for 1900, 1950 and 1998. Administration on Aging (U.S. Census Bureau) projections for 2050
* Life expectancy estimates based on the U.S. Census Bureau's 1996 middle series projections
** Life expectancy estimates based on the U.S. Census Bureau's 1996 high series projections

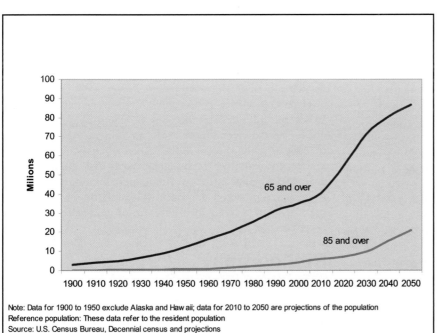

Figure 2. Older population growth trends 1900 to 2050.

Note: Data for 1900 to 1950 exclude Alaska and Hawaii; data for 2010 to 2050 are projections of the population
Reference population: These data refer to the resident population
Source: U.S. Census Bureau, Decennial census and projections

(2.9 million procedures were performed in 2006). However, ophthalmologists should expect a dramatic increase in the number of patients requiring cataract surgery over the next 2 decades (Figure 3).

In addition, refractive errors affect approximately one-third of Americans over age 40, and as baby boomers have discovered (much to their horror), by age 55 the incidence of presbyopia is virtually 100%. The emergence of the new PC-IOLs offers additional benefits for patients undergoing traditional cataract surgery as well as aging baby boomers that have not yet developed a cataract. Given this generation's desire to pursue new interests, new careers, and even new relationships well into their retirement, the prospects of a life free from spectacles is very appealing.

Of course one of the major hurdles to adoption of this new technology is price, with out-of-pocket expense to the patient ranging from $2000 to $5000 per eye. While the high cost has contributed to more modest market volume of PC-IOLs than lens manufacturers had hoped for, recent forecasts are more optimistic. There are many reasons for the increased demand for PC-IOLs, but chief amongst them are the relative affluence of the baby boomer generation and the personality traits that make them the ultimate consumers.

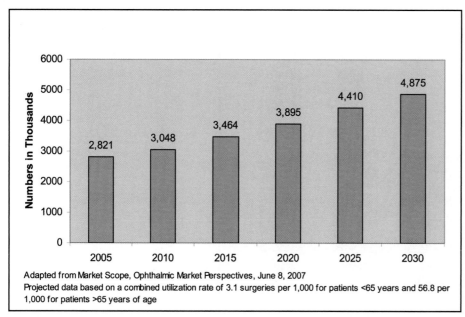

Figure 3. Total US cataract procedures 2005 to 2030.

Adapted from Market Scope, Ophthalmic Market Perspectives, June 8, 2007
Projected data based on a combined utilization rate of 3.1 surgeries per 1,000 for patients <65 years and 56.8 per 1,000 for patients >65 years of age

The Consumer Generation

No single generation personifies consumerism quite like the baby boomers. Because of the sheer size of this cohort, they have seemingly been the perpetual "target audience" for all manner of advertising beginning in the 1960s and 1970s.

A strong work ethic and high educational attainment (boomer's are twice as likely as their parents to be high school and/or college graduates) have provided the economic underpinning to support this generation's quest for high-quality goods and services. Currently boomers spend a staggering $2.3 trillion in annual household expenditures (twice the amount of 18-to-39 year olds) and control $750 billion in discretionary income. With an average income in households headed by 50-to-59 year olds of $75,000, boomers are 71% more likely than their younger counterparts to try new products and services, especially goods and services that help them look and feel better. They place value on premium products and are not afraid of technology. Unlike the Depression-era generation that preceded them, baby boomers feel a sense of entitlement—they do not see their conspicuous consumerism as indulging in luxuries but more as a reward for all their years of dedication and hard work. One need only look at the record numbers associated with plastic surgery, health and beauty products, and spas to realize that PC-IOLs will be an attractive option for boomers wishing to be free from the inconvenience and "age-defining" stigma of wearing glasses.

Looking Ahead

So what do the current trends tell us about future demand for these new lenses? The volume of PC-IOLs is forecast to climb to just over 150,000 units in 2007, a 20% gain over last year's totals. This projected growth has 2 main causes: 1) an increase in the number of patients opting for PC-IOLs versus standard IOLs for cataract surgery and 2) an increase in the number of patients (primarily 55 to 65 years old) undergoing refractive lens exchange (RLE) procedures to correct a combination of refractive error and presbyopia. In fact, based on current projections, it is not unreasonable to expect that within the next 2 decades, the volume of cataract surgery performed in the United States using PC-IOLs will exceed that of standard IOLs. Continuing evolution in lens technology will afford patients even greater benefits and provide a much-needed source of additional practice revenue for ophthalmologists coping with a constrained Medicare payment system. While the full effect of the baby boomers' consumerism will not be felt for several more years, any practice that is looking to "capture" this segment of the market would be wise to assess how well it will meet the boomers' needs over the next 2 to 5 years and adapt accordingly. Any opportunity costs that result from such a proactive approach will surely be rewarded many times over by a large, loyal infusion of new patients into the practice.

Bibliography

1. Adler J. The boomer files. *Newsweek.* November 14, 2005. http://www.msnbc.msn.com/id/9939304/site/newsweek/page/0/. Accessed September 11, 2007.
2. Bergman M. Impact of baby boomers anticipated. U.S. Census Bureau News. March 9, 2006. http://www.census.gov/Press-Release/www/releases/archives/aging_population/006544.html. Accessed September 11, 2007.
3. Covino RM. A "booming" opportunity. Confectioner.com. http://www.confectioner.com/content.php?s=CO/2006/06&p=24. Accessed September 11, 2007.
4. de Mesa A. Don't ignore the boomer consumer. brandchannel.com. http://www.brandchannel.com/features_effect.asp?pf_id=373. Accessed September 11, 2007.
5. Dugdale J. Senior momentum: can design and technology deliver a golden age of aging? *Business Week.* May 1, 2007. http://www.businessweek.com/innovate/content/may2007/id20070501_690761.htm. Accessed September 11, 2007.
6. Facts for Features. Oldest baby boomers turn 60! U.S. Census Bureau. http://www.census.gov/Press-Release/www/releases/archives/facts_for_features_special_editions/006105.html. Accessed September 11, 2007.

7. Facts for Features. Older Americans month: May 2007. U.S. Census Bureau. http://www.census.gov/Press-Release/www/releases/archives/facts_for_features_special_editions/009715.html. Accessed September 11, 2007.

8. Freeman W. Ophthalmic market perspectives. *Market Scope.* 2007; 12(6):1-4.

9. Glauber B. Active lives defy aging. *Milwaukee Journal Sentinel.* May 6, 2006. http://www.jsonline.com/story/index.aspx?id=421541. Accessed September 11, 2007.

10. Centers for Disease Control and Prevention. Healthy aging for older adults. June 20, 2007. http://www.cdc.gov/aging/. Accessed September 11, 2007.

11. Hiemstra G. Population myths, trends and transportation planning. futurist.com. http://www.futurist.com/articles/future-trends/population-myths-trends-and-transportation-planning. Accessed September 11, 2007.

12. Moos B. Ads target empty nests, full wallets. *The Dallas Morning News.* December 11, 2005. http://www.sfaa.com/sharedcontent/dws/bus/stories/121105dnbusboomertising.29c7e45.html. Accessed September 11, 2007.

CHAPTER 4

REFRACTIVE SURGERY AND IOLS— FUTURE TRENDS

I. Howard Fine, MD

With recent improvements in new phacoemulsification technology, which include sophisticated power modulations and new and improved fluidics, in addition to partial optical coherence methods for measuring axial length, cataract and lens extraction has become incredibly safe and efficacious. We have dramatically improved outcomes with an almost immediate return of excellent uncorrected vision, from the utilization of lower energy, smaller incisions, and adjunctive astigmatic correcting techniques, and as a result, we see the natural evolution of lens surgery into refractive surgery.

There are certain limitations of laser in situ keratomileusis (LASIK). High hyperopes, myopes, and presbyopes are not good candidates, and certainly cataract patients, even those with early lenticular changes, are not good patients for corneal-based refractive surgery. Furthermore, because the spherical aberration in the cornea is constant throughout life but there are changes in the aberration of the lens as the patient ages, anything done to the cornea as a refractive modality—including the most sophisticated, customized shaping—will be degraded by changing spherical aberration in the lens as the patient ages. As a result, I believe that lenticular-based refractive surgery (ie, refractive lens exchange) will become the dominant procedure in ophthalmology.

In addition, the recent development of improvements in multifocal intraocular lenses (IOLs) and a whole armamentarium of new accommodative IOLs, including lenses that move in the eye, dual-optic IOLs, and deformable optic IOLs, are giving surgeons new options for presbyopia-correcting, lenticular-based surgery. There are also enormously innovative new technologies such as light adjustable IOLs; the Liquilens (Vision Solutions Technologies, Rockville, MD); and pixi-lated-optic IOLs, which promise even greater ability for us to achieve excellent results for our refractive lens patients.

My ideal future lens would be a lens that is biocompatible, gives a full field of vision, is aberration free, allows for continuous acuity from distance to near, has an adequate amplitude of accommodation to avoid accommodative fatigue, has an appropriate filter for unwanted light rays, and will either prevent posterior capsular opacification or allow for YAG laser posterior capsulotomy, all while being implantable through an incision of 3.0 mm or less. Some of the new technology is close to achieving these goals, and we can anticipate that within the future these goals will, indeed, be a reality.

Today, children with refractive errors wear spectacles, teenagers wear contact lenses, young adults get refractive surgery, middle-aged adults use bifocals, and senior citizens get cataract surgery. I believe that in the not-too-distant future refractive lens exchange will eliminate all but the use of spectacles in children and contact lenses in teenagers.

This will represent a quadruple win. Patients can enjoy a predictable refractive procedure, with a rapid recovery, that can address all of their refractive errors, including presbyopia, and never develop cataracts. Surgeons will be able to offer these procedures without the intrusion of private or government insurance and be able to establish less stressful relationships with their patients. The industry will get a greater return on their investment in IOL research and lens extraction technology. Finally, the government will be the biggest winner because it will enjoy decreased financial burden from the expense of cataract surgery for the ever increasing ranks of baby boomers, as more and more of these patients opt for lens exchange to address their refractive surgery goals, ultimately reaching Medicare coverage as pseudophakes.

CHAPTER 5

REFRACTIVE SURGERY AND IOLs— FUTURE TRENDS

Richard L. Lindstrom, MD

Sir John Maddox wisely stated, "The most important discoveries of the next 50 years are likely to be ones of which we cannot now even conceive."

In spite of this prudent observation, in the following paragraphs I will present my personal thoughts regarding some possible future trends in refractive cataract surgery and refractive lens exchange. The thoughts discussed are based on 35 years dedicated to advancing the art and science of this field and a fertile imagination. I do not intend to provide references to substantiate the ideas presented and suspect much of what I prognosticate will come to pass in totally unexpected ways that no one today could anticipate. My musings should be considered a personal communication. The primary focus will be on the United States and similar developed countries, where I currently practice, but similar trends can be anticipated throughout the advanced world as emerging country economies develop and adequate manpower and financial resources become available worldwide.

I see refractive cataract surgery and refractive lens exchange continuing to grow until they are replaced by medical therapy, anti-aging therapy, and genetic engineering. Today, approximately 3 million lens implants are performed following these 2 procedures in the United States alone, and nearly 15,000,000 worldwide. In the United States, the aging population, the affluence of the American "baby boomer" generation, and the ability of surgeons to bill for a premium refractive outcome will drive significant growth in this lens-based refractive surgery sector.

The standard intraocular lens (IOL) channel will grow at 3% to 4% per year but the "premium" channel will grow at a significantly higher rate, at least 10% per year and perhaps as high as 20% per year in dollars.

The IOL market will segregate into 3 channels that will each have a very different future. These will include a standard optic IOL channel, a multifocal optic IOL channel, and an accommodating optic IOL channel.

The standard optic IOL channel, which dates its origins to Harold Ridley in 1949, today represents 95% of lenses implanted by US surgeons. The standard monofocal IOL channel will be slowly but continuously eroded by the multifocal IOL and accommodating IOL channels until lens-based surgery disappears in 2100 and beyond. The multifocal IOL channel, which dates its origins to the early 1980s when the IOLAB center surround bulls eye and 3M diffractive multifocal IOLs were launched in Europe and parts of Asia, will experience a 5- to 15-year surge in popularity before being nearly totally replaced by the continuous development of improved accommodating IOLs.

The accommodating IOL channel will grow relentlessly in popularity and market share as continuous innovation and invention increases achievable accommodative/pseudo accommodative amplitude to over 10 D. Patients after lens implantation will be able to achieve the vision of a 20- to 40-year-old emmetropic patient: seamless vision distance through intermediate to near, normal, or even supra-normal quality of vision, an absence of significant dysphotopic or night vision symptoms, good stereopsis with both eyes targeted for plano, and a full visual field will become the standard outcome.

By the year 2030, mid career for the ophthalmic surgeon entering practice today, the majority of patients in affluent countries will opt for a lens exchange with an accommodating IOL as their preferred method of visual rehabilitation when their natural lens becomes dysfunctional through natural aging with loss of transparency, induced aberrations, or reduced accommodation. The decision to undergo surgery will occur at an earlier and earlier age until it becomes routine between ages 45 to 55. Refractive lens exchange with placement of an accommodating IOL will over take corneal surgery as the most common method for correction of refractive errors and will become the preferred modality in all presbyopic patients.

Additional vision-enhancing features will be bolted on to each of the 3 primary channel implants: monofocal, multifocal, and accommodating. Customization of optic power and optic shape to correct myopia, hyperopia, astigmatism, and higher-order aberration will become routine. Early generation accommodating IOLs will have their optic shape optimized for increased depth of focus until accommodative amplitudes grow to over 3 D. Ultraviolet, violet, and blue light transmission will become further understood and optimized for quality of vision, optimal color perception, and retinal/macular safety.

Photochromic lenses will emerge as a viable option. Enhancements for the continuously decreasing number of patients with a residual refractive error will be achieved by adjusting the IOL implant's optic shape or refractive index and not through corneal surgery. Capsular opacity will be eliminated through a combination of medical therapy and advances in lens implant design and material, likely through surface modification and drugs impregnated in the optic itself. Capsular elasticity will be better retained postoperatively, further enhancing accommodating amplitude of the lens implant. While first emulating a 40-year-old pre-presbyopic emmetrope, advancement toward simulating the normal lens at the age of 20 will occur. Infection and inflammation will nearly disappear through the use of a combination of antibiotics and anti-inflammatories injected into the eye at the time of surgery or impregnated into the lens implant optic and/or viscoelastics. Endothelial cell loss will become history as growth factors leave the endothelial cell count higher after surgery than before. By the year 2050, as the generation of currently training ophthalmic surgeons wind down their careers, the typical patient with a normal macula will experience 20/10 vision with a quality of vision and accommodative amplitude superior to that of an emmetropic 20 year old after undergoing a 5-minute procedure with minimal morbidity and complications.

The raging controversy will be whether or not it is ethical to perform surgery on a 40-year-old emmetropic patient with 20/20 vision at distance and J1 at intermediate and near who wishes the increased accommodative amplitude and enhanced quality of vision afforded by the latest generation of refractive lens exchange with an accommodating lens implant. The most advanced lens implants will be accommodating, biconvex, 9 mm in diameter, customized, and repeatedly adjustable in power, toricity, and higher-order aberration, and insertable through a 1- to 2-mm incision. The lens will be delivered inside an insertion device. The IOL will not only emulate the 20-year-old natural human lens, but its optic power, toricity, higher-order aberration correction, and light transmission will be repeatedly adjustable as the patient's cornea and retina ages, and his or her needs or environment changes.

The surgeon experience will evolve as well. All eye surgery will be office based. It will be performed on a surgical work station that incorporates enhanced three-dimensional imaging. Surgical microscopes will be a historical memory. Multiple laser delivery systems and surgical interventions will be controlled through computer software and robotics. The incision size will be 2 mm or less and created by a laser. The anterior capsule will be opened and the lens softened with a combination of laser energy and therapeutic agents. The lens material will simply be aspirated.

The surgeon will customize the procedure for each individual patient and cognitive skills and ability will dominate over procedure. Outcomes will become consistent from one patient to the next and one surgeon to the next as the procedure becomes progressively more automated.

Patients who underwent cataract surgery prior to the development of this advanced generation of accommodative IOLs will seek upgrades for their own visual systems. Piggyback and replacement lenses will evolve that can simulate accommodation through a range of 4 to 6 D using refractive index change controlled by sensors and small batteries with a 100-year life implanted in the ciliary muscle. Ciliary muscle contraction occurring in response to the normal accommodation will generate an accommodation-like response by increasing the refractive index of the lens optic.

A high quality of vision and the absence of dysphotopsia will be retained. Implantation of these lenses will also be performed using a multilaser three-dimensional video image–based robotic surgical workstation, but the surgery will be less automated and require more of the classical surgeon skills.

As the technology advances, the population ages, and surgeon numbers decline with the retirement of the baby boomer generation of ophthalmic surgeons, a significant manpower shortage of ophthalmic surgeons with the required cognitive and procedural skills will occur. Eye care delivery will be organized into integrated eye care delivery systems utilizing ophthalmic surgeons, medical ophthalmologists, optometrists, ophthalmic technicians, and administrators as efficiently as possible to meet the enormous demand these advances generate.

Some time before 2050 the ability to retard and even reverse the aging process of the natural lens will emerge. Individuals under the age of 50 will have their natural lens rehabilitated to normal transparency and elasticity through a combination of laser application and topical, transcleral, or systemic application of a reducing agent containing medication. What we today call cataracts and presbyopia will no longer develop. Refractive errors will continue to occur, and lens-based surgery will be primarily performed to treat myopia, hyperopia, astigmatism, and presbyopia.

By 2100 genetic engineering will eliminate ametropia as well. The application of genetic engineering as it pertains to the eye will remain the domain of the ophthalmologist, whose practice on the refractive side will be dominated by genetic testing of pregnant women and infants followed by gene modifying treatments that prevent the development of ametropias. The lifelong ophthalmology/patient relationship of today will be retained as the ophthalmologist applies advanced diagnostic and therapeutic strategies to prevent disease and aging of the eye. Retention and enhancement of quality vision will dominate over today's emphasis on vision restoration and the treatment of disease. Vision will continue to be the most valued of the senses, and practicing ophthalmology will remain a rewarding, well-compensated, and honorable profession.

CHAPTER 6

REFRACTIVE SURGERY AND IOLs— FUTURE TRENDS

Lee T. Nordan, MD

The future of intraocular lens (IOL) surgery can be summarized by the following axiom: "Refractive mentality with IOL technology."

The following are my basic beliefs with respect to presbyopia and IOLs:

* Moderate to severe presbyopia is better corrected by an IOL than by corneal surgery.

* Keratorefractive surgery can create an aspheric cornea (with resulting increased depth of field) and can also create monovision. These are reasonable alternatives, but only until a superior binocular solution for presbyopia is provided.

* Current multifocal IOLs are acceptable for cataract/IOL patients but because younger presbyopes are more discerning, more widespread use of phakic IOLs will require a multifocal IOL with less glare.

* A fully functional accommodating IOL should represent the gold standard for the correction of presbyopia, but it is very uncertain as to whether and when a truly accommodating IOL can be achieved. Once the integrity of the capsular bag is compromised, filling the bag with a material capable of accommodation tends to create a sphere, not a lenticular shape.

* Current iris-fixated phakic IOLs are too difficult to implant and will be limited in popularity as a result.

* Current "accommodating IOLs" provide some increased depth of field, perhaps a limited degree of accommodation secondary to IOL movement. Not enough accommodative amplitude is provided, however, to serve as a full-fledged correction of pseudophakic presbyopia.

If the aforementioned statements are accepted (varying opinions are possible), then some interesting concepts with respect to the future of IOL's may be derived.

The correction of presbyopia is the greatest driving factor in new IOL development. Sophisticated diffractive optics allow for consistently thin optics, virtually no chromatic aber-

ration, and minimal glare compared to the current multifocal IOLs. These new optics will be employed in phakic and as piggyback posterior chamber (PC)-IOLs that correct pseudophakic presbyopia.

Thicker, multicomponent pseudophakic multifocal IOLs will have to demonstrate their efficacy in clinical trials. In order to gain popularity (assuming acceptable function), surgeons must be able to easily insert them through a small incision.

PC phakic IOLs function well optically, but the true risk of cataract formation in the 3 to 7 year postoperative period is still not fully known. A multifocal PC phakic IOL should be forthcoming.

Anterior chamber (AC) phakic IOLs will become more popular in the future because they can be removed easily and they carry a much lower risk of cataracts compared to a PC phakic IOL. An AC IOL, however, requires a very sophisticated and effective haptic design in order for the optic to be consistently positioned in the posterior third of the AC. The phakic IOL must not cause any significant long-term endothelial cell damage. Successful AC phakic IOL implantation will require precise preoperative measurement of the AC diameter by technology such as the Zeiss Visante OCT (Jena, Germany) or high-frequency ultrasonic biomicroscopy. This instrumentation ideally could also be used intraoperatively to document the precise location of the IOL at the conclusion of surgery.

An improved multifocal phakic IOL would be preferable to clear lensectomy plus a pseudophakic multifocal IOL for several reasons: excellent accommodation could be maintained at various distances, excellent preoperative distance visual acuity is uncompromised, and the incidence of complications is potentially much lower than with clear lensectomy.

Most importantly, cataract/IOL surgeons must develop a refractive surgical mentality. Why is this so important? The current complication rate for phaco/IOL surgery is probably 5% to 6%, despite the general belief that it is much lower.

A successful refractive surgeon must have a minor complication rate in the 1% range, especially if intraocular surgery is performed. Therefore, not only must the IOL technology improve, which it certainly shall, but so must surgical technique as well. Cataract surgeons must be prepared to transition from operating on patients with eye pathology to operating on healthy eyes. These latter patients have higher expectations compared to a cataract patient.

The anatomic results of IOL surgery can be seen at the slit lamp and objectively measured as visual acuity. Therefore, the success or failure of a procedure should be readily obvious. Studies suggest that virtually all refractive surgeons will make the transition to using a phakic presbyopic IOL, and about one-third of current cataract surgeons will do the same.

I believe that all cataract and refractive surgery will be re-defined in the future as being "quality anterior segment surgery." It will not be possible to otherwise differentiate between cataract surgery and refractive IOL surgery. The surgeon will help the patient choose which keratorefractive and/or IOL procedure best suits his or her needs. Often, several sequential procedures might be performed to obtain the best results. Cataract surgeons are not used to planning for more than one surgery, but this is a common practice in refractive surgery.

The surgeon should refrain from considering keratorefractive surgery and IOLs as being competing technologies. Rather they should be thought of as complementary means for achieving a desired goal. The choice of surgical procedure will be based upon an evaluation of the risks and benefits for that patient, plus the surgeon's comfort level with a given procedure.

Conclusion

In the future we will witness a great rise in the popularity of phakic and piggyback PC pseudophakic IOLs for the correction of ametropia and presbyopia in particular. Meanwhile, as the quest for a truly accommodative IOL continues, multifocal diffractive optics will improve for both phakic and pseudophakic IOLs. Another possibility will be the development of a long-acting pharmaceutical agent that could increase the power of the ciliary body (without brow ache or severe miosis). This approach to correct presbyopia could become available well before a totally functional accommodating IOL.

CHAPTER 7

WHAT IS A PREMIUM IOL WORTH?

J. Andy Corley

Cataract surgery is the most successful procedure in all of medicine and has the lowest complication rates. Cataract surgery through its evolution and without the benefit of a formal announcement became refractive surgery. Surgeons and patients expect a refractive outcome after successful cataract removal and a lens implant. The delivery of this wonderful procedure has produced billions of dollars in value for everyone associated (ie, patients, surgeons, insurers, and industry).

Most recently the bar has been raised again with the introduction of presbyopia-correcting intraocular lens (Pr-C IOL). Now the patient expects successful cataract removal, elimination of any ametropia, and the treatment of presbyopia. The introduction of PIOLs, the IOL Master (Carl Zeiss Meditec, Jena, Germany), and improved formulas to calculate lens power, have led every surgeon participating in this new premium channel to try his or her best to achieve the refractive target. Greatly reduced spectacle dependence is now routinely a part of the surgeon-patient discussion. Success in the operating room no longer equates to successfully meeting patient expectations. It is the refractive outcome that will receive the most scrutiny and ultimately determine the success of the procedure.

I was very interested when Dr. Chang asked me to contribute this chapter on the value of cataract surgery. I attribute the reason for this request to the fact that, as a member of the ophthalmic industry for the past 29 years, I have observed the devaluation of cataract surgery. In this chapter I will examine how that happened. How could the most successful operation known to man sink to such low value in the eyes of governments and the health care insurers of the world? What had to be done to re-establish the value? Lastly, how can the value produced be protected in the future? These are questions that must be answered if we are to avoid the mistakes of the past and preserve the value of this modern miracle for both patients and surgeons.

There are many definitions of value, but for purposes of thinking about modern cataract surgery I have chosen the following: *the worth of something in terms of the amount of other things for which it can be exchanged or in terms of some medium of exchange.* I think this definition better than any other puts the value of cataract surgery into perspective. If you had a progressive visual disorder that reduced your quality of life and would ultimately blind you, what would you exchange in order to have it corrected? Yet how many patients and surgeons think of modern cataract surgery in those terms? Due to the standards of excellence achieved every day in operating theaters around the world, the miracle of cataract surgery has become routine. I hope this chapter will help all of us remember the incredible value of modern cataract surgery to the patient and to the surgeon who delivers the care.

How Was Value Lost?

In the mid 1980s, Medicare willingly paid for the exciting new miracle operation. Cataract surgery was provided primarily to patients in their late 70s and 80s and surgeons were satisfied with the economics around the new procedure. Surgical technique and technology flourished in this emerging market. Over 20 companies vied to supply their innovation to the market. As the procedure improved, surgeons felt comfortable providing it to younger patients, dramatically expanding the market for cataract surgery. Medicare now had a rapidly growing procedure that was extremely safe and effective fueled by satisfied patients. It was a good time for both surgeons and patients. However, the cost accelerated with increased usage and ophthalmology found itself tagged with the most expensive line item in Medicare Part B. In the early 1990s, budget pressure affected all of Medicare; the unavoidable response to the popularity of cataract surgery was to reduce remuneration for both surgeon and facilities. Thus began the commoditization of cataract surgery. Unfortunately, surgeons had become more dependent on Medicare over this period of time. When Medicare began to reduce payments, surgeons were forced to focus on cost reduction. It was in this period that the value began to drift into the background and everything was first evaluated as a cost. Value had become a second class citizen in

Medically-Mediated Consumer Decisions in Healthcare 2007: Surgical Experience, Recovery, and Benefit						
Procedure	Indication	Patient Surgical Experience	Recovery	Length of Benefit	Price*	Outcomes
Face lift	Improved appearance	2- to 3-hour surgery under general anesthesia	2 to 6 months, pain	7 to 15 years	$12,000 to $25,000[1]	Variable
Elective athletic surgery	Improve athletic performance (ie, shoulder)	2- to 3-hour surgery under general anesthesia	6 to 18 months of physical therapy	10 years to permanent	$12,500 to $15,000[3]	Good
Dental implants	Improved appearance and function	Multiple surgeries over 4 to 5 months	Pain immediately postoperative	5 years to permanent	$5000 to $10,000[2] per tooth	Good 5% to 10% of implants fail within 6 months
Canine cataract	Prevent blindess	30-minute surgery	1 month	Permanent	$2500[4]	Patient tail wags
Standard cataract surgery	Preserve and improve vision	20-minute surgery	1 week	Permanent	$4000[5 for] both eyes	Highly predictable
PIOL cataract surgery	Greatly reduce spectacle dependance Preserve and improve vision	20-minute surgery	1 week	Permanent	$10,000 to $12,000[6] for both eyes	Highly predictable

[1] www.ienhance.com; [2] www.yourdentistryguide.com/implants; [3] Thomas C. Hopkins, MD; [4] CareCredit; [5] David Chang, MD; [6] eyeonics data on file 2007.
*Includes surgeon fee, anesthesia, facility fee

Figure 1. Medically medicated consumer decisions in health care 2007: Surgical experience, recovery, and length of benefit.

the world of reimbursement and surgeon thinking.

Modern cataract surgery was indeed a victim of its own success, and the value proposition was far removed from the person who enjoys the benefit the most, the patient. When distanced from the value proposition by insurers, it was the beginning of a long decline. Why did the value decrease in spite of improved outcomes, improvements in safety, and improvements in surgeons' skill as well as technological advancements? Over time the answer became painfully clear: there was only one buyer. One buyer has set the rules for both publicly and privately insured patients—Medicare. That buyer could no longer afford the value of modern cataract surgery.

What Had to Be Done to Regain Value?

With all the advancements in modern cataract surgery, how did the value become so depressed? To answer that question, you must first ask, "Who derives the most value from cataract surgery?" The answer is obvious: the patient. The patient had to be reinserted into the value proposition. After 20 years of dependence on third parties to reimburse for cataract surgery, there is suddenly a new paradigm, the premium channel, where the patient pays for the enhanced value he or she receives. This brings us to the premium channel and why you have purchased this book. Ophthalmology is extremely fortunate to have new technologies that are elective in nature and outside the covered service plan of insurers. Thus the benefit of reduced spectacle dependence offered by PIOLs is a service that your patients may "choose" to enjoy. Premium channel patients will pay the majority of your procedure charges and that requires some adjustments, which are described thoroughly in this book, by you and your staff. No longer will the majority of your professional fee come from faceless insurers;

your customer is sitting right in front of you and will now have a say in the market value of your service. As mentioned earlier in this chapter, the bar has been raised again; the demands on you and your staff to deliver the best possible refractive outcomes are now real time.

With the birth of the premium channel, cataract surgery has evolved to a medically mediated consumer decision. Rarely do patients find themselves in a complete state of debilitation before electing to have the surgery. Therefore, cataract surgery compares favorably to other medically mediated consumer decisions like shoulder and knee surgery for better athletic performance or facelifts for better appearance. Baby boomers have made it quite clear that they will not go quietly into older age; they will choose procedures and technologies to help extend the youthful, active lifestyle that they enjoy. Ophthalmology is perfectly positioned to enjoy serving the baby boomers, but we must be prepared to compete with other lifestyle decisions being made by the boomers. Let us compare modern cataract surgery to some of the other medically mediated consumer decisions in 3 ways: surgical experience, recovery, and length of benefit (Figure 1).

SHOULDER SURGERY

1. Surgical experience—Full anesthesia, 1- to 2-hour operation, discomfort postoperatively

2. Recovery—3-month rehabilitation period

3. Length of benefit—10 to 15 years, sometimes permanent

FACE LIFT

1. Surgical experience— 1- to 2-hour surgery

2. Recovery—Excruciating pain postoperatively for up to 6 months

3. Length of benefit—10 to 15 years

MODERN CATARACT SURGERY

1. Surgical experience—10-minute operation

2. Recovery—Return to work the next day

3. Length of benefit—Permanent

The premium channel is in its infancy. The cataract procedure is highly competitive with other lifestyle choices that baby boomers will make. It is up to the profession and industry to make sure that John Q. Public is well aware of how effective our offering is for patients. Indeed baby boomers will seek rejuvenation like no other group. Cataract removal with PIOL does serve this need for rejuvenation better than other medically mediated procedures.

Maintaining Value in the Future

The value lesson of the first 35 years of modern cataract surgery can be summed up simply: ophthalmology and industry surrendered the surgeon-patient relationship to third-party insurers. It was economically satisfactory for a short period and then a steady state of continuous fee reduction was slowly ground into the culture of everyone involved. The expectation became that the slow drumbeat of reduced value was unavoidable despite incredible improvements in outcomes and safety. Unfortunately for standard cataract surgery, the modern miracle that it is, the drum continues to pound due to pressure on the system. Luckily ophthalmology has the premium channel, a method of differentiating services, and allows us the opportunity to reverse these troubling trends. The solution to maintaining future value is quite simple. We must learn to meet the needs of the individual patient/consumer. In modern ophthalmology, the demanding patient is our best friend. Learning to satisfy the needs of the patient who pays privately for the majority of his or her treatment will ensure that the value proposition is not handed off to third parties again. As a profession and industry we must resist the temptation to have insurers interject themselves into the premium channel. The value proposition belongs to the patient receiving the care. As long as it remains there, ophthalmology will enter into a new golden age in which the incredible advances in surgery and technology can continue to flourish and be enjoyed by all who participate.

CHAPTER 8

What Is a Premium IOL Worth?

Kay Coulson, MBA

Almost every surgeon believes that the "other" guy—down the street, across the country, or in a different medical specialty—has figured out a secret to elective fee-setting that he or she has not. How many conferences have we attended where someone says, "Let's learn from the cosmetic surgeons. They've figured out how to get top dollar for their services. Why can't we be like them?"

Truth #1: LASIK Surgeons Lead the Way in Setting Fees for Elective Medical Procedures

It is time to reorient our thinking. In 2006, the average LASIK patient paid just over $4000 for bilateral laser in situ keratomileusis (LASIK). This compares to $3495 for the top 5 surgical cosmetic procedures, which include breast augmentation, blepharoplasty, liposuction, rhinoplasty, and abdominoplasty. These 5 procedures account for 75% of all cosmetic surgical procedures.

A good deal of attention has been paid, and advertising committed, to the newer, minimally invasive procedures in the cosmetic and dental industries. However, these procedures yield only $400 to $500 per occurrence, which is well within everyday, discretionary budgets for many lifestyle-motivated consumers (Figure 1).

Truth #2: Ophthalmologists Perform More Surgery on More Patients Than Other Elective Specialists

Adding LASIK and lens procedures together, ophthalmologists perform surgery on roughly 2.3 million people annually. If we perform our task well, we will not see these patients back in the laser suite or ambulatory surgery center (ASC). Conversely, cosmetic surgeons perform a huge number of procedures on the same repeat patients. In 2006, 40% of cosmetic patients had repeat procedures, and 41% had multiple procedures during the same visit. The only growing area of cosmetic surgery is BOTOX (Allergan, Irvine, CA) and fillers (Figure 2). Have they figured out something that we have not? No. What they have is a tightly targeted, tightly marketed demographic that can be repeatedly served. The vision surgeon must continue to reach out across a much broader spectrum of the population for his or her surgical volume to grow.

Truth #3: Elective Vision Fees Should Reflect Vision Value Received

There are 2 ways to evaluate reasonable fees for elective vision services. The first is based on perceived value. What is the value of the vision you deliver? How do your patients assess this value? We have solid bookends of value in the vision marketplace. Roughly 9 million cataracts are diagnosed annually, but only 3 million proceed to surgery. The typical cataract patient will pay approximately $400 per eye out-of-pocket to have cataract surgery and still need glasses afterward. At the other end of the spectrum, we have a predictable history of 1.4 million LASIK surgeries annually at $2000 each, with virtually 100% expecting 20/20 vision and no glasses ever again. Every LASIK surgeon in the country works to increase this $2000 fee through technology innovations, surgeon expertise, outstanding outcomes, and an improved customer experience. In reality, we may have hit the "vision value" ceiling. We have our bookends: monofocal lens surgery at $400 and LASIK surgery (distance and/or monovision) at $2000.

How much better is the vision delivered by upgraded presbyopia-correcting and toric intraocular lenses (IOLs)? Is this presby-IOL vision worth an extra $2000 per eye? $3000?

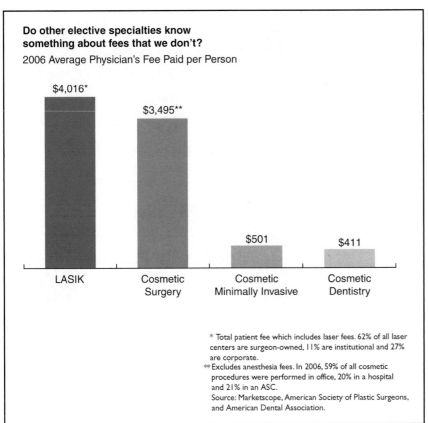

Figure 1. Patient payments for selected US elective procedures show LASIK surgeons lead in their ability to set fees.

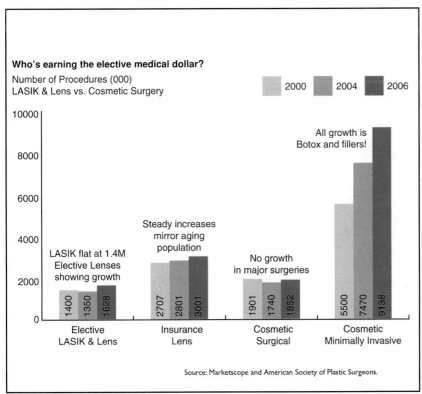

Figure 2. Comparison of LASIK and LENS procedures versus cosmetic procedures show flat to minimal growth, other than BOTOX and fillers.

$4000? I have seen 2 consistent trends in the practices where I consult. Cataract patients will choose upgraded lenses at high levels (25% to 40%) at up to $2000 above insurance coverage per eye. The improvement in glasses-free (or glasses-reduced) vision versus insurance vision appears to be worth an out-of-pocket expenditure similar to fees paid for LASIK.

A 55- to 64-year-old clear-lens candidate responds positively to the single-surgery option an upgraded lens provides and will pay up to $1000 more per eye than what he or she expected for custom LASIK because of the permanent benefit a lens provides.

Figure 3. Fee-setting must take into consideration both market-driven and cost-driven perspectives.

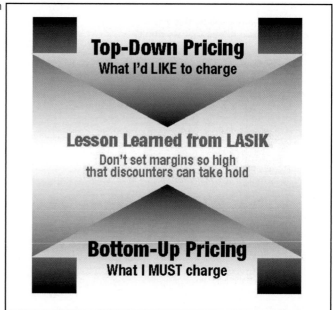

Are there exceptions to this pricing? Sure. Surgeon reputation and limited providers in a market can increase fees. But I ask you to consider the vision improvement you are delivering today to this patient, and set fees accordingly. Many surgeons are tempted to try to correct reimbursement compression on the backs of early lens-upgrade adopters. Many of these same practices are experiencing poor conversions and wonder whether the market for upgraded lenses really exists. You must ask yourself, "How much better is the upgraded IOL vision I am delivering versus monofocal lenses and LASIK?" It will help you set fees that make sense to the patient, accurately reflect the vision delivered by the technology, and result in more surgery for you.

Truth #4: Elective Vision Fees Should Deliver Reasonable Margins

The second pricing methodology to consider is bottom-up or cost-plus pricing (Figure 3). LASIK went wrong in the late 1990s because of our greed. Simple supply and demand dictate that any business with bottom-line margins of 50%+ will attract competition. We attracted the discounters and corporations to LASIK because we set exorbitant fees. We do not want a repeat in the lens marketplace.

A commodity business has margins in the 2% to 5% range. Lucrative businesses yield 15% to 25% margins. Think about your fee from the standpoint of what it actually costs you to deliver the service and add a reasonable margin to this total.

When determining fees, include costs for the ASC, anesthesia, the lens, increased YAGs, and increased LASIK enhancements. Add an incremental physician's fee to cover the increased cost of testing, the increased physician time for counseling and postoperative care, and any staff increases required to service this patient. This becomes your clear lens fee for lifestyle IOLs.

For cataract surgeries, look at the increased lens cost and additional testing required for upgrade lenses. For most practices, the fees outlined in Figure 4 for cataract upgrades are within reason of the $2000 per eye the market has accepted for LASIK. For clear lens, the fees are generally within the "custom LASIK + $1000 for permanence" that people have demonstrated a willingness to pay. Overall, I find these fees to be logical from both a top-down and bottom-up perspective, generating increased practice profitability, without attracting aggressive discounter competition.

Setting elective vision fees is fact-based, quantifiable, and ultimately market driven. Your customers will tell you when your fees and/or vision delivery are out of line simply by proceeding with or foregoing surgery. The key to elective vision fees is to objectively look at today's market and today's consumer and set fees that generate response. What you used to earn, what you used to be reimbursed, and what you think you are worth have no bearing on how the customer today will behave.

Ophthalmologists are leading the way in elective medicine. There is no other specialty that has had more success in educating, persuading, and involving the customer in surgical care. Look no further. You are the expert.

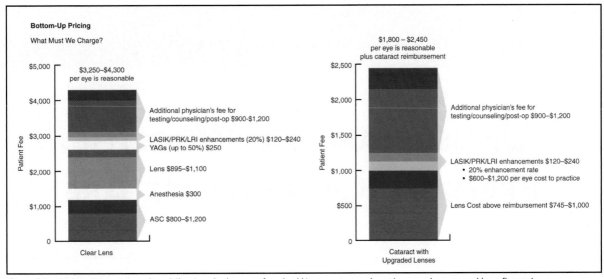

Figure 4. Establishing Cataract-Upgrade and Clear Lens Replacement fees should incorporate actual practice costs plus a reasonable profit margin.

CHAPTER 9

UNDERSTANDING WHO THE PREMIUM IOL PATIENTS ARE

Shareef Mahdavi, BA

To gain an understanding into the patients who are the best candidates for a premium intraocular lens (IOL), it is helpful to put this technology into the context of other advances in health care and medicine. For the past few decades, significant advances have been made to improve all aspects of life and its quality. Pharmacological and surgical interventions are allowing people to lead active lives into their 80s and 90s, and the number of people in the United States 100 years of age or older is projected to reach 131,000 by the year 2010.[1] Modern cataract surgery is a prime contributor to extended quality of life, restoring vision to millions of people en route to becoming the single most commonly performed surgical procedure, in large part due to its high level of both efficacy and safety. Widespread coverage of the procedure by Medicare and private insurance helped cement its popularity. The paradigm for patients has been relatively straightforward: with symptoms of decreased vision, go see a doctor. If 65 years or older, the government pays to have your lens removed and a new one put in. Glasses are prescribed to handle residual refractive error and/or induced astigmatism. End of story.

Arguably, the advent of laser vision correction for non-therapeutic surgical intervention has helped IOL technology developers see beyond that traditional paradigm just described. Laser in situ keratomileusis (LASIK)'s popularity as a means of creating spectacle independence has allowed it to become the single most commonly performed elective surgical procedure in the United States since the first excimer laser was approved in 1995. What LASIK demonstrated to the ophthalmic community is that patients will pay out of pocket for the benefits of medical technology and will not necessarily wait for a third party to pick up the tab. LASIK, with near-instant results and a similar efficacy and safety profile to cataract surgery, has raised the bar in the minds of patients and surgeons as to what would be defined as an acceptable outcome for either refractive and cataract surgery. This, in turn, has served as a stimulus to develop better IOLs with greater refractive functionality.

Demographics

Who is likely to step up and want a premium IOL? It would be tempting to draw a line dividing patients according to age and simply proclaim that "older" patients will not consider a premium IOL and "younger" ones will. Although there is some merit to this concept, it is not an exact science. We might describe the traditional cataract patient as someone in his or her late 60s or older, with poor preoperative visual acuity and reasonable expectations. Often described as part of the "World War II Generation," this patient profile largely expects (courtesy of Medicare and private insurance) their healthcare needs to be covered by a third party. In return, they expect less and are more accepting of the surgical and refractive outcome.

Contrast this with a younger population of patients in their 40s to early 60s. This group, defined by demographers as the "baby boomer" generation, accounts for 78 million Americans and has created economic shifts at each stage of their lives. As kids and teenagers, they created demand for fast food, amusement parks, malls, and music. As adults, they are responsible for entirely new industries: health clubs, mutual funds, and luxury travel, to name a few. This population has been known to behave differently from their parents, approaching life with a different set of needs and desires. There is a demanding tone observed in their consumer behavior, with much higher expectations being set for the delivery of goods, services, and, increasingly, experiences.[2]

When applied to the realm of eye surgery, the demands and expectations of this generation for cataract surgery actually resemble more closely what surgeons anticipate for those looking into LASIK: good to excellent preoperative (corrected) visual acuity and high expectations for results. Because they are paying out-of-pocket, they expect more in terms of the technology (what the IOL can do for them), the service (how well they are treated by the surgeon and staff), and the overall experience (because there is competition for how the consumer will spend the discretionary dollar in the first place).

Psychographics

Even with these clear but generalized distinctions in place between the 2 generations, there are exceptions. LASIK surgeons can name numerous patients they have operated on who are in their 60s and even 70s. Similarly, some younger patients may be satisfied to have the same cataract procedure that was performed on their parents, especially knowing the cost is covered by a third party. Thus, it is equally important to consider other characteristics of a patient profile, typically boiled down to these 3 questions: Is he or she an active participant in the game of life? Does he or she want to control/manage health and related decisions? Does he or she want to achieve spectacle independence after having a new lens implanted? Answers of "yes" to these 3 questions are likely a strong indicator of interest in a premium IOL.

Additionally, it is important to understand the impact of vision on the patient's self perception. Ophthalmologists already know and appreciate the importance of vision, which is often termed the single most valued of all the senses. Going further, we can draw a relationship between 2 of the most common conditions of an aging eye and life milestones. As described by Donnenfeld,[3] the first sign of "middle age" for many people is the onset of presbyopia. "I must be getting older, as my arms are too short and I can't read the paper without glasses," is a common refrain. Ten to 20 years later, the majority of the population will develop cataracts, a visible sign of "old age" in these same patients. When these 2 milestones are overlaid on top of the demanding nature of baby boomers (Figure 1), the situation begs for a solution to help this generation in its attempt to look, feel, and stay "young."

Economics

With the regulatory ruling in 2005 that allows surgeons to offer and charge for premium IOLs above and beyond what Medicare allows for traditional cataract surgery, cataract surgeons were given an opportunity to act in a free-market environment similar to LASIK surgeons, plastic surgeons, and other providers of elective medical procedures.

For many cataract surgeons, this is a difficult chasm to cross. For them to be successful, they are going to have to directly charge and collect from patients rather than wait for third-party reimbursement. As described earlier, the patient who is willing to pay for elective surgery also carries higher expectations in terms of product (what the IOL will do) and process (how they will be treated throughout).

Surgeons considering investing in the necessary staffing and skills to be successful should know that the next generation of cataract patients does in fact have the means to afford the $4000 to $10,000 fees that will need to be paid. Research has shown that[4] the baby boomer population controls 75% of the nation's wealth with a household net worth of $19 trillion. Each year, more than $1 trillion is spent on goods and services

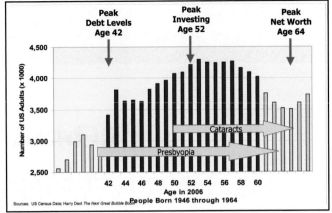

Figure 1. Milestones for the boomer. The baby boomer generation will experience a number of major milestones that positively impact their desire and ability to afford premium IOLs.

by this group, accounting for 80% of all luxury travel, 60% of all healthcare spending, and 41% of all new car purchases.

Actuarial studies have shown that this population is also ideally suited from the standpoint of wealth accumulation.[5] The typical American is at their peak debt levels at age 42 and through investing and saving during their 40s and 50s builds his or her own personal net worth to a peak at age 64 (see Figure 1).

Conclusion

The world for surgeons has changed with the introduction of the premium IOL. Building on decades of innovation in traditional cataract surgery, this new category of lenses offers a new level of functionality beyond correction of distance vision. What LASIK has shown is that the traditional paradigm for the doctor-patient relationship in the cataract surgery model needs to change in order to gain market acceptance of these lenses. Consumers who want and are willing to pay for spectacle independence will be equally demanding when it comes to levels of service from the surgeon and his or her staff. The demographic, psychographic, and economic factors surrounding the next wave of cataract patients all support market acceptance for premium IOLs.

References

1. Midrange estimate from Centenarians in the United States, US Census Bureau, 1999.
2. Pine BJ, Gilmore JH. *The Experience Economy.* Cambridge, MA: Harvard Business Press; 1999.
3. Donnenfeld E, Presentation at 2006 Refractive IOL Symposium; December 2, 2006; Las Vegas, NV.
4. Entrepreneurs Getting Hip on the Graying of America/Marketing Machine Out to Mine Gold in Boomers' Wallets," *San Francisco Chronicle,* May 11, 2005.
5. Dent Jr. HS. *The Next Great Bubble Boom.* Free Press; 2004.

CHAPTER 10

PREMIUM IOLS—
RE-ENGINEERING YOUR PRACTICE

Darrell E. White, MD

The next revolution in cataract surgery is here and it is here RIGHT NOW. The advent of the premium intraocular lens (IOL) channel in cataract surgery will define every anterior segment practice in the United States. The question that is now being asked of cataract surgeons is, "Do you offer implants that will let me see both far away and near?" Very soon the question that will be asked is, "Are you a premium cataract practice?" It will not be enough to simply offer premium channel IOLs to your patients; you will have to offer a premium level of service to every patient who walks through your door. If you wish to do anything more than dabble in this new IOL technology, nothing short of a re-engineering of your practice will do. And very soon is likely to feel like tomorrow!

Ophthalmologists, especially cataract surgeons, have rightfully earned the reputation of running the most efficient practices in all of medicine. Through the innovative use of wave scheduling and physician extenders we have been able to see prodigious numbers of patients. We have whittled down the time necessary to see, test, educate, and book surgical patients, and our personal involvement as the surgeon in that process is managed in such a way that we are ever more protected from interruptions and bottlenecks. In short, the modern cataract practice is centered on the cataract surgeon. The premium cataract practice must be centered on the patient and the patient's experience while making sure that our hard-won efficiencies are not lost.

Do this thought experiment before you embark on the re-engineering process. Take a blank piece of white paper and put a patient in the middle. What will attract her to your practice initially? Once she has come to your practice what will encourage her to choose a premium IOL when she has cataract surgery? Now build the practice flow around the answers to those questions, being careful to keep the patient (and not you!) in the center of the paper. Every practice will have specific answers to those questions that take into account local customs and expectations. There are certain characteristics that underlie these local answers that are necessary building blocks of the premium practice.

By giving our patients the opportunity to choose a premium IOL we are changing the dynamic of their experience. Whereas a traditional cataract surgery is simply a solution to a medical condition, a premium IOL is also a solution to a lifestyle. This choice adds a new dimension to our patient's experience in that he or she is now also buying a service, and because this service is not covered by insurance, she is truly buying it herself. Because this service is expensive they will compare it with other premium service businesses with which they have come in contact. Fill in the rest of that blank piece of white paper with an experience that will remind your patient of the most recent wonderful consumer service experience they had rather than their last doctor's appointment. Create an experience that reminds them of a trip to Nordstrom's or an overnight at the Ritz Carlton.

Create an atmosphere of "total immersion" in the Premium experience. We should learn not only from our refractive and plastic surgery colleagues but also from those very best consumer service businesses. Each patient who telephones your office may be a premium IOL patient, or a patient who will refer your next premium IOL patient. Your operators should have script guidelines that promote the Premium image of the entire practice. Your lobby should invoke the same type of feeling that one has when they walk into the lobby of a Four Seasons Hotel, or when they enter Nordstrom's from a crowded mall. Elegance, confidence, and quality should be all around your patient as she or he walks through the door. It should be immediately evident that you intend to make her or his experience a special one. Surround your patient with information about premium IOLs. The education and awareness process takes place in the lobby (handbills and larger photos) (Figures 1 and 2), while dilating (brochures or DVDs), and in the exam room (videos and staff education). Every step of the visit and every staff member is another opportunity to raise the awareness of premium IOLs.

Assume that every patient who has a cataract will choose to undergo Premium cataract surgery. The goal should be to allow your process to winnow out those patients who will choose a traditional IOL before they are in the exam chair

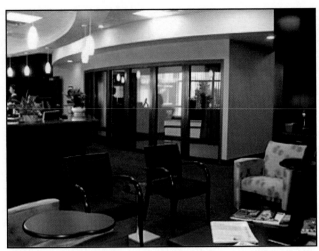

Figure 1. Our refractive lobby. You can see the glass wall of the laser room to the left.

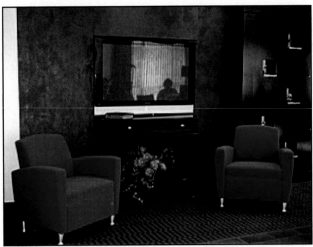

Figure 2. Patient view upon entering our office through the main entrance; the 52-inch screen plays loops of educational material from Eyemaginations.

in front of the surgeon. The conversation about premium IOLs should start at the time of the first telephone call to the practice. Your operator can mention that yours is a premium practice. Each patient should be asked questions that determine if she or he might have a cataract and information about premium IOLs should be either sent to the patient before the visit or presented to her when she arrives at the office. Think of the patient's visit as if it was a voyage on a train, one having many interactions with the crew (front desk, tech, OD, counselor) and one on which there are many stations (lobby, preexam, dilation, preoperative testing, surgery scheduling). At each station someone comes in contact with the patient and a little more information can be given. The patient then chooses whether or not to stay on the Premium train. By the time the patient has reached her destination (you, the surgeon), she has either switched to a traditional IOL, or has stayed on the Premium Express and it is time to talk about WHICH premium IOL will be received.

It is important to realize at this point that you are no longer having a traditional cataract conversation with this patient; you are now having a REFRACTIVE conversation. Your interactions with your premium IOL patients will have much more in common with your interactions with your laser in situ keratomileusis (LASIK) patients than your traditional cataract patients. Now it is time for you (and your IOL counselor) to educate your patient about her particular implant. In addition to a standard cataract informed consent each patient will need to know what to expect from the specific premium IOL that has been chosen. Now is the time to review the potential side effects of the selected lens and to set appropriate expectations for the outcome. Agree on a shared definition of success for this patient and write it down for posterity. Every part of your patient's voyage should have exceeded expectations so far. Be sure to agree on reasonable expectations so that you can continue your winning streak.

On to surgery. Whew! Finally something with which we are familiar. Not so fast, though. This is not traditional cataract surgery where + or −1 D is OK because we can clean it up with glasses. The Premium experience that you have provided to your patient has to be backed up by premium surgery. Accurate measurements using state of the art equipment must produce results that are + or −0.25 Ds. Meticulous, safe, and repeatable surgical technique has to occur for each and every case. Got cylinder? Get a solution. Be prepared to perform limbal relaxing incisions or laser vision correction for levels of astigmatism that you would have previously ignored. Be willing to correct small degrees of cylinder with LASIK or photorefractive keratectomy.

The "total immersion" process does not end after surgery. Remember that your patient is in the middle of your process and she would like you to be a part of it. Play a role in the postoperative experience, even if it is a small role, even if you do not do so for traditional cataract surgeries. Success is now measured by your patient. How is she doing in the "real world?" How often is she wearing glasses and for what activities? Did the two of you achieve your goal? If so, congratulate yourselves! Revel in the success. This was a great experience for both of you!

Are you a premium cataract practice? This is the question that will define every anterior segment practice in the near future. The answer lies in re-engineering your practice to provide a Premium level of experience that your patients will compare with their best experiences in other service businesses. The standard is not their best office visit experience but their very best service experience anywhere. Every patient who walks through your door could be your next premium IOL patient. The revolution has already started. Your patient is coming tomorrow!

CHAPTER 11

THE REFRACTIVE IOL PATIENT'S JOURNEY

Stephen S. Lane, MD

The preoperative process of preparing a patient for a presbyopia-correcting intraocular lens (IOL) (or lifestyle IOLs as I like to call them) can be considered as stops along the "road" of the patient's surgical "journey." By following these steps, surgeons can often achieve better overall patient satisfaction postoperatively.

There are 6 stops along the road:

1. Change the physician mindset.
2. Educate your staff and develop the process.
3. Educate your patients even before they come in to see you.
4. Technical assessment of the patients' physical candidacy and examination of personal vision preferences.
5. The surgeon's exam and discussion of options.
6. The direct hand-off to the scheduler/counselor.

Stop 1: Physician Mindset

Surgeons must be willing to accept and embrace change in their practice model. Surgeons must switch from the Medicare model of treatment, which consists of high volume, high efficiency, and low cost, to the patient model, which emphasizes high quality of personalized care that aims to meet patients' expectations.

The mindset of the presbyopic refractive patient is different from that of the traditional patient with cataracts. The former is interested in lifestyle, not in the pathology. Refractive patients are happy to pay for an enhanced quality of life.

An important shift needs to occur in the doctor-patient relationship, with the surgeon committing to deliver the best individualized treatment possible. This should start in the waiting room (Figure 1).

You need to create an office environment that exudes comfort and professionalism and in which the patient hopes that he or she is a candidate for some of these procedures as soon as he or she walks in. This can be due to something as simple as the furniture, the art hanging on the wall, and the magazines that you have on your shelves. Every patient who comes through your office should know that you perform refractive IOL surgery. The optimal office environment is uncluttered and stylish (Figure 2). Small details, such as reading material in the waiting room, can be important, and internal marketing should begin in the waiting room. Wall art testimonials, "brag books" with successful cases, and practice brochures should be posted throughout the office so that patients can learn about the practice before even entering the examination room. The overall impression created by these details is an invaluable marketing tool.

Stop 2: Educate Staff

The only way for an office to run efficiently is if every employee has a clear understanding of his or her role. We use a flow sheet in my office to prevent confusion among staff (Figure 3). By having the process written out, staff members know what their next step is or what they need to do.

Staff activities should be monitored to ensure that employees are performing tasks as needed. You should develop a field guide, if you will, for your staff. You have to talk to your staff and make sure that the necessary education is spread throughout every division—from your waiting room to the front desk and all the way to the back office. You should require that each staff member understands and is able to perform his or her specific role and understands what the process is, making the patient visit as smooth and seamless as possible.

Stop 3: Educate Patients

Surgeons should send out brochures to patients before their first appointment to begin the education process and reduce the "shock factor" of various facets of the procedure. I recommend providing the address of the practice Web site, which should include information about the lenses you use and the surgical procedure itself.

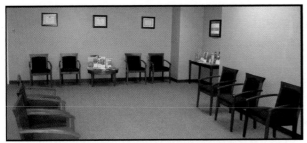

Figure 1. Example of a drab and uninviting "cold" waiting room.

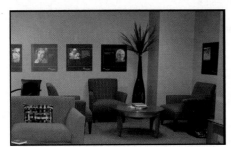

Figure 2. Warm inviting waiting room with informational wall hangings and reading materials.

Once patients enter the office, the front desk should provide them with a vision requirements survey (like the Dell survey) (Figure 4) so the patients can consider what kind of visual outcome they desire before even entering the examination room. Such surveys can assist in measuring a patient's personality, desire, and candidacy for the procedure.

At any point while the patient is in the office, educational brochures, educational videotapes or DVDs, or other materials one might have should be offered to patients to better inform them and increase their awareness of the technology. There should be as little idle time as possible during their office journey, and educational materials are an excellent way to fill time.

Stop 4: Technical Assessment

The technician should assess a patient's physical candidacy by collecting information such as lens measurements, amount of corneal cylinder, biometry, and IOL calculation. Technicians should also elicit, in greater detail than the preoperative survey did, the patient's personal vision preferences. Staff members should determine what is most important to the patient, including whether he or she wants sharp vision at distance, intermediate, or near or if driving at night is important. All of this information should be given to the surgeon. This not only streamlines the patient visit but also aids the surgeon in directing questions and comments toward the most relevant aspects of the patient's desires and demands.

I also encourage the use of the IOL Counselor (Patient Education Concepts, Houston, TX), which includes surgical and refractive error simulations/animations that can assist patients in understanding IOL implantation and final outcomes (Figures 5 and 6).

Stop 5: Surgeon Exam

Surgeons must be up-to-date on the latest IOL technology. They need to know to what degree patients want to be spectacle free and should be concerned with pre-existing astigmatism and contrast sensitivity issues.

It is important that physicians speak to patients at length about the different lens options, including the mixing and matching of different lenses. They should then recommend the procedure that they think would work best based upon the patients' specific needs and desires.

You have to provide specific lens recommendations based upon your interaction with the patient. Patients want to know what you would do, and if you leave it too open-ended, the options can be too confusing. You should introduce the options by saying for example, "I would recommend this individual lens because you told me this is what you want, and this lens performs in this way to take care of that issue."

The surgeon's time with the patient is important because the chair time you spend before surgery helps ease patient expectations. In contrast, chair time spent after the surgery places the patient and surgeon on the defensive and gives the perception of a complication when in fact none is present. The more chair time you spend before surgery, the less you will spend after surgery.

Stop 6: Office Scheduler

Scheduling, finalizing the decisions, and reassuring the patient is the key last stop. In a streamlined fashion, the surgeon should direct the patient to the office counselor or scheduler to arrange a surgery date and to finalize selection of the lens that will be implanted. Schedulers and counselors should be clear on payment matters at this time.

You need to have finance plans available so that options exist that make it easy for your patients to have the surgery they desire. Your process should not become one of the patient's problems. This portion of the patient's visit needs to flow quickly and easily.

The opportunity offered by lifestyle IOLs for the ophthalmic surgeon is tremendous, but change will be necessary to realize its significance. By following these steps, the transition to making lifestyle IOLs a significant part of your practice will be eased.

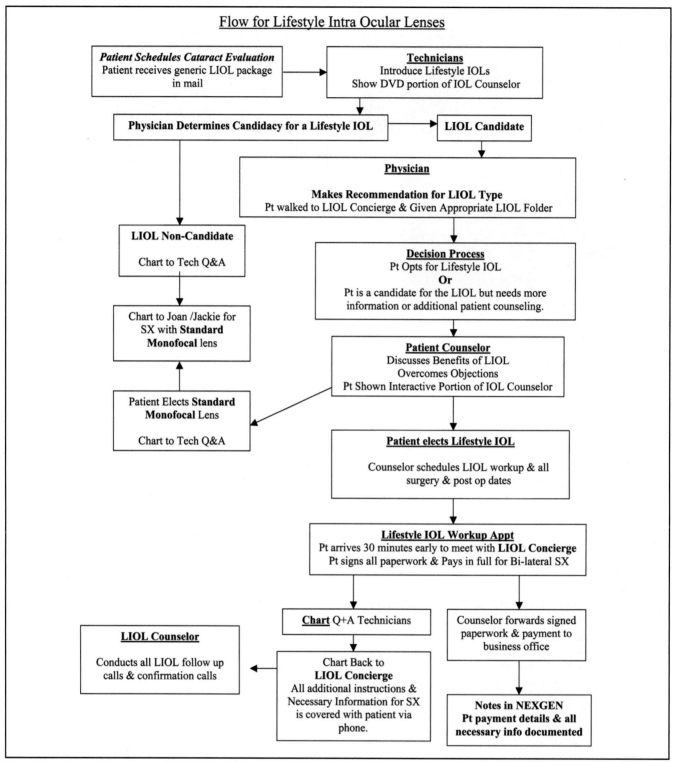

Figure 3. Flow sheet outlining staff responsibilities and processing of the patient.

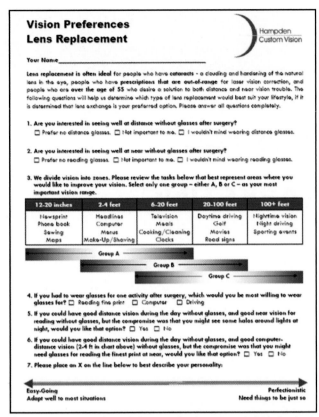

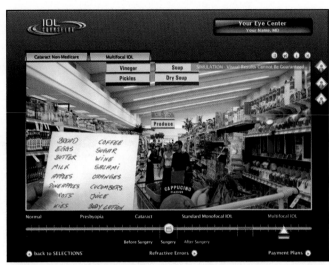

Figure 6. IOL Counselor demonstrating to the patient a simulation of what vision would be like after multifocal IOL implantation.

Figure 4. Modification of the Dell Survey used to determine an individual patient's visual demands.

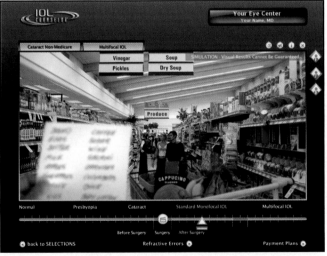

Figure 5. IOL Counselor demonstrating to the patient a simulation of what vision would be like after monofocal IOL implantation.

CHAPTER 12

PREMIUM IOLs— EXTERNAL MARKETING

Michael W. Malley, BA

Some surgeons refer to it as the "unofficial resurrection of cataract surgery." Other cataract surgeons refer to it as "their day of enlightenment—and entitlement."

In either case, since the pivotal moment of the Centers for Medicare & Medicaid Services (CMS) ruling allowing cataract and refractive surgeons to charge a premium fee for new presbyopia-correcting intraocular lenses (IOLs), 2 major developments have occurred that continue to change the course of how these lenses are marketed to patients: patient expectations following "custom" cataract surgery have dramatically increased and the need for pre- and postoperative patient education and staff training was greatly underestimated, causing patient flow challenges and staffing shortages.

Early on, the CMS ruling also caused some anxious surgeons to over promise—and under deliver—their postoperative results. But here is the good news. In the past 2 decades, no other product line has offered the ophthalmic industry more promise for patients—and more financial potential for surgeons—than refractive IOLs. Not only is the target audience for these lenses burgeoning beyond belief, the same sector also controls more than 70% of the wealth in the United States. Match these demographics with an "anti-aging" psychographic mindset of the baby boomers and it has set itself up to be the perfect ophthalmic storm.

From a medical marketing standpoint, it simply does not get any better than this. However, as in all areas of medicine, nothing is perfect and results may vary. Therefore, great caution must be taken in all areas of marketing refractive IOLs to potential patients. This includes your patient educational packets, internal signage, back-office collaterals, patient videos, general patient correspondence, and absolutely all of your conventional external advertising, including the Internet. (Yes, this target audience is actively engaged on the Internet and will be covered later in the section.)

Experienced Refractive Practices Versus Conventional Cataract Practices

Marketing refractive IOLs falls into 2 categories of surgeons: experienced refractive surgeons and traditional cataract surgeons. The marketing also falls into 2 distinct categories of patients: the traditional cataract (Medicare) patient and the baby boomer presbyope.

Those practices that have seen the earliest success with refractive IOLs have generally been the experienced refractive practices that understand the "service economy" mantra of focusing on the overall "experience" of refractive office exams. Marketing refractive IOLs to your patients requires an extraordinary level of patient service, education, and the ability to raise the perceived value of your refractive IOL of choice to match that of your actual asking price. This requires additional staff training and education in not only the risks and benefits of the new lenses, but also marketing and sales training aimed at helping patients make a more informed decision about their lens and lifestyle options following surgery.

It might help you from a marketing viewpoint to compare "shopping" at your practice for a $9000 refractive IOL to that of visiting the Apple store for a $5000 computer system. Or on a lesser note, visiting your favorite coffee shop for a $4 latte. Service, ambience, atmosphere, ease of browsing and buying, and courteous, efficient staff all matter in today's marketing world.

Savvy refractive practices understand that presbyopes and cataract patients are not required to spend $8000 to $9000 on premium IOLs and have much lower-priced options such as reading glasses or monofocal lenses. They understand the need to help patients understand the value of these lenses by listening to their desires and lifestyle traits and reminding them how these new lenses will help them continue to lead the lifestyle they desire.

They also know the value of allowing patients to have a comfortable, private area (versus the examination rooms) to discuss lens options and ask the difficult financial questions. They know the value of a free bottle of water to a patient who has been in the office nearly 2 hours is much more than the $0.99 it costs the practice. From the smell of the reception area to the age of the carpet and the color on the walls—it all matters in marketing.

In contrast, most traditional cataract practices were based mainly on billing insurance companies and Medicare for patients receiving the standard monofocal lens. There was never really a need to ever "upgrade" patients to a premium product line outside of perhaps limbal relaxing incisions. Surgical schedulers were accustomed to taking patients' insurance and Medicare information and arranging a date for cataract surgery, which normally occurred for some reason on a Monday; not exactly the best day for today's patients to have refractive surgery. These traditional cataract practices were fully capable of seeing massive numbers of cataract patients in a single day (as many as 30 to 40 in an afternoon), but they were totally lacking in the training and staffing required to successfully promote a premium line of cataract lenses.

Initially, most surgeons simply assumed their brief educational efforts in the exam rooms would be satisfactory to convince patients of the need to upgrade their cataract or refractive procedure to a premium lens implant. What they quickly discovered, however, was that the vast majority of patients were simply not converting to the new lenses as expected. The out-of-pocket expense was the major hurdle that many very qualified surgeons found themselves unable to get patients over. Despite their best efforts, patients' "perceived" value of the new lenses did not match the $4500 asking price.

In addition to an initial lackluster conversion factor, surgeons soon found themselves spending inordinate amounts of "exam time" answering questions, alleviating fears, and discussing increased procedural fees. The increased surgeon time in the exam rooms could possibly be overlooked if it resulted in a higher percentage of patients converting to the premium lenses. Unfortunately it did not, which is why some surgeons seemed less than enthusiastic about promoting the new lenses to patients.

Marketing to Presbyopes Versus Cataract Patients

Fortunately, a comprehensive marketing approach is today enabling all practices to enjoy extremely high patient satisfaction (and conversion) rates with refractive IOLs. Practices need to understand the need to initiate patient marketing early and often in the refractive IOL arena. A combination marketing/educational process needs to occur at every possible stage of the visit, including the pre-exam at-home stage. It also needs to be divided into 2 distinct categories: presbyopes and cataract patients.

In recent focus group studies with postoperative refractive IOL patients ranging in age from 50 to 65, the vast majority of patients were adamant that they had NOT undergone "cataract" surgery. They were quick to point out they had a name-brand lens put in their eye to help them see better without glasses, but they were convinced they did NOT have cataracts, which they associated with a much older demographic.

From a marketing standpoint, this is a key message that should not be under appreciated. If you are targeting 55- to 60-year-old presbyopes with cataracts, your message should NOT be geared toward cataracts. Instead, it should be directed at the frustration with reading glasses and bifocals. In contrast, if you are targeting Medicare-age cataract patients, the 2 key words to use in your marketing are "Medicare-approved" and "cataracts." Medicare patients covet and understand the benefit of Medicare-approved services when it comes to their insurance coverage. By age 65 or 70, they are probably already well aware they have at least the beginning of a cataract.

Practices both young and old— cataract or refractive— need to also understand the important marketing role that staff members play in converting patients from monofocal to refractive IOLs. Surgery counselors, as opposed to surgery schedulers, are needed. Specially trained staff will also need dedicated rooms to show patient marketing videos like the IOL Counselor and other multimedia presentations that should be utilized in the closing process. The same room can be used to discuss the all-important financial responsibilities associated with these lenses.

Initial Marketing Steps

The perfect place to start your refractive IOL marketing is with easy-to-read printed information to all potential presbyopes and cataract patients prior to their first visit. These can be in the form of a 4-color, trifold brochure; a simple coupon envelope stuffer; or a letter on practice stationary. Remember, marketing materials to presbyopes should focus on reading glasses, bifocals, and the restoration of more youthful vision. Collateral pieces to cataract patients need to have the words Medicare-approved and cataracts prominently displayed.

"Medicare-Approved" does NOT mean that these lenses are "completely covered" by Medicare. It simply means that Medicare has delivered its gold standard seal of approval to these lenses, which is a huge factor in the minds of Medicare patients. This gives your practice the opportunity to inform patients about what portion of the costs Medicare does and does not cover. The absolute best way to discuss Medicare coverage of the new refractive IOLs is to first tell patients that they are fortunate to have Medicare covering a portion of the new lenses. Tell patients that were it not for this fact, their out-of-pocket expense would be dramatically higher. (Be specific here if you know the difference.)

Although product-specific marketing materials are available, practices should consider customizing these information pieces for a more personal feel. Initial marketing pieces should be limited to themes like "Great News For Cataract Patients: Now You Have Options!" or "Do Reading Glasses Make You Look Older Than You Feel?" Save the detailed information for in-practice patient education. These pieces are simply designed to generate interest in the new lenses and create a general awareness that they are now available.

In additional to simple mailers, letters, and inserts, you should also take every opportunity to reinforce this message at the front desk at the time of patients' initial visits. Not only should simple countertop displays be strategically placed on the front desk, but wall posters and videos should also be prominently placed in the reception area.

Proper signage promoting "Cataracts? Now You Have Choices" should be prominently displayed. Countertop displays offering relief to all patients "Frustrated With Reading Glasses and Bifocals" should also be strategically located. Every potential refractive IOL patient should be properly informed, educated, and motivated before ever seeing the surgeon, thereby dramatically reducing the amount of surgeon time needed in the exam lanes.

Successful refractive practices understand the value of multiple levels of patient education and how this can elevate the perceived value of refractive IOLs. They know the important role a good technician can play in helping patients understand their options before meeting the surgeon. They know there was a need to identify a patient's chief complaint before his or her actual office visit, which helps the staff to properly prepare for his or her exam.

Perhaps most importantly, refractive-based practices understand how to help patients overcome their financial hurdles. With increased fees—in some cases well over $5000 per eye—refractive surgeons know that raising the patient's perceived value of his or her refractive IOL procedures is not enough. They may actually need to make these lenses seem affordable. Zero percent patient financing has come to the rescue of the refractive IOL market just as it did for the car industry and the laser in situ keratomileusis (LASIK) industry.

Cataract patients and presbyopes are embracing patient financing with the same enthusiasm as LASIK patients. They understand the value of interest-free financing and low-entry payment options that can easily be modified to fit their budget. That is why many of today's successful refractive practices are financing upwards of 50% of all refractive IOL procedures.

External Advertising Campaigns

Compared to marketing to the elusive and younger LASIK patient, marketing refractive IOLs to baby boomers and senior citizens is a much more conventional process. A large percentage of both of these target audiences watches television on a daily basis. A large percentage also continues to read the news-paper. Most presbyopes are still working, so radio advertising is proving to be an effective medium for this group. Seniors continue to read more junk mail than younger target audiences and are responding favorably to practice newsletters and invitations to health and vision screenings. Internet marketing should be reserved for the baby boomers, but senior citizens are not far behind them in their desire to get up to speed on the Web.

A combination of radio, newsprint, and Internet advertising would be most appropriate for presbyopes. In terms of frequency, utilize no fewer than 2 radio stations and target mainly news/talk and sports/talk AM radio stations. Run an average 6 commercials per day for 3 days per week for a minimum of 2 weeks. Use small newspaper ads (8 column inches or less) but utilize a large type headline such as "Readers Got You Down?" or "Bifocals A Drag?" Run print ads in the business section for more affluent readers and in the lifestyle section for a variety of readers Your Internet campaign should include buying keyword searches in your area on Google, Yahoo, and MSN for cataracts, presbyopia, and any brand-specific lens you choose. Be prepared to spend from $500 to $2500 a month on Internet marketing.

Cataract patients are among the "slowest moving" advertising target audiences in the marketing world. They are very predictable and much more sedentary in their habits. Since they drive much less than presbyopes, expensive radio campaigns are not advisable. Since the majority of cataract patients are not yet online, divert your Internet budget to direct mail campaigns and printed newsletters rather than an electronic newsletter. Since these patients stay home and watch more daytime TV than any other target audience, narrow your television media buy to affordable daytime programming as opposed to prime time rates.

From a medical and marketing standpoint, there has never been a better time to be a patient considering a lens implant procedure. There has also never been a better time to be a refractive lens implant surgeon. That does not mean today's refractive IOLs are perfect. They are not, but they are improving everyday and there are exciting new lens implants in the production pipeline. The market segment for these lenses will continue to grow as the capabilities of these lenses also continue to grow. Finally, thanks to the CMS ruling, there may never be a better time to market refractive IOLs to potential patients than right now. Do your homework. Know your limits. Understand your patients' expectations. Deliver the desired result. Watch your practice grow!

CHAPTER 13

Premium IOLs— External Marketing

Shareef Mahdavi, BA

In this chapter, I hope to address 2 types of surgeons: those who want to promote their services, and those who want to provide services yet shy away from promoting them.

For most surgeons, the thought of marketing one's services cuts against the grain of what motivated them to enter medicine in the first place. Marketing smacks of retailing—a far cry from what was taught in medical school and residency. However, the rise of laser in situ keratomileusis (LASIK) and refractive surgery has caused this procedure to be part of a new category of elective medicine that has been described as medical retail.[1] This merging of these 2 different worlds requires the surgeon to consider the marketing requirements as carefully as the clinical ones in order to be successful.

What is marketing? Too often, it gets oversimplified as representing a single activity (such as advertising) or a single event (such as placing an ad in a newspaper). In reality, marketing is a complex activity that encompasses nearly everything that happens outside the exam room and surgical suite. Marketing's role is to influence consumer behavior both beforehand (to purchase your services) and afterward (to recommend you to others). Advertising, a form of promotion in which you pay another party to showcase or describe your offering, is simply one form of marketing.

Another common error is the belief that one must advertise in order to successfully attract patients. This belief typically takes root after a surgeon becomes certified to perform a procedure, and advertising is viewed as the next challenge in the process. For sophisticated marketing firms with well-designed systems to capture and convert interest in their products or services, this is true. But for most surgeons, this is a recipe for frustration and failure. Let me illustrate: soon after Doctor Smith became certified to insert the new fangled techno lens, he urged his administrator to place a series of ads in the local newspaper. His enthusiasm was bolstered by the nice-looking logos and advertising templates supplied by the manufacturer during the course. The administrator, wanting to please her boss, did as told. But when the phone rang, the receptionist had no clue what the new lenses were about. Only slightly

more knowledge was imparted to the caller after they were transferred to a back office technician. After 2 weeks, only 3 people had come in to learn about the new lens and how it could help them. The clinical exam indicated they were candidates, but no one knew how to discuss financing. Thus, only 1 of those 3 patients actually agreed to move forward with surgery.

This scenario occurs all too often in ophthalmic practices looking to incorporate premium intraocular lenses (IOLs). Because no one has sufficiently trained staff members to answer questions about the new offering, both staff and patients end up confused. Because so few people had surgery, Doctor Smith blames the advertising. In fact, the problem lies within the internal structure and systems of the practice, not with the external advertising. The point here is simple: advertising is the last thing you should do.

Taking an "Inside-Out" Approach

In approaching the marketing challenge of attracting new patients, it is more helpful to focus on what can be done inside the practice to market to existing patients. For example, the person answering the telephone should be viewed as the Director of First Impressions. Long before they meet with a surgeon, patients first interact with the staff member(s) in charge of answering the phone. Studies have shown[2] that poor telephone skills often prevent consumers from moving forward and scheduling a consultation for refractive surgery. This should come as no surprise. Ironically, the person entrusted to influence consumer behavior (ie, marketing) at the point of first contact is typically the least experienced, lowest paid, and least knowledgeable employee in the practice.

Thus, for most surgeons, an appropriate pathway for the marketing of refractive IOLs would be as follows:

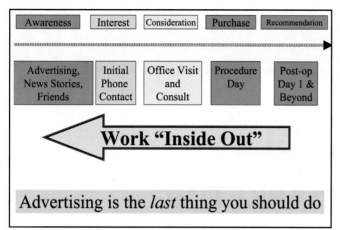

Awareness	Interest	Consideration	Purchase	Recommendation
Advertising, News Stories, Friends	Initial Phone Contact	Office Visit and Consult	Procedure Day	Post-op Day 1 & Beyond

Work "Inside Out"

Advertising is the *last* thing you should do

Figure 1. Consumer decision process: All consumer purchases follow a path that begins with awareness of the product or service. These stages align to specific steps in the process of considering premium IOLs. Once surgeons become certified in doing procedures, they should next work to perfect their consultation skills, followed by how their staff answers questions from interested patients. Advertising and external marketing are last on the list.

* Become clinically competent in the procedure.
* Define the key benefits for your patients and convert this list into a script that can be used during the consultation process.
* Decide what specific role the surgeon will have in the consultation and what role the technicians and counselor will perform (eg, decide who will be talking about money and financing).
* With the staff, brainstorm all the different opportunities that can be used to inform and educate patients while they are in the office. This should be a comprehensive look at all steps during the patient's visit from reception through checkout. Additionally, consider how to inform and educate "influencers" (eg, adult children of patients).
* Select and train the most appropriate staff members to speak either in person or over the telephone with patients who express interest.
* Create a protocol for your scheduling staff to ask patients scheduling a cataract consultation if they would be interested in achieving spectacle independence. Have materials in place that can be sent or viewed on your Web site to begin the education process.
* Put educational tools in place, such as DVDs in the reception area and the IOL Counselor (Patient Education Concepts, Houston, TX) in the consultation room, that can educate patients about what premium IOLs can do for their vision and for their lifestyle.

External marketing has intentionally been left off of this list. Practices that focus on doing these steps correctly and continuously improve how they interact with patients at every step will typically find little need to move externally to promote their services, in part because few of today's cataract practices are following these 7 steps. The experience that patients have when exposed to these 7 steps will probably be unique enough (relative to other doctors' appointments) that the word-of-mouth referrals will lead to increasing interest in both the procedure and your practice (Figure 1).

When Is External Marketing Appropriate?

Once internal systems are in place, tested, and refined, the practice wishing to increase its surgical volume may be in a position to reach outside to attract more patients. As described earlier, advertising is but one form of promotional medium that includes direct mail, professional relations with referral sources, public relations, event sponsorship, and seminars.

By itself, advertising is a risky proposition for 3 reasons. First, it is expensive and puts pressure on the practice to create a return that justifies the original investment. Second, it automatically sets expectations among the target audience due to the fact that the procedure is being promoted. For some consumers, seeing an advertisement implies that the procedure is proven and failsafe. For other consumers, advertising creates a negative perception of the procedure and/or the provider (eg, "I would never go to a doctor that has to advertise"). Finally, the public is becoming increasingly resistant to advertising messages as evidenced by the popularity of the digital video recorder for TV and satellite radio mediums that allow you to bypass or eliminate exposure to commercials. In effect, the consumer that you are trying to reach with advertising is becoming harder to reach.

In contrast to the "broadcast" approach offered by newspaper, radio, and television advertising, a narrower "target" approach can be more effective both in terms of generating patient leads and reaching the target audience. The prime example of a targeted approach is the use of direct mail, which gives you the opportunity to segment the population by age, income, gender, and lifestyle interests, and communicate directly with a more refined target population. Another targeted approach is to have a booth at a specific event, such as a golf or tennis tournament, that would attract many individuals who are in or approaching the ideal demographic for a premium IOL.

As an alternative to paid promotion, the use of a local public relations (PR) firm can be effective in gaining exposure for the practice via local media coverage. The benefit of using PR is that it is much more credible to read about a surgeon in a news story than to see that surgeon in an advertisement. The downside is that the practice has little or no control over if and when such stories will appear. That is the role of the PR firm, but no firm can guarantee that their media outreach efforts will result in publicity for the practice.

For those that remain convinced that external marketing is right for their practice, I offer 2 pieces of advice. First, do not abandon a focus on the internal systems described earlier. As can be seen in Figure 2, it is the internal infrastructure that must convert any interest generated from advertising into consultations and procedures. Improvements made in how patients are handled during the decision process will be manifest in higher conversion rates to premium IOL surgery. Poor conversion rates can be viewed as "leaky plumbing"; it does not matter how far you turn on the faucet (spend on advertising) if the pipes are broken (weak internal systems).

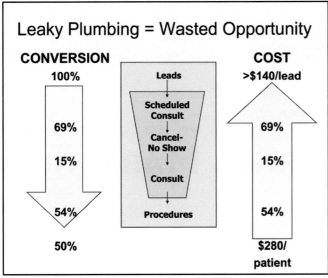

Figure 2. Conversion versus cost: These ratios and costs of marketing refractive surgery to consumers show the expensive nature of external marketing. With only 1 of every 2 inquirers to a practice eventually having refractive surgery (LASIK historicals), it makes more sense to improve how you communicate and educate interested patients rather than increase the amount spent on external marketing.

Second, every practice that advertises should have a system in place to track the source of every phone call. At a minimum, every new caller should be asked, "How did you hear about us?" This metric is essential in understanding how patients are finding you and evaluating the effectiveness of any money spent on external marketing.

Conclusion

Marketing is a complex task that seeks to influence consumer behavior. Most practices will succeed if they focus on internal marketing to create a better experience for patients at every step in the process, beginning with the first telephone call. Once those fundamentals are solid, it may make sense for some practices to move beyond their own walls to conduct external marketing in the community. External marketing may include advertising but can also include other forms of promotion and/or PR. Every practice that conducts marketing should track how new patients and callers find out about them.

Reference

1. Mahdavi SA. Strand of pearls. *Cataract and Refractive Surgery Today.* 2003;January:68-69.

2. Mahdavi S. Telephone improvement project. A skills assessment of refractive surgery providers. March 2006 (published by SM2 Consulting; available at www.sm2consulting.com)

PREMIUM IOLS—INTERNAL MARKETING

Kay Coulson, MBA

"It is not the strongest of the species that survives, nor the most intelligent, but the one most responsive to change."—Charles Darwin

"Thanks to a creative leap, something that was once mundane becomes noticeable."—Jean-Marie Dru

Something occurs every day in your practice. Done well, it educates patients, creates higher referrals, motivates employees, and helps your office run smoothly. Done poorly, it deters referrals, alienates potential patients, disillusions even the most loyal existing patient, and fosters employee cynicism. I am talking about internal marketing.

It is commonly believed that the most critical role of marketing is to sell your services outwardly to potential customers. In fact, the first and most urgent job of marketing is often to sell inwardly to the patients and employees who have already demonstrated a commitment to your practice.

What is internal marketing? It is many things, from the way your receptionist answers the phone to the cleanliness of your exam lanes. It is the structure of your appointment calendar to the knowledge your staff conveys about surgical results. Internal marketing is simply how you advertise, wittingly and unwittingly, positively and negatively, audibly and visually, to the patients and employees who are inside your doors.

Ophthalmology is at the forefront of change in the medical profession. Our landscape shifted in May 2005 when Centers for Medicare & Medicaid Services (CMS) allowed practices to offer and incrementally charge for presbyopia-correcting intraocular lenses (Pr-C IOLs). The trend solidified with similar approval for toric IOLs in January 2007. I believe that ophthalmology's future will be built not as refractive or comprehensive practices, but rather as elective or insurance practices. Now that IOLs and phakic lenses have moved into the elective domain, many practices are confused about how to introduce private-pay services to their insurance-oriented patient base.

Yesterday's refractive center was focused on laser in situ keratomileusis (LASIK). How should they add elective lenses into their mix? The new lens patient—often older—might not fit with the LASIK patient they have cultivated. Surgeons and facilities need to be credentialed by insurance panels, as most lens patients have cataracts and expect the benefit of partial insurance coverage. How will the LASIK center adjust to space needs, enhanced testing, stringent charting requirements, and protracted fee collection?

Yesterday's comprehensive ophthalmology practice was built around insurance assignment and maximum patient-throughput. Packed appointment schedules, long patient-wait times, diverse pathology and treatment requirements, and surgeons confounded by the thought of introducing even one more event into their day characterize this performance model. How will the comprehensive practice become more service-oriented and patient-friendly? Can a process-driven, specialized employee become an excellent utility player on the elective vision team? How will you learn to discuss fees, payment plans, and patient choice without feeling uneasy about this 2-tiered fee system?

What I have learned in working successfully with various refractive and comprehensive ophthalmology practices is that there are common reasons we fail to build vibrant, viable elective vision service lines. Many surgeons and administrators say, "My practice is different" or "My patients are different." I respectfully refute this notion. The problems I have seen, and the patients I have counseled and interviewed, confirm commonality rather than dissimilarity. Using the "We're different" excuse really means, "I won't change." But that would be a serious practice-limiting mistake. Ophthalmology is leading the way in elective medical services. No specialty has done a better job of educating and collecting fees than ophthalmologists performing LASIK. We have a huge new market open to elective vision choice with presbyopic, toric, and phakic lenses (which collectively I refer to as lifestyle IOLs). Elective vision now covers corneal and anterior segment surgery. Indeed, the defining distinction of elective vision is really permanent vision. What can we offer at various life stages to allow people to be glasses-free as much as possible throughout their day? Practices that understand the power of glasses-free—through

LASIK, lifestyle IOLs, and all the technologies yet to come—will prosper in the elective vision world.

Convincing Yourself

ARE LIFESTYLE INTRAOCULAR LENSES WORTH IT?

The first step in internal marketing is to determine for yourself whether the addition of lifestyle IOLs is desirable for your practice; desirable in the vision benefit delivered to patients and desirable in the financial reward offered to you.

DO PATIENTS WANT GLASSES-FREE VISION?

More than 10 million excimer laser procedures (LASIK, photorefractive keratectomy [PRK], et al) have been performed in the United States between 2000 and 2007,[1] more than any other elective medical procedure during that timeframe. Elective Medical Marketing (EMM) research indicates 65%[2] of the 18- to 44-year-old glasses-wearing population desires LASIK and roughly 14% of those have had the procedure. The primary motivation for these patients? Reduce or eliminate the need for glasses and contacts. While the research is not yet well established for cataract patients, recent EMM research shows 75% of diagnosed cataract patients say glasses-free vision would be a significant motivator to them in moving forward with cataract surgery. Is it a leap to assume a similar 15%+ would upgrade to lifestyle IOLs? We think not, especially as the population that drove the LASIK boom reaches cataract age and has demonstrated their willingness to pay for improved healthcare.

IS THE FINANCIAL BENEFIT SUFFICIENT?

Most practices have more cataract surgery walk out the door than sign up in any given week. Not in your practice, you say? Then consider the numbers (Figure 1). If you are an average comprehensive practice seeing 50 patients per day, roughly 30% of those are complete exams on patients age 50+. We know cataract incidence among the general population of 50- to 74-year olds is 6%,[3] yet it is closer to 30% by the time they reach your exam chair. We know presbyopia incidence among this same population is virtually 100%. So of the roughly 40 complete exams performed per week (3 clinic days weekly), you may perform 12 cataract surgeries. This 15% conversion to surgery means the remaining 85% enter your recheck pool. Why is surgical conversion so low? Two reasons. First, why would someone let you operate on his or her eyes when it will cost him or her approximately $800 (average copay/deductible for 2 eyes) in what you characterize as a risky procedure, where he or she will still need glasses 100% of the time afterward?

Most patients wait until their vision is significantly compromised before proceeding with the feared nonbenefit of cataract surgery! Second, they do not proceed because you have not recommended they should. Your recommendation compels action. Your lack of recommendation compels inaction. For a practice increasing surgical conversion from 15% to 25% and increasing upgrades from 5% to 35% at average

national physician fees, surgical revenue will increase between $300,000 and $400,000, more than 75%! There is not a more significant opportunity for revenue increase, via drugs, devices, or techniques, available to the lens surgeon today.

ARE YOU SABOTAGING LIFESTYLE INTRAOCULAR LENS SUCCESS?

Take this quiz to see if you are unwittingly sabotaging your internal marketing efforts.

1. My patients are different.

   Yes _____ No _____

   They are not. Patients are remarkably similar across the country; it is your practice that is different.

2. My patients like wearing glasses.

   Yes _____ No _____

   This is what the 10-eye-per-month LASIK surgeon said while the practice across town did 100 cases. Learn to identify the services that appeal to a niche segment of your patient base and offer them. Do not fall into the trap that if all cannot choose or afford the upgrade procedure, none should be offered it.

3. I close the majority of my exams to surgery.

   Yes _____ No _____

   Easy enough to calculate: eyes per month/1.8 eyes per person/average exams aged 50+ per week = surgery conversion. Most comprehensive practices average 10% to 15%. Great practices average 20% to 30%.

4. I am a (rural, suburban, urban, new, established, working class, inner city, depressed geography, other) practice and my patients cannot afford an upgraded lens.

   Yes _____ No _____

   As a realistic goal, you are striving for 1 out of 4 patients to choose an upgraded Pr-C IOL or toric IOL. Most cannot or will not choose them, but I have seen successful practices convert 30% to 60% of cataract surgeries to upgrades by focusing on the benefit of patient-desired glasses-free vision.

Challenge yourself to develop an accurate practice conversion assessment, and establish realistic performance expectations so that you truly commit to lifestyle IOLs before persuading staff or patients to do the same.

Persuading Your Staff

The second step in internal marketing is persuading your staff that lifestyle IOLs should be a significant practice offering. Did you return enthused from an industry convention and announce at a staff meeting the addition of lifestyle IOLs? Have you placed free manufacturer brochures in the exam lanes and waited to see if patients would ask for the lenses? Remember that while you have evaluated and opted for or against certain lenses over the years, your staff has not. Lens selection has traditionally been 100% driven by the surgeon. You have evaluated lens choice with a manufacturer's representative behind the closed doors of the operating room, through clinical trial results, and through shared discussion with other surgeons. Lens features and benefits are not widely

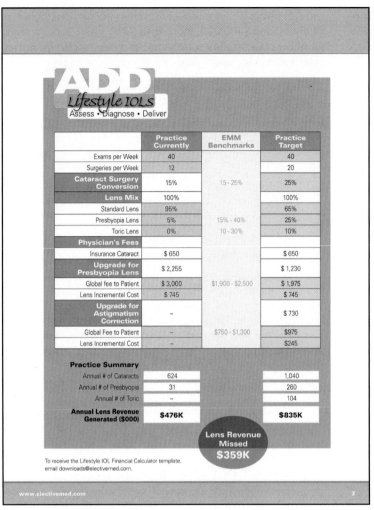

Figure 1. Evaluate cataract conversions and upgrade IOL potential using the Lifestyle IOL Financial Calculator.

understood by your staff and have never been presented as a choice to the patient. Be mindful of the seismic shift that lens choice represents for your technicians, surgical schedulers, and refractive counselors and create an internal marketing effort that increases their knowledge and wins their support.

CREATE A VISION SPA

Start with a realistic perspective of the experience you provide. Nobody wants to visit the eye doctor—ever! We visit because we must. Our prescription is expired or seems to be changing rapidly. Overnight it seems we cannot see a menu or our cell phone. Our children insist we stop driving, or limit night driving, because we have missed a few too many turns. We have had an accident or fear recent vision changes mean impending blindness. Very few people visit an ophthalmologist when they are seeing well. We are a nation that seeks health care when we have a problem. So how do you disrupt the typical medical office experience? How do you alleviate the apprehension? How do you convey your practice is different, better, and worth recommending?

Alter the environment from the minute they open your door. Create a vision spa. Invest in updated furniture arranged in seating pods, rather than straight-backed chairs arranged in lines. Have attractive countertop finishes with all "Don't" and "You Must" signs removed. Paint the walls a soothing color

and introduce natural and lamp lighting. Remove barriers from your check-in desk and outfit front-office staff in solid-color business clothing instead of scrubs. Turn off the TV and turn on nature videos and comforting, commercial-free music. Throw away the expected magazines and provide aspirational magazines. Even better, introduce interesting books that help the prospective patient enjoy your reception lounge. Assist them in forgetting about daily life. Allow them to start thinking about the better life, and better vision, they desire. Give them a visual, tactile reason to support the notion that you can change their world (Figure 2).

RESTRUCTURE YOUR APPOINTMENT CALENDAR

The appointment calendar governs a medical practice. Without meaningful adjustment to the master template, you will not see real staff or patient changes. We have found template modification to be absolutely critical in insurance-oriented practices, where appointment slots are stacked with multiple patients and vague visit-type definition. The trend over the last 10 years is to see more patients per day and spend less time per patient as insurance reimbursements have declined. This method often leaves large numbers of patients stacked up at various stages in your office—in the waiting room, in exam lanes, in testing, in sub-waits. We have disguised the process of

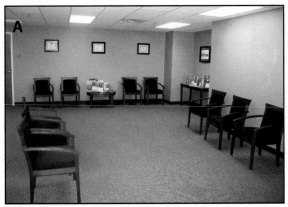
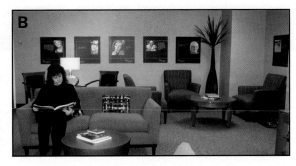

Figure 2. (A and B) Vision for Life, before and after. (Courtesy of Dr. Jeffrey Horn, Nashville, TN.)

actually getting to the doctor by moving patients frequently, allowing multiple technicians to interact with each patient while testing, and showing instructional videos and procedure DVDs to shorten patient conversations. The process is built for patients to wait, so that surgeons never have to.

Any practice looking to grow elective vision will recognize and structure their schedule around the patient, not the surgeon.

* Elective patients should not wait. They must be seen on time, and equally important, released on time. We encourage block days for cataract consultations when this is the only visit-type seen. The entire staff, from receptionist through scheduler, focuses on a single need and optimizes surgical conversions. Eliminating varied visit-types and shifting emergency visits to other physicians allows the practice to run on-time and achieve a rhythm in work-ups, testing, and scheduling.

* Elective patients must be given time before the surgeon exam to consider options. We revise client templates so there is a specific cataract evaluation appointment. Schedulers are instructed to slot patients into this visit if they have been diagnosed with a cataract previously or are age 50+ and have symptoms consistent with a cataract. Printed materials are mailed before the appointment so the patient is educated about cataracts, their cause and cure, and the lens options available. This step shifts the in-office discussion from, "Should I have surgery?", to "Which lens should I choose?"

* Elective patients must have time to consult with and agree to treatment with their surgeon. We extend the surgeon-to-patient time from approximately 5 minutes in an insurance exam to 10 to 15 minutes in upgraded IOL consults. This extra time benefits the practice in 2 ways: overall surgical conversions increase (typically 5 to 10 percentage points) and approximately 25% to 40% of patients will choose upgraded lenses.

MEASURE YOUR RESULTS

What percentage of your cataract patients do you enhance? Most surgeons will tell me that, outside of limbal relaxing incisions during surgery and YAGs postsurgery, their enhance-

ment rate is less than 5%. Many surgeons are concerned about the expected increase in enhancements with lifestyle IOLs. However, I will venture you enhance almost 100% of your cataract patients currently because you expect to put them all in glasses postsurgery! Measuring and optimizing your results with lifestyle IOLs is the most significant step you can take in internal marketing. The ±1-D result with residual astigmatism that is tolerable for an insurance patient expecting glasses afterward is completely unacceptable to an elective lens patient hoping to be virtually glasses-free. To be a best-in-class lens surgeon over the next 10 years, you must track outcomes for each and every eye treated. You must optimize surgeon factors and/or A-constants at least every 6 months. You must measure and track distance and near vision acuities to develop outcomes that can be shared with patients considering these lenses. The benchmark of future success in lens surgery will be measured by the percentage of time a patient lives glasses-free. Establish systems today to measure and report that outcome (Figure 3).

Educating and Converting Your Patients

The final rung in internal marketing is educating patients about the benefits and drawbacks of lifestyle IOLs and converting these patients to surgery. If you have attended to changes that persuade yourself and your staff that lifestyle IOLs are a priority for the practice, then expansion into patient education becomes the most rewarding and self-perpetuating activity in elective vision success.

EDUCATION IS A PROCESS, NOT AN EVENT

Get the right patient into the right appointment slot by making sure you have a specific cataract evaluation visit-type and that the patient has been slotted based on past cataract diagnosis or appropriate age and expressed cataract symptoms.

Mail or email educational materials before the visit. These should include a procedure overview, lens options, fees, patient testimonials, and frequently asked questions (Figure 4).

Figure 3. Report outcomes and expected vision improvement in your patient materials.

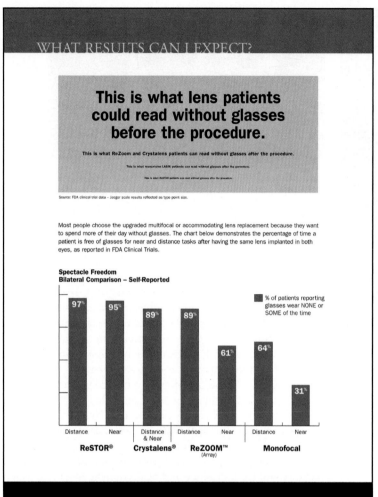

* Use subtle promotional material upon check-in to further educate all practice patients.
* Use printed clipboards to highlight what is new in cataract surgery.
* Instruct front-desk staff to attach a bookmark to the clipboard of every patient checking in if they appear over age 50. While these lenses might not be right for them, they can take the bookmark home for another family member or friend.
* Move your patient testimonials out of the waiting room brag book and onto your walls. We have developed 2-ft x 2-ft wall art capturing a key word and illustrative sentence from patient testimonials and feature these in our wait lounges, exam lanes, even the rest rooms (Figure 5)!

DELIVER THE VISION PATIENTS WANT

One of the most significant shifts a practice must make in delivering elective vision to the 40+ audience is to accept that Plano is not always the right answer. Each patient has varied needs and preferences for near, intermediate, and distance vision. Most presbyopic, astigmatic, and cataractous patients understand that there is no perfect solution to make their eyes age 20 again. It is critical to probe the vision they want and where and when they will be tolerant of glasses within their lifestyle.

An effective tool for initiating this conversation is the Vision Preferences Checklist, which we've modified from the Dell Refractive IOL Questionnaire (Figure 6). Sent in a mailing before the appointment, or filled out upon check-in and reviewed by the technician during work-up, it prompts a patient to consider and decide, "What vision do I really want?" Practices routinely prescribe a distance-optimized, progressive lens solution for our age 50+ patients without asking enough about their reading, computer use, and driving. Often, patients are tolerant of some distance vision trade-off if it means reduced need for glasses at intermediate or near. We must ask the questions and listen to that patient's unique answers to decide upon the appropriate surgical treatment.

RECOMMEND IS NOT A FOUR-LETTER WORD

One of the most basic tenants of selling is to ask for the business. Too often in our practices, especially if we have been insurance-oriented, we think selling is beneath the medical profession. I have been in countless exam lanes where the surgeon never recommends a solution—in effect, never closes the sale. When queried, the surgeon often believes he or she did recommend surgery. Usually this occurs because they are relating all of the options aloud, and expect the patient to understand which option is the recommended choice. Alternatively, physicians feel they should not recommend,

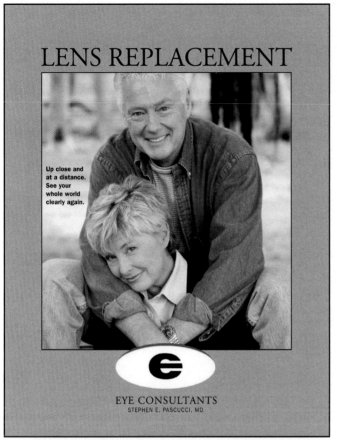

LENS REPLACEMENT

Up close and
at a distance.
See your
whole world
clearly again.

EYE CONSULTANTS
STEPHEN E. PASCUCCI, MD

ABOUT LENS REPLACEMENT

Why can I not see as well up close as I did when I was younger?

All of us notice an important change in our vision sometime around the age of 45. It seems like we wake up one day and can't focus up close. Perhaps this change was more gradual — it became difficult to see menu or credit card statements in a dimly-lit restaurant, or price tags and caller ID weren't as clear, but as long as we held our arms out a little further, we could read. But one day, we ran out of arm length, and reading glasses or progressive lens glasses became a constant companion. This condition is called presbyopia, and comes from the gradual hardening of the lens in the eye. As we age, the lens doesn't flex well to shift focus between distance and near, and reading becomes difficult without magnification. Presbyopia afflicts everyone over the age of 45.

Why does my vision seem cloudy, and why do I have more trouble with glare?

Our eye functions much like a camera. The natural lens focuses images onto the back of the eye so we can see clearly, much like the lens of a camera focusing images onto film for a clear picture. At birth, our natural lens is clear, but as we age it yellows and hardens. In addition, the lens may become cloudy. This condition is called a cataract, and is usually a result of the natural aging process. Everyone over the age of 60 will at some point develop cataracts. As the lens becomes cloudier, vision becomes more blurred.

Symptoms that could indicate the presence of a cataract include a gradual dulling of colors, halos around lights or glare when driving, difficulty reading in low light, blurred or double vision, and a frequent need to change your glasses prescription.

A cataract can progress until eventually there is a complete loss of vision in your eye. Surgery is the only way a cataract can be removed. You should consider surgery when cataracts cause enough loss of vision to interfere with your daily activities.

What are my lens replacement options?

There are many different types of intraocular lenses (IOLs) to choose from to correct a cataract. In addition, many people with clear lenses are opting for lens exchange with newer options to improve near and distance vision.

Lens replacement remains the most frequently performed surgery in the U.S. and is one of the safest as well. You have two options today in choosing a lens replacement solution for your vision needs.

Correcting Distance Vision with a Monofocal IOL
A monofocal IOL is designed to provide clear distance vision. This means you will be able to see objects far away. However, you will need glasses for reading and any type of close, detailed work. Monofocal IOLs have been the standard implant used for decades to help patients after a cataract is removed. Millions of these lenses have been successfully implanted providing cataract sufferers with clear distance vision. New monofocal lens technologies are a step up from the type of lenses you may know of from years ago when a friend or family member had cataract surgery. These lenses incorporate unique optics to compensate for specific deficiencies in your vision. The Tecnis® wavefront lens corrects for spherical aberration that increases as you age. The Tecnis lens is designed to mimic the performance of the average 20-year-old eye and should provide you with sharper, clearer vision, restoration of vibrant colors and better contrast in dim light.

Correcting Distance Vision and Astigmatism
Astigmatism Management is a vital new area of cataract surgery. Astigmatism is a common condition where your eye is out-of-round, shaped more like a football than a basketball. Your vision is potentially affected by two types of astigmatism — corneal and lenticular — and we can correct both with new astigmatism management tools. Today's cataract patient demands excellent vision after surgery, and wants their astigmatism and refractive error corrected at the same time. There are two ways we correct pre-existing astigmatism during cataract surgery. The most advanced method uses a new type of lens implant, called a Toric lens, which incorporates unique optics to compensate for specific deficiencies in your vision. Toric lenses greatly reduce the likelihood of needing a second procedure after cataract surgery to correct residual astigmatism. For those patients who suffer from astigmatism so pronounced that they are outside the power range of the Toric lens, we recommend a combination treatment of lens replacement and relaxing incisions that delivers both improved vision and astigmatism correction. Once we fully understand your level of astigmatism, and desire for improved distance vision and/or near vision, we will recommend the appropriate lens implant option for you.

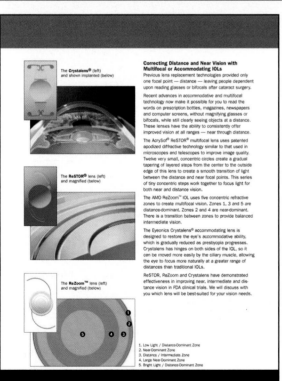

The **Crystalens®** (left) and shown implanted (below)

The **ReSTOR®** lens (left) and magnified (below)

The **ReZoom™** lens (left) and magnified (below)

1. Low Light / Distance-Dominant Zone
2. Near-Dominant Zone
3. Distance / Intermediate Zone
4. Large Near-Dominant Zone
5. Bright Light / Distance-Dominant Zone

Correcting Distance and Near Vision with Multifocal or Accommodating IOLs
Previous lens replacement technologies provided only one focal point — distance — leaving people dependent upon reading glasses or bifocals after cataract surgery.

Recent advances in accommodative and multifocal technology now make it possible for you to read the words on prescription bottles, magazines, newspapers and computer screens, without magnifying glasses or bifocals, while still clearly seeing objects at a distance. These lenses have the ability to consistently offer improved vision at all ranges — near through distance.

The AcrySof® ReSTOR® multifocal lens uses patented apodized diffractive technology similar to that used in microscopes and telescopes to improve image quality. Twelve very small, concentric circles create a gradual tapering of layered steps from the center to the outside edge of this lens to create a smooth transition of light between the distance and near focal points. This series of tiny concentric steps work together to focus light for both near and distance vision.

The AMO ReZoom™ IOL uses five concentric refractive zones to create multifocal vision. Zones 1, 3 and 5 are distance-dominant. Zones 2 and 4 are near-dominant. There is a transition between zones to provide balanced intermediate vision.

The Eyeonics Crystalens® accommodating lens is designed to restore the eye's accommodative ability, which is gradually reduced as presbyopia progresses. Crystalens has hinges on both sides of the IOL, so it can be moved more easily by the ciliary muscle, allowing the eye to focus more naturally at a greater range of distances than traditional IOLs.

ReSTOR, ReZoom and Crystalens have demonstrated effectiveness in improving near, intermediate and distance vision in FDA clinical trials. We will discuss with you which lens will be best-suited for your vision needs.

Figure 4. Address cataract symptoms and the full range of lens options in patient materials provided before the office visit.

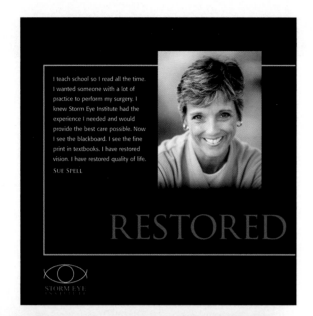

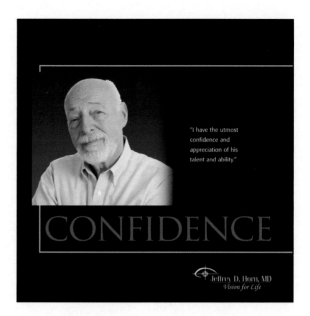

Figure 5. Bring patient testimonials alive by showcasing their words on your walls.

even with a clear medical diagnosis of the cataract, because this will somehow reflect negatively on them in the event of a surgical complication. My experience is if you do not recommend how they proceed, they will not. They are waiting for your expert opinion. You are compounding congestion and low surgery counts by retaining these patients in the recheck cycle. Today's lenses, whether aspheric, toric, multifocal, or accommodating, all provide improved vision versus a cataract. People want to live healthy, uncompromised lives to the greatest extent possible. There is simply no reason, with the safety and accuracy of today's cataract surgery, to delay a return to good vision.

EMBRACING THE LIFESTYLE IOL OPPORTUNITY

Embracing the internal marketing opportunity presented by lifestyle IOLs means you genuinely understand and value the quest for glasses-free vision. You are prepared to reap the benefit with increased surgical fees. You appreciate that

patients want to understand choices and participate in treatment decisions. Internal marketing means shifting the focus of your practice from the surgeon to the patient. Then you will have truly embraced elective vision.

References

1. Marketscope Ophthalmic Market Perspectives, subscription newsletter for the ophthalmic marketplace. www.market-scope.com.

2. Patient Awareness Phone Survey among 400 known glasses/contact lens wearers with 100% awareness of laser vision correction within the 7-county Denver Metro area. 2000.

3. Tan AG, Wang JJ, Rochtchina E, Mitchell P. Comparison of age-specific cataract prevalence in two population-based surveys 6 years apart. *BMC Ophthalmology.* 2006;6:17.

Figure 6. Use the Vision Preferences Checklist to encourage patients to think about the type and range of vision they desire before they see you.

Vision Preferences Checklist

EYE CONSULTANTS
STEPHEN E. PASCUCCI, MD

Your Name ____________________ Date ____________

The term "cataract" refers to a cloudy lens within the eye. When a cataract is removed, a lens implant is placed inside the eye to replace the cloudy human lens. Occasionally, clear lenses that have not yet developed cataracts are also removed to reduce or eliminate the need for glasses or contacts. If it is determined that surgery is appropriate for you, this questionnaire will help us provide the best treatment for your visual needs. Please fill this form out completely and return it to us.

❶ If surgery is recommended for you, would you be interested in seeing well without glasses in the following situations?

- **Distance Vision**: driving, golf, tennis, other sports, watching TV.
  - ☐ Prefer no Distance glasses
  - ☐ I wouldn't mind wearing Distance glasses
- **Mid-range Vision:** computer, menus, price tags, cooking, board games, items on a shelf.
  - ☐ Prefer no Mid-Range glasses
  - ☐ I wouldn't mind wearing Mid-Range glasses
- **Near Vision:** reading books, newspapers, magazines, detailed handwork.
  - ☐ Prefer no Near glasses
  - ☐ I wouldn't mind wearing Near glasses

❷ Please check the **single** statement that best describes you in terms of **night vision**:

- ☐ Night vision is extremely important to me, and I require the best possible quality night vision.
- ☐ I want to be able to drive comfortably at night, but I would tolerate some slight imperfections.
- ☐ Night vision is not particularly important to me.

❸ If you **had** to wear glasses after surgery for one activity, for which activity would you be **most** willing to use glasses?

- ☐ Distance Vision
- ☐ Mid-range Vision
- ☐ Near Vision

❹ If you could have good Distance Vision during the day without glasses, and good Near Vision for reading without glasses, but the compromise was that you might see some halos or rings around lights at night, would you like that option?

☐ Yes ☐ No

❺ If you could have good Distance Vision during the day and night without glasses, and good Mid-Range Vision without glasses, but the compromise was that you might need glasses for reading the finest print at near, would you like that option?

☐ Yes ☐ No

❻ How many hours per day do you spend:

________ On the computer

________ Reading books, newspapers, typed documents or small print

________ Driving

❼ Please list up to three favorite hobbies:

____

____

____

❽ Please place an "X" on the following scale to describe your personality as best you can:

☐————☐————☐

Easy going — Perfectionist

Please Sign Here ____________________

Internal Marketing

Jim Denning, BS

What is marketing? My favorite definition is "meeting needs profitably." EBay is a perfect example of a company that turned a need into a profitable business. To have success in the free market the following components must be present: the right product, in the right place, at the right time, and at the right price. Radial keratotomy (RK) was a successful surgical procedure for the reduction of myopia in the 1980s. If it was introduced after the approval of the excimer lasers circa 1995, it would have failed on every criteria of a successful product. Another example of a product that meets the needs of customers profitably is the iPod (Apple, Cupertino, CA). The iPod created a new market by integrating the Internet with Bluetooth (Bluetooth SIG, Bellevue, WA) and other wireless technology.

The following 4 questions should be asked and answered when executing an internal marketing program:

1. Who are our customers?
2. What are their needs?
3. How can we fulfill their needs?
4. Why should they choose us?

The 78 million baby boomers moving through the system will represent the customers for presbyopia-correcting intraocular lenses (IOLs). The laser vision correction market has already benefited from this powerful market segment. In 1995 to 1996, when excimer lasers first got approval, the leading age of the baby boomer population was 52, the average age was 41, and the trailing age was 30. The sweet spot for laser vision correction procedures peaked around 2001. The baby boomers have now moved out of the laser vision correction market and are heading toward the premium IOL market. In 2008, the leading age of the baby boomer population is 62, the average age is 53 and the trailing age is 44 (Table 1 and Figure 1).

Premium IOLs are the new kind of "eye pod." The baby boomer will want to see well at all distances: far, intermediate, and near without glasses, which is especially true for those who have already undergone laser vision correction. The premium IOL market is huge and has only begun the growth path. Every 7 seconds a baby boomer reaches age 53, (the average age of this demographic segment), which is now well past the laser

Table 1

DEMOGRAPHIC MOVEMENT OF BABY BOOMERS

Year	1996	2008	2011	2021
Leading Age	50	62	65	75
Average Age	41	53	56	66
Trailing Age	32	44	47	57

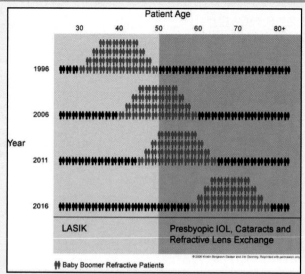

Figure 1. Demographic movement of baby boomers.

vision correction sweet spot. This is good news for the premium IOL market. Baby boomers account for more than half of all spending in the United States. We need to market what we are selling—premium IOLs and premium services—to our patients and our staff.

It is important to go back to the basics and think of marketing as a way of communicating. Whether it is internal or external, we are sending a message about our practice. Internal marketing is as or even more important than external marketing. The bottom line is you cannot promise or promote superior customer service before your staff is trained to provide it. Train your staff to provide premium customer service through internal marketing. Internal marketing can be a very simple formula. Communicating your business strategy to your employees will motivate them to serve customers. All employees have to be on the same page. It is a mistake to over look the potential of your employees because they can be a huge sales force. Induce your employees to sell premium IOL services. If they understand and believe in the premium IOL product, they will become an effective sales force. How do we get everyone on the same page? We hire and train, motivate and communicate, reward and give feedback; 365 days of 1-day training. First, it is important to hire and train employees who want to serve customers. Some of the best staff you can hire are waiters or waitresses. If you think about it, the premium IOL channel and the food industry have the same goal... providing a good customer experience.

Motivate and communicate standards for performance: do not assume that every employee knows what you are trying to accomplish. Taking the time to tell them what you are doing and involving them in the process makes employees feel valued and they will take more pride in what they are doing. You can spend as much money as you want on internal marketing, but if the patient has a bad customer service experience, your investment goes down the drain.

It is important to make sure that the office environment is consistent with your marketing efforts. Provide educational materials for your staff and patients. There are companies such as i-Port Media (Chicago, IL) and Eyemaginations (Towson, MD) who develop educational video loops that run on large monitors in your reception areas. These types of internal media formats are very powerful in educating your existing patients about the services you provide. Finally, reward and give feedback. There are always employees who will not respond, just like there are ads that will not capture the attention of every consumer. Facilitating a consistent environment of motivation, communication, and feedback will help to get most of your staff on board.

CHAPTER 15

LESSONS LEARNED FROM MARKETING COSMETIC SURGERY*

Marie Czenko Kuechel, MA

Premium intraocular lenses (IOLs). Premium outcomes. Premium dollar. Premium patients. Premium perks. Welcome to a new era in medicine and a new business venture, where success equally requires clinical and business knowledge. Premium IOLs represent something heretofore unknown to many patients and physicians: the opportunity to subsidize covered medical services for the benefit of a better medical outcome. This is not cosmetic medicine: purely out-of-pocket and sought-after to improve appearance. This is not elective medicine: the patients you see will be in need of some form of treatment to improve or preserve sight. This is not the current business model of medicine: services are billed and reimbursed at a rate the Federal Government or corporate America (the insurers) predetermines your services to be worth. This is an entirely new era, where you must decide whether and how to offer your patient a premium service, convince your patient of premium outcomes, and persuade your patient to personally and directly bear a significant portion of the cost. Refractive IOLs have born the business of "premium medical services."

While this era of refractive IOLs may present a whole new paradigm in medicine, in your quest to succeed there are lessons to be learned from the business of cosmetic medicine: aesthetic plastic surgery and nonsurgical, medically based procedures. The closest thing in plastic surgery to the new era in ophthalmology is nose surgery prescribed to improve breathing function (a reimbursed surgical procedure) by a patient who also desires an aesthetic improvement (not a reimbursed surgical procedure). This is a patient who presents with the need for functional correction and the desire for aesthetic improvement. Your patient, who presents with the need for improved vision, will have the option of electing and paying for a premium upgrade.

When I wrote my book, *Aesthetic Medicine: Practicing for Success*, in 2004, I stated in the prologue:

This guide is designed to help you be competitive—to set and realize attainable business goals to build a successful non-payor services practice or segment of your practice. It won't give you a predetermined plan to follow; it will help you define a plan best for you and your market. It won't tell you how to build or operate your practice; it will provide background, strategies and cases to consider in defining your practice and building your business model.

A successful practice is not one modeled after another successful practice; it is one uniquely designed to fit market and client demographics, that upholds ethical medical standards and patient safety, and is led by a medical/business professional who is both a passionate provider and an active proprietor.

You did not think of yourself as a proprietor? If you plan on succeeding in premium medicine, you had best start thinking, strategizing, and acting like both physician and a business person. Are you expecting me to give you a marketing plan to follow? Cookie cutter marketing is an enterprise called "franchising." McDonalds failed at offering premium meals along side the Big Mac.

Instead of cookie cutter marketing, what I do offer is the concept of "total patient satisfaction" and the following supposition: You must not view the premium IOL patient's journey through your practice as a linear one with a distinct beginning and end, but rather as a cyclical relationship. With aesthetic surgery, even when one performs a procedure that does not need repeating, the notion must be that patient relationship endures—the physician is remembered, respected, and generates referrals.

Diagnosis and a prescribed treatment whose success depends on a good clinical outcome is merely a process. To be successful, your approach must result in success with each patient through every aspect of his or her journey while receiving premium medical services. This journey is shaped by 3 key phases: recruitment, conversion, and retention.

---

*"Cosmetic surgery" in this context defines the category of elective procedures that enhance appearance; cosmetic surgery in this context does not define a medical specialty.

Recruitment: Needs and Expectations

Recruitment for premium IOL patients will result from 1 of 4 sources:

1. Ideal candidates from within your own practice
2. Candidates referred to you by another physician
3. Candidates referred to you by another patient
4. Candidates who find you as a result of external marketing/communications

The first 3 sources are the most successful means to recruit patients, but they are by no means effortless.

PATIENT RECRUITMENT FROM WITHIN

Patients from within your own practice must not feel they are being "upsold" to IOL, but rather must feel that you are adding value to the treatment for their cataract. When recruiting patients from your own practice consider:

* Demographics: Is this person of an age and lifestyle, and healthy enough to benefit from a premium IOL?
* Economics: Can this person afford or finance a premium IOL without jeopardizing present or future lifestyle?
* Interests: Does this person have an interest in value, or simply want a basic fix?

It would be unfair not to present the IOL option to clinically appropriate patients, but it would be equally unfair to encourage premium IOLs simply to make money. Unlike aesthetic surgery where the patient knows he or she will be fully paying out of pocket, the premium IOL candidate may be surprised to know he or she must dig deeper beyond insurance reimbursement to achieve the best possible outcome. Therefore, patients must know that you have their best interests in mind, whether or not they can or are willing to spend on premium services.

PATIENT RECRUITMENT BY REFERRAL

Whether referral comes from another physician or another patient, there are several rules to live by:

* You must ask for what you want. If you do not ask for referrals, you will not get them.
* You must also show gratitude for what you get, and be gracious when you are turned away. Although you may not get the referral today, a gracious reply will be remembered in the future. If you are not thankful for what you get, do not expect to get it again in the future.

Candidates referred by another physician do not come to you educated and willing; they come to you to investigate options. The essentials to successful recruitment from referring physicians include:

* Educating your referring physicians about the service you provide, and what defines good candidates
* Educating your referring physicians about patient benefits
* Regularly communicating with your referring physicians

* Establishing clinical and administrative points of contact in your office who will regularly communicate with and support your referring physicians
* Making the transition and the communications between the 2 practices as seamless as possible
* Providing appropriate referral materials and keeping these materials current and stocked
* Giving back the patient referred to you, with gratitude

Word of mouth travels, and your happiest patients and referral sources will bring you new referrals. Strive for total patient satisfaction, generate only the happiest patients, ask for referrals, and you will get referrals. ("Total patient satisfaction" is defined later.)

PATIENTS FROM EXTERNAL MARKETING/ COMMUNICATIONS

Reach out, but not too far. Know the demographics and economics of your market. Relate to this population based on lifestyle and interests. These are the keys to reaching patients on the outside, not snappy headlines or expensive ads:

* Visibility—a means for others to find you
* Information—a means for others to learn about you or your specialty and safety
* Education—a means for others to learn about the services you provide that may interest them or that they may desire
* Traffic—a means to get people through your door

Conversion: Education

Regardless of the source of patients, the most critical point in the success of your IOL practice will be conversion to your premium service. You must educate the patient about a premium service, and then meet expectations and achieve total patient satisfaction. If you have not recruited patients well, conversion will be an uphill battle. You will either have poor candidates that you cannot convert, misinformed candidates you must re-educate, or impulse buyers who will never be happy. If you have selected your market well, presented your message effectively, and recruited properly, conversion should be a matter of formalizing, rather than closing the sale. No matter how eager or confident you or the patient may be, conversion occurs at the conclusion of the consultation, which includes the following key elements.

Patient assessment: You and your patient must determine that this is clinically and personally the right lens implant for him or her, and that he or she is someone who will readily enjoy the added value of a premium IOL. This may initially be uncertain, but by the end of the consultation, it should be readily apparent to you and your patient.

Benefits: No matter how committed your patient is to any one option, you should impartially demonstrate the benefits of the premium IOL versus other available options. Emphasize that the benefits of premium IOLs are not simply a recovery of vision, but rather long-term, life-long improvement in lifestyle. Try to relate the visual benefit and the cost of the IOL to a relative tradeoff in life. (For example, the benefits of BOTOX (Allergan, Irvine, CA) have been demonstrated as being equivalent to the cost of a latte each day. Instead of a daily caffeine high, you will look progressively younger over time.)

Risks: You cannot expect a patient to experience total satisfaction if they are not educated about potential risks. A patient who experiences a risk, was educated and fully understood the potential for risk, and whose complication is addressed immediately will usually still be a satisfied patient. Informed consent is as much a legal tool as it is a conversion tool. Do not rattle off the risks quickly and without making eye contact. Make certain your patient fully understands what is communicated and ask if he or she has any unanswered questions. Education is not frightening; it is the unknown that is frightening to your patient.

Options: Options include more than just whether to have a standard or premium IOL. Options include the times when surgery can be scheduled. Options include the comfort and convenience of surgical locations, not just for your patient but also for his or her family and caregivers. Options include payment choices such as credit cards or patient financing.

Process: Process is what must be accomplished, step-by-step, medically and administratively when a patient undergoes IOL surgery. Educate your patients about each step of the process. Outline the preoperative, operative, and postoperative expectations, instructions, experiences, and treatment events. Outline chronologically all the administrative requirements necessary for surgery. Assign one person in your office to be an "IOL coordinator," to guide your patients through all the paperwork, approvals, testing, and pre-certification. Create checklists that help your patients stay on track and avoid surprises. Make the entire medical and administrative process evident, efficient, organized, and easy to comply with. Cross train your staff, so that if someone becomes ill or leaves your practice, the transition is seamless for you and your patients.

Experience: Process is fundamental. The patient's experience is indelible. From the moment your premium IOL patient is connected with your practice, a positive experience stems from excellent service. Your patients will remember the staff members who were kind, polite, organized, and compassionate. They will remember who held their hand, who updated family about surgical status, who offered them a drink. Your patients will remember the doctor who looked them in the eye; who was direct with responses; who was understanding of their concerns; and who was pleasant, polished, and never pompous. You and I both know there are difficult patients, but the most difficult patients who do not compromise the experience of others can become your biggest advocates. Your patients will remember the clean and efficient office, the warm and comfortable exam chair, the soft smell of ginger or vanilla rather than alcohol, and the comforting sounds of acoustic guitar rather than clanging metal, ringing phones, and office chatter. Your patients will remember how short their waiting time was, how interesting and relevant the reading materials were, and they will never forget how long you kept them waiting without the courtesy of an apology or an update. A good experience can overcome a bad process. A bad experience can make even the best process regrettable.

Cost: What to charge? These new IOLs are a premium product, but that does not mean their price is yours alone to define. The market sets the price range, and you determine where within that range you want to fall. The price should consider the cost of the lens, the cost of the office overhead, the cost of your time and skill as a surgeon, and the cost of the experience (without making the experience indulgent) relative to what you believe your patients are willing to pay. Never itemize these costs to your patient unless you want each item to be open to question. Simply define the reimbursed amount and point out that this is a premium medical service. Use the term *out-of-pocket costs* for items such as deductibles, but not for premium IOLs.

Never compete on price or you may start a price war. You want your patient to choose you because of trust—not because of a lower price. You never want a prospective patient to disregard your service because of a published price, so avoid giving out prices up front until the time of the consultation. During the consultation, you, the physician, should never discuss price. Cost is an administrative element that belongs in the hands of the appropriate administrative staff member who guides the process. The IOL coordinator should be the one name, the one face, and the one person your patient will come to know and trust, and this person should define the price and guide the process.

Follow these steps and converting patients to premium IOLs should be easy. It should pleasantly become second nature for you, your staff, and your patients. Your premium IOL service is a valuable experience that the right candidates will accept without hesitation. Those who are looking for a deal, or who question your value will move on to become someone else's thorn. Remember that how you attract and how you educate your patients will ultimately deliver exactly the type of patient (and sometimes the problems) you deserve.

SALESMANSHIP

When I began consulting in aesthetic medicine, there was a marketing concept that some still preach today, which is simply absurd when applied to elective or premium medicine. It is the ultimate concept in salesmanship—how to turn "no" into "yes."

Overcoming objections is reasonable, but not without first identifying the source of the objections. You may find your patient is uninformed, misinformed, confused, or simply objectionable. Some things you can correct, but other times you must simply let go and move on to the next patient.

There is no value, however, in ignoring objections. Keep track of the patients you lose and cannot convert. Ask your patients why they did not opt for a premium IOL. By reviewing the reasons you mind find a problematic pattern. Every problem offers the opportunity for a solution and improvement. For example, maybe the person scheduling the appointments is providing incorrect information. Maybe your patient educational materials are not consistent with what you say in consultation. Maybe your referring physicians are steering poor candidates to you. Pay attention to the prospective patients you lose, only insofar as to learn how to do better. However, never pressure a "no" decision into a "yes" that you, your staff, and your patient will later regret.

Retention: Outcomes, Satisfaction, and Referral

Good outcomes do not always result in happy patients. In order to achieve total patient satisfaction, you must accomplish the highest of ratings for both process and experience. Your patient must perceive that the premium IOL not only functions well, but was part of an overall positive experience. In all of medicine, but especially with premium and elective procedures, outcomes are judged by the entire service experience, and not just by the clinical result.

In medicine, unexpected problems can happen. Apologize, correct the problem, and continue on a path of highest quality. In life, mistakes happen. Apologize, correct the mistake, and continue on a quality path. Even with poor outcomes or complications, a good experience can still result in patients who are ultimately happy.

Satisfaction

Your goal is simple: to achieve total patient satisfaction. Do not wait for a new patient referral to find out if you have achieved total patient satisfaction. At that "final" postoperative visit, look your patient in the eye, and ask if he or she is pleased with both the outcome and process. Listen. Then tell the happy patient, "If a family member, a friend, or a neighbor ever has a question, I hope you will refer them to me. Please tell anyone you send my way to share your name, because I want always to be reminded of you." This will only take 30 seconds to do, if the process and the experience have been crafted to achieve total patient satisfaction.

You can, and should, also use a formal survey to measure satisfaction several weeks later. Send your patients a letter and a brief informal survey. Ask him or her to put down the current best seller (he or she is now able to clearly read and enjoy) for just a moment, to rate your practice so that you can continue to strive for "total patient satisfaction." The survey can be anonymous or patients can disclose their identity so that you can follow up and address any areas where the service fell short. There are wonderful online survey services, and I offer templates in my book, *Aesthetic Medicine: Practicing for Success,* that you can tailor to premium IOL surgery.

Retention and Referral

You must still retain satisfied patients for life. You should reach out on the anniversary of their IOL surgery with a card that marks the occasion. You should send an annual newsletter about ocular health and other topics of interest. You should notify them when you have a change in status, location, or service. You should stay connected because the satisfied patient is your ambassador. He or she is more influential than the best advertising or the most prolific referring physician. Stay visible, stay connected, and you will receive qualified referrals in the future from this person. A personal endorsement is priceless: it will win you a patient who trusts you without meeting you, and it should demonstrate the power of total patient satisfaction to you.

Top 10 Musts for Succeeding With Premium IOLs

1. Know your market. Define your patients, clinically and demographically. Relate to them. Define your brand and identity based on your market.

2. Forget cookie cutter strategies. Strive for marketing and communications that highlight visibility and education, and complement your market and their buying and lifestyle preferences.

3. Educate your referral sources (physicians and patients) and stay connected.

4. Avoid guerilla marketing. Do not create a revolving door or a price war.

5. Get organized and stay polished. Strive for the best in outcomes, process, and experience for your patient, yourself, and your staff.

6. Assign an IOL patient coordinator to manage everything but the clinical details. Be the surgeon and let someone else manage the patient process.

7. See conflict as an opportunity to learn, improve, and grow.

8. Put salesmanship aside. Remember, your tactics will earn you the patients you deserve.

9. Strive for total patient satisfaction, not a pre-defined revenue stream.

10. Your relationship with your patients is cyclical. For as long as you are in practice, and for as long as your patients are alive, find a way to stay in touch.

www.czenkokuechel.com

CHAPTER 16

PREMIUM IOLs AND THE ROLE OF YOUR STAFF

R. Bruce Wallace, III, MD, FACS

Refractive intraocular lenses (IOLs) have only recently become available to most surgeons and in some ways have presented staff members with a significant paradigm shift in regard to effective patient selection, patient education, and postoperative care. Today's successful lens surgery practices have quickly learned how important their staff is to success with the new premium IOLs. I depend heavily on my team's expertise and experience for every step toward desired refractive outcomes for our patients.

Following is a partial list of important lessons we have learned in order for our staff members to maximize their effectiveness in caring for patients who choose a premium IOL in order to reduce their dependency on glasses.

Involve the Entire Office Staff in the Process

We have provided a number of educational seminars on refractive IOLs for everyone in the practice, and not just the ophthalmic technicians. Every member of our team understands the important role they play in achieving the visual results our patients have learned to expect. They are made aware of the variety of products available and their unique differences. There is a sense of pride for each staff member, whether they be front office, technician, or business office staff, that takes place when they hear about a happy postoperative patient because they know they played a part in the care of that patient.

Encourage Staff to Look for Good Refractive IOL Candidates and Warn of Potentially Poor Choices

Experienced staff members develop a sixth sense for who would make a great refractive IOL patient and maybe more importantly, who is not. Listening to their assessment of potential candidates and acting on their recommendations verifies their valuable position in the process.

Clear the "Terminology Fog"

The terminology surrounding refractive IOLs and biometry can be confusing to staff members. Some commonly used nomenclature may need clarification:

* The basic difference between diffractive and refractive multifocal IOLs
* How accommodating IOLs differ
* IOL constants—often generically referred to as A-constants, which only apply to the SRK family of formulas, lens constants are actually variables and need to be personalized to the surgeon and the methods of preoperative biometry. Some modern IOL formulas such as the Holladay II, Hoffer Q, and Haigis use "ACD" for the lens constant. However, this is different from the measured anterior chamber depth—see how a staff member could be confused?

Provide the Best Technology

Fortunately, biometry has been greatly enhanced with immersion A-scan and the advent of the IOL Master (Carl Zeiss Meditec, Jena, Germany), now with an important software upgrade.[1] The latest in corneal topographers, wavefront aberrometers, and optical coherence topography have also helped staff members assist us in objectively measuring parameters of ocular health that are important for achieving expected surgical results. The best technology includes not just exam equipment but telephones, computers, educational materials, and informational Web sites.

Watch Out for Tear Dysfunction

Especially important for multifocal IOL patients, an inadequate tear film can cause a significant increase in unwanted visual sensations. Many older patients have marginal tear function preoperatively that can be made worse with surgery and medications. To maximize quality multifocal vision, our team encourages aggressive treatment of dry ocular surface with lubricants, Restasis (Allergan, Irvine, CA), and punctual occlusion.

Be Happy With 20/Happy

Our staff knows to avoid the "20/20 trap." The scenario of happy postoperative patients coming in for an exam very satisfied because of their wonderful visual improvement and leaving unhappy because a technician shared with them that their vision was "good but not 20/20" is not an infrequent event in some practices. What really matters to patients is visual functionality (a term I learned from Dr. Charles "Skip" Bechert) and not what size letters they can read on a Snellen chart. Our staff records what visual tasks patients can perform now without glasses that they could not before surgery, such as reading, sewing, or using the computer.

Encourage Neuroadaptation

Especially important for recently implanted multifocal patients, our staff frequently needs to reinforce how important visual cortical neuroadaptation is in order to achieve functional multifocality. For some patients this process is rapid, but for others it may take many months. Our staff plays a key role in encouraging patients to be patient and "practice" near tasks with their new vision system.

Add a Patient Satisfaction Program

Our Patient Satisfaction Program, which began over 15 years ago, is an outcomes measuring device to monitor IOL power calculations and astigmatism reduction. Our goal has been to be within 0.50 D of our spherical target and less than 1.0 D of astigmatism after lens surgery. We have shared our results regularly with the entire staff. By doing this exercise on a regular basis, our staff is constantly reminded of how important their participation in biometry, refractions, and so on is to achieving desired outcomes.

Take Advantage of Troubleshooting

Whenever an unexpected result in refractive error occurs, troubleshooting to find the cause by re-evaluating the preoperative data and, if necessary, repeating the biometric measurements helps our staff to avoid future miscalculations.

Celebrate Success

In a busy cataract practice, ignoring the incredible value lens refractive procedures can provide to so many people can creep into the mindset of many care providers. Praising staff members for their effectiveness in providing the refractive outcomes patients are hoping to achieve and encouraging the office team to celebrate with the patients is a "win-win." Patients will appreciate the staff members more for their role in the process and the staff will be encouraged to continue to provide excellent care for future patients.

Conclusion

Lens surgeons are likely to see greater demand for their services as baby boomers age. A natural consequence will be more responsibility for patient care falling on the shoulders of talented and well-trained staff members. Encouraging staff involvement in the refractive lens surgery process can greatly improve patient care and desired results.

Reference

1. Fang JP, Hill WE, Wang L, Chang V, Koch DD. Advanced intraocular lens power calculations. In: Kohnen and Koch, eds. *Essentials in Ophthalmology—Cataract and Refractive Surgery*. Berlin: Springer-Verlag; 2007.

CHAPTER 17

Premium IOLs and the Role of Your Staff

Kevin L. Waltz, OD, MD

Implanting premium intraocular lenses (IOLs) is a team sport. The surgeon is the captain of the team. On the surgeon's team are the patient and the surgeon's staff. On the opposing team are fear and lack of education. The staff is a key element in winning with premium IOLs. Educate and reward your staff in order to succeed with premium IOLs. In return, your staff will educate your patients and promote premium IOLs.

The surgeon sets the tone. The surgeon needs to be confident, well-informed, and prepared. The staff needs the same level of confidence and knowledge to educate the patient about the pros and cons of premium IOLs. For example, the staff must consistently achieve accurate biometry. The surgeon uses the biometry data to make an accurate premium IOL selection. The surgeon and the patient depend on the staff and benefit from this team work. A smart surgeon will make every effort to educate his or her staff and support them with the best equipment. This includes investing in staff education at regional and national meetings.

My practice began using multifocal IOLs in 1998. We did not call them premium IOLs, but we treated them like a premium service. We worked hard to achieve optimal outcomes with them. We also learned the importance of educating our staff and involving them in clinical decisions. Imagine the reaction of my staff in 1998 when I told them we were going to remove "clear" lenses and replace them with a multifocal IOL. They were afraid. There was a fear of acting inappropriately and harming the patient. They did not understand my decision. Once my staff understood the decision and they worked with the patients postoperatively, they were excited to be involved with premium IOLs. We also closely tracked our outcomes. I realized very quickly that contact A-scan biometry and manual keratometry were not going to be sufficient to make the most of multifocal IOLs. I discussed the situation with my staff, and I purchased a topographer and an IOL Master (Carl Zeiss Meditec, Jena, Germany). We leveraged the investment in premium IOL services to improve the care for all of our cataract patients. I expect the best from my staff, and they

deserve the best tools available to achieve my goals.

The staff requires 3 things from the surgeon to make premium IOLs successful: clinical education, appropriate tools, and good outcomes. The surgeon provides the initial clinical education, buys the tools for the staff, and creates the surgical outcomes. However, the staff is the key to the surgeon's success with premium IOLs. In most cataract practices in the United States, the surgeon and the staff benefit from a general level of knowledge of the patients. The patients have multiple friends who have had cataract surgery with a monofocal IOL and the typical patient knows the routine. *It won't hurt. There won't be a patch. The patient will need glasses after the surgery... The insurance will cover everything.* This is a blessing and a curse. It makes informed consent for cataract surgery with a monofocal IOL very straightforward. It makes educating a patient about the benefits of a premium IOL a deviation from the normal, expected preoperative consultation. The surgeon's staff is the key to bridging this gap. I have been working with my staff to optimize this process for 10 years. We are good at it, but we still have room for improvement. The surgeon working with premium IOLs should recognize that it is a long journey and the staff is a traveling companion to be treated with respect, support, and education.

The patient needs to be educated about the pros and cons of premium IOLs to make an informed decision. This can be a lengthy, time-consuming process. Your staff makes this process efficient and productive for all concerned. The staff responds to the tone the surgeon sets and then communicates that tone to the patient. The message the practice sends to patients about premium IOLs begins with marketing materials and the initial phone contact. The message never ends. The surgeon should define the message and the staff should deliver it consistently.

My own staff is very comfortable and confident with premium IOLs, and they know that we have the best interests of the patient in mind at all times. They are encouraged to speak to patients about the *benefits and downsides* of premium IOLs. We do not over emphasize the upside nor overlook the downside.

My staff will look a patient in the eye and tell him or her that halos after premium IOLs are normal and expected. They will do this preoperatively and postoperatively and they will not apologize for it because they understand that they are normal. Likewise, my staff is comfortable with our pricing for premium IOLs.

My practice does not make pricing decisions in a vacuum. The practice management understands that the added charges for premium IOLs are a significant investment of time and money for the patient, the staff, and the surgeon. The staff must believe there to be value in premium IOLs for the patient. The staff works in a medical environment but also lives outside of the practice of medicine. They have to deal personally with the issues of covered and noncovered benefits in their own care and in the care of their loved ones. The staff is the toughest sell the surgeon will have with premium IOLs. Once the surgeon has educated the staff about the value of premium IOLs, the staff will educate the patient.

I strongly favor external professional education for premium IOLs for the surgeon and the staff. Educating the staff about premium IOLs is a challenging process. I have been lecturing on premium IOLs and providing external education to other practices for years. I still find it very helpful to send my own staff to outside educational programs on premium IOLs. It validates what I tell them internally and they return with new ideas and enthusiasm. There is still a great deal to be learned about premium IOLs. Obtaining outside help and support in staff training is one of the cornerstones of the educational process.

CHAPTER 18

ASCRS PRESBYOPIA EDUCATION TASK FORCE—CHALLENGE AHEAD

John Ciccone

The American Society of Cataract and Refractive Surgery (ASCRS) conducts public and patient education activities under the auspices of the Eye Surgery Education Council (ESEC) of the ASCRS Foundation. In the fall of 2006, the Foundation determined that there was a need for the development of public education materials on presbyopia-correcting intraocular lenses (Pr-C IOLs) that are accurate and balanced in explaining the benefits these lenses offer. The factors that contributed to this decision were 1) the availability of lenses—the approvals by the U.S. Food and Drug Administration (FDA) of the Eyeonics, Inc Crystalens (Aliso Viejo, CA), the Alcon ReSTOR lens (Fort Worth, TX), and the availability of the Advanced Medical Optics ReZoom lens (Santa Ana, CA); 2) the decision in May 2005 by the Center for Medicare and Medicaid Services to allow patients to select premium lenses and pay for their additional costs out of pocket; 3) the large population of presbyopic baby boomers; and 4) growing interest of the general news media in presbyopia management.

The Foundation's first expedition into public education activities grew from the need to address public concerns about the safety of laser in situ keratomileusis (LASIK). In 2000 and 2001 there were numerous TV and print media stories about patients who had had unsatisfactory LASIK outcomes. This coverage, largely a thing of the past, led ASCRS to launch the Eye Surgery Education Council and charge it with developing balanced and accurate information on the risks and benefits of laser vision correction.

The main product of the Council at that time was the development of a Web site and patient screening guidelines for LASIK, and a media campaign targeted to patients and media opinion leaders. The guidelines include a description of eye examinations, and profiles of ideal, less-than-ideal, and noncandidate patients. In addition, the guidelines stressed the need for patients to be well informed and have realistic expectations for outcomes. Given the environment of a public controversy and intense media interest in the subject, the guidelines received extensive media coverage when they were launched in 2002. That coverage helped to dampen the safety concerns and further educate potential patients about the benefits of LASIK.

Although the campaign was a success, it is recognized that several other factors contributed to reducing the safety concerns about LASIK. LASIK is an excellent procedure. Since the time of its introduction in the mid 1990s there has been considerable technical progress (most notably with the introduction of wavefront guidance and femtosecond laser flap formation). Surgeons have made substantial progress in clinical techniques and patient selection. Laser vision correction is a mature technology that yields immediate and substantial contributions to patient quality of life. Finally, there has been a constant drumbeat of advertising and marketing by surgeons in their local communities. It has been estimated that since LASIK was introduced, surgeons have invested more than $100 million dollars in local advertising.

Today, ophthalmologists can offer a variety of surgical options for managing presbyopia—premium IOLs, conductive keratoplasty (CK), monovision, and soon to be approved multifocal ablations—in addition to traditional reading glasses and multifocal contact lenses. However, the public's lack of understanding of presbyopia and its management options are a hindrance to acceptance.

To get a better understanding of that problem, the ESEC commissioned a Harris Interactive survey in the fall of 2006. The survey looked at what the general population already knew about presbyopia, the different surgical treatment options that were available, and what types of treatment options they would consider. The results of survey are available at the ASCRS presbyopia education Web site, www.readclearlyagain.org.

The survey polled 500 adults between the ages of 45 and 65 (general population) and 250 patients who have Pr-C IOLs implanted either as part of cataract surgery or as a clear lens replacement option (ASCRS patients). Among the key findings:

✳ Lack of understanding of presbyopia

 ❖ 62% of the general population and 70% of the ASCRS sample have experienced presbyopia.

 ❖ 79% of the general population and 56% of the ASCRS sample are not at all knowledgeable about presbyopia. This finding was particularly interesting in light of the fact that the ASCRS sample is composed of patients who opted for Pr-C IOLs or took part in FDA trials of the lenses. Differences in ways that doctors talked to their patients about presbyopia, the advanced age of some patients, and the time interval between the date of the procedure and the date of the survey may be contributing factors.

 ❖ 9% of the general population and only 10% of the ASCRS sample could describe presbyopia as "beginning at middle age, the need to use reading glasses to read or focus at near distances."

 ❖ 50% of the general population and 48% of the ASCRS sample are not sure of the correct definition, even when definitions were read to them.

 ❖ This lack of understanding makes the ophthalmologist's job of educating patients more difficult, and may short change individuals who may be interested and good candidates, but simply do not know about their options. Despite the obvious lack of understanding about presbyopia and surgical management options, many of those polled indicated a willingness to have a surgical management option, but safety remains a concern.

 ❖ 66% of the general population is at least somewhat willing to get an artificial lens if the procedure was FDA approved.

 ❖ Obstacles to having vision correction surgery include: "you don't know enough about the procedure" (55%); "you are comfortable wearing reading glasses to improve your vision" (54%); "it's too costly" (51%); "you are worried about potential complications" (51%).

  As expected, many in the general population (aged 45 to 64) sample say they also do not know much at all about IOLs. Following from this, in terms of managing presbyopia, the general population thinks prescription glasses would be most effective whereas nearly one third are unsure how effective an IOL would be.

 ❖ 58% of the general population does not know much at all about a "bifocal lens permanently implanted onto the eye."

 ❖ 70% of the general population thinks that "prescription glasses or bi-focal lenses" would be very effective or effective in managing presbyopia. 33% say the same about a "bifocal lens permanently implanted onto the eye," with 31% being unsure of its effectiveness.

✳ Impact on quality of life

 ❖ The ASCRS Survey found that a majority of the 45- to 64-year-old general population has difficulty with tasks that require them to focus on near objects.

 ❖ 43% of the general population currently have a great deal of difficulty with "reading ordinary print in newspapers or magazines without glasses"; 39% have a great deal of difficulty with "reading a menu at a restaurant without glasses"; 34% have a great deal of difficulty with "doing work or hobbies."

 ❖ 77% of the general population wears glasses now or did so in the past.

 ❖ 81% of the general population says focusing on objects up close has/would have some impact on their lives (38% say major impact).

  For the ASCRS patient sample, prior to surgery, a majority of the patients had the same kinds of difficulties with vision as the general population, and most think that not being able to focus on close objects had some impact on their overall quality of life. Not surprisingly, then, a majority believes their surgery has had a major positive impact on their quality of life.

 ❖ Prior to surgery, 70% of the ASCRS patient sample had a great deal of difficulty "reading ordinary print in newspapers or magazines without glasses"; 57% had a great deal of difficulty with "reading a menu at a restaurant without glasses"; 55% had a great deal of difficulty with "driving without glasses"; 50% had a great deal of difficulty with "doing work or hobbies."

 ❖ After surgery, 49% of the ASCRS sample have no difficulty "reading ordinary print in newspapers or magazines without glasses"; 51% have no difficulty with "reading a menu at a restaurant without glasses"; 71% have no difficulty with "driving without glasses"; 51% have no difficulty with "doing work or hobbies."

 ❖ 81% of the ASCRS sample says being able to focus on objects close had some impact on their lives (42% say major impact).

 ❖ 64% of the ASCRS sample says that vision correction surgery/cataract surgery had a major positive impact on their lives.

Education

Aggressive public education and industry-supported promotion and marketing campaigns may have the unintended effect of raising patient expectations beyond what current technology and outcomes can justify, especially among mid-life emmetropic presbyopes. Experts note that "we must under promise and over deliver if we are to avoid some of the problems encountered in the early years following the introduction of LASIK."

To help in the task of educating the public, the ESEC developed the www.readclearlyagain.org Web site. The site was developed under the direction of the Presbyopia Education Task Force whose members include Samuel Masket, MD, chair; David Chang, MD; Steven Dell, MD; Natalie Afshari, MD; and Stephen Lane, MD. The site explains presbyopia through text and video animations, and provides a description of the surgical means for managing it. Although ASCRS feels the site is a helpful tool, more needs to be done. Ongoing educational activities will include expansion of Internet-based patient education resources, exploitation of print and broadcast news opportunities, and development of a Web-based resource library. To be housed on the ASCRS Web site, the library will include focus group–tested educational and marketing materials that surgeons can use in their offices to educate patients.

SECTION II

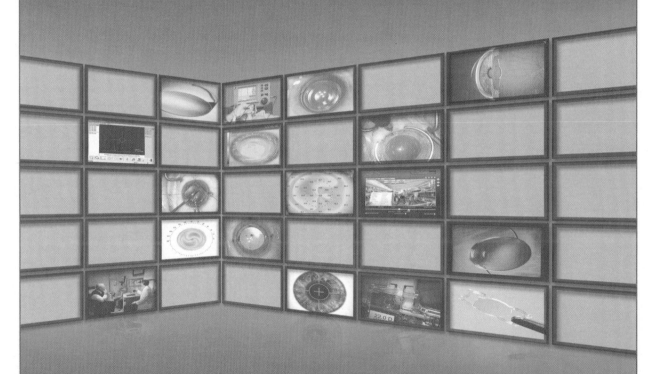

Transitioning to Presbyopia-Correcting IOLs

CHAPTER 19

LESSONS LEARNED FROM KERATOREFRACTIVE SURGERY

Louis Probst, MD and John Lehr, OD

The perceptive reader may ask why 2 professionals that specialize solely in refractive corneal surgery are writing the chapter on patient candidacy in a textbook on refractive cataract surgery. Although the authors deal with the cornea, and this textbook addresses lens surgery, the common ground is the "refractive" component of the surgery, which generally requires private payment as refractive corrections are not medically necessary. Because the authors have specialized in refractive surgery for 100% of their practice for 10 years, we have considerable experience with the refractive patient. The obvious advantage of refractive surgery is the physician can improve the patient's functional vision while earning additional income. Along with these benefits comes the sometimes less obvious challenges that are the subject of this chapter.

Medical Versus Retail Patients

MEDICAL PATIENTS

With a vision-threatening disease, a patient tends to follow the system dictated by his or her insurance or health system. Patients that are treated within the medical system can expect to wait for up to an hour in "waiting" rooms, the staff is courteous but curt, the system is effective but impersonal, and the emphasis is on rules and regulations rather than customer care. All this is accepted by the patient as he or she has been trained to expect it from his or her earliest visits to the "doctor" as a child.

Once seen by the surgeon, an explanation of the diagnosis, the surgery, the likely prognosis, and potential complications usually results in the patient proceeding to surgery. Arrangements for the surgery may include several more visits for preoperative testing and an inflexible surgery date at some time in the future. Success is defined as an uncomplicated procedure. Even ambulatory surgery centers that specialized solely in cataract surgery have many of the characteristics just outlined. If the reader is a cataract surgeon, he or she may won-

der what is unusual or wrong with this approach. If the reader is a refractive surgeon, he or she knows that this model would be a refractive surgery disaster.

RETAIL PATIENTS

Refractive surgery patients are voluntarily paying for a functional improvement in their vision with discretionary spending. This means that their mode of thinking is transformed into the retail mindset in which the customer is king (or queen). People do not like to wait before making a $10 purchase at MacDonald's so they certainly do not want to wait in a "waiting" room before spending $4000 dollars. They expect reasonable customer care and appreciate excellent care. At our centers, the staff introduce themselves and shake the patient's hands. Patients are offered food and drinks. Comments are positive and never negative. Our staff is personable, respectful, confident, effective, and enthusiastic. No reasonable request is denied as we need to keep the atmosphere positive so the patient will choose us for his or her procedure. The number of visits to the center is minimized so the potential barriers to have the procedure are minimized. If we create a poor impression, there are lots of other providers that would be very happy to take our business. We aim to make the visit to our center as close to enjoyable as possible. Success with a retail patient is defined as an encounter that results in the referral of another patient, creating "word of mouth" business growth.

Surgeons interested in getting involved in refractive surgery will appreciate these characteristics of the retail patient and will make the necessary adjustments. The challenge often lies with the office staff, which initially has the same approach and mannerisms for every patient.

Expectations for Refractive Surgery

Expectation management in refractive surgery is critical. The best philosophy is "under promise and over deliver."

Because they are paying for the surgery, patients often assume that they will have perfect uncorrected vision of 20/20 after the surgery. This impression has been re-enforced by the advertisements of the laser vision correction business. Make sure that the patient understands the limitations of the procedure. As a clinician, we may be very pleased with a result of 20/40 uncorrected vision following a clear lens extraction on a patient who was –14.00 D all of her life, but was the patient aware that he or she would probably not achieve an uncorrected "20/20" or "perfect" vision? Does the patient truly grasp that all near vision would be compromised? The expectations of patients are just as high for a preoperative patient with a –10 D prescription with 3 D of astigmatism as they are for someone with a simple –2 D myopia. The authors have had many patients that demand enhancements for less than 1 D of sphere or astigmatism after enormous initial corrections. No matter how thorough your informed consent is, it is critical to chart all discussions involving special needs and risks pertinent to each individual, including the need for reading glasses.

Presbyopia

Presbyopia is one of the most complicated issues for patients to understand. At least one third of all patients do not understand that refractive surgery will not inherently solve all of their distance, intermediate, and near vision needs. Progress in lens design, wavefront analysis, and multifocal lenses have certainly brought us closer to this goal, but all these new advancements also come with a certain amount of compromise. Helping patients understand the limitations of the refractive modality you are proposing prior to surgery will save much time and effort after surgery. Be sure to specifically mention, and illustrate as accurately as possible, what a patient can expect from his or her new vision. Presbyopic patients usually understand that they will need glasses to read a book but do not realize that their dashboard and the food on their plate will also be blurred after surgery. It is not intuitively obvious to them that surgery will affect their computer vision at 20 to 36 inches. Because many patients spend the majority of their work day in front of the computer, this is not an issue to ignore or just assume they understand.

Educating patients about realistic outcomes following monovision or multifocal visual results is one of the most time-consuming aspects of expectation management. Every patient who wants to pursue monovision correction should first successfully complete a contact lens trial prior to having surgery. Due to problems with anisometropia, treatments are best limited to no more than +1.50 D of near vision when the fellow eye is to be corrected for distance. This provides good intermediate vision, decent near, and does not significantly impair the brain's ability to see well at a distance at the same time. Multifocal implant options are becoming more advanced and allow for better functionality at most distances but still represent a compromise in the quality of vision. Experience with multifocal contact lenses has shown us that these new intraocular lenses (IOLs) are not a "cure" for presbyopia. Patients complain that they have "O.K." distance vision and serviceable intermediate ability, but do not have great vision at any distance. A multifocal contact lens trial may be one way for a patient to experience and accept these limitations prior to surgery.

Consent

In the medical environment, consent is obtained by informing patients of their risks and asking them to sign a consent form. Because the patient has a problem such as a cataract, the small risks associated with the procedure seem justified in order to have the problem corrected. Although complications are not expected, if they do occur they are generally accepted as being a part of having the procedure.

In the retail refractive surgery environment, patients often do not have a medical problem or disease. This makes the risks of surgery much less acceptable. It is an art form to educate patients about complications while ethically promoting the procedure. Although the appropriate risks and forms should be addressed, the goal is not to scare the patient so he or she decides not to proceed with surgery. In this, the "information age," it can be assumed that the patient has at least done some Internet research into the procedure and the associated risks. The patient should be given the consent form prior to surgery to carefully read at his or her convenience, and he or she should have an opportunity to ask questions about the risks and the consent form. All complications that are discussed should be followed by a discussion of the treatment that would correct the problem so the patient can see that there are solutions to the complications. The informed consent with the surgeon should ideally be ethical and honest but at the same time concise and positive.

Who Is a Good Candidate for Refractive Surgery?

On the most simplistic level, the best refractive candidates are those that would benefit from refractive correction and are willing and able to pay for it. If the patient is eager to have the procedure performed yet he or she has a minimal correction, the surgeon should be cautious about proceeding as the patient will likely not be impressed with the outcome. Unhappy refractive patients will not grow your refractive business and will be an emotional and financial drain on your practice. As refractive surgery has become more mainstream, we encounter more patients who are good refractive surgery candidates that are unable to afford the procedure even with fairly liberal financing arrangements.

The best patients for refractive surgery are those who are educated about how their procedure will benefit them, realistic about their visual function after surgery, and are aware that, even with a perfect surgery, they may not have a perfect result. Patients that bring up questions about risks and expectations are usually ones that have been doing research on their own. This shows that they are taking the appropriate steps to educate themselves and are taking the process seriously.

Although the Internet can be a source of misinformation and a forum for patients who have experienced poor outcomes, it is still a useful tool. Refractive surgery Internet sites are roughly split between those promoting various procedures and sites that detail the negative aspects of surgical vision correction. Even if it was just black and white, without a nonbiased view to be found, most prospective patients will be able to form an opinion, either for or against, without even visiting a doctor's office. If someone reads the worst-case scenarios outlined on some of the more aggressive sites and still proceeds with surgery, the doctor can be assured that this patient is making an educated decision.

From a strictly medical standpoint, a healthy patient is the best candidate for elective surgery. The surgeon who performs elective refractive procedures is held to a higher standard of care. Because of this, detailed testing and more thorough diagnosis of all related and unrelated visual and structural issues are required. Careful patient history and thorough examination of the eyes are critical to proper patient selection. Advanced instrumentation that may not otherwise be standard is the norm when evaluating refractive patients.

Who Is a Poor Candidate for Refractive Surgery?

Lee Nordan, MD (personal communication) has facetiously said that "the best way to identify a poor refractive candidate is to operate on them." The wisdom in this statement is that those patients that often seem like they would be hard to please generally do well after surgery, whereas the unhappy postoperative patients may have seemed normal prior to surgery. However, there are some guidelines that are helpful to allow for the intelligent screening of refractive patients.

Patients that will experience only a minimal benefit from the procedure will not be happy with the outcome. Unhappy patients will eventually destroy a refractive practice as they will not produce word of mouth referrals; instead, they will diminish the reputation of the surgeon and the practice, and will strain the resources of the surgeon and the office to address the postoperative concerns. The successful refractive surgeon will only perform elective refractive corrections when they honestly believe that there is a 99% chance of making the patient happy regardless of the patient's willingness to pay for the procedure.

If a patient cannot afford the refractive procedure, they would initially seem to be a poor candidate. However, there are a number of credit services available that will not require the patient to pay the full cost immediately. Although credit cards are the simplest method of financing, financing companies such as MBNA and Care Credit also may provide attractive arrangements with lower monthly payments. Practices are discouraged from "self" financing arrangements as this could create an adversarial relationship between the patient and the surgeon in the future that could increase the risk of legal problems if the outcome is not perfect.

The patient's psychological and emotional status needs to be evaluated. Assessing the patient's candidacy for surgery based on these issues can be difficult. If there is a question as to whether a patient understands and accepts the risks or limitations of a procedure, proceed with caution. If a patient is overly confrontational or challenging during their consultation, be wary. Patients who repeatedly question every minute detail and belabor the rarest of complications may not be ready to proceed. Conversely, the patient who does not ask any questions and downplays or ignores all negative risks may be difficult to work with if the surgical results do not meet their expectations. Excessive nervousness, fidgeting, and abnormal anxiety are good indicators of an unprepared patient.

Because it is elective surgery, refractive surgery is held to a higher medicolegal standard than procedures that are medically necessary. Therefore, the surgeon should always be wary of any sign that the patient is litigious. An obvious example would be a patient coming to your practice for advice or assistance after an unsuccessful result with another surgeon. This patient may even indicate that they have already sought the opinion of an attorney. Refusal to sign the consent form or an arbitration agreement is another obvious sign of higher risk. The authors have seen patients that have called their attorney while in the consultation room to discuss the consent form; any patient that has their attorney's phone number programmed into their cell phone is a concern. Conversely, the authors have successfully performed refractive procedure on many attorneys and even malpractice attorneys without adverse legal consequences.

There are those patients who are very motivated for surgery and are good physical candidates, but, for various reasons, you do not want to offer them surgery. A blunt refusal can be misconstrued as an attack on a patient's character or personality and will not generate good will toward you or your practice. In denying someone surgery, a tactful approach is required. For good candidates, one would usually focus on the positive aspects of surgery without unduly focusing attention on the rare, potentially negative outcomes. For patients that do not have realistic expectations or for some other reason are deemed poor candidates, it may be useful to have a detailed discussion regarding potential risks. Take advantage of any hesitation or indecision from the patient to reinforce that this is an elective procedure and is not necessary. Often patients get so caught up in the minutiae surrounding surgery that they forget that glasses and contacts are still good options.

Ocular Contraindication for Refractive Surgery

Refractive surgery is not recommended for patients with unstable refractions. If an eye has changed more than 0.5 D in the last 12 months, surgery should be postponed until it is stable. If there is an abnormal corneal condition, such as corneal scarring, it may affect the quality of the vision following refractive surgery. A history of injury or surgery to the cornea (radial keratotomy [RK], photorefractive keratectomy [PRK], laser in situ keratomileusis [LASIK], retinal surgery, or strabismus surgery) can make an individual a poor candidate for the procedure and could result in an unstable outcome.

Corneal diseases such as keratoconus and pellucid marginal degeneration are, for obvious reasons, contraindications to most elective corneal procedures. Thinning of the cornea can cause further attenuation of the cornea with the need for a corneal transplant. Much attention is given to Orbscans (Bausch & Lomb, Rochester, NY) and topography to diagnose forme fruste keratoconus and subclinical corneal changes that can result in ectasia years after surgery. A cautious approach is the best approach.

Patients with very poor vision due to amblyopia are not good candidates. If one eye does not have 20/40 or better corrected vision, it is not appropriate to risk elective surgery on the sole eye with good vision. If a rare complication of the procedure causes loss of uncorrected vision in the "good" eye, the amblyopic eye would not be sufficient to allow the patient to continue normal activities and particularly driving without a restricted license.

A common question is whether or not a partial correction should be attempted. A good example would be the very near-sighted patient who was told that he was not a good candidate for surgery because his prescription exceeds the parameters for the type of refractive procedure in question. Despite this the patient would still like to have "as much correction as I can get." No matter how eager a patient is for surgery, if the expectation is not to reach a full correction no surgery should be performed. Experience has shown that all patients end up wanting full correction of their vision even when they are convinced preoperatively that a partial correction will be sufficient. When they are told that they cannot have further correction, they are disappointed and unhappy. If the ultimate goal is to leave a person in glasses or contact lenses, albeit with a lesser correction, it is better to avoid surgery.

Medical Contraindications for Refractive Surgery

There are many precautions and contraindications for surgery that need to be assessed prior to successful surgery, but in general, the best patients are those with the fewest mitigating health problems. Patients with stable or medically controlled conditions and healthy eyes should get a letter of clearance from their internist prior to proceeding with elective surgery. This demonstrates a conscientious approach, confirms the patient is indeed stable, and provides supportive medical documentation in the event of future legal action. Patients with unstable or uncontrolled medical conditions should have surgery postponed until they are stable.

Patients will often seek out a second opinion if they are denied surgery. Patients should be informed that you have their best interests in mind and that you are very cautious in your approach to surgery. Patients have a hard time finding fault with taking the more conservative route when it comes to their eyesight. Once you have stated your hesitation to proceed, most patients will not insist that you continue, but you should still offer to re-evaluate the situation in a few weeks or months. Simply postponing their decision can emphasize that you are being cautious but not abandoning them.

Conclusion

Surgical procedures continue to evolve, providing better visual outcomes and less risk for both patients and doctors. Careful evaluation of both physical and psychological aspects of each patient will enable us to best choose who is a good candidate for surgery. Comprehensive education regarding realistic expectations and the possibility of complications is critical to a successful refractive practice. The old adage "an ounce of prevention is worth a pound of cure" describes the best approach to evaluating and counseling refractive patients. Happy postoperative refractive patients will build a successful practice.

CHAPTER 20

Transitioning From Cataract to Refractive IOL Surgery

Kevin Denny, MD

Despite my San Francisco location (and geographic proximity to certain famous athletes), I do not have a surgical practice "on steroids." Mine is a comprehensive ophthalmology practice with mostly internally generated surgical patients plus a good mix of complex cataract surgical referrals from other ophthalmologists, both subspecialist and comprehensive. Like some anterior segment surgeons, I have also maintained an interest in purely refractive surgery since starting practice. It has been fascinating to watch these 2 previously separate interests merge together.

The focus of this chapter will be on the general concepts and specific practice modifications that have enabled me to successfully participate in the challenging and evolving area of refractive IOL surgery. The message I want to leave with you is if I can do it, so can you.

Some Basic Requirements

During my residency training, I became enthralled by the elegance of cataract surgery and committed myself to developing expertise. As part of this process, I continuously evaluate my results and regularly make the little improvements that enable success. Having the right equipment is a big help. I have an IOL Master (Carl Zeiss Meditec, Jena, Germany) for biometry, a topographer for evaluating corneal shape, and current generation IOL calculation formulas for optimizing my surgical results. Just as important as the equipment is an attitude that every detail can make a difference. Preoperatively, I personally review the data for every surgical case, and I will bring the patient back for remeasurement if there are any doubts about the validity of the information.

I believe the limbal relaxing incision (LRI) procedure to correct astigmatism is the gateway procedure for refractive IOL surgery. Every cataract surgeon should learn this technique but it is mandatory for refractive IOL patients because even the smallest amount of residual astigmatism may reduce their satisfaction with the visual result.

I started doing LRIs more than 15 years ago and have always charged patients for this additional benefit. Along with my staff, I have had to learn to select the right patients, explain the benefit and risks, and justify the additional out-of-pocket charge. This is excellent preparation for the transition to refractive IOLs since it involves many of the same issues and skills.

My experience with LRIs has been overwhelmingly favorable. I estimate that 75% of my patients to whom the offer is made choose to have the procedure. Most patients are pleased to be offered this opportunity, do not mind spending the extra money, and—so far—have not expressed the slightest dissatisfaction with their results, which is an indication of the forgiving nature of the procedure, properly performed. Patients frequently mention that they thought the LRI cost would be much higher than it actually is given their perception of the benefits.

Building on Current Assets

It is fair to say that we all have acquired a tremendous amount of knowledge during our careers from everyday experience, focused study, and colleagues generous enough to teach us. We have also established a measure of credibility with our patients and within the medical community in which we practice. Our surgical skills have evolved and improved concurrent with better techniques and technology. These assets are the cornerstone for making the transition to refractive IOL surgery, but they are unfortunately not, by themselves, sufficient.

By far, the most important changes in the transition to refractive IOL surgery take place in the office, not the operating room. Of course, we must deliver optimal surgical results. But to be successful providing these services and—more importantly—for the patient to obtain the full benefit of refractive IOLs, we need to develop new systems. At the core of this new approach is a focus on the patient experience, also termed *patient-centered care*. I cannot speak about how high-volume practices try to accomplish this. My practice is more on the low-volume, high-touch end of the spectrum.

Facility and Staff

A clean, attractive office supported by personable and knowledgeable team members will, at the very least, persuade the patient to continue through the exam process with a positive mindset. It does not need to reach the level of cosmetic surgeons with interior design touches and enhanced assistants, but it should convey that you care about your patients' comfort and have stayed current. Posters and well-placed pamphlets demonstrating your interest in the latest developments in cataract surgery will confirm that your patients are in the right office.

I have been fortunate to have the services of a particularly professional and motivated surgical coordinator who has learned to assess patients' goals and expectations. She is able to introduce available options, provide materials, and answer logistical questions. We make good use of the Dell questionnaire, with minor modifications, to separate out those who are interested in being less dependent on glasses after cataract surgery from those who do not value this option. Whenever possible, we try to start this informational process even before the patient comes for his or her visit. What needs to become absolutely clear is that you, as the physician, do not want to be the first person to mention refractive IOLs while in the exam lane.

While it is invaluable to have a designated lead team member to assist patients through the decision process, it is important to elevate the knowledge of your entire staff as well. I try to set an educational theme each month and allocate office time for the purpose of instruction. These sessions allow me to probe the knowledge level of my team and formulate our answers to commonly asked questions. Audiovisuals are readily available from multiple sources, but it is helpful for you to be there to explain the nuances not necessarily included in the marketing materials provided by the various companies.

Getting to Know the Refractive Intraocular Lens Patient

A major obstacle still to be overcome is that most patients are not yet familiar with the concept of the premium refractive IOL. Perhaps this is due to still relatively low penetration and a minimum of external marketing in my geographic area. The consequence is that we must assume the responsibility of educating our patients.

While the surgical coordinator can assess a patient's interest level, only the ophthalmologist can determine whether the patient is suitable and which IOL is most likely to meet the patient's needs. The inescapable fact is that this takes time, well beyond the norm. Do not think your usual scheduling patterns will suffice. I carve out 2 half days primarily for refractive IOL and refractive surgery pre- and postoperative visits during which patients are scheduled at half the usual pace.

My experience suggests that the refractive IOL patient tends to be younger, either chronologically or in outlook about life. They lead active lives, travel extensively, and consider glasses a limitation. Their personalities are positive and trusting but not naïve. They believe that newer technology can offer better options and results. Finally, this patient group is successful and can purchase what seems best for them. Cost alone does not break the deal for them.

These characterizations are simply generalizations, and it is a mistake on several levels to decide not to offer these premium products to patients who seem to have more modest means. Appearances can be deceiving, and you do not want to have one of your patients ask you later why you did not offer him or her the latest technology. Patients understand that this lens is going to be with them for the rest of their lives and many will invest in something that is of value to them.

My mindset is that I am presenting my patients with an opportunity to expand their range of focus beyond what is possible with a standard IOL alone. I clearly state that our goal with refractive IOLs is to reduce their dependence on glasses. I do not "sell." I offer "good options," including monofocal IOLs. Be careful to avoid having a manufacturer's brochure make promises that you may not be able to deliver. Each patient needs to be told what he or she can reasonably expect to achieve given his or her particular circumstance.

It is useful to get off to a good start with your early cases. A hyperope with bilateral cataracts, low astigmatism, and many of the above personality characteristics would be ideal. While it is likely that this patient might be quite happy with monofocal IOLs, refractive IOLs can provide an even better result.

It is equally important to know who is generally not an ideal refractive IOL patient. I would urge a cautious approach toward the patient with unilateral cataract with borderline symptoms. Myopes with a history of functional reading vision may not sufficiently appreciate their improved distance vision if their reading is not equal to their presurgery state. Avoid the patient with a "glass half empty" outlook. You may hear him or her obsess on every limitation while ignoring the excellent distance vision and functional near vision.

Do not be afraid to tell a patient that he or she does not seem to be a good refractive IOL candidate. Most patients will appreciate your candor. I even had one 40-year-old, PDA-toting patient become more insistent that she should have a refractive IOL after I told her that her unilateral cataract, lack of experience with presbyopia, and her own self-assessment of her personality as "beyond perfectionist" suggested that she would not be accepting of the compromises of a refractive IOL. After putting her off for 6 months, and against my better judgment, I finally implanted a multifocal and prepared for the worst. At day 1, she was 20/20 uncorrected distance and near and has not uttered a peep about haloes, glare, or computer problems. I think the lesson here was not just the luck of the Irish but that she wanted the refractive IOL more than I wanted to give it to her and she was determined not to prove my original assessment correct.

Selecting the IOL and Setting Patient Expectations

While it seems tempting to use the same refractive IOL for all situations, I think doing so is lazy intellectually and fails to acknowledge that these lenses have differences and people have different needs. Long-armed computer users will do better with one refractive IOL than short-armed readers with small pupils. Our obligation is to the patient and not to any particular product manufacturer.

Based on my experience, it is usually a mistake to mention all the available lens designs with their particular qualities and expect the patient to make a decision. This most often leads to endless repetitive loops of discussion without resolution, mostly because the patient is striving for the "perfect" choice rather than the "better" choice.

With the patient's modified Dell survey in hand, I try to understand what he or she does and the relative importance of these activities. Clearly, this is not always a linear process but often the "better" choice emerges and at that point I make my recommendation.

Coming to the recommendation does not mean you can leave the exam room yet. At this point, I start setting the expectations. Since the IOL to be implanted is not perfect—like a youthful natural lens—I tell the patient that it will take a period of adjustment, often several months, for him or her to learn how best to use it. I try to impart the concept that the patient needs to play an active role in achieving optimal function. I make clear that we are going to support him or her through this adaptation period and that he or she should not expect to perceive the full benefit of the lens until his or her second eye is done and the brain has had at least a month to integrate the 2 eyes in this new way of seeing. It is difficult to know exactly what patients retain of this counseling, so it is imperative that these cautions are reflected in the written material handed to them as well.

This is the first part of the valuable adage "under promise, over deliver." I think this moment is quite similar to our discussions with the cataract patient who has coexisting diabetic retinopathy or macular degeneration. We acknowledge the challenges but communicate how we are going to do the very best we can and work together while reserving final judgment for at least 3 months after surgery.

Final Details/Dry Run

There are a myriad of details that need to be nailed down before your first refractive IOL patient. A printed sheet should be prepared for the patient indicating costs, preoperative testing, correction of astigmatism, postoperative care period, and additional costs, if any, for enhancements. Your consent form needs to be modified to include this new option. You will need to negotiate with your surgical facility as to how much will be charged for providing the refractive IOL. Your billing department and that of your ASC need to become familiar with these new products and services.

Postoperative Care

I see my refractive IOL postoperative patients at 1 day, 1 week, 4 weeks, and any time in between if it seems they need some additional hand-holding (and believe me, some of them will need it). I try to be supportive; look for dry eye, drug toxicity, and astigmatism; and remind them that it takes time to adjust and that visual performance improves considerably when both eyes get fixed. With multifocal IOLs, patients generally have good distance vision early but often the near vision will "kick in" after several weeks when the patient figures out how to alternate between images. I often will do the second eye a month after the first eye. If the patient has misgivings, I prefer to wait until he or she is comfortable moving forward.

Near or intermediate vision tends to be the challenge that takes up the most time. By far, the single-most useful demonstration that addresses these concerns is to have the patient look at a reading card and then hold a −3 lens in front of the refractive IOL eye while I tell him or her that this is how he or she would have seen without the refractive IOL. This often helps the patient to recognize the benefit, better accept the imperfect, and move on to their other eye.

Conclusion

Adding refractive IOL surgery to your practice is within the capability of most conscientious cataract surgeons. It does require making adjustments to your previous office standard operating procedure. Sharing with the staff your motivation and enthusiasm for this exciting new service can help turn your plans into reality.

CHAPTER 21

Transitioning From Cataract to Refractive IOL Surgery

Sandra Yeh, MD

My personal journey into the realm of presbyopic lenses came in the summer of 2005 when, thanks to the tremendous efforts of Eyeonics, Inc's president, J. Andy Corley, Centers for Medicare & Medicaid Services (CMS) made a historic decision that allowed Medicare patients to choose presbyopic lenses. I do not perform clear lens extraction and have only used presbyopic lenses on my cataract patients.

I have always been a devoted user of Alcon products, so I greatly anticipated the arrival of the ReSTOR lens (Alcon, Fort Worth, TX). I was in fact the first surgeon in my town to take the certification course and was the first to implant one. Based on my understanding of the course, I thought I chose an excellent patient: a 55-year-old-female with bilateral cataracts who was a −5.50 myope with very little corneal astigmatism and who did virtually no night driving. I placed a ReSTOR without complications, but postoperatively I was quite stunned to find an extremely unhappy 20/30 uncorrected patient. Although she recalled that I had warned her about halos at night, she felt that everything had a haze or ghost image around it. I tried to refract her and could not get any improvement beyond 20/30. I even did optical coherence tomography (OCT) but found no cystoid macular edema (CME). I was very uncomfortable with the prospect of placing a second ReSTOR in this patient who was already so unhappy with her first, so we later made a joint decision to explant the ReSTOR implant and replace it with a monofocal lens. In hindsight, this was partly due to my inexperience, my own feeling of helplessness, and my inability to resolve her complaints. My patient lost confidence in me and I lost confidence in multifocal lenses.

A few months later, I encountered a cataract patient also in her fifties who asked for the Crystalens by name. She told me that her brother had cataract surgery the year before in California, had Crystalenses placed, and that he just "loves them." When I informed her that I had never implanted a Crystalens, she very kindly told me that she would wait until I took the certification course. Two months later, I took the Crystalens certification course and placed a Crystalens in her and 2 other patients 5 days later. The next postoperative day I had 3 happy patients with uncorrected visions between 20/20 and 20/30 and J2 to J4, even with their eyes dilated with Cyclogyl (Alcon). (I cannot explain how this is possible, but it is). I knew that day that I had found my presbyopic lens of choice. Since then, I have implanted more than 400 Crystalenses and I have not had to explant a single one.

The advantages of the Crystalens are numerous. The most important one to me is the crisp quality of vision that patients mention. I very rarely hear complaints of glare and halo; no more than with a monofocal lens. The predictability of the new 5-0 Crystalens when using the IOL Master is excellent, and I am able to obtain postoperative results within 0.25 D from the target. Another advantage is that the Crystalens works quite well in just one eye when the patient has a monofocal lens or an insignificant cataract in his or her fellow eye. In fact, some of my happiest patients are those with a monofocal lens in their dominant eye and who are already emmetropic. They already understand the limitations of near vision with monofocal lenses and easily grasp the advantage of seeing better at near again. I generally target −0.50 to .−0.75 in the other eye and they are delighted with their new found range. Also, we have patients who truly want near vision but cannot afford 2 Crystalenses IOLs. I can offer a Crystalens in just one eye and still give them useful near vision.

The only disadvantage I have found with the Crystalens is that it only accommodates about +1.50 D (more in patients age 40 to 55). However, mini-monovision works very well and unlike traditional monofocal monovision, patients who are −0.50 with a Crystalens generally will typically have 20/30 distance vision, 20/20 intermediate vision, and J2 at near. I have never been able to achieve such results with a monofocal monovision lens. In fact, I do not recommend monofocal monovision unless the patient has already tried it in contact lenses and is certain that he or she can adapt. I hate having to explant a monofocal lens to reverse monovision in patients who later discover they cannot tolerate the anisometropia.

Implanting the Crystalens has been greatly improved with the new 5-0 injector. Great care should be taken with preoperative measurements. I recommend doing both manual and IOL Master K-s. I recommend having your best technician do all of the presbyopic IOL measurements because consistency is key. Corneal astigmatism needs to be looked at carefully, and anything over 0.50 D needs to be addressed. For some unknown reason, patients with 1 D of astigmatism see quite well with a monofocal IOL but not as well with a Crystalens. We also do a Pentacam (OCULUS, Inc, Lynwood, WA) evaluation and corneal topography on all presbyopia-correcting IOL patients to confirm the axis of astigmatism. We also want to be certain that there are no other conditions, such as an early undetected keratoconus, that may affect the quality of their vision. It is essential to be proficient with limbal relaxing incisions (LRI) or astigmatic keratotomy which I perform at the 7-mm optical zone.It is very helpful to be able to perform laser in situ keratomileusis (LASIK) enhancements or to refer such patients to colleagues who perform it at a discount. I generally do astigmatic keratometry (AK) for 0.50 to 2.50 of astigmatism. Above that I recommend LASIK correction and I cut the flap first, perform the cataract surgery, and then lift the flap 30 days postoperatively to correct the residual astigmatism.

A water tight wound is an absolute requisite for the Crystalens. I do a scleral wound under topical anesthesia with a technique I learned from Dr. Lisa Arbisser. I put topical lidocaine jelly in the eye at the beginning of the surgery, inject a small bleb of preservative-free lidocaine, and enter the superior conjunctiva. I have the patient look slightly downward and do the traditional scleral tunnel. I replace the conjunctiva at the end of the case and cauterize the ends of the conjunctiva together. This is a very forgiving wound, which virtually never leaks, and is not associated with any increase in endophthalmitis. It is important to have a well-centered, symmetrical 6-mm capsulorrhexis, and I usually use a 6-mm photorefractive keratectomy (PRK) marker lightly touched onto the cornea to guide me. I would avoid the Crystalens in patients with severe glaucoma who may need a trabeculectomy in the near future and in patients with any history of iritis, even years ago. Patients with strabismus or prism in their glasses, patients with significant diabetic retinopathy or extensive retina history, patients who have been on Flomax (Boehringer-Ingelheim, Ingelheim, Germany) (they may be poor dilators and have a poor accommodative amplitude), and patients with significant unstable zonules are also poor candidates for this IOL. However, I have implanted a Crystalens after a Mentor capsular tension ring and it has worked well. Finally, one should avoid the mentally unstable, highly critical, and unrealistic patient.

While good surgical technique is important, making presbyopia-correcting IOLs a successful part of your practice requires a team effort. My technicians attended the training course from Eyeonics so that they would have a strong understanding of the mechanism of the lens. Each delighted patient (and we have many) added to their confidence and enthusiasm. We also use visual aids. Patients who qualify are shown an educational DVD provided by Eyeonics in a portable DVD player and the technicians introduce it. By the time I enter the room, the patient generally knows what the Crystalens is and how it works. After explaining cataract surgery, I am usually very direct with my approach to the IOL options. I tell the patient that there are 3 different distances in life: far, intermediate, and near. I explain that the traditional lens gets them only one out of 3; usually the patient opts for distance and will require glasses for intermediate and near. I tell them that the Crystalens would give them the best 2 out of 3 (actually it does more than that) and that with their dominant eye, I target far and intermediate and with the nondominant eye I target intermediate and near.

I explain that in this way, they will be able to see all 3 different distances with 2 eyes. The patients seem to understand this very well. I ask them point blank whether they "love" their glasses or whether they would like to read again without their glasses on. In those who really want this freedom, you will see an instant spark of interest. Once they have decided on this lens, it is important to limit their expectations by saying that at this time, there is no lens that can guarantee that they will NEVER wear glasses under any circumstances. They may require some glasses for night driving and they may have to use eyeglasses for the very small near vision items, such as threading a needle or reading the stock quotes in the paper. Reasonable patients are always accepting of this; unreasonable patients who do not accept this should be noted and probably avoided.

I remember when refractive surgery first began and I was trying to decide whether to get into this new and exciting area. I took numerous RK courses in which instructors talked about equipment, financing, and technique, and I found this to be terribly monotonous. One day, I had the great fortune of taking a course by Dr. Spencer Thornton, who is also an amateur magician. Unlike everyone else, he spoke about the "magic" of refractive surgery. He talked about the joy, the excitement, the sheer exhilaration of restoring sight to those who have never been able to see the world clearly with their own eyes. This is why I became a refractive surgeon... this is why we all became surgeons.

Ophthalmology is on the verge of an exciting new era; the technology is changing, the world is changing, and we must change with it. We now have the power not only to improve our patients' sight but to change their lives. I truly believe this new technology will continue to improve and should be made available to all patients requiring cataract surgery. Our patients should be able to choose how they see and how they live.

CHAPTER 22

TRANSITIONING FROM CATARACT TO REFRACTIVE IOL SURGERY

Timothy B. Cavanaugh, MD

My journey as an intraocular lens (IOL) surgeon began in 1987 when I started my ophthalmology residency and learned extracapsular cataract surgery. Although we successfully treated the disease and improved patients' best-corrected vision, it always bothered me that we were still leaving patients with dysfunctional vision without glasses. Too often, patients had several diopters of induced astigmatism from large incisions and sutures as well as residual myopia or hyperopia due to inaccurate IOL calculations. To add insult to injury, our cataract patients were completely reliant upon reading glasses.

When I completed my corneal fellowship and entered practice, I was surrounded by forward-thinking partners and our group became involved in multiple research projects involving small-incision phacoemulsification techniques and innovative IOLs. At the same time, I began performing refractive surgery and participated in clinical trials for many laser companies including Summit, Autonomous, and Bausch & Lomb. I realized very early on that cataract surgery had the potential to be the ultimate refractive surgery if things were handled correctly. The advent of small-incision, foldable IOLs as well as improved A-scan techniques and IOL formulas provided the tools to bring cataract surgery closer to refractive surgery. With this in mind, I made a commitment in my practice to change the way we looked at cataract surgery and issued a challenge to my staff to provide refractive cataract surgery (RCS) for every patient.

✳ Redefining success
  ❖ Past → successful cataract removal and use glasses to correct refractive error
  ❖ Now → successful cataract removal and better functional uncorrected vision at all distances—far and near
✳ View cataract surgery not as treatment of a disease but as an opportunity to enhance one's quality of life by providing enhanced vision without glasses.

With this new attitude, we began providing patients with excellent distance vision without glasses. We abandoned contact A-Scan biometry for immersion to increase accuracy and began using the IOL Master (Carl Zeiss, Jena, Germany) as soon as it was available. Advanced IOL calculation formulas such as the Holladay II further added to our precision. At that time, astigmatic keratotomy was the procedure of choice for astigmatism control but was later replaced by limbal relaxing incisions. In my opinion, mastering surgical astigmatism correction is a prerequisite for truly achieving emmetropia and the kind of outcomes needed for your procedure to qualify as true refractive cataract surgery.

Although I was very happy with the care we were delivering compared to other surgeons in our community, there was still something missing. I realized that I had only addressed one half of my patient's refractive surgery needs in providing good distance acuity but had completely ignored his near vision needs. I honestly believe I had underestimated the impact of near vision deficit as I was only in my 30s at that time and was many years away from experiencing presbyopia myself. We began to offer monovision correction to patients but this was received with varying degrees of enthusiasm. It bothered me that we were still compromising on near vision and I began to search for other options and alternatives.

In the mid 1990s, technology was introduced that seemed able to solve this last piece of my RCS puzzle. Allergan Surgical (Irvine, CA) introduced the Array Multifocal IOL and my group quickly became involved in the Array clinical trials. I was involved as an assistant investigator. Like other surgeons with similar interests, we monitored the study results with skeptical enthusiasm and reviewed the data. The small group of clinical investigators were excellent surgeons with a commitment to making the technology work. As a result, the data submitted to the Food and Drug Administration (FDA) were acceptably good and with great excitement, we all waited in anticipation of FDA approval, which came in late 1997. Surgeons began training by using the identical Allergan SI40 platform (Irvine, CA), in order to personalize their surgeon factors for the Array. The next step was to review the lens parameters as well as the marketing information and materials with the Allergan sales representatives. With the marketing hype generated by Allergan and the mounting excitement on the part of both surgeons and patients, we enthusiastically began implanting the Array in numerous patients. The other factor adding to the Array's initial strong acceptance by patients was that this advanced technology was offered to patients without a premium price up-charge.

Some of the highest volume cataract surgeons began implanting the Array with very little change in their practice habits compared to traditional monofocal IOLs. Having started with the clinical trials, we enjoyed a head start in our market and implanted the lens aggressively as well. For the first few months we enjoyed initial success and had many happy patients. As time went on, however, we began to have some negative experiences similar to what other surgeons nationwide began to report. The optical shortcomings of the Array IOL left many patients and surgeons disappointed. It seemed that our "White Knight" that had been sent to rescue our patient's near vision had a chink in the armor. Patients complained of poor near vision, nighttime glare and halos, and even some poor-quality distance acuity. As a consequence, I performed explantation and IOL exchange in 2 Array patients. I then reviewed similar negative experiences with other surgeons and reluctantly abandoned using the Array altogether.

Although I mourned the loss of my "White Knight," I began to examine what went wrong. I not only looked critically at Allergan and the implant itself but also at myself and our processes. The main causes of failure really boiled down to several key factors:

 * Inadequate understanding of the IOL's characteristics
 * Improper patient selection
 * Poor management of patient expectations
 * Failure to consistently achieve emmetropia and to fully correct astigmatism
 * Failure to allow enough time for adjustment and neuro-adaptation

In addition to the medical failures, I became disenchanted by the marketing hype associated with the debut of the Array lens. At the time of introduction, Allergan decided to undertake a fairly aggressive marketing program aimed directly at patients. As a consequence, patients came in asking for this lens and many surgeons implanted the Array in patients who were not the best candidates. With television and print advertising driving patient demand, surgeons were sometimes pressured into using the Array rather than risk seeming "behind the times." In retrospect, this type of patient-directed marketing campaign served to undermine the success of the product as it bypassed the doctor. A careful product roll out would have been much more effective in the long run.

After I stopped using the Array, I continued doing RCS to the best of my ability but there was still that void for near vision that weighed heavily on my mind. I did not feel as though I had given multifocal IOLs my best effort. Perhaps it was the dawn of a new millennium, but in the year 2000 I decided to revisit the Array. There were several reasons but the most notable were

 * I hate to fail!

 * True refractive cataract surgery demands multifocality in some patients
 * We needed better alternatives for presbyopic hyperopic refractive surgery patients
 * Multifocality takes over where monovision falls short

In my refractive practice, I was still not satisfied with the menu of choices I was able to offer my hyperopic patients and especially my hyperopic presbyopes. Although hyperopic laser in situ keratomileusis (LASIK) worked in some, it was not accurate and predictable for higher levels of hyperopia and I noted visual quality issues at those more aggressive levels of treatment. With LASIK, the hyperopic presbyope was still faced with monovision as the only choice for near vision. As luck and fate would have it, there was a groundswell of several like-minded surgeons nationwide who also felt there was a place for the Array lens in hyperopic refractive surgery patients. Drs. Kevin Waltz and Bruce Wallace organized this group of surgeons and coined the term *PRELEX* or presbyopic lens exchange to describe the use of the Array Multifocal IOL for refractive surgery purposes. Many surgeons became interested in this "off-label" use of the lens and the Array was reborn! My journey back to multifocal technology had begun. Over the next couple of years, I participated in stand-alone PRELEX courses as well as those held in conjunction with national meetings. To reintroduce the Array to my practice, I began with extensive study so that I truly understood the nuances of multifocality. I further reviewed things with colleagues as well as the Allergan-Advanced Medical Optics representatives and scientists so that both I and my staff were prepared. Allergan-Advanced Medical Optics learned their lesson from the initial Array roll out and launched their efforts in PRELEX with a refocus on success through proper patient selection and education, rather than through marketing.

Out of this rebirth came some very important principles that guided the success of PRELEX and the Array. Very simply put, to ensure success with PRELEX, I initially did surgery only on hyperopic presbyopes and higher hyperopes if prepresbyopic. I specifically avoided surgery on emmetropic presbyopes, myopic presbyopes, and nonpresbyopes. Furthermore I followed a set of guidelines for patient selection that were precursors to those principles we now recognize as being essential for success with the newer multifocal IOLs such as ReZoom (Advanced Medical Optics, Santa Ana, CA) and ReSTOR (Alcon Laboratories, Fort Worth, TX). These important guiding principles that were developed under the auspices of the PRELEX educational system and have been adopted for use with other types of presbyopia-correcting IOLs are the following:

 * Hyperopia and presbyopia make for the best refractive indications
 * Patients should have a strong desire for independence from glasses most of the time
 * Patients should have a willingness to undergo bilateral implantation and to work with surgeon for up to 3 months until final outcome is determined
 * Patients must have reasonable expectations for functional vision, and must understand that halos are the tradeoff for achieving a full range of functional vision

* Patients should have a compatible attitude, occupation, and lifestyle

As one of the early adopters of multifocal IOLs, Dr. Howard Fine refined and popularized the use of 3 simple questions that were also developed by Kevin Waltz and Bruce Wallace to screen for Array candidates and to eliminate those who should not have the technology. The 3 questions he asked were

1. If you could have an implant that would significantly reduce your need for near spectacles, would you be interested?

2. If such an implant caused you to see "glow" around lights, would you still be interested?

3. Will you agree to allow 3 months for adaptation, and to have both eyes done, prior to addressing any visual symptoms?

Armed with these new revelations and tools, I enjoyed good success with the Array for refractive lens exchange and even began to use it again in cataract patients with good success.

We then fast forward to 2005 and the FDA approval of 2 excellent new multifocal IOLs. The ReZoom lens was a redesign of the Array that addressed many of its shortcomings. The ReSTOR lens represented new technology with its apodized diffractive multifocal optic. For many younger surgeons and for those who never embraced the Array, the process of incorporating multifocal IOLs into an already busy practice can sometimes be a daunting one. For me, the transition to the new multifocal IOLs was seamless. I applaud both Alcon and Advanced Medical Optics for their approach to the clinical introduction of ReSTOR and ReZoom. I was pleasantly surprised that Alcon did not make the same mistake that Allergan-Advanced Medical Optics did in beginning direct consumer marketing right away. Although the potential sales volume brought in by such marketing would have directly benefited the company's bottom line, Alcon felt it was important to roll out the product slowly in order to ensure success. The process started with physician and staff education followed by excellent support materials as well as interaction with knowledgeable sales and technical people. I now enjoy a thriving cataract and refractive surgery practice that comfortably and confidently embraces multifocal technology. I can now say that we truly have an office that focuses on genuine refractive cataract and lens surgery. Adding these new generation multifocal IOLs has filled in the missing pieces in my practice. From our experience over the years, we now know that success with multifocal IOLs depends on

* Knowledge of IOL design parameters and performance
* Proper patient selection
* Patient education and management of expectations
* High-quality small-incision surgery
* Astigmatically neutral incisions with adjunctive treatment of astigmatism using limbal relaxing incisions
* Consistently achieving emmetropia with excellent biometry
* Surgeon and staff commitment

The bottom line in this formula for success is that you simply have to pick the right patient and use the implant the right way. With this approach I have enjoyed steady growth in my refractive IOL practice and feel that the multifocal IOL has become an essential tool in refractive lens implant surgery.

CHAPTER 23

TRANSITIONING FROM KERATOREFRACTIVE TO REFRACTIVE IOL SURGERY

Jay Bansal, MD

As a laser in situ keratomileusis (LASIK) refractive surgeon for the past 11 years and having performed only laser vision correction, I have been very pleased professionally with my specialty choice. However, over the past several years, I have seen my surgical volume not only plateau, but actually decline. I believe the following factors have led to this downswing:

* An increase in corporate and private LASIK centers with discount fee structures.
* An overall plateau in patient interest in laser vision correction (LVC).
* A growing baby boomer population with early lenticular changes better suited for intraocular lens (IOL) technology rather than LVC.
* More patients demanding better distance and near vision.
* More borderline patients from both a legal and medical standpoint.

Cogitating over the aforementioned conditions, I realized that I must act proactively to push my practice and patient care to the next level. I had reached a crossroad in my career—I could continue my position as a corneal-based surgeon or step outside of my comfort zone and build my practice as a cataract surgeon to the same level of success I had attained over a decade in the LASIK industry. Both options would present significant long-lasting effects on the growth of my practice and sense of professional fulfillment as a surgeon. Motivated to better serve my patients and reach out to even more potential candidates, it was clear that I needed to expand my range of treatment options and include new premium multifocal IOLs and phakic IOLs in an effort to better address the expanding visual needs of a growing presbyopic population.

Making the actual transition to include cataract surgery in my practice has been daunting and challenging at times. Most of my patients specifically come to me for my refractive experience and they expect nothing less than top technology paired with quality care. However, my decision to perform lens-based surgeries pushed me back to where I was more than a decade ago when I started training as a LASIK refractive surgeon. I was inundated with and reminded of a series of emotional experiences I had undergone over the first years of my training. I was motivated by the prospect of becoming a better-rounded surgeon yet constantly challenged by the fear of failure that loomed over me. Over the years, I have been a mentor for numerous fledgling LASIK surgeons but now the roles were about to be reversed. With any surgeon in training, the rite of passage is to make your share of mistakes before you develop your surgical style and finesse. Looking back, it seemed rather unrealistic at the time, but I tried to push myself to become as confident with cataract surgery as I was with LASIK procedures in a short period of time.

I began the educational process by watching countless surgical videos, taking numerous wet lab courses at ophthalmology meetings, observing many leading cataract surgeons and their techniques, and talking with representatives from major IOL manufacturers. I surrounded myself with every type of learning opportunity and resource available to try and soak in all the information. I quickly learned that phacoemulsification surgery has progressed greatly in both surgical equipment and technique over the past decade since I had last performed one. For example, mastery over the fluidics of phaco equipment is not only crucial but also necessary to achieve excellent surgical outcomes. In addition, increasing popularity of the phaco-chop technique due to reduced surgical time has largely replaced the standard divide-and-conquer approach, which I had learned back in residency. Again, I was faced with the challenge of pushing myself out of my comfort zone as soon as I realized that I needed to expand my repertoire of surgical techniques in order to improve and excel as a cataract surgeon. With each procedure, I became more comfortable, which has allowed me to significantly reduce my total ultrasound time and consequently, maximize early postoperative visual outcome. Although it was a small step up on the learning curve, it was leaps and bounds for my burgeoning confidence as a cataract surgeon.

However, not everything has been a smooth ride, and I have definitely struggled through my share of setbacks. So far, I have already experienced dropping the nucleus, breaking the capsule due to nonoptimal settings on the phaco machine, emulsifying part of an iris due to intraoperative floppy iris syndrome (IFIS), and experiencing a near ocular perforation with a patient who tried to get up in the middle of his procedure. Needless to say, it was like residency all over again in which anxiety ran high the night before surgery and periodic panic attacks became a ritual I quickly grew accustomed to.

I still remember my first cataract surgery, which I had carefully selected. The patient was an amblyopic esotrope who spoke little to no English. The biggest challenge I faced was to demonstrate the same degree of confidence to a cataract patient as I would with my LASIK patients, knowing very well that this was my first cataract surgery on my own since 1995. To make matters worse, there were no attending surgeons in the room to fall back on in case of a major catastrophe. I hardly slept the night before and constantly reminded myself not to rush through the methodical steps that I had played repeatedly countless times in my head. As a dyed-in-the-wool overachiever, I had set a goal for my surgery time; therefore, I had to constantly remind myself not to get too fixated on speed. The surgery itself went well, with significant corneal edema the next day, which was something I could live with given the array of other serious complications that could have occurred.

Feeling more energized and confident after my first procedure in a long time, I allowed myself to slip a little and forgot to appreciate or remember the importance of phaco settings. In one particular case, I proceeded to remove the final quadrant of lens nucleus under high vacuum setting and found vitreous instead. Again, this was another humbling learning experience that taught me to never overlook something as basic as phaco settings and the importance of pacing myself through each sequential step without self-imposed time pressure.

Having learned from yet another mistake and moved forward, I found myself in another startling situation. We have all seen multiple slides of what IFIS looks like but when the situation presents itself under your microscope, it takes on a completely different meaning. During the procedure, I realized that I was unable to maintain a well-dilated iris as the procedure progressed and suddenly, a portion of the iris was vacuumed into my phaco port. I remember feeling desolate and wondered why I was putting myself through this self-inflicted stress when I could be teeing off at the course with my friends. Fortunately, I was able to finish the case successfully and afterwards, I did a complete assessment of what I could have done differently to prevent similar cases besides a thorough review of the patient's medical history. After that day, I immersed myself with what various leading cataract surgeons recommend in terms of preventative and restorative measures when dealing with IFIS. I developed a comprehensive plan to ensure that I would be much better prepared to deal with those challenges ahead.

As I have progressed and become more comfortable as a cataract surgeon, real world surprises have continued to challenge my skills and perseverance in every conceivable capacity. Most recently a patient tried to get up from the operating table in the middle of the procedure. Before I had a chance to even process and mull over the situation, I instinctively removed the phaco needle faster than I could blink my eye. My first thought was that I might have gone through the capsule and possibly much deeper. Again, I wondered why I had chosen to inflict all this stress upon myself and for the next protracted minute, I could not hear anything in the room except my accelerated heartbeat. I remember considering canceling my surgeries for the rest of the day, and possibly for good. It was not until the patient became repositioned under the microscope again that I was able to rationalize that everything was going to be all right. Miraculously, all the ocular structures remained intact, and I was able to finish the case without any complications. The patient simply said, "Doc, I'm sorry I moved. Did I mess anything up?" Like in most difficult situations, by telling patients the truth about what occurred during surgery and finding the proper course of action to take, I have managed to steer clear from any major issues so far.

After facing a series of challenges and setbacks, I realized that keeping myself abreast of the latest advanced surgical technique and technology, performing umpteen wet lab courses, or attending all the relevant conferences probably would not have prevented these incidents. It did not take very long after I embarked on my transition from a LASIK to cataract surgeon to accept that not every case will turn out textbook perfect and not every patient will be brimming with joy and gratitude. Inevitably, these challenging cases will initially chip away the very foundation of confidence you have arduously built up over the years, but these are the same lessons that will shape you to become a more skilled and composed surgeon.

Despite hitting a few bumps along the road, there are some benefits to having an established LASIK practice. For example, we had already built a substantial database of prospective patients who were interested in alternative presbyopic treatment options besides monovision with LASIK or conductive keratoplasty (CK). Extensive patient education and counseling on the benefits of premium technology lenses has made the transition from standard to multifocal IOLs easier than expected. Because my practice was already a fee-for-service elective surgical center, we did not require significant staff training to incorporate this new service. Regardless of the direction IOL technology seems to follow, patients are demanding more from their surgeons to reduce dependence on glasses and/or contacts. Being a refractive surgeon with his own excimer laser has been another great advantage because I have the capability of performing minor postcataract surgery touch ups in-house when necessary.

My experience of diving back into cataract surgery has been both a challenge and a blessing. The surgical skills that I have honed and learned from cataract surgery have and will continue to help me with every type of eye surgery that I perform. In addition, I feel more confident now as a better-rounded surgeon because I am able to provide a wider range of quality customized treatment options to the majority of prospective patients. Gone are the days when I felt frustrated because I was not capable of treating a high myope or hyperope whose prescription was beyond the ideal parameters of laser vision correction. Furthermore, I can now offer multiple treatment options to presbyopic LASIK candidates with/without significant cataracts. I can make my recommendations with even greater confidence and certainty because I can offer them what is truly best for them, and isn't that what it is really about at the end of the day?

CHAPTER 24

TRANSITIONING FROM KERATOREFRACTIVE TO REFRACTIVE IOL SURGERY

Marguerite B. McDonald, MD, FACS

The introduction and growing popularity of multifocal and accommodating intraocular lenses (IOLs) presents unique challenges for anterior segment surgeons. Although we all learned a broad array of surgical skills in medical school and residency, many of us have specialized during our careers in cataract surgery or keratorefractive surgery.

For many years, my practice consisted primarily of keratorefractive surgery, with a smaller percentage of "classic" corneal procedures such as penetrating keratoplasties (PKPs) and Gunderson flaps. With LASIK, LASEK, epi-LASIK, IntraLASIK, PRK, CK, AK, and LRIs, there was plenty to learn and plenty of work for me as a refractive surgeon. In addition, in the 1980s, my department chairman at the university had asked the faculty members to stop performing cataract surgery, as it was the "bread and butter" operation of our referring doctors. Therefore, I "exited" from cataract surgery just before phacoemulsification became the standard of care.

It makes sense for a refractive surgeon to implant the new refractive IOLs. We are accustomed to high expectations for a perfect refractive outcome. Our staff is used to dealing with the more demanding "retail" patient who is paying out of pocket for elective services. We already offer special perks in the waiting room and have staff with sales training. We can easily handle the corneal refractive enhancements that may be required.

But—and it is a big but—the central skills of lens emulsification and IOL implantation are ones that we laser surgeons have not learned, or practiced, for years. Returning to the risks of intraocular surgery (eg, dropped nuclei, retinal detachments, endophthalmitis, TASS, etc) is extremely daunting. The experienced keratorefractive surgeon is well aware of the consequences of a complication in a demanding baby boomer patient.

People have resolved this dilemma differently. There are prominent examples in our field of surgeons who successfully do both lenticular and keratorefractive surgery and those who have taken a team approach, specializing in one type of surgery while their partner performs the other.

Personally, I decided several years ago that the time had come to return to cataract surgery. I wanted to be active with the latest refractive technology, whether the site of surgery was the cornea or the anterior chamber, and I wanted to be able to offer my patients a comprehensive range of refractive solutions.

Learning the Ropes

A sabbatical to learn phaco was unrealistic given my practice and academic commitments. Instead, I began by studying American Society of Cataract and Refractive Surgery (ASCRS) surgical videos from the experts. I spent hours watching Howard Fine, Skip Nichamin, Sam Masket, Steve Brint, Roger Steinert, Dick Lindstrom, Doug Koch, Paul Koch, David Chang, Bobby Osher, and others perform surgery from the comfort of my own office or living room.

It is helpful to ask colleagues for advice or visit them and observe surgery live. I would suggest that keratorefractive specialists open their minds to learning as much as possible from nonsurgeons, as well.

For instance, I spent time with the phaco manufacturers' representatives, practicing techniques in the office after hours. These individuals have a wealth of knowledge and can help you learn from other surgeons' successes and mistakes.

Operating room or ambulatory surgery center (ASC) technicians can also be extremely helpful. I would encourage those returning to cataract surgery to do as I did and throw yourself at the mercy of the technicians. Encourage them to speak up during surgery; a hand signal or subtle warning can prevent you from making costly errors.

First Cases

Do everything you can to "stack the deck" in your favor. For your first few cases, choose cataract patients with a legitimate reason for general anesthesia, such as those with a

Table 1

TRANSITIONING BACK TO PHACO

- Educate yourself
- Watch experts' phaco videos
- Practice with device representatives
- Rely on operating room technicians for assistance
- Watch yourself on video and eliminate unnecessary movements
- Choose initial cases wisely
- For your very first cases, pick those that require general anesthesia; then suggest headphones/cotton in ears when the patients are awake
- Pick easy cases
- Anatomically normal
- Reasonable expectations
- Set yourself up for success
- Book cases at the end of the day
- Give complete informed consent
- Tape the patient's head before prepping for extra stability

history of psychosis, uncontrollable movements or speech, or someone who is non-English speaking. Other than these factors, choose cases that are not unusual or difficult in any way. Avoid patients with previous refractive surgery, long or short eyes, or unreasonable expectations. Even after your first few cases under general anesthesia, when you have "graduated" to using a retrobulbar/peribulbar block or topical/intracameral anesthesia, avoid patients who have difficult lying still due to arthritis or other systemic problems.

Give very complete informed consent, spending time on what will happen if there is a complication, since complications may be more likely to occur in your first few cases. It is always a good policy to under promise and over deliver; this is particularly true for the beginning phaco surgeon. Tell the patient that recovery will take several weeks. Be honest about the potential for spectacle independence and the financial details related to enhancements should they be necessary.

Book your cases at the end of the day so your colleagues are not waiting for you to finish. Ask your device representative to be with you in the operating room for as many of those first surgery days as you can possibly negotiate. It is difficult to get physician colleagues to assist in surgery, as it means the loss of income-producing time for them. In any case, you may find that the representative is more patient than fellow surgeons!

Make the cases easier on yourself by taping the patient's head before prepping to eliminate as much movement as possible. If the patients are not sedated, give them headphones or put cotton in their ears (to "catch the irrigating solution") to increase your own comfort level, as you may need to chat quietly with the technicians or representatives.

Be sure to use armrests; take a moment or two to position them carefully and to tighten the height adjustment screws so that they do not collapse suddenly during the case.

Immediately after your initial cases and on an ongoing basis thereafter, you should watch the experts' tapes again, and your own surgical videos as well. I watched for and tried to eliminate unnecessary movements, especially inside the eye, to improve my own efficiency and to achieve better results for the patient in the immediate postoperative period.

Transitioning back to phacoemulsification (Table 1) was one of the hardest things I have done in recent memory, but the results have been absolutely worth the stress and time commitment involved.

I have the satisfaction of being able to perform a wider variety of surgical procedures that benefit my patients. I can participate in clinical trials for the newest refractive technologies and still assist my colleagues by performing postphaco laser enhancements. Perhaps most importantly, I experienced the joy of learning something new and the humility of being a student again. As anyone who teaches knows, the single most distinguishing characteristic of a good teacher is that he or she remembers what it was like to be a student.

Keratorefractive surgeons have the staff and infrastructure for refractive procedures in place. We need only change ourselves to be ready to implant refractive IOLs.

CHAPTER 25

TRANSITIONING FROM KERATOREFRACTIVE TO REFRACTIVE IOL SURGERY

Jose L. Güell, MD; Merce Morral, MD; Oscar Gris, MD; and Felicidad Manero, MD

During the last 20 years, laser corneal refractive surgery (laser in situ keratomileusis [LASIK], photorefractive keratectomy [PRK], EpiLASIK, or laser-assisted epithelial keratomileusis [LASEK]) has been used to correct a wide range of refractive errors, and has been proven effective and safe in most cases.[1] However, despite the use of highly optimized and customized laser-based treatments such as with wavefront technology, physical limitations of corneal thickness and curvature, as well as biomechanical behavior, limit the range of indications for a safe corneal refractive procedure.[2] Moreover, the optical quality of the outcomes may not be as good as desired, especially when treating patients with higher refractive errors, or large mesopic pupil sizes.[3-5] A considerable number of patients that would have had LASIK 10 years ago are now being excluded from this procedure because of these concerns about safety and quality of vision.

Although LASIK provides better predictability, less regression, and less corneal haze than PRK,[6] the choice of LASIK to correct hyperopia should be made with caution in light of potential complications, such as regression,[7] undercorrection,[7,8] epithelial ingrowth,[8] glare, or dry eye.[9]

When keratorefractive surgery is not the best approach for a patient, we should consider either phakic intraocular lens implantation (Ph-IOL) or clear lens extraction (CLE) with intraocular lens (IOL) implantation.

Phakic IOL Implantation

Although there have been several Ph-IOL models in the international market during the last few years, only the Visian Implantable Contact Lens (ICL, STAAR Surgical Inc, Monrovia, CA) and the Artisan (Ophtec B.V., Groningen, The Netherlands)—Verisyse (AMO, Santa Ana, CA) iris-claw Ph-IOL have been approved by the Food and Drug Administration (FDA) (December 2005 and September 2004, respectively).

In our experience, implantation of iris-claw Ph-IOLs has shown excellent long-term efficacy, stability, and safety for the correction of myopia, hyperopia, and/or astigmatism, provided that certain requirements are met (Figure 1).[1,10,11] These prerequisites are central anterior chamber depth (measured from the corneal epithelium to the anterior surface of the crystalline lens) ≥ 3.2 mm, central endothelial cell count >2300 cells/mm^2, scotopic pupil size >4.5 mm and normal pupil function, intraocular pressure between 8 and 21 mmHg, and the absence of anterior segment or retinal pathology. Ph-IOLs are our choice in young patients because they preserve accommodation.[12]

As far as the acquisition of surgical skills is concerned, it will be easier for those surgeons with previous experience in cataract surgery. However, specific training courses and the guidance of experienced surgeons in Ph-IOL surgery is mandatory.

To date, as multifocal optics may decrease contrast sensitivity and data does not allow us to consider accommodating IOLs as a valid dynamic substitute for the natural lens, CLE should be avoided in patients still able to accommodate. However, in presbyopic patients, CLE with IOL implantation may be considered a better option.

Clear Lens Extraction

CLE with posterior chamber IOL implantation has proven to be a safe and effective procedure for the correction of moderate to severe myopia[13-16] and hyperopia,[17-21] especially in the presbyopic age range. There are 3 main types of IOLs: monofocal, multifocal (refractive or diffractive), and accommodating. Personally, we prefer the monofocal-monovision approach for both hyperopic or myopic patients. The details of each kind of IOL are beyond the scope of this chapter and will be discussed thoroughly in later chapters.

Although new phacoemulsification techniques have made this procedure very safe, every refractive surgeon should be aware of potential complications. Posterior capsule opacification is especially common in younger patients. Meticulous

Figure 1. (A and B) Clinical photograph and Visante optical coherence tomography (OCT) of a Veriflex PIOL 12 months postoperatively. (C and D) Clinical photograph and Visante OCT of a Verisyse Toric PIOL 3 years after its implantation.

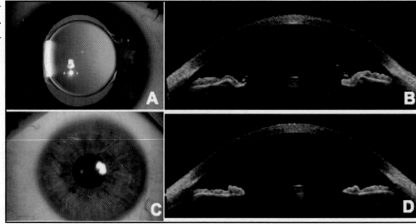

Figure 2. Clinical photographs of both eyes of the same patient. (A) Right eye: Relaxing corneal limbal incisions (optical zone 10 mm) were performed at the same time of cataract surgery to correct a corneal astigmatism of −1.7 D (41.3 × 43.0 @ 60 degrees). (B) In the left eye, arquate keratotomy (optical zone 7 mm) was chosen to correct a corneal astigmatism of −4.4 D (39.8 × 44.1 @ 125 degrees).

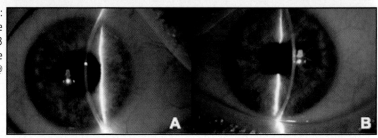

surgical technique, careful elimination of the equatorial cells of the capsular bag, and the use of acrylic and silicone sharp-edged optics may prevent this complication.[22,23]

One of the main concerns when performing CLE in high myopic eyes is the increased risk of retinal detachment (RD), especially in younger patients (<55 years old), and in those eyes with longer axial lengths (>26 mm).[15] The incidence of this complication after CLE is variable, ranging from 0% to 8%.[13-15,24-28] The following factors have been associated with a higher risk of RD: younger age, longer axial length, history of RD in the contralateral eye, surgical technique and preservation of the posterior capsule, and longer follow-up time after surgery. On the other hand, a history of detachment of the posterior vitreous is inversely related to the risk for RD. It is of utmost importance to treat high risk predisposing lesions in the periphery of the retina prior to CLE surgery.[13] In the case of hyperopia, RD is not much of a concern, and CLE can be safely performed in younger patients (age group 45 to 55 years old), except for eyes with extreme hyperopia such as patients with nanophthalmos. Nevertheless, hyperopic eyes with a smaller axial length, small anterior chamber, and small corneal diameter are more vulnerable to intraoperative complications.

Nowadays, cataract surgery has 2 main goals (increasing visual acuity and a best refractive result), and surgeons should be able to satisfy both. Enhancements with corneal refractive surgery, either laser ablations or incisional surgery (arcuate keratectomy or relaxing limbal incisions), may be necessary, and may require collaboration between cataract and refractive surgery specialists (Figure 2).

Conclusion

At present we should consider other options besides keratorefractive surgery to treat moderate to high refractive errors, namely Ph-IOL implantation in younger patients, and CLE at the presbyopic age groups. When correctly indicated, these procedures have proven to be both effective and safe.

References

1. Malecaze FJ, Hulin H, Bierer P, Güell JL, et al. A randomized paired eye comparison of two techniques for treating moderately high myopia. LASIK and Artisan Phakic Lens. *Ophthalmology.* 2002;109:1622-1630.

2. Pepose JS, Feigenbaum SK, Qazi MA, et al. Changes in corneal biomechanics and intraocular pressure following LASIK using static, dynamic, and noncontact tonometry. *Am J Ophthalmol.* 2007;143(1):39-47.

3. Seiler T, Holschbach A, Derse M, et al. Complications of myopia photorefractive keratectomy with the excimer laser. *Ophthalmology.* 1994;101:153-160.

4. Seiler T, Koufala K, Ritcher G. Iatrogenic keratectasia after laser in situ keratomileusis. *J Refract Surg.* 1998;14:312-317.

5. Artal P, Navarro R. Monochromatic modulation transfer function of the human eye for different pupil diameters: an analytical expression. *J Opt Soc Am A Opt Image Sci Vis.* 1994;11:246-249.

6. Ditzen K, Huschka H, Pieger S. Laser in situ keratomileusis for hyperopia. *J Cataract Refract Surg.* 1998;24:42-47.

7. Göker S, Hamdi E, Kahvecioglu C. Laser in situ keratomileusis to correct hyperopia from +4.25 to +8.00 diopters. *J Refract Surg.* 1998;14:26-30.

8. Sanders DR, Martin RG, Brown DC, et al. Posterior chamber phakic intraocular lens for hyperopia. *J Refract Surg.* 1999;15:309-315.

9. Albietz JM, Lenton LM, McLennan SG. Effect of laser in situ keratomileusis for hyperopia on tear film and ocular surface. *J Refract Surg.* 2002;18:113-123.

10. Güell JL, Morral M, Gris O, et al. Five-year follow-up of 399 phakic Artisan®-Verisyse® implantation for myopia, hyperopia and/or astigmatism. *Ophthalmology.* 2007 Oct 31; [epub ahead of print].

11. Güell JL, Vazquez M, Malecaze F, et al. Artisan toric phakic intraocular lens for the correction of high astigmatism. *Am J Ophthalmol.* 2003;136:442-447.

12. Güell JL, Morral M, Gris O, et al. Evaluation of Verisyse and Artiflex phakic intraocular lenses during accommodation using Visante™ Optical Coherence Tomography. *J Cataract Refract Surg.* 2007;33(8):1398-1404.

13. Güell JL, Rodriguez-Arenas A, Gris O, et al. Phacoemulsification of the crystalline lens and implantation of an intraocular lens for the correction of moderate and high myopia: four-year follow up. *J Cataract Refract Surg.* 2003;29:34-38.

14. Fernandez-Vega L, Alfonso JF, Villacampa T. Clear lens extraction for the correction of high myopia. *Ophthalmology.* 2003;110:2349-2354.

15. Goldberg MF. Clear lens extraction for axial myopia: an appraisal. *Ophthalmology.* 1987;94:571-582.

16. Colin J, Robinet A. Clear lensectomy and implantation of low-power posterior chamber intraocular lens for the correction of high myopia. *Ophthalmology.* 1994;101:107-112.

17. Colin J, Robinet A. Clear lensectomy and implantation of a low-power posterior chamber intraocular lens for correction of high myopia: a four-year follow-up. *Ophthalmology.* 1997;104:73-77, discussion 77-78.

18. Kolahdouz-Isfahani AH, Rostamian K, Wallace D, et al. Clear lens extraction with intraocular lens implantation for hyperopia. *J Refract Surg.* 1999;15(3):316-323.

19. Preetha R, Goel P, Patel N, et al. Clear lens extraction for hyperopia. *J Cataract Refract Surg.* 2003;29(5):895-899.

20. Kohnen T. Advances in the surgical correction of hyperopia [editorial]. *J Cataract Refract Surg.* 1998;24:1-2.

21. Siganos DS, Pallikaris IG. Clear lensectomy and intraocular lens implantation for hyperopia from +7 to +14 diopters. *J Refract Surg.* 1998;14:105-113.

22. Lyle WA, Jin GJC. Clear lens extraction to correct hyperopia. *J Cataract Refract Surg.* 1997;23:1051-1056.

23. Cheng JW, Wei RL, Cai JP, et al. Efficacy of different intraocular lens materials and optic edge designs in preventing posterior capsular opacification: a meta-analysis. *Am J Ophthalmol.* 2007;143(3):428-436.

24. Lyle WA, Jin GJ. Phacoemulsification with intraocular lens implantation in high myopia. *J Cataract Refract Surg.* 1996;22:238-242.

25. Colin J, Robinet A, Cochener B. Retinal detachment after clear lens extraction for high myopia: seven-year follow-up. *Ophthalmology.* 1999;106:2281-2284.

26. Jacobi FK, Hessemer V. Pseudophakic retinal detachment in high axial myopia. *J Cataract Refract Surg.* 1997;23:1095-1102.

27. Javitt JC, Tielsch JM, Canner JK, et al. National outcomes of cataract extraction. Increased risk of retinal complications associated with Nd:YAG laser capsulotomy. The Cataract Patient Outcomes Research Team. *Ophthalmology.* 1992;99:1487–97, discussion 1497-1498.

28. Fritch CD. Risk of retinal detachment in myopic eyes after intraocular lens implantation: a 7-year study. *J Cataract Refract Surg.* 1998;24:1357-1360.

CHAPTER 26

REFRACTIVE IOLs IN A RESIDENCY PROGRAM—CAN IT WORK?

Thomas A. Oetting, MD; Jeffrey J. Caspar, MD;
Bonnie An Henderson, MD; and Terry Kim, MD

The simple answer to this question is "Yes."

Why Can It Work?

Incorporating refractive intraocular lenses (IOLs) into the curriculum of residency programs is an excellent opportunity for 4 reasons. First, unlike keratorefractive surgery, becoming a competent cataract surgeon is mandatory for comprehensive ophthalmologists completing a residency program. Therefore, systems and resources have already been developed in all training programs to ensure surgical competency in lens extraction procedures used for placing refractive IOLs. There is minimal additional technical training involved with these "premium" lenses. Instead, the additional training for refractive IOL surgery is centered on proper and complete knowledge of the IOL technology, the preoperative testing, patient and IOL selection, and postoperative care. These topics can and should be mastered during residency training. Second, caring for refractive IOL patients will improve the resident's communication and interpersonal skills. Effective communication skills are critical for identifying appropriate candidates for these lenses and avoiding the hypercritical patients who may have unrealistic expectations. These skills must also be used to educate patients about these IOL options, such as the different lens designs, mechanisms of action, and their respective advantages and limitations. Residents must also learn how to gauge, set, and manage the expectations of these patients, which is one of the most crucial components of the preoperative patient assessment. For example, ophthalmology training programs can establish a rotation where residents can observe and shadow experienced faculty as they evaluate potential candidates for refractive IOL surgery. They can witness first hand the informed consent process, the interactive dialogue, and the various factors involved in the decision-making process. These roles can then be reversed where the resident can take the patient through the evaluation process with faculty observation. Videotaping these sessions can demonstrate the positive and negative aspects of the interaction, which can sometimes be very subtle.

Clearly, one of the most difficult components of incorporating refractive IOL technology into a residency training program involves teaching these interpersonal and communication skills and does not even require that the resident perform the surgery. Emphasis on this aspect of training is valuable for residency programs where it may be more complicated to actually have the resident perform refractive cataract surgery with a premium IOL. Furthermore, residents will benefit from learning the importance of preoperative patient selection, communicating the options and consent, and finally, the postoperative communication, counseling, and follow-up of the patient. This last phase may involve reassuring the patient about various side effects of presbyopia-correcting (Pr-C) IOLs.

Third, preoperative and postoperative patient counseling is more extensive for refractive IOL procedures than for standard cataract patients with monofocal lenses. Much more "chair time" is needed to discuss these IOL options, potential risks, and anticipated postoperative refractive outcomes. In general, compared to attending physicians, residents have more time allotted to spend with these patients. Because of this, a thorough, unhurried discussion can take place between the resident and patient. This in-depth discussion will create a stronger doctor–patient relationship between the resident and this future surgical patient. This strong relationship will help foster trust and will yield a greater likelihood that the patient will allow this resident to perform the surgery.

Fourth, the Accreditation Council for Graduate Medical Education (ACGME) has mandated the use of six competencies for resident education, including medical knowledge, patient care, practice-based learning and improvement, systems-based practice, professionalism, and interpersonal and communication skills.[1] The introduction of new-technology IOLs provides a great opportunity for residency programs to emphasize the more difficult nonclinical and nonmedical knowledge competencies. These new IOLs provide an opportunity to teach residents the difficult competencies of systems-based competency, practice-based improvement, professionalism, and communication. Although these lenses have significantly advanced the range of patient options, the actual surgical procedure is not that different from cataract surgery with a standard monofocal IOL. However, the other issues involving patient management (ie, patient selection, patient education, and setting/management of expectations), preoperative corneal and axial measurements, IOL selection, and postoperative counseling and follow-up become the more challenging topics to master and therefore teach. As a result, the prospect of incorporating new refractive IOL technology provides a great opportunity for residency training programs to expand education into these areas so that mandated educational goals can be met while providing refractive IOL competency at the same time.

How Can It Work?

Ophthalmology residency training programs across the country continue to strive to train residents that feel competent and comfortable upon graduating and entering clinical practice. One of the major challenges in structuring the surgical curriculum lies in when and how to incorporate new procedures and technologies as they are developed and introduced into our field. With the arrival of refractive IOLs, such as toric, multifocal, and accommodating IOLs, we now must decide how to incorporate these technologies into a residency training program.

STEP 1: PREOPERATIVE PATIENT CARE AND MEDICAL KNOWLEDGE

The resident must have an intimate knowledge of the methodology used by his or her department to obtain axial length measurements, whether by partial coherence interferometry (IOL Master; Carl Zeiss Meditec, Jena, Germany) or immersion A-scan biometry. This process requires an understanding of how such measurements are obtained and the ability to assess the accuracy and consistency of these measurements.

Measuring keratometric astigmatism is a critical part of the preoperative assessment and requires knowledge of a variety of measurement modalities such as corneal topography, and manual and automated keratometry. Patients should have keratometric measurements performed by 2 different methods with consistently comparable results. Corneal topography is critical to success with both Pr-C and toric IOLs, and residents should be comfortable interpreting topographic scans for evidence of irregular astigmatism.

The resident must have demonstrated the ability to produce accurate postoperative refractive results in straightforward cataract surgery cases. Preferably, he or she should have derived a customized A-constant or surgeon factor for the monofocal version of the lens used. At the very least, the resident should have tracked their previous surgical results and demonstrated accurate postoperative refractive outcomes. They should also have experience with the most common IOL formulas and know the ideal postoperative refractive target for the Pr-C IOL that they are implanting.

No matter what a resident's experience level is, each surgical candidate should be reviewed by a faculty member expe-rienced with refractive IOL surgery to ensure that the patient is a good candidate.

STEP 2: SURGICAL SKILLS

Residents must first be accomplished surgeons, comfortable with all aspects of routine phacoemulsification. They must be able to reliably perform a well-centered capsulorrhexis of appropriate size for the IOL to be used. They must be familiar with the characteristics of the refractive lens to be used and, in the case of multifocal lenses, should be very experienced with implantation of the monofocal version of the lens.

Patient selection is particularly critical for the surgeon's first patients. Pre-existing astigmatism is the greatest hurdle to patient satisfaction and, as such, beginning surgeons should limit their cases to those with less than 0.75 D of corneal astigmatism. Residents must also have an appreciation for the astigmatic effect of their surgical incision. Ideally, they shall have determined the astigmatic effects of their surgery through postoperative analysis by a program such as the Surgically Induced Astigmatism Calculator.[2]

They should also understand the principle of on-axis surgery and be familiar with techniques of surgical correction of astigmatism. While their initial cases should not require surgical correction of astigmatism, this should ultimately become an integral part of Pr-C IOL surgery, and the resident will want to choose a nomogram to follow for limbal relaxing incisions or astigmatic keratotomy.

Due to high patient expectations, the limitations of current technologies, and the patient costs involved, implantation of refractive IOLs leaves little margin for error. Improper patient selection, inaccuracy of IOL power, small amounts of residual astigmatism, and other postoperative complications (ie, dry eyes, cystoid macular edema, posterior capsular opacification, etc) will result in poor outcomes that could necessitate further surgical intervention. Because of this, implantation of these IOLs requires a smooth, consistent surgical approach, and implantation of such lenses should not be considered until the resident feels very comfortable with routine cataract surgery. Furthermore, residents need to be prepared to address the treatment options (ie, YAG laser capsulotomy, excimer laser refractive surgery, incisional astigmatism management, etc) that may be required to optimize patient outcomes after implantation with these IOLs.

STEP 3: PRACTICE-BASED LEARNING, SYSTEMS-BASED PRACTICE, PROFESSIONALISM

Practice-Based Learning and Improvement

Physicians must be able to investigate and evaluate their current patient care practices, appraise and assimilate scientific evidence, and use this to improve patient care. Practice-based learning and improvement is "how you get better at medicine." It is an extremely important practice for any ophthalmologist who intends to keep pace with the continual progression of advancing technology.

Residency training programs should develop a mechanism to check on the competency of their surgeons-in-training prior to their departure into clinical practice. The goal is to ensure that they can consistently produce excellent surgical results with cataract surgery using a monocular lens.[3] Residents can track the results of their cataract surgeries in a manner consistent with the ACGME's practiced-based learning and improvement competency using organized systems such as OASIS.[4] Alternatively, residency programs can develop systems to track resident surgical outcomes on their own. By establishing certain refractive outcome goals that need to be met with cataract surgery using standard IOLs, residency programs can then determine whether such trainees are ready to evaluate and offer implantation of the newer refractive IOLs.

The use of refractive IOLs provides an excellent opportunity for residents to develop practice-based learning and improvement. This experience can serve as a model for learning to use new techniques and devices in the future. As newer technologic breakthroughs challenge ophthalmologists to use tools with which they have little or no experience, the ability to assess such technology and incorporate it into one's practice becomes critical.

Systems-Based Practice

The ACGME describes competency in systems-based practice as demonstrating "an awareness of and responsiveness to the larger context and system of health care and the ability to effectively call on system resources to provide care that is of optimal value."[5] Residents often do not understand the larger issues involved in medical decision making, such as financial impact to the society, resource allocation, and interdependencies of the different factors in healthcare.

The introduction of refractive lens implants is accompanied by a host of macro- and micro-system issues that are quite interesting.[1] Macro-system issues, such as the rules regarding reimbursement for Medicare and the advocacy work that has been done by organized ophthalmology to bring about this change, come into sharp focus when discussing multifocal and toric IOLs. This precedent provides a great opportunity for residency programs to introduce the concepts of organized medicine as agents able to change the Medicare system. This issue provides an opportunity to introduce the concept of services that are, and are not, covered under Medicare, and thus, must be billed separately.

The use of refractive lenses is also an opportunity to teach the differences between private and public insurance agencies and the relationship between them. The resident may witness the different methods that various insurance companies use to handle refractive IOLs. Although private companies are not regulated by Medicare, many follow the standards set by Medicare regarding reimbursement policies whereas others do not. In learning about the use of these lenses, residents may learn about reimbursement issues such as obtaining prior authorization.

Micro-system issues within the department are also relevant to refractive IOLs. It is important for the resident to understand how the various measurements are obtained, how patients flow through the clinic, how a bill is generated, and how the system has been modified for these new IOLs. Additionally, systems are needed to ensure that the proper lens is ordered and delivered to surgery in time. Postoperatively, systems must be in place to monitor the efficacy and quality of the surgery.

As a result, the introduction of refractive IOLs provides residency programs with an opportunity to address the difficult-to-teach area of systems-based learning, including both the macrosystems involved in healthcare delivery such as Medicare and the micro-system of delivery of care within their own department.

Professionalism

The introduction of toric, multifocal, and accommodating lens technologies brings with it a host of ethical and professionalism issues that pertain to every resident. Surveys of graduating residents have confirmed our suspicion that they feel ill-prepared for the business of medicine.[6,7] The billing issues surrounding the use of these IOLs must be dealt with in a very direct manner with patients, which allows residents-in-training to gain exposure in this area. Articles and lectures on the economics of refractive IOLs provides residents with important and needed exposure to business issues. Advocacy by our professional organizations, such as the American Academy of Ophthalmology (AAO) and the American Society of Cataract and Refractive Surgery (ASCRS), have helped to make it possible for billing a premium outside of the Medicare system for these Pr-C IOLs. This achievement emphasizes the importance of organized ophthalmology's role in our profession to our residents. Ethical issues regarding these premium lenses are equally important and include inappropriate patient selection for monetary gain, miscommunication of consent, risks and benefits, and improper use of comanagement.

Conclusion

We believe that refractive IOLs could play an important role in the current curriculum of residency programs (Table 1). Achieving a successful outcome with a refractive IOL patient is similar to passing an end-of-the-semester final examination for competency on cataract surgery. In order to have a successful outcome with a refractive IOL patient, the resident must master the preoperative evaluation, must perform surgery competently, and must proficiently care for the patient postoperatively while addressing all of the patient's concerns. If the resident "passes" this refractive IOL test, then he or she has shown competence in the major skills needed to care for any lens extraction patient, refractive or otherwise. Training residents to become competent in the care of refractive IOL patients can be beneficial to all parties.

References

1. Lee AG, Carter KD. Managing the new mandate in residency education: a blueprint for translating a national mandate into local compliance. *Ophthalmology*. 2004;111:1807-1812.

2. Hill W. Surgically Induced Astigmatism Calculator: http://www.doctor-hill.com/physicians/download.htm, accessed on October 10, 2007.

3. Oetting TA, Lee AG, Beaver HA, et al. Teaching and assessing surgical competency in ophthalmology training programs. *Ophthalmic Surg Lasers Imaging*. 2006;37(5):384-393.

Table 1

REFRACTIVE IOL CURRICULUM

1. Preoperative Measurements

a. Axial length measurement (ie, immersion A-scan biometry, partial coherence interferometry)
b. Keratometry (ie, manual/automated keratometry, corneal topography)
c. Acquisition, interpretation, and assessment of accuracy

2. Cataract Surgical Skills

a. Consistent incision location and construction to provide reproducible effects on corneal astigmatism
b. Creation of a properly-sized, well-centered capsulorrhexis
c. Proper surgical technique to minimize intraoperative and postoperative complications
d. Experience with implantation of monofocal version of refractive IOL (if available)
e. Corneal astigmatism management (ie, limbal relaxing incision (LRI), astigmatic keratotomy (AK), on-axis surgery)

3. Preoperative Communication

a. Patient education on different refractive IOL options
b. Gauging/setting/managing patient expectations
c. Identification of appropriate candidates for surgery
d. Consent process for refractive IOLs

4. Preoperative Assessment

a. Astigmatism assessment (corneal versus lenticular)
b. Nomogram selection and customization for incisional astigmatism management
c. Surgical plan (ie, LRI/AK versus toric IOL, selection of appropriate Pr-C IOL)
d. Appropriate refractive target for type of Pr-C lens used
e. Practice-based learning
   i. Personalized A-constant for single-piece and multipiece acrylic IOLs
   ii. OASIS or other system to track outcomes[4]

5. Postoperative Follow-Up

a. Techniques and skills in dealing with happy and unhappy patients (ie, reassurance, −3.00 D spectacle test, neuroadaptation, etc)
b. Diagnosis for suboptimal outcome (ie, residual refractive error, dry eyes, posterior capsular opacification, cystoid macular edema, etc.)
c. Treatment options for suboptimal outcomes (ie, excimer laser refractive surgery, incisional refractive surgery, YAG laser capsulotomy, etc)
d. Discussion of option of IOL exchange

6. Other Core Competencies

a. Systems-based practice
   i. Lectures/reading materials on Medicare, private insurance
   ii. Lectures/reading materials on methods of delivering care (eg, this book)
   iii. Observation of system to order/deliver IOLs
b. Professionalism
   i. Lectures on ethics of refractive IOLs
   ii. Lectures on business of refractive IOLs
   iii. Role of AAO and ASCRS in new refractive IOLs

4. Cremers SL, Ciolino JB, Ferrufino-Ponce ZK, Henderson BA. Objective assessment of skills in intraocular surgery (OASIS). *Ophthalmology.* 2005;112(7):1236-1241.

5. ACME Project, http://www.acgme.org/outcome/e-learn/introduction/SBP.html, accessed on October 10, 2007.

6. Lee A, Beaver H, Boldt H, et al. Teaching and assessing professionalism in ophthalmology residency training programs. *Surv Ophth.* 2007;52:300-314.

7. McDonnell P, Kirwan T, Brinton G, et al. Perceptions of recent ophthalmology residency graduates regarding preparation for practice. *Ophthalmology.* 2007;114(2):387-391.

CHAPTER 27

REFRACTIVE IOLs
IN A MANAGED CARE SETTING

William Jerry Chang, MD

Refractive Cataract Surgery

As discussed in great detail in this book, cataract surgery is increasingly becoming refractive surgery in this modern era. In the not too distant past, patients were content to have their cataract removed and experience improved vision. Wearing glasses was an acceptable condition of surgery and indeed an expectation. Patients are now becoming increasingly aware of new surgical options and, as informed consumers, are beginning to expect not only excellent vision, but also freedom from eyeglasses. In short, patients want to regain the clarity and range of vision they once enjoyed in their youth.

Surgeons performing modern cornea-based refractive surgery have long recognized the powerful ability of modern technology to transform patients' ametropia to emmetropia with startling speed and comfort. Surgeons and patients alike have understood the value of this surgery, which, when performed well in the right patient, is well worth the time and expense from the perspectives of both parties. Generally speaking, laser refractive surgery has not been a covered benefit by insurance plans, and patients have become accustomed to paying significant out-of-pocket fees to gain the "magic" of refractive surgery.

By contrast, cataract surgery has been a benefit covered by Centers for Medicare and Medicaid Services (CMS) or insurance plans. Patients have grown to expect that cataract surgery will be covered by insurance with little or no out of pocket expense. Although the economics of health care is beyond the scope of this chapter, it is clear that the marriage of cataract surgery and refractive surgery can be a difficult one in our current era. Physicians and patients alike will experience growing pains as our field evolves.

Managed Care—
General Context

The economics of health care has evolved tremendously in the past several decades, and there are legitimate concerns about the cost and delivery of health care in the United States today. Several models of managed care have emerged throughout the country, such as Staff-Model, Group-Model, Network-Model, and Independent-Practice Association (IPA). Comments in this chapter on "managed care" are made from the perspective of a Group-Model managed care organization, although many of the issues are shared in the various models. Managed care is most successful in settings where there is a strong integration and inter-accountability between physicians and insurer. Such collaborative partnerships foster a culture of cooperation toward common goals in both clinical and financial arenas. A well-organized, integrated managed care system optimizes high clinical quality, service, patient safety, and affordability through systems that provide consistency of care. Care decisions are evidence-based and outcomes are monitored for quality. Efficiency and productivity are continually examined and refined but not at the expense of quality of care.

Whether a physician is working in a traditional private setting or managed care, the goal is the same: do the right thing for the patient. The route in a managed care setting is more global in nature because the managed care organization, and thus the physician, takes a population view in addition to the more narrow single patient view.

Refractive IOLs in Managed Care

PATIENTS

In managed care settings, as in other health insurance systems, certain services are defined as covered benefits. These benefits are often comprehensive and inclusive, as in the arena of functional impairment from cataract. Although this typically can include the cost of a traditional monofocal intraocular lens (IOL), the cost of a premium refractive IOL is generally not covered, at least at the time of this writing. Significant patient education must occur about the financial cost of the lens in addition to the usual clinical aspects. Patients who have been part of a managed care setting for a long period can be sometimes surprised that the cost of these new IOLs is not covered and that they face a significant out-of-pocket expense. This provides a challenge as well as an opportunity to educate patients about the advantages of the new premium IOLs so that patients can make an informed decision.

No matter what the financing arrangements are—traditional fee for service or managed care—refractive IOLs are not for every patient. Sometimes a patient's decision to decline a premium IOL is based on his or her personal finances, but often patients are counseled away from these IOLs due to patient specific factors such as ocular comorbidities, occupational or recreational visual needs, or unusual visual expectations.

SURGEONS

Just as these premium refractive IOLs are not for every patient, they are also not for every surgeon.

In any clinical setting not yet incorporating refractive surgery, the transition to refractive lens technology is a significant undertaking. Surgeons must fully understand what the technology can and cannot provide and be able to communicate this to the patient so that a truly informed decision can be made. In addition, surgical skills must be raised to a higher and more consistent level in order for the surgery to be successful. Cataract surgeons with experience in cornea-based refractive surgery such as laser in situ keratomileusis (LASIK) will have a much easier time transitioning because they already have an understanding of the discerning nature of the refractive personality. They already know and practice the concept of "under promise and over deliver" and most importantly, they understand that selecting good candidates sometimes is best thought of in reverse: know on whom to not operate.

SYSTEMS

In a managed care setting, a well-organized system helps manage patient interactions with physicians and staff effectively and efficiently but in a high touch, personalized manner. Setting up an efficient but personal system for refractive IOLs is not a trivial task, in part because the technology is complex and there is much patient education needed to ensure thorough understanding and informed consent.

Patient Education

Every refractive surgeon knows how much chair time is commonly devoted to refractive patients. Now cataract surgeons involved with refractive cataract surgery will experience the same phenomenon, and similar systems need to be developed to keep patient flow moving efficiently.

Optometry colleagues need to be informed and engaged in the process of patient education so that referred patients are prepared with significant knowledge of IOL options before they arrive for their surgical consultation.

In the office, it is helpful to engage staff so they can participate in patient education. Often it is useful to create a refractive staff specialist role whose time is dedicated to refractive surgical matters. Their scope can include, in addition to patient education, handling of finances, surgery scheduling, and maintenance of outcome databases. The staff specialist should have a full array of materials at hand for patient education, including patient handouts, posters placed in strategic areas, and electronic education materials. All clinic staff should be engaged to the point of having a 2 or 3 line simple description or a prepared script to respond to interested patients. They can then be directed to the staff specialist for further information.

Although external media naturally reaches many patients, it is important for the physician office infrastructure to make patient information freely available. As refractive IOLs become more mainstream, it is arguable that all cataract patients should be made aware of these new IOL options. If such education does not take place, a patient receiving a traditional monofocal lens implant might later complain that they might have preferred and chosen a premium IOL if the option had been made available to them before surgery.

Patient information must be current and written in an accessible style. Information can take the form of a Web presence or patient handout materials that are available at appointments or mailed to potential candidates. Although vendor-supplied information can be helpful, patients often trust a nonbranded source of information, and the physician office has the opportunity to promote its integrity by providing a balanced, nonhyped perspective on these new technology lenses. In a managed care setting, commonly there is an evidence-based organization-wide position on the technology, which is observed by all participating surgeons.

Ideally, when the patient arrives at his or her surgical consultation, he or she should be already fully informed and able to make a decision on implant type. This preparatory work will save significant chair time and improve surgeon efficiency in the clinic. Patient education is thus a shared team effort, not just the time-consuming activity of the surgeon. Time that would have been otherwise spent on basics of lens options can now be spent in more meaningful ways to optimize the physician–patient relationship, which is of great importance in all surgeries, especially refractive surgeries.

Surgical Excellence

Systems are needed to support surgeons to obtain the most accurate measurements preoperatively. Technology must be brought up to date, and the most current IOL calculation formulae must be utilized. Consistency of biometry is particularly critical, and staff education and staff deployment must be optimized to ensure accuracy.

Systems are also needed to be sure surgical technology is up to date. This may involve upgrading to the best and most current equipment, including the most advanced phaco technology and related instrumentation. As is well known and discussed elsewhere in this book, the stakes with refractive IOL surgery are much higher than with traditional monofocal IOLs and the tolerances for surgical variability are much narrower. Systems are needed to allow the surgeon to perform at the highest level in the operating room.

A good and accurate surgical outcome is obviously important for each patient. Systems must be set up by the surgeon to monitor outcomes of all postoperative patients over time. Cataract surgeons who do not yet track their outcomes will need to set up such a system to be sure results are optimized. Long-term surgical success requires consistent outcomes.

In a large managed care setting, the transition in such systems as equipment, staff deployment, staff education, and even surgeon education is not trivial. A method that may prove helpful is that of a "centers of excellence" approach to organize strategic core groups of surgeons with their teams. With this approach, the highly skilled and motivated surgeons and their teams can be the initial pioneers and other surgeons can follow after the success of the initial core group. In a managed care setting, surgeons and teams are collaborative, not competitive, so sharing learning is a natural and effective tool to spreading best practices.

Conclusion

As IOL options continue to evolve and multiply, new opportunities for patients and surgeons abound. Because so many new and complex options exist, it is critical to develop systems to promote efficient patient education, improve surgical skills, and optimize patient outcomes. Managed care at its best can accomplish these goals efficiently while maintaining excellent personalized physician–patient relationships.

CHAPTER 28

REFRACTIVE IOLs IN A COMANAGED OPTOMETRIC NETWORK

Paul Ernest, MD

Comanaging refractive intraocular lens (IOL) patients is both challenging and rewarding, and establishing an OD network takes a lot of time and diligence. However, it has benefits for both doctors and patients.

The relationship between the ophthalmologist and the referring ODs must be based on trust and respect. Ophthalmologists need to remember to do the simple things, such as sending letters to optometrists or calling to keep them informed about patients.

Ophthalmologists also need to take care of referred patients in a way that reflects well on the optometrist because we are a reflection on them. If we do high-quality work and provide honest care in a timely fashion, the patient will thank the optometrist for referring him or her to a particular ophthalmologist.

When an optometrist sends me a patient, I strive to get the best possible result and really show the patient that he or she is first and foremost in my thoughts and concerns, no matter how many other patients I am also taking care of that particular day.

Financial Arrangements

Determining the financial arrangements is an important consideration in a comanaged network. First, I do not believe in buying referrals. Even if you are successful, it is a very short-lived arrangement. The price will continue to rise, and you may find yourself in a bidding war with another ophthalmologist. You will end up either spending more money than it is worth or losing referrals because you cannot spend enough money. I have seen colleagues enter into these relationships, and they are not long-lasting.

I also do not believe that ophthalmologists should collect a fee and then pay the optometrist a percent of that fee. The ophthalmologist should set the fee schedule for his or her services, and the optometrist should set the fee schedule for his or her services. Each should collect his or her own fee. Some

practices offer more services to patients and should be able to charge accordingly. The optometrist's fee is not our concern and in fact, incorporating the optometrist's fee into the ophthalmologist's fee can result in a bidding war. Having separate fees also protects practices from the Office of the Inspector General. Both doctors benefit from this arrangement.

Comanaging Premium IOLs

Ophthalmologists should reassure optometrists that offering premium IOLs is best for their patients. Some optometrists are concerned that these IOLs may eliminate patients' need for glasses. However, many of the patients implanted with these lenses still need glasses for certain activities. Offering premium IOLs is part of high-quality care, and if they are not offered by a particular optometrist, the patient may think that the optometrist is not on the leading edge of technology. Many patients who feel this way will take their business elsewhere.

How Comanagement Works

I receive referrals from more than 100 optometrists. Typically, the optometrist will refer the patient to me for cataract surgery. Follow-up care after the surgery is performed can be handled in several ways.

If the optometrist has trained with me in follow-up care, then I will refer patients back to him or her. If not, then I do the follow-up care. However, the patient has the last word on who he or she sees for follow-up care, and the decision may be based on convenience. A patient may live far from my office but closer to the optometrist, so he or she may choose to have the optometrist do the follow-up care.

In cases in which the optometrist sees the patient for the 1-day follow-up visit, I require that the optometrist fax me a form so that I can see the postoperative result. I check the vision, the pressure, and the refraction, among other things. I want to see everything on that patient that day. All of us go

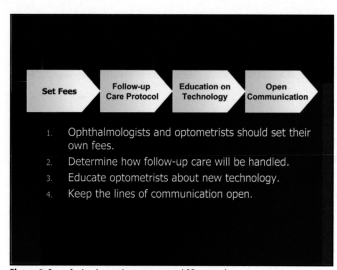

1. Ophthalmologists and optometrists should set their own fees.
2. Determine how follow-up care will be handled.
3. Educate optometrists about new technology.
4. Keep the lines of communication open.

Figure 1. Steps for implementing a comanaged OD network.

into that visit with the understanding that if anything is out of the ordinary, the patient will come to my office immediately.

Education

We educate our optometrists through letters, fax blasts, and booklets to ensure that they are up-to-date on our patient selection criteria as well as the newest technology. Additionally, we schedule private meetings, lunches, dinners, and seminars. It is a very methodical, ongoing process.

We have seminars a minimum of twice a year, and we will schedule additional seminars if something important comes up. The seminars can be set up so that the optometrists receive continuing education credits for attending, which can help boost attendance.

During the programs, we cover topics such as patient selection for premium lenses, managing patient expectations, managing patient outcomes, patient criteria for new technologies and treatments, new treatments in IOLs, advances in surgical techniques, advances in refractive and retinal surgeries, and any changes to practice offerings, such as new products.

Keeping the Lines of Communication Open

To keep the process running smoothly for both the doctors and patients, the lines of communication must be kept open. My office keeps track of our referrals, and if we are not receiving referrals from a particular optometrist, I will schedule a lunch or dinner with that person to understand why the number of referrals have declined.

I have an open-door policy, and I encourage optometrists to call me to discuss any concerns. Unfortunately, one bad experience can ruin a relationship, so it is important that both parties feel comfortable discussing any issues that may arise. We have a fairly large organization with a lot of doctors, and we have staff members whose job it is to call referring optometrists and monitor the relationship. These staff members are always available to talk to an optometrist if he or she calls with a concern. While ophthalmologists may not always be immediately accessible by phone, we never want to give the impression that we are too busy to care.

Conclusion

The networking relationship between ophthalmologists and optometrists requires a lot of time and effort. It is not something that you can buy. Both parties must establish trust and confidence in what they are doing as professionals. Optometrists must trust you and believe that you are sincere. Additionally, ophthalmologists can institute safeguards for the occasional episode that will inevitably happen. This relationship is really no different from any other business relationship.

SECTION III

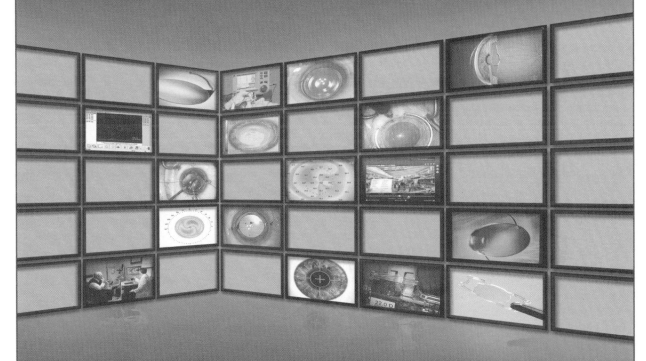

Transitioning to Presbyopia-Correcting IOLs: Quick Start Guides

CHAPTER 29

HOW DO I GET STARTED WITH THE REZOOM?

George Beiko, BM, BCh, FRCS(C)

By the year 2010, the United States Department of Health and Human Services estimates that there will be 40 million individuals aged 65 and over, with this increasing to 55 million by the year 2020.[1] In addition, the Framingham Eye Study[2] indicates that the prevalence of cataracts increases with age from 4% in those aged 52 to 64, to 50% in those 65 to 74 years, and more than 90% in those aged 75 to 85 years. These factors will likely drive the current 3 million cataract operations performed annually in the United States to much higher levels.

In March 2005, the US Food and Drug Administration (US FDA) approved the ReZoom intraocular lens (IOL) (AMO, Santa Ana, CA). This multifocal IOL offers patients the promise of both near and far visual acuity with limited or no reliance on corrective lenses. However, in order for this promise to become a reality, clinicians need to properly select the patient in addition to having meticulous surgical technique. This chapter reviews the ReZoom multifocal IOL, summarizes characteristics of the ideal multifocal IOL patient, provides a "how-to" guide on matching lens options to meet a patient's lifestyles and vision needs, and discusses strategies to consider in patients who may not be "ideal" but may still benefit from implantation of the ReZoom lens.

The ReZoom IOL is a refractive, distance-dominant multifocal IOL that enables good visual acuity through a range of distances. Its design is based on the 5-zone Array multifocal lens that was approved by the US FDA a decade ago. Like the Array, the ReZoom design also includes 5 optical zones to focus light on the retina at all pupil diameters: Zones 1, 3, and 5 are distant dominant, Zones 2 and 4 are near dominant, and the aspheric transition between zones provides balanced intermediate vision. This design enables distance-dominant vision with a near add of 3.5 D in the plane of the IOL (+2.5 D at the spectacle plane), which results in a slightly longer working distance for reading vision as compared to other multifocal IOLs. The ReZoom lens is hydrophobic acrylic with a posterior sharp square-edged optic design so as to reduce the development of posterior capsular opacification and thus

maintain clear visual acuity. As compared to the Array, the ReZoom IOL has a triple-edge design (OptiEdge design) that reduces edge-related glare and halo. The 3 edge components are a rounded anterior edge to reduce internal reflections, a sloped side edge to reduce edge glare, and a squared-off posterior edge to facilitate contact with the posterior capsule. The foldable ReZoom lens is designed for capsular bag placement following standard phacoemulsification cataract surgery, using a 2.8 mm posterior limbal incision centered on the axis of plus cylinder.

In a multicenter Canadian study of the ReZoom multifocal IOL implanted bilaterally, investigators found that the lens provided excellent distance, intermediate, and near vision, postoperatively, and it was observed that there was continued functional improvement at all distances over time.[3] The study design allowed inclusion of patients with cataract, with hyperopia, with myopia, with presbyopia, with astigmatism that could be corrected, and/or with significant refractive error who sought clear lens extraction. Those with significant dry eye, corneal scarring, mild to moderate myopia, a pupil size of <2.5 mm, a monofocal implant in the first eye, uncorrected postoperative astigmatism >0.5D, and unstable capsular support were excluded. Postoperative refraction was targeted at emmetropia to +0.50 D so as to provide good distance vision for driving. Of the 159 patients who completed the preoperative vision, 106 were available at the 6-week follow-up (55% female, 45% male) and 98 completed the 6-month follow-up (60% female, 40% male). Two-thirds or more of patients completing each evaluation time point were 61 years of age or greater. As illustrated in Figures 1 through 3, patients' visual acuity improved over time: at the 6-month follow-up 97%, 100%, and 84% had uncorrected distance, intermediate, and near visual acuity of 20/30 or better, respectively. Spectacle independence (defined as never or seldom needing corrective eyeglasses) was reported by 94.3% of patients at the week 6 visit and by 91.0% of those at the month 6 visit. The bother from halos and glare also dissipated over time: at week 6, 77% and 82% reported having none to mild bother from halos and glare, respectively,

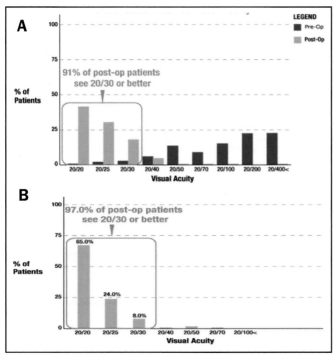

Figure 1. Preoperative and postoperative uncorrected distance visual acuity.

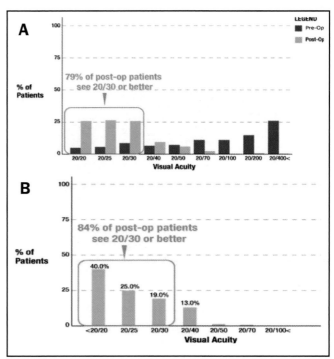

Figure 3. Preoperative and postoperative uncorrected near visual acuity.

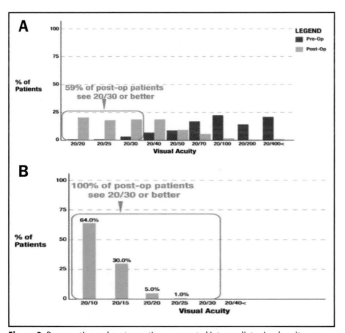

Figure 2. Preoperative and postoperative uncorrected intermediate visual acuity.

whereas at month 6, 82% and 87% reported having none to mild bother from halos and glare, respectively. Nearly 2 of 3 patients reported improvement in dysphotopic symptoms from 6 weeks to 6 months postoperatively. Overall, 88% at week 6 and 86% at month 6 reported being satisfied with their bilateral implantation of the ReZoom lens.

An interesting finding of the study was that although near visual acuity was reported to be similar in all age groups, reported spectacle independence decreased with age (higher percentages of spectacle independence was noted in those

between 46 and 50 years of age [86%] as compared to other age categories; 70% in those 51 to 60 years, 50% in those 61 to 65 years, 65% in those 66 to 70 years, and 52% in those >70 years).

The study was designed to provide a real world view of the outcomes with the ReZoom lens, as the group of investigators included not only those experienced in the use of multifocal IOLs, but also a number of novice surgeons. This study found that excellent outcomes were attained not only by the experienced but also by those who were new to the use of multifocal IOLs.

In another study, a retrospective analysis of contrast sensitivity was undertaken in 20 patients implanted with the ReZoom multifocal IOL and 20 patients implanted with the Tecnis Aspheric Monofocal IOL (AMO, Santa Ana, CA).[4] This study found that the ReZoom multifocal IOL has aspheric qualities that are more evident in photopic conditions (see Figures 4 and 5).[4] In this single-surgeon analysis, patients were similar postoperatively with respect to spherical equivalent (-0.05 ± 0.33 versus -0.19 ± 0.78, $p = .532$), visual acuity (0.86 ± 0.13 versus 0.77 ± 0.16, $p = .095$), and corneal spherical aberration (0.25 ± 0.07 versus 0.29 ± 0.08, $p = .125$). Distance corrected contrast sensitivity was measured at 4 or more weeks postoperatively using Stereo Optical VI 1600X.

Comparison of visual results with the ReZoom and the ReSTOR IOL (Alcon, Fort Worth, Texas) has found poorer near vision in low-light conditions and a lower reading speed under mesopic conditions in the ReSTOR patients (reading speed of 72 words per minute with ReSTOR versus 115 words per minute with ReZoom).[5] Another study found that the ReZoom IOL provided better average distance vision than the ReSTOR (average of 20/20 versus 20/25) and better intermediate vision (J 2.15 versus J 3.85, respectively).[6]

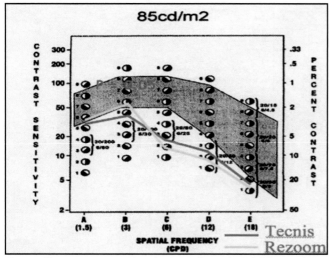

Figure 4. Photopic contrast sensitivity showing similar results with ReZoom and Tecnis IOLs.

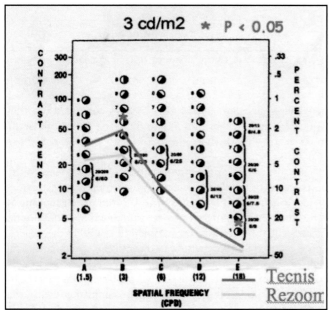

Figure 5. Mesopic contrast sensitivity showing superior results with Tecnis IOL at 3 and 18 cps.

Ideal Candidates for ReZoom Multifocal IOLs

Identifying the ideal candidate for implantation with a multifocal IOL is key to success with this lens. To this end, Stephen J. Dell, MD has developed a questionnaire (see Appendix A), which is in widespread use due to its ability to identify a patient's visual function desires, and to highlight a patient's personality. This useful tool should be considered by surgeons thinking about any lens-based refractive surgery.

Specifically for ReZoom lens implantation, I continue to make use of a series of questions designed to determine which patients should be targeted for possible multifocal lens surgery. These questions allow the surgeon to determine a patient's interest in multifocality and the patients' tolerance of short-

Table 1

IDEAL CANDIDATES FOR MULTIFOCAL IOLs

- Patients with realistic expectations and noncritical personalities.
- Patients who are motivated to reduce their dependency on eyeglasses.
- Individuals who understand that attaining near-vision may come with some sacrifice of quality in their distance vision and the potential for glare or halos.
- Patients with vision needs primarily in normal light levels and who do not perform a significant amount of nighttime driving.
- Hyperopic patients with presbyopia and some degree of cataract.
- Patients without ocular pathology that may preclude normal visual potential.
- Younger patients.

comings of the technology. Although these 3 key questions were originally introduced with the AMO Array multifocal IOL, I continue to use them in my practice for selecting potential ReZoom patients. These questions are as follows:

1. Following cataract surgery, would you like to be less dependent on your eyeglasses or are you happy the way you are?

2. This new procedure may produce glare or halos around lights at night that the brain adapts to within several months. Would that bother you?

3. Would you accept the use of glasses for certain limited occasions?

A primary advantage to the implantation of a multifocal IOL is the opportunity to eliminate or significantly reduce one's dependency on eyeglasses. Of the many characteristics that define the "ideal" multifocal lens patient (Table 1), a key criterion is the patient's desire for freedom from spectacles. The patient should have an active lifestyle with a desire to decrease dependency on glasses; he or she should be motivated with an accepting and adaptable personality. The fussy, obsessive, introspective patient who is not accepting of an adaptive period should be avoided.

Word-of-mouth and the widespread availability of medical information have resulted in many patients considering postoperative spectacle independence as a necessity rather than a mere bonus of this technology. Ideally, those considering multifocal IOLs should not only understand and desire functional vision, but should also have an awareness and acceptance of the possible compromises. Patients whose occupation involves significant night driving or working in low-light conditions (such as a pilot) should be discouraged due to the decreased contrast vision under mesopic conditions with multifocal IOLs. Significantly, an answer in the negative for any of the 3 key questions would tend to disqualify the patient for ReZoom lens implantation.

In order to improve postoperative outcomes, surgeons need to provide proactive patient counseling and align the patient's expectations with the anticipated outcome. All patients should

Table 2

IOL FORMULAS AND AXIAL LENGTH, SHOWING DEGREE OF ACCURACY (FROM WARREN HILL, MD)

AI in mm	Haigis only a0 Optimized	Haigis a0, a1, & a2 Optimized	Hoffer Q ACD Optimized	Holladay 1 SF Optimized	Holladay 2 ACD Optimized	SRK/T A-constant Optimized
18.00 – 19.99	0.50 D	0.50 D	0.50 D	1.00 D	0.50 D	2.00 D
20.00 – 21.99	0.25 D	0.25 D	0.25 D	0.50 D	0.25 D	1.00 D
22.00 – 25.99	0.25 D	0.25 D	0.25 D	0.25 D	0.25 D	0.25 D
26.00 – 27.99	0.25 D	0.25 D	0.50 D	0.25 D	0.25 D	0.25 D
28.00 – 30.00	0.50 D	0.25 D	0.50 D	0.25 D	0.25 D	0.50 D
Minus power IOLs	1.00 D	0.50 D	1.00 D	0.50 D	0.50 D	1.00 D

be made aware that "freedom from eyeglasses" is accompanied by the potential for night glare and loss of contrast, which may be perceived as reduced distance quality. It should be emphasized that a patient's perception of these nighttime halos will likely diminish over time.

Once it is found that a patient is interested in multifocal IOL surgery and has the "ideal attitude," the next step is to ensure that the patient has the "ideal eye." Ideally, there should be a significant cataract, as these patients are more appreciative of their vision postoperatively. A significant hyperopic or high myopic refraction is preferable to a low myopic one as the former patients appreciate the new-found uncorrected distance and near vision with a multifocal IOL. Low myopes tend to have good near vision without spectacles preoperatively and have this as a basis for comparison postoperatively; thus, the potential for dissatisfaction is high. The patient should also have normal eyes with no evidence of significant tear dysfunction; of corneal pathology such as significant astigmatism greater than 1 D, scarring, dystrophy, dysplasia, ectasia, or history of corneal refractive surgery; of capsular or zonular abnormality; or of retinal problems. The pupil diameter should be larger than 2.5 mm so that at least 2 of the refractive zones of the ReZoom are exposed by the pupil in order to gain full benefit from the multifocal technology. Finally, as younger patients (50 to 70 years old) adapt more quickly and have been found to have greater spectacle independence, they may be better candidates than their older (eg, 80-year-old) counterparts.

Having identified the "ideal patient" with the "ideal eye," it is also necessary to perform the "ideal surgery." Accuracy in biometry is imperative. To this end, the staff member doing the biometry should be experienced. Either immersion biometry or the IOL Master (Carl Zeiss Meditec) should be used to determine the axial length; these instruments should be regularly calibrated. The surgeon factor should be optimized; an initial A constant can be obtained from the IOL Master User Group Website (www.augenklinik.uni-wuerzburg.de/eulib/const.htm) and this should then be optimized by collect-

ing data on all initial patients implanted. Twenty patients can be used for a preliminary adjustment, and then further adjustment should be made as more patients are implanted. The formula used for IOL calculation should be varied according to axial length measurement. Table 2 gives a recommendation with the most accurate formula on the top of the list for each axial length.

The refractive endpoint depends on the patient's needs. For most patients, the recommendation is to target plano to +0.50 D. This optimizes distance vision, minimizes dysphotopsias, and reduces the near blur circle. However, in patients who want to maximize near vision and who *are not concerned* with night driving, a target of –0.50 D should be considered. If the refractive target is not met, then adjustment either by IOL exchange or laser refractive corneal surgery should be considered. This can be done once refractive stability has been documented and can be as early as 4 weeks postoperatively. It should be borne in mind that not all patients necessarily desire a secondary procedure, and that in some, in particular elderly patients, a weak pair of corrective glasses may be acceptable. Prior to further surgery, options should be fully explored with the patients.

The surgery should be flawless in execution. Small incision surgery so as to minimize induced astigmatism should be performed. The capsulorrhexis should be centered and made 0.5 mm smaller than the optic so as to ensure an overlapping capsulorrhexis edge. All cortical material must be aspirated to prevent the formation of secondary cataract, and the IOL should be placed in the capsular bag. All preoperative corneal astigmatism should be addressed with limbal relaxing incisions, astigmatic keratotomy, or subsequent laser corneal refractive surgery; astigmatism of as little as 0.5 D can deteriorate the image significantly. This correction can be done intraoperatively or postoperatively. An excellent example of an astigmatic correction normogram is listed in Figure 6.

In the postoperative period, the posterior capsule should have pristine clarity. Any decrease in clarity or any wrinkling of the capsule can result in degradation of the vision,

For With-the-Rule and Oblique Astigmatism

Astigmatism (in diopters)	40 – 50yo	50 – 60yo	60 – 70yo	70 – 80yo	80 + yo
1.00 – 1.50	60°(1)	50°(1)	50°(1)	40°(1)	30°(1)
1.50 – 2.00	70°(1)	70°(1)	70°(1)	60°(1)	60°(1)
2.00 – 2.50	60°(2)	60°(2)	60°(2)	70°(1)	70°(1)
2.50 – 3.00	70°(2)	70°(2)	70°(2)	60°(2)	60°(2)
3.00 – 4.00	80°(2)	80°(2)	80°(2)	70°(2)	70°(2)

For Against-the-Rule and Astigmatism

Astigmatism (in diopters)	40 – 50yo	50 – 60yo	60 – 70yo	70 – 80yo	80 + yo
1.00 – 1.50	60°(1)	50°(1)	40°(1)	40°(1)	30°(1)
1.50 – 2.00	70°(1)	60°(1)	60°(1)	60°(1)	40°(1)
2.00 – 2.50	60°(2)	80°(2)	80°(2)	70°(1)	60°(1)
2.50 – 3.00	70°(2)	70°(2)	70°(2)	60°(2)	60°(2)
3.00 – 4.00	80°(2)	80°(2)	80°(2)	70°(2)	70°(2)

(1) – denotes one (1) incision
(2) – denotes two (2) incisions

When using nomogram, if age/astigmatism at dividing point:
  – choose shortest incision length
  – choose one incision over two

*Wallace LRI Nomogram / Developed by R. Bruce Wallace III, M.D.

Figure 6. R Bruce Wallace II AK normogram.

especially the near vision. In these circumstances, a capsulotomy should be performed.

In the postoperative period, the patient may be slow to adapt to the simultaneous vision. If this is the case, counseling and encouragement should be offered to the patient; occasionally, dilute pilocarpine drops or –1.0 D spectacles may also be temporarily employed. These symptoms usually resolve over a period of 6 months.

If glare and halos are intolerable, "hand-holding" encouragement should be proffered to the patient. The patient should be reassured that the symptoms diminish over time and they should not become too obsessed with them. If the patient is particularly unhappy, then temporizing maneuvers may be tried. Alphagan (Allergan, Irvine, CA) or dilute pilocarpine drops to constrict the pupil, turning on the dashboard lights during night driving, polarized lenses, or –1.0 D spectacles have all been used with varying success.

For the patient who still does not adapt to dysphotopsias after 6 months, ReZoom lens explantation should be considered. However, the patient should be informed of the potential disadvantages of this secondary procedure. It is my experience that the majority of patients when informed of and shown the loss of near vision (by having the patient read unaided, and then through a –3.00 D lens to see the implications of replacement with a monofocal IOL) will opt not to be explanted.

Remember that not all complaints of dysphotopsias are bad. Many patients when confronted with the complaint and asked if it is bothersome will offer that it was more of an observation rather than a complaint. One prime example of this is given in Figure 7, in which the patient admitted to bragging about his new vision.

Matching Lens Options to Patient's Lifestyle and Vision Needs

Several strategies have been developed over the years to increase patient satisfaction following cataract extraction and lens implantation. One that is gaining widespread acceptance is that of "Staged Implantation" of multifocal or accommodative lenses (as reviewed in Table 3).

Staged implantation requires the surgeon to review patient characteristics so as to determine and implant the best IOL in the first eye. The lens choice should be based on several key considerations with distance vision being a primary consideration. The next consideration should be the patient's requirements for visual range; the patient should be questioned regarding the level of activity or inactivity that is normal for him or her; if there is a requirement for near vision for work- or leisure-related activities; and if spectacle independence is desired for computer or near activities.

In patients with cataracts, implantation should be performed on the dominant eye first, except in cases where there is a significant best-corrected visual acuity difference between the eyes. In these cataract cases, it is recommended that the worst eye is implanted first. In patients who are "pre-cataract," ocular dominance should also be determined with the primary lens implanted in the dominant eye first.

Following implantation of the first lens, patients should be re-examined after 1 to 2 weeks and assessed for vision satisfaction. For those who are not satisfied with their primary lens, every

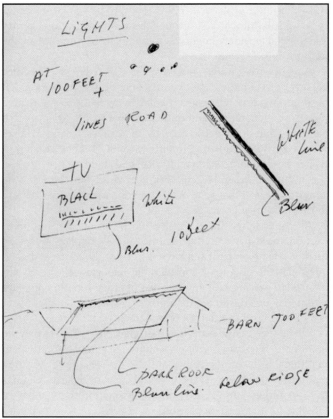

Figure 7. Dysphotopsias noted by a patient who was not bothered but felt compelled to draw his new vision.

effort should be made to determine the exact cause of their dissatisfaction (ie, dissatisfied with near-, intermediate-, distance-, or night-vision; or with the perception of halo and glare). IOL selection for the second eye should be based on the patient's satisfaction and vision with their first IOL. Figure 8 illustrates a "staged implantation" scenario staring with the ReZoom IOL in the first eye, with subsequent lens selection based on the patient's 1 to 2 week postoperative visit assessment.

There are several benefits to the use of a staged implantation strategy. First and foremost, it allows patients to actively participate in their care as well as the customization of IOL selection to their individual lifestyle and vision needs. It also allows clinicians an extra opportunity to maximize patient satisfaction with their implanted IOLs.

In clinical practice, I have found that the majority of my patients are satisfied with bilateral ReZoom IOL implantation. Implantation of a second, different IOL is offered in exceptional cases in which the ReZoom lens is found to be inadequate in the first eye.

Non-Ideal Patients and Situations

Before considering the use of a ReZoom multifocal IOL in compromised conditions or eyes, the limitations of its use must be considered. Although a multifocal IOL can provide superior intermediate and near vision compared to a monofocal IOL, this comes at a price, which is the loss of some contrast

Table 3			
SELECTED LENSES USED IN STAGED IMPLANTATION			
	*ReZoom**	*ReSTOR***	*Crystalens****
Diameter	6.0 mm	6.0 mm	4.5 mm
Material	Hydrophobic, acrylic, UV blocking	Acrylic, blue light, or UV blocking	Silicone
Diopter range	6.0 to 30.0 D with 0.5-D increments	10.0 to 30.0 D with 0.5-D increments	10.0 to 27.0 D with 0.25-D increments
A-constant	118.4	118.1	119.24
Near add	+3.5 D at lens plane, +2.6 D at spectacle plane	+4.0 D at lens plane, +3.2 D at spectacle plane	+1.0 D of accommodative power
Haptics/design	3-piece 13-mm overall length Triple edge design	1-piece	1-piece with hinged plate haptics, 11.5 mm overall length
Spectacle independence (per package inserts)	92% "never" or only "occasionally" wear glasses By visual need: 93% never needed glasses for distance or intermediate and 81% never needed glasses for near	80% across all distances	25.8% never wear spectacles 73.5% never or almost none of the time

*AMO, Santa Ana, CA; **Alcon Laboratories, Fort Worth, TX; ***Eyeonics, Aliso Viejo, CA

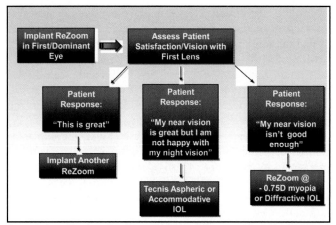

Figure 8. Staged implantation. (Figured reproduced from materials on file at Advanced Medical Optics.)

sensitivity. Fortunately, under bright light conditions, there is no difference in distance contrast sensitivity between these 2 groups. This finding may be explained by the previous reports that as pupil size diminishes, the effect of spherical aberration on contrast sensitivity is minimized, and photopic pupils tend to be small. However, under mesopic conditions, distance vision is decreased under higher spatial frequencies. With near vision, compared to corrected near vision with a monofocal IOL, multifocal IOLs provide decreased contrast sensitivity for all spatial frequencies and illuminations.[7]

With respect to contrast sensitivity, it should be remembered that patients with cataracts have reduced contrast sensitivity prior to cataract extraction. This may explain why these patients, when implanted with a multifocal IOL, do not appreciate any decreased contrast sensitivity.

The following discussion reviews studies that have looked at multifocal IOL use in unusual situations. The majority of these studies were with the zonal refractive IOL, the AMO Array. The ReZoom is also a zonal refractive IOL, but with significant design improvements. Although studies with the ReZoom have not been reported for these situations, I have encountered many of them and had the opportunity to use the ReZoom with comparable excellent results.

ReZoom in Patients With Concurrent Disease

Multifocal IOLs have traditionally not been advocated in patients who have concurrent eye disease. This recommendation is similar to that which was originally given for IOLs when they were introduced into mainstream cataract surgery. In fact, package inserts for most IOLs still list concurrent ocular diseases as a contraindication for IOL implantation. However, recent experience has expanded the boundaries and it is now acceptable to implant an IOL in almost any patient undergoing cataract surgery. In a similar fashion, multifocal IOL indications will likely also expand as experience is amassed.

As clinical experience with multifocal IOLs has increased, their benefit has been reported in a meta analysis of 10 clinical trials.[8] Visual acuity, visual satisfaction, spectacle dependence, glare, and contrast sensitivity were compared with standard

IOLs. Distance visual acuity was found to be similar in monofocal and multifocal IOL groups; however, near visual acuity and spectacle independence was found to be superior in the multifocal IOL group.

A prospective study[9] looked at the effectiveness of multifocal IOLs in 111 patients with concurrent disease, including diabetic retinopathy, glaucoma, ocular hypertension, age-related macular degeneration, and optic neuropathy. Of 133 eyes that were implanted, 81 eyes received an Array IOL and 52 eyes received a standard IOL. No difference in distance visual outcomes was found between multifocal and standard IOL groups; the multifocal group had superior near vision and there was no compromise in management of the concurrent ocular disease in the multifocal group.

As contrast sensitivity is affected by glaucoma, one must caution these patients that multifocal IOL implantation may further impair contrast sensitivity. In a poorly controlled glaucoma patient, this is of considerable importance. For a well-controlled patient with minimal loss of visual function, implantation may be considered for a properly counseled patient who is motivated to have decreased spectacle dependence.

Of further consideration is that glaucoma patients may be monitored by scanning laser technologies, and the effect of multifocal IOLs on the ability of these devices to register their readings is unknown. Thus, it would be wise to take readings prior to surgery, and shortly after implantation so as to have a baseline for further comparison.

In patients with age-related macular degeneration, the use of multifocal IOLs *may be* contraindicated if the goal of surgery is to restore driving vision because contrast sensitivity will be diminished compared to a monofocal aspheric IOL. However, if the goal is to improve reading vision, a multifocal IOL may provide additional magnification. If the surgical outcome is plano, and a +3.00 reader is used, magnification of 1.5× occurs at the near focal point; with a −2.00 result, and a +3.00 reader, magnification of 2× results. These magnifications can make it possible for a patient with 6/9 to 6/18 compromised vision from age-related macular degeneration to read (R. Lindstrom, personal communication).

In cataract surgery complicated by vitreous loss, multifocal IOLs may be implanted into the sulcus with good outcomes. In a study of 15 eyes, it was found that subjective and objective visual results were good; 93% of patients had improved vision, 73% had 6/12 or better distance vision, and 80% had at least J2 BCNVA.[10]

In these cases, it is important that the IOL remains centered. Decentration of 1.0 mm can result in vision decreasing below 6/12. Thus, the creation of an anterior capsulorrhexis of 0.5 mm less in diameter than the optic is of paramount importance in these cases for maintenance of centration. In complicated surgery, attempts should be made to capture the optic behind an intact anterior capsulorrhexis and to place the haptics in the sulcus. A smaller, well-centered capsulorrhexis should capture the optic and afford excellent centration.

If it is not possible to place the optic behind the capsulorrhexis, the IOL may still be placed in the sulcus. Stability of the optic in the sulcus may be tested by performing the spring back test; a Sinsky hook is used to displace the IOL by a few millimeters, and then released to see if the optic "springs back" into position. If it does not, then the likelihood of the

IOL decentering is high and the multifocal IOL should be removed.

Because eyes complicated by vitreous loss are at higher risk for further surgical intervention, in particular vitreoretinal procedures, there may be concerns that the surgical view may be compromised by multifocal IOLs. In order to investigate this possibility, rabbit eyes were implanted with either a monofocal or a multifocal IOL.[11] It was found that vitrectomy with retinal surface maneuvers was possible through both IOL types; visualization of posterior segment structures was adequate in both fluid-filled and air-filled eyes.

In addition, it has been reported that laser photocoagulation of the retina and macula is not compromised in patients with multifocal IOLs.[9]

Pupil Less Than 2.5 mm

The ReZoom multifocal IOL is a zonal refractive lens; in order for it to work, the light has to pass through the various zones. Pupil size needs to be assessed. It should be borne in mind that the measured pupil size is about 15% greater than the true pupil size due to the magnification of the anterior optical system of the eye (this is true for an eye with an average anterior corneal curvature and anterior chamber depth; significant deviations from this will affect the value).[12]

Near vision with the ReZoom can occur either through the use of the pinhole effect or through the use of the near vision zones. To utilize the pinhole effectively, a pupil measuring less than 1.9 mm is needed. However, the ideal conditions for near vision occur with the ReZoom when the pupil is larger than 2.5 mm, and ideally at 3.8 mm. In an average-sized anterior chamber, these pupils sizes correspond to the diameter of the second zone of the IOL, after adjustment for corneal magnification.

If the pupil diameter is too small for effective near vision, laser pupilloplasty can be employed to enlarge the pupil by 0.5 to 1.0 mm. Using an Argon laser, the initial series of 8 to 12 burns should be applied for 360 degrees, near the papillary margin. These spots should be 300 μm in size to start, and applied for an exposure of 0.2 sec (which can be increased to 0.5 sec) at 0.15 watts power, to produce this effect. The power can be increased if no contraction of the pupil muscle occurs, but too high a setting should be avoided as this can produce thermal necrosis of the iris. A second ring of burns outside the first row should also be applied, but the spot size should be increased to 500 μm. Once again, the power setting may need to be adjusted to produce the desired effect of pupil contouring.

If the pupil is eccentric, then Argon pupilloplasty can be used to realign and reshape the pupil by placing the burns in an arcuate pattern in the direction in which the pupil needs to be moved (K. Waltz, personal communication).

Needed IOL Power Outside Available Range

For patients who are highly hyperopic or myopic, if the calculated ReZoom IOL power is not available, then piggyback IOL implantation can be considered. As with any piggyback procedure, one IOL should be placed in the capsular bag, within a centered capsulorrhexis, which is smaller than the optic in size, and the piggyback IOL should be placed in the sulcus. The monofocal IOL should be placed in the capsular bag, and the ReZoom should be placed in the sulcus, as the refractive zones are on the anterior surface of the lens. Sulcus placement of the ReZoom has been previously discussed, and the guidelines given should be followed.

Good results have also been reported with the piggybacking of multifocal IOLs.[13] Similarly, in a patient with anisometropia, multifocal IOL implantation may require piggyback implantation in the eye with greater refractive error. This combination of a single multifocal IOL in one eye, and a piggyback solution in the second anisometropic eye has been reported with good effect.[14]

One further situation in which a piggyback may be considered is in pseudophakic individuals who were originally implanted with a monofocal IOL. A multifocal IOL can then be placed in the sulcus, if the patient desires multifocality at a later date. The power of the piggyback IOL can be selected so as to compensate for any residual refractive error. Unfortunately, the ReZoom is not available in low powers; thus it cannot be used in situations that require a low power or when a zero power multifocal is to be used in emmetropic pseudophakes.[15] The AMO Array is available in low powers for this purpose.

Second Eye Surgery if Monofocal IOL in First Eye

Traditionally, the advice has been to implant a monofocal IOL in the second eye. However, more recent experience suggests that implantation of a multifocal IOL may be beneficial in this situation. In a prospective study involving monofocal and multifocal IOLs, 123 patients were identified who had a multifocal in one eye and a monofocal in the other eye.[16] It was found that mean uncorrected distance visual acuity were similar in monofocal and multifocal IOL eyes, but the multifocal IOL had a mean 2-line increase in uncorrected and distance corrected near visual acuity. Although low contrast visual acuity was measured to be decreased by 1 line of Snellen acuity in the multifocal eyes, no perceived disadvantage was apparent to the patients.

Ocular dominance has an influence on the outcome with a unilateral multifocal IOL. Implantation of a multifocal IOL into a dominant eye results in 80% spectacle independence for near vision compared to 22% if a nondominant eye is implanted.[17] However, there are some limitations to unilateral implantation of a multifocal IOL. Compared to bilateral implantation of multifocal IOL, unilateral cases have less stereopsis, more aniseikonia, and less spectacle independence for near vision.[17]

Unilateral Cataract

In a study of 95 pre-presbyopic patients with a unilateral cataract, 54 patients were implanted with a multifocal IOL.[18] Distance vision was similar in the multifocal and monofocal groups; however, uncorrected near visual acuity and stereopsis were significantly better in the multifocal IOL eyes. Similar findings were reported in patients presenting with traumatic cataracts. Eyes implanted with a multifocal IOL had superior results compared to those implanted with a monofocal IOL for near vision and for stereopsis.[19]

IOL Implantation in Children and Young Adults

It is only recently that IOL implantation in aphakic children and young adults has become accepted practice. However, it is still controversial to consider multifocal IOL implantation in this patient group. It has been reported that multifocal implantation in a cohort of 35 eyes of 26 children, aged 2 to 14 years, resulted in 71% having 6/12 or better, and 31% with 6/7.5 or better vision.[20] Although these results may seem low, one must remember that this is a group of patients in whom occlusive amblyopia due to congenital cataracts is common. Stereopsis was also improved following surgery in this group. Ten eyes required a second surgical procedure; 4 eyes required a membranectomy; and 6 required IOL repositioning. These secondary procedures are not uncommon in IOL implantation in children.

In a study of transcleral IOL fixation in 26 aphakic children and young adults, aged 6 to 29 years, 12 patients were implanted with a multifocal IOL.[21] The distance vision was similar in both groups; however, near vision (uncorrected and distance corrected) and stereopsis were significantly better in the multifocal IOL group. There was no difference in complications between the 2 groups. Similar findings were also reported in another study on aphakic pediatric patients implanted with scleral fixated multifocal IOLs.[22]

Conclusion

The ReZoom multifocal IOL is a significant addition to the armamentarium of the cataract and refractive surgeon. Knowledge of its design, mechanism of action, and limitations is essential for its effective and potentially extensive use. The ReZoom provides excellent distance and intermediate vision, and very good near vision. Reading vision and stereopsis are significantly improved with this lens. The issue of dysphotopsias is minor and tends to significantly diminish with time.

Acknowledgment

The author respectfully acknowledges the editorial assistance of Susan Ruffalo, PharmD, of MedWrite, Inc, Newport Coast, California.

References

1. Population Resource Center/U.S. Bureau of the Census. The demographics of aging in America. Available at www.prcdc.org/summaries/aging/aging.html.

2. Leibowitz HM, Krueger DE, Maunder LR, et al. The Framingham eye study monograph: an ophthalmological and epidemiological study of cataract, glaucoma, diabetic retinopathy, macular degeneration, and visual acuity in a general population of 2631 adults, 1973–1975. *Surv Ophthalmol.* 1980;24(Suppl):335-610.

3. Beiko G. Canadian Multicentre Evaluation of AMO ReZoom Multifocal IOL. Presented at the Congress of the European Society of Cataract and Refractive Surgeons; September 9-13, 2006; London.

4. Beiko G. Patients with AMO ReZoom Multifocal IOL or AMO Tecnis Monofocal IOL—comparison of quality of vision. Presented at Congress of the European Society of Cataract and Refractive Surgeons: Stockholm, 2007.

5. Huetz WW. Reading acuity and speed with different multifocal IOLs. Presented at Congress of the European Society of Cataract and Refractive Surgeons: September 9-13, 2006, London.

6. Akaishi L, Fabri PP. PC IOLS mix and match technologies: Brazilian experience. Presented at World Ophthalmology Congress; February 19-24, 2006; Sao Paolo, Brazil.

7. Montés-Micó R, España E, Bueno I, Charman WN, Menezo JL. Visual performance with multifocal intraocular lenses: mesopic contrast sensitivity under distance and near conditions. *Ophthalmology.* 2004;111(1):85-96.

8. Leyland M, Pringle E. Multifocal versus monofocal intraocular lenses after cataract extraction. *Cochrane Database Syst Rev.* 2006;(4).

9. Kamath GG, Prasad S, Danson A, Phillips RP. Visual outcome with the array multifocal intraocular lens in patients with concurrent eye disease. *J Cataract Refract Surg.* 2000;26(4):576-581.

10. Aralikatti AK, Tu KL, Kamath GG, Phillips RP, Prasad S. Outcomes of sulcus implantation of Array multifocal intraocular lenses in second-eye cataract surgery complicated by vitreous loss. *J Cataract Refract Surg.* 2004;30(1):155-160.

11. Lim JI, Kuppermann BD, Gwon A, Gruber L. Vitreoretinal surgery through multifocal intraocular lenses compared with monofocal intraocular lenses in fluid-filled and air-filled rabbit eyes. *Ophthalmology.* 2000;107(6):1083-1088.

12. Waltz KL, Rubin ML. Capsulorrhexis and corneal magnification. *Arch Ophthalmol.* 1992;110(2):170.

13. Donoso R, Rodríguez A. Piggyback implantation using the AMO array multifocal intraocular lens. *J Cataract Refract Surg.* 2001;27(9):1506-10.

14. Mejía LF. Piggyback posterior chamber multifocal intraocular lenses in anisometropia. *J Cataract Refract Surg.* 1999;25(12):1682-1684.

15. Clare G, Bloom P. Bilateral ciliary sulcus implantation of secondary piggyback multifocal intraocular lenses. *J Cataract Refract Surg.* 2007;33(2):320-322.

16. Steinert RF, Aker BL, Trentacost DJ, Smith PJ, Tarantino N. A prospective comparative study of the AMO ARRAY zonal-progressive multifocal silicone intraocular lens and a monofocal intraocular lens. *Ophthalmology.* 1999;106(7):1243-1255.

17. Shoji N, Shimizu K. Binocular function of the patient with the refractive multifocal intraocular lens. *J Cataract Refract Surg.* 2002;28(6):1012-1017.

18. Jacobi PC, Dietlein TS, Luke C, Jacobi FK. Multifocal intraocular lens implantation in prepresbyopic patients with unilateral cataract. *Ophthalmology.* 2002;109(4):680-686.

19. Jacobi PC, Dietlein TS, Lueke C, Jacobi FK. Multifocal intraocular lens implantation in patients with traumatic cataract. *Ophthalmology.* 2003;110(3):531-538.

20. Jacobi PC, Dietlein TS, Konen W. Multifocal intraocular lens implantation in pediatric cataract surgery. *Ophthalmology.* 2001;108(8):1375-1380.

21. Jacobi PC, Dietlein TS, Jacobi FK. Scleral fixation of secondary foldable multifocal intraocular lens implants in children and young adults. *Ophthalmology.* 2002;109(12):2315-2324.

22. Kumar M, Arora R, Sanga L, Sota LD. Scleral-fixated intraocular implantation in unilateral aphakic children. *Ophthalmology.* 1999;106(11): 2184-2189.

CHAPTER 30

HOW DO I GET STARTED WITH THE ReSTOR?

Richard Tipperman, MD

This quickstart guide is written to allow the surgeon beginning to perform multifocal intraocular lenses (IOLs) in general (and the ReSTOR lens [Alcon, Fort Worth, TX] specifically) a broad overview of clinical issues so that the more detailed information in the subsequent chapters can flow smoothly and logically. In its simplest terms, success with presbyopia-correcting (Pr-C) IOLs hinges on 3 main conditions: 1) appropriately selecting and counseling patients, 2) utilizing the selected presbyopic platform appropriately, and 3) managing any patient concerns in the postoperative period.

This quickstart guide is not meant to be a substitute for the wonderfully comprehensive information that can be found in each particular chapter; in fact, I have tried whenever possible to reference specific chapters of the remainder of this book, which will provide more comprehensive discussions of particular clinical concerns. It is hoped that by providing this broad overview, the more specific information available in each section and chapter will be more meaningful.

There could potentially be many ways to determine which presbyopic platform is best; however, one objective way is to examine market share. It is clear in ophthalmology that surgeons will utilize clinical products and procedures that they believe will produce the best possible results. This was evident with the rapid adoption of technologies such as foldable lenses, topical anesthesia, and clear corneal surgery. At the time of this writing, the ReSTOR IOL is utilized 60% of the time in the United States, the ReZoom IOL (Advanced Medical Optics, Santa Ana, CA) 30%, and the Crystalens (Eyeonics, Inc, Aliso Viejo, CA) 10%.

I was fortunate to be one of the original core investigators for the ReSTOR IOL and have also had the opportunity to utilize the aspheric version of this lens as well. In this chapter I would like to describe my basic clinical approach to the ReSTOR IOL.

Patient Selection: Picking the First Few Patients

The best initial ReSTOR patients have both significant bilateral cataracts and significant spherical refractive errors with minimal astigmatism. Although hyperopic patients are often described as the easiest to please with any presbyopic platform, my experience is that moderately to highly myopic patients are just as easy to "make happy" with the ReSTOR IOL.

Surgeons should avoid multifocal IOL surgery in patients with low myopia who are comfortable reading without correction. Because these patients are used to excellent uncorrected near vision preoperatively (and often do not notice the blur in distance without correction), they are very difficult to make happy with any Pr-C IOL platform.

There are 2 initial steps in the patient selection process: 1) determining if the patient can be educated about the advantages (and potential disadvantages) of the ReSTOR IOL, and 2) the patient indicating that he or she desires increased functional near vision following cataract surgery.

If the answer is "yes" to both of the above, then the patient may be a good ReSTOR candidate. If the answer is "no" to either, then it is not likely they would be a good candidate for any Pr-C IOL. (A detailed description of this education and counseling process is found in Chapter 99, Managing Patients Expectations)

The main details I want the patient to understand during the preoperative counseling process for the ReSTOR IOL are as follows:

* Their functional near vision will be much better with a ReSTOR IOL than it would be if they had chosen a conventional monofocal IOL.

* They will function best and be happiest once their second eye is implanted and they should view ReSTOR cataract surgery as a bilateral procedure.

* Early on, the "sweet-spot" for their near vision will be closer than they might normally hold something (I physically take their hands and show them where their reading will be clearest at 14 to 18 inches away). However, over time the range of vision will expand.

* Their best uncorrected vision will be for distance and near—they will function well at intermediate and the intermediate vision will improve over time, but it will not be as strong as their near or distance vision.

* There is the potential for glare and halo at night with a multifocal IOL and indeed any IOL. I explain that the majority of patients do not notice any difficulties with glare and halo. A small minority notice glare and halo and a smaller subset of these patients find it bothersome. This improves over time for most but not all patients. (This is even less of an issue with the aspheric ReSTOR IOL.)

* They may still wear glasses for some visual tasks—but they will still be better than they would have been had they chosen a conventional monofocal IOL.

* The procedure is "reversible." Conceivably if they are severely dissatisfied with their vision, the IOL can be replaced with a conventional monofocal IOL.

Patient Selection: Who Is Not a Candidate?

It is just as important to exclude certain patients as it is to select appropriate patients. Some patients will not be candidates because of unreasonable expectations whereas others will have ophthalmic contraindications.

The easiest way to determine if a patient has unreasonable expectations is if a patient wants a "guarantee" of spectacle independence or tells me he or she will only be happy if he or she "never wears glasses again." In both of these instances I do not believe these patients would be good candidates for any Pr-C IOL platform. I tell these patients, "I would not recommend surgery with these IOLs for you. The only guarantee I can give is that I will take the best care of you that I possibly can and that I will make things better than they would be if you had selected a monofocal IOL. Even with a ReSTOR IOL you may still wear glasses on occasion."

In many instances after hearing the above the patient will rephrase their position by saying something such as, "I'd like to not have to wear glasses but I understand now I may wear them for some activities…. still, all in all this seems like the best option for me."

If, as described above, the patient indicates a clear understanding of the potential need for occasional spectacle wear, then I tell him or her that as long as we both agree on this point I would consider him or her a candidate. I explain to the

patient that I will note this in the chart and remind him or her of it in the postoperative period as well.

The main ophthalmic contraindications to multifocal IOL usage would include any condition that could lead to a reduction in best-corrected visual acuity. Common entities include corneal abnormalities such as irregular astigmatism, significant keratitis sicca, advanced glaucoma, or any significant retinal disorder. Most surgeons consider even a subtle epiretinal membrane in the fovea as a contraindication to ReSTOR IOL implantation. This is not only because the induced metamorphopsia negatively affects the overall visual quality but also because they are at higher risk for cystoid macular edema.

Preoperative Planning

Section IX of this book contains chapters on ocular assessment with comprehensive articles on biometry, targeting emmetropia, and IOL calculations, all written by experts in these areas. It is critical reading regardless of the presbyopic platform being utilized.

With the ReSTOR IOL I personally target emmetropia and will modify my incision to treat corneal astigmatism of 0.5 D. Above 0.5 D and up to and including 2 D of corneal cylinder, I will perform limbal relaxing incisions (LRIs). (Surgical management of astigmatism is covered in Section X, Managing Astigmatism.) For patients with greater than 1.50 D of astigmatism, I explain that I cannot always reliably eliminate their entire astigmatic error and they may need a secondary procedure; I especially reinforce this for patients with greater than 2 D of astigmatism. I will still perform LRIs in these patients in an attempt to "de-bulk" their astigmatism so that there is less to correct with the laser platform.

Implantation of the ReSTOR IOL

The approach and management of the patient's intrinsic corneal cylinder will dictate the cataract incision location and sizing. Appropriate sizing of the capsulorrhexis is important for success with the ReSTOR IOL both because it allows for greater predictability of the IOL power and also because it allows the maximum portions of both the refractive and diffractive optic to be utilized.

If the capsulorrhexis is too small, then the peripheral portion of the ReSTOR IOL (which is purely refractive and transmits much of the light energy for the distance image) will be inhibited. This can lead to poor-quality distance vision as well as poor-quality night vision. If the capsulorrhexis constricts enough, it will conceivably interfere with the near vision by obscuring the outer portion of the apodized diffractive rings. (Capsulorrhexis sizing and complications of capsulorrhexis sizing are covered in Chapters 182 and 227)

Surgeons familiar with implantation of the 1-piece AcrySof IOL (Alcon) will find that their insertion technique readily transfers to the ReSTOR IOL. However, one distinction is that although haptic orientation is not critical with a monofocal IOL with the ReSTOR IOL, most surgeons will leave the haptics oriented vertically in the capsular bag (ie, from 12 o'clock to 6 o'clock). This is done to allow for best centration of the apodized rings when the pupil is in its normal physiologic state. When patients are pharmacologically dilated for cataract surgery, they typically have a centroid shift, which causes the geometric center of the dilated pupil to be more temporal than it would be in its resting state. By having the haptics oriented vertically, the surgeon can "nudge" the IOL optic nasally by approximately 1 mm to account for the centroid shift when the pharmacologic dilation resolves.

Postoperative Management

The postoperative management of ReSTOR patients is similar in many respects to that of conventional cataract patients; however, there are some important differences that the transitioning surgeon should be aware of. For example, the vision on the first postoperative day (POD) will often be reduced because of factors such as residual pupillary dilation, corneal drying, or other normal "POD 1" changes. This is especially true for the near vision. I inform my patients of this preoperatively and tell them that either myself or my staff will remind them of this detail postoperatively. (This is much less of an issue with the aspheric ReSTOR IOL and it is more common to see patients with a "wow factor" on POD 1. Nonetheless I still educate patients in this manner to establish realistic expectations.)

After the first eye has been done, patients will typically be re-evaluated in 5 to 7 days. At this point they are usually happy with the visual function in their first eye but may have questions about specific observations they are making with regard to their visual function.

In my experience, 85% to 90% of patients are quite pleased with their visual function and interested in proceeding quickly with their second eye surgery. The next subset of patients (10% to 12%) fall into the category I term "good, but not great." They are functioning well for distance but feel the near vision is not as good as they would desire. This is the group of patients who benefit the most from proceeding with their second eye because of the phenomenon of binocular summation. I remind these patients that we discussed preoperatively that they should view their surgery as a bilateral procedure and that they would be happiest when their second eye was implanted.

The remaining small subset of patients (2% to 3%) not only are not happy with their visual function but they may actually be dissatisfied. The most common reason for this is a residual refractive error. In some multifocal patients, residual cylinder of even 0.5 D can lead to unsatisfactory vision. Depending on the patients' expectations and desires, I will either 1) proceed with the second eye with the goal of helping them function so well bilaterally that they are no longer symptomatic with regard to the residual refractive error in the fellow eye, or 2) perform an appropriate refractive procedure to improve the uncorrected vision in the first eye.

The remaining patients in this "dissatisfied" subgroup will be patients with dysphotopsias or unwanted optical images. In these cases I personally recommend against proceeding with multifocal IOL implantation in the fellow eye until the situation has come to resolution. In many instances the images are not that bothersome or improve overtime. These patients can proceed to ReSTOR implantation in the fellow eye.

If the patient has good visual acuity for distance and near but finds the unwanted optical images persistent and bothersome, then I will consider placing a monofocal IOL in the fellow eye. Often that will allow good distance vision with suppression of the unwanted optical images.

If the patient is significantly dissatisfied with their vision for any reason, I will offer him or her the option of an IOL exchange. In my personal experience, the need for this is fortunately extremely rare.

CHAPTER 31

How Do I Get Started With the Tecnis Multifocal?

Julian D. Stevens, MRCP, FRCS, FRCOphth

The Tecnis multifocal lens implant (Advanced Medical Optics, Santa Ana, CA) was once described by one of my patients as a "double lens implant" and for the recipient of such lenses this is how it appears to function. The lens is a very effective multifocal in the clinical setting.[1-3] The key optical feature of the Tecnis multifocal lens is the aspheric optic,[4] as the lens is based on the successful Tecnis monofocal lens platform with a modified prolate anterior surface.

The aspheric design tightens both the distance and near focus, aiming for higher contrast and a better quality of perceived vision. The aspheric optic and the diffractive design are key features in ensuring the lens' function has considerable independence from pupil size.[5] Both the current Tecnis multifocal with low refractive index silicone and the future acrylic Tecnis multifocal provide a far distance focus and a +4.0 D near add equivalent.

The Tecnis multifocal lens has a strong distance and near (+4.0 D) focus with relatively little in between (Figure 1). It is therefore suitable for those who wish to read well—in particular smaller text or music. Currently it is often combined with the refractive multifocal ReZoom lens in the opposite eye, which provides for significant intermediate focus. This "custom matching" is very popular, allowing for a spread of vision when neural adaptation has taken place.[6] In my own practice, currently most Tecnis multifocal lenses are used as custom matching with the ReZoom being placed in the non-dominant eye.

Preoperative Assessment

The preoperative assessment is critical. The surgeon has to make a decision as to whether monofocal, monovision, multifocal, or accommodating lenses are to be used. This is based on the consultation, vision measurement, visual potential, and also very much on the patient's occupation, interests, and future possible needs.

It is important to clarify for both patient and surgeon the patient's expectations and to manage this so that these are acceptable to the patient.

Some occupations have restrictions regarding which intraocular lenses (IOLs) can be used. Currently commercial pilots are prevented from having multifocal lens implants. When the patient is a professional driver, such as a bus or truck driver, and there may be considerable need for night driving I discourage the use of multifocal lenses or monovision.

Age is also an important consideration because with increasing age (>75 years) there may be coexisting disease, such as glaucoma and macular degeneration. Patients are then less able to deal with the halos and visual phenomena associated with multifocal lenses. When there is cataract in the prepresbyope or in the early emerging presbyope or where there is clear lens exchange in the 45-year-old presbyope, then the visual phenomena can appear to be quite a surprise. It is important to advise that it may take 3 months for neural adaptation to occur.[6] Fortunately, considerable neural adaptation in the visual system occurs even by 1 week.[7]

There is no single approach that I use for all patients. In discussing what to do, let us consider the following different categories of patients presenting either for cataract or clear lens surgery.

* Pre-presbyopia cataract
* Emerging presbyopia (up to mid 50s)
* Post-presbyopia (55+), often with the beginnings of lenticular change and increasing high-order aberration
* Elderly (>75 years)

Cataract Versus Refractive Lensectomy

Where there is cataract and there has been a longstanding deterioration in visual quality the visual phenomena and halos associated with multifocal lens implants are usually well tolerated. The patient's perception will be that his or her vision got better with surgery. The Tecnis multifocal lens with its excellent distance and near focus provides for a dramatic reversal of presbyopia for the patient.

Figure 1. The Tecnis multifocal lens has a strong distance and near (+4.0 D) focus with relatively little in between. (Reproduced with permission from Advanced Medical Optics.)

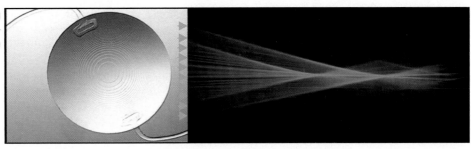

In contrast, with a refractive lens exchange for presbyopia the patient is exchanging good corrected vision for pseudophakic multifocal vision. These patients may have considerable symptoms of halos, glare, and visual phenomena in dim illumination early on. This is especially the case during night driving and many of these patients report that the reduced contrast and optical phenomena make them cautious with night driving in this early postoperative period. There is a powerful process of neural adaptation over time and patients begin to feel more confident as they become used to their new vision. It is my practice to most often use the ReZoom lens in the dominant eye and to perform this surgery first. I would then implant the Tecnis multifocal lens in the nondominant eye most commonly a week later. If the patient is not happy with the first lens implant, I delay performing the second eye surgery.

It is important therefore to discuss with patients that achieving spectacle independence with multifocal lenses will lead to some light phenomena at night. This is difficult for people to grasp, as it is an abstract concept for many people unless they have already used multifocal contact lenses. Many patients can be hesitant as it is a leap of faith to accept having such visual phenomena.

Postpresbyopia (55+) Often With the Beginnings of Lenticular Change and Increasing High-Order Aberration

This is the most common group of patients in which I use multifocal lenses and the Tecnis multifocal in particular. There is often early lenticular change, with progressive reduction of contrast sensitivity in dim light. In this situation I am reluctant to consider a laser procedure such as wavefront-guided laser in situ keratomileusis (LASIK), due to the reduced contrast and the potential future instability of the refraction due to lenticular change. The human eye appears to tolerate a certain degree of aberration and forward scatter to the retina. The retinal cones have wave-guide properties[8,9] (Stiles-Crawford effect) but rods have much less.[10] As a result, there can be perceived photopic glare despite good scotopic vision.

Where there is forward scatter from prior corneal laser refractive surgery or corneal irregularity I avoid multifocal lenses. If the scatter exceeds the threshold where it can be tolerated, then the patient will probably have excessive symptoms. Adding a diffractive multifocal lens behind an irregular cornea would lead to symptomatic reduced quality of vision.

The Elderly

Reduced macular function often accompanies advanced age. The typical visual deterioration associated with advanced aging is macular/visual system in origin. Age-associated straylight scatter in the human eye may also be a factor.[11] The elderly eye appears to be less able to image process the forward scatter inherent in the multifocal lens and there may be issues with reduction in contrast sensitivity. I therefore prefer using monofocal lenses in this age group. It can be very difficult to assess the retina and macula on slit-lamp examination through a significant cataract. If one performs macular optical coherence tomography (OCT) imaging in the elderly, one might commonly find an early epimacular membrane. There may be mild amblyopia in one eye, which was not recalled by the patient in the initial history due to longstanding cataract. Implanting a multifocal lens in an amblyopic eye already with reduced contrast sensitivity can lead to dim and poor quality vision.

I screen carefully for the following:

* Corneal irregularity (eg, previous keratorefractive surgery where there is high corneal aberration)
* Keratoconus or significant ectasia where there is high corneal aberration
* High corneal astigmatism ($\geq$3.0 D)
* Diabetes
* Macular disease
* Lack of stereopsis/strabismus
* Amblyopia
* Decentered preoperative pupil or tonic dilated pupil
* Unrealistic expectations and reluctance to accept postoperative optical phenomena

The Consultation

The consultation is supplemented with Steven Dell's patient questionnaire, which every patient completes (Appendix A). I have made only small modifications to this, specifically for U.K. patients. This is complemented by detailed information about phaco surgery and the options available. After initial detailed assessment by my technician, optometrist, and cataract fellow, I review the options with the patient. At this stage the patient has been pre-assessed, has had time to consider the options available, and I can provide further guidance. Patients commonly are already clear as to whether they will opt for multifocal lenses or monofocal distance-distance or monofocal monovision.

Those used to contact lens monovision most commonly opt to retain this with monofocal IOL monovision. Those who could not tolerate monovision or who have never tried it can consider multifocal lenses. A contact lens trial of monovision can be attempted preoperatively, but often this is not possible because of cataracts.

High Astigmatism

When there is a high amount of corneal astigmatism it is difficult to completely correct this with limbal relaxing incisions (LRI). For lesser amounts of astigmatism (3.0 D or less) I perform LRI, often in both eyes at the time of the original phaco surgery. Performing bilateral LRI in this way allows me to review the residual corneal cylinder for both eyes using topography prior to the second surgery. This provides an opportunity to refine either astigmatic result with additional LRI when the second operation is scheduled. Longer term additional LRI refinement can also be done at the slit lamp using a nasal mini lid speculum, slit-lamp guarded diamond blade, and angulation marker (Duckworth & Kent Ltd, slit-lamp LRI set). This instrument set is excellent for performing minor cylinder adjustment in an outpatient setting.

Excimer Laser Keratorefractive Surgery

Excimer laser keratorefractive surgery is very effective for treating residual low-order (sphere and cylinder) aberration and can also treat some high-order aberration after phaco surgery. Currently a wavefront-guided laser application cannot be performed if there is a refractive multifocal lens in situ as the system will attempt to apply a multifocal correction to the cornea (to offset that of the multifocal IOL). A wavefront-guided treatment can be performed, however, when there is a Tecnis multifocal lens in situ.

The wavefront sensor has 2 zones of focus and these are discreet. It is straightforward using the VISX WaveScan (Santa Clara, CA) to obtain the spherocylinder consistent with manifest refraction and then to apply a wavefront-guided laser treatment. This can be very helpful if there is defocus present. The diffractive rings do not cause difficulties with the keratorefractive surgery.

A key decision with excimer laser enhancement is whether to perform LASIK/IntraLASIK or surface ablation. If a yttrium-aluminum-garnet (YAG) capsulotomy has been performed, I tend to perform surface ablation. LASIK/IntraLASIK involves the application of suction to the eye with applanation of the cornea. This can distort the anterior segment and may cause the IOL to move slightly, which could affect focus or aberration. In addition, there may be a risk that vitreous could prolapse around the edge of the IOL after YAG laser capsulotomy and sufficient applanation pressure.

Where there is a clear, intact posterior capsule, the Tecnis multifocal IOL is stable within the capsular bag and there is no contraindication to the application of suction pressure to the eye, then IntraLASIK is very effective, fast, and efficient in improving the unaided vision.

I perform surface ablation whenever I wish to avoid suction pressure and patients normally tolerate this well. The older patient appears to tolerate surface treatment (wavefront-guided laser-assisted epithelial keratomileusis [LASEK]) very well using modern bandage contact lenses such as PureVision (Bausch & Lomb, Rochester, NY) or Night&Day (CIBA Vision, Duluth, GA).

I do not commonly perform bioptics, where an IntraLASIK flap is created prior to phaco surgery, as only a small proportion of these eyes will require laser refractive surgery when pseudophakic. Careful LRI surgery can reduce pre-existing astigmatism considerably.

There are commonly some induced aberrations from laser refractive surgery. When these are combined with the forward scatter from a LASIK flap interface, they may interfere with the patient's ability to image process aberration through a multifocal lens implant. In the future this will be an area of much research interest.

Corneal Topography

All patients have corneal topography during the initial consultation because multifocal lenses are contraindicated if any corneal irregularity is present. Topography is also used to assess the corneal spherical aberration such that the Tecnis multifocal IOL can also be used to compensate for any positive corneal spherical aberration.[12] Corneal topography is also performed after surgery to assess for residual corneal and lenticular cylinder.

Biometry and Residual Refractive Error

Attention to detail with preoperative biometry is important to minimize unintended postoperative ametropia. The lens constant for the Tecnis (silicone) multifocal is 119.0 or 118.9.[13] Surgeons using Wolfgang Haigis' excellent formulae should perform the necessary optimization. I use the IOL Master (Carl Zeiss Meditec, Jena, Germany) together with a comparison review of corneal topography. This is to ensure the autokeratometry is consistent with dedicated corneal topographers. The preoperative anterior chamber depth is important because an unusually deep or shallow anterior chamber may lead to a less predictable final axial IOL position. It may be worth emphasizing the possible need for a laser refractive procedure to the patient if there is postoperative spherical defocus. The Holladay IOL Consultant (Holiday II formula), Wolfgang Haigis' formula on the IOL Master, the SRKT, and Hoffer-Q formula are used. I normally calculate the lens using multiple formulae and compare the recommendations. When the results are concordant, there is good confidence. If there are discrepancies, then a decision has to be made as to which formula to use. Critical attention to detail with the choice of formula and using correct and optimized personal lens constants all contribute to a good refractive outcome.

The limitations of biometry, IOL calculation, and the final axial position of the IOL affect the precision and refractive predictability of the procedure. Both the low-order aberration sphere and cylinder and higher-order aberrations contribute to blur.

Preoperative Surgical Technique

When implanting the Tecnis multifocal IOL, as with all multifocal IOLs, I modify my surgical technique slightly. I take great care to ensure that the capsulorrhexis is as close to a 5.0-mm diameter as possible. It should be as regular and as well centered as possible. Although it can be argued such rigor should be present for all surgeries, it is with a multifocal IOL that lens centration and lack of any tilt is most important. A corneal imprint marker can help the surgeon during capsulorrhexis creation.

Since there is a (small) potential for multifocal IOL intolerance, there is always the possibility that a lens implant exchange may potentially be required. I therefore use a capsular tension ring in all eyes. This facilitates lens exchange even years later as the haptics are not entombed within a contracted capsular bag.

Careful attention to corneal cylinder is made during wound placement and construction. I favor a clear corneal approach with LRI, as this is both efficient and well tolerated.

Anesthesia is normally topical with sedation or with a small (1.5 mL) single quadrant posterior sub-Tenon irrigation.[14]

Postoperative Complications and Issues

It is common postoperatively to develop some dry eye from use of preoperative povidone-iodine conjunctival irrigation and preserved eyedrops.[15] Dry eye and altered tear composition is associated with reduced visual quality as the tear film breakup time becomes lower. Use of topical tear film supplements (especially hyaluronic acid-based products) is very effective in improving visual quality in the postoperative period.

Centration with the Tecnis multifocal IOL is simple to determine by checking how well the concentric rings align with the pupil. Because the IOL is geometrically centered within the capsular bag, it may not align with the center of the pupil. Significant decentration may induce coma[16,17] but pupil centration is one aspect that should be assessed preoperatively.

The unhappy patient who does not tolerate the multifocal lens can have an IOL exchange and the presence of a capsular tension ring facilitates this.

Posterior capsular opacification is managed as with any other lens implant. For the Tecnis silicone multifocal IOL, the lens is soft. It is critical not to pock the posterior lens surface and YAG pulses should be applied peripheral to the central optical zone. During the YAG procedure the posterior capsule tends to stick to the silicone optic and some patience is required to allow the capsule to separate from the posterior lens surface in the normal manner. The future acrylic Tecnis multifocal IOL will likely behave like the 1-piece Tecnis monofocal acrylic IOL that is available in Europe when a YAG capsulotomy is performed.

Long-Term Follow-Up

For routine monofocal IOL cataract surgery I normally discharge happy patients after a routine postoperative clinical and refractive assessment. For multifocal lens patients I examine them 3 months postoperatively after neural adaptation has occurred. Overall, patients are normally delighted with their vision but often have some longer-term questions, which can be answered at that time. This also provides an opportunity to assess whether a slit-lamp based outpatient LRI should be performed for any residual corneal cylinder. Alternatively, excimer laser options may need to be considered for residual refractive error. Currently 5% of my patients undergo an excimer laser enhancement after multifocal lens implantation.

Conclusion

The Tecnis multifocal 3-piece lens is very effective in providing clear distance and near vision. The reading distance is around 25 to 33 cm and for some patients they find this to be too close for their liking. Therefore, as with many other surgeons, I combine this lens with a ReZoom IOL in the second eye to provide for more intermediate focus. This custom matching facilitates use of a computer monitor or workstation. The Tecnis provides near vision for reading e-mails on a BlackBerry (Research in Motion, Waterloom, Ontario) and small text on smartphones.

The acrylic Tecnis multifocal IOL will offer new future possibilities, as the defocus curve is tighter for the acrylic model. This will provide even more light to be focused for distance and near. The enhanced separation of the distance and near foci should further improve patient acceptance of these lenses.

The Tecnis multifocal lens when used appropriately provides for very happy patients and is rewarding for the surgeon.

References

1. Denoyer A, Le Lez ML, Majzoub S, Pisella PJ. Quality of vision after cataract surgery after Tecnis Z9000 intraocular lens implantation: effect of contrast sensitivity and wavefront aberration improvements on the quality of daily vision. *J Cataract Refract Surg.* 2007;33:210-216.

2. Munoz G, Albarran-Diego C, Montes-Mico R, Rodriguez-Galietero A, Alio JL. Spherical aberration and contrast sensitivity after cataract surgery with the Tecnis Z9000 intraocular lens. *J Cataract Refract Surg.* 2006;32:1320-1327.

3. Toto L, Falconio G, Vecchiarino L, Scorcia V, Di Nicola M, Ballone E, Mastropasqua L. Visual performance and biocompatibility of 2 multifocal diffractive IOLs: simonth comparative study. *J Cataract Refract Surg.* 2007;33:1419-1425.

4. Kasper T, Bühren J, Kohnen T. Visual performance of aspherical and spherical intraocular lenses: intraindividual comparison of visual acuity, contrast sensitivity, and higher-order aberrations. *J Cataract Refract Surg.* 2006;32:2022-2029.

5. Montes-Mico R, Espana E, Bueno I, Charman WN, Menezo JL. Visual performance with multifocal intraocular lenses: mesopic contrast sensitivity under distance and near conditions. *Ophthalmology.* 2004;111:85-96.

6. Sugita Y. Global plasticity in adult visual cortex following reversal of visual input. *Nature.* 1996;380:523-526.

7. Richter H, Magnusson S, Imamura K, Fredrikson M, Okura M, Watanabe Y, Långström B. Long-term adaptation to prism-induced inversion of the retinal images. *Exp Brain Res.* 2002;144:445-457.

8. Marcos S, Burns SA. Cone spacing and waveguide properties from cone directionality measurements. *J Opt Soc Am A Opt Image Sci Vis.* 1999;16:995-1004.

9. Pask C, Stacey A. Optical properties of retinal photoreceptors and the Campbell effect. *Vision Res.* 1998;38:953-961.

10. Alpern M, Ching CC, Kitahara K. The directional sensitivity of retinal rods. *J Physiol.* 1983;343:577-592.

11. Van Den Berg TJ, Van Rijn LJ, Michael R, et al. Straylight effects with aging and lens extraction. *Am J Ophthalmol.* 2007;144:358-363.

12. Beiko GH. Personalized correction of spherical aberration in cataract surgery. *J Cataract Refract Surg.* 2007;33(8):1455-1460.

13. Gale RP, Saldana M, Johnston RL, Zuberbuhler B, McKibbin M. Benchmark standards for refractive outcomes after NHS cataract surgery. *Eye.* 2007 Aug 24; [Epub ahead of print]

14. Stevens JD. A new local anesthesia technique for cataract extraction by one quadrant sub-Tenon's infiltration. *Br J Ophthalmol.* 1992;76:670-674.

15. Li XM, Hu L, Hu J, Wang W. Investigation of dry eye disease and analysis of the pathogenic factors in patients after cataract surgery. *Cornea.* 2007;26(9 Suppl 1):S16-S20.

16. Altmann GE, Nichamin LD, Lane SS, Pepose JS. Optical performance of 3 intraocular lens designs in the presence of decentration. *J Cataract Refract Surg.* 2005;31:574-585.

17. Piers PA, Weeber HA, Artal P, Norrby S. Theoretical comparison of aberration-correcting customized and aspheric intraocular lenses. *J Refract Surg.* 2007;23(4):374-384.

CHAPTER 32

HOW DO I GET STARTED WITH THE CRYSTALENS?

D. Michael Colvard, MD, FACS

Over the past several years, the Crystalens (Eyeonics, Inc, Aliso Viejo, CA) has become an integral part of my clinical practice. I prefer the Crystalens for presbyopia correction over multifocal options for one very fundamental reason—visual quality. The Crystalens' greatest strength is that it offers patients an improved range of visual function without a reduction in visual quality. Neuroadaptation is not required, dependence on spectacles is reduced, and there is nothing difficult for the Crystalens patient to get used to.

Success with the Crystalens, however, requires attention to detail. Intraocular lens (IOL) surgery for presbyopia correction is intrinsically a refractive procedure. The implantation of the Crystalens requires the same appreciation for detail that we afford our keratorefractive patients. Good patient selection, careful counseling, sound surgical technique, and optimization of refractive outcomes are all necessary to achieve the highest level of patient satisfaction.

Choosing Patients: Who Is a Candidate for the Crystalens?

The ideal initial Crystalens candidate is the hyperope, 55 years or older, with a visually significant cataract, who requires surgery in order to maintain an acceptable quality of life. The Crystalens affords approximately 1.5 to 2.0 D of accommodation for most patients. The average age of cataract patients in my practice is 72 years of age. The chances are very good that a hyperopic patient of this age, who has been without useful accommodation for years, will be thrilled with the accommodative boost provided by the Crystalens. As the surgeon's experience with the Crystalens grows, the refractive range of candidates can be expanded. Emmetropes and high myopes over the age of 55 are also very likely to be happy with the vision afforded by the Crystalens, if the desired refractive target is achieved.

Poor candidates for the Crystalens are myopes who like to read without their glasses, successful monovision contact lens wearers, and younger patients who still have useful accommodation. Patients with pseudoexfoliation are not good candidates for the Crystalens because of potential problems with capsular support and anterior capsular phimosis. Also, patients who dilate poorly and patients with a history of Flomax (Boehringer Ingelheim, Ingelheim, Germany) use should be approached with great caution because of potential problems with creation of the anterior capsulotomy and probable difficulties with visualization of the anterior capsular margins during implantation. Clearly, patients who do not have the potential for good uncorrected vision (eg, those with significant maculopathy) are poor candidates for the Crystalens because they will not be able to appreciate the benefits of the technology.

Preoperative Evaluation and Planning: What to Look For and What to Think About

In addition to all the standard aspects of preoperative evaluation, careful attention should be paid to ocular dominance, mesopic pupil size before and after mydriasis, and manual keratometry.

Ocular dominance is important to establish for 2 reasons. First, a little "mini-monovision with the Crystalens" helps to enhance reading vision and is very well tolerated. In most cases, the ideal refractive outcome is plano to –.25 sphere in the dominant eye and –.50 to –.75 sphere in the nondominant eye. Second, it is helpful, but not essential, to perform surgery on the nondominant eye first. The refractive outcome of the nondominant eye is sometimes useful in refining the uncorrected distance vision of the dominant eye.

Mesopic pupil testing before mydriasis helps identify patients who may be at greater risk to experience postoperative glare and halo. The Crystalens has an optic size of 5 mm.

In my experience this is seldom an issue in older patients who generally have smaller pupils in mesopic conditions. Younger patients, however, who have larger pupils in low levels of illumination, are more likely to experience glare and halos with the smaller optic.

Pupil measurement after mydriasis helps to identify patients who may present intraoperative challenges with the creation of the anterior capsulotomy or with implantation of the Crystalens.

Manual keratometry helps define the corneal component of astigmatic error. Corneal astigmatism of .75 D or less can be managed effectively by simply placing the incision on the steep axis. Astigmatic errors up to 2.00 D generally can be managed with limbal relaxing incisions. Corneal topography is very helpful in directing the placement of these incisions. Patients with corneal astigmatism of greater than 2.00 D are much more difficult to correct with limbal relaxing incisions, especially if the cornea is steep horizontally. Patients with these higher levels of astigmatism are less likely to achieve the desired uncorrected refractive outcome, and generally are not ideal candidates for the Crystalens unless keratorefractive surgery is also part of the preoperative plan.

The importance of accurate biometry cannot be over-emphasized. The benefits of the Crystalens simply cannot be realized unless the patient achieves a desirable refractive outcome. Immersion ultrasound or IOL Master (Carl Zeiss Meditec, Jena, Germany) measurements provide the most reliable biometric data, and up-to-date lens calculation formulae help us to select the best possible IOL power. In our facility we use the IOL Master whenever the "noise to sign ratio" is low and immersion ultrasound when the ratio is high (as with denser lenses). We use the Hoffer Q formula for axial lengths of less than 22 mm, the Holladay 1 for lengths between 22 and 25 mm, and the SRK/T for eyes with lengths greater than 25 mm.

How to Counsel Crystalens Patients

Careful preoperative counseling is a critical element to success with the Crystalens. Setting realistic expectations may be the most important thing a surgeon can do to ensure patient satisfaction. The good news is that it is easy to tell a Crystalens patient what to expect. Here is a step-by-step approach to patient counseling that I have found very useful.

1. Explain That Cataract Surgery Is Actually a Lens Exchange Procedure

   I begin the discussion by explaining that the eye works very much like a camera. Sitting next to the patient, holding a model of the eye, I discuss in simple terms how the eye works and how a cataract affects vision. Even very intelligent, well-informed patients need to hear that the cataract is not just a cloudy film over the eye. Patients must understand that a cataract is cloudiness in the focusing lens of the eye and the only way to improve their vision is to remove the cloudy lens and replace it with "a new clear lens." This 2-minute discussion helps the patient understand why an IOL is necessary and is a natural segway into a discussion of the differences between a "standard monofocal IOL" and "the new Crystalens."

2. Discuss the Differences Between the Standard Monofocal Lenses and the Crystalens

   If a patient is a good candidate for the Crystalens, I then explain that we are fortunate today because "we have 2 excellent types of intraocular lenses to replace the cloudy cataract lens—the standard lenses and the newer Crystalens. Our standard lens is one that we have used successfully for over 20 years. This standard lens is called a monofocal lens because it provides a single focal point of best vision. This lens usually provides good distance vision without glasses, but glasses are generally needed in order to see the computer screen clearly or to read most printed material."

   "The new Crystalens gives vision at distance that is comparable to the standard monofocal lens, but it also offers an improved range of vision. The Crystalens provides better intermediate vision—computer vision—and helps with the reading as well." I explain that "the new Crystalens is a soft, flexible lens that uses the eye's natural focusing muscles to provide a better and more youthful range of vision." I carefully emphasize that "the Crystalens will not allow you to read like you did when you were 29. Most Crystalens patients are able to do the majority of their routine daily activities without glasses but many still use a little pair of over-the-counter reading glasses to see very small print, to read for prolonged periods, or to read in poor lighting." This is a clear, understated message that I am comfortable with, and most of my cataract patients find both reasonable and very appealing.

3. Explain That Presbyopia Correction With the Crystalens Is an Elective Upgrade and That It Is Expensive

   Next, I discuss the additional cost of presbyopia correction with the Crystalens. I want patients to know about the expense of the new technology before, not after, they have decided that they want it. "The big problem with this new lens," I point out, "is that it costs a lot more."

   I explain that "Medicare and other insurers have recognized that this new lens provides significant benefits, but they view it as an elective upgrade and they will not pay for it." "If you chose to upgrade to the new Crystalens lens," I explain, "you will have to pay the extra costs out of pocket. If, on the other hand, you chose the standard monofocal lens, there is no additional charge."

   I finish by saying, "So that's the way it is. Both lenses are excellent, and I think that you will notice a big improvement in your vision with either one of them. The Crystalens certainly offers advantages, but it costs a lot more. Just give it some thought, and we'll go with whatever ever you decide."

4. Reemphasize Realistic Expectations Before You Proceed

   The approximately 50% of our cataract patients who are presented with this option decide immediately that they would like to have the new lens. At this time I want to

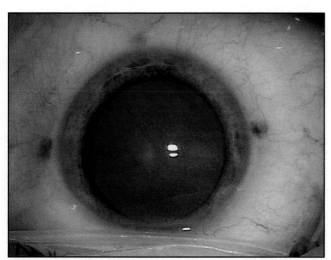

Figure 1. In the management of astigmatism, it is useful to mark the 0-, 90-, and 180-degree axis preoperatively while the patient is in a sitting position. This helps to eliminate the effects of cyclotorsion.

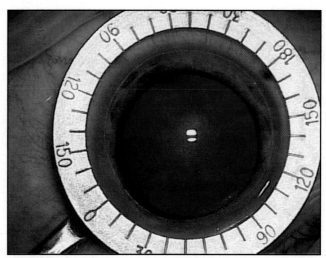

Figure 2. An axis indicator aids the surgeon in identifying the precise location of the steep axis.

be sure that the patient's expectations are realistic and that the patient is choosing the new lens based on the information that I have just reviewed and not on something else that they have read, heard elsewhere, or imagined.

I reiterate that glasses will still be needed for small print, prolonged reading, or reading in poor illumination. I explain that "since the Crystalens depends on the natural focusing muscles of the eye, improvement in reading vision with the Crystalens takes some time to develop." I point out that "the focusing muscles in the eye haven't done much for quite a few years, so it'll take some time for these muscles to get strong again." I also explain that "the reading muscles will get stronger the more they are used after surgery and that data from clinical studies show that reading vision without glasses often continues to improve over time."

I emphasize that "although most Crystalens patients have very good quality of vision postoperatively, it is possible to experience glare and halos after surgery and sometimes a second procedure is necessary to fine tune the distance vision after the initial operation." This point is particularly stressed with post-laser in situ keratomileusis (LASIK) or radial keratotomy (RK) patients and with high hyperopes, but all patients are made to understand that it is a possibility.

Aside from the basic consent information regarding the general risks of cataract surgery, I say very little else.

I feel very positive about the Crystalens technology. Patients sense this, but also realize that I have their best interest at heart. I believe that a key element to success with any surgery, and the Crystalens in particular, is not to sell it. An honest, straightforward description of the benefits of the Crystalens will allow patients to make a decision that is best for them.

Implantation of the Crystalens

MANAGEMENT OF ASTIGMATISM

The optimization of refractive outcomes requires the careful management of astigmatic errors. This begins with preoperative planning. I find it helpful to make detailed notes and drawings that describe the planned incision location, and the placement and size of limbal relaxing incisions as directed by manual keratometry and corneal topography. For every patient, I review these notes, which I tape to the wall next to my microscope, just before beginning the case.

To insure proper placement of the primary incision and limbal relaxing incisions, it is important to mark the 0- and 180-degree axis, as well as the 90-degree axis, while the patients is in a sitting position (Figure 1). This is easily done on the gurney just before surgery. The axis of the planned incision and that of limbal relaxing incisions, if needed, can then be marked under the microscope using an axis indicator (Figures 2 and 3).

MANAGEMENT OF INCISIONS

It is important that all incisions are absolutely solid and water tight at the end of the case. Any decompression of the anterior chamber in the early postoperative period will lead to forward vaulting of the Crystalens and the induction a myopic shift in the postoperative refraction. This is easy to prevent, but if it occurs, secondly intervention is often necessary to correct the vault.

The primary incision should be sutured, if it is corneal, or a scleral tunnel incision can be made. A well-constructed scleral tunnel incision usually does not require a suture (Figures 4 and 5). Side port incision(s) should be small, beveled, and well hydrated at the end of the case. All incisions should be checked rigorously before completing the case to ensure that they cannot be made to leak.

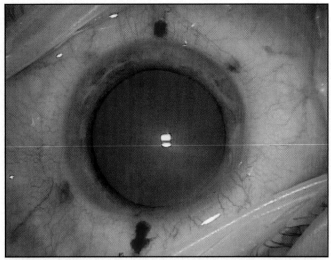

Figure 3. Marking of the steep axis insures more accurate placement of the primary incision and limbal relaxing incisions,

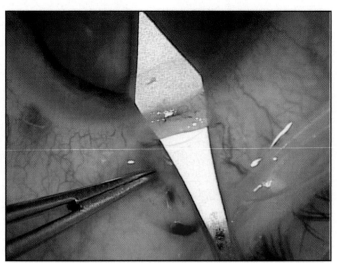

Figure 5. The length of internal flap of the incision should be as long as the width of the external incision in order to ensure maximum stability.

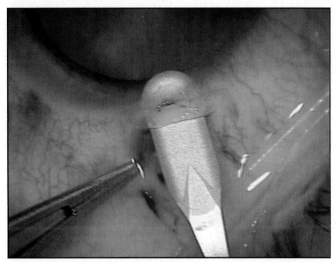

Figure 4. All incisions in a Crystalens procedure must be absolutely water tight. A scleral tunnel incision helps to ensure competency of the primary incision.

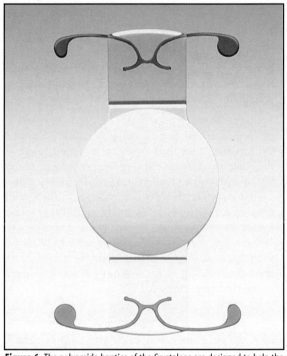

Figure 6. The polyamide haptics of the Crystalens are designed to help the surgeon to identify the "right side up" of the lens. The rounded knob of the lead haptic should always be on the right.

CAPSULORRHEXIS

The capsulorrhexis should be central, circular, and between 4 to 6 mm in diameter. If the capsulotomy is too small, it is difficult to insert the proximal haptic in the capsular bag. If the capsulotomy is very large or eccentric, it is possible for the lens to dislocate.

CRYSTALENS INSERTION AND POSITIONING

The Crystalens is implanted through a 2.7- to 3.0-mm incision with an injector, using a cohesive sodium hyaluronate viscoelastic material to fill the capsular bag. Care must be taken not to place the Crystalens upside down in the capsular bag. This can happen if the lens is loaded incorrectly in the injector or if the lens rotates in the injector during insertion. Implantation of an upside down lens can be avoided easily by inspecting the flat circular knobs at the ends of the polyamide haptic of the lens during insertion. The lens is designed so that, with the proper side up, the knob to the right is rounded

(round on right) and the knob to the left is oval. During insertion it is advisable to pause for a moment, just as the distal haptics unfurl in the anterior chamber (Figures 6 and 7). If the right knob is oval, and not rounded as it should be, the injector should be rotated 180 degrees, so that the IOL anterior-posterior orientation is corrected.

Once the IOL is placed in the capsular bag, I like to lift the optic forward slightly using lens hooks. I then rotate the lens to a 12-to-6 position, with the lens lifted slightly so that the polyamide haptics do not engage the capsule during this maneuver. The cohesive viscoelastic material is then removed completely. This should allow the Crystalens to settle into perfect position with both haptics symmetrically placed in the

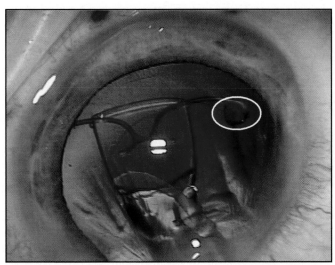

Figure 7. During insertion, it is advisable to pause for a moment to make sure that the IOL is properly oriented before placement of the lens in the bag. An adjustment, if necessary, can be made easily by simply rotating the inserter.

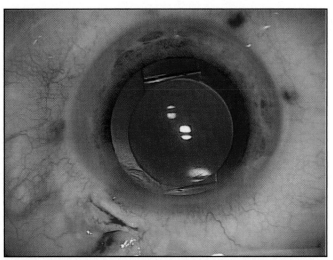

Figure 8. Crystalens should be positioned with both haptics symmetrically placed in the equator of the capsular bag and the optic vaulted in a slightly posterior location.

equator of the capsular bag and the optic vaulted in a slightly posterior position (Figure 8). If the IOL does not seem to position itself perfectly, viscoelastic should be used to refill the bag and anterior chamber, and these positioning maneuvers should be repeated.

POSTOPERATIVE MANAGEMENT

In my experience, the postoperative management of the Crystalens patient is far easier than that of the multifocal patient. The multifocal lens patient is faced with the challenge of adapting to an inherently unphysiologic light-splitting optical system. Sometimes this goes well, but often, it does not. A patient who finds it difficult to adjust to vagaries of multifocality requires a lot of encouragement, a great deal of hand-holding, and frequent postoperative visits. The management of the Crystalens lens patient is generally far less problematic. Complaints of reduced visual quality are rare, patients do not tend to tend to balk at having their second eye done, and small residual refractive errors, especially small astigmatic errors, are far better tolerated with the Crystalens than with multifocal lenses.

Still the level of patient satisfaction is highly dependent on the success in achieving a desired refractive outcome.

When a Crystalens patient presents postoperatively with a refractive outcome that is less than optimal, a cycloplegic refraction should be performed. The magnitude of hyperopic errors, especially, can be underappreciated in the Crystalens patient because of the accommodative action of the lens. Lower levels of residual hyperopia may lead to underperformance of uncorrected near vision and yet be masked by good uncorrected distance vision. This is a very frequent and often overlooked cause for poor uncorrected near vision with the Crystalens.

SPECIAL POSTOPERATIVE INSTRUCTIONS

Patients should be instructed not to read without glasses during the first 2 weeks of the postoperative period. Patients who exercise their accommodation excessively too early in the postoperative period tend to develop a myopic shift in their refraction. This can be avoided by asking patients to use a pair of +2.50 readers for reading during the first 2 weeks after surgery. If a myopic shift occurs and is undesirable, correction is generally not difficult.

Residual Myopia

A low level of myopia caused by excessive reading early in the postoperative period can sometimes be corrected by simply placing the patient on a cycloplegic of several days. If the refractive error is not corrected with cycloplegia, rotation and repositioning of the Crystalens is often successful. Residual myopia, caused by forward vaulting of the Crystalens early in the postoperative course, is often the result of suboptimal incision closure. This can be managed before capsular fibrosis has occurred by simply suturing the incision and repositioning the optic more posteriorly.

Astigmatic and Spherical Errors

Residual refractive errors not caused by lens malposition are best managed by a keratorefractive procedure, IOL exchange, or a "piggy-back" IOL.

A keratorefractive procedure is the treatment of choice for a patient with significant residual astigmatic error. LASIK is a very good option for younger patients but may not be the ideal for many older patients. Recovery from LASIK in older patients can be slow and associated with severe dry eye symptoms. Photorefractive keratectomy (PRK) paradoxically may be more comfortable and predictable for older patients who require a keratorefractive procedure.

An IOL exchange is an excellent option for correction of spherical errors, but this procedure should be performed before there is an opportunity for the polyamide loops of the Crystalens to become fibrosed within the capsular bag. Healon 5 (Advanced Medical Optics, Santa Ana, CA), which is a high-molecular-weight sodium hyaluronate viscoelastic material, is especially useful in expanding and maintaining the capsular bag during lens removal. Special care must be taken, however, to aspirate all of this material after the replacement IOL is in position. If several months have passed before secondary intervention is taken, a "piggy-back" IOL is a very good option for the correction of spherical errors.

With both IOL exchange and "piggy-back" IOL implantation, preoperative topography is very helpful. Topographic analysis allows the surgeon to reduce the likelihood of inducing a new astigmatic error though the secondary intervention.

Conclusion

The Crystalens provides a full range of visual function, utilizing an accommodative optical system that is physiologic, effective, and well accepted by patients. Implantation of this lens is easy, but special attention to detail is essential to ensure the highest level of patient satisfaction. Careful patient selection, thoughtful preoperative evaluation, good counseling, and a dedication to achieving the best possible refractive outcome are all necessary components of a successful Crystalens procedure.

SECTION IV

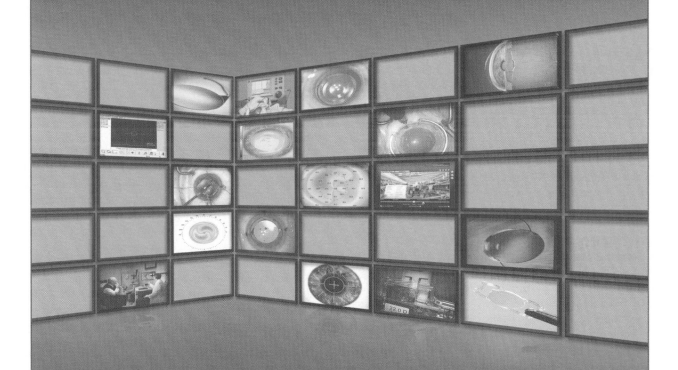

Presbyopia-Correcting IOLs Today

CHAPTER 33

AMO ReZoom Multifocal— Clinical Pearls

R. Bruce Wallace III, MD, FACS

Recent design improvements for the ReZoom refractive multifocal lens (Advanced Medical Optics, Inc., Santa Ana, CA) translate to benefits for both surgeons and patients. The ReZoom IOL provides quality multifocal vision, including intermediate vision, which patients require for daily activities such as computer work. Clinically, this 3-piece lens offers surgeons more versatility compared to 1-piece lenses. For example, the ReZoom may be placed in the ciliary sulcus if the posterior capsule is ruptured, thereby saving the procedure. This is especially important if a ReZoom has already been implanted in the fellow eye.

Function and Design

The ReZoom refractive multifocal lens has a 6-mm optic and an overall length of 13 mm. It features Balanced View Optics Technology, which uses zones proportioned to provide good visual function across a range of distances in varying light conditions. The 5 zones (rings) use all the available light that travels through the optic to provide distance, intermediate, and near visual acuity (Figure 1).

The design of the ReZoom's optic differs from that of the Array multifocal IOL (Advanced Medical Optics, Santa Ana, CA), in that its second and third zones have been enlarged and the fourth has been reduced in size. Zones 1, 3, and 5 are distance-dominant, whereas zones 2 and 4 are near-dominant. An aspheric transition between the zones provides balanced intermediate vision. This design lessens any noticeable halo effect at night; in fact, patients from the lens' initial investigation reported less halos compared to Array patients.

The ReZoom's optic is made of a hydrophobic acrylic material rather than silicone. It has a near power that is similar to the Array's (3.50 D add in the near portion of the IOL optic, and 2.57 D add at the spectacle plane).

The ReZoom also employs an OptiEdge triple-edge design, where the edge of the optic is round on the anterior side and square on the posterior side. It provides an uninterrupted 360-degree barrier of protection against posterior capsular opacifi-

cation and is designed to minimize edge glare (Figure 2). The triple-edge design lessens the chance of edge reflection than if there were a fully squared edge.

Quality of Vision

In my experience, patients' uncorrected near vision with the ReZoom has been quite good and appears to be better than with the Array. More than 70% of ReZoom patients stated that they did not use spectacles for any task postoperatively, although in the initial phase, some patients who read avidly benefited from reading glasses from time to time.

Spectacle usage was dependent on each individual's visual activity. For example, in the Food and Drug Administration (FDA) studies, spectacle independence was in the 60% range for the Array and is now reported at approximately 80% and beyond with the ReZoom for all levels of distance, intermediate, and near vision. Some studies are showing even higher numbers. Granted, postoperative uncorrected visual acuity (UCVA) is very much dependent on other factors such as accurate IOL calculations, astigmatism reduction, adequate tear function, and the quality of the patient's macula.

The ReZoom lens provides particularly good intermediate vision, such as for computer work and other tasks such as reading the speedometer. For many patients, their intermediate visual function improves with time.

Lens Refractive Procedures

Refractive lens exchange patients generally have high expectations when they enter an ophthalmologist's office, often based on the experiences of friends and relatives who have undergone a similar procedure. When I discuss the ReZoom lens with patients, I talk of "spectacle reduction" rather than "total spectacle independence." Therefore, those patients who achieve independence are even more satisfied. It is always better to under promise and over deliver.

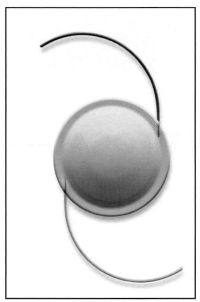

Figure 1. The ReZoom uses all the available light that enters through the optic to provide distance, intermediate, and near acuity.

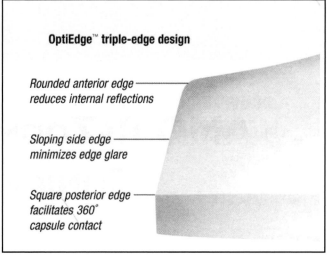

Figure 2. The edge shape of the ReZoom provides uninterrupted 360-degree barrier protection and is designed to minimize edge glare.

Patient Selection

We discuss the availability of presbyopia-correcting IOLs (Pr-C IOLs) with all patients undergoing cataract surgery and for refractive lens exchange patients (where the lenses are implanted "off label" for an FDA-approved device). We offer all FDA-approved Pr-C IOLs and are currently enrolling patients for FDA trials for the AMO Tecnis multifocal IOL and the Visiogen Synchrony (Irvine, CA) accommodative IOL. We consider the AMO ReZoom as our "go to" Pr-C IOL because it provides excellent distance visual acuity and good intermediate and near vision.

When discussing IOL choices with a patient, we try to determine just how motivated they are to reduce their dependency on glasses. We discourage patients who have other ocular pathology such as active retinal disease or glaucomatous nerve damage. We avoid Pr-C IOLs in patients who appear to have unrealistic expectations. If a low myope answers "yes" to the question "Do you read in bed without your glasses?" we spend extra chair time explaining the compromise of near vision of the ReZoom lens compared to the reading ability associated with bilateral myopia. Some of our patients in this category have benefited from a ReSTOR multifocal IOL in the fellow eye.

Case Study

One of our female patients, aged 74, had bilateral ReZoom multifocal implantation and 2 months later saw 20/20 bilaterally without glasses. She was able to read small print (J1) well, although she was still learning how to use the optic's near vision. She would visualize and work at kitchen counter distances as well as see her watch without a problem. She occasionally needed reading glasses when reading for longer periods of time (a somewhat common situation during the early postoperative stage).

This patient was also dealing with a previous dry eye condition while adjusting to her new lens. Dry eye is usually not an issue for people who receive a monofocal lens because that type of IOL does not split the light, and therefore any dryness on the surface of the cornea does not typically lead to a visual problem. However, when the light rays are split (ie, for distance, near, and intermediate viewing), dry eyes can add to visual disturbances. Patients with a compromised tear film may notice near vision trouble because this distant-dominant lens does not allocate as much light transmission for near vision. This patient started using artificial tears more frequently, and her near vision improved.

Future Outlook

My experience with the ReZoom lens has been very positive. I believe in the technology and am confident that most patients will be satisfied with this lens and their resulting vision.

CHAPTER 34

AMO ReZoom Multifocal—
Clinical Pearls

Farrell Tyson, MD, FACS

The ReZoom multifocal implant by Advanced Medical Optics (Santa Ana, CA) is 3-piece, square edge, acrylic posterior chamber intraocular lens (IOL). It achieves its 2 primary focus points by the use of 5 alternating concentric zones. The central zone is for distance. The second zone is for near with the third zone providing distance vision. Zones 4 and 5 have been reduced in relation to the previous-generation Array multifocal lens (Advanced Medical Optics). This reduction in zone areas 4 and 5, in addition to an overlapping capsulorrhexis, effectively makes the ReZoom implant a 3-zone lens. This leads to a reduction in nighttime glare and improved near vision when compared to the Array lens.

Proper patient selection is the most important step when deciding to implant the ReZoom lens. I have found that it is best to identify patients with low amounts of astigmatism. I tend to limit this lens to patients with 1.5 D of astigmatism or less, as I can accurately achieve correction at this level with limbal relaxing incisions (LRIs). The treatment of higher levels of astigmatism with a bioptic laser in situ keratomileusis (LASIK) procedure has to be weighed against increased contrast loss, increased dry eye issues that can lead to glare, and the additional cost to the patient. Another factor to consider during patient selection is dry eyes. All patients should be screened preoperatively for dry eyes and treated with punctual plugs or Restasis (Allergan, Irvine, CA). Dry eyes cause ocular surface irregularities that can exacerbate or cause symptoms of glare and halos. Re-evaluation of patients who experience glare and halos during the postoperative period is warranted, as cataract surgery can temporarily induce ocular surface disease.

Selecting the right patient also involves determination of the ideal personality type. It is better to avoid implanting the ReZoom lens in patients who are pessimistic, but rather to find patients with a "glass half-full" mentality. The patient's nighttime driving needs are another key consideration. These needs may vary by geographical region as daylight lasts a little longer in Florida, while it gets darker slightly earlier in the North. These and other patient characteristics and preferences can be determined with the help of a preoperative questionnaire.

I prefer to spend enough face-to-face time with the patient to fully understand his or her needs and expectations.

No one presbyopia-correcting IOL is right for all patients. Surgeons will get the best results and the happiest patients when they pick the right lens for the right patient. The ReZoom implant seems to be ideal for patients who prefer the progressive style bifocal and those who have an active lifestyle and want a range of functional vision. Our society is moving more toward a lifestyle in which intermediate vision is very important, such as for using the computer or playing cards. Patients with flat-top bifocals tend to do better with one of the diffractive multifocal IOLs as they have already adjusted to having limited intermediate vision but good distance and near vision. Patients with minimal lens opacity tend to do better with the ReZoom lens because diffractive multifocal IOLs have greater loss of contrast sensitivity, which is perceived by patients as dimness of vision. This is not a problem with either lens design in patients with mature cataracts. Patients who need only to undergo unilateral IOL implantation are best served with the ReZoom lens as it is less dependant on bilateral implantation for success. I find bilateral implantation with ReZoom lenses gains the patient 1 line of visual acuity compared to my ReSTOR patients who gain 1.5 lines of visual acuity with bilateral implantation.

A good preoperative workup is essential to achieving success. If you find that you are not getting good refractive outcomes with your monofocal IOLs, you will certainly have difficulty with your multifocal IOLs. One should either use immersion A-scan or the IOL Master (Carl Zeiss Meditec, Jena, Germany) to measure axial length. The use of contact A-scan is too variable and inconsistent for multifocal lens implantation. Surgeon optimized third-generation formulas or the Haigis or Holladay II IOL calculation formulas are very effective with multifocal IOLs as they work well over a large range of axial lengths. I generally aim for plano or if necessary a little bit of minus with the ReZoom. A little minus will leave room for an LRI if necessary. Even though LRIs will supposedly keep you spherically equivalent, the patient is going to perceive a hyperopic shift. I have found that staggering refractive targets between the 2 eyes reduces best uncorrected binocular vision due to reduced cerebral summation and thus should be avoided.

The preoperative consultation is your opportunity to set the patient's expectations. I warn all of my multifocal patients about the possibility of having glare or halos in the early postoperative period, which then disappear in the majority of my patients by 3 months after surgery. We discuss that best distance and near vision will not be obtained until after the second eye is implanted. The possible need for a secondary enhancement procedure, such as an LRI, is explained to the patient. It is better to spend a little more time informing your patients preoperatively than spending a lot of time postoperatively quelling their concerns.

I have had very good success with the ReZoom implant. My uncorrected near vision results are 15% achieving J1+, 53% achieving to J1, 82% achieving to J2, and 98% achieving J3. Uncorrected binocular distance vision is equally good with over 99% of my patients being able to read the 20/30 line or better. I can tell my patients with confidence that they have a 98% chance of using both eyes to read the newspaper and drive a car without glasses.

When considering the impact of age, I find that younger patients tend to have better distance and reading vision. These same younger patients, however, also tend to be the most critical and demanding. I attribute this to better retinal health. Once patients reach 60 to 70 years of age, the visual outcomes start to flatten out, but even patients in their 80s are achieving 20/25 vision on average at distance and near.

It is a good practice to accentuate the positives after surgery. Patients may not be sure what to expect, so they expect perfection. You need to let them see with (−)3.0-D glasses that they truly have gained the ability to see up close. Treating small amounts of posterior capsular opacification (PCO) with a YAG capsulotomy early on can be very beneficial, as even slight PCO will readily decrease contrast. Small amounts of residual cylinder (over 0.75 D) should also be treated. Both slight PCO and slight astigmatism tend to cause a significant decrease in near vision performance, and treatment can therefore produce a surprising degree of improvement in near vision. When patients are complaining of glare and halos, rechecking for and treating dry eyes will solve many cases. If glare symptoms persist, I have found that eyeglasses with DriveWear lenses (Younger Optics, Torrance, CA) can be very beneficial. These lenses are polarized and photochromatic. They darken with visible light in the car and then lighten in dim conditions. The yellow to amber tint also improves contrast.

With proper patient selection and education and a thorough preoperative workup, the ReZoom IOL can result in excellent outcomes and satisfied patients.

CHAPTER 35

AMO ReZoom Multifocal— Clinical Pearls

Rosa Braga-Mele, MD, MEd, FRCSC

Multifocal intraocular lenses (IOLs) are increasingly becoming part of a cataract surgeon's armamentarium. Multifocal IOLs allow surgeons to correct presbyopia as well as cataracts, and most patients are grateful. Still, this is a relatively new field for ophthalmology, and questions linger. Who makes the ideal patient for a multifocal IOL? What are the visual benefits to a refractive or diffractive multifocal IOL? Are there visual aberrations after surgery, and if so, how should the surgeon manage them?

This chapter will address those questions as they apply to the ReZoom IOL (Advanced Medical Optics, Santa Ana, CA), a refractive multifocal lens that offers superior distance and intermediate vision and good near vision.

Patient Selection— Who Is the Ideal Patient for a Multifocal IOL?

The best patients for multifocal IOLs are realistic, motivated, and accepting. Over time and with a few tools, it becomes easier to determine which patients should not receive a multifocal IOL. These lenses are good for both refractive lens exchange in younger, presbyopic patients and for cataract surgery patients.

I have found patient selection questionnaires to be helpful in determining what type of vision is a priority for the patient. Two that are often mentioned are from Drs. William Maloney[1] and Steven Dell (see Appendix A).[2]

The key selection criteria should include the patient's personality, visual expectations, lifestyle, pupil size and mobility, general eye health, and dominant eye. The patient questionnaires help identify what areas of vision the patient values the most, the likelihood of spectacle wear acceptance, and what tolerance, if any, the patient would have to unwanted visual

phenomena postoperatively. It is important to disclose all possible risks with implantation of these IOLs, including glare, halo, and the possibility that they will still require glasses for some tasks. It is best to make these an expectation rather than a complication.

There are relative contraindications for multifocal IOL implantation. Patients with severe dry eye that is refractory to treatment, corneal scarring, small pupils (under 2.5 mm) and/or immobile pupils, monofocal implants in the first eye, or unstable capsular support, such as loose or broken zonules or torn anterior capsulorrhexis, are my general rule of thumb contraindications.

Why a Refractive Versus Diffractive Multifocal Lens?

There are now 5 options for surgeons with respect to refractive cataract surgery, and this will increase as different types of IOLs are introduced in the coming years. For now, surgeons have the option of implanting bilateral refractive IOLs, bilateral diffractive IOLs, bilateral accommodating IOLs, mixing IOL types (ie, refractive in the dominant eye and diffractive in the nondominant eye), and aspheric monofocal IOLs with monovision.

I personally prefer to implant bilateral refractive IOLs, as I find refractive lenses give the greatest range of vision for the majority of my patients. With refractive IOLs, the parallel rays that pass through the distance rings provide excellent distance vision, essentially without degradation. Further, they do not aberrate the light as much as a diffractive lens does, which helps improve the patient's visual quality (Figure 1). In short, they provide an excellent range of vision based on the lens design.

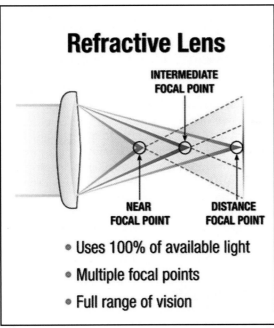

Figure 1. Refractive lens.

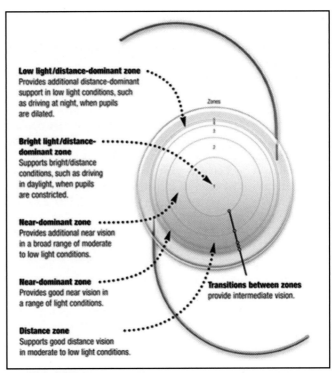

Figure 2. ReZoom IOL zones.

ReZoom: A Second-Generation Refractive IOL

The ReZoom lens is based on AMO's Array platform, but it has significant improvements over the earlier generation. The ReZoom uses hydrophobic acrylic biocompatible material, whereas the Array was based on a silicone platform. The ReZoom incorporates "balanced view optics," with the zones proportioned to provide good visual function across the range of distances under varying light conditions. Zones 1, 3, and 5 are distance dominant, with zones 2 and 4 being near dominant; an aspheric transition between zones provides balanced intermediate vision (Figure 2). The truncated optic edge helps reduce the risk of posterior capsule opacification (PCO) by providing 360-degree barrier protection. This is important because any amount of PCO in these eyes rapidly degrades the uncorrected vision and also amplifies any halo and glare. The rounded anterior optic edge reduces internal reflections. The sloping side-edge minimizes edge glare, and the square posterior edge keeps 360 degree capsule contact. The lens is a 3-piece design with polymethylmethacrylate (PMMA) haptics. Three-piece designs promote contact between the optic and posterior capsule and this helps stabilize the IOL in the bag. Centration is of paramount importance with any multifocal IOL. The ReZoom has a 6-mm diameter optic and a total diameter of 13 mm. The technology provides expanded distance-dominant zones; the near-dominant zones provide +3.5 D of add power at the IOL plane, which provides an effective near add greater than the 2 D needed by most adults over 50.

All of the improvements in the design from the Array to the ReZoom have been aimed at optimizing optic zone size and light direction so as to reduce halo and glare and improve the range of vision and visual quality.

Surgical Approaches to Maximize Success

Bilateral cataract surgery is typically a staged implantation, with one eye completed several weeks before the fellow eye. In multifocal IOL surgeries, staging the implantation allows surgeons to customize the lens selection to patient lifestyle, helping to give the patient the best possible outcome. It also provides the surgeon with a safety net of sorts by allowing the opportunity to monitor patient progress in between surgeries. The optimal surgical spacing is about 3 weeks with multifocal implantation.

It is best to implant the dominant eye first. If there is a significant difference, however, in best-corrected visual acuity at baseline in cataract patients, one can implant the worst eye first. Since every patient tends to expect excellent distance vision, one should aim for emmetropia in the first eye. I choose a refractive multifocal IOL (ReZoom) for the distance dominant eye. I adjust the second eye depending on what the patient experiences at about 1 to 2 weeks postsurgery.

The follow-up conversation with the patient after the first IOL implantation will yield 1 of 3 responses. If the patient responds that the vision is great for both near and far and he or she has no issues, then I will pick the same type of IOL for the second eye and again aim for emmetropia.

The patient may respond that his or her near and far vision is great, but he or she is having some night vision issues; this is a patient with which you need to spend a bit more time. If the halos are severe and intractable, you may want to postpone the second eye indefinitely until the patient experiences some improvement. If, however, no improvement occurs, you may want to discuss possible IOL exchange with an accommodating IOL or a monofocal IOL. If the halos are mild to moderate, the patient will likely get better with implantation of the second eye and one may chose either a diffractive or refractive IOL.

The third response may be that the patient complains the near vision is not nearly what was expected. In this case, I plan either a ReZoom aiming for about −0.5D to provide mini-monovision, or I plan on implanting a Tecnis MF (Advanced Medical Optics) or ReSTOR. The majority of my patients have received bilateral ReZoom.

I recently conducted a pilot study of bilateral ReZoom implantations with a total of 25 patients (11 men, 14 women). All patients had follow-up through 6 weeks, and 11 had follow-up through 6 months.[3] Preoperative visual acuity ranged from −10.25 D to +4.25 D. At 6 weeks, 80% had uncorrected distance visual acuity of 20/25 or better, with none of the patients seeing worse than 20/30; 88% saw 20/30 or better at intermediate vision, and 96% saw 20/30 or better at near.

By 6 months (n = 11), none of the patients saw worse than 20/40 at any distance; 81% had 20/25 or better vision at near, 91% had 20/25 or better at intermediate, and 91% had 20/25 or better distance vision.

Halos, Glare, and Astigmatism

It is important to be able to correct any corneal astigmatism either intraoperatively with limbal relaxing incisions and/or incision placement or postoperatively with bioptics such as photorefractive keratectomy (PRK) or laser in situ keratomileusis (LASIK).

A good percentage of patients will experience halo and glare, and in rare instances, the side effects may be significant. I have found that with proper patient counseling, these patients will neuroadapt to the halos and glare in about 6 months. It is especially important to inform patients about halos preoperatively, thereby making such symptoms an expectation rather than a complication.

The most common patient concerns before and after surgery include blurry distance vision, monocular diplopia, object glow, ghosting, and night halos. There are numerous methods to treat and/or manage these concerns. I suggest looking for and treating the patient's dry eye with multiple dosage lubricating drops and/or Restasis (Allergan, Irvine, CA.).

Correcting any outlying astigmatism is important. Check for residual astigmatism or PCO, as these can both exacerbate the situation. Pharmacologic miosis (with Alphagan P [Allergan]) may be an appropriate early treatment method, and I usually instruct the patient to instill one drop 30 minutes before night driving. Again, counsel and remind the patient that he or she needs to allow adequate time to adapt to the new visual system that these lenses provide.

Interestingly, in my pilot study,[3] 56% of patients complained of mild halos at 6 weeks, and 36% said the halos were severe. By 6 months, only 9% considered their halos severe, with a large majority (82%) noting only mild halo. Likewise, at 6 weeks, 28% said they had severe glare (36% said they had mild glare); by 6 months, only 9% said they had severe glare and 64% said they had no/barely noticeable glare. There was an improvement in 64% of the eyes in terms of neuroadaptation and halos, and 45% improved in terms of glare at 6 months.

Other Pearls

Patients should avoid using readers for the first few weeks so they can find the different near, intermediate, and distance vision points. I have found that if spectacles are used too soon after surgery, the patient may miss out on being able to fully adapt to the lens. Advising patients to delay using spectacles can help them to reduce their dependence on readers in the future after they have better trained themselves to adapt.

Please remember that not every lens is perfect for every patient, nor is this procedure perfect for every patient. Select your IOL and patient carefully.

References

1. Maloney WF. Presbyopia success depends on comprehensive preop evaluation. *Ocular Surgery News*. http://www.osnsupersite.com. Accessed June 28, 2007

2. Dell SJ. Screening and evaluating presbyopic patients. *Cataract and Refractive Surgery Today*. http://www.crstoday.com/PDF%20Articles/0307/CRST0307_18.php. Accessed June 28, 2007.

3. Braga-Mele RM. Patient selection criteria for multifocal IOL technologies to optimize patient satisfaction and range of vision. Paper presented at: American Society for Cataract and Refractive Surgery, April 29, 2007; San Diego, CA.

CHAPTER 36

ALCON RESTOR MULTIFOCAL— CLINICAL PEARLS

Robert J. Cionni, MD

The introduction of the ReSTOR apodized diffractive intraocular lens (IOL) (Alcon, Fort Worth, TX) represents a tremendous advance in our ability to provide patients with the possibility of spectacle freedom following cataract surgery. The Food and Drug Administration (FDA) study demonstrated that 80% of patients were completely spectacle free after bilateral implantation of the ReSTOR IOL. This represents about a 2- to 3-fold improvement over previous presbyopia-correcting intraocular lens (Pr-C IOL) designs. Still, no single IOL is ideal for each and every patient. Selecting the patients who are most likely to do well with a Pr-C IOL and matching those patients to the best Pr-C IOL for them is an art well worth learning. Pearls for selecting and educating patients about Pr-C IOLs are also discussed in my chapter on patient selection for refractive IOLs (Chapter 95). In addition to selecting and educating your patients, several other factors are important in achieving success. These include a detailed examination, proper IOL selection, accurate power determination, uncomplicated surgery, and appropriate follow-up. I will expand on these components in more detail in this chapter.

Who Are Good Candidates for ReSTOR IOLs?

Undoubtedly, when the ReSTOR IOL is placed in a patient best suited for this style IOL, and the postoperative refractive goal is attained, the result is a "grand slam" for the patient. So, how do we decide who will do best with a ReSTOR IOL? The answer is multifactorial and depends on both objective and subjective information.

PUPIL SIZE

Patients with small pupils do exceedingly well with bilateral ReSTOR IOLs at all distances and the ReSTOR IOL is clearly the lens of choice for most of these patients. The benefit of this IOL in patients with larger pupils is a lower risk for significant

halos and better contrast sensitivity because the vast majority of light rays will be directed to the distance focus point. However, patients with large pupils under normal lighting conditions may have more difficulty with near and intermediate vision and these patients need to understand this compromise before coming to a decision about IOL choice. For patients with larger pupils topical Alphagan (Allergan, Irvine, CA) will slightly constrict the pupils in the evening and may improve their near and intermediate vision. Educating those patients with larger pupils concerning the possible need for glasses at the computer and in dim light situations before they make a lens choice is imperative.

ASTIGMATISM

Any patient who has more than 0.50 D of astigmatism after surgery is far less likely to be happy with their vision with any style of Pr-C IOL. The surgeon needs to be able to reduce the patient's astigmatism to less than 0.50 D with either a limbal relaxing incision (LRI) or a laser refractive procedure.

TEAR FILM

Pr-C IOLs do not perform well whenever the ocular surface is less than perfect. Patients with irregular corneal astigmatism or other ocular surface abnormalities may not do well with a ReSTOR IOL. Those with an insufficient tear film need to be treated aggressively if a ReSTOR IOL is planned. This includes the use of preservative free artificial tears, punctual plugs, topical cyclosporine A, and omega-3 fatty acids.

OTHER OCULAR PATHOLOGY

Patients with epiretinal membranes, diabetic macular edema, significant age-related macular degeneration (ARMD), advanced glaucoma, or other pathology that would preclude the potential for good postoperative central vision are not good candidates for any multifocal IOL (MFIOL). Some surgeons recommend obtaining an optical coherence tomography (OCT) on every patient considering a Pr-C IOL to better evaluate the macula and screen out those patients who may not do well. The one exception may be the patient with ARMD who has a vision potential of 20/30 to 20/100 and a goal of better reading ability, rather than spectacle freedom in particular. Richard MacKool, MD and Johnny Gayton, MD have a series of patients like this in whom they have implanted ReSTOR IOLs while purposely leaving the patients myopic. Their results seem to indicate an improvement in uncorrected and best correct reading ability due to increased magnification and field of view provided by the ReSTOR add power combined with intended myopia.

UNDERSTANDING THE PATIENT'S VISUAL NEEDS (FAR, INTERMEDIATE, NEAR)

This means getting to know the patient in terms of his or her occupation, hobbies, and lifestyle. A vision preference questionnaire and an appropriate amount of time spent with the patient in consultation will help the surgeon determine which Pr-C IOL will likely work best for the patient. If the patient's main daily tasks involve distance vision, such as driving, and near vision, such as reading books, then they will likely do very well with bilateral ReSTOR IOLs. If, however, they spend the vast majority of their time at a desktop computer or working at arm's length as does a car mechanic, they may not get what they expect with the current ReSTOR IOL. These patient needs to know up front that they are more likely to need glasses for those specific tasks if they receive bilateral ReSTOR IOLs. Providing they understand this completely and still desire the ReSTOR IOL to take advantage of its other characteristics, they will likely be happy with this lens design.

PATIENT CONCERNS ABOUT HALOS

Although the apodized nature of the ReSTOR IOL minimizes halos, it is best to tell all patients who are considering any MFIOL that they will see halos around lights. Patients who are significantly concerned about the possibility of halos while driving at night for social reasons or for their occupation may not be best suited for any MIOL.

REALISTIC EXPECTATIONS

The single most important factor that will lead to patient satisfaction is making certain the patient understands what he or she is getting and will be able to accept any compromises that the Pr-C IOL may have. Therefore, the aforementioned factors should be discussed with the patient to help them better understand the benefits and limitations of the ReSTOR IOL. Certainly, as the technology of these lenses improves with time the relative benefits and limitations will likely change. A perfect example is the introduction of the ReSTOR aspheric IOL (Alcon Model SN6AD3). Bench studies of this aspheric IOL demonstrate superior modulation transfer function with small and large pupils, meaning that the quality of vision at all distances should be significantly better than that found with the initial ReSTOR IOLs (Figure 1).[1,2] I always finish my discussion with the patient by saying that nothing I can offer him or her is as good as the lens he or she was born with but what we can provide for him or her today is far better than our limited choices even a few years ago.

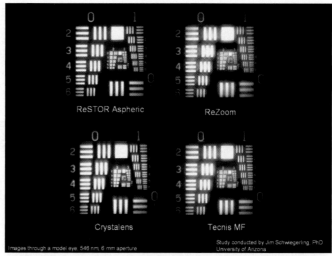

Figure 1. Airforce bar targets study conducted by J. Schwiegerling, PhD at the University of Arizona demonstrating the high image quality of the Aspheric ReStor Apodized Diffractive IOL compared to other Pr-C IOL models. (Reprinted with permission of Jim Schwiegerling, University of Arizona.)

Preoperative Exam

So let us assume that we have chosen a good candidate for a ReSTOR IOL based on our objective and subjective findings and the patient's understanding of the benefits and limitations of the IOL choice. Now we need to choose the proper IOL power. Accurate axial length measurements are crucial. It is strongly recommended to measure the axial length with either an IOL Master (Carl Zeiss Meditec, Jena, Germany) or an immersion A-scan. Contact A-scan measurements tend to be too variable and operator dependent to be reliable enough for these premium IOLs. Keratometry values are obtained using 3 different methods including manual keratometry, IOL Master, and topography. These readings must agree with each other. If they do not, repeat them until they do agree. The IOL power is then calculated using a newer generation formula such as the Holladay II. Aiming for a refractive result of about +0.10 to +0.25 in each eye seems to yield the best vision at all distances with this particular IOL.

Surgery

Only a few details need to be elaborated relating to the surgical technique for implanting the ReSTOR IOL. As mentioned previously, the surgeon needs to limit astigmatism to less than 0.50 D to maximize the level of patient satisfaction. Therefore, small amounts of preoperative corneal astigmatism should be addressed with LRIs or astigmatic keratotomy. A small amount of cylinder can often be reduced by placing the incision on the steep axis when possible. I have found it difficult to reliably eliminate cylinder in excess of 1.50 D with a LRI and I prefer to either suggest a toric IOL for these patients or refer them to a laser refractive surgeon for a more predictable astigmatic laser in situ keratomileusis (LASIK) or photorefractive keratectomy (PRK) postoperatively.

The surgeon should strive to make the anterior capsulorrhexis (CCC) larger than the diffractive rings yet smaller than the optic edge. A 5.0 to 5.5 mm CCC is ideal. A surgeon who makes a consistently sized CCC will find that his or her A-constant is quite predictable. Because the pupil in its natural state tends to rest slightly nasal, it may be a good idea to fashion the CCC slightly nasal as well. Doing so allows the surgeon to position the single-piece IOL slightly nasally within the bag while assuring overlap of the CCC edge on the anterior surface of the optic for 360 degrees.

The only caveat concerning IOL implantation is to place the IOL in the bag and orient the haptics vertically. This allows the surgeon to more easily nudge the IOL slightly nasal of center so that it will rest in the center of the pupil after surgery. Be certain to remove all viscoelastic from behind the IOL to avoid capsular bag distention syndrome and unexpected myopia.

Postoperative

Just as pre-existing macular pathology would have challenged the vision in patients with MFIOLs, so will postoperative macular problems. Therefore we need to do all we can to prevent cystoid macular edema (CME). Studies have clearly demonstrated the benefit of combining a topical nonsteroidal anti-inflammatory drug (NSAID) with a topical steroid drop in reducing the risk of CME.[2-4] Most believe the NSAID should be started 1 to 3 days before surgery to better stabilize the blood aqueous barrier before surgery begins. Because these patients do best after both eyes are implanted, it is recommended to proceed with the second eye within 3 weeks of the first.[5]

I believe it is very important for the surgeon to follow these patients until they are happy with their results. Scheduling additional postoperative chair time with these patients allows the surgeon enough "unrushed" time to address any concerns and answer all questions.

Finally, the surgeon should track his or her results in terms of achieving the postoperative refractive goal for sphere and cylinder, binocular uncorrected visual acuity at distance, near and intermediate, spectacle independence, glare symptoms, and so on. With this information, the surgeon will be able to fine tune the procedure in terms of such variables as A-constant, effect of LRIs and IOL choice. Additionally, a postoperative questionnaire can be very helpful and should be completed for all refractive IOL patients.

Without a doubt, some of the happiest patients in my practice today are those with bilaterally implanted ReSTOR IOLs. Proper attention to details preoperatively, intraoperatively, and postoperatively will help to ensure patient satisfaction with this tremendous technological advance in surgical eye care.

References

1. Cionni R. Aspheric presbyopia correcting IOL outcomes. Presented at the American Academy of Ophthalmology Annual Meeting, 2008, New Orleans, USA

2. Schwiegerling J. The aspheric apodized diffractive IOL. Presented at: The European Society of Cataract and Refractive Surgery Annual Meeting 2007.

3. Samiy N, Foster CS. The role of nonsteroidal anti-inflammatory drugs in ocular inflammation. *Int Ophthalmol Clin.* 1996;36(1):195-206.

4. Wolf E, Braunstein A, Shih C, Braunstein R. Incidence of visually significant pseudophakic macular edema after uneventful phacoemulsification in patients treated with nepafenac. *J Cataract and Refract Surg.* 2007;33;1546-1549.

5. Cionni R. Strategies for Multifocal IOLs. Presented at the American Society of Cataract and Refractive Surgery Meeting 2007.

CHAPTER 37

ALCON ReSTOR MULTIFOCAL— CLINICAL PEARLS

David Allen, BSc, FRCS, FRCOphth

I regard the ReSTOR apodized diffractive intraocular lens (IOL) (Alcon, Fort Worth, TX) as a third-generation presbyopia-correcting bifocal IOL. The first-generation multifocal IOLs were the early pioneer implants of the late 1980s. The mid 1990s saw much improved second-generation implants such as the Pharmacia 811E diffractive bifocal (Pfizer, Inc, New York, NY) and the Array refractive multifocal IOL (Advanced Medical Optics, Santa Ana, CA). The ReSTOR is one of the latest generation multifocal IOLs that has benefited from advances in IOL technology and design.

Patient Selection

The ReSTOR gives much better reading vision with fewer unwanted visual effects compared to first- or second-generation bifocal/multifocal IOLs. Although it is still important to select patients carefully, in my opinion, the selection criteria can now be wider than with earlier lenses. However, as with other clinical decisions requiring careful patient selection, the first and most important step is to identify individuals who are clearly not suitable for this IOL (Table 1).

PATIENTS TO AVOID

Because pseudoaccommodative IOLs are always going to have certain compromises, it is first of all important to select patients who truly wish to be free from spectacles. Until we have more experience, we should probably not place multifocal IOLs in individuals who are professional night-time drivers. Avoid patients who demand visual perfection and, therefore, might not tolerate even the mild degree of night-time halo that some patients report with this IOL. Such patients might also have complained of intolerable halos with monofocal IOLs. However, if they received a bifocal IOL, they will certainly blame their symptoms on the decision to have a multifocal, or more importantly on you for convincing them to do so. Another example of this type of perfection seeking is the patient who wishes to have refractive surgery to correct only 1 D of refractive error.

You should also reject patients in whom you are not confident in achieving a low amount of postoperative astigmatism. In the formal study used to obtain Food and Drug Administration (FDA) approval of the lens, and similar studies,[1] <1 D of preoperative keratometric astigmatism was a requirement for inclusion in the study. It is, however, the postoperative astigmatism that is the deciding factor. I would now recommend that you should only use this IOL in patients in whom you can reasonably expect to have <1 D of postoperative astigmatism (either immediately after surgery or after any postsurgery enhancement you may be able or willing to offer).

SUITABLE PATIENTS

Patients who have age-related cataract and who are also hyperopic are the easiest patients to begin with, as they will be delighted simply with achieving unaided distance vision for the first time. When they also get unaided near vision as well, they will be particularly happy and will not stop telling their friends and relatives about it! I recommend that surgeons begin using the ReSTOR in these patients so as to build up their experience and confidence with the lens. Later, you can move to the more challenging patients such as low myopes who always had good unaided near vision until their cataract developed.

A 4 D add at the IOL plane (around 3.2 D at the spectacle plane) has been incorporated into the ReSTOR. One reason for having this relatively large add is that the increased spatial separation of the 2 images decreases the influence of the out-of-focus image on the focused one. A quick look at the math will show that this gives a best reading distance of about 31 to 32 cm. Cataract patients over the age of 60 years have become accustomed to absolute presbyopia and a fixed reading distance of about 36 cm (with a typical 2.5 or 2.75 spectacle reading add) and should therefore adapt fairly easily to a slight reduction in their reading distance. Our clinical experience with the ReSTOR, however, has been that the reading distance does gradually extend out a little and after a few months is probably closer to 34 or 35 cm. The reason for this is unclear. Although

Table 1
PATIENTS TO AVOID
• Those who are happy to continue wearing reading glasses.
• Those who dislike their glasses because of dysphotopsia.
• Visual perfectionists.
• Professional night-time drivers.
• Degree of postsurgery astigmatism >1 D.

Table 2
PATIENT COUNSELING
• Twenty percent increased chair time before surgery equals 100% decreased chair time after surgery.
• Warn in advance about reading distance.
• Warn in advance about computer screen distance.
• Warn in advance about halos.
• Warn in advance about unsettling problems when only one eye has been operated.
• Then, when symptoms prove not to be so bad, you are a hero!

many hypothesize that "neuro-adaptation" occurs, we do not really know what this is. The improved functional reading distance may be related to the fact that the uncorrected reading vision is so good (averaging better than J1 in the ReSTOR FDA study). Thus, patients gradually adapt or gravitate to a more comfortable reading distance, even if it means being unable to read the smallest print at this distance.

This naturally leads to the thorny question of "intermediate vision." It is sometimes said (usually by surgeons who do not have extensive experience with bilateral ReSTOR implantation) that the ReSTOR provides poor "intermediate vision." Although what is meant by intermediate vision is often unclear, the task usually cited is computer use, and of course an increasing proportion of cataract patients use computers. However, in my experience, if patients are first warned of the possible need to adjust the placement of their computer screen and also told that visual function will improve over the first several months, there is no real problem. Laptop computers can be positioned at any distance, and modern desktop flat-screens can also be more easily placed at a convenient distance compared to the old cathode ray tube (CRT) monitors. The intermediate vision improves with time, just as the ease of reading does .

I believe that binocular summation is important in order to achieve the best visual acuity and the best contrast sensitivity. It therefore theoretically does not make sense to mix different multifocal lens technologies (refractive and diffractive) as well as different working distances in the 2 eyes. While this is only anecdotal, I can report that my wife had refractive lens exchange with bilateral ReSTOR implantation 2 years ago. She works full time in an office environment. Initially, she had a pair of +1.25 reading glasses placed by the computer for computer work, but she never used them for anything else. After about 1 year, she found that she only uses the readers for prolonged computer use. For her, simply needing +1.25 readers at her desk for prolonged computer use only is a small price to pay for the unrivalled unaided distance and near vision she now has.

Patient Counseling

Having selected a potential surgical candidate, the next important step is counselling the patient about what to expect from the lens, and more importantly what not to expect (Table 2). It is a truism that the more chair time you spend with the patient before surgery, the less you will need to spend after surgery. It must be made clear to the patient that the bifocal implant represents a compromise and that some side effects are inevitable. Tell him or her that he or she will see halos around lights at night, but at the same time emphasize that they will not cause confusion, they will not be troublesome, and they will decrease in both size and intensity over the first few weeks/months.

Tell the patient that he or she will have a reading distance that is a little closer than what he or she currently has (and show them where 31 cm is), but tell him or her that this reading distance will gradually increase with time. Tell them that if he or she has a computer, he or she will need to move the screen a little closer than where he or she normally has it, but tell him or her that this distance will also increase with time. Remind the patient that he or she can always increase the font size of documents or Web pages. I learned from Robert Kaufer of Buenos Aires that you should tell the patients to expect disappointment and possibly confusion between the 2 eyes as long as only one has been operated on. He tells them that he will not listen to complaints about the multifocal lens until both eyes have been implanted. This only works if you tell patients this before the first surgery and not after it! I would recommend performing both surgeries as close together in time as possible, perhaps 1 week apart. Some even advocate bilateral immediately sequential surgery because of the discomfort and visual confusion experienced when only one eye has the multifocal technology.

Surgical Considerations

Binocular implantation of the ReSTOR IOL is recommended. Most measures of visual function improve when measured binocularly, and patients are generally more comfortable when both eyes have broadly similar function. We have found with the ReSTOR that binocular distance and reading performance is approximately 1 line better than the best monocular result. However, there is no absolute contraindication to monocular implantation in binocular patients, but both the surgeon and patient need to be aware that the results will probably not be quite as good.

Surgeons wishing to use the ReSTOR implant should already have a consistently good surgical technique and be familiar with using the AcrySof SA60/SN60 platform (Alcon, Fort Worth, TX). They and their team should be confident that they can consistently achieve the predicted refractive outcome from their surgery. In order to achieve spectacle independence with the ReSTOR, surgeons must already be consistently achieving distance spectacle independence in their monofocal patients. Use of the correct A-constant is important. Whereas Alcon Laboratories recommends an A-constant of 118.4 for ultrasound biometry and the SN60AT, the recommended A-constant for the ReSTOR (SN60D3) is 118.1. A similar adjustment (ie, reduce by 0.3) should be made to surgeons' own individualized A-constant when switching from the SN60AT to the ReSTOR. This change is needed because the posterior surface of the ReSTOR has a small degree of asphericity to improve the optical image quality. The newly released ReSTOR aspheric IOL will of course have a different A-constant.

It is recommended that surgeons aim for a postsurgery refraction that is slightly hyperopic (0 to +0.5). This outcome tends to increase the reading distance (while retaining excellent unaided distance vision) and also reduces the unwanted night-time images even further (the near image is even more out of focus).

The surgical technique is the same as that for a standard AcrySof SN60 IOL implantation. The capsulorrhexis should be round, centered, and 5 to 5.5 mm in diameter. This allows the anterior capsule to overlap the anterior edge of the IOL, which will reduce PCO. The Monarch injector with a "C" cartridge (Alcon) is recommended for implanting the ReSTOR. When removing the IOL from its packaging and transferring it to the cartridge, care should be taken to grasp the haptic or, if necessary, the optic close to its edge, so as to avoid any possible damage to the diffractive grating (which occupies the central 3.6-mm diameter of the anterior IOL surface). This cartridge will easily pass through a 2.75-mm corneal incision and can also be carefully used with a 2.2-mm incision. The newly released "D" cartridge is part of Alcon's Intrepid microcoaxial system, and this is the ideal cartridge to use for 2.2-mm incisions. While the AcrySof IQ IOL (Alcon) is validated for the D cartridge, at the time of this writing the ReSTOR aspheric IOL has not been. It is of course important to ensure that the IOL sits securely within the capsular bag and that all viscoelastic material has been removed. It is not necessary to directly aspirate behind the IOL optic with a traditional cohesive viscoelastic provided the latter is rocked and nudged during viscoelastic aspiration. If a retentive agent such as Viscoat (Alcon) has been used, this should be directly aspirated from behind the optic. My experience with DisCoVisc (Alcon) has been that this also needs to be aspirated from behind the IOL, but it is very easy to see the fracture lines in this viscoelastic as it is removed in "fragments." Once the haptics have fully returned to their preinsertion configuration, it is important to ensure that the IOL optic is centered because the position of the lens will not change postoperatively. In terms of the pseudoaccommodative properties of the lens, perfect centration is not really important because decentration of up to 1 mm does not degrade optical function. However, in general terms it is important to center the ReSTOR optic.

Reference

1. Kohnen T, Allen D, Boureau C, Dublineau P, et al. European multi-centre study of the AcrySof ReSTOR apodized diffractive intraocular lens. *Ophthalmology*. 2006;113:578-84.

CHAPTER 38

ALCON RESTOR MULTIFOCAL— CLINICAL PEARLS

Samuel Masket, MD

Given appropriate patient selection, meticulous surgery, attainment of emmetropia, and postoperative "optical enhancement" as needed, marked success and spectacle independence can be achieved with the ReSTOR apodized diffractive multifocal intraocular lens (IOL) and its new partner, the Aspheric ReSTOR (Alcon, Fort Worth, TX). This chapter describes the author's experience in achieving the desired outcome with this product. Although the material is organized in a "Ten Step" approach, no facet is more important than another, as all are necessary key elements.

#10: Understand How the Lens Works

The surgeon should have a clear understanding of how the lens provides multifocality and the effects of pupil size and ambient lighting on the optical performance of the device. These factors will also be important as one considers patient selection.

The optic consists of a 6.0-mm lens with the central 3.6 mm containing the apodized diffractive component and the peripheral portion providing monofocal distance correction. (The newer aspheric model features 10 μm of negative asphericity on its anterior peripheral surface.) As such, when the pupil is small, light energy is approximately equally divided between distance and near functions. This is an intuitive design concept, as the pupil constricts during the near reading synkinesis. Likewise, during distance tasks, such as night driving, the pupil dilates, allowing more of the light energy to be employed for distance vision. The "wishbone" distribution of light energy, as seen in Figure 1, illustrates these concepts. Approximately 20% of light energy is "lost" due to scattering in a diffractive optical system. Knowing this, the ReSTOR should not be expected to work as well in eyes that have reduced contrast sensitivity function. Moreover, patients with atypically large pupils may have difficulty with reading, a fact that should be considered when selecting this device.

Another interesting observation regarding visual function with the ReSTOR IOL (and presumably other multifocal IOLs) is neuroadaptation. In a study from Souza et al,[1] patients demonstrated improved visual function over time with the ReSTOR multifocal, but not with the monofocal control. This phenomenon was well demonstrated in the investigation as the eyes that received the multifocal were noted to have improved vision for both far and near 4 to 6 months after surgery, while the eyes with the monofocal control IOL revealed no change in visual function over time.[1]

#9: Implant the Same Intraocular Lens in Both Eyes

It must be recognized that all present presbyopia-correcting IOLs (Pr-C IOLs) represent a compromise between the quest for best vision and the desire for spectacle independence. As such, none of the products can offer perfect vision over the full range of functional distances; this may be termed *seamless vision*. In my view, it is best to allow each product to perform to its maximum potential in order to provide the best quality of vision for as many tasks as possible, and supplement with spectacle correction for those visual tasks that are not adequately managed without additional optical tools. Cerebrocortical summation of binocular vision input allows the 2 eyes to achieve a higher quality of vision than either eye alone can provide. However, summation is lost if the 2 eyes have different images. Loss of cortical summation is deleterious to quality of vision, affecting those with monovision or "mixing and matching" of Pr-C IOLs. The advantages of summation may be noted in Figures 2 and 3.

As can be seen in the graphs, there is a marked improvement in visual acuity with ReSTOR IOLs when the patient uses 2 eyes, rather than 1 eye.

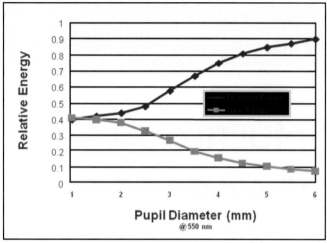

Figure 1. Theoretical total energy balance at 550 nm for AcrySof ReSTOR apodized diffractive optic.

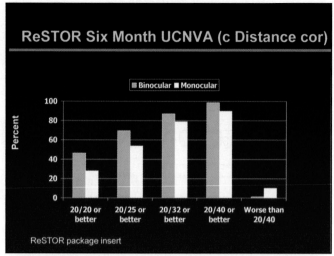

Figure 3. ReSTOR 6-month uncorrected near visual acuity (with distance correction).

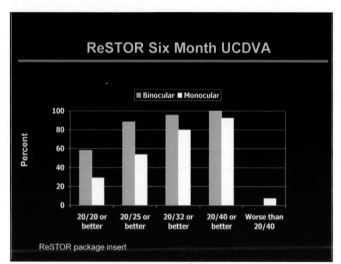

Figure 2. ReSTOR 6-month uncorrected distance visual acuity.

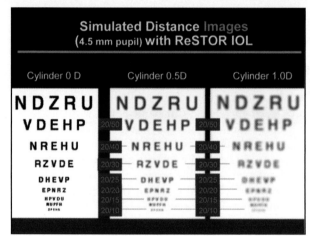

Figure 4. Simulated distance images (4.5-mm pupil) with the ReSTOR IOL.

#8: Correct For or Control Astigmatism

Given that any multifocal IOL divides light energy between distance and near visual functions, there is an understandable loss of contrast sensitivity and an increased requirement for emmetropia. Figure 4 demonstrates the simulated loss of clarity through a ReSTOR IOL with a pupil aperture of 4.5 mm; the example on the left represents emmetropia. The negative effect of 0.5 D and 1.0 D of astigmatism are demonstrated.

Obviously, cylinder must be addressed for appropriate performance with the ReSTOR IOL. The great majority of eyes do not require adjustment of presurgical corneal astigmatism. However, significant degrees of surgically induced corneal astigmatism risk conversion from an acceptable to an unacceptable amount of postoperative astigmatism. For that

reason, I prefer to take advantage of the single-piece platform of the AcrySof IOL (Alcon) and routinely remove the cataract and implant the ReSTOR through a 2.2-mm temporal incision, employing microcoaxial phacoemulsification. I have found that 2.2-mm incisions induce significantly less cylinder than 3.0-mm incisions, as can be noted in Table 1.

Given that it is essential to eliminate virtually all astigmatism (and ametropia, for that matter), patient selection comes heavily into play. Pre-existing astigmatism, up to 2 D, may be approached during surgery with peripheral corneal relaxing incisions (Figure 5), which may need to be repeated postoperatively. Alternatively, patients with greater degrees of presurgical corneal astigmatism will likely require laser vision correction after the healing period in order to achieve good results. That fact must be explained to the patient prior to surgery. In some cases, it might be appropriate to consider raising a microkeratome flap in advance of cataract surgery; in this manner, the flap may be lifted as early postoperatively as desired, avoiding a prolonged optical correction.

Table 1

SIA RESULTS: 22 PATIENTS (44 EYES)

	2.2 mm	3.0 mm	p Value
AlgA	0.10 D (SD – 0.08)	0.32 D (SD – 0.20)	0.0002
VecA	0.35 D (SD – 0.21)	0.67 D (SD – 0.48)	0.006

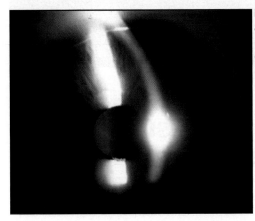

Figure 5. Pre-existing astigmatism, up to 2 D, may be approached during surgery with peripheral corneal relaxing incisions.

Table 2

PERSONAL ENHANCEMENT EXPERIENCE

- Limited to ReSTOR
- 300 ReSTOR IOLs
- 30 procedures in 23 eyes—7 eyes had 2 enhancements
- 2 eyes scheduled for or need enhancement
- Approximately 10%

Enhancement Procedures

- PCRI (LRI)—14
- LASIK/PRK—8
- Piggyback IOL—2
- Epithelial debridement—2
- EOM surgery—1
- IOL exchange—3 (remove/replace for monofocal)

#7: Accurate Biometry and Use of Latest Generation Intraocular Lens Power Formulae Are a Must

As mentioned previously, owing to the nature of the diffractive optic, best results with the ReSTOR require that emmetropia be achieved for each case. Partial coherence interferometry (PCI) with the IOL Master (Carl Zeiss Meditec, Jena, Germany) proves to be the most reliable device to measure axial length, although immersion A-scan ultrasonography is also very accurate.

I use the axial length value to determine which IOL power formula to apply. In general, I prefer the Hoffer Q for eyes that are shorter than 22.5 mm, the SRK-T for eyes that are longer than 24.0 mm, and the Holladay I for eyes of average length. However, the Haigis formula, which is available with the IOL Master, is valuable for all axial lengths, as is the Holladay II.

I do not hesitate to employ the ReSTOR in patients who have had prior laser vision correction and will employ my personalized regression formula for those patients whose laser vision correction data are available, while the Haigis-L formula is applied when laser treatment details cannot be obtained.[2]

#6: Be Willing and Able to Adjust or Enhance the Optical Results of Surgery

All IOL power formulae are potentially flawed, and a given percentage of patients will require an additional procedure(s) in order to achieve spectacle independence, the primary goal for the use of the ReSTOR IOL. In general, this figure will fall somewhere between 10% and 20%.

Enhancements may include any procedure designed to achieve spectacle independence. Table 2 reveals 30 enhancement procedures that I performed in 23 eyes of approximately 300 implants. Excimer laser vision correction for the ReSTOR patient may be achieved with traditional algorithms or by custom treatment, assuming that a wavefront analysis can be obtained. Note that not all procedures were for ametropia. Patients and surgeons must be aware that enhancement is an integral part of success with Pr-C IOLs.

I have found that some patients may have simple optical errors that are not easily discernible with standard clinical refraction. However, use of wavefront analysis has helped to uncover optical errors in a few cases. In my experience, in the absence of pathology, emmetropic patients will uniformly see well at far and near with the ReSTOR. A wavefront analysis could be revealing should the visual results of surgery be less than expected, pathology fully excluded, and refraction not helpful. I have come to recognize that so called "waxy vision" that some have attributed to the ReSTOR IOL most likely represents unrecognized ametropia rather than higher-order aberration.

Surgeons who offer a full array of refractive procedures will be able to personally manage most enhancement needs.

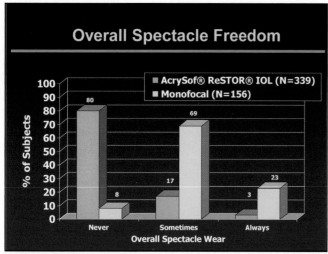

Figure 6. Overall spectacle freedom.

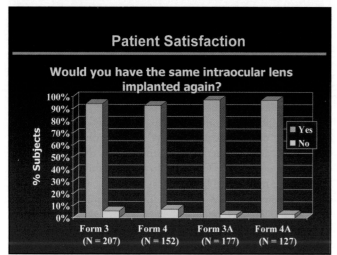

Figure 7. Patient satisfaction.

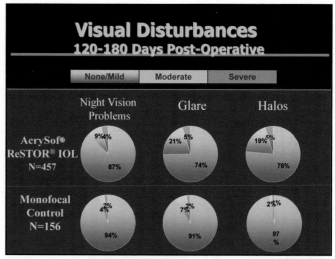

Figure 8. Visual disturbances.

#4: Explain the Strengths and Weaknesses of the ReSTOR IOL to the Patient

The patient needs to have an objective view of the benefits and drawbacks to any IOL technology, particularly when he or she will be paying a premium for any given device. This "consumerism" cannot be avoided and is one facet of implanting "premium" IOLs. With regard to the ReSTOR IOL, I inform patients of the US Food and Drug Administration (FDA) trial results in terms of spectacle independence, patient satisfaction, and incidence of undesired optical imagery (Figures 6, 7, and 8) .

#3: Establish Credibility With Both Staff and Patients: They Want to Hear From You!

Although there are a number of valuable teaching aids for patients presented in a variety of formats, they should serve only a partial role in the process of patient education regarding "premium" IOLs. Patients appreciate hearing from the physician about the devices and whether they are well suited for the patient in the doctor's opinion. Often patients inquire whether I would implant the device in my relatives. Indeed, I have implanted my sister's eyes with ReSTOR IOLs, a fact that I readily share with prospective surgical candidates. Knowing that I believe in the device sufficiently to have placed it in a relative adds much to the patient's confidence and to my credibility. Likewise, it is prudent to have educational seminars for the office staff so that they are fully aware of the device and that you believe in it. Where possible and appropriate, it could be very beneficial to implant a staff member or his or her close relative.

However, for those who do not, it will be necessary to share patient management with other specialists.

#5: Know the Patient

Working knowledge of the patient's lifestyles, hobbies, employment, etc are essential to success, particularly in regard to patient selection. As an example, those who spend much of their life driving at night are not ideal candidates.

Similarly, careful and complete ocular evaluation is necessary to rule out certain, and sometimes subtle, conditions that could make the outcome less than desirable. Examples include corneal anterior basement membrane dystrophy, significant heterophorias that require prism correction, epiretinal membrane, diabetic maculopathy, significant optic nerve damage from glaucoma, unusually large pupils, etc.

Personality profile is another individual feature that should be ascertained prior to final determination of a patient's candidacy for the ReSTOR IOL. In general, highly demanding or negative personality types are not ideally suited.

#2: Do Impeccable Surgery— Do Not Allow the Surgery to Be the Limiting Factor of a Successful Outcome

The quality of surgery can have a definite impact on surgical outcomes and, in turn, patient satisfaction. Surgeons must have careful control of induced astigmatism and employ strategies to limit postoperative corneal astigmatism to less than 0.5 D in all cases. Surgeons, therefore, need to measure outcomes with regard to mean surgically induced astigmatism of their incisional method and create reproducible, clean incisions that hopefully will not require sutures, as the latter also have an effect on postoperative astigmatism.

The capsulorrhexis must be well centered and correctly sized (approximately 5.0 mm) so that the lens edge is fully covered by the anterior capsulorrhexis. This helps maintain IOL centration, retards posterior capsular opacification, and helps to achieve consistent optical results of surgery.

Surgeons should strive carefully to avoid rupture of the posterior capsule as the single-piece AcrySof ReSTOR cannot be implanted in the ciliary sulcus. While a 3-piece ReSTOR model is available, outcomes are likely to be less predictable unless the surgeon has considerable experience with this device.

It is also beneficial to align the center of the optic with the patient's visual axis. After the viscoagent has been removed at the end of the surgery, I request that the patient look directly toward the microscope light filament (it is a good idea to reduce the brightness at this stage of the surgery) and I nudge the IOL with a small cannula through the side-port incision to facilitate the process. The eye is then gently pressurized and wound closure is completed. Typically, it is necessary to move the IOL slightly nasally and inferiorly; the lens generally stays where it is placed, as the tackiness of the IOL surface enables it to "stick" to the posterior capsule.

#1: Under Promise and Over Deliver: Be a Strong Patient Advocate

The physician should be cognizant that a new relationship is forged when patients pay a premium for Pr-C IOL devices; consumerism may have a meaningful effect on the patient's view of the procedure. Furthermore, some patients may not adapt rapidly to the nuances of the surgery, particularly until second eye surgery has been completed, and a significant percentage of cases will require enhancement surgery for best results. Consequently, the operating surgeon needs to have a comfortable, nonadversarial relationship with the patient. The patient should feel confident that the physician is concerned about his or her welfare, capable of managing problems, and able to adjust the optical outcome of surgery should it be needed. There should be no attempt to hide information from the patient prior to surgery, as the more consultative chair time the surgeon spends prior to surgery, the less will be needed afterward. The patient and surgeon should have the sense that they are embarking on a cooperative mission, with each doing his or her part to reach a successful outcome.

References

1. Souza CE, Muccioli C, Soriano ES, et al. Visual performance of AcrySof ReSTOR apodized diffractive IOL: a prospective comparative trial. *Am J Ophthalmol.* 2006;141:827-832.
2. Masket S, Masket SE. Simple regression formula for intraocular lens power adjustment in eyes requiring cataract surgery after excimer laser photoablation. *J Cataract Refract Surg.* 2006;32(3):430-434.

CHAPTER 39

ASPHERIC ReSTOR— WHAT IS DIFFERENT?

Paul Ernest, MD

The designs of the AcrySof ReSTOR intraocular lens (IOL) (Alcon, Fort Worth, TX) and the AcrySof ReSTOR aspheric IOL are similar. Both contain 3 optical systems—apodization, diffraction, and refraction—to provide patients with a range of vision. The lenses provide one optical lens power for near vision and one optical lens power for distance vision.

While these lenses share some properties with full-optic diffractive lenses, they also have some unique characteristics. The ReSTOR lenses have a 3.6-mm diffractive region that consists of 12 diffractive steps. The largest diffractive step (1.3 µm) is at the lens center.

The "add" power of the lens is determined by the locations of the steps. The height of each diffractive step controls the amount of light that is directed to the 2 primary lens powers. While the step heights are the same for the full-optic diffractive lenses, the AcrySof ReSTOR and ReSTOR aspheric lenses have step heights that decrease with increasing distance from the lens center (1.3 to 0.2 µm), which is called apodization. As the pupil diameter changes, apodization gradually changes the amount of energy directed to the 2 primary images. The apodized diffractive design of both lenses complements the pupil and compensates for changes in light intensity and activity.

The AcrySof ReSTOR optic is designed to match the needs of the patient. For example, while people need to have good vision at all distances, they rarely need to read or do other close work in dimly lit conditions when their pupils are dilated. Typically, patients can add light for near work.

With ReSTOR, the energy directed to the near image stays constant as the pupil dilates outside the diffractive area. However, patients occasionally experience visual disturbances when looking at bright light sources at night. This can occur because the defocused image from the second lens power may be visible as a halo. The occurrence of this phenomenon is much less with both ReSTOR lenses than with other multifocal technologies.

With the AcrySof ReSTOR lens, the apodized diffractive region is limited to the central part of the lens. For larger pupils, more energy is directed to the outer part of the lens, which provides distance vision. The limited diffractive region reduces the size and energy of a halo surrounding a light source at night.

The ReSTOR IOL's add power is +4 D at the lens. This provides approximately +3.2 D of add power at the spectacle plane. The IOL's location in the eye is responsible for the lower add power at the cornea, and the ReSTOR's add power makes the second image as defocused and faint as possible.

The only difference between the AcrySof ReSTOR and the AcrySof ReSTOR aspheric is the sphericity of the lens. The AcrySof ReSTOR aspheric IOL model SN6AD3 is designed with negative spherical aberration. The negative spherical aberration compensates for the positive corneal spherical aberrations, resulting in enhanced image quality and, ultimately, contrast for the patient.

Benefits of the ReSTOR Aspheric Intraocular Lens

Spherical aberration occurs when marginal rays are over-refracted, resulting in a region of defocused light, which can decrease image quality (Figure 1).

Aspheric optics align the light rays to compensate for positive corneal spherical aberration, resulting in enhanced image quality (Figure 2).

Most patients have very good results with the AcrySof ReSTOR IOL. However, a small percentage of patients were not happy due to visual disturbances described as halos and glare or fuzzy vision.

In my experience, the ReSTOR aspheric was like a breath of fresh air. With this lens, halos are reduced by 70% to 80%, and contrast sensitivity is improved. I have not had any patients complain about the Aspheric ReSTOR. It is important to note that I limit preoperative cylinder to 0.75 D or less.

My early 1-month postoperative results (24 eyes) are shown in Figure 3.

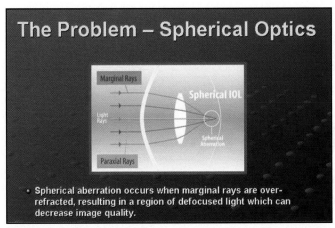

Figure 1. The problem: spherical optics.

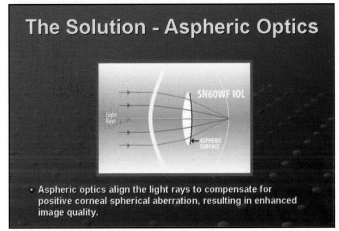

Figure 2. The solution: aspheric optics.

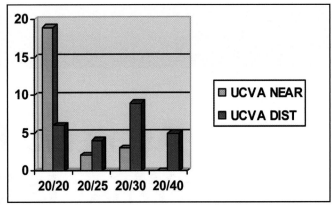

Figure 3. Early 1-month postoperative results.

Patient Selection

When evaluating a patient for the ReSTOR lens, my practice uses a lifestyle questionnaire that assesses a patient's wish list. Then, I evaluate his or her corneal astigmatism. If it is approximately 1 D or more, I do not consider the ReSTOR lens. Instead, I encourage an AcrySof toric IOL.

If a patient has less than 1 D of corneal astigmatism and no diseases precluding him or her from ReSTOR implantation, I will discuss the ReSTOR lens. This will certainly change when a lens that combines the benefits of both the ReSTOR and toric lens is introduced.

When implanting the ReSTOR lens, it is important to under promise and over deliver. I tell every patient to expect to wear glasses for some tasks. People will be free from glasses approximately 90% of their day. I tell every patient to expect to see halos and glare. However, less than 2% of our patients report seeing halos and do not consider this as being problematic. I also tell them that they may need a laser procedure. This has not been necessary with the preoperative restriction on corneal astigmatism.

I typically leave the nondominant eye undercorrected (hyperopic), and I ensure that the lens is centered.

Conclusion

The ReSTOR aspheric IOL is a valuable addition to our armamentarium because it reduces the incidence of glare and halos and improves contrast sensitivity.

CHAPTER 40

ASPHERIC RESTOR—
WHAT IS DIFFERENT?

Robert P. Lehmann, MD, FACS

Today, the ReSTOR Aspheric intraocular lens (IOL) (Alcon, Fort Worth, TX) has essentially replaced the original spherical ReSTOR first available in the United States. Although I have had personal extensive and quite successful experience with the original lens, there can be no doubt that the optical qualities of the aspheric design outperform the spherical optic in bench testing and clinical performance. I anticipate that ongoing studies will demonstrate the same improvements in quality of visual performance for the aspheric ReSTOR lens as did comparative evaluations of the spherical monofocal AcrySof (Alcon) compared with the aspheric monofocal lens with regards to contrast sensitivity, night driving, and visual performance (AcrySof IQ).[1]

In a study of 44 subjects, the aspheric monofocal (AcrySof IQ) demonstrated superior functional performance in contrast sensitivity in a night driving simulator. Testing was conducted in both city and rural situations for detection and identification of warning signs, pedestrians, and text in fog, glare, and normal conditions. The aspheric lens consistently performed better than the spherical monofocal control (AcrySof single-piece IOL) from detection to identification of targets in both city and rural situations, resulting in improved functional vision and increased stopping distance for our patients.

In a city setting, eyes implanted with the AcrySof IQ lens identified pedestrians in fog and glare conditions, and road signs at least a half of second earlier than the spherical monofocal control group. A half second of increased reaction time is equivalent to 25 feet. In the rural setting, they identified warning signs in fog, glare, and normal conditions at least a full second before the control group. Long term, I expect that the addition of asphericity to the ReSTOR lens will lead to similar results for our patients and their safety as the addition of asphericity did for monofocal lenses.

In comparing the ReSTOR to the ReSTOR aspheric IOL, I have found that my patients are happier postoperative day 1. I am finding that my patients are looking forward to receiving the lens in the second eye, which allows them to take full advantage of the technology through binocular summation.

Personally, I think this result is due to the improved quality of distance vision that my patients receive due to addressing corneal spherical aberrations.

With the original ReSTOR lens, we saw the lowest number of patient complaints for visual disturbances in a multifocal design due to the apodized diffractive optic. The apodized diffractive optic optimally manages light energy depending on the situation, which minimizes the amount of glare and halos a patient may experience. In my practice, the Aspheric ReSTOR lens has further reduced the amount of visual disturbances my patients are experiencing because it compensates for corneal spherical aberrations, which ultimately leads to happier patients sooner in the postoperative period.

Like its monofocal counterpart, the one exception to use of the aspheric optic remains the posthyperopic laser in situ keratomileusis (LASIK) patient. In such patients, a standard spherical optic is preferred in order not to induce additional spherical aberrations for these patients.

I will assume that the reader by this time understands the importance of patient selection for successful outcomes with presbyopia-correcting IOL technology. I specifically decline use of multifocal technology in patients with significant corneal guttata, postradial keratotomy (RK) patients, and patients who lack the potential for good postoperative visual recovery.

The "best candidates" for the aspheric ReSTOR IOL are patients with realistic expectations who can accept the possibility of nocturnal rings or halos (which typically diminish over time), and who understand that any residual ametropia may require refractive "touch up" (either limbal relaxing incisions [LRIs], photorefractive keratectomy [PRK], or LASIK). Patients should never be told that there is any guarantee that they will "never need glasses," but may be assured that the majority of the time most patients will see well for their daily tasks without correction. My own data confirm that nearly 90% of ReSTOR patients never wear glasses for any task. To achieve these results, a surgeon must address postoperative issues such as dry eye, subclinical cystoid macular edema

(CME), and residual refractive cylinder of as "little" as 0.75 D, which can have a very significant impact on quality of vision in the multifocal patient.

Achieving these results requires more than excellent patient education and selection. Meticulous care is taken in measuring corneal curvatures and axial lengths and in choosing the appropriate IOL power. All of my premium IOL patients undergo measurements with the upgraded IOL Master (Carl Zeiss Meditec, Jena, Germany) and immersion biometry. In eyes with average axial length, I prefer the SRK-T formula or the Holladay 2. Warren Hill has long been my "go to guru" for both the easy and the complicated IOL selections (see www.doctor-hill.com). I personally review and select the target IOL power in every eye and generally target emmetropia. I have found that the most satisfied patients will be those with less corneal cylinder preoperative and in whom a nearly spherical outcome can be accomplished.

Finally, meticulous surgery is essential to success. A capsulorrhexis overlapping the optic is beneficial with this technology, and thus a 5.5-mm size is ideal. I make certain to remove all viscoelastic from behind the IOL and to be sure that the IOL is centered and seated against the posterior capsule at the completion of the case. I do not constrict the pupil with a miotic and generally find little or no decentration of the ReSTOR optic.

Although I have several hundred patients with the original spherical ReSTOR IOLs in both eyes, I believe that the eye surgeon who is new to multifocal technology is now better equipped to select for success. The aspheric multifocal technology provides a higher level of visual performance and should, when used in the appropriate patient, yield excellent patient and surgeon satisfaction. With extensive experience with both multifocal and accommodative technologies available, I prefer to use similar optic designs in both eyes in the vast majority of my patients. With the technologies available today, it is finally possible to achieve a new level of patient satisfaction and spectacle independence, but not without careful patient education and selection, precise measurements and calculations, surgical excellence, and postoperative management.

The introduction of the ReSTOR lens with asphericity is simply the first of many new product introductions for these presbyopia-correcting lenses. I believe that, long term, we will have the opportunity to offer presbyopia-correcting IOLs on the same platform that provide a patient with the option of near vision at different distances through alternative add powers. Additionally, we will ultimately be able to treat both presbyopia and astigmatism in a lens with aspheric optics.

References

1. Lehmann R. Functional performance of the AcrySof IQ IOL: night-driving simulation and contrast sensitivity using the FACT chart. Presented at the ASCRS ASOA Symposium & Congress, San Diego, April 28, 2007.

CHAPTER 41

ReSTOR Designs—
Past, Present, Future

Satish Modi, MD, FRCS(C), CPI

Ever since its approval by the Food and Drug Administration (FDA) (international release 2003/2004) in March 2005 and its widespread commercial availability in May 2005, the ReSTOR multifocal lens (Model SN60D3) (Alcon, Fort Worth, TX) has quickly become the most widely implanted presbyopia-correcting intraocular lens (IOL) in the world, with over 325,000 implanted worldwide as of this writing.

After having implanted several hundred of these first-generation ReSTORs myself, my patients and I have been both very pleased with the results. The patients' near acuities and their consequent ability to read without glasses have been both unparalleled and hitherto unattainable. Providing keratometric cylinder is attended to, and due attention is paid to pupil size (both scotopic and accommodative), these patients have excellent distance acuities.

About 5% of my patients complain of halos and poor night time vision, especially those with small scotopic pupils, and so they have to be counseled preoperatively. I practice in IBM country, and everyone has a personal computer; these patients often complain about the lack of crisp intermediate "computer" vision and are initially displeased with the foreshortened (near vision) distance of about 13 inches. We warn them of this preoperatively, and those patients that cannot adapt by moving closer to the computer monitor, do well with an over-the-counter (OTC) pair of +1.50-D readers. This amount of reading add serves them well until cortical adaptation "kicks" in. We find that the vast majority of these patients have discarded their computer glasses by 6 months postoperatively. In fact, about 95% of our ReSTOR patients function without corrective lenses.

In an effort to try and gain more immediate intermediate vision, ophthalmologists have attempted, and enjoyed success with a "mix and match" approach. Typically, a ReSTOR is put into the nondominant eye, and a ReZoom (Advanced Medical Optics, Santa Ana, CA) or Crystalens (Eyeonics, Inc, Aliso Viejo, CA) is put into the dominant eye in an attempt to gain better intermediate vision in that eye. After having done a "mix and match" approach on 20 patients, I have come to the following conclusions:

* A number of patients complain of a qualitative difference in vision between the 2 eyes.
* Patients with large scotopic pupils complain of more night time halos with the ReZoom eye.
* There is only a 2 to 3 inch difference in reading distance between eyes (ReSTOR 13 inches, ReZoom 15 inches), and even at that distance the ReZoom eye does not see as clearly.

Because of these results, I have stopped mixing and matching different technology implants. A vast majority of patients prefer bilateral ReSTOR lenses. For the few patients that are not big readers and do most of their work at arm's length (an excavator I did recently comes to mind), a bilateral ReZoom implantation works best; however, ALL of these bilateral ReZoom patients need an OTC +1.25 D pair of readers to do close work.

The second generation of ReSTOR implants, the Aspheric ReSTOR (Model SN6AD3), became commercially available in the United States in July 2007. Since spherical aberration is the single largest higher-order aberration responsible for decreased quality of vision in older patients, this lens, with its negative spherical aberration on the posterior surface, is a welcome change. It has quickly, in 4 months, accounted for over 60% of sales of all ReSTOR lenses, and with good reason (Figures 1 and 2).

I was involved in a Postmarketing Study in which 40 patients were bilaterally implanted with ReSTOR aspheric (Model SN6AD3) or ReSTOR regular IOLs (Model SN60D3). Follow-up was 3 months after the second eye surgery. Postoperative evaluation included logMAR visual acuity testing at various distances, patient reported outcomes, and contrast sensitivity measured with the CSE-1000E (VectorVision Inc, Dayton, OH).

At postoperative day 1, only 6% of the regular ReSTOR patients saw 20/20; a full 43% of the aspheric ReSTOR

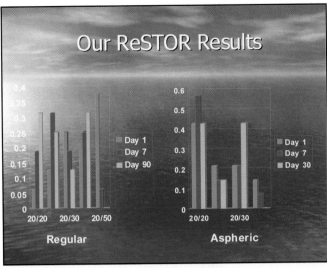

Figure 1. ReSTOR results.

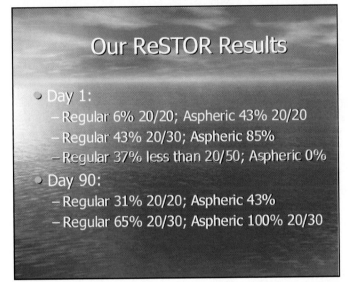

Figure 2. ReSTOR results.

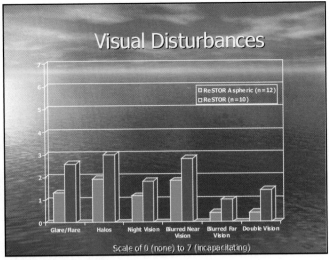

Figure 3. Visual disturbances.

patients saw 20/20, significantly increasing the "wow" factor. Eighty-five percent of the aspheric ReSTOR patients saw at least 20/30. We see our ReSTOR patients in the afternoon the day after surgery, which allows their pupils to return to normal. A vast majority of these patients were reading Jaeger 1 on postoperative day 1.

At 3 months postoperatively, 100% of patients were seeing 20/30 or better and reading Jaeger 1 in the aspheric group. Moreover, visual disturbance ratings on a scale of 0 (none) to 7 (debilitating) consistently favored the aspheric ReSTOR implant (Figures 3).

The aspheric patients had less glare and halos and better overall vision both for near and far. We took wavefront measurements on these patients. The differences with a 3.5-mm pupil are miniscule, but they are very apparent with a 5.0-mm pupil, as the accompanying pictures show (Figures 4, 5, 6, and 7). The amount of spherical aberration with a 5.0-mm pupil size is 2.3 times less in the aspheric group as compared to the regular group. This translates into better overall vision and happier patients.

The next generation of ReSTOR lenses is going to introduce further improvements on the same platform. Studies are already underway for the ReSTOR 3.0, which has a +3.0 D add at the IOL plane and translates to a +2.25 D add at the spectacle plane. This should theoretically give good near vision at a distance of 17 to 18 inches, thereby satisfying the need for both near and computer vision and obviating any need for glasses even in the early months before cortical adaptation has fully occurred. I suspect that this third-generation lens shall suffice for over 90% of our patients' visual needs.

Unfortunately, none of these 3 generations of ReSTORs helps patients with significant amounts of astigmatism; these patients right now need bioptics or a separate refractive corneal procedure to give them unfettered vision. With this in mind, I am sure that on the horizon, we will see the amalgamation of all of Alcon's technologies, with the introduction of an aspheric, toric, and ReSTOR lens all in one platform. This should meet the needs of all our patients that want premium IOLs in one fell swoop. I, for one, cannot wait.

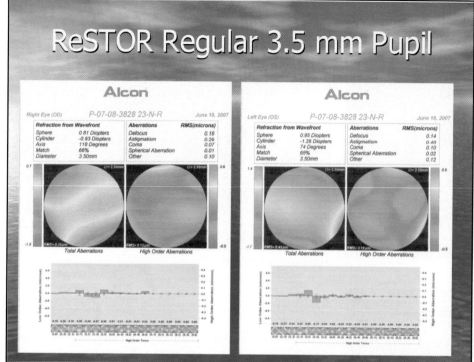

Figure 4. ReSTOR regular 3.5-mm pupil.

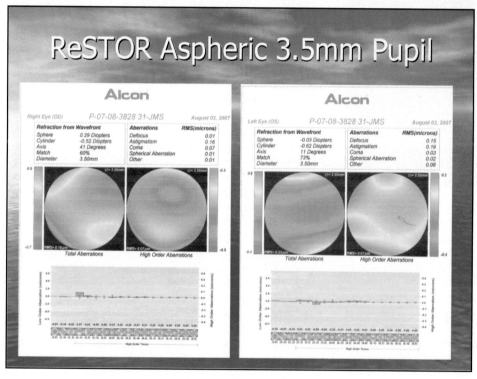

Figure 5. ReSTOR aspheric 3.5-mm pupil.

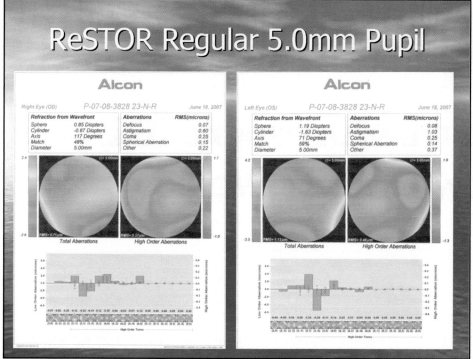

Figure 6. ReSTOR regular 5.0-mm pupil.

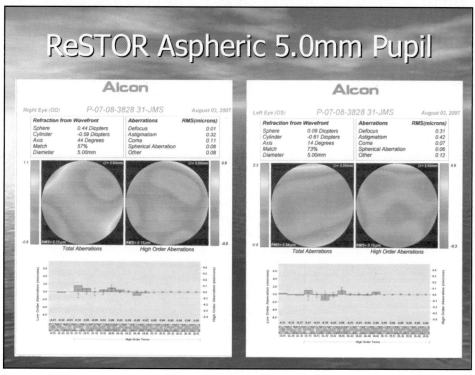

Figure 7. ReSTOR regular 5.0-mm pupil.

CHAPTER 42

DIFFRACTIVE MULTIFOCAL IOL— HOW DOES IT WORK?

James A. Davison, MD, FACS

Although light travels in a straight line, when it encounters the edge of an obstruction, it slows and spreads out slightly. This effect is called diffraction. It cannot be adequately explained with a ray-tracing model because ray tracing should only be applied to smooth and continuous optical surfaces. Rays are normally perpendicular to a wavefront at every point, but, if the wavefront encounters an edge, simple ray tracing gives misleading results because diffractive effects become dominant.

The AcrySof ReSTOR refractive-diffractive intraocular lens (IOL) (Alcon, Fort Worth, TX) uses a set of circular zones to focus light at 2 foci. The far focus is at the foveola, and the near focus is approximately 1 mm in front of the foveola. There are a number of discontinuities, also known as diffractive steps or zone boundaries. There are zones between the discontinuities, but these do not act like the zones of a refractive multifocal IOL. That is, they do not alternate far-near-far-near. Instead, the diffractive effects created by the geometry of the steps combine with the refractive lens properties to create a unique design.

The Design in Detail

The ReSTOR's construction is inherently difficult to represent in a simple fashion for 2 reasons. First, there are the distractions of too much detail, such as the thickness of the optic, the range of wavelengths for visible light, the refractive indices of the media, and the anatomy of the fovea. Second, there are numerous light waves involved. Ignoring those distractions, Figure 1 schematically represents the distance from the lens to the foveola (19 mm) and the distance from the lens to the point of near focus (18 mm) in an emmetropic model eye.

The distances can be measured in wavelengths of light as well. Using green light as an example, there are approximately 46,000 wavelengths of 550-nm light in the vitreous from the lens to the foveola (the far image) and about 44,000 wavelengths from the lens to the add-power focus (the near image), which is approximately 1 mm in front of the foveola. Starting

at the first diffractive step of the ReSTOR lens and moving radially outward, the location of the second zone boundary is where the difference of the distances between the 2 foci changes by just one wavelength on the IOL's optic. The other 11 zone boundaries are placed at increasingly peripheral locations of 1 wavelength of change. As it turns out, in order to keep the same 2 points of focus (far and near) as zones are added, zone boundaries become progressively closer together peripherally. If the add power were lower, the second focus would move closer to the foveola (eg, it would be at 18.5 mm for a 2.00-D add), and the family of zones would move outward on the lens to maintain the 1-wavelength requirement.

The magnitude of these numbers seems incredible, but changes in the optical path length of 1 wavelength of relating points that are thousands of wavelengths away specify the widths of the optical zones that lie within the zone boundaries. The engineering of the IOL with regard to these numbers is equally fascinating. That is, the company had to develop a cast-molding process that can reliably produce plastic lenses out of foldable AcrySof lens (Alcon) material that have step heights of approximately 1.3 µm and gradually decrease in a stepwise fashion to 0.2 µm peripherally. As 1.3 µm equals 1300 nm, this is little more than 2 wavelengths of green light in air, or about 3 wavelengths in aqueous. Two tenths of a micron is 200 nm or one half a wavelength of blue light in air.

Diffractive Steps

The diffractive steps introduce phase delays for light at the zone boundaries. The height of the step is a measure of the phase delay, although the entire zone surface changes if the step height is altered. The reason is that, although the optical zones themselves have generally spherical surfaces, they each are composed of individually different curvatures that also differ from the underlying optical base curve of the lens. The characteristics of a diffractive IOL can be seen in the ReSTOR lens' surface (Figure 2). The shape of the surface profile of each zone determines the predominant direction of light

Figure 1. Light travels slower on the plastic side of the step of the lens compared with the speed at which it moves through aqueous. The resultant phase delay creates 2 points of focus, one for distance and one for near. (Reprinted with permission from Davison JA. Deciphering diffraction: How the ReSTOR's apodized, refractive, diffractive optic works. *Cataract Refract Surg Today.* 2005;June:42-46.)

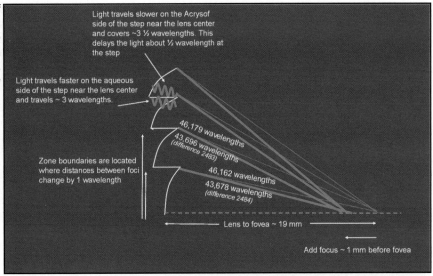

passing through the zone, whereas tiny steps at the zone boundaries adjust the phase of the light. The combination of the zone boundary's placement, the zone's surface profile, and the phase delay at the steps creates the overall optical properties.

The step height can be used as a simple descriptor of the overall optical properties of the ReSTOR IOL. If there were no steps at the zone boundaries, for example, it would be a monofocal lens, and all the light would go to its base power. If the step heights all increased the optical path by 1 wavelength, then the lens would be monofocal, with all the light going to the add power; in this case, the curvatures of the individual zones would all be identical and similar to those of a refractive lens.

Something that is less obvious is that if the step heights all increased the optical path by half a wavelength, then approximately 41% of the light would go to each of the 2 primary lens powers. This is theoretically and practically the best division of light that can be achieved by diffraction alone for 2 lens powers, and it results from the complex interaction between the zone boundaries' locations and the zonal structure. The step height essentially determines how much light goes to each image and provides control over energy balance. The additional light energy goes into other lens powers of −4.00, +8.00, −8.00, and +12.00 D, powers that are related to other image distances that geometrically have integral multiples of optical path distance (3 wavelengths, 5 wavelengths, etc). The images are not perceived because they are extremely defocused and their energy is very low.

Apodization

Apodization refers to the change of a property across the optical surface from the center to periphery. The term could apply to a filter that is clear in the center and becomes increasingly opaque toward the periphery. In the case of the ReSTOR's optic, the diffractive structure is apodized in order to control light energy's contribution to the distant and near foci. This concept is illustrated in Figure 3, which compares the exaggerated surface with the approximate energy balance

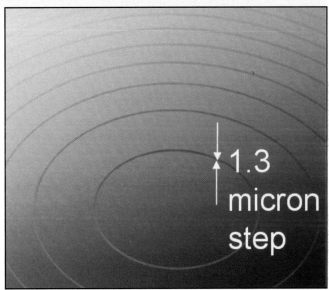

Figure 2. On the apodized diffractive anterior surface, the steps become progressively shorter, from 1.3 to 0.4 μm. (Reprinted with permission from Davison JA. Deciphering diffraction: How the Restor's apodized, refractive, diffractive optic works. *Cataract Refract Surg Today.* 2005;June:42-46.)

between the 2 images. Previous diffractive lenses have used the same step height for all the zone boundaries, a design that also makes all the zone curvatures similar to each other. For the ReSTOR lens, with small pupils, the phase delay at the central steps is approximately half a wavelength, which divides the light energy fairly equally between the base and add powers. As pupils become larger, additional zones are used, with the step heights becoming progressively smaller and the zones less steeply curved. The phase delay at the steps is less because the step heights get shorter, which results in less light going to the add power and correspondingly more light being used for far vision. The step heights actually straddle the base curve so that the calculation of the zone boundary's location is not affected by changes in step height.

Two factors are complementary when considering the design: the situations where near vision is used and the visibility of photic phenomena. In general, near vision is important

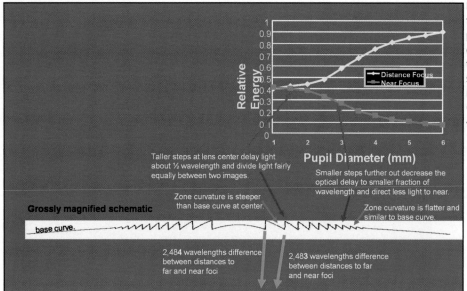

Figure 3. The ReSTOR's apodization virtually equalizes the portions of light for distance and near with small pupillary diameters and increases the contribution for distance vision as the pupil becomes larger and more of the peripheral optic is utilized. (Reprinted with permission from Davison JA. Deciphering diffraction: How the Restor's apodized, refractive, diffractive optic works. *Cataract Refract Surg Today.* 2005;June:42-46.)

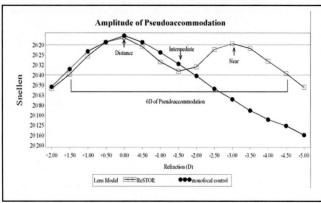

Figure 4. The monofocal IOL's peak performance is with 0 D in the phoropter. The ReSTOR IOL has 2 performance peaks, one with 0 D and the other with −3.00 D dialed into the phoropter because the lens possesses a plano correction and a +3.00-D correction. The ReSTOR lens has a pseudoaccommodative range of 6.00 versus 3.50 D for the monofocal IOL. (Reprinted with permission from Davison JA. Deciphering diffraction: How the Restor's apodized, refractive, diffractive optic works. *Cataract Refract Surg Today.* 2005;June:42-46.)

diffractive pattern to maintain the 2 focal points, foveal and 1 mm anterior to the fovea.

Range of Focus

The ReSTOR lens has 2 fixed primary powers where retinal focus is sharpest and best acuity can be achieved. It also provides good visual acuity for 2 ranges of object distances. The midpoint of each range is each of the primary best-focusing distances. Figure 4 shows defocus curves measured in the phoropter that compare the ReSTOR lens to a monofocal control. Far-vision ranges are comparable for both lenses, but the ReSTOR lens provides an additional range of vision around the best near focus of 32 cm. Both primary lens powers of the ReSTOR lens contribute to intermediate distance vision. With the ReSTOR, the expanded performance of near and intermediate depths of field improves patients' vision of everything within arm's length.

The change in the intensity of defocused light varies with the type of object and other parameters. For a point source, the light from the second power has less than 1% of the intensity of the focused spot. For a line or other object, it may be 2% to 3%. The human visual system is designed to pick out structure in a scene and to ignore other optical phenomena, which arise normally in the phakic eye due to corneal tear film effects, dryness, and swelling; floaters; and other phenomena. Faint, secondary, defocused light is rarely noticeable, although it is more likely to be visible at night, when there are bright point sources against a dark background.

ReSTOR patients do not report a loss of light, although the energy's focus is split between the 2 images. Human vision is very tolerant of the continual changes in light energy upon fluctuations in pupillary diameter and in illumination. The eye seeks details of interest and ignores modest changes in intensity. Objects are visible under luminance changes of more than a factor of 1 million, from a lighted office to outdoor sunshine. An intensity change of a factor of 2 normally is not noticeable.

primarily when the pupil is smaller because of normal illumination levels for near work and the accommodative reflex. Photic phenomena due to the second image are more likely at night when the pupil is larger. The apodization profile for the ReSTOR lens equally distributes energy between the 2 primary images for smaller pupils, but more light goes to the far lens power as the pupil becomes larger.

The peripherally decreasing step heights reduce net-energy contribution to near, which by definition simultaneously increases net-energy contribution to distance. That is, the zone surfaces and the step heights at the zone boundaries determine how much light goes to each of the 2 primary images.

The zone pattern of zone boundaries determines the 4.00-D add power in the optic plane (3.20 D in the spectacle plane). The fact that the space between boundaries gets progressively smaller from the optic's center to its periphery is necessary to define the 2 focal points consistently across the optic. That is, the pattern of decreasing step widths is the necessary

Analogies

Two analogies can describe diffraction. The first is sound waves traveling down a hall, encountering a corner, and then slowing and spreading out so that the sound wave travels around the corner and is heard 90 degrees from the wave's original direction. The second analogy is not exactly correct but may be used to conceptualize light in its particulate form as photons and to compare it to atmospheric gas molecules as air. An air-vent diffuser in an automobile dashboard that directs air straight outward without deflection is analogous to distance vision, where the light is directed to the distance focal point at the fovea (Figure 5). The diffusers can be aimed downward to deflect the air stream in that direction, similar to if most of the light were deflected toward the shorter near focal point 1 mm in front of the fovea. The diffuser can be placed in an in-between position so that half of the air is directed straight outward and half of it is deflected toward the near lower point. The ReSTOR's refractive-apodized diffractive optic accomplishes the same objective in its most central zones by dividing the light wavefront so that half of it goes to the distance foveal focus point and half of it goes to the near point 1 mm in front of it.

The ReSTOR IOL represents a revolutionary integration of apodized diffractive structure on a platform with which we are all familiar. This technology combined with the consistent centration of the AcrySof single-piece IOL architecture can dramatically improve the quality of distance, near, and intermediate focus after lens replacement surgery, in almost immediate fashion for almost all patients.

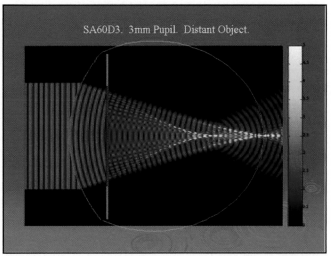

Figure 5. An eye with a 3-mm pupil sees a distant object through the ReSTOR. Half of the light is projected to the foveola, and half is focused at a point 1 mm anterior to the fovea. The latter projection is so far forward that the patient cannot perceive a near image. (Reprinted with permission from Davison JA. Deciphering diffraction: How the Restor's apodized, refractive, diffractive optic works. *Cataract Refract Surg Today.* 2005;June:42-46.)

Acknowledgments

This chapter has previously appeared as an article in *Cataract & Refractive Surgery Today* and it is reprinted with their permission.

CHAPTER 43

AMO Tecnis Multifocal— Clinical Pearls

Pietro Giardini, MD and Nicola Hauranieh, MD

The Tecnis MF intraocular lens (IOL) (Advanced Medical Optics, Santa Ana, CA) is part of the newest generation of multifocal IOLs (MIOL). This diffractive MIOL combines the anterior prolate surface of the well-known Tecnis monofocal optic with a posterior surface diffractive optic. The entire posterior surface is covered by the 32 rings (Figure 1). This lens represents a new approach in the field of multifocal optics. We have over 10 years of experience with MIOLs, including the Array MIOL (Advanced Medical Optics).[1] We understand that they all have some "side effects" that vary in their intensity and severity from patient to patient. We believe that the Tecnis MF best minimizes the side effects of multifocality and provides a consistently excellent outcome. We all know that the best IOL would be the one that reproduces the natural movement of the crystalline lens, but so far, accommodating lenses have not been able to give us the expected results. Multifocal lenses are therefore our best option currently.

Some of these clinical pearls come directly from the experience of the "pioneer" surgeons who starting using the Array more than 10 years ago. Many of these surgeons are now able today to say, "If I follow these very simple guidelines and with the help of some clinical pearls, I am very confident of a safe and stable result." Today, it is possible to follow these guidelines and to be confident of the results. The growing number of MIOLs being implanted in Europe is evidence of this. In Italy, where surgeons were initially distrustful of multifocal implants it has become more popular to use them. If the surgeon treats these patients like other refractive patients, performs careful preoperative screening, formulates a detailed and precise surgical plan, and follows some very straightforward rules, he will consistently achieve good results.

A refractive or diffractive multifocal optic will always have some problems such as halos, glare, and loss of contrast sensitivity, which are inherent to multifocal optics. When an optic creates multiple images to accomplish multiple functions, there will be a tradeoff in the quality of vision (Figure 2). The international studies of MIOLs with long term follow-up confirm that a significant percentage of patients have blurred vision or halos at night.[2-5] These same studies also confirm that after a period of adjustment or "neural adaptation," these same patients adapt to their vision and do not complain anymore. After a period of time, most patients with MIOLs are pleased with the overall compromise solution that they have chosen.

When compared to the excellent visual quality of a monofocal IOL, the Tecnis MF offers the best compromise in terms of a MIOL that can provide good distance and near vision. Although the diffractive optic causes some loss of contrast sensitivity, the anterior prolate surface creates a very sharp image that is free of spherical aberration in most patients. This creates a better contrast image, especially at night, while still providing the multifocal benefits. The lens also has a 4.00 D add, which provides excellent near visual acuity and the fastest reading speed of any presbyopia-correcting IOL we have measured (see Chapter 67). The new acrylic Tecnis platform should be available soon. It is made with a hydrophobic acrylic material that is among the most carefully studied and commonly implanted worldwide. This lens produces an even faster reading speed than the silicone Tecnis MF.

Another advantage of this IOL is excellent centration. We all know that a MIOL needs to be well centered to provide refractive stability and to minimize halos and glare. The Tecnis MF haptics have been specifically designed to provide great centration. The diffractive optic has 32 rings over the entire optic and is NOT pupil size dependant (Figure 3).

It is very important for the surgeon using MIOLs to understand both the unique properties of each lens and the best patients in which to implant them. First, recognize that these patients are refractive surgery patients, even if they have cataracts. They are paying for and expect to receive premium services. This includes the time spent in preoperative and postoperative counseling. Even in the best of cases, patients receiving a MIOL are relatively intolerant of residual refractive error. It is critical to minimize postoperative refractive surprises and to have a plan to enhance or adjust the final refractive outcome, if needed. This might include a laser vision enhancement, an

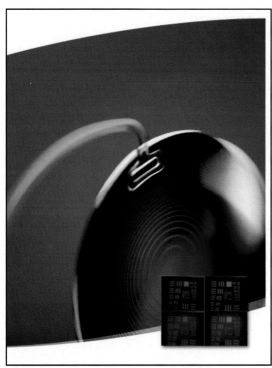

Figure 1. The Tecnis MF is a full optic diffractive IOL.

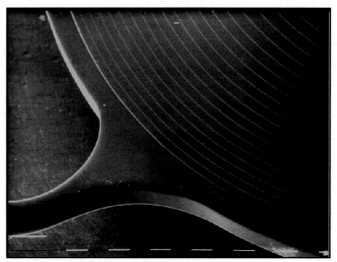

Figure 3. Microscopy image of the diffractive surface of the Tecnis MF IOL.

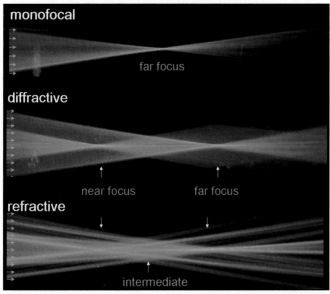

Figure 2. Demonstration of the difference between monofocal and multifocal lens image quality.

IOL exchange, or a piggyback IOL. Precise IOL calculation is one of the most important factors for success with these lenses. This includes using the most up-to-date formulas, obtaining accurate keratometry, and a precise and accurate axial length.

You also need to understand the psychology of each patient. How do you choose the "right" patient? If we believe that neural adaptation is a cortical mechanism, we may have to exclude patients who are not very perceptive or who are too inflexible to adapt to the optical compromises of the lens. Such patients will tend to complain about any small change in their vision. These subjective complaints may impair the quality of vision more than physical side effects such as residual refrac-

tive error. Remember that when some patients describe their visual symptoms (eg, "I see halos"), they just want to make sure that this is normal. It is important for the surgeon to listen and to acknowledge the patient's symptoms, and to recognize they are observations and not necessarily complaints.

Proper patient selection also requires having a good understanding of the different MIOLs on the market. Knowing the pros and cons of each IOL design and their unique optical characteristics and differences enables us to decide which IOL is best suited for a particular patient. A diffractive IOL is, by definition, bifocal. This is the reason why the Tecnis MF provides patients with better near vision. A refractive multifocal such as the ReZoom (Advanced Medical Optics) can produce more foci on the retina and the patient will have better intermediate vision, but at the "cost" of some loss of contrast. Poor candidates for the Tecnis MF are those patients who favor intermediate vision or those who need a distance dominant MIOL and have a small pupil. The best candidates for a Tecnis MF are those who need the best near vision and are willing to accept distance vision that is slightly less sharp in return. Perfect Tecnis candidates would be individuals who generally do not require intermediate vision as much. Patients with small or poorly mobile pupils need a presbyopia-correcting MIOL that is not pupil dependent, and are also better candidates for the Tecnis MF than the ReZoom.

Surgeons today have many choices. There are many new options such as prolate and other aspheric optic surfaces, different haptic designs for greater stability, microincisional lenses, and IOLs preloaded into injectors. When the patient is sitting in front of us, it can be very challenging to decide which IOL to implant. It has also become difficult to distinguish between a cataract surgeon and a refractive surgeon. In Europe, cataract surgeons are now becoming more like refractive surgeons, and refractive surgeons are doing more cataract and lens-removal surgery. This trend has given birth to the combined cataract-refractive surgeon and we must adopt this new mentality.

MIOLs in general, and the Tecnis MF in particular, represent one of the most important options for presbyopic patients who want to read without glasses. There are many patients

50 years of age or older who want to be free of glasses, and we finally have the opportunity to help them. We must approach these cases exactly as we do for refractive laser procedures: follow the guidelines and good results will follow.

While many of these considerations might seem very obvious for some colleagues in the United States, it has to be mentioned that the evolution of MIOLs has been slightly different in Europe. We have a different healthcare system that is publicly funded in most countries. This means that our IOL options are limited by the administrative departments of our hospitals due to cost controls, resulting in a short delay in the adoption of some products such as MIOLs. However, today our market seems to be ready for these refractive IOLs. We have entered the era of "customization" of services for patients, and with the mix and match technique we have the opportunity to provide more of our patients with a life without glasses.

References

1. Dick HB, Gross S, Tehrani M, Eisenmann D, Pfeiffer N. Refractive lens exchange with an Array multifocal intraocular lens. *J Cataract Refract Surg.* 2002;18:509-518.

2. Mester U, Hunold W, Wesendahl T, Kaymak H. Functional outcomes after implantation of Tecnis ZM900 and Array SA40 multifocal intraocular lenses. *Cataract Refract Surg.* 2007;33:1033-1040.

3. Häring G, Dick HB, Krummenauer F, Weissmantel U, Kröncke W. Subjective photic phenomena with refractive multifocal and monofocal intraocular lenses. *J Cataract Refract Surg.* 2001;27:245-249.

4. Auffarth GU, Hunold W, Wesendahl TA, Mehdorn E. Depth of focus and functional results in patients with multifocal intraocular lenses: a long-term follow-up. *J Cataract Refract Surg.* 1993;19:685-689.

5. Dick HB, Krummenauer F, Schwenn O, Krist R, Pfeiffer N. Objective and subjective evaluation of photic phenomena after monofocal and multifocal intraocular lens implantation. *Ophthalmology.* 1999;106:1878-1886.

CHAPTER 44

AMO TECNIS MULTIFOCAL— CLINICAL PEARLS

Frank Jozef Goes, MD

In my clinical practice, a private praxis in Antwerp, Belgium, I have gathered experience with several types of multifocal lenses over many years. I started using the 3-piece, 6-mm, polymethylmethacrylate (PMMA) 3M multifocal intraocular lens (IOL) (St. Paul, MN) in 1985. From 1992, I was involved in the one-piece refractive PMMA Storz True Vista study (Storz Instrument Co, St. Louis, MO). In 2002, I began using the Alcon ReSTOR lens (Fort Worth, TX). I have also implanted the Crystalens IOL (Eyeonics, Inc, Aliso Viejo, CA).

In 2004, I switched exclusively to the Tecnis ZM900 multifocal IOL (Advanced Medical Optics, Santa Ana, CA), and in 2006, I began combining it with the ReZoom IOL (Advanced Medical Optics) (Figure 1). The Tecnis MF is my current presbyopia-correcting (Pr-C) IOL of choice because of its intrinsic qualities and excellent outcomes. Since ReZoom is well known in the United States, I will concentrate my comments on the Tecnis MF lens. I now have experience in implanting 600 Tecnis lenses bilaterally and another 90 mixed with the ReZoom.

Product Description— Tecnis ReZoom Lens

The **Tecnis ZM 900** IOL (Figure 2) is a foldable, 3-piece IOL of high-quality silicone with a near/far light distribution of 50/50. The diffractive component is on the back surface of the lens and provides an optical power add of 4 D corresponding with 3.2 D at the corneal plane. It comes in a power range of +5 to +34 D in 0.5-D steps. The −0.27-prolate anterior surface compensates for the positive spherical aberrations of the typical cornea. The refractive effect is pupil independent and the lens has the Z-SHARP optic edge technology, delaying early posterior capsular opacification (PCO) while minimizing edge glare. The overall diameter of the lens is 13 mm, with a 6.0-mm optic. The lens is available in a hydrophobic acrylic

material in Europe, and United States availability is anticipated in 2008 or 2009.

Understanding the Candidates

There are 2 groups of candidates or interested patients.

The first group consists of cataract patients. Some have heard about the possibility of implanting lenses that correct far and near vision; some have friends or relatives who had the procedure done with successful outcomes. These people are very interested in discussing this option.

Some cataract patients have never heard about this premium refractive lens concept. Experience has taught us that it is impossible for the surgeon to decide which patient can afford the extra cost associated with the lens. If we do not mention the option of a Pr-C IOL, some of our patients will be upset later on when they find out that they have missed the opportunity to have one.

The second group consists of refractive patients who specifically come in for refractive surgery: high hyperopes (greater than +5 D), moderate to low hyperopes with incipient reading problems at age 45 and older, and presbyopic patients who have good distance vision but want to eliminate their reading glasses.

We would not advise lens replacement surgery in presbyopic myopes with a clear lens since sooner or later a YAG laser capsulotomy will have to be done, and we feel that the risk of complications (eg, retinal detachment) is higher in myopes. We have experience in performing at least 500 YAG laser capsulotomies in our private practice in moderate to high hyperopes and have never seen a retinal detachment following a YAG capsulotomy.

Generally speaking, the cataract patient group is less demanding than the refractive group. The ideal candidate to start with is a moderate hyperope (2 to 5 D) between 50 and 60 years old. Be aware of emmetropic presbyopes with good distance vision because they are usually very demanding.

Figure 1. Reading speed with different multifocals.

Better Reading Acuity and Reading Speed

Comparison of Multifocal IOLs

DESCRIPTION	Reading Acuity (logMAR)		Reading Speed (words per minute)	
	Bright Light (100 cd/m²)	Low Light (6 cd/m²)	Bright Light (100 cd/m²)	Low Light (6 cd/m²)
TECNIS™ Multifocal IOL ZM001	0.1	0.3	174	142
TECNIS™ Multifocal IOL ZM900	0.15	0.35	160	125
Array™ IOL	0.35	0.4	87	68
AcrySof™ ReSTOR	0.15	0.4	138	72
ReZoom™ IOL	0.35	0.4	90	115
Acri.Twin™	0.15	0.35	135	140

Hutz W, et al. Reading ability with 3 multifocal intraocular lens models. *J Cataract Refract Surg.* 2006;32:2015-2021.
Hutz. Reading Acuity at Intermediate Distances. Presented at ASCRS, April 2007

TECNIS
MULTIFOCAL IOL
DIFFRACTIVE ASPHERIC

Figure 2. Characteristics of the diffractive Tecnis multifocal IOL.

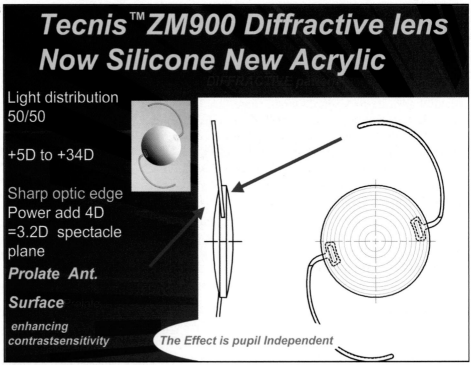

Tecnis™ ZM900 Diffractive lens Now Silicone New Acrylic

Light distribution 50/50

+5D to +34D

Sharp optic edge
Power add 4D
=3.2D spectacle plane
Prolate Ant.
Surface
enhancing contrastsensitivity

The Effect is pupil Independent

Patient Expectations

General advice such as "under promise and over deliver" and "more chair time before surgery means less chair time after surgery" are well known, but what do these statements actually mean? It is a fact that our patients will always remember the very first things we say during our discussion. They should feel that we are confident but that we do not want to "oversell" the product. I tell them that, in the huge majority (over 95%, and I give them my data) patients will be spectacle free after the procedure for all distances—far, intermediate, and near.

I tell them that some will need time (1 to 3 months) to adjust to seeing at all distances. Some will get used to working closer to their desktop and/or laptop computer and only a minority will need to wear glasses for intermediate distances (Figure 3). In our latest series of customized mixing approach (Tecnis MF-ReZoom) in 45 patients followed for 3 months, not one single patient required glasses (Figures 4 and 5).

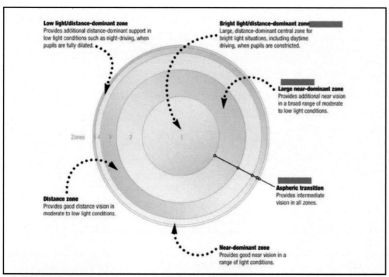

Figure 3. Characteristics of the refractive multifocal ReZoom IOL.

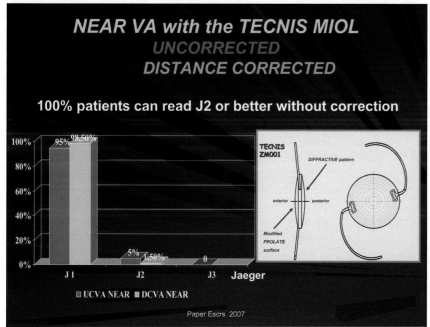

Figure 4. Results near vision with Tecnis MP.

Patient Selection

Of course patients should be motivated and interested in becoming spectacle free or less spectacle dependent. They should be willing to be patient with the process, recognize that it may take time to adapt to the new visual system, and have the means to pay for the added cost of Pr-C IOL surgery.

My chief problem is, "How can we filter out those patients who will be unhappy at the end of the journey?" This may have more to do with the patient's personality than with the type of accommodative or multifocal lens implanted because unhappy patients will usually blame the procedure. We are involved in some international studies wherein patients have to undergo some psychological and psychometric testing with the hope of finding some correlation between degree of satisfaction, personality, and expectations.

Much has been said regarding neuroadaptation but at this point we do not have a way to measure this function before implanting a lens. A surgeon with experience in laser refractive surgery has a tremendous advantage in this area since he or she is accustomed to trying to sense whether the patient's expectations and motivation will overcome and offset the potential side effects.

Informed Consent

We always mention that some patients may experience problems like halos and glare, that we never know who will experience them, and that most patients will get used to them and will not be bothered by them after 1 to 3 months, or as long as 6 months in exceptional cases.

We also tell our patients that the lens can later be exchanged if necessary. Of course we also discuss the patient's hobbies and activities such as driving and computer work. Patients should enter the process with a firm understanding of possible side effects, and we let them make the final decision. However,

Figure 5. Results distance vision with Tecnis MP.

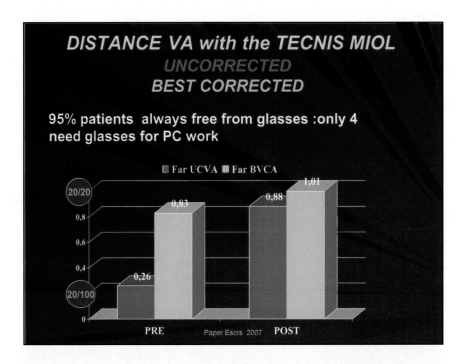

we recently did surgery on 2 bus drivers with custom mixing of ReZoom-Tecnis multifocal and they experienced no problem with night driving!

Generally speaking, the disturbing subjective complaints may decrease in many patients after a touch-up for residual refractive errors, after implantation of an IOL in the second eye, or with time due to neuroadaptation. Halos and unwanted images remain significant for approximately 5% of patients. These patients can still drive at night although they may not like to do so. Since many such complaints diminish with time, encouragement and waiting may be helpful.

Preoperative Testing

It is logical that prospective candidates for a multifocal lens should have normal and healthy eyes. Diabetes (under medical control) and other systematic general conditions are not exclusion criteria. Accurate biometry and IOL power calculation is a "conditio sine qua non."

The use of the IOL Master (Carl Zeiss Meditec, Jena, Germany) with laser interferometry measurement of the optical axis to within ±0.3-μm accuracy is advisable, especially for long myopic eyes where there is a staphyloma, and in short eyes where differences of 0.1 mm have far more impact on the IOL power calculation.

We use at least 2 formulae for multifocal IOL calculation: the Holladay II and the Haigis formula (not as well known in the United States; see User Group for Laser Interference Biometry [ULIB] Web site at www.augenklinik.uni-wuerzburg.de/scripts2/ulist.php).

Both formulae are excellent for all axial lengths; the SRK T is excellent for long myopic eyes and the Hoffer Q formula is outstanding for short hyperopic eyes.

A-constants are constantly updated on his Web site by Prof. Haigis and are currently at 119.8 for the Tecnis ZM900 and 118.8 for the ReZoom lens.

With the Tecnis IOL, the target should be +0.25 D to plano since a myopic outcome will bring the reading distance too close. It is much better to err on the plus side than on the minus side. Intentionally one could also aim for +0.5 with the Tecnis ZM in order to obtain a better intermediate vision. The refractive target should be plano with the ReZoom IOL.

Preoperative astigmatism of more than 1.5 D should be a relative exclusion criterion for novices since the immediate effect of the multifocal lens would be diminished. Laser in situ keratomileusis (LASIK) enhancement or limbal relaxing incisions (LRIs) can solve this problem, but the patient should be informed of that beforehand. We charge separately for an enhancement (only 40% of the normal LASIK fee) and tell the patient this at the initial examination. For experienced surgeons, astigmatism will not be an exclusion criterion.

Surgical Technique

We do the surgery in our private freestanding outpatient surgical center under topical anesthesia with the supervision of an anesthetist. The patient is examined day 1, day 14, and day 30 postoperatively. We do not use subconjunctival injections at the end of the procedure. We choose the incision site according to the pre-existing astigmatism; superiorly when the astigmatism is 0.75 D or more with-the-rule, and temporally for all other cases. We will make the corneal incision more anteriorly when we have 2 D of astigmatism. Since LRIs are not predictable enough, we perform them only when the pre-existing astigmatism is significant (more than 4 D). We use a 3.0-mm clear corneal incision fashioned with a diamond knife.

The capsulorrhexis should be 5.5 to 6.0 mm in diameter and preferably circular (although this is not mandatory). The Tecnis ZM centers remarkably well by itself due to the broad C-haptics, even with an oval or asymmetric capsulorrhexis. We never suture the wound unless we have had to enlarge it.

Enhancements and Complications

When a touch-up for residual refractive error (spherical or astigmatic) may be advisable, we demonstrate the difference to the patient and let him or her decide. We prefer to use LASIK or EpiLASIK (in case of a thin or irregular cornea) and wait until at least 3 months after surgery. We have never had any complications with the LASIK touch-up; our present enhancement rate is 15%.

Eventual Intraocular Lens Exchange—When?

Up to this point, we have never been forced to explant either the Tecnis or ReZoom. When faced with an extremely unhappy patient, one should exclude all other possibilities before considering an IOL exchange.

A subjectively unsatisfactory outcome for the patient may be the result of residual refractive error, posterior capsule opacification that can be cured with YAG laser capsulotomy, or a subtle retinal abnormality that can be demonstrated with optical coherence tomography.

Even when you are convinced that the multifocal optic is the cause of persistent complaints, try to postpone doing an IOL exchange for as long as possible (at least 6 months). We have personal experience in 2 cases where the patient decided to keep the lens and declined explantation after adjusting to the lens over an 8-month time period.

Waxy or hazy vision with the Tecnis ZM is very unusual and was only observed in 2 eyes in our series to date. These patients eventually adapted to the vision without requiring explantation.

Tecnis Multifocal Implantation Technique

For transitioning surgeons, IOL loading should be done by the surgeon under the microscope using the Silver Series Unfolder (Advanced Medical Optics). The different steps are nicely highlighted in the company brochure (Figure 6) but attention should be paid to the following points:

* Always have a back-up lens available; a novice surgeon will have to discard some lenses (around 5 to 10% in the first 20, this will drop to 1% with experience) because of damage during the loading procedure.
* Take your time loading and folding the lens. It is more time consuming and more difficult than some other IOLs.
* Carefully ensure that the lens presents itself nicely with the leading haptic protruding toward the tip when you advance the knob. If you feel too much resistance, something is wrong. Advance the lens in the injector to make sure that the leading end of the haptic is moving freely

and does not stick to the optic. In the case of a haptic sticking to the optic, deliver the lens on the table and load the back-up lens or reload the same lens if you are experienced.

* Use sufficient viscoelastic material such as Healon GV or Healon 5 (Advanced Medical Optics) to fill the capsular bag. With the present model and material (silicone), the lens can unfold with a spring-like action when released too quickly. The viscoelastic will act like a shock absorber, preventing damage to the capsular bag.
* Insert the cartridge tip into the incision bevel down and turn it slightly to the left so that the leading haptic is directed under the capsulorrhexis (be sure that this is the case) and pointed to the left as the lens unfolds. This is done by turning the mouth of the injector also toward the left.
* Turn the knob slowly to advance the lens and again take your time to let the lens unfold in the eye. Slowly release the IOL as you would turn a pancake around. Once the optic becomes visible, proceed very slowly and the lens will unfold itself. Thanks to the C-haptics, the IOL centers extremely well.
* If the lens unfolds upside down due to mishandling, no damage will be done if enough viscoelastic is in place; however, the result will be a.-1.0 D myopia. Once the optic is in the capsular bag, retract the plunger of the unfolder and use a Sinskey hook to deliver the trailing haptic into the capsular bag. Since you will have used a lot of viscoelastic take care to thoroughly aspirate it out and go beneath the IOL with the irrigation-aspiration tip as well. There is no need to use miotics (miostat or miochol) at the end of surgery with the Tecnis MF lens except in complicated cases. The wound should of course be watertight at the end of the case. This is easily achieved by hydrating the corneal incision and the side-port site (see Figure 6).

Staged IOL Selection

Since we have a diffractive lens (Tecnis ZM900) that provides good distance vision and excellent near vision and a refractive lens (ReZoom) that provides excellent distance and intermediate vision but performs weaker for near in our armamentarium, we should select the multifocal lens by considering the hobbies and professions of our patients. Therefore, we prefer a staged implantation of the 2 eyes (Figure 7).

A frequent computer user may be better off with bilateral ReZoom to provide good intermediate range. A professional car or truck driver who must also drive at night will be best off with a Tecnis aspheric monofocal IOL in both eyes. An avid reader, such as a librarian, will be better off with a Tecnis multifocal in each eye. An outdoor enthusiast or golfer might be better of with a ReZoom in each eye. A person with strong motivation for complete spectacle dependence will be a candidate for a mix and match.

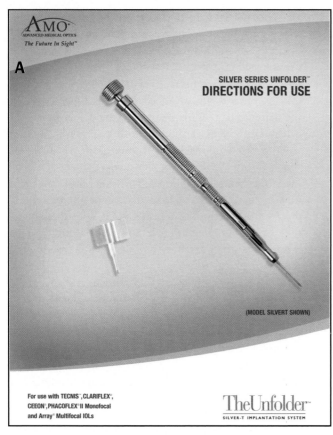

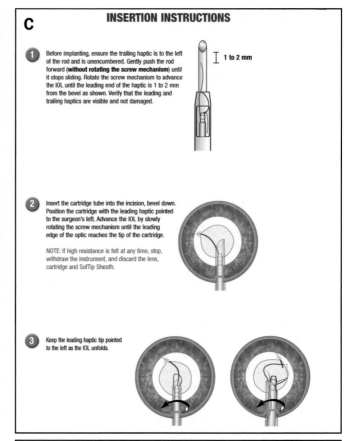

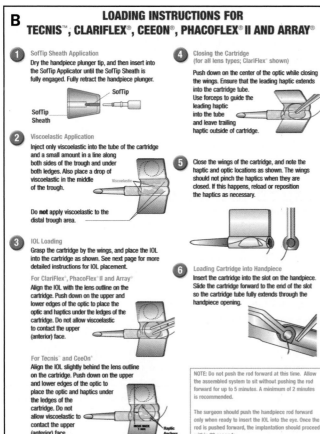

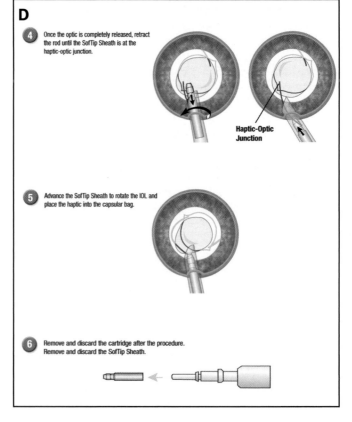

Figure 6. (A to D) For transitioning surgeons, IOL loading should be done by the surgeon under the microscope using the Silver Series Unfolder. The different steps are nicely highlighted in the company brochure. (Reprinted with permission of Advanced Medical Optics.)

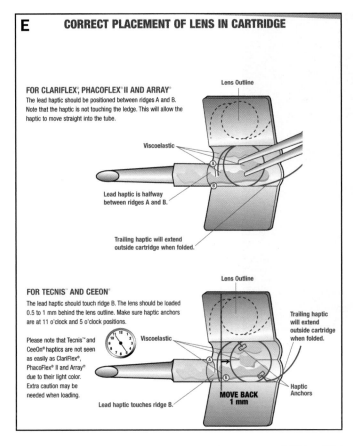

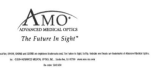

Figure 6. (E to F) For transitioning surgeons, IOL loading should be done by the surgeon under the microscope using the Silver Series Unfolder. The different steps are nicely highlighted in the company brochure. (Reprinted with permission of Advanced Medical Optics.)

Custom Mixing

First, we determine the dominant eye by having the patient point toward a distance target with both eyes open and then close each eye alternatively. This will nearly always disclose which eye is dominant.

Surgery is done first in the dominant eye, with the plan of operating on the second eye within 1 to 2 weeks. Which lens in which eye?

If the major activities are distance dominant, ReZoom is implanted in the dominant eye. If the major activities are near dominant, Tecnis multifocal is implanted in the dominant eye.

We evaluate the first eye outcome after 7 to 10 days and query the patient about his or her satisfaction. If he or she is completely happy, we choose the same lens for the other eye. If a ReZoom patient complains of inadequate near vision, we implant a Tecnis multifocal in his or her second eye. Finally, if a Tecnis multifocal patient complains of inadequate intermediate vision, we may implant a ReZoom in his or her second eye.

Conclusion

Although it is sometimes reported that the Tecnis multifocal IOL does not give excellent distance vision, all my Tecnis patients are very satisfied with their distance vision. After a customized mix and match approach, some of my patients spontaneously state that the ReZoom eye is their "computer" eye with better intermediate vision. Our data show that all of our mix and match patients are spectacle free. Unwanted optical effects are more pronounced with the ReZoom but the difference was not statistically significant.

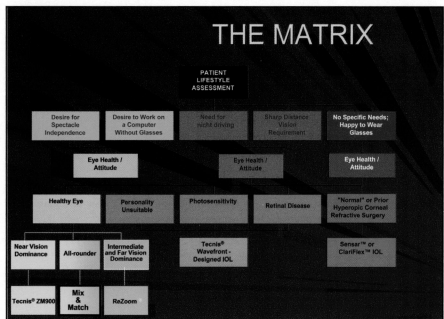

Figure 7. Matrix for staged implantation.

CHAPTER 45

AMO Tecnis Multifocal— Clinical Pearls

Y. Ralph Chu, MD

The Tecnis Multifocal (Advanced Medical Optics, Santa Ana, CA) offers the advantages of both asphericity and multifocality for the refractive intraocular lens (IOL) patient. The lens combines a full diffractive posterior surface (Figure 1) with a wavefront-designed aspheric anterior surface.

Light distribution through the lens is 50/50 for near and far. The diffractive surface of the lens is pupil-independent (Figure 2) so the quality of vision is not compromised in dim lighting, as it can be with an apodized diffractive surface.

The optical power add is +4.0 D at the IOL plane, which translates to a +3.0-D add at the spectacle plane, to optimize acuity at the typical preferred reading distance of 33 cm.

By press time, data from the clinical trials conducted to support U.S. approval of the silicone Tecnis Multifocal IOL (ZM900) will have been submitted to the Food and Drug Administration (FDA). This lens has the same squared-edge design (Opti-Edge) found in AMO acrylic lenses available internationally. An acrylic version of the Tecnis Multifocal IOL (ZMA00) with the same squared-edge design would likely be available in 0.5-D power increments from +5.0 to +34.0 D. It is currently available in some countries, including the European Union, and is undergoing approval in others.

This chapter reports on results of the completed clinical trial that is 1 of 2 studies that will be submitted to FDA by press time.

Asphericity

Like the Tecnis monofocal lens, this presbyopia-correcting (Pr-C) IOL reduces spherical aberration (SA), which is most clinically relevant in the aging eye. Wavefront aberration analysis confirms that the average human cornea has +0.27 μm of SA throughout life.[1] Lenticular SA grows and becomes increasingly positive as the eye ages. Higher amounts of positive SA degrade the optical quality of images (Figure 3).

Multiple studies have shown that peak visual performance occurs around age 19, when the average total SA is 0.0 μm.[2,3]

In other words, the cornea's 0.27 μm of positive SA is perfectly balanced by 0.27 μm of negative SA in the lens of the young adult eye, resulting in zero net SA. The Tecnis monofocal and multifocal lenses aim to restore zero SA to the pseudophakic eye by countering the cornea's positive SA.

The advantages of asphericity in the Tecnis monofocal lens, including improved functional vision and night driving simulator performance, are well established among cataract surgeons. The Tecnis monofocal aspheric lens was granted "new technology IOL (NTIOL)" status for reduced postoperative SAs and improved night driving simulator performance compared to lenses with spherical optics.

Diffractive Multifocality

Increasingly, presbyopic patients want to be able to function well at all distances without glasses after cataract/IOL surgery. We have a variety of multifocal and accommodating IOLs, as well as lenticular monovision options, to help patients achieve this goal of spectacle independence.

Diffractive multifocal IOLs have always offered excellent near vision acuity and have been considered ideal for patients who do significant amounts of reading or other near work. A disadvantage of the currently available apodized diffractive multifocal lens, however, is its dependence on pupil size. As the pupil diameter increases in dim light, optical quality (as measured by modulation transfer function [MTF]) at both near and distance declines with ReSTOR multifocal lenses (Alcon, Fort Worth, TX), but remains about the same with the new diffractive Tecnis Multifocal IOL (Figure 4).[4] MTF is the way that optical scientists measure the performance of an optical system.

Laboratory testing shows that the Tecnis Multifocal provides better image quality than other diffractive multifocal IOLs in both low and bright light (Figures 5 and 6).[5]

I have experience implanting all the commercially available IOLs that correct presbyopia and, in my opinion, the Tecnis Multifocal IOL will be the best multifocal diffractive IOL

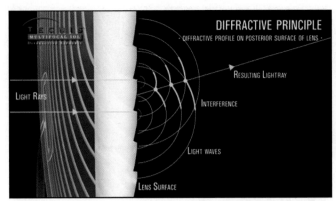

Figure 1. The lens combines a full diffractive posterior surface with a wavefront-designed aspheric anterior surface.

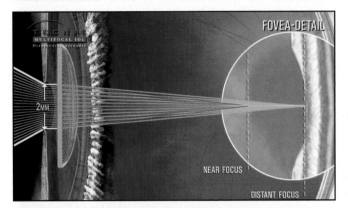

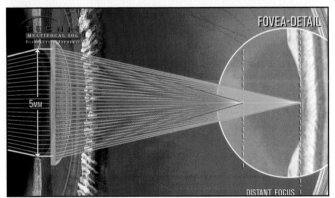

Figure 2. The diffractive surface of the lens is pupil-independent so the quality of vision is not compromised in dim lighting, as it can be with an apodized diffractive surface.

20/20*	E	E	E	E
Average Corneal SA	+.27	+.27	+.27	+.27
Lens SA	-.27	-.17	0.0	+.15
Total Residual SA	0.0	+0.10	+0.27	+0.42

*Images simulated using ZernikeTool, created by George Dai, PhD

Figure 3. Higher amounts of positive SA degrade the optical quality of images.

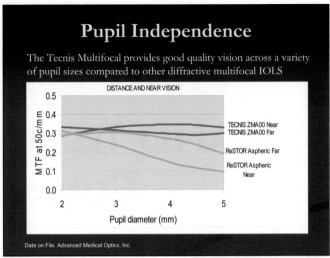

Figure 4. As the pupil diameter increases in dim light, optical quality (as measured by MTF) at both near and distance declines with ReSTOR multifocal lenses, but remains about the same with the new diffractive Tecnis Multifocal IOL.

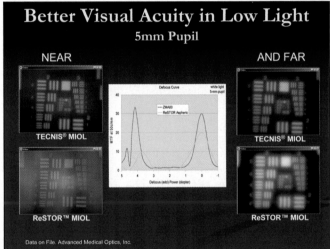

Figure 5. Laboratory testing shows that the Tecnis Multifocal provides better image quality than other diffractive multifocal IOLs in both low and bright light.

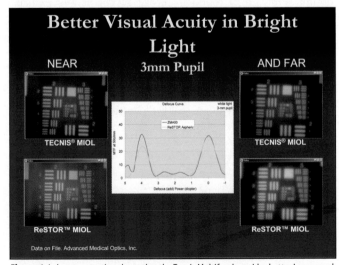

Figure 6. Laboratory testing shows that the Tecnis Multifocal provides better image quality than other diffractive multifocal IOLs in both low and bright light.

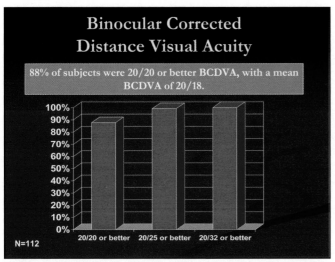

Figure 7. Eighty-eight percent of patients had best-corrected distance vision of 20/20 or better.

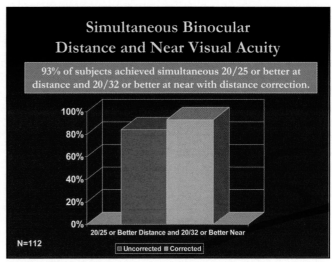

Figure 9. Nearly all subjects (93%) achieved simultaneous binocular vision of 20/25 or better at distance and 20/32 or better at near with distance correction.

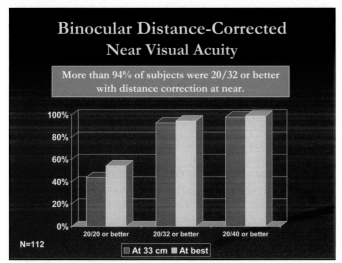

Figure 8. Binocular distance-corrected near acuity was 20/32 or better in more than 94% of patients.

when available. It provides the easiest reading vision and the highest quality of vision for near and far vision. As with all multifocal IOLs, some patients may require a little extra time for neuroadaption.

For patients enrolled and treated in our center, there were no complaints of waxy vision or "Vaseline vision," nor have we experienced a significant increase in night vision complaints of glare and halo. We also have not seen any dissatisfaction with the quality of the distance vision with this lens. In more than 41 eyes implanted with this lens in my practice, none has needed to be explanted. It is important to note that these are results from our center, and that outcomes from other centers and the overall study outcome could vary.

US Clinical Trial

A multicenter, evaluator-masked comparative clinical evaluation was conducted at 13 investigational sites around the United States. Patients were not randomized, but were assigned to multifocal or monofocal IOLs based on their own preferences. In all, 121 bilateral multifocal and 122 bilateral monofocal subjects were enrolled. One-year results include follow-up on 114 multifocal subjects. This evaluation and another subsequent study that will be completed at press time comprise the clinical data set that will be submitted to the FDA for approval of this IOL in the United States.

At 1 year, the mean best-corrected distance visual acuity was 20/18. Eighty-eight percent of patients had best-corrected distance vision of 20/20 or better (Figure 7). Binocular distance-corrected near acuity was 20/32 or better in more than 94% of patients (Figure 8).

Nearly all subjects (93%) achieved simultaneous binocular vision of 20/25 or better at distance and 20/32 or better at near with distance correction (Figure 9).

The majority of the multifocal subjects reported being able to function comfortably without glasses at all distances (Figure 10). Nearly 85% of subjects report that they never wear glasses. The rest wear glasses occasionally (13.4%) or always (1.8%).

In a test that measures real-world near abilities, the MNREAD distance-corrected reading test demonstrated that the multifocal group had statistically significantly higher reading acuity and reading speed compared to the monofocal group. The multifocal patients could see 20/20 at a reading distance of 33 cm, compared to only 20/47 acuity at 41 cm for the control group. The multifocal group could read smaller print faster, reading 148 words/minute compared to 117 words/minute in the control group.

Most importantly, fully 94.6% of patients said they would choose the Tecnis Multifocal IOL again. To me, this is an indication that the lens met patients' expectations for spectacle independence and visual quality.

The rate of IOL-related adverse events was very low. Five lenses had to be explanted. One patient in the clinical trial underwent pupilloplasty and then bilateral lens explantation due to halos and glare. Three lenses were removed due to incorrect lens power, and one IOL was explanted due to incorrect lens type.

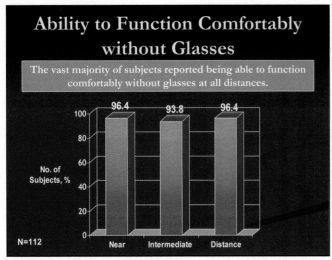

Figure 10. The majority of the multifocal subjects reported being able to function comfortably without glasses at all distances.

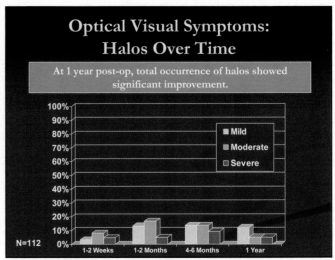

Figure 11. Halos were reported but improved considerably over the course of the first year.

Halos were reported but improved considerably over the course of the first year (Figure 11).

In summary, the US clinical trial demonstrated that the Tecnis Multifocal can correct near and distance acuity, with 93% of subjects achieving simultaneous 20/25 or better distance and 20/32 or better near vision without glasses. The Tecnis Multifocal provides statistically significantly better reading acuity and speed compared to monofocal IOLs and offers high rates of patient satisfaction.

Implantation Pearls

The target refraction with this IOL should be emmetropia ±0.25 D. In general, the closer one can get to plano, the more successful patients are with the lens. However, targeting a slightly hyperopic result can extend the range of focus without compromising quality of vision for those patients who might have trouble with the close focal point for reading. In contrast, myopic outcomes theoretically increase the risk of glare and halo and should not be targeted. In our clinical experience, when patients have been slightly undercorrected, small degrees of myopia have been well tolerated despite the theoretical risk.

As with all the Pr-C IOLs, correcting astigmatism is critical. For an optimal outcome, the patient should have less than 0.75 D of astigmatism postoperatively. Anything above that should be corrected at the time of surgery or, if necessary, postoperatively. A small cataract incision that induces minimal astigmatism is important.

The surgeon should also make a capsulorrhexis that is neither too small nor too large. The ideal capsulorrhexis should be between 5.5 to 6.0 mm in diameter, which provides good contact and sealing of the lens inside the capsular bag without increased risk of capsulophimosis or obstruction of the optical zone.

The Tecnis Multifocal is injected through a standard Advanced Medical Optics Silver Series Injector, using a standard implantation technique. It centers well without any additional attention to centration. In the rare case of a disparity between the center of the visual axis and the center of the pupillary axis, pupilloplasty with an argon laser is a possible course of action.

Adequate cortical cleanup, as with all the Pr-C IOLs, is critical. I typically use bimanual irrigation/aspiration instrumentation, and take care to clean up subincisional cortex and to carefully polish the posterior capsule and anterior capsular rim so that the capsule is absolutely pristine. All multifocal lenses are very sensitive to posterior capsular opacification (PCO) and thickening of the capsule. Early PCO may affect reading vision first, leading to complaints of decreased vision despite good distance Snellen acuity. In such cases, a Nd:yttrium-aluminum-garnet (YAG) capsulotomy often resolves the complaints.

The Tecnis Multifocal IOL provides another important addition to our growing armamentarium of refractive IOLs. I am excited about the potential for this lens in my practice, given the very high rates of patient satisfaction and the excellent near and distance acuity at all light levels.

References

1. Holladay JT, Piers PA, Koranyi G, et al. A new intraocular lens design to reduce spherical aberration of pseudophakic eyes. *J Refract Surg.* 2002;18:683-691.
2. Artal P, Alcon E, Villegas, E. Spherical aberration in young subjects with high visual acuity. Free paper, ESCRS 2006.
3. Holzer M. Free paper, DOC, Nuremberg, Germany, 2006.
4. Data on file, Advanced Medical Optics, Inc.
5. Data on file, Advanced Medical Optics, Inc.

CHAPTER 46

COMPARISON OF
DIFFRACTIVE MULTIFOCAL IOLS

Ulrich Mester, MD and Hakan Kaymak, MD

The use of multifocal intraocular lenses (MIOL) has been very limited in the past due to several drawbacks and limitations.[1] Surgical techniques were not as refined and predictable as they are today, and accurate biometry to achieve emmetropia was challenging. Moreover, independence from glasses could not be achieved in all patients, particularly for near vision. Many patients complained of photic phenomena,[2,3] and driving was impaired due to reduced contrast sensitivity under mesopic conditions.[4,5]

A new generation of MIOLs has been developed and has been investigated in clinical studies. Several new optical concepts were incorporated in theses lenses.

With the application of a diffractive optic, the visual performance became independent of the pupil size, which was one major drawback of the previous MIOL generation with refractive optics.

The introduction of an aspheric lens design enhances contrast vision, which could be demonstrated previously in clinical studies with monofocal IOLs.[6-8]

Another new concept is unequal light distribution for distance and near vision, based on the consideration that most patients prioritize distance vision.

A further development aims to improve distance vision by apodization of the central diffractive optic of the IOL and the combination with a peripheral monofocal zone due to the greater pupil diameter for far distance, particularly under dim light conditions.

To reduce the complaints due to stray light, smooth steps within the diffractive pattern were engineered.

Three models of the new MIOL generation gained widespread acceptance: The *Acri.LISA (*Acri.Tec, Henningsdorf, Germany), the AcrySof ReSTOR (Alcon, Fort Worth, TX), and the Tecnis ZM900 (Advanced Medical Optics, Santa Ana, CA). The characteristics of these 3 MIOLs are summarized in Table 1.

We performed clinical studies with these 3 MIOLs, comparing the Tecnis lens with a first-generation MIOL, the Array lens (Advanced Medical Optics). The *Acri.LISA was compared to results gained with the first-generation MIOL from *Acri.Tec, the *Acri.Twin. Our results with the ReSTOR lens were gained with the conventional model. Actually, we investigated the newly developed aspheric ReSTOR.

*Acri.LISA

Twenty patients with bilateral implantation of the *Acri. LISA were examined 6 weeks after surgery of the second eye; 15 of the 20 patients were re-examined after 1 year.

Monocular and binocular visual acuity (VA) (uncorrected and best corrected) at the 6-week control are shown in Figure 1 and the results after 1 year in Figure 2. Despite the dominance for far distance of this MIOL, near visual acuity (VA) was also very satisfying (uncorrected monocular 0.85, binocular 1.05 under photopic conditions, 350 cd/m²) (Figure 3).

The defocus curve demonstrates the drop of VA at intermediate distance, but it does not exceed the critical limit of 0.5 (Figure 4).

Overall patients satisfaction was 8.3 using a scale from 0 to 10 after 1 year. The superiority of the *Acri.LISA compared to the first-generation MIOL from *Acri.Tec (*Acri. Twin) becomes visible when comparing the contrast sensitivity assessed with the Functional Acuity Contrast Test (FACT) instrument (Figure 5).[9,10] When asked about photopic phenomena 6 weeks after surgery, 16 out of the 20 patients reported moderate halos under dim light conditions, but none were overly concerned by them.

Tecnis

Twenty-three patients with the Tecnis MIOL (46 eyes) and 24 patients with the Array MIOL (48 eyes) were re-examined at the 6-month control. The mean spherical equivalent at the last follow-up visit (120 to 180 days) was 0.1 ± 0.4 D (mean ± SD, Tecnis) and 0.2 ± 0.6 D (mean ± SD; Array). This difference was not statistically significant.

Table 1

CHARACTERISTICS OF THREE MULTIFOCAL INTRAOCULAR LENSES

*Acri.LISA

- Hydrophobic surface of hydrophilic acrylic material
- Full diffractive optic with smooth steps
- Light distribution 65% for far and 35% for near (both eyes)
- Aspheric

Tecnis ZM900

- Silicon second generation
- Full diffractive optic
- Light distribution 50% for far and 50% for near
- Aspheric

Acrysof ReSTOR

- Hydrophobic acrylic
- Central optic (3.7 mm) diffractive
- Apodization
- Peripheral monofocal zone
- Aspheric

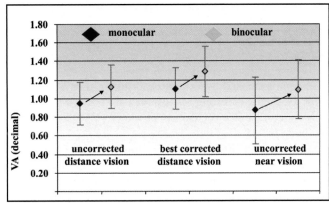

Figure 1. Impact of binocularity on VA 6 weeks after surgery with *Acri.LISA (Early Treatment of Diabetic Retinopathy Study [ETDRS]-charts, C.A.T.).

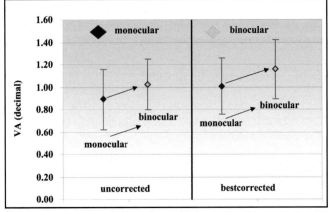

Figure 2. Impact of binocularity on distance VA 1 year after surgery with *Acri.LISA (ETDRS-charts).

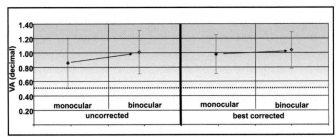

Figure 3. Impact of binocularity on near VA 1 year after surgery with *Acri.LISA tested with C.A.T.

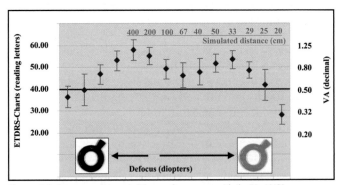

Figure 4. Defocus curve (binocular) 1 year after surgery with the *Acri.LISA.

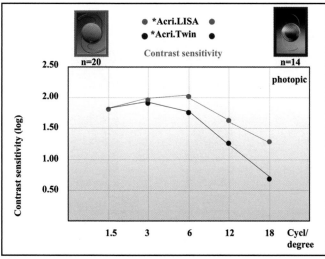

Figure 5. Contrast sensitivity measured with Functional Acuity Contrast Test (FACT) under photopic conditions (results of 2 different studies).

Table 2

DISTANCE UNCORRECTED VISUAL ACUITY AND BEST-CORRECTED VISUAL ACUITY AT DAYS 120 AND 180 ASSESSED BY ETDRS-CHARTS (NUMBER OF LETTERS)

	Tecnis N = 23		Array N = 24	
	EDTRS-Score	VA	ETDRS-score	VA
Uncorrected	48.2 ± 4.2	0.71	49.4 ± 6.8	0.77
Best corrected	52.2 ± 6.3	0.87	52.9 ± 5.4	0.91

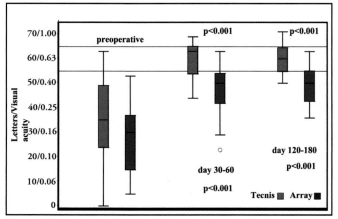

Figure 6. Uncorrected near VA 6 months after surgery measured with Contrast Acuity Test (C.A.T.) (40 cm).

Binocular uncorrected and best corrected distance VA did not show a statistically significant difference between the 2 groups at all follow-up visits (Table 2). In contrast, uncorrected as well as distance-corrected near vision revealed sig-

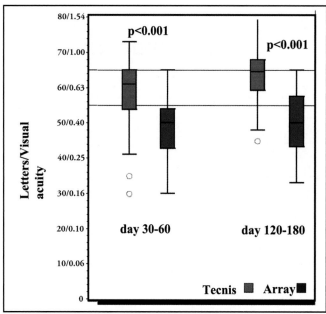

Figure 7. Distance corrected near VA 6 months after surgery measured with Contrast Acuity Test (C.A.T.) (40 cm).

Table 3

CONTRAST VISUAL ACUITY ASSESSED AT DAYS 120 AND 180 WITH ETDRS-CHARTS (DISTANCE) AND WITH C.A.T. (NEAR) (NUMBER OF LETTERS)

	Tecnis N = 23	Array N = 24	P-value
Near			
25% contrast	41.7 ± 9.9	36.3 ± 6.3	P<0.05
12.5% contrast	35.8 ± 9.5	30.4 ± 7.5	P<0.05
Far			
25% contrast	45.4 ± 6.8	47.5 ± 5.6	n.s.
10% contrast	37.0 ± 8.9	38.9 ± 5.8	n.s.

nificantly superior performance of the Tecnis MIOL compared to the Array MIOL ($P < 0.001$) (Figures 6 and 7). At 40 cm distance and under photopic conditions, the Tecnis MIOL group performed also significantly better than the Array MIOL group at 25% (P<0.001) and 12.5% (P<0.001) contrast levels but not at far distance. Data are summarized in Table 3.

The questionnaire survey at the last follow-up visit revealed a major difference between the 2 groups in terms of spectacle independence: 82.6% of patients with the Tecnis MIOL versus 33.3% of patients with the Array MIOL reported not wearing glasses. This difference was predominantly due to the need for reading glasses in the Array group; only 1 patient in the Tecnis MIOL group needed near correction versus 12 patients (50%) in the Array MIOL group (Table 4). The most frequent photic phenomenon reported by our patients was halos, which were more often associated with the Array MIOL. However, 9 out

Table 4

SPECTACLE DEPENDENCE

	Tecnis	Array
Glasses Prescribed?		
No	19 (82.6%)	8 (33.3%)
Yes	4 (17.4%)	16 (66.7%)
Type of Glasses Prescribed		
Distance	3 (75.0%)	4 (25.0%)
Near	1 (25.0%)	6 (37.5%)
Bifocals	0	6 (37.5%)

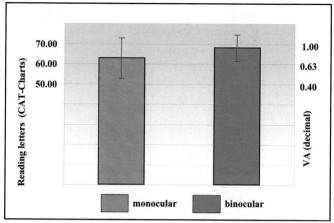

Figure 9. Impact of binocularity on uncorrected near VA 3 months after implantation of the AcrySof ReSTOR.

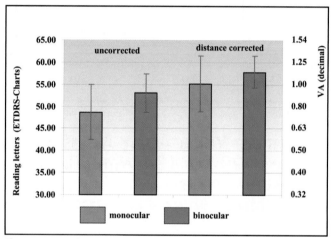

Figure 8. Impact of binocularity on VA 3 months after surgery with AcrySof ReSTOR.

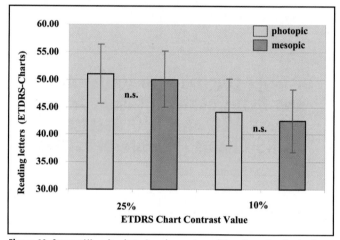

Figure 10. Contrast VA under photopic and mesopic conditions 3 months after implantation of the AcrySof ReSTOR. There was no loss of VA under mesopic conditions.

of 23 patients with the Tecnis multifocal lens also reported halos but without serious complaints after 6 months.[11]

AcrySof ReSTOR

In a prospective study, 30 patients received the AcrySof ReSTOR after bilateral phacoemulsification.

The postoperative spherical equivalent was 0.24±0.4 D after 3 months. Mean binocular distance vision was 1.0 uncorrected and 1.18 best corrected (Figure 8), uncorrected near VA was 0.93 (Figure 9). Contrast visual acuity was 0.83 (25%) and 0.6 (10%) under both photopic and mesopic conditions (Figure 10). Contrast sensitivity measured with FACT was within the normal range.

The defocus curve showed a pseudoaccommodation range of 5.5 D with a bifocal profile (Figure 11). The intermediate vision was sufficient for daily life activities for most of the patients; 91.0 % of patients were satisfied with their vision at the intermediate zone. The questionnaire survey revealed that 83.0% of the patients were completely spectacle independent. This finding is supported by other investigations.[12]

As the light distribution of the ReSTOR MIOL depends on pupil size, we looked for the relationship between pupil size and visual performance. A larger pupil correlated significantly

with better uncorrected distance VA and smaller pupils with better near and intermediate VA (Figure 12). (Results presented at the ASCRS meeting, San Diego, 2007).

Only 1 patient complained seriously of halos 3 months after surgery.

Discussion

Our differing experiences with 3 models of the latest generation of MIOLs stem from different study designs. Therefore, we cannot use these studies as a valid functional comparison of the MIOLs mentioned. Nevertheless, the following conclusions can be drawn:

* VA for distance is good with all 3 MIOLs and comparable to that of monofocal IOLs (at least under photopic lighting conditions).

* Near vision is also sufficient, even with the *Acri.LISA despite the unequal light distribution in favor of the far distance.

* Contrast vision is within the normal range.

* There is a significant drop of VA at the intermediate distance with all 3 MIOLs. This stems from the bifocal optical design of all 3 MIOLs. Therefore, we should

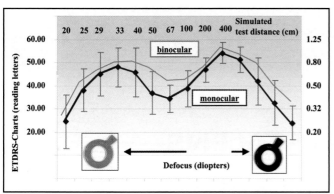

Figure 11. Impact of binocularity on defocus curve 3 months after implantation of the AcrySof ReSTOR.

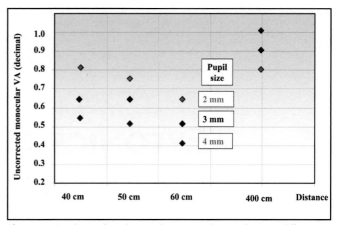

Figure 12. Correlation of pupil size with uncorrected monocular VA at different distances with the AcrySof ReSTOR (ETDRS-charts and Contrast Acuity Test (C.A.T.)) AcrySof ReSTOR.

speak of "bifocal" intraocular lenses instead of "multifocal" lenses to avoid disappointing patients who might otherwise imagine that their intraocular lenses will perform like progressive-add glasses. On the other hand, the drop of VA in the intermediate distance did not exceed 0.5, which was sufficient for daily life activities for most patients.

✳ More than 80.0% of patients gained complete spectacle independence with all 3 MIOLs. This represents enormous progress compared to the Array lens in which only one-third of patients were free of glasses.

✳ Even with the new MIOL designs, photic phenomena, particularly halos, has not been totally eliminated. These effects seem to be inherent in MIOLs as a result of creating multiple images with simultaneous focus. Fortunately, most patients are usually not disturbed by these optical effects and report that they become less noticeable over time.[13,14] All the results in our studies were achieved without additional refinement of postoperative refraction using photoablative procedures. Laser vision correction would likely further improve the attainable results.

✳ Precise biometry is crucial. Therefore, we use 3 different formulas to get as close to emmetropia as possible. We do not recommend MIOLs for patients who are expected to have more than 1 D of postoperative astigmatism and are not willing to undergo a second laser procedure for refinement. Toric MIOLs may better address the problem of astigmatism in the future.

✳ A second crucial step is patient selection. Studies to determine how to best identify suitable MIOL patients are underway.

References

1. Leaming DV. Practice styles and preferences of ASCRS members—2002 survey. *J Cataract Refract Surg.* 2003;29:1412-1420.

2. Dick HB, Tehrani M, Brauweiler P, et al. Complications with foldable intraocular lenses with subsequent explantation in 1998 and 1999: result of a questionnaire evaluation. *Ophthalmologe.* 2002;99:438-444.

3. Mamalis N, Davis B, Nilson CD, et al. Complications of foldable intraocular lenses requiring explantation or secondary intervention—2003 survey update. *J Cataract Refract Surg.* 2004;30:2209-2218.

4. Auffarth G, Hunold W, Breitenbach S, et al. Contrast and glare sensitivity in patient with multifocal IOLs: results two years after lens implantation. *Klin Monatsbl Augenheilkd.* 1993;203:336-340.

5. Steinert R, Aker B, Trentacost D, et al. A prospective comparative study of the AMO Array zonal progressive multifocal silicone intraocular lens and a monofocal intraocular lens. *Ophthalmology.* 1999;106:1243-1255.

6. Bellucci R, Scialdone A, Buralto L, et al. Visual acuity and contrast sensitivity comparison between Tecnis and AcrySof SA60AT intraocular lenses: A multicenter randomized study. *J Cataract Refract Surg.* 2005;31:712-717.

7. Kershner RM. Retinal image contrast and functional visual performance with aspheric, silicone, and acrylic intraocular lenses: prospective evaluation. *J Cataract Refract Surg.* 2003;29:1684-1694.

8. Mester U, Dillinger P, Anterist N. Impact of a modified optic design on visual function: clinical comparative study. *J Cataract Refract Surg.* 2003;29:652-660.

9. Mester U, Dillinger P, Anterist N, Kaymak H. Functional results with two multifocal intraocular lenses (MIOL). Array SA40 versus Acri.Twin. *Ophthalmologe.* 2005;102:1051-1056.

10. Kaymak H, Mester U. Erste Ergebnisse mit einer neuen aberrations-korrigierenden Bifokallinse (*Acri.LISA), *Ophthalmologe.* In press.

11. Mester U, Hunold W, Wesendahl T, Kaymak H. Functional outcomes after implantation of Tecnis ZM900 and Array SA40 multifocal intraocular lenses. *J Cataract Refract Surg.* 2007;33:1033-1040.

12. Kohnen T, Allen D, Boureau C, et al. European multicenter study of the AcrySof ReSTOR apodized diffractive intraocular lens. *Ophthalmology.* 2006;113:578-584.

13. Dick HB, Krummenauer F, Schwenn O, et al. Objective and subjective evaluation of photic phenomena after monofocal and multifocal intraocular lens implantation. *Ophthalmology.* 1999;106:1878-1886.

14. Pieh S, Lackner B, Hanselmayer G, et al. Halo size under distance and near conditions in refractive multifocal intraocular lenses. *Br J Ophthalmol.* 2001;85:816-821.

CHAPTER 47

EYEONICS CRYSTALENS— CLINICAL PEARLS

Jack A. Singer, MD

The Eyeonics Crystalens (Aliso Viejo, CA) has unique characteristics with which the surgeon must become familiar in order to achieve optimal outcomes and minimize unpleasant surprises. I will discuss preoperative pupil size and target postoperative refractions before focusing on surgical considerations.

For Crystalens models AT-50SE and AT-52SE, when the scotopic pupil measures 6.5 mm or greater, I inform the patient of an increased risk of halos or seeing the intraocular lens (IOL) outline. However, this is no different than with standard monofocal IOLs, and I have implanted the Crystalens with scotopic pupils as large as 6.75 mm without any problems.

As with any IOL, the postoperative refractive target should be tailored to each patient's visual needs. That being said, the Crystalens lends itself well to a mini-monovision approach, with −0.50 to −0.75 in the nondominant eye and plano to −0.25 in the dominant eye. I call this "accommodative blended vision" and make sure patients understand this approach before surgery. I may skew this toward greater myopia in myopes or toward plano in low hyperopes, depending on individual needs.

Since the Crystalens is designed to vault farther posteriorly in the capsule, the shape and size of the anterior capsulotomy is one of the most important factors for good outcomes. The lens functions best when the capsulorrhexis is larger than the optic and outside the hinges. The reason for this is that you want the anterior and posterior capsules to adhere to each other, with closure of the capsular bag periphery. This gap will close, the refraction will be stable, accommodation will increase over time, and the peripheral capsule will stay clear with a proper capsulorrhexis. Because the lens vaults so far backwards, if the capsulorrhexis is too small, you will have a persistent gap between the anterior and posterior capsule that may not close. Over time, lens epithelial cell proliferation may fill this gap and reduce accommodation.

Typically, sealing of the capsular bag periphery will occur within the initial 2 weeks postoperatively, and a capsular sleeve with parallel sides will form around the plate haptics (Figure 1). Presumably, the plate haptics glide within this sleeve during accommodation. If the capsulorrhexis does not cover at least half of the plate haptic length, then the normal posterior vault may be reduced, resulting in a myopic surprise. I aim for an anterior capsulotomy of 6.0 x 7.0 mm for the crystalens AT-50SE and AT-52SE, which equates to a capsulorrhexis just outside of the hinges and about a millimeter wider than the optic on each side (Figure 2). The following pearls will help in safely achieving such a large capsulorrhexis in a reproducible fashion:

* First, you want a maximally dilated pupil that will facilitate visibility of zonules. I use a neurosurgical "patty" soaked with a dilating solution (Figure 3).

* Use a high-cohesive viscoelastic. I use Healon GV (Advanced Medical Optics, Santa Ana, CA) routinely. For smaller pupils, shallow chambers, and positive vitreous pressure, I use Healon 5 (Advanced Medical Optics) (with a layer of balanced salt solution [BSS] just over the anterior capsule). For intraoperative floppy iris syndrome (IFIS) cases, I use Steve Arshinoff's method of combining Viscoat (Alcon, Fort Worth, TX) over the iris, Healon 5 in the center to hold the Viscoat over the iris, and a layer of BSS just over the anterior capsule.

* Keep the incision small for the capsulorrhexis and then enlarge for phaco if necessary (I use a 2.5-mm incision for both capsulorrhexis and phaco/IOL).

* Use cross-action capsule forceps, such as Inamura Capsule Forceps (Duckworth & Kent, Hertfordshire, England), which will fit through a smaller incision (I use Utrata capsule forceps [Katena Products, Inc, Denville, New Jersey] for most cases and reserve the Inamura forceps for challenging cases and for a posterior capsulorrhexis).

* Do not fixate the eye, which can increase posterior pressure and shallow the chamber. Be ready to release the capsule quickly if the patient moves.

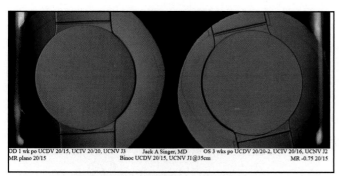

Figure 1. Crystalens 5-0 at 1 week and 3 weeks.

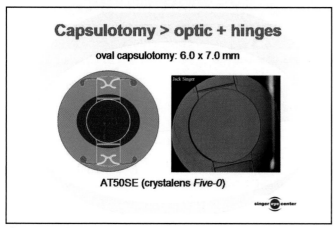

Figure 2. Crystalens AT50 capsulorrhexis.

* If you have zero-degree illumination (or near-zero) in your microscope and use topical anesthesia, have the patient fixate on the light and then center the capsulorrhexis on the light reflex. I have found that the Crystalens will nearly always be centered on this same light reflex after it is properly positioned in the bag.

* Use high magnification and focus precisely. This requires that you also move the y position to keep the area of the tear centered and focused.

* As you approach the anterior insertion of the zonules, begin curving the capsulorrhexis into a smaller radius. Keep the capsule flap folded over and pull in the direction you wish to go.

* Do not hesitate to stop and inject more viscoelastic if you loose any control. If that does not help, then switch to Healon 5.

* If you need to make a sharp turn inward, stop and regrasp the capsule adjacent to the point of tearing and pull directly toward the center of the pupil.

* The most challenging part is making the capsulorrhexis wide enough under a temporal clear corneal incision. It would be easier to make the oval with its long axis vertically, but I prefer to position the Crystalens as close to the vertical axis as possible (to avoid patients visualizing the hinges).

* As I approach the limit of how wide I can go temporally by pulling the folded flap of capsule in the direction of travel, I regrasp the capsule adjacent to the point of tear

Patties are prepared by soaking them in a specimen container with the following:

			Actual Concentration
10.0%	Neo-Synephrine	2.5 ml	1.9%
1.0%	Mydriacyl	2.5 ml	0.2%
0.3%	Ciloxan	5.0 ml	0.1%
0.03%	Flurbiprofen	2.5 ml	0.006%
0.5%	Tetracaine	1.0 ml	0.04%

* When previous patient is transferred to the operating room (or 30 min preoperatively for the first patient of the day), instill a dollop of 2% preservative-free lidocaine jelly into the superior temporal area (under the upper lid) of the operative eye.

* Place one saturated surgical patty into the superior-temporal conjunctival fornix (the space behind the upper eyelid) of the operative eye using sterile forceps 10 minutes following the instillation of lidocaine jelly.

* Instill a dollop of 2% preservative-free lidocaine jelly into the inferior conjunctival fornix (the space behind the lower eyelid) 10 minutes following the insertion of the saturated patty.

Supplies:

* Neuray Surgical Patties, Ref #80-03099, ¼″ x ¼″
  10 Patties per sterile pack
  Made by Martland Healthcare, Waterford, CT
  Distributed by XOMED, Jacksonville, FL

* 2% preservative-free lidocaine jelly
  20 ml, 400 mg, 20 mg/mL
  IMS International Medical Systems Ltd
  South El Monte, CA

Figure 3. Preoperative patties.

and slowly pull in the direction of travel. This will give a wider passage of the tear underneath the incision.

* Finally, pull the flap back toward the beginning to complete the capsulorrhexis.

* If you employ a cystotome through a very small incision, it will be easier to maintain the chamber.

* You can also use an instrument such as the Ahmed Duet with a 23-gauge Fine/Hoffman capsulorrhexis head (MicroSurgical Technology, Redmond, WA) through a side port incision for enhanced control of the chamber.

* If you get caught in the zonules, do not force or continue the tear. Stop and make a fresh cut with Vannas

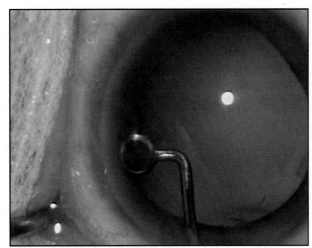

Figure 4. Capsule polisher.

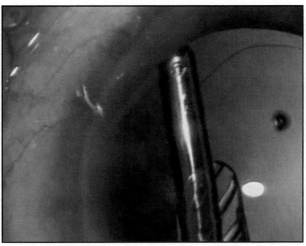

Figure 5. Ultrasound I/A tip.

or other microscissors (Hoffman/Ahmed, MicroSurgical Technology) before continuing. I have done this and still successfully implanted a Crystalens.

❋ At the end of the case, rotate the Crystalens to give a maximal gap between the sides of the optic and the anterior capsule.

It is well accepted that meticulous removal of lens cortex combined with postoperative anti-inflammatory drops for 6 to 8 weeks will help prevent capsule contraction. In addition, meticulous removal of lens epithelial cells (LECs) from the anterior capsule will prevent contraction of the capsulorrhexis over time.[1,2] This will also help to maintain good visualization of the peripheral retina, and will facilitate late reopening of the capsular bag should an IOL exchange become necessary. Removing anterior capsular LECs will also reduce fibrotic posterior capsule opacification (PCO) but will not prevent regeneratory PCO.[3] Contraction of the capsulorrhexis may cause an undesirable refractive shift and may limit accommodation over the long term.

The 360 degrees of the anterior capsular leaflet can be cleaned with Shepherd capsule polishers (Momentum Medical, Tampa, FL). First fill the bag and anterior chamber (AC) with viscoelastic. Next scrape the undersurface of the anterior capsule, moving centrally from the peripheral fornix (Figure 4). This is very useful with small pupils, and you will often be surprised at how much material can be scraped off what appeared to be a clean anterior capsule following cortical cleanup.

I also use a curved ultrasonic irrigation/aspiration (I/A) tip with a 0.2-mm port on a 50-kHz ultrasound handpiece with free-flow infusion and outflow (Figure 5). The free-flow fluidics allow me to alternate (with the footswitch) between using gravity only inflow/outflow and using the pump. To my knowledge, these features are only available on the Ocusystem Advantage phaco machine (Surgical Design, Armonk, NY).

Before I aspirate viscoelastic, I hydrate the incision (preaspiration hydration) to prevent chamber shallowing when I withdraw the I/A tip (while injecting BSS through the side port). This in turn will prevent the Crystalens from vaulting forward.

At the end of the case I instill approximately 0.5 cc of Miostat (Alcon) (diluted 5 parts BSS to 1 part Miostat) in the AC. I use no cycloplegia postoperatively other than for dilated postoperative exams.

The Crystalens requires absolutely watertight incisions to prevent anterior lens vaulting during the early postoperative period. Suture when in doubt about incision integrity.

With the AT-50SE and AT-52SE lenses it is not as crucial to keep the patient from accommodating during the first 2 postoperative weeks as compared with the Crystalens AT-45SE. Nonetheless, I still have patients use +1.50 over-the-counter readers for the first 2 weeks postoperatively. Alternatively, they may use their own eyeglasses with the lens for the operative eye popped out. I like to see closure of the peripheral capsule before I let them start to accommodate. This will typically occur within 2 weeks, during which time the anterior capsule rim can be seen becoming adherent to the posterior capsule, particularly around the polyimide loops and distal half of the plate haptics.

In order to appreciate the posterior vault at the slit lamp, wide dilation certainly helps. Have the patient gaze in the direction of the long axis of the lens and then perpendicular to the long axis. You should be able to appreciate an angle between the hinged plate haptics and the optic when the Crystalens is properly posteriorly vaulted.

References

1. Hanson RJ, Rubinstein A, Sarangapani S. Benjamin L, Patel CK. Effect of lens epithelial cell aspiration on postoperative capsulorrhexis contraction with the use of the AcrySof intraocular lens. *J Cataract Refract Surg.* 2006;32(10):1621-1626.

2. Tadros A, Bhatt UK, Karim MN, Zaheer A, Thomas PW. Removal of lens epithelial cells and the effect on capsulorrhexis size. *J Cataract Refract Surg.* 2005;31(8):1569-1574.

3. Menapace R, Wirtitsch M, Findl O, Buehl W, Kriechbaum K, Sacu S. Effect of anterior capsule polishing on posterior capsule opacification and neodymium:YAG capsulotomy rates: three-year randomized trial. *J Cataract Refract Surg.* 2005;31(11):2067-2075.

CHAPTER 48

EYEONICS CRYSTALENS—
CLINICAL PEARLS

James P. Gills, MD and Pit Gills, MD

We have witnessed the evolution of today's presbyopia-correcting lenses over the past 10 years. While we originally addressed the objective of simultaneous near and distance vision with multifocal technology, patients now have other options. Multifocal lenses, by their very design, require a substitution of near acuity for contrast acuity. In addition, patients must accept that both near and distance vision will be slightly compromised. While acceptable by a relatively small number of patients, we have dealt with many patients of our own and from other surgeons who, despite careful selection, complained bitterly about their lost contrast. With the Crystalens (Eyeonics, Inc, Aliso Viejo, CA), we have a means to provide our patients with near and distance vision without sacrificing quality of vision.

The idea of pseudoaccommodation is not a new one.[1] One of us (JG) was an avid user of silicone plate intraocular lenses (IOLs) back in the late 1980s. We observed at that time that 25% of our patients had functional reading acuity despite having been focused for distance vision. Observations and theories about accommodation by Stuart Cumming, Spencer Thornton, and others led Dr. Cumming to develop the first version of Crystalens.[1,2] The original design has undergone 5 modifications over the last 9 years, culminating in the AT-50 SE model (Figure 1). This model, which was introduced in November 2006, has a 5-mm optic and square edge design and is available in 11.5 mm and 12 mm lengths depending on the power required.

We have found one of the most important advantages of Crystalens over other lens technology is that it provides a full spectrum of visual acuity—from distance to near without compromising quality. Too often, we focus on clarity at near or distance. However, the intermediate range—our functional vision—is what patients appreciate most, and we believe that this is one of the most important features of Crystalens.

Prescreening and Patient Selection

Incorporating presbyopia-correcting lens technology into the cataract practice can be a challenging one. It requires a change in both the surgeon's and staff's mindset to adopt a "retail medicine" approach. In fact, engaging staff is absolutely essential for success. Our staff is instrumental in establishing the patient's goals and presenting us with critical information that allows us to make a recommendation in a short period of time. Following the surgeon's recommendation to the patient, the staff explains the Crystalens technology to the patient, along with pricing considerations.

Setting patient expectations is another important consideration. We intentionally set low expectations and emphasize that Crystalens will not guarantee complete independence from glasses. In fact, patients understand that they will need glasses for night driving and also for very fine print. All of the staff throughout the practice are trained to reinforce this message.

Other Considerations

Crystalens certainly is not appropriate for every patient. We offer 4 types of premium lenses: Crystalens, STAAR Toric (STAAR Surgical Co, Monrovia, CA), Tecnis (Advanced Medical Optics, Santa Ana, CA), and Collamer (STAAR Surgical) (Table 1). Each lens has specific indications, and we base our recommendation not only on the patient's motivation for spectacle independence but also on medical considerations. There are 2 critical components that are absolutely required for evaluating Crystalens candidates: evaluation of retinal disease with optical coherence tomography (OCT) and topography analysis to measure pre-existing astigmatism.

Figure 1. Crystalens AT-50 SE.

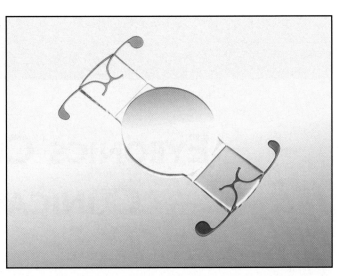

Table 1

INDICATIONS AND CONSIDERATIONS FOR PREMIUM LENSES

Crystalens	Tecnis	Collamer	Toric
Ideal for patients motivated to have minimal spectacle dependence	Premium contrast sensitivity	Biocompatibility	Ideal for astigmatics who do not opt for Crystalens
Patients must be willing to pay a premium for state of the art technology	Endorsed by the Food and Drug Administration for improving reaction time for night driving	Ideal for diabetic patients/retinal disease	Close follow-up with surgeon required
More chair time required		Fixes tightly to the capsule	Can be performed with relaxing incisions to correct higher amounts of astigmatism
Requires "refractive" surgery mindset		Results in hyperopic shift in some patients	Requires rotation in some cases

Patients who present with diabetes or any retinal disease that would result in substandard postoperative acuity are probably not good candidates for Crystalens. We order an OCT for any patient who falls into this group. A large number of these patients are diabetic and are predisposed to activation of their diabetic retinopathy postoperatively, resulting in longer visual recovery.[3] James Gills prescribes a nonsteroidal anti-inflammatory drop for his cataract patients 3 times a day for 1 week prior to surgery. This is particularly important for diabetic patients. We also recommend administering a steroid and nonsteroidal every 15 minutes on the day of the procedure for diabetics. In some cases, pretreating the patient with an intraocular injection of anti-vascular endothelial growth factor (VEGF) and steroid to minimize reaction and release of VEGF is appropriate prior to cataract surgery. This reduces recovery time and, particularly in the case of diabetic patients, can maximize their outcome. We typically use a Collamer lens for patients in this group because of its biocompatibility.

Astigmatism analysis is the second key component for screening Crystalens candidates. Neglecting to address pre-existing astigmatism diminishes the patient's return on his or her investment and can result in a very unhappy patient. We perform topography on all Crystalens patients not only to evaluate astigmatism but also to assess corneal health prior to surgery. Corneal assessment and analysis are included in the patient's out-of-pocket expense for Crystalens. Topography is absolutely required for identifying potential pitfalls such as irregular astigmatism secondary to keratoconus, corneal scars, pterygia, and previous refractive surgery.

Identifying and correcting astigmatism in Crystalens patients is critical to their satisfaction and success postoperatively. We treat as little as 0.50 D with limbal relaxing incisions and have corrected up to 5 D.[4] Corneal and limbal relaxing incisions are both important components of astigmatism correction. Limbal relaxing incisions have less coupling effect and tend to create a hyperopic shift. This is an important consideration and should be taken into account when selecting the IOL power.[5] Corneal relaxing incisions on the other hand create a greater coupling effect when performed in a 15- to 20-degree arc and produce a multifocal cornea with an increased depth of focus.

Biometry

Another important factor to any practice's success with Crystalens is biometry and the process for selecting the appropriate power. Taking the time to analyze postoperative data, customize IOL constants, and evaluate mean absolute error are essential functions for excellent outcomes.

Using the IOL Master (Carl Zeiss Meditec, Jena, Germany) and immersion biometry are absolutely essential for accuracy. IOL Master is effective for most patients; however, certain patients with dense cataracts still require biometry with immersion ultrasound. Applanation has been supplanted by both immersion and IOL Master because of its inaccuracy.[6,7] Measurements can be highly variable from one technician to another. With current technology, tolerance for biometry error should be 0.1 mm.

The importance of keratometry is often overshadowed by the emphasis we place on axial length measurements. Technicians should be trained to perform manual keratometry, but improvements in technology have made the keratometry function in the IOL Master and many topography units reproducible and accurate.

We use the Marco OPD topography system (Marco, Jacksonville, FL). We conducted a comparative analysis between a single experienced technician performing manual keratometry measurements and keratometry from the Marco OPD topography unit, and the difference was negligible. By implementing this technology, we have saved time, improved our reproducibility, and eliminated variability between technicians. We now rely on the topography measurements for calculations. Our standard protocol is to perform keratometry with IOL Master and compare the results to our topography measurements. If the 2 measurements do not correlate, the topography is repeated. In cases where fixation is a problem or there is a question of accuracy with either method, manual keratometry is used.

Intraocular Lens Selection

Prior to surgery, the staff discusses each patient's goals in detail. The primary goal for the majority of patients is not to see perfectly but to have a wide spectrum of vision, from distance to near. They wish to be able to watch television while working on a computer and make the transition from distance vision to intermediate or near vision seamlessly without changing glasses. Even with the visual spectrum that Crystalens provides, we still tailor the IOL selection according to each patient's needs to further enhance the effect. Generally speaking, we target the first eye for approximately −0.50. Targeting patients for a −0.50 gives a broad range of vision initially.

The target for the fellow eye is dependent on the patient's perception of his or her visual acuity and personal demands for more precise near or distance vision. We also take into consideration the patient's preoperative refractive error when selecting the lens for the fellow eye. For example, myopes tend to have less of an accommodating effect from Crystalens than hyperopes and tend to require a more myopic result to appreciate near vision. Hyperopes, on the other hand, tend to have a greater accommodating effect and function well without near correction even when targeted for distance. Some believe reading exercises can increase the accommodating effect; however, there is not sufficient evidence to indicate its effectiveness. It is typical, however, to see near acuity improve over time in these patients.

For those who have a high demand for near work, particularly myopes, we target the first eye for −1.00. This target, combined with a distant target on the fellow eye, provides the broadest range of vision. Because of the accommodative effect of the Crystalens, in some cases, even when focused for −1.00, distant acuity can be 20/25 to 20/30. This combination of near and distant targets allows us to "fine tune" near vision without causing a significant degradation of distant acuity. Discriminating patients do notice the difference between the distant acuity of their eyes, so this approach should be used only for patients who are counseled preoperatively and have appropriate expectations.

When evaluating the postoperative outcome, it is important to verify the postoperative refraction. It is easy to "over minus" when refracting Crystalens patients, and the refractions can be somewhat variable. A cycloplegic refraction may be required to obtain the most accurate result postoperatively.

When selecting the lens power for the fellow eye, the most accurate approach is to base the lens power on the empirical data from the first eye. If the patient's postoperative refractive error is off-target on the first eye, it should be considered when selecting the IOL for the fellow eye. We use a simple method for selecting power on the fellow eye:

* Change the sign of the postoperative spherical equivalent (PSE).
* Add the PSE to the target refraction of the first eye.
* That sum is the corrected target refraction for the fellow eye.
* Select the lens that is less than the corrected target refraction for the fellow eye.

Example:

Lens 1: IOL	Pred Ref	Lens 2: IOL	Pred Ref
20.0	+0.45	20.0	+0.32
20.5	−0.1	20.5	−0.14
21.0	**−0.43**	21.0	−0.47

In this case, a 21.0-D lens was selected for a target refraction of −0.43 on the first eye. The patient's outcome was −0.75. The process for selecting the IOL for the fellow eye is as follows:

* Change the sign of −0.75 to +0.75.
* Combine target refraction on the first eye with PSE (−0.43 + 0.75 = +0.32).
* The adjusted target is +0.32, and a 20.0 D IOL should be selected for the fellow eye.

The example above assumes the patient's refraction is stable and does not account for the myriad of factors that can potentially impact the postoperative outcome. That is where the art of IOL selection comes in. Of particular importance with the

Table 2

CALCULATE CORNEAL CURVATURE METHODS

History Method

This method uses pre- and postrefractive data to calculate the change in corneal curvature. When using this method, the most recent refraction should be used before any myopic shift from nuclear sclerotic cataract has occurred.

- Determine preoperative spherical equivalent and PSE.
- Correct the refraction for 0 mm vertex distance/corneal plane. (This is not necessary if less than 4 D of refractive error.)

> Formula: Corrected sph. equ. = $\dfrac{1000}{\dfrac{1000}{\text{sph. equ.}} - \text{vertex dist. mm}}$

> Example: Spherical equivalent = –6.0 vertex distance = 12 mm
> $$CSE = \dfrac{1000}{\dfrac{1000}{-6.0} - 12} = -5.6$$

- Determine the change in spherical equivalent
  Formula: Corrected pre-RK sph. equ. – post-RK sph. equ.

- Calculate correct K-reading
  Formula: Corrected K = preop K average – change in refraction

Contact Lens Method

The contact lens method is based on the following rationale:
- If there is a myopic shift in over-refraction, then the contact lens is *stronger* than the cornea.
- If there is a hyperopic shift in refraction, then the contact lens is *weaker* than the cornea.
- The contact lens method loses reliability when the vision is less than 20/50 or if the cornea is too flat to obtain a good contact lens fit. Use a plano power rigid gas permeable contact with a base curve that provides the most stable fit. If it is impossible to get a stable refraction due to poor fit of the contact lens, this method should not be used.

> Formula: Corrected K = (Post-RK sph. equ. – over-refraction sph. equ.) + Base curve

> Example:
> RGP base curve = 40.0 D
> Post-RK refraction = –0.5 - 0.5 x 180 (–0.75 SE)
> Over refraction = –2.0 - 0.50 x 180 (–2.25 SE)
> The refractive change is –3.0
> Because there was a myopic shift, the contact is stronger than the cornea.
> Corrected K-reading: 40 – 3.0 = 37 D

Crystalens is to compare the uncorrected near and distance acuity and make sure that it matches the refraction.

Previous Refractive Surgery

The baby boomer patients who underwent refractive surgery over the last 20 years are typically the same patients who want Crystalens. Their expectations are high, and their memory of the "wow" factor from refractive surgery is still fresh. These patients can be some of the most difficult to satisfy; however, if their expectations are set appropriately, Crystalens is an excellent option. Unlike monofocal lenses, the range of vision provided with Crystalens makes it forgiving for these postrefractive patients and, in many cases, an ideal option.

The biggest pitfall in performing cataract surgery on postrefractive patients is calculating the IOL power.[8] These patients can absorb a tremendous amount of chair time that is required not only to give them realistic expectations but in measuring and calculating for the lens. The true curvature of the cornea is in question. Refractive surgery, by its very nature, changes the corneal architecture, and therefore the assumptions made by manual keratometry are invalid. We use 3 methods to calculate corneal curvature: the history method, hard contact lens method, and corneal topography (Table 2).

Postoperative management of these patients can be challenging, and the staff and patient should be prepared. The biggest problem in the early postoperative period is the variability of the corneal shape, particularly for post-RK patients. It can take several weeks for the edema to resolve and to determine a stable postoperative refraction. It is typical to find a hyperopic shift resulting from corneal flattening following cataract surgery. Our protocol is to place these patients on sodium chloride ointment up to 4 times per day for the first week. The objective is to minimize corneal edema in the early postoperative period.

We closely follow the postoperative refractions of these patients and monitor corneal topography at each postoperative visit. Typically, the cornea flattens initially, and over several weeks, it returns to approximately the previous shape. When preoperative measurements have been correctly obtained, most patients are within a reasonable tolerance of their target refraction. In some cases, however, the cornea permanently flattens, leaving the patient with a postoperative hyperopic shift. In these cases, we offer the patient an IOL exchange if necessary to correct the refractive error.

Crystalens is the first IOL that has provided surgeons the ability to address presbyopia without compromising best corrected acuity or binocularity. Offering a solution to the loss of the broad range of vision associated with presbyopia has not only improved patient satisfaction, but in many cases, has allowed patients to return to a lifestyle they have not enjoyed in years. By addressing the cataract along with presbyopia, our patients enjoy a superior quality of vision and a better quality of life.

References

1. Thornton, SP. Accommodation with monofocal IOLs. *Ophthalmology.* 1992;99(6):853-860.

2. Cumming JS, Slade SG, Chayet A. Clinical evaluation of the model AT-45 silicone accommodating intraocular lens: results of feasibility and the initial phase of a Food and Drug Administration clinical trial. *Ophthalmology.* 2001;108(11):2005-2009.

3. Kim SJ, Equi R, Bressler NM. Analysis of macular edema after cataract surgery in patients with diabetes using optical coherence tomography. *Ophthalmology.* 2007;114(5):881-889.

4. Gills JP, Wallace RB, Miller K, et al. Reducing astigmatism with limbal relaxing incisions. In: Gills JP, ed. *A Complete Surgical Guide for Correcting Astigmatism.* Thorofare, NJ: SLACK Incorporated; 2003:99-120.

5. Gills JP, Rowsey JJ. Managing coupling in secondary astigmatic keratotomy. In: Gills JP, ed. *A Complete Surgical Guide for Correcting Astigmatism.* Thorofare, NJ: SLACK Incorporated; 2003:131-140.

6. Rose LT, Moshegov, CN. Comparison of the Zeiss IOL Master and applanation A-scan ultrasound: biometry for intraocular lens calculation. *Clin Experiment Ophthalmol.* 2003;31(2):121-124.

7. Hoffman PC, Hutz WW, Eckhardt HB, Heuring AH. Intraocular lens calculation and ultrasound biometry: immersion and contact procedures. *Klin Monatsbl Augenheilkd.* 1998;213(3):161-165.

8. Holladay JT. IOL power calculations for the unusual eye. In: Fine IH, Packer M, Hoffman RS, eds. *Cataract Surgery: The State of the Art.* Thorofare, NJ: SLACK Incorporated; 1998:197-206.

CHAPTER 49

EYEONICS CRYSTALENS— CLINICAL PEARLS

Robert Jay Weinstock, MD

For centuries, eye doctors have been puzzled and the general public has been frustrated by the natural aging process of the eye. In particular, the biological process of presbyopia has been a continuing challenge with little or no surgical remedies until the last few years. Historically, the only available solution for presbyopia has been the use of reading glasses, bifocal contacts, or monovision contact lenses. It has only been in the last decade that surgical alternatives have arisen. These options were limited until 2003 and include multifocal implants and surgically targeted monovision.

More recently, a revolutionary implant has become available that corrects presbyopia in a more physiological and natural way than monovision or multifocal lenses. This implant is called the Crystalens implant and is manufactured by Eyeonics (Aliso Viejo, CA). In 2003, their first-generation implant—the Crystalens AT-45—was introduced, which for the first time offered a truly accommodative solution to presbyopia at the time of cataract surgery or clear lensectomy (Figure 1).

The original model was quickly updated to a square-edge design in order to reduce posterior capsule opacification. Although the Crystalens AT-45 significantly improved pseudophakic accommodation, there were a variety of unpredictable refractive surprises that occurred. Due to the flexing nature of this implant and its 4.5-mm optic size, abnormal postoperative capsular contractile forces led to capricious shifts in the position of the lens within the capsular bag, resulting in refractive abnormalities and some surprising outcomes. Although this did not occur often, it motivated the manufacturer to create a more stable platform for improved refractive stability inside the capsular bag. In November 2006, Eyeonics released an improved version, called the Crystalens AT-50 which is also known as the Crystalens Five-0 (Figure 2).

For over 1 year, this newer design has been implanted worldwide with outstanding success. Data have shown that this accommodative flexing implant provides significant independence from reading glasses after lens replacement surgery. Most importantly, the Crystalens provides excellent binocular distance visual acuity with minimal to no nighttime or low-light visual dysphotopsias, which are so common and frustrating for patients with multifocal implants.

The Crystalens Five-0 has dramatically changed the landscape of cataract- and lens-based surgery. For the first time, cataract surgeons have a viable and reliable weapon against presbyopia for cataract and refractive patients that does not produce the undesirable side effects of glare, halos, and loss of contrast sensitivity. This chapter will discuss the Crystalens Five-0 and detail its use and applications.

Implant Properties

The Crystalens AT-50 is made of a third-generation silicone material called Biosil. It is a modified plate-style implant with a 5-mm optic and overall loop-to-loop length of 11.5 mm. A longer 12 mm version is available for lens powers below 19 D. It has 2 small polyimide loop haptics at the end of each plate. The tip of one haptic is round while the other is oval to facilitate the correct anterior/posterior positioning of the lens. There is a hinge at the junction of the optic and the plate on each side, which enables forward vaulting of the implant with accommodation. There is a 360-degree square-edge design to the optic to impede posterior capsule opacification (Figure 3). Besides a larger optic size, differences between the AT-45 and the Five-0 include a 27% wider arc of the haptic loops and a more rectangular shape to the plates. These changes improve centration and provide greater torsional fixation in the bag and greater accommodative function compared to the original version (Figures 4 and 5).

Although the full mechanism of action has not been fully explained for the Crystalens Five-0, current consensus is that the flexing nature of the lens is responsible for its accommodative effect. Whether you believe in Helmholz's, Tschernings, or Schachar's theory, it is thought that the ciliary body constricts during accommodation, releasing tension on the zonules and capsular bag, allowing the Crystalens to bow forward. This movement results in an accommodative effect as the effective dioptric power of the lens increases. Furthermore, wavefront

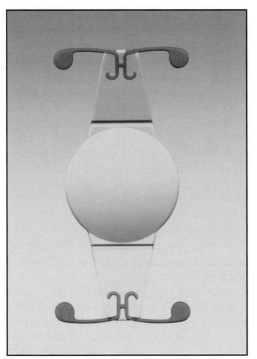

Figure 1. Crystalens AT-45.

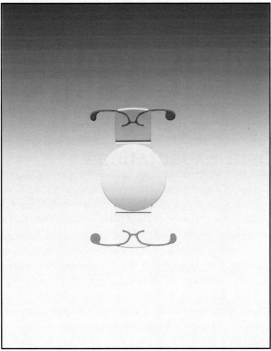

Figure 2. Crystalens AT-50 (Five-0).

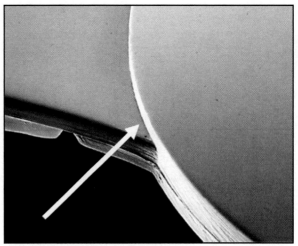

Figure 3. High magnification of the posterior surface of the Crystalens showing the 360-degree square-edge design.

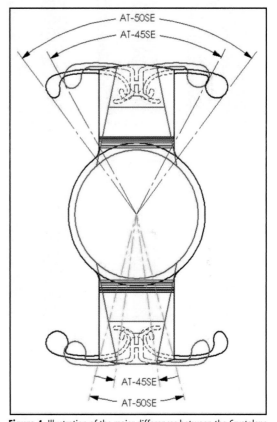

Figure 4. Illustration of the major differences between the Crystalens AT-45 and Five-0. Note that the Five-0 has a wider loop arc length and a wider plate haptic.

analysis studies performed by Kevin Waltz, MD and done under accommodative stress have also revealed a steepening in the curvature of the central optic, additionally increasing the effective near power of the lens. The exact influence and the amount that each mechanism is responsible for has yet to be determined.

Patient Selection

A key component to success with the Crystalens Five-0 is proper patient selection. Although it would be nice to be able to offer an accommodating implant to all cataract and refractive surgery patients, it is not possible to apply this technology in all situations. The ideal candidates for the Crystalens are

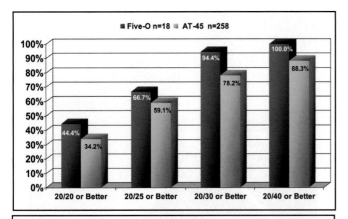

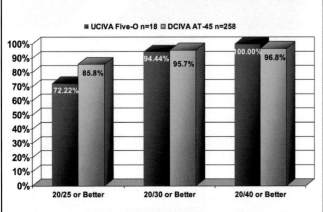

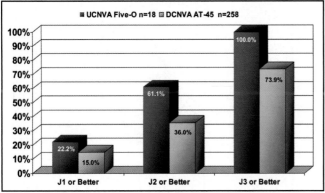

Figure 5. Comparison of visual results with the Crystalens AT-45 and Five-0.

patients who have a history of no previous intraocular surgery, trauma, or severe ocular conditions. For example, patients who have a history of progressive diabetic retinopathy, macular degeneration, advanced glaucoma, retinal surgery, or previous vitrectomy are probably not those best suited for the Crystalens. It is best to stick with routine, healthy eyes with no underlying ocular conditions such as pseudoexfoliation syndrome or Fuchs' endothelial dystrophy.

In regards to the preoperative refractive status, the best Crystalens patients are moderate to high hyperopes or myopes with low amounts of astigmatism. They tend to benefit the most from the technology. Patients with very high hyperopia or myopia may also do well with the Crystalens, although the chances of an unexpected refractive outcome are increased due to the difficulty in biometric analysis and lens selection formulas in these outlying cases. The surgeon must be ready to

address the imperfect refractive status postimplantation with additional refractive procedures at the appropriate time.

Patients with significant amounts of preoperative corneal astigmatism pose an additional challenge for targeting emmetropia for Crystalens candidates. Two D or less of astigmatism can often be managed with intraoperative limbal relaxing incisions, but patients should still be counseled about possibly needing additional refractive surgery in the postoperative period to treat any residual astigmatism. This is usually performed at the 3-month mark when the patient's refraction has stabilized and the corneal wound is well-healed. Either photorefractive keratectomy (PRK), epi-LASIK, laser in situ keratomileusis (LASIK), or additional limbal relaxing incisions can safely be performed at this point.

If it is determined preoperatively that the patient has a very high amount of corneal astigmatism—in the order of 2.5 D or greater based on corneal topography measurements—then it may be best to avoid using the Crystalens. A toric intraocular lens (IOL) may be a more practical choice to ensure good distance vision with a single procedure. Alternatively, some surgeons prefer a bioptics approach with a Crystalens implant followed by LASIK or surface ablation 3 months later.

Other issues regarding patient selection that the surgeon must carefully evaluate are personality traits and characteristics. Overly demanding patients or those with extremely nervous or obsessive personalities may not be best suited for refractive cataract surgery with the Crystalens. These patients end up being more trouble in the postoperative period than the surgeon wishes to deal with and are never happy regardless of their objective results. There are a variety of preoperative patient questionnaires that can be used to screen patients and identify their goals, expectations, and personalities to help the surgeon qualify them as good or poor candidates.

Patient Expectations

Another key to ensuring successful cataract surgery with the Crystalens, as with any procedure, is to set patient expectations properly at the time of the initial consultation. Continued reaffirmation of these expectations by the rest of the surgical and clinical team should continue afterwards. It is imperative to disclose to the patient that the Crystalens accommodative implant is not guaranteed or designed to completely eliminate the need for glasses after cataract or lens replacement surgery. Cumulative data have shown that the Crystalens can consistently provide up to 1.5 D of accommodation postoperatively. This still leaves the need for approximately +1 D power of additional strength for Jaeger 1 near vision at 14 inches. Therefore, Crystalens patients should be counseled appropriately and told that there will most likely be a need for a light pair of over-the-counter reading glasses after the procedure.

Some patients do experience complete spectacle independence postoperatively, but it is best to tell the patients that this is not the norm. Under promising and over delivering allows the surgeon some flexibility in his or her postoperative results and also helps with targeting the refractive error. The patient can be told that intermediate vision, such as computer and car dashboard range should be excellent with the Crystalens and no glasses should be needed. Patients should be told that the goal of the Crystalens implant is to provide sharp distance visual acuity in the daytime and night time with sharp intermediate vision. It can be explained to the patient that the Crystalens allows the patient to be free of glasses in 2 out of 3 ranges of vision versus the traditional monofocal implants that only allow spectacle independence for one range of vision (leaving 2 ranges that require spectacles).

Setting patients' expectations too high by trying to promise complete spectacle independence will only backfire, resulting in unhappy patients and postoperative dissatisfaction. If the patient demands complete spectacle independence and is not willing to wear a light pair of reading glasses after cataract surgery, then the Crystalens may not be a good choice for that patient. This type of patient may be better suited for a monovision or multifocal contact lens trial prior to lens-based surgery to see if he or she can gain more complete spectacle independence with other surgical and implant strategies.

Preoperative Testing and Surgical Planning

Success with the Crystalens demands very thorough preoperative evaluation, testing, and surgical planning. Some preoperative diagnostic tools that can prove to be extremely useful for not just the Crystalens but all IOLs are immersion A-scan, IOL Master (Carl Zeiss Meditec, Jena, Germany), corneal topography, manual keratometry, wavefront aberrometry, and retinal optical coherence tomography (OCT) (to rule out any retinal pathology). The information gained with all of these diagnostic modalities will give a very accurate assessment of the refractive and optical status of the eye for proper lens power selection and targeting. More specifically, the type and amount of astigmatism, as well as very accurate axial length and corneal power measurements, are crucial to success for Crystalens usage.

Current recommendations call for the use of the SRK-T formula for eyes with axial lengths greater than 22 mm and the Holiday II formula for axial lengths of 22 mm or less. Many surgeons find it very helpful to perform 2 different types of A-scans. For example, immersion A-scan biometry can be compared with the IOL Master reading to ensure proper lens selection. If the 2 scans call for different implant powers, careful attention must be paid to the source of the difference. If it is the K-readings that differ, then it may be prudent to obtain a third keratometry measurement based on a corneal topography device. If the axial length measurements vary between the 2 machines, then a third independent axial length measurement should be obtained to corroborate either of the first 2 readings. The doctor can make certain that the proper lens is being selected for the patient by using both technologies. Corneal topography and wavefront analysis can be used for additional keratometry readings, astigmatism analysis, and identification of abnormal aberrations of the optical system.

Lens Power Selection and Targeting

Several strategies can be applied when targeting patients for postoperative emmetropia, as well as planning for adequate

near vision with the Crystalens. One strategy consists of targeting the dominant eye for distance and performing this cataract or lens replacement surgery first. Once the surgery has been performed, the patient is evaluated several days to 1 week postoperatively to confirm the postoperative refractive status of the eye. If the patient is indeed emmetropic, then the nondominant eye can be targeted to be −0.50 myopic. This enables the surgeon to provide excellent binocular distance visual acuity, although the dominant eye may see slightly sharper than the nondominant eye. With this mild amount of anisometropia, however, the patient should still not be aware of any significant difference in distance visual acuity between the 2 eyes and should enjoy good binocular fusion. In addition, this mildly myopic target in the nondominant eye will allow a slightly broader functional range of vision for near. Alternatives to this strategy have been employed by some surgeons where the nondominant eye is performed first with a mildly myopic target of −0.50. If this target is achieved after the initial surgery, then the fellow dominant eye can be performed with a target of plano. With either strategy, if the refractive target is not exactly where the surgeon intended it to be for the first eye, the second eye's lens power selection can be slightly modified to further provide and ensure good postoperative vision with minimal need for reading glasses. For example in the first strategy where the dominant eye is performed first with an emmetropic target, consider what to do following a mildly myopic result of −0.5. One could then target emmetropia or even a slightly hyperopic target of +0.25 for the second eye even though it is nondominant.

Some surgeons take a less complex route and target emmetropia in both eyes. This is an excellent strategy as long as the patient accepts the fact that there may be greater reliance on low power reading glasses for fine print.

Operative Considerations

In addition to careful preoperative planning and proper lens power selection, successful Crystalens use is highly dependent on proper intraoperative management. It is essential to create astigmatically neutral incisions and to address preoperative corneal astigmatism at the time of cataract surgery. Limbal relaxing incisions to reduce preoperative corneal astigmatism are routinely accomplished at the beginning of the case after viscoelastic is placed in the anterior chamber. However, it is also acceptable to perform them at the end of the case prior to removal of the viscoelastic material (Figure 6).

Initially, Crystalens AT-45 use was accompanied by a recommendation for either a scleral tunnel incision or a clear corneal incision with suture placement. After significant experience with the Crystalens Five-0, it is apparent that standard clear corneal incisions are adequate in maintaining chamber integrity and preventing anterior displacement of the Crystalens. If there is any doubt about the seal, however, a suture should be placed.

Cataract removal with anticipation of Crystalens implant placement should be done carefully and methodically with special attention to not disturbing the zonular capsular apparatus. The Crystalens Five-0 is highly dependent on an intact capsular zonular system and any aggressive manipulation

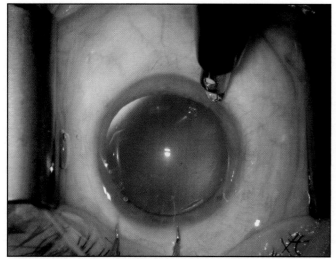

Figure 6. Limbal relaxing incision being performed to reduce astigmatism at 180 degrees.

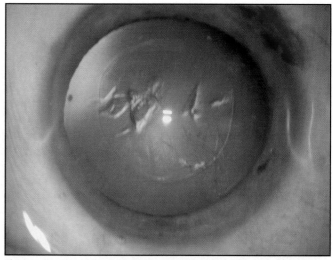

Figure 8. View of a 6-mm capsulorrhexis prior to nucleus removal.

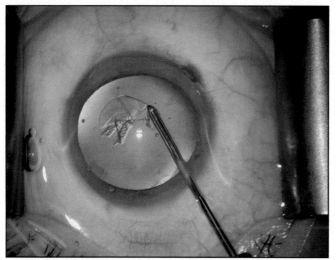

Figure 7. Microcapsulorrhexis forceps being used to initiate a 6-mm capsulorrhexis.

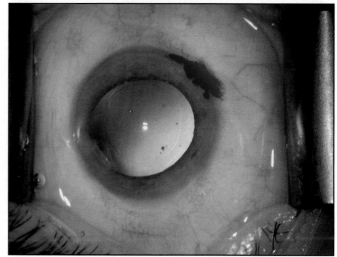

Figure 9. View of a completely empty and clean capsule fully filled with viscoelastic material prior to Crystalens implantation.

of the zonules or the capsule can affect its accommodative function or its centration postoperatively. This is especially important during cortical clean-up, where it is not uncommon to inadvertently grab the capsule and strip zonules with the irrigation-aspiration (I-A) instrument. The surgeon may want to proceed more cautiously and slowly during the cortical clean-up portion of the procedure to avoid zonular stress and to ensure that the capsule is left in pristine condition. Meticulous attention should be paid to removing all cortical material and lens epithelial cells.

Initially, a very small capsulorrhexis was recommended with the Crystalens AT-45. However, experience over the last few years has shown that with the AT-45 and the Five-0, a larger 5.5- to 6-mm capsulorrhexis is a better size for good postoperative centration and visual results. Although the Crystalens will work fine with a slightly smaller or larger capsulorrhexis, most surgeons are using this moderate diameter because it has significantly reduced the incidence of capsular contraction syndrome (Figures 7 and 8).

Situations can arise where a surgeon may decide not to implant the Crystalens contrary to the initial surgical plan.

Situations such as obvious zonular compromise, zonular stripping, or capsular instability would call for aborting Crystalens placement and using a back-up standard, monofocal IOL. The same holds true for cases with inadvertent tears in either the anterior or posterior capsule. The surgeon may wish to consent the patient preoperatively with regards to these potential complications.

When the Crystalens AT-45 was first introduced, smooth forceps were used to grasp the lens and place it into the capsular bag. There was no folding or injection of the implant. This required an approximately 4.0-mm incision. The Crystalens Five-0 is designed to be folded and injected, thereby avoiding this larger incision. The lens is able to be injected through an incision as small as 2.8 mm. Having the capsular bag fully expanded and filled with viscoelastic greatly facilitates IOL placement. One should never hesitate to inject additional viscoelastic if needed (Figure 9).

Injector systems from STAAR Surgical, Advanced Medical Optics, and Bausch & Lomb can all be used successfully with the Crystalens Five-0. Regardless of which injector system is used, inserting the Crystalens with the right side up is

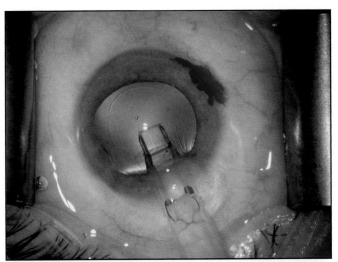

Figure 10. Bausch & Lomb softport injector system being used to implant the Crystalens Five-O. Note how the injector tip is placed well into the eye and in the capsular bag.

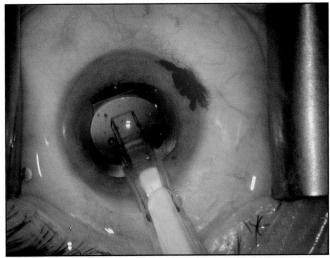

Figure 12. The optic of the Crystalens is injected into the capsular bag and in the center of the eye.

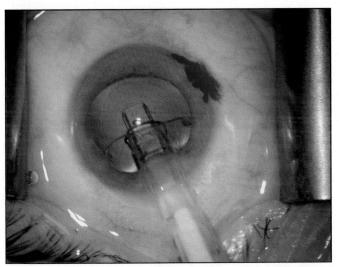

Figure 11. The leading haptics are aimed deep into the capsular bag. Note the round haptic is on the right and the oval-shaped haptic on the left.

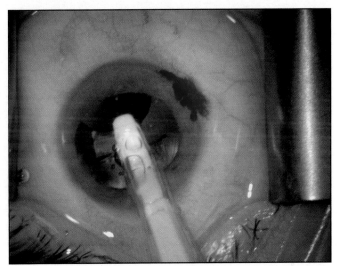

Figure 13. Trailing plate and haptics are delivered directly into the capsule. Note how far the optic is able to be displaced toward the capsule sulcus.

paramount for proper functioning and positioning of the lens since the hinge is cut with a groove on the anterior surface. The proper anterior-posterior orientation of the Crystalens is maintained by keeping the round leading haptic on the right and the oval on the left while the trailing oval haptic is on the right and the round on the left, as viewed from the surgeon's perspective. If the lens happens to flip upside down inside the eye during injection, it is very easy to place additional viscoelastic material inside the eye prior to using a Kuglen or Sinskey hook to gently rotate the implant and flip it into the proper orientation.

Most surgeons aim the injector cartridge tip down through the capsulorrhexis so that the leading plate haptic is delivered directly into the capsular bag. At this point, the trailing plate haptic can either be injected into the capsular bag or left in the anterior chamber (Figures 10 to 14). Sometimes the hinged leading plate haptic will bend down toward the posterior capsule and other times it will flex up toward the anterior capsule. Either situation is acceptable, and once the trailing plate and haptics are inside the bag, the lens will drift into its desired

position (Figure 15). Sometimes a hook or the I-A handpiece can be used to gently push the optic posteriorly, which allows the plate haptics to fully expand into the fornix of the capsular bag.

If the Crystalens cannot initially be injected completely into the capsular bag, then a Sinskey or Kuglen hook can be used to gently push the optic posteriorly at the junction of the optic and the plate. This will allow the lens to move posteriorly so that the trailing plate and haptics will be delivered into the capsular bag. At this point, the lens should assume a well-centered position, providing that there is no residual cortex or nuclear debris within the capsular bag or viscoelastic trapped beneath the lens (Figures 16 and 17).

I-A can then be used not only to remove the viscoelastic from the capsular bag and anterior chamber but also to gently spin the Crystalens 360 degrees inside the capsular bag. This spinning maneuver does several things. First, it allows the haptics to fully expand into the capsular bag fornix. It also allows the surgeon to confirm that there is no remaining cortex hidden in the capsular fornices that might adhere to or constrain

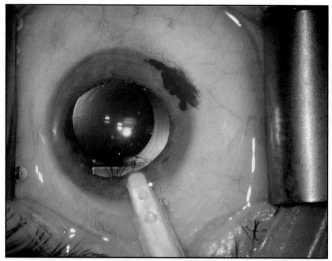

Figure 14. The Crystalens implant centers itself once it is completely inside the capsule.

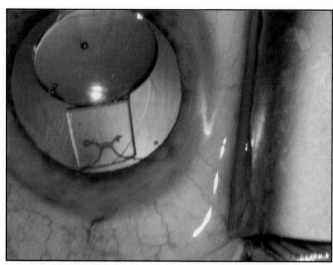

Figure 16. View of the Crystalens Five-0 with the leading plate/haptics inside the capsule and the trailing plate and haptics in the anterior chamber angle after initial delivery into the eye.

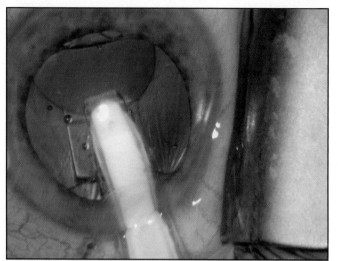

Figure 15. View of the Crystalens Five-0 being injected and the leading plate/haptic complex folding posterior into the capsule. Its position will usually rectify itself and become planar once the entire lens is inside the capsule.

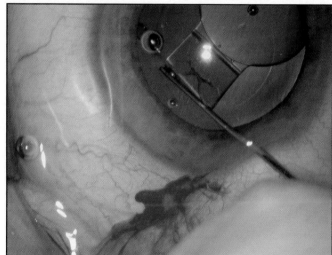

Figure 17. A Kuglen hook is used to place the trailing plate and haptics into the capsule.

the Crystalens. Finally, it allows all of the viscoelastic to be expressed out of the capsular bag and removed from the eye.

Most surgeons feel that it is important to place the I-A tip behind the Crystalens to remove any viscoelastic that is trapped there. This allows the Crystalens to fully expand posteriorly into its natural desired anatomical position (Figure 18). If the Crystalens is not centering properly at the end of the case, the surgeon should reinflate the capsular bag with a cohesive viscoelastic material and again spin the Crystalens 180 to 360 degrees with the I-A tip until the lens takes a more natural and centered position.

If the Crystalens is still not centered adequately following multiple attempts with this maneuver, it may be prudent to remove and exchange it with a standard monofocal implant. Once the Crystalens is well-centered with good posterior vaulting and all of the viscoelastic is removed, it is very important to ensure a well-sealed incision at the end of the case. This will guarantee that the Crystalens will remain in its posterior position throughout the postoperative period. Although particular orientation of the axis of the 2 plates is not required,

some experienced Crystalens surgeons find the implant sits in a more stable and centered position when the plates are oriented vertically and away from the wound (Figure 19).

If the wound is not well-sealed and there is a postoperative leak, there is the possibility that the Crystalens will vault forward, causing a myopic shift. If there is any question as to whether the incision is well-sealed, it is certainly prudent to place a 10-0 suture to ensure secure closure.

Postoperative Management

With the more stable platform of the Crystalens Five-0, postoperative management is more straightforward and uneventful compared to the original Crystalens AT-45 model. Some patients developed capsular contraction syndrome with a resultant posterior displacement of the AT-45 IOL (Figure 20). Additionally, due to the flexing nature of the AT-45 Crystalens implant, some patients experienced unexpected myopic or hyperopic shifts during the postoperative period.

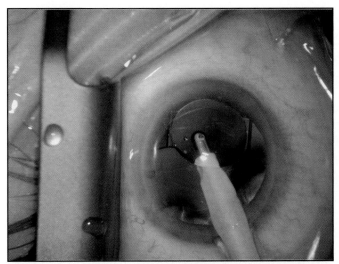

Figure 18. Coaxial I-A handpiece is placed under the implant to remove trapped viscoelastic material.

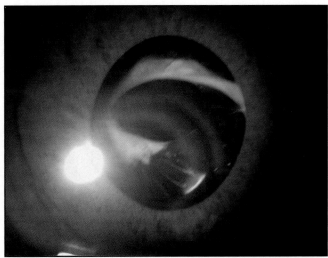

Figure 20. Capsular contraction syndrome with ovalization of the capsulorrhexis seen with the Crystalens AT-45.

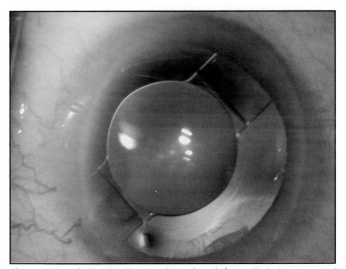

Figure 19. View of a Crystalens Five-0 implant at the end of a case. Notice its more vertical plate orientation and it posterior vault with no striae in the posterior capsule.

Patients also needed to be cyclopleged for an extended period of time postoperatively.

The design and shape of the Crystalens Five-0 provides a tremendous amount of refractive stability postoperatively but yet incorporates the beneficial accommodative effects of its being flexible. If proper preoperative assessment and targeting are done, it is very easy to obtain consistently accurate postoperative results within 0.25 D of the intended target. Postoperative cycloplegia is not required any longer although some surgeons still like to use one drop of atropine immediately after surgery. This allows the surgeon to view the lens well on the first postoperative day and may help to keep the lens vaulted posteriorly.

The Crystalens Five-0 comes in 0.25-D steps to further refine the refractive target appropriately. It is good practice to check the outcome of the first eye prior to proceeding with the second eye. This allows the surgeon to see if the intended target is indeed achieved and to make minor adjustments on the second eye's implant power selection to further minimize spectacle reliance.

Very few complications are seen in the immediate postoperative period. However, in situations where the incision is not well-sealed or is leaking postoperatively, there can be a collapse or shallowing of the anterior chamber and resultant flexing of the implant anteriorly into the iris plane. If this is seen, it is best to take the patient back to the operating room, reinflate the eye, and place a suture in the wound to keep the anterior segments deep and well-formed with the IOL in a posteriorly vaulted position. Mild chamber shallowing or myopic IOL shift in the early postoperative period can also be treated with cycloplegic eyedrops, which may return the IOL to a more posterior vault. There is also a very rare event where the IOL is vaulted too far posteriorly due to improper expansion inside the capsular bag, resulting in a hyperopic result. If this is seen, the patient should then be taken back to the operating room to have the lens rotated into a more planar orientation. Another less invasive strategy would be to try a short course of pilocarpine drops to see if it can reduce the exaggerated posterior vault. Fogged and/or cycloplegic refractions can be helpful in identifying the source of visual complaints and any residual ametropia in the early or late postoperative period.

In the event that there is a significant refractive error identified postoperatively despite a normal lens position, many surgeons choose to wait approximately 3 months and then perform excimer refractive surgery to the cornea to treat residual astigmatism, myopia, and/or hyperopia. Three months provides adequate time for the refraction to stabilize and for the wound to heal completely. PRK, epi-LASIK, or LASIK can be done at this time. If needed, YAG posterior capsulotomy should be done prior to excimer laser treatment to fully stabilize the intraocular component of the refraction.

As with all IOLs, posterior capsular opacification is often seen postoperatively. Once opacification becomes visually significant, a standard YAG posterior capsulotomy can be performed. Surgeons sometimes prefer to keep this posterior capsular opening slightly smaller in accordance with the decreased optic diameter of the Crystalens Five-0. This prevents vitreous prolapse around the optic and also decreases the risk of posterior dislocation of the implant into the vitreous

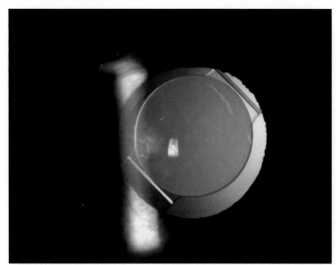

Figure 21. A typical well-centered Crystalens Five-0 as seen at the slit lamp with retroillumination on postoperative day 1.

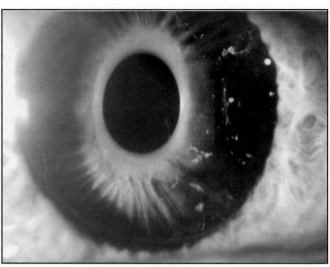

Figure 22. An example of capsular contraction syndrome with severe anterior capsule phimosis probably caused by too small of a capsulorrhexis.

cavity. Although this complication occurred in the past with plate-style lenses, it has not occurred with the Crystalens.

Unlike the Crystalens AT-45, the Crystalens Five-0 has enjoyed a very low rate of capsular contraction syndrome with resulting displacement and malposition of the optic. However, if this is noted postoperatively, it is most likely due to residual cortex, lens epithelial cells, or a too-small capsulorrhexis (Figure 21). If an abnormal IOL position is clinically significant or asymmetric vaulting is present, selective YAG capsulotomy—either to the anterior capsule or posterior capsule in the area of contraction—can be performed to resolve the problem. If the anterior capsulotomy assumes an oval shape due to contraction, then the YAG laser can be used to make small nicks in the edge of the anterior capsule to release the tension. This should allow the capsulorrhexis to take a larger and more rounded shape, reducing capsular tension on the IOL and shifting it into a more natural position inside the capsular bag.

Additionally, abnormal asymmetric striae and contraction in the posterior capsule are usually located beneath one or both of the plates of the IOL. If this is seen, the YAG laser can also be used to create small holes and nicks in the striae, which will release the tension in that area. This can be performed simultaneously with treating posterior capsular opacification by making the posterior capsule opening slightly decentered towards the area of striae. It is advisable not to YAG the anterior capsule and the posterior capsule at the same time because it may induce too much of a shift in the IOL position. It would be better to do it in a staged fashion where the surgeon can monitor the changes in the lens position and refraction

before deciding to perform additional YAG laser treatments as needed.

The Crystalens AT-45 has a very low incidence of night time halos or dysphotopsias. Its increased optic size also provides high quality scotopic vision. Patients and surgeons alike are generally extremely satisfied with the quality of uncorrected vision (Figure 22).

With proper patient selection, preoperative testing, surgical technique, and postoperative management, surgeons are now able to offer their patients superior visual outcomes with an improved level of spectacle independence for a greater quality of life.

Bibliography

Cumming JS, Colvard DM, Dell SJ, et al. Clinical evaluation of the Crystalens AT-45 accommodating intraocular lens: results of the U.S. Food and Drug Administration clinical trial. *J Cataract Refract.* 2006;32:812-825.

Doane J. Crystalens refractive lens replacement for high myopia, hyperopia and astigmatism. Paper presented at 23rd Annual Congress of ESCRS; September 11, 2005; Lisbon, Portugal.

Kernian G, Martin Davies J, Doane JF, Pepose JS. Accommodating IOLS in the real world. *Review of Ophthalmology.* 2007.

Lindstrom RL. Providing a full spectrum of vision: an assessment of clinical options of treating presbyopia with IOLS. *Cataract & Refractive Surgery Today.* 2005;69-70.

Macsai MS, Padnick-Silver L, Fontes BM. Visual outcomes after accommodating intraocular lens implantation. *J Cataract Refract Surg.* 2006;32:628-633.

Slade SS. Accommodating IOLS: design technique. *Review of Ophthalmology.* Supplement July 2005.

CHAPTER 50

CRYSTALENS 4.5 VERSUS 5.0— WHAT IS DIFFERENT?

James A. Davies, MD, FACS

The Crystalens AT-50 intraocular lens (IOL) (Crystalens Five-0) (Eyeonics, Inc, Aliso Viejo, CA) was introduced in the fourth quarter of 2006. In order to increase refractive predictability and to provide a more stable placement in the capsular bag, particularly in high myopes, the Crystalens was redesigned and modified. The haptic design was changed from earlier versions of the Crystalens and the optic was enlarged to Five-0 mm in diameter. The square-edge design of the Crystalens AT-45 S.E. lens was retained because this significantly reduced the risk of posterior capsular opacification and eliminated the occurrence of asymmetric lens vaulting (Z-syndrome) occasionally seen with the original AT-45 design.

The Crystalens Five-0 is a biconvex lens implant manufactured from a third-generation silicone material (Biosil; Carpenteria, CA) (Figure 1). This accommodating IOL has a Five-0-mm optic with flexible-hinged plate haptics designed to allow movement and/or changes in shape of the lens optic in response to accommodative effort. The loop design is 11.5 mm in length and provides a 27% wider arc of the lens loops (Figure 2). The haptics fold inward, allowing for ease of use with injectors. More stable positioning and predictability are provided by the 90% increase in plate arc length and the 17% greater area of surface contact between the lens optic, plates, and the capsular bag (Figures 3 and 4). Refractive predictability is 66% greater with the Crystalens Five-0 compared to the first and second designs (Figure 5).

Although the AT-45 was always "well behaved," as lens implants go, those surgeons with significant experience with that model have been uniformly impressed that the Crystalens Five-0 feels much more "substantial" than the AT-45. The additional 0.5 mm of optic diameter, wider plate haptics, and extended reach of the haptic loops serve to give the Five-0 a more robust feel.

Unlike standard silicone or acrylic IOLs, the volume of the capsular bag is an important factor in determining optic axial location and refractive results. A large capsular bag (as in those with higher degrees of myopia) may cause the lens to be less vaulted and further anterior than expected, resulting in more myopia than anticipated. Conversely, a smaller capsular bag will result in greater posterior vaulting and a hyperopic shift. Fortunately, the IOL power calculation nomograms take this factor into consideration, and as more data are collected and entered into the SurgiVision DataLink IOL Registry (Scottsdale, AZ; see Figure 4), refractive predictability will continue to improve.

Given the wider arc of capsular bag contact with the loop extension of the Crystalens Five-0, the incidence of IOL "propellering" occasionally experienced with the AT-45 is substantially reduced or eliminated. Although optic centration was not an issue with the original design, the slightly larger Five-0 tends to retain its position somewhat better. Additionally, the Five-0 is manufactured with a 12.0-mm overall diameter in powers from 4.0 D to 16.75 D (versus the 11.5-mm diameter in powers from 17.0 D to 33.0 D). The estimated lens position is more predictable with this larger diameter.

CRYSTALENS AVAILABLE POWER RANGE (AS OF 2007)
4 to 10.0 D in 1-D steps
10 to 16.0 D in 0.50-D steps
16 to 27 in 0.25-D steps
27 to 33 in 0.5-D steps
4 to 16.75 D in 12.0 mm length
17 to 33.0 D in 11.5 mm length

The power range for the 12.0 mm length is 4 D to 16.75 D, and for the 11.5-mm length, the range is 17 D to 33.0 D.

Figure 1. The Crystalens Five-0 is a biconvex lens implant manufactured from a third-generation silicone material (Biosil; Carpenteria, CA) .

	AT-45	**AT-50**
Diameter	4.55 mm	5.0 mm
Shape	Biconvex	Biconvex
Material	Biosil	Biosil
Powers	4.0D - 10.0 in 1.0D steps 10.0D - 33.0 in 0.50D steps 16.0D - 27.0 in 0.25D steps	4.0D - 10.0 in 1.0D steps 16.0D in 0.50D steps 16.0D - 27.0 in 0.25D steps 27.0D - 33.0 in .50D steps 4.0D - 16.75D available in 12.0mm length 17.0D - 33.0 available in 11.5 mm length
A-Constant	119.24	119.00
Refractive Index	1.428	1.428
Theoretical AC Depth	5.69	5.55
Overall Length	11.5	11.5
Material	Polyimide	Polyimide
Nomogram	Yes	Yes
Incision-Forceps	3.0 mm 3.2 mm	3.2 mm - 3.5 mm
Incision-Staar Blue Injector	5 mm- 5.5 mm	5 mm - 55.5 mm
Rhexis		

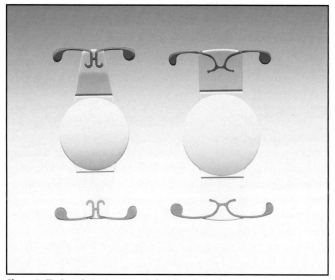

Figure 2. The loop design is 11.5 mm in length and provides a 27% wider arc of the lens loops.

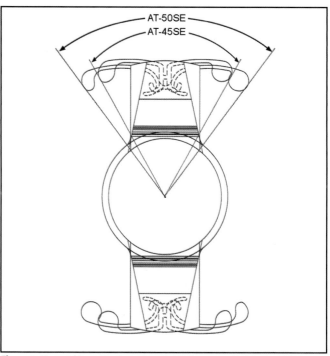

Figure 3. More stable positioning and predictability are provided by the 90% increase in plate arc length and the 17% greater area of surface contact between the lens optic, plates, and the capsular bag.

Surgical Pearls

Several important steps during surgery serve to increase refractive predictability with the Crystalens. Of course, one cannot overemphasize the importance of accuracy in biometry, but proper surgical technique is also critical once the correct IOL is selected.

Creating a well-centered anterior capsulotomy of appropriate size is an important first step. This is done more easily if a Five-0-mm optical zone marker is utilized to make a mark centered on the visual axis. The corneal mark can serve as a guide to both the size and centration of the capsulorrhexis. My own preference is to use a 5.0- to 6.0-mm horizontally oval capsulorrhexis. With the IOL vertically oriented at the completion of the procedure, the capsule will cross the IOL at or near the hinges superiorly and inferiorly. The medial and lateral edges

of the lens are exposed, but the anterior and posterior leaflets of the capsule are usually fused within 2 weeks.

Since patients are willing to pay for a premium lens implant, their expectations of a good result are higher than with standard cataract surgery. For this reason, those experienced with limbal relaxing incisions will typically utilize this technique as needed to control astigmatism. The cataract is removed in the usual manner through a temporal clear corneal incision or in the steep axis of astigmatism. After cortical removal, the silicone sleeve of the irrigation and aspiration tip can be advanced

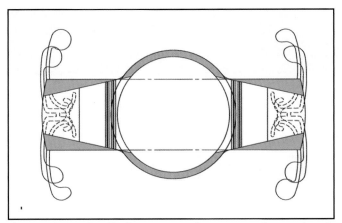

Figure 4. The Crystalens AT50 has 17% more surface area contact between the optic, plates and the capsular bag and 90% greater plate arc length allowing for more capsular bag support.

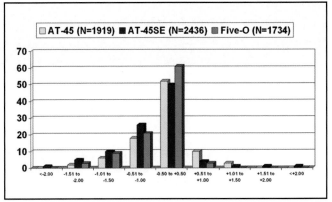

Figure 5. Refractive predictability is 66% greater with the Crystalens Five-0 compared to the first and second designs.

so as to cover the aspiration port. The posterior capsule and subcapsular areas can be vacuumed in this manner, and a Terry Squeegee (Alcon, Fort Worth, TX) or similar device can be carefully used as necessary for fine polishing of the central capsule.

After inflation of the capsular bag with viscoelastic, Shepard curettes to the right and left (Momentum Medical, Idaho Falls, ID) are used to polish the subcapsular leaflets. This assists in prevention of phimosis and likely reduces postoperative inflammation by reducing the lens epithelial cell load.

The Crystalens is then implanted in the normal fashion, with either an injector or with Cumming lens forceps (Eyeonics, Inc). A #10-0 nylon suture is placed in the corneal incision prior to removal of viscoelastic to ensure complete incision closure and viscoelastic is removed by irrigation and aspiration. It is important to irrigate behind the IOL to assure complete removal of viscoelastic.

The Crystalens should be rotated 2 or 3 times at this point to remove any peripheral cortical remnants, and the lens is left in a vertical orientation. The corneal suture is tied and the knot buried. Stromal hydration of the corneal and side port incisions is done to prevent loss of aqueous and to maintain the proper position of the Crystalens in the capsular bag. It is critical to carefully observe the IOL position in these final steps. If there is any shallowing of the anterior chamber, the Crystalens will vault anteriorly and the proper position of the lens in the peripheral capsular bag may be compromised, resulting in an unexpected refractive result and diminished accommodative amplitude. If any anterior chamber shallowing is noted, balanced salt solution is injected through the side-port incision and the Crystalens is rotated 180 degrees to ensure proper placement in the capsular bag. A moistened fluorescein strip can then be used to ensure complete incision closure.

It is advisable to place a drop of cyclopentolate in the eye upon completion of surgery. The pupil will remain dilated the first day, allowing for a reasonably accurate refraction as well as confirmation of proper orientation and vaulting of the Crystalens. The use of a miotic during surgery is likely to artificially enhance the range of vision over the first several days and may lead to patient disappointment as its effect diminishes. It also tends to mask an underlying refractive error that will not be measured until the second postoperative visit.

With the Crystalens AT-50 accommodating lens implant, careful attention to detail at every step in the surgical process has given us a powerful tool in allowing our patients to see well at multiple distances.

CHAPTER 51

CRYSTALENS HD—EARLY RESULTS

John A. Hovanesian, MD; Y. Ralph Chu, MD; James A. Davies, MD;
John F. Doane, MD; and Roger V. Ohanesian, MD

The first-generation Crystalens accommodating intraocular lens (IOL) (Eyeonics, Inc, Aliso Viejo, CA) first became Food and Drug Administration (FDA) approved in November 2003 and has since undergone 2 revisions. The first involved modification of the lens optic to have a "square" rather than smooth edge in order to reduce the incidence of asymmetric capsular fibrosis, which could cause capsular contraction and IOL tilt. The second revision involved enlarging the lens optic to 5.0 mm, modifying the haptic plates to a more square shape for more capsular support, and increasing the arc length of the haptics for greater stability. Each of these revisions provided greater stability and predictability.[1] In order to increase functional near vision with this lens, a third revision was made, known as the Crystalens HD. In lab testing, this lens provided greater depth of field than the parent AT-45 lens (Figure 1) with no reduction in modulation transfer function, an objective measure of contrast (Figure 2). The purpose of this study was to determine surgical outcomes with this lens and whether it would degrade contrast acuity in human subjects.

After IRB approval of the study protocol, a total of 125 primary eyes were implanted with the Crystalens HD. Inclusion criteria were age at least 18, presence of a visually significant cataract, less than 1.0 D of corneal astigmatism, and the potential for best corrected visual acuity of 20/25 or better in both eyes. Exclusion criteria were more than 1.0 D of corneal astigmatism, any anterior segment pathology (chronic uveitis, iritis, iridocyclitis, rubeosis iridis, corneal dystrophy, poor pupil dilation), uncontrolled glaucoma or need for current treatment for glaucoma, or with visual field loss as a result of glaucoma, any visually significant retinal pathology or a history of retinal detachment, proliferative diabetic retinopathy, macular degeneration, or other degenerative visual disorders, congenital bilateral cataracts, marked microphthalmos or aniridia, only one functioning eyed, no potential for visual acuity of 20/25 or better in each eye, lack of intact binocular vision, a non-intact capsulorrhexis and posterior capsular bag at the time of cataract removal and lens implantation, damaged zonules, or zonular rupture during cataract removal.

Surgery was performed using standard phacoemulsification techniques, and the lens was implanted using an injector system.

Postoperatively, patients were evaluated at 1 day, 7 to 14 days, 1 to 2 months, and 4 to 6 months. The following parameters were measured: uncorrected distance visual acuity, uncorrected intermediate visual acuity measured at 32 inches (80 cm), uncorrected near visual acuity measured at 16 inches (40 cm), manifest refraction, cycloplegic refraction, best corrected distance visual acuity, intermediate visual acuity at 32 inches (80 cm), measured through the distance correction, near visual acuity at 16 inches (40 cm), measured through the distance correction, best corrected near visual acuity (with the best spectacle distance correction and minimal reading add to achieve best-corrected near visual acuity [BCNVA]) at 16 inches (40 cm), contrast sensitivity with pupil size, mesopic 3 cd/m^2 with and without glare, photopic conditions 85 cd/m^2 with and without glare.

For analysis of uncorrected and distance-corrected visual acuity we selected patients who achieved a target refraction within 0.5 D of the intended target. We also conducted comparison of monocular uncorrected and distance-corrected near visual acuity with results a randomly selected, similar-sized group of patients from prior studies of the parent lens AT-45 and third-generation AT-50.

Sixty eyes had reached follow-up of 4 to 6 months and were within 0.5 D of intended target. Mesopic contrast sensitivity testing both without (Figure 3) and with glare (Figure 4) revealed no significant difference between Crystalens HD eyes and eyes tested previously[2] with the AT-45 parent lens. Monocular uncorrected visual acuity at distance of 20/40 was achieved by 100% of patients, 20/32 by 86.6%, 20/25 by 61.6%, and 20/20 by 41.6% of patients (Figure 5). Monocular uncorrected intermediate acuity of 20/40 was achieved in 100% of patients, 20/32 by 96.6%, 20/25 by 93.3%, and 20/20 by 80% of patients (Figure 6). Monocular uncorrected near acuity of J3 was achieved by 100% of patients, J2 by 80%, and J1 by 55% of patients (Figure 7). Through distance correction,

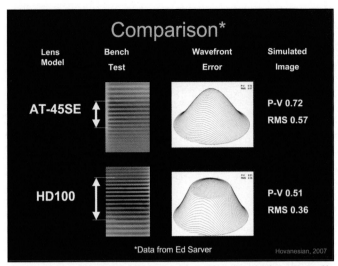

Figure 1. Photography through the Crystalens HD provides greater depth, as measured by more black bars falling into focus than the parent Crystalens AT-45. The wavefront error of the Crystalens HD also has a lower RMS value than the AT-45.

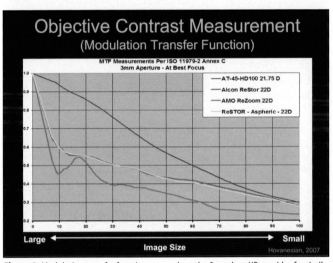

Figure 2. Modulation transfer function curves show the Crystalens HD provides for similar contrast measurements to the AT-45.

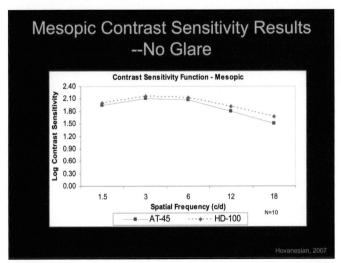

Figure 3. Mesopic contrast sensitivity without glare is similar with the Crystalens HD and AT-45.

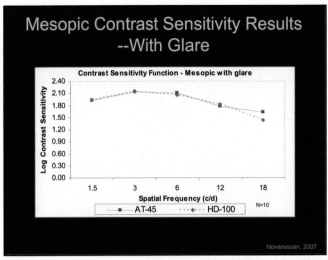

Figure 4. Mesopic contrast sensitivity with glare is similar with the Crystalens HD and AT-45.

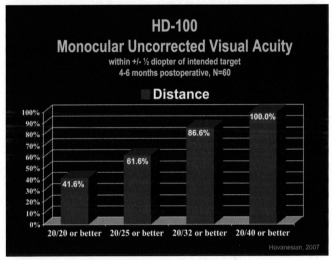

Figure 5. Monocular uncorrected distance visual acuity.

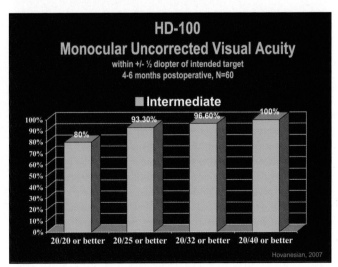

Figure 6. Monocular uncorrected intermediate visual acuity.

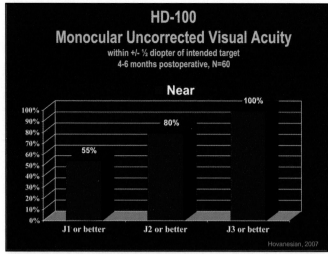

Figure 7. Monocular uncorrected near visual acuity.

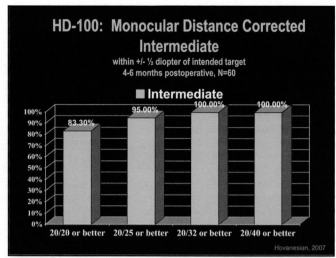

Figure 9. Monocular distance corrected intermediate visual acuity.

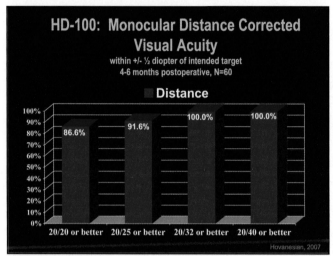

Figure 8. Monocular best corrected visual acuity at distance.

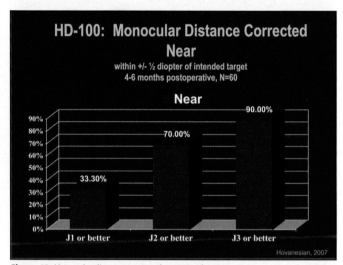

Figure 10. Monocular distance corrected near visual acuity.

100% of patients had distance vision of 20/32, 91.6% achieved 20/25, and 86.6% 20/20 (Figure 8). Distance-corrected intermediate vision was 20/32 in 100%, 20/25 in 95%, and 20/20 in 83.3% (Figure 9). Distance-corrected near vision was J3 in 90%, J2 in 70%, and J1 in 33.3% (Figure 10).

A comparison was made of the aforementioned results of the Crystalens HD with previously collected data on 60 randomly selected patients with the parent AT-45 and the third generation 5.0-mm optic (Crystalens Five-0). Monocular uncorrected near visual acuity improved with each successive generation of the lens (Figure 11). Similarly, distance corrected near visual acuity also improved with each successive generation (Figure 12).

This study demonstrates that the fourth-generation Crystalens HD accommodating IOL provides excellent results for both monocular uncorrected visual acuity and distance corrected visual acuity at distance, intermediate, and near. The effective range of near vision with this lens was improved over prior generations, and the optic modification did not result in a loss of contrast sensitivity in these patients.

Not all patients in this study achieved 20/20 corrected distance visual acuity. Some of these patients may have had

minor posterior capsule opacity at the time of measurements. Others may have had maculopathy that was not detectable at the time of preoperative examination through the cataractous lens. Whatever the cause, the data support the idea that the lens implant did not cause a loss of best corrected vision.

The Crystalens HD studied here had a 4.5-mm optic and the same haptics as the original AT-45. This was a requirement of the FDA, which requested an "apples to apples" comparison of the new lens optic to the original AT-45. However, this lens body has been well known to provide less refractive predictability than the more recent Crystalens Five-0 with its larger 5.0-mm optic and broader haptics.[3] It is on this more predictable lens platform that Eyeonics plans to release the Crystalens HD. For purposes of this study, we performed statistical analysis only on patients whose refractive outcome was within 0.5 D of target refraction. To report our results without selecting these patients out, including those with unintentional myopia, would artificially skew the data toward better uncorrected near vision.

This study demonstrates that a modification to the optic of the Crystalens can significantly increase the range of functional near vision without sacrificing contrast acuity or distance

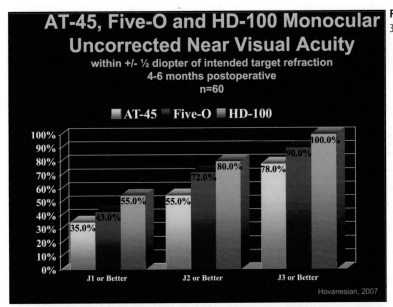

Figure 11. Comparison of monocular uncorrected near visual acuity with 3 models of the Crystalens: AT-45, AT-50, and Crystalens HD.

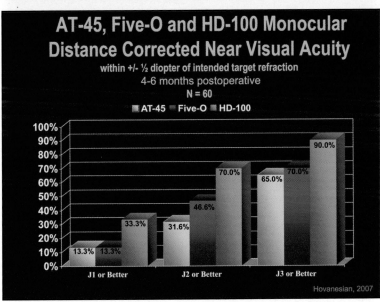

Figure 12. Comparison of distance corrected near visual acuity with 3 models of the Crystalens: AT-45, AT-50, and Crystalens HD.

vision. After FDA approval, which is anticipated in the second half of 2008, further studies on greater numbers of patients will help us establish this lens' capabilities. These initial results, however, suggest that the HD optic should allow surgeons to move a significant step closer toward targeting emmetropia in both eyes of patients undergoing Crystalens implantation.

Acknowledgments

This material was presented at the American Academy of Ophthalmology meeting, New Orleans, LA, November 2007.

This study was funded by a grant from Eyeonics, Aliso Viejo, CA.

References

1. Data on file, Eyeonics, Inc.

2. Data on file, Eyeonics, Inc.

3. Data on file, Eyeonics, Inc.

CHAPTER 52

CRYSTALENS—
WHAT IS THE MECHANISM?

Kevin L. Waltz, OD, MD

The Crystalens (Eyeonics, Inc, Aliso Viejo, CA) was the first accommodating intraocular lens (IOL) approved for use in the United States. It was approved for use in the United States in November 2003.[1] Since that time, there has been considerable controversy surrounding the accommodative efficacy of the Crystalens. Does it really accommodate? If so, how much does it accommodate? What is the mechanism of action of the accommodation? The controversy has continued well into 2007 and is likely to be a topic of discussion for the foreseeable future. In this chapter, I will discuss several proposed mechanisms of action of the Crystalens and consider their strengths and weaknesses.

The original proposed and patented mechanism of action of the Crystalens is a posterior to anterior translocation. This movement resulted in a change in the effective lens position of the Crystalens and an increase in the effective focusing power of the lenses. This is based on the same principle that a lens in the ciliary sulcus will have a greater effective power than the same lens in the capsular bag. This posterior to anterior movement has been documented in a number of studies.[2,3] There are also studies that show minimal axial movement or even a retrograde movement of the Crystalens during accommodative effort.[4,5] In any case, it is unlikely that a posterior to anterior movement of a low-power IOL will result in sufficient refractive power change to be clinically meaningful in a low-power Crystalens, such as a +6.00-D lens. Yet, in the Food and Drug Administration (FDA) trial, and subsequently after the trial, the apparent accommodation as measured by the ability to read has been observed in patients implanted with low-power Crystalens. There must be alternate mechanisms of action beyond the posterior to anterior movement to account for the observed ability to read in those patients implanted with a low-power Crystalens.

One explanation for this apparent discrepancy is pseudoaccommodation. Pseudoaccommodation is commonly defined as improved near vision due to multifocality, increased depth of field due to pupillary constriction, and/or induced optical aberrations. Holladay has proposed the improved near vision in the Crystalens is due to the smaller optic diameter.[6] This was based on the then-current design of the lens with a 4.5-mm optic. There has been no change in the observed near vision with the new 5.0-mm optic suggesting the optic diameter was not a critical factor in the Crystalens' near visual performance.

There is a wavefront-based explanation for the apparent discrepancy between the observed good reading vision of eyes implanted with a low-power Crystalens and the minimal amount of power change expected from axial displacement of a low-power IOL. It is possible for the lens to flex or arch in response to contraction of the ciliary body. The lower power Crystalens is thinner and more flexible than a higher power lens. It would be expected to respond more to a bending force than a thicker, less flexible lens.

I have called this flexing or bending accommodative arching.[7] Accommodative arching occurs in the normal crystalline lens and in the Crystalens.[8-11] It will likely also occur in other accommodating lenses. Wavefront analysis clearly shows significant power variations within the crystalline lens and the Crystalens with accommodative effort. The wavefront changes have been documented to be in proportion to expected accommodative responses based on direct electrical stimulation of the Edinger-Westphal nucleus.[11] A typical example of an accommodative arching wavefront change with a Crystalens patient is seen in Figure 1. Accommodative arching has been shown to be a dynamic process that can change rapidly over a relatively short time course. A series of wavefront images from the same eye are shown in Figures 1A-F. Note the time marked on each image and circled in red.

At first, it is difficult to imagine how bending or arching a flexible lens could cause such an asymmetric response. There is a simple way to imagine how accommodative arching might work in a pseudophakic eye. Assume that you have a 20-D IOL with symmetrical power and curvature on both sides. You then apply force to side A. In response the lens flexes or arches toward side B. Side A increases in convexity and the surface becomes more taut. Side B decreases in convexity and the

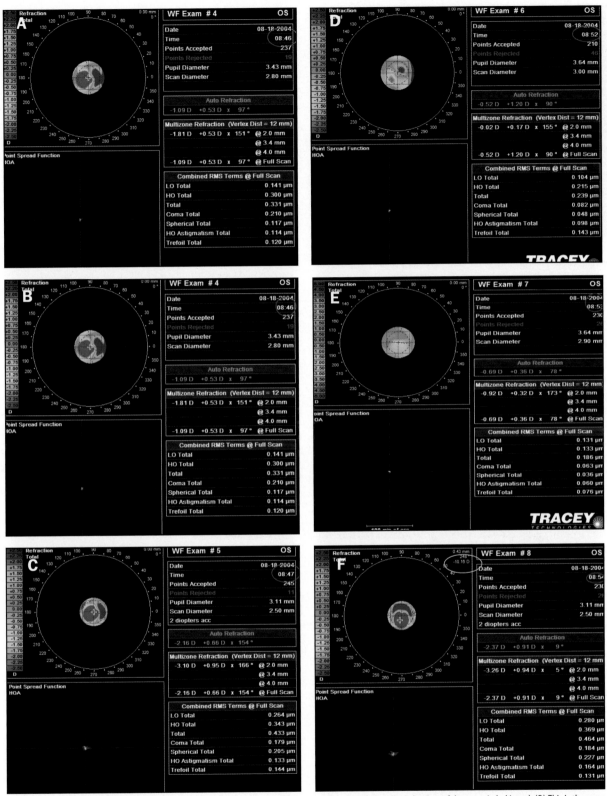

Figure 1. (A) This is the first in a series of images of the same eye. This image is while the eye is focusing at near. Note the time of the scan circled in red. (B) This is the same eye as in A. The image is taken 1 minute later. Note the similarity between the images. They are identical even though they were taken 1 minute apart. (C) This is the third image in the series. It was taken 1 minute after the last image. It is no longer identical, but it is very similar. The patient is focused on a near target. The red hot spot has a maximum focusing power of 10 D. This image was taken 7 minutes after the first image. The patient is trying to relax his accommodation, but there is still some arching of the lens. (E) This image is taken 1 minute after the previous image. The patient's lens is now fully relaxed and the image is focused for distance with a very precise dot in the middle of the point spread function image at the lower left. (F) This is the final image in the series. It is done 1 minute after the previous image. The eye is once again focused at near. It is possible to do a point by point measurement with the Tracey device. In this image I have placed the cursor within the red hot spot to measure the power at that point. The power is indicated within the yellow oval as 10.10 D.

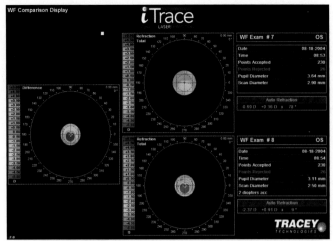

Figure 2. The upper right image is the wavefront of the eye while focused at distance. The spherical equivalent is about −0.5 D. The lower right image is the wavefront of the eye while focused at near. The spherical equivalent is about −1.90 D. Although this seems to indicate accommodation of about 1.4 D, it does not take into account the dramatic increase in focusing power within the red hot spot. The peak focusing power within the red hot spot is 10.0 D. The image to the left is an electronic subtraction image of the two images to the right.

surface becomes less taut. In fact, as the lens arches it creates a mismatch in the surface areas of the 2 sides. The 2 sides began as symmetrical convex surfaces. When you arch the lens away from side A, it stretches the lens surface smooth. When you arch the lens toward side B, it tends to subtly fold onto itself because of the excess surface area. If this were true, in addition to the accommodative arching you would expect an associated area of compensatory flattening of the lens surface with a decrease in the effective power. This is exactly what you see with a Crystalens when it arches.

Please examine Figure 2. Notice the image to the top right compared to the bottom right. The top right is the distance image. The bottom right is the near image. There is a striking red "hot spot" of increased power in the bottom right image. However, there is also evidence of compensatory flattening or a blue area around the hot spot. The compensatory flattening is most pronounced superior to the red hot spot. It is in a crescent shape that is very characteristic for this associated area of flattening around an area of increased curvature. It is also the shape you would expect from a wave created in the surface as it arches and has an excess of surface area that needs to be distributed over a limited circumference. You will

notice a similar process occurring in Figure 1A to C and F and the dynamic, variable nature of those changes.

The Crystalens works. It creates better near vision than a monofocal IOL. The exact mechanism of action is still unclear. It appears unlikely that the optic size makes much difference in the near vision based on equivalent or better near vision with the new 5-0 version of the Crystalens versus the now obsolete AT-45 with a 4.5-mm optic. The Crystalens is likely to produce its accommodative effect through several different mechanisms of action, including axial translation and accommodative arching. This makes sense because the normal prepresbyopic phakic eye also produces accommodation using several different mechanisms of action, some of which are similar to the Crystalens.

References

1. Food and Drug Administration approval letter. Available at: http://www.fda.gov/cdrh/pdf3/P030002a.pdf. Accessed May 6, 2005.
2. Cumming JS. Crystalens accommodating intraocular lens. Presented at European Society of Cataract and Refractive Surgery; September 11-14, 2004; Paris, France.
3. Colvard DM, Dell SJ, Doane J, et al. Accommodation with the Crystalens accommodating intraocular lens. White paper published by Eyeonics. 2006.
4. Findl O, Leydolt C. Meta-analysis of accommodating intraocular lenses. J Cataract Refract Surg. 2007;33(3):522-527.
5. Kriechbaum K, Findl O, Koeppl C, et al. Stimulus-driven versus pilocarpine-induced biometric changes in pseudophakic eyes. Ophthalmol. 2005;112:453-459.
6. Holladay JT. Selecting IOLs for presbyopic correction. J Cataract Refract Surg Today. March 2006. Available at: http://www.crstoday.com/PDF%20Articles/0306/CRST0306_F9_Holladay.html. Accessed October 22, 2007.
7. Waltz KL. The Crystalens changes its radius of curvature. J Cataract Refract Surg Today. June 2005. Available at: http://www.crstoday.com/PDF%20Articles/0605/CRST0605_F9_Waltz.htm. Accessed October 22, 2007.
8. Ninomiva S, Fujikado T, Kuroda T, et al. Changes in ocular aberrations with accommodation. Am J Ophthalmol. 2002;134:924-926.
9. Cheng H, Barnett JK, Vilupuru AS, et al. A population study on changes in wave aberrations with accommodation. J Vis. 2004;4:272-280.
10. Findl O, Baikoff G, Cummings S, et al. Presbyopia: is surgery able to compensate for loss of accommodation? Presented at XXII Congress of the European Society of Cataract and Refractive Surgery; September 11-14, 2004; Paris, France.
11. Vilupuru AS, Roorda A, Glasser A. Spatially variant changes in lens power during ocular accommodation in a rhesus monkey eye. J Vis. 2004;22(4):299-309.

CHAPTER 53

CRYSTALENS—
WHAT IS THE MECHANISM?

Stephen B. Wiles, MD

Understanding the mechanism of action of accommodating intraocular lenses (IOLs) will become increasingly important with the growing demand for this technology by baby boomers. Much has been learned about the mechanism of action of the Eyeonics Crystalens (Aliso Viejo, CA), the first Food and Drug Administration (FDA)-approved accommodating IOL. Studies have indicated that the primary mechanism of action of the Crystalens is its forward movement resulting from contraction of the ciliary muscle that subsequently redistributes the muscle's mass posteriorly.[1,2] This movement leads to an increase in vitreous cavity pressure. Simultaneously, there is a decrease in anterior chamber pressure. These pressure changes in turn push the optic anteriorly toward the iris (Figure 1). The redistribution of the ciliary muscle mass during contraction has been documented in studies using magnetic resonance imaging (MRI)[3] and UBM.[4]

The degree of axial movement exhibited by Crystalens has been evaluated using immersion A-scan ultrasound to measure either vitreous cavity length (VCL) or the anterior chamber depth (ACD). Dr. Steven Dell[5] reported on 10 Crystalens eyes 3 years after implantation. A-scan measurements were obtained after the patients were administered 1% Cyclogyl (Alcon, Fort Worth, TX) then repeated 3 weeks later after administration of 6% pilocarpine. The difference between the 2 measurements represents the movement of the optic with chemical stimulation of the ciliary muscle simulating accommodation. In this population, the mean anterior movement was 0.84 mm (SD 0.16, range 0.53 to 1.11 mm), corresponding to a power increase of 1.79 D. Other researchers have found similar results with lens movement of 1.44 mm and 1.1 mm, significantly more than the standard IOL lens movement of 0.12 mm (Figure 2).[6-8]

Axial movement has been shown without the aid of pharmacological agents as well. Dr. DiChiara demonstrated the forward movement recorded by the IOL Master (Carl Zeiss Meditec, Jena, Germany), which used the average of 5 ACD measurements at each of 2 distances— 15 cm and 3 mm. The mean movement of Crystalens was 1.13 mm versus the mean of a standard lens of 0.12 mm (Figure 3).[7]

Since FDA-approval of the Crystalens in 2003, the degree of axial movement necessary to achieve visual outcomes for near vision has been a topic of interest in the ophthalmic community. Since then, much has been learned. Optic flexure, or accommodative arching,[9] which was first described in 2004 by Dr. Kevin Waltz, is described as the secondary mechanism of action of the Crystalens, which explains why some patients implanted with a Crystalens see better at near than might be predicated based on IOL power and lens movement alone.[10,11] Wavefront patterns of this optic flexure or bowing of the Crystalens are similar to that of the crystalline lens.

Although the restoration of accommodation may be accomplished through anterior displacement of the Crystalens, not all studies support this theory. One report evaluated mean axial shift of the Crystalens using laser interferometric measurements under stimulation with pilocarpine and physiologic near point targets. With pilocarpine stimulation the Crystalens paradoxically demonstrated a small posterior shift, and under physiological near-point stimulation, no shift was seen.[12] The exact mechanism of action for accommodative IOLs is currently unknown and remains a strong interest for ongoing research.

The theorized axial shift mechanism of action of the Crystalens is dramatically shown in a case report of traumatic aniridia in the left eye of a 52-year-old patient following a motor vehicle accident 2 months after cataract extraction with Crystalens implantation (Figure 4).[13] One month following the procedure and before the accident, the patient's uncorrected distance visual acuity was 20/20 in the right eye and 20/25+ in the left eye. Near vision was J3 in both eyes.

The patient was unable to recall details of the accident, but he believes he hit his head on the steering wheel or dashboard. Following the accident, the patient presented with hyphema and traumatic aniridia of the left eye and left-sided skin lacerations. IOLs in both eyes remained well centered in the capsular bag. A complete inspection of the capsular bag and zonular apparatus of the left eye was possible, and no zonular dehiscence or capsular tear was present. Pigment was identified at the internal aspect of the clear corneal incision and the globe suffered no lacerations. We postulate that the

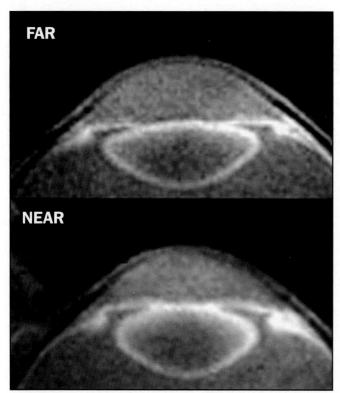

Figure 1. MRI from a young patient demonstrating bulging of the ciliary muscle into the vitreous cavity.

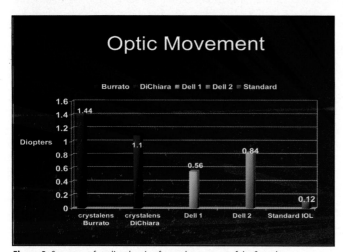

Figure 2. Summary of studies showing forward movement of the Crystalens.

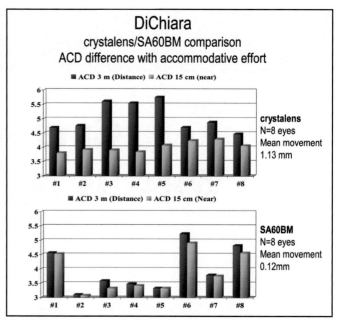

Figure 3. Results of DiChiara movement study using ACD difference.

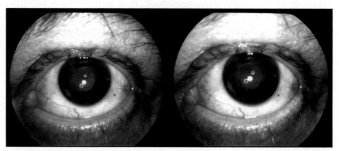

Figure 4. The theorized axial shift mechanism of action of the Crystalens is dramatically shown in a case report of traumatic aniridia in the left eye of a 52-year-old patient following a motor vehicle accident 2 months after cataract extraction with Crystalens implantation.

iris was expulsed through the clear corneal incision, which self-sealed following the injury and required no suturing. One month following the accident, the Crystalens implant remained stable and the patient's visual acuity returned to 20/20 (distance) and J5 (near). Slit lamp inspection of the implant provided an excellent opportunity to observe the Crystalens during accommodative effort. Anterior displacement of the implant was noted when the patient fixated on a near target.

References

1. Cumming JS, Colvard DM, Dell SJ, et al. Clinical evaluation of the Crystalens AT-45 accommodating intraocular lens. *J Cataract Refract Surg.* 2006;32(5):812-824.
2. Macsai MS, Padnick-Silver L, Fontes BM. Visual outcomes after accommodating lens implantation. *J Cataract Refract Surg.* 2006;32(4):628-632.
3. Strenk SA, Semmlow JL, Strenk LM, et al. Age-related changes in human ciliary muscle and lens: a magnetic resonance imaging study. *Invest Ophthalmol Vis Sci.* 1999;40:1161-1169.
4. Marchini G, Mora P, Pedrotti E, et al. Functional assessment of two different accommodative intraocular lenses compared with a monofocal intraocular lens. *Ophthalmology.* 2007;2038-2043.
5. Data on file, eyeonics.
6. Buratto. 2002.
7. DiChiara. 2003.
8. Dell. 2002.
9. Waltz K. The Crystalens changes its radius of curvature. *Cataract & Refractive Surgery Today.* 2005;66-68.
10. Charters L. Additional mechanism of action possible in accommodative lens. *Ophthalmology Times.* 2005;30(14).
11. Dell SJ. The Crystalens accommodating IOL. *Cataract & Refractive Surgery Today.* 2004;1-3.
12. Menapace R, Findl O, Kriechbaum K, et al. Accommodating intraocular lenses: a critical review of present and future concepts. *Graefes Arch Clin Exp Ophthalmol.* 2007;245(4):473-89.
13. Wiles S, Tischinski R. Traumatic aniridia. *EyeNet Magazine.* 2006:74. 2006:82.

SECTION V

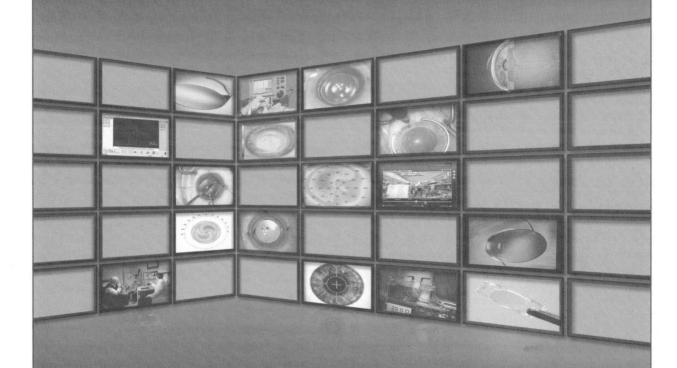

Presbyopia-Correcting
IOLs in the Future

CHAPTER 54

OVERVIEW OF ACCOMMODATING IOLs

George Beiko, BM, BCh, FRCS(C)

Although multifocal intraocular lenses (IOLs) may provide good distance and near vision, the drawback is the reduction of quality of vision.

Contrast sensitivity has been measured to be significantly reduced in patients with multifocal IOLs compared to those with monofocal IOLs; in patients with monofocal IOLs, contrast sensitivity reduction is already estimated to be 25% less than in young phakic adults and no better than age-controlled phakic patients with similar Snellen acuity.[1,2] In addition, dysphotic phenomenon such as glare, halo, and night vision problems are greater than with monofocal IOLs.[3,4]

In the 1980s, Stuart Cummings made the observation that patients with silicone plate haptic IOLs were able in some instances to read well through their distance correction. Using A-scan ultrasound, he demonstrated optic movement of 0.7 mm. This was later confirmed by Spencer Thornton.[5] This realization has generated much interest in lens displacement as a mechanism for achieving accommodation, and several lens designs have been proposed.

In addition to accommodation, pseudoaccommodation has also been proposed as an explanation for pseudophakic near visual acuity.

Arguably, the effects of accommodation and pseudoaccommodation are superimposed in functional near vision in phakic and pseudophakic individuals; their separation is academic and serves only to aid in the understanding of the design of IOLs.

Definitions

Accommodation is defined as the process by which the eye is able to clearly image objects at different distances onto the retina; this is accomplished by a change in the eye's refractive power.

Accommodation as a process, involves the contraction of the ciliary body, which moves the apex of the ciliary body forward and inward. According to the Helmholtz theory of accommodation,[6] this process produces the release of the resting tension of the zonular fibers, resulting in an increased lens curvature both anteriorly and posteriorly (thus, increasing the refractive power of the lens); increased lens thickness (this has been measured to be 0.30 mm and equals 6 D of accommodative effect)[7]; and anterior displacement of the lens. Alternatively, according to Tscherning, the contraction of the ciliary muscle increases tension on the zonule, which alters the shape of the lens without changing the thickness.[8] More recently, Schachar et al have resurrected this latter theory.[9] Another theory of accommodation has been proposed as Coleman's hydraulic theory, which states that the ciliary body contraction may result in changes in vitreous pressure causing the lens to be displaced forward.[10]

The change in shape of the lens is also accompanied by an increase in spherical aberration of the eye as measured by wavefront aberrometry.[11]

Accommodation could theoretically also occur if there was a change in the refractive index of the structures involved in imaging.

The dynamic process of a change in the lens curvature and/or movement of the natural lens result in a shifting focus and allow the eye to image the object of regard, at any distance, onto the central retina.

In a 20 year old, the amount of accommodative power has been measured at 6 to 8 D. For near vision, 3 D would be required and 6 to 8 D allows for sustained near vision without fatigue.[12]

Accommodation, convergence, and miosis are all components of the synkinetic near reflex. With age, accommodation decreases, miosis increases, and convergence remains relatively unchanged. Factors that impact on one of these components may also influence the others. For example, blocking convergence by occluding one eye will result in decreased miosis and accommodation.[13] This must be borne in mind when evaluating measurements of accommodation in clinical studies.

Accommodation decreases with age due to mechanical (including progressive enlargement and hardening of the natural lens) and elastic property changes in the lens and its capsule, weakening and atrophy of the ciliary muscle, and loss of zonular elasticity.[14,15]

Figure 1. An example of recognition, from research done at Cambridge University.

fi yuo cna raed tihs, yuo hvae a sgtrane mnid, too. Cna yuo raed tihs? Olny 55 plepoe tuo fo 100 anc.

i cdnuolt blveiee taht I cluod aulaclty uesdnatnrd waht I was rdanieg. The phaonmneal pweor of the hmuan mnid, aoccdrnig to a rscheearch at Cmabrigde Uinervtisy, it dseno't mtaetr in waht oerdr the ltteres in a wrod are, the olny iproamtnt tihng is taht the frsit and lsat ltteer be in the rghit pclae. The rset can be a taotl mses and you can sitll raed it whotuit a pboerlm. Tihs is bcuseae the huamn mnid deos not raed ervey lteter by istlef, but the wrod as a wlohe.

Figure 2. Depth of field and depth of focus.

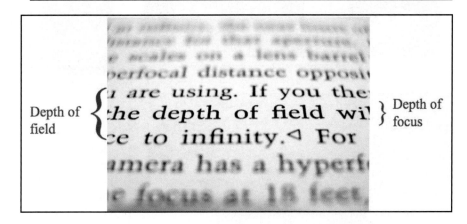

Although all these factors are important in causing loss of accommodation, ciliary body function has been found to decrease less with age than previously thought, and studies suggest that ciliary body contractility is retained throughout life.[16-19] It should be no surprise that ciliary body action remains intact with age as the accommodative process is part of the synkinetic near reflex that is active throughout life; the ciliary muscle receives parasympathetic stimulation, as does the iris sphincter, when the eyes converge to look at near objects.

The implications of this finding are that ciliary body contraction may be able to effect pseudophakic lens changes, which should restore accommodation; the challenge is to design a lens that is able to do this.

Laser scanning studies have supported the conclusion that crystalline lens ageing is the main determinate of loss of accommodation in presbyopia.[20] Lens hardness is most likely to be most responsible for loss of accommodation. There is a 1000-fold increase in lens hardness over a lifetime.[21]

Pseudoaccommodation is the ability of patients to attain functional perception of objects at different distances without focusing. Factors that aid in pseudoaccommodation include residual myopia, the pinhole effect of miotic pupils (2 D of pseudoaccommodation with a pupil 2.5 mm), mild with the rule astigmatism (according to Dr. Chris Huber, a refraction of −1.00 +1.00 × 90 gives 20/30 at both distance and near by straddling the conoid of Sturm), corneal asphericity, which produces corneal multifocality, corneal coma, neural processing, visual potential (any concurrent ocular pathology can impair this), recognition of word/visual patterns (Figure 1), and patient motivation. Whether or not patients are encouraged to guess or to try harder can have significant effect on the results.

Depth of field (Figure 2) is the distance in front of and beyond the object of regard that appears to be clear, while depth of focus is the distance in front of and beyond the object of regard that appears to be in focus. The depth of field is necessarily larger than the depth of focus.

Pseudoaccommodation can provide 1.5 to 2.0 D of accommodative power in most eyes.[22,23] Pseudoaccommodation is not dependent on the presence of an IOL, as it occurs in phakic, pseudophakic, and aphakic individuals.[24-28]

True pseudophakic accommodation must, by definition, be able to demonstrate pseudophakic movement and/or change in optical power of the IOL with accommodative effort.

The physiological decrease in amplitude and speed of accommodation with age, accompanied by compromised near vision, is what defines presbyopia. At age 10, the amplitude of accommodation is about 14 D and decreases to zero by age 52.[29-32]

Measures of Accommodation

The greatest challenge in evaluating and comparing the accommodation of various IOLs is the current lack of standardized psychophysical and objective techniques. Various subjective techniques have been employed to study accommodation, and the limitation of subjective measures should be considered when these data are reviewed.

Subjective

Accommodative amplitude is the change in lens power as measured in D. A number of methods may be used to measure

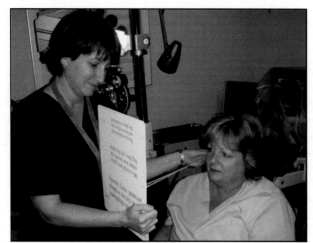

Figure 3. Near point of accommodation or Donder's push-up method.

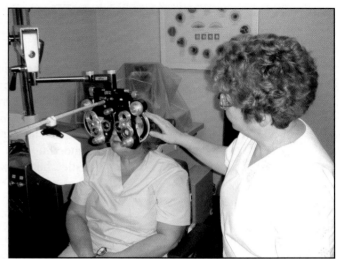

Figure 5. Method of spheres.

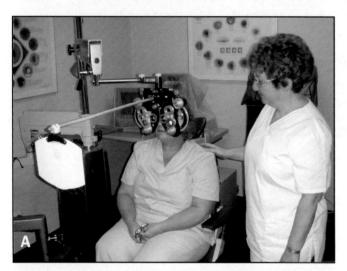

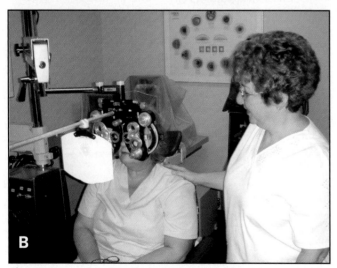

Figure 4. Accommodation/Prince's rule, recording near and far points.

this, including "near point of accommodation" or "Donder's push-up method" (Figure 3); "accommodative rule" or "Prince's rule" (Figure 4); and "method of spheres" (Figure 5).

In both the near point of accommodation and Donder's push-up method, the near point of clear vision is recorded. However, this is not the near point of accommodation, but rather describes the near depth of field and defines the near point of acuity. It is dependent on accommodation as well as the pupil size, the optical aberrations and multifocality of the eye, and neural processing; thus, it is a culmination of the contributions of accommodation and pseudoaccommodation.

Near reading cards, for the reasons already revealed with near point of accommodation, do not distinguish between accommodation and pseudoaccommodation. Most near reading cards are not scaled to the Snellen system, resulting in overestimation of the near visual acuity by the Jaeger system. An example is that the J1 on the Rosenbaum card corresponds to 20/33 on the Birkhauser chart.[33]

Reading speed is determined by using an EDTRS chart or newspaper print size of log RAD 0.4, at 40 cm, and timing the number of words per minute. This is a good measure of a patients level of functioning but it does not distinguish accommodation from pseudoaccommodation.

Accommodation or Prince's rule involves using a scaled accommodative ruler. Normally, a +3.00-D sphere is also used. The reading chart is moved slowly toward and away from the patient to locate the near and far points of clear vision. The same limitations as with near point of accommodation apply.

Method of spheres uses minus and plus spheres to blur the reading chart. The point of blur is recorded as the greatest value of sphere employed. The difference from largest plus and largest minus is the accommodative amplitude. However, this method can underestimate the amount of accommodation as there is a lack of proximal stimuli to accommodation, as the patient's interpretation of the blur is not standardized, and as there is the confounding factor of image minification and magnification. Despite these limitations, this is the tool which has been used by the Food and Drug Administration (FDA) for approval of some IOLs.

Defocus curves (Figure 6) are derived by plotting the information gained from an accommodative rule or method of sphere measurement. The level of visual acuity for a given distance or spherical dioptric equivalent is plotted.

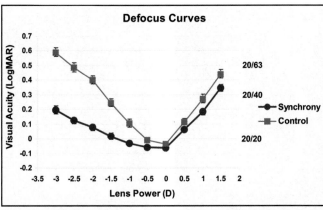

Defocus Curves chart showing Visual Acuity (LogMAR) versus Lens Power (D), with Synchrony and Control curves.

Figure 6. Example of a Defocus curve. (Courtesy of L. Vargas, MD.)

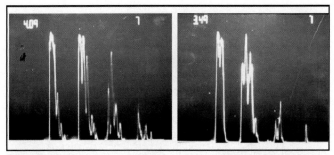

Figure 7. An example of ultrasound biomicroscopy demonstrating anterior displacement of a 3-piece IOL with accommodation. (Reprinted with permission of S. Thornton.)

Figure 8. High-definition ultrasound biomicroscopy of Synchrony (Visiogen, Inc, Irvine, CA) dual optic IOL demonstrating increased lens separation with accommodation (Courtesy of Ivan Ossma.).

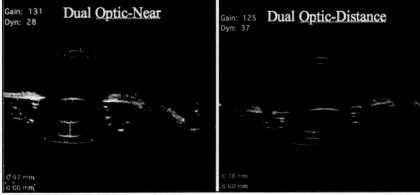

Dynamic retinoscopy involves the use of a retinoscope to measure the refractive power of the eye for distance and near vision. It is able to measure the degree and speed of accommodation, and detect any irregular light reflexes from the cornea or lens. Unfortunately, this test relies on the subjective interpretation of the clinician and can be inconsistent.[35]

Subjective measures of accommodation in single piece conventional IOLs have been reported to be an average of 0.42 to 1.08 D.[36,37]

Objective

Instruments that measure lens displacement include continuous ultrasound biometry, ultrasound biomicroscopy (Figures 7 and 8), partial coherence interferometry (Figure 9), optical coherence tomography, Scheimpflug slit-lamp imaging (Figure 10), and high-resolution magnetic resonance imaging (MRI) (Figure 11). The accuracy of these displacement measurements is limited by their precision and resolution; for ultrasound techniques, this is 150 to 200 μm, whereas for dual beam partial coherence interferometry it is 4 to 10 μm.[28] An axial movement of 600 to 720 μm is required to effect 1 D change in refraction at the spectacle plane.[38-40]

Displacement measurements may employ pilocarpine and cyclopentolate instillation. Cyclopentolate 1% relaxes the ciliary muscle and is used to get baseline measurements. Pilocarpine 2% mimics the lens thickness changes of young phakic eyes during near point fixation; thus, it is meant to simulate accommodation. Some authors think that pilocar-

pine-induced displacement may be greater than physiologically possible.

High-resolution MRI has also been used to objectively image accommodation in human and animal subjects. It has demonstrated ciliary muscle contraction with decrease in zonular tension and lens equator diameter, and an increase in lens thickness and curvature; thus, supporting some of Helmholtz's theory (personal communication with SA Strenk and LM Strenk).

Lens displacement measurements may have some limitations. Measurements performed with the patient looking straight ahead may be decreased compared to head tilt down, which has the potential for gravity aiding in the movement of the lens-capsule complex. Measurements requiring the supine position may underestimate movement as gravity will act against any displacement anteriorly.

Measurement performed with the patient looking straight ahead may be decreased compared to head tilt down, which has the potential for gravity aiding in the movement of the lens-capsule complex. Measurements requiring the supine position may underestimate movement as gravity will act against any displacement anteriorly.

Displacement measurements may employ pilocarpine and cyclopentolate instillation. Pilocarpine 2% mimics the lens thickness changes of young phakic eyes during near point fixation; thus, it is meant to simulate accommodation. Some authors think that pilocarpine-induced displacement may be greater than physiologically possible. Given this limitation, the value of pilocarpine is that it may give the maximum potential for displacement of an IOL. Cyclopentolate 1% relaxes the

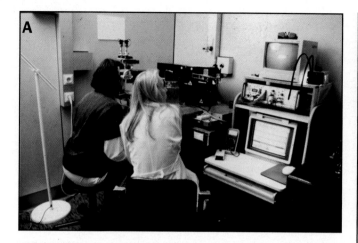

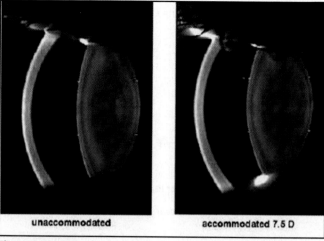

Figure 10. Scheimpflug Photography of a 29 yo human lens, demonstrating 0.35 mm of lens thickness change with accommodation. (Courtesy of Michiel Dubbelman, VUMC Univ Amsterdam.)

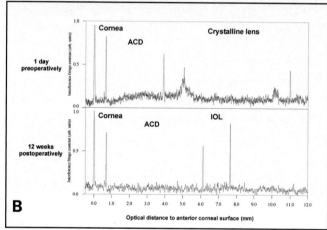

Figure 9. Partial coherence interferometry, which has a precision of greater than 10 fold of ultrasound (Courtesy of O. Findl.).

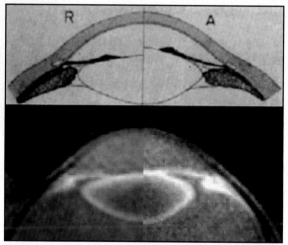

Figure 11. High resolution MRI of lens before and after accommodation, showing lenticular changes, compared to original drawing from Helmholtz.

ciliary muscle and is used to get baseline IOL measurements.[28]

Using pharmacological stimulation, standard monofocal IOLs have been reported to move forward 0.25 to 0.42 mm.[41,42]

Another significant observation is that there is a change in the position of the IOL during the first few months following implantation due to capsular shrinkage and fibrosis. With the 1 CU, this has been reported to be as much as 0.300 mm in the first 3 months; this is most pronounced in the first week. Comparatively, a standard IOL moves anteriorly about 0.100 mm, with the most significant amount occurring in the first week postoperatively.[43,44] Thus, any measurements of effect should not be considered until after this time when things have presumably stabilized.

Infrared optometers and wavefront aberrometers (Figure 12) are also able to objectively measure accommodation by measuring the refractive power of the eye.

Infrared optometers, autorefractors, and video refractometers use the Scheiner principle to measure the refractive power of the eye. Instruments that use photoretinoscopy can rapidly measure distance refraction as well as binocularity. These latter optometers calculate an average refraction for the entire pupil. Alignment is important and small amounts of optical irregularity may cause unreliable readings. These instruments

may underestimate the degree to which accommodation increases the amount of optical aberrations.[45]

Using photorefraction, the accommodative amplitude of single piece conventional IOLs has been found to be 0.35 ±0.26 D.[36]

Autorefractors have been validated for phakic accommodation studies but not for pseudophakic measurements.[45,46] Autorefractor and video refractometer measurements may be impacted upon and confounded by Purkinje images III and IV, which arise from the higher refractive index of the IOLs compared to natural lenses; by the spherical nature of the IOL compared to the aspheric crystalline lens; and by posterior capsular opacification, which can produce optical aberrations.[47]

Most wavefront aberrometers use the Hartmann-Shack principle to measure the shape of the wavefront of light exiting the eye as it reflects from a point source on the retina. These instruments are able to measure the exact amount of accommodation by determining the refractive power of the eye both before and during accommodation. Thus, objective and quantitative measurements can be obtained. The use of

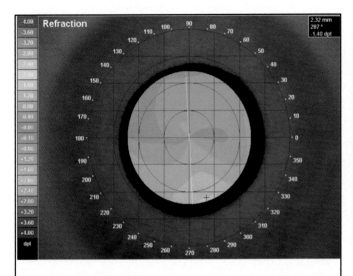

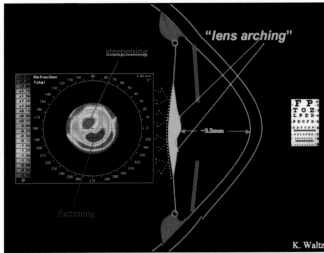

Figure 13. The concept of lens arching as proposed by K. Waltz.

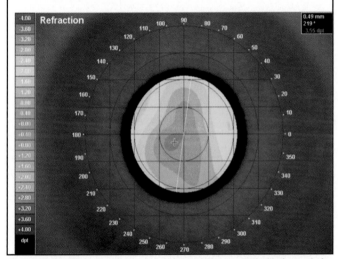

Figure 12. Wavefront aberrometry of a 19 year old phakic individual before and after accommodation; a great deal of power variation over the pupil area is seen and a dramatic increase in HOA is associated with accommodation. (Personal communication with K. Waltz.)

phenylephrine, which dilates the pupils, allows for accurate measurements without affecting accommodation.[48]

At distance, wavefront aberrometry measurements have minimal higher-order aberrations (HOAs). At near, the accommodative demand is equal to the power spread over the pupil; the measured pattern shows increased HOAs, which may be family specific. There is also significant asymmetry between distance and near wavefronts suggesting asymmetry in contraction within the ciliary body and zonules (personal communication with K. Waltz).

Wavefront aberrometry has revealed that IOLs respond to accommodation by flexing with a nonsymmetrical response resulting in a characteristic wavefront pattern and an increase in HOAs with accommodation. An area of steepening and a compensatory area of flattening are typically seen. This concept has been termed *lens arching* (Figure 13) by Kevin Waltz (personal communication) and has been used to explain how IOLs may affect accommodation.

Animal Models

Animal modeling of accommodation is difficult. Cats and raccoons accommodate by axial translation of the lens; rabbits and dogs do not accommodate; and birds accommodate by squeezing the lens and effecting a lens curvature change. Monkeys are the only animals with an accommodative system similar to humans; however, monkey eyes are relatively small compared to human eyes so the IOL must be scaled down for trial implantation.[49]

Accommodative Effect in Non-Accommodative IOLs

When considering the following studies and chapters remember that, as previously mentioned, nonaccommodative IOLs provide some pseudoaccommodative effect. Accommodative IOLs must surpass this standard in order to be able to claim a true accommodative effect.

In the 3M diffractive IOL study, 40% of the uncorrected monofocal eyes achieved J4 or better, and in the multicenter Array study, 43% of monofocal eyes achieved J3 or better with best distance correction.[50,51] Thus, proposed accommodative IOLs, when corrected for distance, should be able to provide better than J3/J4 near vision in order to substantiate their efficacy.

References

1. Nio YK, Jansonius NM, Geraghty E, Norrby S, and Kooijman AC. Effect of intraocular lens implantation on visual acuity, contrast sensitivity, and depth of focus. *J Cataract Refract Surg.* 2003;29(11):2073-2081.
2. Steinert RF, Aker BL, Trentacost DJ et al. A prospective comparative study of the AMO Array zonal-progressive multifocal silicone intraocular lens and a monofocal intraocular lens. *Ophthalmology.* 1999;106:1243-1245.

3. Schmitz S, Dick HB, Krummenauer F, Schwenn O, Krist R. Contrast sensitivity and glare disability by halogen light after monofocal and multifocal lens implantation. *Br J Ophthalmol.* 2000;84:1109-1112.

4. Pieh S, Lackner B, Hanselmayer G, et al. Halo size under distance and near conditions in refractive multifocal intraocular lenses. *Br J Ophthamol.* 2001; 85:816-821.

5. Doane JF. Accommodating intraocular lenses. *Curr Opin Ophthalmol.* 2004;15(1):16-21. Review.

6. Helmholtz H. Ueber die Accommodation des Auges. *Allbrecht von Graefes Arch Ophthalmol.* 1855;1(2):1-74.

7. Baikoff G, Lutun E, Ferraz C, Wei J. Static and dynamic analysis of the anterior segment with optical coherence interferometry. *J Cataract Refract Surg.* 2004;30:1843-1850.

8. Tscherning, M. The theory of accommodation. *Ophthalmic Rev.* 1899;18:91-99.

9. Schachar RA, Cudmore DP, Black TD. Experimental support for Schchar's hypothesis of accommodation. *An Ophthalmol.* 1993;25;404-409.

10. Coleman DJ. On the hydraulic suspension theory of accommodation. *Trans Arch Ophthalmol Soc.* 1986;84:846-868.

11. Dick HB. Accommodative intraocular lenses: current status. *Curr Opin Ophthalmol.* 2005;16(1):8-26. Review.

12. Duane A. Normal values of the accommodation at all ages. *JAMA.* 1912;59: 1010-1013.

13. Parsa, CF. Accommodative spasm (spasm of the near reflex) in Fraunfelders FT, Roy FH eds. *Current Ocular Therapy*, 5th ed. Philadelphia: WB Saunders; 2000:507-508.

14. Croft MA, Glasser A, Kaufman PL. Accommodation and presbyopia. *Int. Ophthalmol Clin.* 2001;41:33-46.

15. Crawford K, Terasawa E, Kaufman PL. Reproducible stimulation of ciliary muscle contraction in the cynomolgus monkey via a permanent indwelling midbrain electrode. *Brain Res.* 1989;503:265-272.

16. Lutjen-Decroll E, Tamm E, Kaufman PL. Age changes in rhesus monkey ciliary muscle light and electron microscopy. *Exp Eye Res.* 1988;47:885-899.

17. Strenk SA, Semmlow JL, Strenk LM et al. Age-related changes in human ciliary muscle and lens: a magnetic resonance imaging study. *Invest Ophthalmol Vis Sci.* 1999;40:1162-1169.

18. Swegmark G. Studies with impedence cyclography on human accommodation at different ages. *Acta Ophthalmol.* 1969;47:1186-1206.

19. Bacskulin A, Gast R, Bergmann U, Guthoff R. Ultrasound biomicroscopy imaging of accommodative configuration changes in the presbyopic ciliary body. *Ophthalmologe.* 1996;93:199-203.

20. Glasser A, Campbell MCW. Biometric, optical and physical changes in the isolated human crystalline lens with age in relation to presbyopia. *Vis Res.* 1999; 39:1991-2015.

21. Weeber HA, Eckert G, Soergel F, et al. Dynamic mechanical properties of human lenses. *Exp Eye Res.* 2005;80:425-434.

22. Would JE, Hu A, Chen S, Glasser A. Subjective and objective measurement of human accommodative amplitude. *J Cataract Refract Surg.* 2003;29:1878-1888.

23. Ostrin LA, Glasser A. Accommodation measurements in a pre-presbyopic and presbyopic population. *J Cataract Refract Surg.* 2004;30:1435-1444.

24. Verzella F, Calossi A. Multifocal effect of against-the-rule myopic astigmatism in pseudophakic eyes. *Refract Coreal Surg.* 1993;9:58-61.

25. Nakazawa M, Ohtsuki K. Apparent accommodation in pseudophakic eyes after implantation of posterior chamber intraocular lenses. *Am J Ophthalmol.* 1983;96:435-438.

26. Oshika T, Mimura T, Tanaka, S, et al. Apparent accommodation and corneal wavefront aberration in pseudophakic eyes. *Invest Ophthalmolo Vis Sci.* 2002; 43:2882-2886.

27. Elder MJ, Murphy C, Sanderson GF. Apparent accommodation and depth of field in pseudophakia. *J Cataract Refract Surg.* 1996;22:615-619.

28. Findl O, Kiss B, Petternel V, Menapace R, Georgopoulos M, Rainer G, Drexler W. Intraocular lens movement caused by ciliary muscle contraction. *J Cataract Refract Surg.* 2003;29(4):669-676.

29. Heron G, Schor C. The fluctuations of accommodation and age. *Ophthalmolo Physiol Opt.* 1995;5:445-449.

30. Heron G, Charman WN, Gary LS. Accommodation responses in aging. *Ophthalmol Vis Sci.* 1999;40:2872-2883.

31. Koretz JF, Kaufman PL, Neider MW, et al. Accommodation and presbyopia in the human eye. II. Aging of the anterior segment. *Vision Res.* 1989;29: 1685-1692.

32. Koretz JF, Kaufman PL, Neider MW, et al. Accommodation and presbyopia in the human eye. I. Evaluation of in-vivo techniques. *App Opt.* 1989;28: 1097–1102.

33. Kuchle M, Nguyen NX, Langenbucher A, Gusek-Schneider GC, Seitz B, Hanna KD. Implantation of a new accommodative posterior chamber intraocular lens. *J Refract Surg.* 2002;18:208-216.

34. Ossma, IL, et al. Synchrony dual-optic accommodating intraocular lens Part 2: pilot clinical evaluation. *J Cataract Refract Surg.* 2007;33:47-52.

35. Whitefoot H, Charman WN. Dynamic retinoscopy and accommodation. *Ophthalmic Physiol Opt.* 1972;12:8-17.

36. Langenbucher A, Huber S, Nguyen NX, Seitz B, Gusek-Schneider GC, Kuchle M. Measurement of accommodation after implantation of an accommodating posterior chamber intraocular lens. *J Cataract Refract Surg.* 2003;29:677-685.

37. Hazel CA, Cos MJ, Strang NC. Wavefront aberrations and its relationship to the accommodation stimulus-response function in myopic subjects. *Optom Vis Sci.* 2003;80:151-158.

38. Olsen T, Gimbel H. Phacoemulsification, capsulorhexis, and intraocular lens power prediction accuracy. *J Cataract Refract Surg.* 1993;19:695-699.

39. Haigis W, Trier HG. Linsenberechnungsformeln. In: Buschmann W, Trier HD, eds., Ophthalmologische Ultraschalldiagnostik. Berlin: Springer-Verlag; 1989:75-80.

40. Holladay JT. Refractive power calculations for intraocular lenses in the phakic eye. *Am J Ophthalmol.* 1993;116:65-66.

41. Hardman Lea SJ, Rubinstein MP, Snead MP et al. Pseudophakic accommodation? A study of the stability of capsular bag supported, one piece, rigis tripos, or soft flexible implants. *Br J Ophthalmol.* 1999;74:22-25.

42. Lesiewska-Junk H, Kaluzny J. Intraocular lens movement and accommodation in eyes of young patients. *J Cataract Surg.* 2000;26:562-565.

43. Findl O, Kriechbaum K, Menapace R, Koeppl C, Sacu S, Wirtitsch M, Buehl W, Drexler W. Laser interferometric assessment of pilocarpine-induced movement of an accommodating intraocular lens: a randomized trial. *Ophthalmology.* 2004;111(8):1515-1521.

44. Koeppl C, Findl O, Kriechbaum K, et al. Changes in IOL position and capsular bag size with an angulated intraocular lens early after cataract surgery. *J Cataract Refract Surg.* 2005;31(2):348-353.

45. Wolffsohn JS, Gilmartin B, Mallen EA, Tsujimura S. Continuous recording of accommodation and pupil size using the Shin-Nippon SRW-5000 autorefractor. *Ophthalmic Physiolo Opt.* 2001;21:108-113.

46. Nakatsuka C, Hasebe S, Nonaka F, Ohtsuki H. Accommodative lag under habitual seeing conditions: comparison between adult myopes and emmetropes. *Jpn J Ophthalmol.* 2004;47:291-298.

47. Langenbucher A, Seitz B, Huber S, Nguyen NX, Kuchle M. Theoretical and measured pseudophakic accommodation after implantation of a new accommodative posterior chamber intraocular lens. *Arch Ophthalmol.* 2003;121(12):1722-1727.

48. Ostrin LA, Glasser A. The effects of phenylephrine on pupil diameter and accommodation in rhesus monkeys. *Invest Ophthalmol Vis Sci.* 2004;45:215-221.

49. Nawa Y, Ueda, T, Nakatsuka, M, et al. Accommodation obtained per 1.00 mm forward displacement of a posterior chamber intraocular lens. *J Cataract Refract Surg.* 2003;29:2069-2072.

50. Steinert RE et al. A prospective comparative study of the AMO ARRAY zonal-progressive multifocal silicone intraocular lens and a monofocal intraocular lens. *Ophthalmology*. 1999;106(7):1243-1255.

51. Rossetti L, et al. Performance of diffractive multifocal intraocular lenses in extracapsular cataract surgery. *J Cataract Refract Surg*. 1994;20:124-128.

CHAPTER 55

OVERVIEW OF ACCOMMODATING IOLs

John A. Vukich, MD

Common to all accommodating intraocular lenses (IOLs) is the concept that mechanical forces generated in the eye can result in movement of the IOL. Single-optic IOLs use hinged haptics that allow translation of the effective lens position in the Z axis. Dual optic IOLs are variably separated under compression within the capsular bag and move apart with accommodative effort. Each of these strategies should in theory yield a net gain in near power, and this is what we see clinically. In practice, however, predictability of the accommodative effect remains a challenge with the current generation of accommodating IOLs. As a principal investigator in the US Food and Drug Administration (FDA) Phase III clinical trials for the single-piece Kellan Tetraflex IOL (Lenstec, Inc, St. Petersburg, FL), the dual optic Visiogen Synchrony (Irvine, CA) along with use of the Crystalens (Eyeonics, Inc, Aliso Viejo, CA), my clinical impressions of accommodating IOL technology are based on data as well as personal experience.

There is little doubt that an IOL that reliably delivers 6 D of peak and 3 D of sustained accommodation will forever alter the paradigm of how we do cataract surgery. The upside potential of having such a lens for pure refractive use in the presbyopic age range is self-evident. Given the vast potential demand for such a device, it is not surprising that multiple lens designs seeking to deliver smooth translation of variable power are under development.

The Crystalens and Tetraflex IOLs have a single-optic design differing primarily in that the Crystalens vaults posteriorly and the Tetraflex is designed to vault anteriorly in the unaccommodated state. Both lenses have haptics that are designed to facilitate movement of the optic, thereby changing the effective lens position in response to intraocular dynamics associated with near stimulus.

One of the surprising aspects of modern ophthalmology is that we are still learning about something as fundamental as the dynamics of near vision focus. The fact that there are unsettled debates over the "theoretical" mechanism of accommodation underscores the challenge of designing IOLs meant to address

this seemingly simple and basic task. Advances in ocular imaging, in particular ultrasonic biomicroscopy (UBM), have allowed us to visualize in real time the mechanics associated with accommodation. In fact what has been observed by many researchers is the relative difficulty in objectively quantifying positional changes of either an IOL or the natural lens within the eye. Even skilled ultrasonographers are often unable to demonstrate lens movement in any given patient, even when selecting for those eyes that have the greatest subjective effect. This has been the case in my experience with all 3 versions of accommodating IOLs that I have used. This is not to say that the IOLs do not move as predicted but rather to point out the challenge of correlating the mechanism of action with physical evidence to support the theory of why accommodating IOLs work.

The central question about the current generation of accommodating IOLs is do they deliver functional near vision and do they provide benefit to the patient. In my experience, the answer is a qualified yes. The majority of patients achieve excellent uncorrected distance acuity, and intermediate vision is typically quite good. For many patients, however, uncorrected near vision with these IOLs is often described as labored. Most patients readily accept a +1.50 D reading correction. Although this is a lower power than would otherwise be expected, these IOLs commonly fall short of total spectacle independence. In my experience this has been the case for both the single and dual-optic accommodative IOLs. The range of focus can be supplemented by adopting a modified monovision strategy. By targeting plano to −0.5 D in one eye and −1.50 D in the other, accommodative IOLs provide a full range of useful vision. In my experience this has been a very effective way to use the Crystalens and it will likely continue to be advantageous to use monovision to supplement the current generation of accommodative IOLs that are being developed. The fact is that accommodating IOLs do work, although not as perfectly or as completely as we would like. They do work well enough for us to offer this to our patients and to reliably describe this option as an advantage over monofocal IOLs.

One of the advantages of accommodating IOLs is that even if the dynamic range of focus falls short of expected, they at a minimum provide similar quality of vision as a monofocal lens. In this regard there is little difference between the single- and dual-optic variety of implant. Above all, these lenses seem to do no harm. Unlike multifocal IOLs of either the diffractive or refractive style, accommodative IOL patients rarely complain about visual quality. These patients are also less affected by minor residual astigmatism than those with multifocal implants.

The single optic accommodative IOLs are designed to be injected through a sub-3-mm incision. Both the Tetraflex and Crystalens use a familiar injector system and the learning curve for either lens is brief. The cataract removal technique for the 2 lenses differs primarily in the size of the capsulotomy. The Tetraflex is designed to use a 5.5-mm capsulotomy whereas the Crystalens works with a 6- to 7.5-mm opening. Both lenses are similar in concept regarding movement of the optic in the Z axis but differ in the angulation of the primary vault. The Tetraflex IOL angulates anteriorly, which is unique from most other IOLs. One of the relative advantages of the Tetraflex over the Crystalens and Synchrony is that there is a high degree of consistency in the neutral resting position of the optic from person to person. In my experience the Tetraflex has had the most accurate IOL power calculations for uncorrected distance acuity of the 3 lens styles.

The dual-optic Visiogen Synchrony is an innovative IOL design that depends on dynamic separation of 2 optics to create a variable accommodative effect. The fact that a reliable injector system has been designed for this lens is remarkable given the complexity of the dual-optic configuration. The injector system is preloaded and requires only balanced saline solution to fill the cartridge. The use of the dual-optic IOL requires a few adjustments in surgical technique compared to a standard IOL procedure. An incision size of 3.6 mm is necessary to handle the bulk of the 2 optics being injected simultaneously. Another unique aspect of the Synchrony is that a precise capsulotomy is a critical component of the surgery. The anterior capsulotomy must be well centered, between 5.0 and 5.5 mm, and free of any notches or irregularities. Recognizing the orientation of the emerging implant as it is gradually injected into the capsular bag is part of the learning curve. In this regard, the dual-optic IOL takes some additional effort to learn to use.

Having used 3 significantly different styles of accommodative IOLs, I am convinced that the strategy of variable focus will be the trend for future development of premium IOLs. The options we have currently provide benefit and are an important first step. There is no doubt that we will continue to see innovation and design improvements.

CHAPTER 56

VISIOGEN SYNCHRONY— CLINICAL PEARLS

Ivan L. Ossma, MD, MPH and Andrea Galvis, MD

The surgical reversal of presbyopia has long been an elusive target for ophthalmologists. Monovision utilizing monofocal intraocular lenses (IOLs), a common practice among the phakic contact lens population, has shown high rates of spectacle independence.[1] Multifocal IOLs allow excellent near vision and provide varying degrees of spectacle independence,[2,3] but the simultaneous foci produced by multifocal IOLs require optical tradeoffs such as decreased contrast sensitivity and unwanted photic phenomena.[4,5]

Truly accommodating devices would overcome many optical compromises associated with multifocal IOLs and allow enhanced functional transition through the intermediate range of visual tasks. In seeking this purpose, numerous devices have recently been developed to achieve active ciliary–muscle-derived pseudophakic accommodation mediated by anterior displacement of the optic leading to myopic shift and improved near vision. These devices have been called accommodating intraocular lenses (AIOLs)

The Synchrony Design

The accommodative efficacy of a single-optic AIOL based on optic shift principles depends on the optical power of the displaced lens.[6]

To overcome the inefficiency of single optic AIOLs, Visiogen Inc (Irvine, CA) has designed a single-piece, dual optic, foldable silicone IOL (Synchrony) that has a highly powered moving anterior optic coupled to a minus-power static posterior optic joined via a spring haptic (Figure 1). Once in the capsular bag, physiologic bag tension compresses the optics, thus reducing their separation. Compressing the lens system stores strain energy in the connecting haptics. Upon accommodative effort, zonular relaxation releases tension in the bag, thus allowing release of the stored energy in the spring system with anterior displacement of the anterior optic.

It is obvious that the biggest hurdle to overcome with this lens design is capsular fibrosis. Visiogen has implemented numerous features in the Synchrony AIOL design to warrant long-term stability and function of the device.

The anterior optic is coupled to a system of flow channels (Figure 2) designed to tent the anterior capsule and avoiding lens-capsule seal while allowing adequate flow in and out of the capsular bag. The leaflets in these flow channels help minimize contact between the anterior capsule and the lens optic thus reducing the potential for anterior capsule opacification.

Biocompatibility studies performed in rabbits with the Synchrony AIOL have shown minimal bag fibrosis and absence of capsular contraction.[7]

Implantation of the Synchrony AIOL is done via the use of a preloaded injector (Figure 3), eliminating the need for IOL manipulation upon implantation as well as avoiding the potential for contamination of the IOL system. The injector system allows implantation through a 3.7-mm incision, and the inner coating of the nozzle has been optimized for slow, controlled release of the whole lens system into the capsular bag.

Choosing the Perfect Candidate

Synchrony AIOL success relies on the patient's ability to use the ciliary muscle-bag complex interaction to generate an accommodative effort that translates into lens movement and thus provides the full range of visual function. Disease states in which there is an involvement of the zonular apparatus, such as pseudoexfoliation, trauma, Marfan syndrome, and homocystinuria, among others, contraindicate the use of the Synchrony AIOL. As we have discovered with other premium IOL technologies, outcomes are far better in patients who are motivated and willing to undergo all postoperative recommendations for success. Bilateral implantation has been shown to provide the best results overall with this technology.

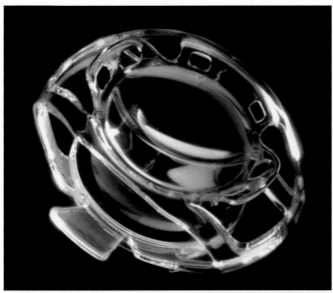

Figure 1. Synchrony Dual Optic Accommodating Intraocular Lens (AIOL).

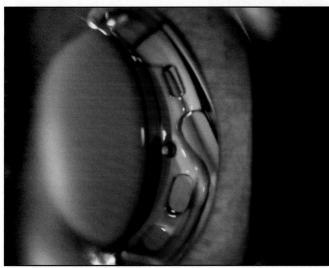

Figure 2. Anterior flow channel system.

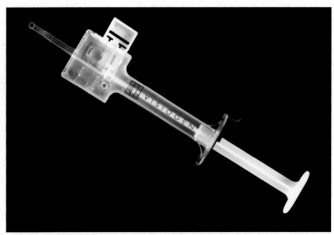

Figure 3. Synchrony AIOL preloaded injector system.

Perfect Surgery/Perfect Outcome

Implantation of the Synchrony AIOL requires all of the following steps in order to achieve success:

* Perfectly centered 4.5 to 5.25 mm continuous capsulorrhexis.
* Fully working zonular apparatus (refrain from implantation in the setting of evident zonular dehiscence).
* Thorough cortical cleanup as well as anterior capsule polishing.
* Intact posterior capsule.
* Complete lens delivery into the capsular bag.
* Complete removal of all remaining viscoelastic between the 2 lens optics.

The 3.7-mm incision required to implant the Synchrony AIOL can be left unsutured, or a single 10-0 nylon suture can be placed depending on the surgeon's preference.

The postoperative pharmacologic regimen includes antibiotic drops as well as prednisolone acetate 1%. Steroids are tapered over the course of 1 month according to the surgeon's individual protocol. Patients are instructed to resume all near work unaided on their first postoperative day, and patients are instructed to avoid or minimize using near vision spectacles in order to use their accommodative apparatus as much as possible.

Clinical Experience With the Synchrony AIOL

To date, more than 260 Synchrony AIOLs have been implanted in our practice. The sole indication for implantation has been cataract, as no cases of clear lens extraction for purely refractive purposes have been performed. Our first implant was performed in July 2003. Our initial implants were performed via the use of forceps, as no injector system was available at that time.[8] Analyses of patients binocularly implanted with the Synchrony AIOL have shown high degrees of spectacle independence as well as outstanding intermediate visual acuities (Figure 4).[9] These results remain stable over time, with all patients maintaining J3 or better near visual acuities at the two-year follow-up visit.

Clinicians and patients have recognized 2 major drawbacks of multifocal IOL technologies—quality of vision and lack of a functional range of vision. It is expected that AIOL technologies will fill the gap in these 2 arenas in order to provide patients with higher satisfaction. Diffractive multifocal IOLs behave like bifocal lenses and provide very good distance and near visual acuities. Their performance for intermediate tasks is not as robust and therefore some surgeons have advocated the mix and match strategy where refractive multifocal IOLs, which have better intermediate visual range, are combined with diffractive multifocal IOLs. Even if mixing and matching were to provide a better range of vision with multifocal IOL technologies, the detrimental effect of multifocality on contrast sensitivity would not be taken care of.

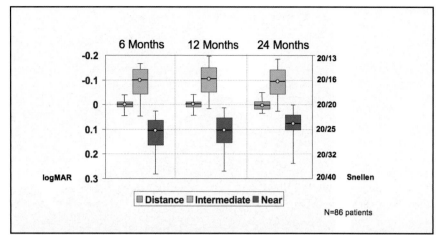

Figure 4. Long-term results, binocular implantation of Synchrony AIOL.

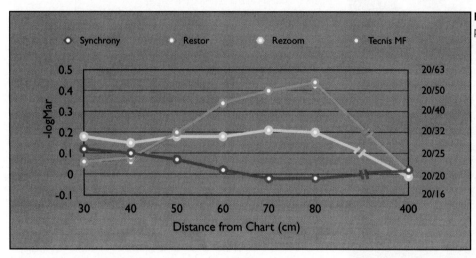

Figure 5. Functional range of vision of 4 different presbyopia-correcting technologies.

Functional Range of Vision

The restoration of a functional range of vision (good unaided distance, intermediate, and near visual acuities) is of paramount importance when assessing the effectiveness of presbyopia-correcting IOLs.

A nonconcurrent comparative case series of 120 patients divided into 4 groups (Synchrony AIOL [Visiogen, Inc, Irvine, CA], ReZoom Multifocal Zonal Refractive Lens [Advanced Medical Optics, Santa Ana, CA], Tecnis Multifocal Diffractive Lens [Advanced Medical Optics], and the ReSTOR Apodized Diffractive Multifocal Lens [Alcon, Fort Worth, TX]) was designed to elucidate the differences in visual outcomes with these 4 technologies.[10] Visual acuities were measured using ETDRS charts with standardized illumination at 85 cd/m^2 testing at various distances ranging from 0.30 to 4 meters. Patients implanted with the Synchrony AIOL showed better intermediate visual acuities (50 through 80 cm), with the results achieving high statistical significance (one-way Anova p < .01). Near visual acuities (30 and 40 cm) were higher for the ReSTOR, Tecnis MF, and Synchrony groups when compared to the ReZoom (Figure 5).

Reading speed measurements have shown that photopic reading speeds are comparable for diffractive multifocal IOL recipients and Synchrony AIOL recipients. Mesopic reading speeds are higher in the Synchrony and Tecnis MF IOL groups compared to ReSTOR or ReZoom.

Capsule Biocompatibility

The incidence of posterior capsule opacification (PCO) in this cohort of patients has been studied with the use of the OSCA System. This system has been previously proven to be both valid and reliable.[11,12] In the OSCA System, standard retroillumination slit lamp photographs are used and merged in such a way that unwanted reflections are removed prior to image analysis.

In a prospective analytical observational study comparing 25 Synchrony AIOL recipients with 75 age-matched Rayner C-Flex monofocal IOL (Domedics AG, Neuenhof, Aargau) recipients, mean PCO scores were lower in the Synchrony AIOL group at all time points from 6 to 24 months. It is important to note that the Rayner C-Flex IOL is a single-piece lens made from hydrophilic acrylic with a square edge all around the optic and haptics thus having a very low propensity toward PCO. At the 2-year follow-up visit the cumulative incidence of clinically significant PCO was 5.1% in the Synchrony AIOL group. Grading of photographs by an ophthalmologist revealed that 88% of the Synchrony subjects had none or mild anterior capsule opacification (ACO) whereas this was true in only 73% of the monofocal IOL recipients.

Figure 6. Digital retroillumination photograph of subject BPG 38 months after implantation with the Synchrony dual-optic AIOL.

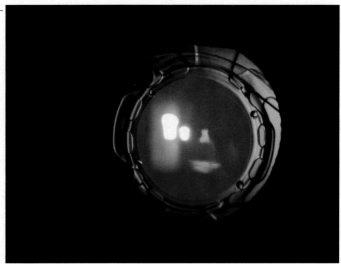

Figure 7. Simonth mesopic contrast sensitivity curves under glare conditions for Synchrony AIOL, Acrysof ReSTOR, and Acrysof SA60AT recipients.

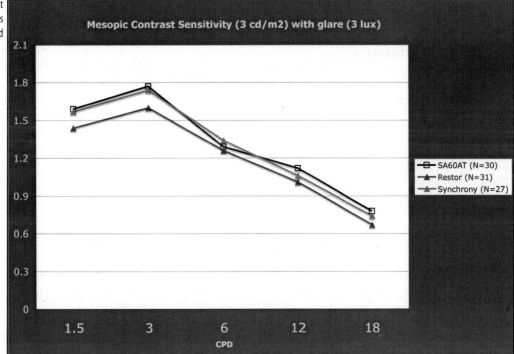

Figure 6 depicts a patient implanted with the Synchrony AIOL after 38 months of implantation. It is important to note the absence of signs of capsular contraction, fibrosis, or opacification in this photograph. It is likely that the low incidence of PCO and ACO with this lens system is due to its ability to minimize the potential for fibrosis by filling the capsular bag and minimizing contact with the anterior capsule.

Contrast Sensitivity

Multifocal lenses, whether diffractive or refractive, provide pseudoaccommodation by focusing incoming light at several fixed distances. As a result, for any given distance brought into the focal plane, only a fraction of the light entering the lens (often <50%) is used to produce the image. Accommodating lenses focus nearly all incoming light at any given point within their accommodative range. The mechanism used to provide simultaneous vision in multifocal IOLs generates detrimental effects on contrast sensitivity. This loss of optical quality could potentially be much more noticeable in younger patients seeking clear lens extraction for refractive purposes.

A comparative study between the Synchrony AIOL, the multifocal Acrysof ReSTOR (Alcon) and the monofocal Acrysof SA60AT (Alcon) showed comparable mesopic contrast sensitivity values under glare at all spatial frequencies between the monofocal and the Synchrony AIOL. All patients were tested on the Optec 6500 device (Stereo Optical Co, Inc, Chicago, IL). The multifocal (Acrysof ReSTOR) IOL exhibited lower contrast sensitivity values at all spatial frequencies (Figure 7).

Table 1

INCIDENCE OF HALOS AT 6 MONTHS AFTER IMPLANTATION WITH FOUR DIFFERENT PRESBYOPIA-CORRECTING IOLs*

Incidence	Synchrony (n = 31)	ReSTOR (n = 27)	ReZoom (n = 28)	Tecnis MF (n = 34)
Mild	2 (6.4%)	3 (11.1%)	5 (17.5%)	4 (11.8%)
Moderate	0	1 (3.7%)	0	2 (5.8%)
Severe	0	0	1 (3.5%)	0
Overall	2 (6.4%)	4 (14.8%)	6 (21%)	6 (17.6%)

* $p = .49$ Chi-Square Test

Halos and Glare

Halos and glare can be very disturbing to the patient. Their incidence after AIOL implantation is related to the diameter of the lens optic in mesopic conditions. On the contrary, halos after multifocal IOL implantation are inherent to the design whereby multiple foci are produced. The incidence of halos of any magnitude is 6.4% with the Synchrony AIOL, in contrast to incidences ranging between 14.8% and 21% with different multifocal technologies (Table 1).

Complications

Over the last 4 years, one patient (0.36%) has undergone lens explantation due to partial subluxation of the anterior optic after an eccentric rhexis of 5.5 mm. Lens subluxation ensued 2 weeks after surgery. Lens explantation was performed under topical anesthesia with unpreserved lidocaine 1% by severing all 4 spring haptic-anterior optic connections and then bisecting the anterior optic to allow its removal through the original 3.7-mm incision. Removal of the posterior optic plus the attached spring haptics was easier because this optic is thinner (low minus power). The lens was replaced with a 3-piece zonal refractive acrylic multifocal IOL to ensure centration in the presence of a 5.5-mm eccentric capsulorhexis.

Conclusion

Synchrony AIOL implantation yields complete spectacle independence in over 83% of patients binocularly implanted. Careful patient selection and strict adherence to the surgical protocol ensure good uncorrected visual acuities from distance to near. Most importantly, the Synchrony AIOL avoids the detrimental effect of a multifocal IOL on contrast sensitivity, and has a much lower incidence of unwanted photic phenomena. Once approved and marketed, the Synchrony AIOL will surely become a mainstream device for presbyopia correction. As phacoemulsification technology evolves into even smaller incisions, one can hope that future designs of injector systems will allow Synchrony AIOL implantation through sub 3.2-mm incisions as well.

References

1. Greenbaum S. Monovision pseudophakia. *J Cataract Refract Surg.* 2002;28:1439-1443

2. Javitt JC, Steinert RF. Cataract extraction with multifocal intraocular lens implantation; a multinational clinical trial evaluating clinical, functional, and quality-of-life outcomes. *Ophthalmology.* 2000;107:2040-2048.

3. Nijkamp MD, Dolders MGT, de Brabander J, et al. Effectiveness of multifocal intraocular lenses to correct presbyopia after cataract surgery; a randomized controlled trial. *Ophthalmology.* 2004;111:1832-1839.

4. Steinert RF, Aker BL, Trentacost DJ, et al. A prospective comparative study of the AMO ARRAY zonal-progressive multifocal silicone intraocular lens and a monofocal intraocular lens. *Ophthalmology.* 1999;106:1243-1255.

5. Dick HB, Krummenauer F, Schwenn O, et al. Objective and subjective evaluation of photic phenomena after monofocal and multifocal intraocular lens implantation. *Ophthalmology.* 1999;106:1878-1886.

6. McLeod SD, Portney V, Ting A. A dual optic accommodating foldable intraocular lens. *Br J Ophthalmol.* 2003;87(9):1083-1085.

7. Werner L, Pandey SK, Izak AM, et al. Capsular bag opacification after experimental implantation of a new accommodating intraocular lens in rabbit eyes. *J Cataract Refract Surg.* 2004;30:1114-1123.

8. Ossma IL, Galvis A, Vargas LG, et al. Synchrony dual-optic accommodating intraocular lens. Part 2: Pilot clinical evaluation. *J Cataract Refract Surg.* 2007;33:47-52.

9. Ossma IL, Galvis A. Binocular visual function after dual optic accommodating intraocular lens implantation. Presented in part at the Annual Meeting European Society of Cataract and Refractive Surgery. London, September 2006.

10. Ossma IL, Galvis A. Binocular performance after implantation of multifocal and dual optic accommodating intraocular lenses. Presented in part at the Annual Meeting European Society of Cataract and Refractive Surgery. Stockholm, September 2007.

11. Aslam TM, Patton N, Rose CJ. OSCA: a comprehensive open-access system of analysis of posterior capsular opacification. *BMC Ophthalmol.* 2006;6:30.

12. Aslam TM, Patton N, Graham J. A freely accessible, evidence based, objective system of analysis of posterior capsular opacification; evidence for its validity and reliability. *BMC Ophthalmol.* 2005;5(1):9.

13. Galvis A, Ossma IL. Comparative study of capsule opacification between accommodating and monofocal intraocular lenses. Presented in part at the Annual Meeting of the American Academy of Ophthalmology. Las Vegas, November 2006.

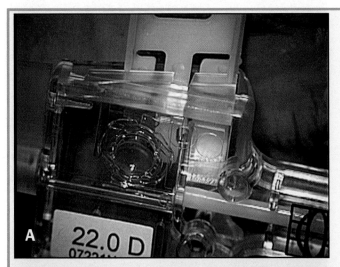
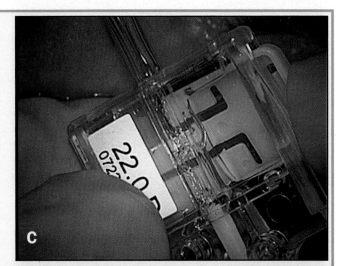
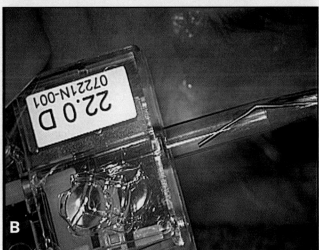
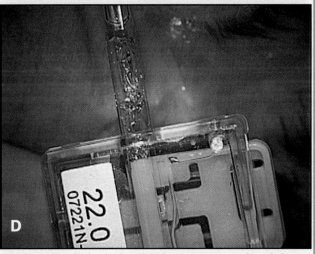

Figure 1. (A) Preloaded injector showing dual optic IOL in chamber. (B) Rear optic is slid forward and cartridge is filled with saline. (C) Both optics are compressed into the lumen. (D) Plunger advances the two compressed optics within the injector lumen.

PEARLS FOR IMPLANTING THE VISIOGEN SYNCHRONY IOL

David F. Chang, MD

The Visiogen Synchrony one-piece silicone intraocular lens (IOL) comes preloaded in a disposable injector (Figure 1). During the Food and Drug Administration (FDA) clinical trial in the United States, I performed these cases under topical anesthesia using a temporal clear corneal incision. Here are 5 pearls for implanting this IOL.

A 3.8-mm opening through Descemet's works best. Because this is longer than most clear corneal incisions, I employ Michael Wong's suggestion of making 2 tiny pockets in the roof of the incision that can be stromally hydrated at the conclusion of surgery (Figure 2) [Chapter 183].

The capsulorrhexis must entirely overlap the edge of the 5.5-mm diameter anterior optic (Figure 3). A capsulorrhexis that is too large or eccentric will allow the forward moving anterior optic to partially prolapse through the opening. Implantation of the Synchrony should therefore be aborted if the capsulorrhexis is either too large or torn. Using a 5-mm diameter optical zone marker may help the surgeon to estimate the proper size. My own preference is to err on the small side, and to secondarily enlarge the opening after the IOL is placed [Chapter 182].

Polishing or vacuuming the undersurface of the anterior capsule makes sense in order to minimize capsular fibrosis for an accommodating IOL. In addition to using a right and left hand paracentesis incision 45 degrees away from the temporal incision, I make an addition paracentesis at the 10 o'clock position. This provides the aspirating handpiece with better access to the subincisional anterior capsule (Figure 4).

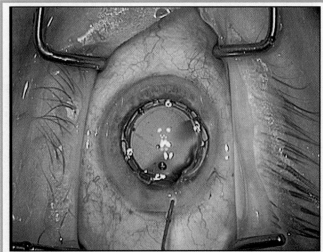

Figure 2. Tiny pocket in the roof of the corneal tunnel is hydrated with saline solution to compress the tunnel.

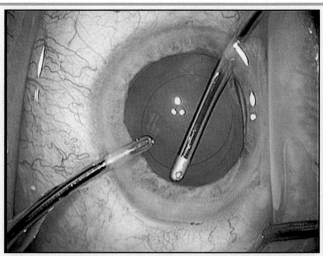

Figure 4. Bimanual irrigation-aspiration (I-A) handpieces remove cortex and vacuum the anterior capsule rim.

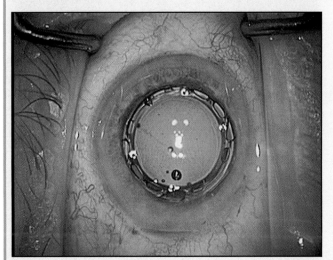

Figure 3. Capsulorrhexis completely overlaps the anterior 5.5-mm Synchrony optic.

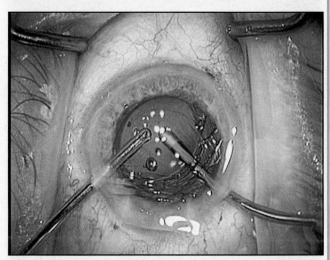

Figure 5. Bimanual I-A handpieces remove Amvisc Plus located between the optics.

Maintaining an inflated capsular bag is of critical importance because of the need to sequentially insert each of the dual optics. One does not want the ophthalmic visco-surgical device (OVD) to burp out too easily for this reason. Once the IOL is in place, it is desirable to remove the OVD between the two optics using bimanual I-A instrumentation (Figure 5). Amvisc Plus (Bausch & Lomb, Rochester, NY) has intermediate rheological properties between those of a cohesive and dispersive agent. It is more retentive than a cohesive OVD, but is more easily removed than a dispersive OVD, and is my agent of choice for Synchrony cases.

When implanting the lens, I enter the incision with the cartridge tip bevel up [Chapter 176]. Injecting the IOL entails a learning curve because of the difficulty in visualizing what part of the lens is emerging from the injector (Figure 6). The posterior minus optic is very thin and will therefore exit the injector very slowly. There are two large finlike tabs on the posterior optic that serve as haptics to center the optic and push it posteriorly. Imagine that the left thumb and pinky finger represent each of these two haptics located 180 degrees across from each other. The rear optic will resemble your pronated left fist as it first starts to exit the injector cartridge. As it emerges, it will be as though your left fist slowly supinates with the thumb extending outward (see Figure 6B). This is the first haptic that can be seen. Slowly opening the supinated left hand will resemble the unfolding of the optic (see Figure 6C). Like the pinky finger, the second haptic is the last structure seen to emerge. The second optic will exit much more quickly because of its greater thickness (>30+ D). It is important to keep the injector tip just beneath the capsulorrhexis plane to assure that the second optic opens within the capsular bag (see Figure 6F).

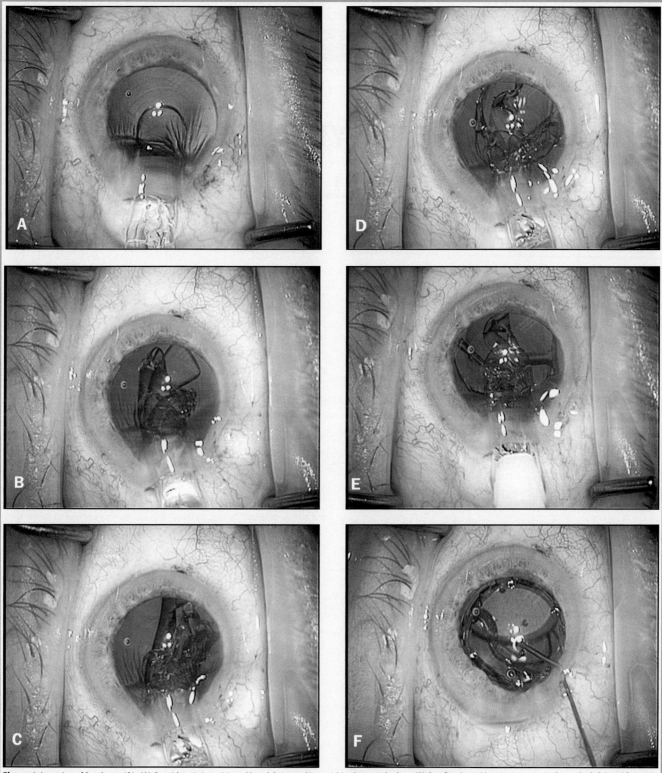

Figure 6. Insertion of Synchrony IOL. (A) Cartridge tip is positioned bevel down and just within the capsular bag. (B) One fin-shaped haptic emerges similar to the left hand fist with the thumb up. (C) Rear optic emerges like a supinated left fist. (D) Rear optic unfolds. (E) Unfolded rear optic slides distally as the anterior optic is injected. (F) Anterior optic unfolds in center of the bag just behind the capsulorrhexis. The rear optic has slid nasally so that its temporal edge is in the middle of the pupil.

CHAPTER 57

VISIOGEN SYNCHRONY— CLINICAL PEARLS

George Beiko, BM, BCh, FRCS(C)

There are currently several viable options for addressing presbyopia correction following cataract surgery and intraocular lens (IOL) implantation. These options include monovision (aiming for emmetropia in one eye for distance activities and mild myopia in the other eye for near vision), multifocal IOL implantation (diffractive, refractive, and mixing/matching), and accommodating IOLs. The advantage of multifocal or accommodating IOL implantation compared to monovision is the potential for improved binocular functions at all distances.

Multifocal lenses are designed to produce at least 2 axially separated focal points that create the "functional equivalent" of accommodation. Many challenges are inherent in the design of such lenses. The demands of minimizing loss of incident light to higher orders of diffraction, minimizing optical aberration, and balancing the brightness of the focused and unfocused images are just some of these challenges.[1]

Current accommodating IOLs provide superior image quality compared to multifocal lenses since they do not have the inherent limitations due to lens design (not only competing images, but also loss of contrast, double vision, glare, and halos). First-generation accommodating IOLs (single optic) work in theory by forward displacement of the lens optic. Theories about how these IOLs work include the concept that the ciliary body directly causes the IOL to vault forward.[2] According to this theory, the ciliary body presses on the lens or the contraction of the ciliary muscle generates a pressure gradient between the aqueous and vitreous, causing anterior displacement of the lens zonule diaphragm with subsequent forward movement of the optic. An alternate theory states that the vitreous creates a positive pressure that causes the anterior displacement of the lens. The accommodative range of a single rigid optic design is dependent on the amount of axial displacement of the optic and on the power of the moving lens (higher diopter IOLs have greater accommodative range).[3]

The Synchrony dual optic accommodating IOL (Visiogen Inc, Irvine, CA) (Figure 1) is a newly developed single-piece accommodating lens manufactured from silicone. This revolutionary lens design has 2 major optic components (anterior and posterior) connected by a bridge through the haptics, which act like a spring. The IOL has a 5.5-mm, high-powered anterior optic (+ 32 D) coupled with a 6.0-mm, negative power optic customized to bring the eye to emmetropia. This dual optic system is designed to work in concert with the capsular bag, according to the traditional Helmholtz's theory of accommodation. When the lens is implanted in the eye, in the unaccommodated state, capsular tension compresses the optics, reducing the separation between the optics. The compression of the lens system stores strain energy in the connecting haptics. Once accommodative effort takes effect, the zonules relax, releasing tension on the capsular bag, thus allowing release of the stored energy in the spring system with forward (anterior) displacement of the front high-plus optic, which results in a change in the effective power of the eye.[4]

The Synchrony IOL incorporates many unique design features that enhance the dual-optic performance. The anterior optic has 2 expansions oriented parallel to the haptic component, which are designed to lift the capsulorrhexis edge and prevent contact of the anterior capsule with the anterior surface of the lens optic. This separation of capsule from optic prevents anterior capsule opacification (ACO).[5,6] These expansions also have channels or fenestrations for fluid exchange between the bag (interoptic space) and the anterior chamber so as to prevent capsular block syndrome and to maintain free aqueous circulation between the open bag and the anterior chamber. The Synchrony lens also has 2 static members (or stabilizers) that originate from the posterior optic. The stabilizers are anteriorly angulated to compensate for capsular bag variations. These stabilizers also maintain the lens's centration within the capsular bag during the accommodation/relaxation process.

I have been implanting the Synchrony IOL since 2005. At the time of writing this chapter, 18 patients and 30 eyes have been implanted with great success. In order to succeed, any presbyopia-correcting IOL (Pr-C IOL) requires careful patient selection and a meticulous surgical technique.

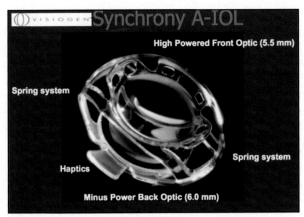

Figure 1. Visiogen Synchrony Dual Optic IOL. (Courtesy of Visiogen.)

Surgery

INCISION

The incisions are designed to enable bimanual phacoemulsification, as this is my preferred method of cataract extraction.

I place the main incision either on the steep axis of astigmatism or in the superotemporal location in spherical corneas. The incision is near limbal and designed to be a Langerman's type. The initial groove is 3.6 mm in length. Two Wong pockets anterior to the groove are created (these are hydrated at the end of the case so as to ensure a tighter incision closure). I use a 1.3-mm diamond keratome to enter the anterior chamber through the main incision. This same diamond keratome is used to create a paracentesis about 100 degrees away from the main incision.

CAPSULORRHEXIS

The capsulorrhexis for this lens needs to be smaller than the anterior optic, centered, and defect free in order to maintain the 2 IOL optics in the capsular bag. The ideal continuous curvilinear capsulorrhexis (CCC) size is circular and between 4.5 and 5.5 mm in diameter. A tool that can help control the size and centration of the capsulorrhexis is a corneal marker (Figure 2). I use a 5.5-mm corneal marker, which will project a 5.0-mm mark on the anterior lens capsule in an average patient (normal Ks and ACD). It is very important to keep the eye centered when using this marker while tearing the capsule; otherwise the mark will appear eccentric, and the CCC might be decentered from the visual axis.

More recently, I have also been using the Seibel Rhexis Ruler (MST, Redmond WA) to help fashion the ideal 5.0-mm diameter capsulorrhexis.

My preferred ophthalmic viscosurgical device (OVD) is Healon 5 (Advanced Medical Optics, Santa Ana, CA) due to its ability to maintain a controlled anterior chamber environment and to dimple the anterior capsule so as to facilitate the creation of the capsulorrhexis.

HYDRODISSECTION

Prevention of capsular fibrosis and capsular shrink-wrapping of the IOL is essential for the proper functioning of the Synchrony accommodating IOL.

Complete hydrodissection is essential for any cataract procedure. Hydrodissection frees the nucleus, which makes the surgery safer, and reduces capsular fibrosis. Among the surgical factors that help to prevent posterior capsule opacification (PCO), hydrodissection with enhanced cortical cleanup is the most important.[7] Faust[8] introduced the hydrodissection technique as a means of expressing the nucleus from the bag for extracapsular cataract extraction. Fine[9] modified and improved the technique to loosen cortical-capsular connections, changing the term to cortical-cleaving hydrodissection. Injecting balanced salt solution (BSS) beneath the anterior capsule to separate the cortex from the capsular bag accomplishes this. Several studies have demonstrated that hydrodissection is an effective, practical, and inexpensive method for

Patient Selection

Patient profiling is perhaps the most important step when evaluating candidates for Pr-C IOL technologies. Patients have different needs, hobbies, and activities. Specifically, age is not as an important factor for Synchrony IOL implantation as one might think. Current data from Colombia, where the average age of implanted patients is in the 60s, and from Canada, where the patients are at least 10 years older on average, reveals that the Synchrony works comparably well for near vision in both groups of patients. Active patients who perform repetitive or numerous activities at all distances (far, intermediate, and near) tend to have superior outcomes. Patients who require intermediate vision (for working on the computer, using the cell phone, writing and reading e-mail, etc) can be confident that this level of vision will be attained easily with the Synchrony lens. Patients who desire spectacle independence for near activities should be able to attain this once they are bilaterally implanted. Preoperative hyperopia is associated with better outcomes, but emmetropes and myopes who routinely accommodate for near also do well. Near vision without spectacle aid improves over time, and patients need to understand that perseverance in near functions improves functioning.

Preoperative Evaluation

As with all other "premium lens" designs, Synchrony candidates undergo a rigorous preoperative evaluation to ensure that the eye is free of any disease or defect that might limit visual performance. The measurement for IOL power calculation requires immersion A-scan or IOL Master (Carl Zeiss Meditec, Jena, Germany) biometry and manual keratometry. Due to its unique dual optic design, Visiogen has its own proprietary formula for calculating the power of this lens. Refractive outcomes have been excellent and very stable over time, with a mean spherical equivalent of −0.09 D at 6 months and −0.08 D at 12 months. About 71% of my patients are within ±0.5 D of emmetropia.

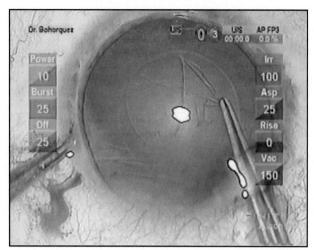

Figure 2. Ideal CCC is demonstrated, using a 5.5-mm corneal marker to indent the corneal so as to provide a template for the capsulorrhexis.

cortex removal, but it alone does not completely eliminate lens epithelial cells (LECs). Using nonpreserved lidocaine solution instead of BSS for hydrodissection has been shown to further decrease LEC proliferation after surgery, and this has been my preferred solution. The rare complications of hydrodissection, such as posterior capsule rupture and nucleus dislocation into the vitreous, are clearly outweighed by the significant advantages.

PHACOEMULSIFICATION

A capsule-friendly technique is recommended. Bimanual sleeveless microincisional phacoemulsification through the 2 1.3-mm incisions as described above is my usual method of cataract removal.

CORTICAL CLEAN-UP

Any technique that allows safe removal of all cortex is indicated. Following cortex removal, attempted complete removal of the LECs is necessary.

The LECs are confined to the anterior surface and the equatorial bow of the crystalline lens. The mean cell density of LECs is between 4000/mm² and 5500/mm², depending on the patient's age with the density decreasing after the age of 80. LECs consist of a single row of cuboidal-cylindrical cells attached to the posterior surface of the anterior capsule, which can be divided biologically into 2 zones with 2 types of cells. Those located in the anterior-central zone (corresponding to the zone of the anterior capsule) consist of relatively quiescent LECs with minimal mitotic activity. The primary response of these A cells is to proliferate and form fibrous tissue by undergoing fibrous metaplasia. These cells are responsible for anterior capsular fibrosis (ACF), and are also essential in creating a shrink-wrap effect around conventional lenses. The second zone is a continuation of the anterior epithelial cells around the equator, forming the equatorial lens bowl, with the germinal cells (E cells). In pathologic states, the E cells tend to migrate posteriorly along the posterior capsule; instead of undergoing a fibrotic trans-formation, they tend to form large, balloon-like bladder cells (Wedl cells). The equatorial cells are the primary source of PCO.

Polishing of the LECs that are located under the anterior capsule is recommended in order to prevent ACF and shrink-wrap formation. Removal of the LEC from the posterior capsule and equatorial capsular bag is undertaken to prevent posterior capsular fibrosis and opacification.

I use bimanual irrigation/aspiration (I/A) for capsular polishing. It is essential to invest enough time to thoroughly vacuum the anterior capsule and polish the posterior capsule.

PRELOADED INJECTOR

One of the most remarkable devices that Visiogen has developed for use with the Synchrony lens is the preloaded injector. The Synchrony lens comes preloaded in a single-use, disposable injector, which avoids the need to load the IOL in the operating room. This minimizes the risk for IOL loading errors and microbial contamination of the lens (Figure 3A). Three easy steps are required to prepare the lens for injection. First, the 2 optics are displaced, one in front of the other, by displacing the lateral white tab (Figure 3B). The posterior (negative powered) optic always will be the leading optic. Second, BSS is injected into the cannula of the injector, allowing fluid to lubricate the injector. Third, the lens is folded by pushing the lateral white tab against the housing of the injector (Figure 3C). The lens, at this stage, is ready for delivery. The injector is syringe-based and is coated with a specially formulated substance to facilitate smooth and consistent release of the IOL as it passes through the delivery cartridge (Figure 4).

IOL IMPLANTATION

The main incision size needs to be enlarged to 3.6 to 3.8 mm; I use a diamond keratome to enlarge the original phaco incision, while ensuring that the configuration remains true to Langerman's description. The anterior chamber is filled with Healon GV (Advanced Medical Optics), and an attempt is made to retain as much BSS in the capsule of the eye rather than replacing it with Healon GV, in essence, the modified soft shell technique of Arshinoff is used. The injector is placed into the anterior chamber through the main incision, and the tip of the cannula is then advanced until it is just beneath the CCC edge. The plunger of the syringe is depressed slowly. The first lens that unfolds is always the posterior (negative power) optic. This optic unfolds completely in a very controlled manner. The surgeon has the ability to control the rate of injection, and if desired, the surgeon can stop the process while the high-plus optic is still within the injector. This enables visualization of the lens prior to complete delivery of the second optic (Figure 5). Once the lens is injected into the capsular bag, the 2 optics may be slightly misaligned, and the lenses may appear to be slightly intertwined. This is easily resolved by separating the lens optics with Sinskey hooks. The lens will then typically center very nicely, without stretching or deforming the capsule.

OPHTHALMIC VISCOSURGICAL DEVICE REMOVAL

All OVD should be removed from the eye in order to avoid intraocular pressure spikes in the early postoperative period. There are 2 main techniques for removal in eyes implanted with Synchrony IOLs:

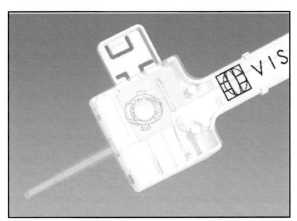

Figure 3A. The Visiogen Synchrony lens comes preloaded in a single-use, disposable injector. (Courtesy of Visiogen.)

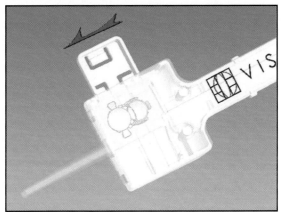

Figure 3B. The 2 optics are displaced, one in front of the other, by displacing the lateral white tab of the injector. (Courtesy of Visiogen.)

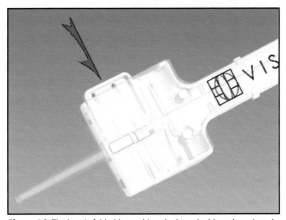

Figure 3C. The lens is folded by pushing the lateral white tab against the housing of the injector. (Courtesy of Visiogen.)

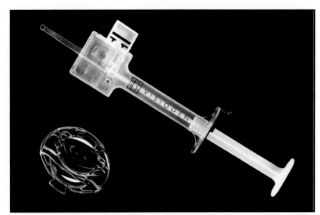

Figure 4. The injector is syringe-based and is coated with a specially formulated substance to facilitate smooth and consistent release of the IOL as it passes through the delivery cartridge. (Courtesy of Visiogen.)

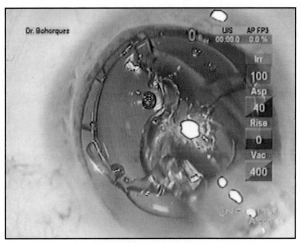

Figure 5. The surgeon has the ability to control the rate of injection and can stop the process while the high-plus optic is still within the injector. This enables visualization of the lens prior to complete delivery of the second optic.

1. The best option is to use bimanual I/A. The surgeon should attempt to go into the space between the 2 optics with a nontextured aspiration tip. I find it easier to approach this by first locating one of the lateral haptics and then pushing the anterior lens 180 degrees away. This provides a gap between the lenses and the CCC edge where the irrigation cannula is positioned and driven into the space between the optics. In some cases, the same approach can be used to go underneath the posterior optic. However, I find this to be a little cumbersome, and usually all OVD can be easily removed with the "between the optics" method.

2. Surgeons who are not comfortable with bimanual I/A or fear capsule damage with the additional manipulation can use a coaxial I/A handpiece to rock and roll the Synchrony IOL in a way similar to removing OVD with a standard 1-piece IOL. The surgeon must move the IOL from side to side and also compress the 2 optics together with the I/A handpiece. This allows OVD from the equatorial region and the interlenticular space to flow into the anterior chamber where it can be aspirated.

INCISION CLOSURE

I hydrate the Wong pockets and the 2 corneal incisions with sterile BSS. In rare cases, a suture (Nylon 10-0) can be used if there is an incision leak. This suture can be removed 1 to 2 weeks after surgery.

Conclusion

Pr-C IOLs are the next logical evolution of IOL designs. Success with these lenses is not only dependent on an extensive preoperative evaluation to properly select patients, but also careful surgical planning and execution. IOL power calculation needs to be as precise as our current technology allows. Surgery should be executed with extreme care.

The Synchrony IOL is a new technology for cataract surgery that allows a patient to achieve functional uncorrected distance, intermediate, and near vision characteristic of multifocal designs without compromising the image quality. Patient satisfaction is high. Long-term data show that this lens is safe and continues to deliver a functional range of vision up to 2 years post-operatively.[10]

References

1. Pieh S, Marvan P, Lackner B, et al. Quantitative performance of bifocal and multifocal intraocular lenses in a model eye. Point spread function in multifocal intraocular lenses. *Arch Ophthalmol*. 2002;120:23-38.

2. Cumming JS, Slade SG, Chayet A, AT-45 Study Group. Clinical evaluation of the model AT-45 silicone accommodating intraocular lens: results of feasibility and the initial phase of a Food and Drug Administration clinical trial. *Ophthalmology*. 2001;108:2005-2009.

3. McLeod SD, Vargas LG, Portney V, Ting A. Synchrony dual-optic accommodating intraocular lens Part 1: optical and biomechanical principles and design considerations. *J Cataract Refract Surg*. 2007;33:37-46.

4. McLeod SD, Portney V, Ting A. A dual optic accommodating foldable intraocular lens. *Br J Ophthalmol*. 2003;87:1083-1085.

5. Werner L, Pandey SK, Izak AM, et al. Capsular bag opacification after experimental implantation of a new accommodating intraocular lens in rabbit eyes. *J Cataract Refract Surg*. 2004;30:1114-1123.

6. Werner L, Mamalis N, Stevens S, Hunter B, Chew JJ, Vargas LG. Interlenticular opacification: dual-optic versus piggyback intraocular lenses. *J Cataract Refract Surg*. 2006;32:655-661.

7. Schmidbauer JM, Vargas LG, Apple DJ, et al. Evaluation of neodymium:yttrium-aluminum-garnet capsulotomies in eyes implanted with AcrySof intraocular lenses. *Ophthalmology*. 2002;109:1421-1426.

8. Faust KJ. Hydrodissection of soft nuclei. *Am Intra-Ocular Implant Soc J*. 1984;10:75-77.

9. Fine IH. Cortical cleaving hydrodissection. *J Cataract Refract Surg*. 1992;18:508-512.

10. Beiko G. Near visual acuity in patients with bilateral implantation of the Synchrony dual optic IOL. Presented at the XXV Congress of the ESCRS, Sept 8-12, 2007, Stockholm.

CHAPTER 58

LENSTEC TETRAFLEX—CLINICAL PEARLS

Paul Dougherty, MD

The Tetraflex accommodating intraocular lens (IOL) (Lenstec, Inc, St. Petersburg, FL) is an exciting new technology that shows great promise for the treatment of presbyopia. Despite the small size of the lens manufacturer, the Tetraflex accounts for more than 30% of the presbyopic IOL market in Europe (data on file with Market Scope, LLC, Manchester, MO). The Phase III FDA Trial of the Tetraflex began in September 2005.

Design and Surgical Technique

The Tetraflex (Figure 1) is a flexible, single-piece, foldable, accommodating IOL that is implanted using a custom-designed 1.8-mm injector system through an incision as small as 2.5 mm. A 1.6-mm pre-loaded injector system is in development. The lens is vaulted 5 degrees anteriorly and has no hinges. The lens' optic is 5.75 mm and is made of a highly biocompatible hydrophilic acrylic material with a refractive index of 1.457. A square-edge design helps minimize posterior capsular opacification. The IOL's 2 haptics (Figure 2), each with 2 footplates, sit posteriorly in the peripheral capsular bag. The lens comes in 0.5 D incremental powers between +5 and +30 D. Because the lens is manufactured with better than ISO tolerances of 0.1 D, the lens is available in +0.2 D increments between +18 and +25 D. The 0.2 D increments allow for more accurate postoperative refractive outcomes.

In loading the lens, care should be taken to make sure that the positioning tab is located in the front right portion of the lens to avoid upside down insertion of the lens in the eye. An upside down lens will result in excellent distance vision, but the loss of accommodative effect of the lens. The surgeon performs his standard capsulorrhexis and phacoemulsification technique. Lenstec, Inc recommends that surgeons create a circular capsulorrhexis up to 5.5 mm in diameter. The lens should only be implanted using a low viscosity viscoelastic like OcuCoat (Bausch & Lomb, Rochester, NY). High viscosity viscoelastics like Healon GV (Advanced Medical Optics, Santa Ana, CA), Healon 5, or Viscoat (Alcon, Fort Worth,

TX) should be avoided, as these products will inhibit proper unfolding of the haptics into the capsular bag. The surgeon should not implant the Tetraflex if a posterior capsular or anterior capsular radial tear is created during surgery. Caution should be used at the time of surgery to visually confirm that the very flexible haptics are properly positioned in the capsular bag by moving the lens optic nasally and temporally with a lens hook. Care should be taken not to overfill the chamber at the end of the case, which could result in posterior positioning of the optic, resulting in unexpected hyperopia. The lens is used internationally for both cataract and refractive lensectomy surgery.

The Mechanism of Action

The mechanism of action of the Tetraflex is not definitively known, but is thought to be multifactorial. On ultrasound biomicroscopy (UBM) the lens can be seen to move forward during accommodative effort (Figure 3). It is believed that this movement occurs due to the contraction of the ciliary muscle that loosens the zonules and also increases vitreous pressure. In addition, the anterior surface of the optic curves more than the posterior surface during anterior vaulting of the lens. This higher radius of curvature of the lens' anterior surface increases the net refractive power of the lens and induces coma. The latter is an important part of the normal accommodative process in the prepresbyopic phakic eye.

United States Clinical Trial

The Tetraflex IOL is currently in phase 3 FDA clinical trials in 12 centers in the United States. To date, more than 450 IOLs have been implanted in this country (data on file with Lenstec, Inc). Of those, 174 eyes of 111 patients have been followed for 6 months or more. Six-month data will be reported here. Sixty percent achieved a distance uncorrected visual acuity (UCVA) of 20/20 or better, and 96% achieved a UCVA of

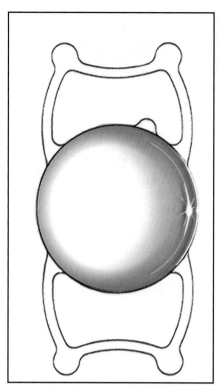

Figure 1. The Tetraflex is a polyHEMA material, 5.75 optic, and refined diopter increment in 0.2 D in the central range of power (18 D to 25 D).

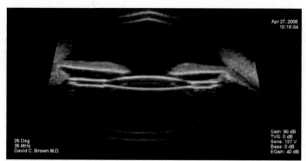

Figure 3. UBM photograph of the Tetraflex IOL in the accommodated (near) position. The anterior portion of the lens has moved closer to the posterior surface of the iris, the anterior chamber depth has diminished by, and the ciliary muscle has thickened compared with the unaccommodated (distance) position. (Courtesy of David Brown, MD and Sonomed, Inc.)

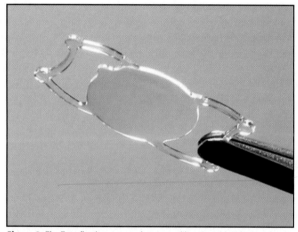

Figure 2. The Tetraflex has patented contoured haptics with 5 degree anterior vault. Note the "nub" on the optic—designed to confirm anterior orientation of optic.

20/40 or better, similar to any competitive monofocal lens. In terms of evaluating the near performance of any accommodating lens, distance-corrected near vision is considered the gold standard. Fifty-two percent of eyes demonstrated a monocular distance-corrected near vision of J6 (print size of stock quotes) or better, and 85% have a monocular distance-corrected near vision of J9 (standard newspaper print) or better. European data of near visual function show that the near performance of Tetraflex is even better when the lens is implanted bilaterally versus monocularly (data on file with Lenstec, Inc). In terms of monocular accommodative amplitude in the FDA study, 91% of those implanted had at least 1 D, and 68% had at least 2 D and 55% had at least 3 D of accommodation at 12 months postoperatively using the "Push Down" amplitude of accommodation test. Currently, none of the patients implanted

with the Tetraflex, either domestically or internationally, have experienced any capsular issues like z-syndrome or decentration. The only adverse events in the study thus far have been 1 eye (0.6%) that required removal and replacement secondary to posterior positioning of the lens resulting in hyperopia, 2 eyes (0.3%) that required lens repositioning due to haptic or optic malposition, and 3 eyes (1%) that required removal and reinsertion due to a lens tear. All eyes achieved excellent UCVA and best-corrected visual acuity (BCVA) after secondary intervention.

My experience as a principal investigator in the FDA trial of this lens has been excellent. So far, I have implanted 60 of these IOLs in 39 patients. When I implant Tetraflex, I usually operate on the nondominant eye first with a goal of −0.37 D to enhance the near effect of the lens. The dominant eye is operated on 3 weeks later per protocol with goal of plano. The only adverse event I have seen is a lens that had posterior positioning of the optic secondary to overfilling the chamber at the end of the case, resulting in hyperopia. Simple wound paracentesis resulted in immediate anterior movement of the optic into appropriate position, which brought the eye back to emmetropia. The lens is simple to implant, has none of the visual side effects (such as glare, halo, and loss of contrast sensitivity) of multifocal lenses, and is consistently giving my patients functional near vision without correction. Because there is a single point of focus through all distances, the quality of vision through the lens is excellent. I consider this lens equivalent in distance performance to any monofocal lens that I use with the fringe benefit of improved near vision. Like any accommodative lens, however, I do not promise that all patients will throw away their reading glasses. Some patients achieve lesser accommodative effect and may require near spectacles part of the time, particularly with low lighting and low-contrast print. I have found that patients with shorter axial lengths tend to have better subjective near vision with the Tetraflex than patients with longer axial lengths. In those that get significant accommodative effect after bilateral implantation, it is not unusual to see the patient reading a magazine without glasses in the exam lane during the postoperative visit, and then look up to read the 20/20 Snellen line on the distance chart.

Thus far, I have not noted any complaints of glare or halos at night in my Tetraflex patients, which is likely due to both the monofocal nature of the lens as well as its 5.75-mm optic. Although I have needed to perform a YAG posterior capsulotomy on only a few eyes after the IOL's implantation (approximately 10% in the first year), the capsulotomy does not seem to negatively affect accommodation, and all lenses have remained in perfect position postoperatively.

Conclusion

Many different lenses are available to treat presbyopia in the United States, including both accommodating and multifocal IOLs. International surgeons in Asia, Europe, and the Middle East have access to many exciting ophthalmic technologies not currently available here. One of these, the Tetraflex IOL, shows significant promise in helping the surgeon to minimize postoperative spectacle dependence in the presbyopic patient. I believe this lens, when and if approved by the FDA, will be the presbyopic-correcting IOL of choice.

CHAPTER 59

LENSTEC TETRAFLEX—CLINICAL PEARLS

Conall F. Hurley, MB, BCh, BAO, FRCSI

Now that the era of presbyopia-correcting intraocular lenses (IOLs) has arrived, surgeons can offer their patients the possibility of variable focus with a pseudophakic eye. The Kellan Tetraflex IOL (Lenstec Inc, St. Petersburg, FL) is a posterior chamber poly-HEMA accommodating IOL that has a 5.75-mm optic with patented 5-degree contoured haptics. This IOL is designed on the basis of the Helmholtz theory of accommodation. Although the exact physiological mechanism that is involved in the process of accommodation has not been fully elucidated as yet, the basic idea behind the function of this IOL is as follows. On attempting to view a near object, changes in the region of the ciliary body result in the anterior movement of the IOL as a unit. A combination of the anterior angle orientation and the design of the haptics (Figure 1) allow the Tetraflex to move anteriorly along with the entire capsular bag. Swelling of the ciliary body combined with movement of the vitreous are the changes that result in the forward movement of the IOL as a whole. Studies have been performed at the Midlands Eye Institute, Solihull, UK by Mr. Sunil Shah that demonstrate that patients achieved an amplitude of accommodation of 3.1 D (±1.5 D) with a range of 1 D to 6.4 D 1 month post-implantation of the Tetraflex. This was 1.7 D (±2.2 D) with a range of 1 D to 6 D at 6 months post-implantation.[1] It is important to remember that with lower powers of the Tetraflex, less potential spectacle magnification is possible than with higher powered implants, as the IOL moves forward. This means that high myopes may achieve less near focus than low myopes, emmetropes, and hyperopes.

However, it would appear that the accommodative property of the Tetraflex is not entirely dependent on the movement of the IOL in that some pseudoaccommodation is also taking place. The combination of both the movement of the IOL and whatever other mechanisms are at work allow a swift return of the IOL to the flat position once the patient resumes viewing objects in the intermediate and distance viewing positions. This gives patients clear vision at these working distances also.

The square edge design of the optic should also reduce posterior lens capsule opacification.

One of the principal advantages of the Tetraflex is that the learning curve for successful implantation of this IOL is practically nonexistent. It can be easily implanted in all the power ranges (ie, +5 D to +36 D) through a 3-mm incision. Lenstec has a reusable titanium injector system that is used in conjunction with a disposable cartridge. The cartridge has 2 sizes for the disposable cartridge (at the time of this writing) that are 1.8 mm and 2.2 mm in diameter. A smaller-gauge cartridge of 1.6 mm is planned for introduction as well. I have injected up to a +25-D Tetraflex with the small-gauge cartridge, while for the upper end of the power range I have used the 2.2-mm cartridge without any difficulty. The Tetraflex centers very well within the capsular bag due to its design (Figure 2). The dimensions of the optic (ie, a 5.75-mm optic) reduce the risk of any postoperative glare and halos considerably, and this is especially so in comparison to multifocal IOL designs that are based on diffractive optics.

I have used the Tetraflex IOL in patients whom I feel are not suited to a multifocal implant. It is most ideally used in emmetropes and hyperopes who have realistic expectations of their outcome. Patients who are more interested in having better distance and intermediate vision and are not overly concerned with being able to read the tiniest print are the most ideal candidates for an accommodating IOL. Patients with severe dry eye disease, ocular infections (such as chronic blepharitis), severe ophthalmic disease (eg, a history of uveitis, glaucoma, or retinal disease), uncontrolled systemic disease (eg, diabetes, hypertension, or cardiovascular disease), or high levels of preoperative astigmatism should not be considered for the Tetraflex. I have used it in patients with lower levels of astigmatism (ie, <2.00 D). It is important to attempt to minimize this patient group's astigmatism by performing on axis surgery with the addition of a pre-placed arcuate keratotomy on their steep corneal axis opposite to the main incision.

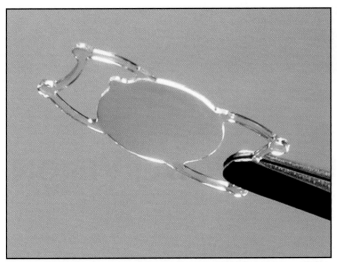

Figure 1. The Tetraflex has patented contoured haptics with 5 degree anterior vault. Note the "nub" on the optic—designed to confirm anterior orientation of optic.

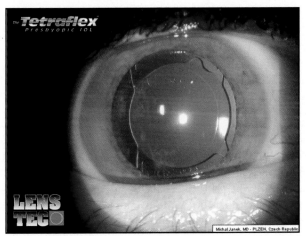

Figure 2. Postoperative photo of a Tetraflex Accommodating IOL. (Courtesy of Lenstec, St. Petersburg, FL.)

The Tetraflex™
Micro Incision Presbyopic IOL with Precision Diopters in .20 Diopter Increments from +18.0 to +25.0

Optic Size:	5.75mm
Optic Type:	Equiconvex
Length:	11.50mm
Haptic Style:	Tetraflex
Angulation:	5 Degrees
Construction:	1 Piece
Position Holes:	0
Optic Material:	Acrylic (26% water content)
A Constant:	118.0
A/C Depth:	5.10mm

Diopter Increments:

Whole	+31.0 to +36.0
Half	+5.0 to +18.0 and +25.0 to +30.0
0.2	+18.0 to +25.0

U.S. Patent No. 6,261,321 B1 July 17, 2001

Square Edge Technology

Figure 3. Illustration of the Tetraflex Accommodating IOL and its design characteristics. (Courtesy of Lenstec, St. Petersburg, FL.)

If a patient is concerned with reading tiny print or if his or her occupational requirements are for really good near acuity, then I would alternatively use a multifocal implant in such a patient. Multifocal IOLs offer the best near vision, but at the expense of intermediate vision. Emmetropic patients can read about J1 or J2 with a multifocal IOL. This is not the case with accommodating IOLs where most patients can easily read only to the J8 to J10 print size. However, I have achieved additional success by instructing patients to perform reading exercises commencing 2 to 3 weeks postimplantation of their Tetraflex lens. If they make this effort, patients can often read to the J4 level. During these exercises, patients cover their nonoperated eyes. However, if they have had both eyes implanted, they use both eyes. First, the patient should find the ideal reading distance for a test type that is easy for him or her to see (eg, J12).

Having found the ideal distance, they should then bring the print slowly toward them until their near vision starts to blur. Patients then move the print out to the ideal reading distance and start over. This exercise allows patients to relearn how to use their accommodation.

In general, I use the Tetraflex in appropriate patients who either need cataract surgery or who are having a refractive lens exchange (Figure 3). In the 18 months prior to this article being written, I had used the Tetraflex in approximately 30% of my lens extraction patients.

Personally, I have chosen the Tetraflex over other accommodating IOLs for many reasons. First, the loading technique with this lens is very straightforward and the Lenstec Web site has PDF files that demonstrate this (see www.lenstec.com/lenstec/tf_surg_info.html). It is critical to remember to have the small nub that the manufacturer has intentionally placed on the optic positioned down and to the surgeon's right side as the lens is injected into the eye. Second, this IOL centers really well. I find it very useful to dip downward as the IOL emerges from the tip of the cartridge. This will cause the leading haptic to move anteriorly as the optic emerges after it. I again dip downward as the trailing haptic emerges, and this usually results in that haptic going directly into the capsular bag. I rarely have to manipulate the IOL with a lens dialing hook with this technique and it centers automatically.

Reference

1. Wolffsohn JS, Naroo SA, Motwani NK, et al. Subjective and objective performance of the Lenstec KH-3500 "accommodative" intraocular lens. *Br J Ophthalmol.* 2006;90(6):693-696.

CHAPTER 60

SHAPE-CHANGING IOLS: POWERVISION

Louis D. "Skip" Nichamin, MD and John A. Scholl, MS

PowerVision, based in the San Francisco Bay Area, California, is currently developing a unique accommodative intraocular lens (AIOL), the FluidVision Lens, which utilizes innate ciliary body forces to transport fluid within the lens in order to achieve accommodative power. This internal fluid transfer results in a shape change, similar to that which occurs in the natural crystalline lens, thus creating an accommodative range equivalent, potentially, to that of a 35 year old.

The prepresbyopic human eye uses a combination of mechanisms to achieve a high amplitude of accommodative power. Convergence and pupillary miosis are known to increase depth of focus. Limited forward movement (50 to 150 μm) of the human crystalline lens has been observed, but this amount of movement accounts for minimal power change.[1] The vast majority of the accommodative power shift is felt to be due to the lens' ability to change its thickness and the resulting curvature of both the front and back surfaces of the lens.

Theoretical studies of other "accommodating" IOLs that function by shifting the position of the lens, or the relative proximity of a pair of lenses indicate that there is, at best, a 2.5 D potential amplitude of accommodation.[2-4]

However, changing the shape or curvature of the optic surface of an AIOL, similar to that of the native lens, should provide a much greater potential amplitude of accommodation. For an optic of 5 mm in diameter, an index of refraction of 1.49 and assuming spherical optical surfaces, a central lens thickness or sagittal height change of .2 mm will result in a 10-D shift (Figure 1). Using slightly aspheric surfaces or smaller optic diameters the movement required to achieve that same high amplitude can be reduced by 30% to 40%.

The FluidVision Lens accomplishes this shape change by moving fluid from the periphery of the lens to a central actuator under the deformable anterior surface of the IOL (Figure 2). The lens consists of anterior and posterior optic surfaces as well as a flexible internal actuator. The spaces between the optic surfaces are filled with fluid that has a matched index of refraction with the polymer layers. The haptics that surround the lens periphery are flexible tubes that are filled with the same index matched fluid. Responsive to accommodative forces in the eye, these haptics are continually reshaped by the enveloping lens capsule to move fluid in and out of the haptics. The haptic fluid communicates with the lens body through channels that allow fluid flow to displace the internal actuator.

Classic theory holds that for distance vision the ciliary muscle relaxes, opening radially, and stretches the zonules and capsular bag. In this relaxed state, the FluidVision Lens design is such that the haptic volume is maximized and fluid is directed into the haptics and away from the lens body. The lens' internal actuator, and with it the central portion of the anterior optic, moves toward the posterior optic layer, flattening the anterior optic and decreasing the lens' power. During accommodation it is similarly believed that the ciliary muscle constricts, which leads to a decrease in the tension on the zonules and the capsular bag. The elasticity of the capsular bag allows it to shrink radially. This reshaping of the capsule compresses the haptics and drives fluid into the lens body, causing it to increase the height of the actuator and thereby increase the curvature and resulting optic power of the anterior surface.

Between the anterior lens element and the actuator lies a second fluid-filled chamber that gently reshapes as the actuator goes through its range of movement. Optical quality is maintained throughout the lens' range of motion by varying the thickness of the anterior lens element centrally and thinning it toward the outer edge. The posterior lens surface incorporates the base power of the lens and does not change shape. The internal fluid channels and lens actuator are rendered invisible by matching the index of refraction of the polymeric components with the fluid, leaving only the outer lens surfaces to refract and focus light coming through the eye.

This AIOL further incorporates design features to specifically direct fluid movement in such a way that deflection at the lens surface will create the greatest optic impact; only very small volumes and pressures are needed to produce a large

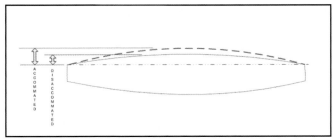

Figure 1. Lens schematic showing how a minor change to the sagittal height or curvature of the anterior lens surface will produce a dramatic optic effect (sagittal height change exaggerated for illustration, not drawn to scale).

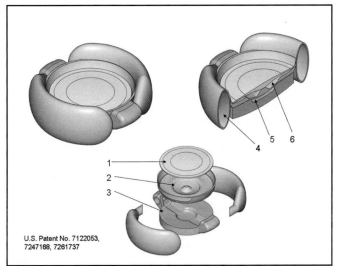

U.S. Patent No. 7122053,
7247168, 7261737

Figure 2. Section and exploded views of the FluidVision lens assembly 1) anterior optic, 2) flexible actuator, 3) posterior optic, 4) fluid-filled haptic, 5) active fluid chamber, 6) passive fluid chamber.

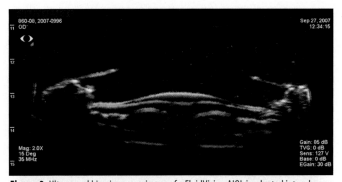

Figure 3. Ultrasound biomicroscopy image of a FluidVision AIOL implanted into a human cadaver eye. (Note: The cornea and iris have been removed for performance testing purposes.)

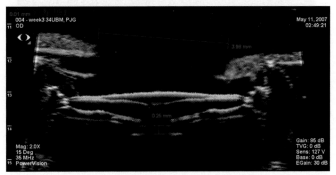

Figure 4. Ultrasound biomicroscopy image of the implanted FluidVision AIOL in patient #004 at the 3 week follow-up period.

accommodative range.

This FluidVision Lens is designed to be implanted in a manner consistent with standard practice in cataract surgery. It is introduced into the eye through a sub–4-mm clear corneal incision and is placed in the capsular bag through a 5.5-mm capsulorrhexis. Implant studies in cadaver eyes demonstrate that lens placement into the bag is very stable and maintains good centration (Figure 3).

The materials of this lens include a novel hydrophobic acrylic biomaterial and a silicone fluid. The key properties of this acrylic are clarity, resistance to fluid diffusion into or out of the lens, high elasticity (low modulus), and responsiveness. The intralenticular fluid is similar to silicone materials that have been used during retinal detachment surgery for many years. Its index of refraction is tailored to match the outer acrylic biomaterial by varying the chemical composition of the side groups attached to the silicone backbone.

Design work and analysis of the FluidVision AIOL has included extensive geometrical, finite element analysis, and optical modeling. Prototype assemblies have been performance tested using bench top test rigs and in cadaver eye studies using published techniques.[5,6] Preclinical testing of the FluidVision AIOL has included implantation of single-piece and nonfunctional but scale-sized devices representative of the lens' final geometry into rabbit eyes. This study demon-

strated biocompatibility, a lack of tissue reaction or inflammatory response, and posterior capsule opacification (PCO) all comparable to leading commercially available 3-piece acrylic IOLs.[7]

Initial clinical evaluations of the FluidVision AIOL have been conducted in a limited number of blind eye subjects using pharmacologic stimuli for both accommodation and relaxation or "disaccommodation," with subsequent imaging using the Visante OCT (Carl Zeiss Meditec, Jena, Germany). Because the AIOL was to be implanted into blind eyes, these lenses were not qualified for optical quality. They were, however, representative from a functional standpoint of early prototype designs and responsive to the movement and forces available within these surgically implanted eyes. The inclusion criteria for the clinical protocol called for patients 45 years of age or older with end-stage glaucoma, a clinically significant cataract in the study eye, and hand movements or worse acuity. Surgery entailed a limbal incision, a 5.5-mm capsulorrhexis, phacoemulsification of the cataract lens, and implantation of the lens into the capsular bag. Patient follow-up included slit lamp exams and measurement of accommodative response. Figure 4 shows a typical ultrasound biomicroscopy image of the implanted FluidVision AIOL 3 weeks postoperatively. Slit lamp exam at 3 weeks postoperative revealed a well-centered lens, quiet anterior chamber, and intraocular pressures that were lower than preoperative levels.

Accommodative response testing followed a previously presented test method[8] using pilocarpine to drive the patients to full accommodation and Cyclomydril (Alcon, Fort Worth, TX) for cycloplegia. Using the height of the active fluid

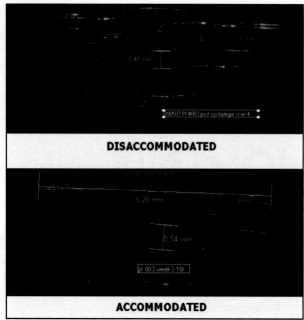

Figure 5. OCT close-up images of the implanted FluidVision AIOL in clinical patient #005 at the week 3 postoperative exam. The position of the lens at both the fully accommodated and disaccommodated positions driven by pharmacological stimulus is shown.

chamber (see Figure 1) as a measure of lens function, a significant response was observed in all subjects. Figure 5 shows a 70-μm response from patient #003 at 3 weeks postoperative.

With this initial clinical experience it has been soundly demonstrated that the human eye is capable of moving fluid in this new AIOL design causing it to reshape, becoming both thicker centrally and creating a more curved anterior lens surface. Testing of more advanced prototypes to this same level of stimulus in cadaver eye testing indicates a potential restoration consistent with 5- to 10-D accommodative amplitude in vivo. Of course, further clinical evaluations will be required to demonstrate fully the safety and efficacy of this new technology; however, the early development work and initial clinical experience have demonstrated the unique potential of the FluidVision AIOL.

References

1. Glasser A. Accommodation: mechanism and measurement. *Ophthalmol Clin N Am.* 2007;19:1-12.
2. Langenbucher A, Reese S, Jakob C, Seitz B. Pseudophakic accommodation with translation lenses—dual optic vs mono optic. *Ophthalmic Physiol Opt.* 2004;24:450-457.
3. McLeod S, Vargas L, Portnoy V, Ting A. Synchrony dual-optic accommodating intraocular lens, part 1: optical and biomechanical principles and design considerations. *J Cataract Refract Surg.* 2007;33(1):37-46.
4. Dick B. Accommodative intraocular lenses: current status. *Curr Opin Ophthalmol.* 2005;16:8-26.
5. Glasser A, Campbell M. Presbyopia and the optical changes in the human crystalline lens with age. *Vision Res.* 1998;38(2):209-229.
6. Manns F, Parel JM, Denham D, Billotte C, et al. Optomechanical response of human and monkey lenses in a lens stretcher. *Invest Ophthalmol Vis Sci.* 2007;48:3260-3268.
7. PowerVision internal document.
8. Scholl J, Gomes A, Turner S, et al. Method to characterize pharmacologically induced accommodation by anterior chamber OCT. ARVO (991/B966) 2007.

CHAPTER 61

Shape-Changing IOLs: NuLens

Jorge L. Alió, MD, PhD; Joshua Ben-Nun, MD; and Paul Kaufman, MD

In order to develop an effective accommodating intraocular lens (IOL) we defined the essential minimal physiological needs necessary to provide stable and consistent vision across all distances (near, intermediate, and far) and independent of capsular bag fibrosis and opacification. Also essential is the connection to the neuroprocessing mechanism that activates and controls the lens performances. Being an artificial device, both biocompatibility and adaptability must also be considered.

Based on these guidelines, we designed and constructed a laboratory model to prove the concept, then tested it in a primate model[1] and, finally, we tested it in an initial prospective pilot clinical study in humans.

Definition and Potential of an Effective Accommodating Intraocular Lens

Our first step was to define the essential characteristics of an ideal accommodating IOL.

* The lens much achieve at least 8 D of accommodation. This number was calculated in the following manner. 1 D for far plane adjustment plus 3 D to bring this plane to reading distance equals a total of 4 D. No system can reasonably operate at 100% capacity for long. We estimated that comfortable accommodation can be achieved by using 50% of the available accommodating forces. This is a common assumption about accommodation of the natural human lens in clinical practice. The accommodative range available in young adults[2,3] supports this assumption.

* The mechanism of action must require minimal movement of the lens. Ideally, this should be less than 500 μm of anterior posterior movement. IOL movements up to 500 μm have been documented.[4,5] Therefore, if move-

ment is needed to operate such an IOL, it should be within this range.

* The lens must overcome issues of capsular contraction and posterior capsular opacification (PCO). Once the lens capsule is opened during the cataract surgery it will naturally scar. PCO is also a byproduct of the surgical injury.[6,7] An effective accommodating IOL must overcome these potential problems, otherwise consistent performance of the accommodating lens will be impossible.

* There must be a real-time control mechanism with a feedback loop. The accommodating process in the lens must follow the brain's commands and neuroprocessing for accommodation must be possible in real time by focusing on the preferred target.

* The lens must be made of biocompatible materials to avoid toxicity effects on the ocular tissue.

NuLens Physical Concept

A simple physical phenomenon was identified as a possible mechanism for an accommodating IOL. A flexible material is contained between 2 rigid plates. The anterior plates have a central, round aperture. When the plates are compressed, the flexible material will be forced into the central aperture of the anterior plate and will "bulge" through the aperture (Figure 1). If the flexible material is transparent, this "bulge" may become a lens that may change in radius of curvature and power in proportion to the pressure applied.

Laboratory Model

A metal ring, 15 mm in diameter and 3 mm in height, was glued to a glass base. A flexible and transparent membrane was attached to the other side of the ring creating a chamber. Through a small valve in the ring the chamber was filled with

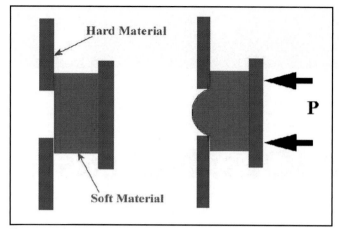

Figure 1. Mechanical model of the lens concept. The flexible material (red color) is being pressed (P) between 2 hard surfaces to create a bulge through a hole in one of these surfaces.

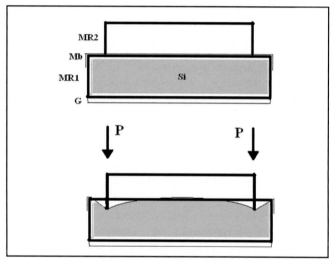

Figure 2. Scheme of the laboratory model of the lens. A large metal ring (MR1) is bounded by a glass (G) surface on one side and a flexible membrane (Mb) on the other side. The space between is filled with silicone fluid (blue). A second metal ring (MR2) smaller in diameter is attached to the flexible membrane. By pressing (P) the smaller ring (MR2) toward the larger ring (MR1) a lens is created within the smaller ring.

a flexible silicone gel (6300M-A, refractive index 1.41, Nusil USA). A second metallic ring, 10 mm in diameter and 3 mm in height was attached to the outer part of the flexible membrane. Gentle pressure on the outer ring created a bulge, generating over 50 D of converging optical power (Figure 2).

Animal Model

The most similar animal model to the human visual system is the monkey; therefore, it is often used for research simulating treatment in human eyes.[6-9] A special force gauge device was implanted first in 8 Macaca fasicularis (cynomolgus) monkeys and was used to obtain essential data regarding the physical characteristics for the proposed concept. This data was also needed to determine if the proposed mechanism of action was feasible and the parameters that affect the IOL design and construction. All the animals are still being followed for assessing long-term effects of postoperative scar-

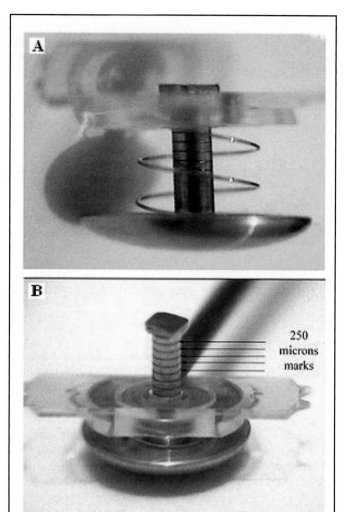

Figure 3. The measurement gauge in open (A) and closed (B) positions. The markings on the center pole are 250 μm apart and can easily be detected by inspection with the surgical microscope.

ring and contraction on the capsular diaphragm. In a second animal investigation (University of Wisconsin, Madison, WI), a similar monkey model was used. Completely iridectomized monkeys were implanted with the investigative device and the performance of the lens was investigated using direct electrical stimulation of the Edinger-Westphal (E-W) nucleus to induce accommodative movements of the ciliary muscle.[10-12]

Measurement Gauge

A special force gauge was constructed to measure the movements and forces that the capsular diaphragm applies along the visual axis (Figure 3). The gauge comprised a base plate, calibrated spring, and a marked rod that moved forward into the anterior chamber (AC) in response to the pressure applied on it by the movements of the capsular diaphragm. This force gauge effectively mimics the operational concept of the proposed IOL. Direct inspection of the AC afforded assessment of the position of the pin above the base plate, which was marked and calculated.

The investigative device was implanted in one eye of 8 monkeys. Each gauge in the implanted device had a spring that

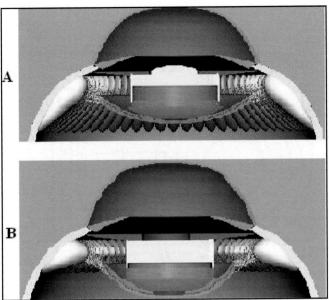

Figure 4. Animated images of the IOL conceptual model as placed in the posterior chamber of the eye. (A) Relaxed ciliary muscle stretches the capsular diaphragm to create a secondary lens (bulge) in the front surface of the lens. (B) Contracted ciliary muscle releases the capsular diaphragm and with no pressure on the flexible material the secondary lens gradually diminishes to a plane surface with zero refractive power.

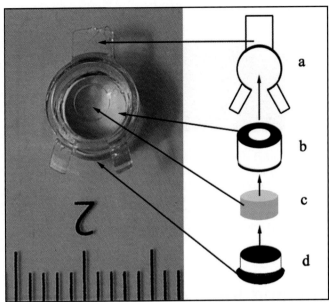

Figure 5. (Left) A constructed prototype of the accommodating IOL. (Right) A scheme of the sub-units that were used to construct the lens: (a) Y-shaped haptic made of PMMA with an open circle in its center to hold the main body of the optic. (b) PMMA cylinder with an aperture in its front surface. (c) silicone gel cylinder that fits the inner side of the PMMA cylinder. (d) PMMA piston that press the silicone to bulge through the aperture in the front face of the PMMA cylinder.

was calibrated to have slightly different elastic properties. The varying elastic properties allow us to test the system against alternate forces. Measurements were taken under 3 different circumstances—total muscle relaxation with the monkey being artificially ventilated, under normal muscle tone, and under pharmacologic ciliary body contraction induced by 2% pilocarpine. All measurements were documented through the surgical microscope on a videotape.

First NuLens Accommodating IOL Prototype

The first prototype was constructed in such way that it would be possible to document the lens dynamics (Figure 4) by ultrasound biomicroscopy (UBM; model P40, Paradigm Medical Industries, Salt Lake City, UT). The dynamic lens had to be formed in the AC because the UBM is limited to effective readouts at up to 3.0-mm depth and also because the UBM cannot produce accurate readings through silicone. The first prototype was constructed from 3 polymethylmethacrylate (PMMA) subunits and a flexible silicone-gel (Figure 5). Due to the large prototype size, it was implanted in 2 stages.

First Monkey Study

This surgery was conducted while the monkey was under general anesthesia, total muscle paralysis, and artificial ventilation. The lens content was removed by microincision surgery (MICS) through a 4.0-mm central capsulorrhexis and the anterior capsule was collapsed on the posterior capsule. The NuLens prototype was implanted in the sulcus with the help of specially designed instruments. After implantation of the

device, pharmacological stimulation of the ciliary muscle was achieved at different times postoperatively by intracameral injection of acetylcholine, topical application of 2% pilocarpine, 1% atropine, 1% cyclopentolate to estimate the range from no muscarinic input to maximum muscarinic input. UBM documented the bulging of the silicone through the anterior hole and measured its radius of curvature. The refractive index was known so it was possible to calculate the dioptric power of the lens formed by the bulging. Because this lens model generated power by direct pressure of the piston on the contained silicone gel, the recovery from anesthesia resulted in increased muscle tone and therefore a more relaxed capsular diaphragm and a reduction in lens curvature that results in reduced power of the secondary lens.

The maximum movement along the visual axis between full relaxation of the ciliary muscle and strong cyclospasm was approximately 800 µm. Induction of moderate ciliary body spasm by 2% pilocarpine or cycloplegia by 1% cyclopentolate resulted in mean movement of 350 µm. Although the initial setup of each device was related to the strength of the spring, the mean movement of 350 µm was consistent for all devices.

The same measurements were taken 3 months postoperatively to test the effect of capsular contraction. The baseline position of the rod under sedation shifted forward approximately 250 µm (Figure 6 [left]). This indicated stretching of the capsular diaphragm due to fibrosis of the capsular bag. Two percent pilocarpine was applied and resulted in ciliary muscle contraction, which caused backward movement of the rod, returning it to the basic position of the gauge 350 µm backwards (Figure 6 [right]), compensating for the forward shift of the rod resulting from the fibrotic process.

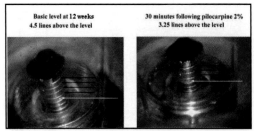

Figure 6. Photograph of the measuring device in the monkey AC 12 weeks after implantation. The original postoperative setup of the gauge was 3 lines above the level (white line). Due to fibrosis of the capsule the pressure on the spring increased and the new setup came to be 4.5 lines above the level. Using topical pilocarpine 2% the new setup returned to the postoperative level, overcoming the effect of the capsular scarring by ciliary muscle contraction.

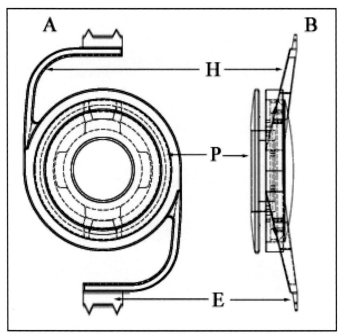

Figure 7. Schematic description of the second-generation accommodating IOL. (A) view from the back. (B) view from the side. Haptics (H) with the fine "end-plates" (E) and the micro-pins that enables stable sulcus fixation. The piston (P) is the back part of the lens and in its center a hole enables the formation of the dynamic lens.

Second Monkey Study

This study evaluated the IOL response to neurostimulation of the E-W nucleus causing maximal contraction of the ciliary body.[13] Animals were prepared by initial surgical removal of the iris[14] from both eyes. Microelectrodes were implanted into the E-W nucleus.[10,12] The whole process takes a few weeks to complete. The force gauge was implanted in one eye and the IOL prototype (Figure 7) in the other. Topical and systemic steroids were given during the early postoperative period and then as necessary to overcome the initial inflammatory response. Measurements were taken beginning approximately 4 weeks postdevice implantation. The animal was anesthetized and the head was held by a supporting device while the examined eye was fixated to avoid eye movements during the stimulation. Stimulation at increasing intensity levels was given, starting at a no response level and growing to a no change level. During stimulation, refraction of the eye with the IOL and video-recording to document the response of the force gauge in the other eye were performed.

The force gauge consistently showed 400-μm movements during 1 year of follow-up. Some forward shift of the gauge from its original position at implantation was noted. Such shift indicates contraction of the capsular diaphragm. The implanted lenses provided an initial 80% of the designed dioptric power of the lens (10 out 12 D). Six months after implantation this early prototype lens was performing at approximately 40% of the designed optical power. This decrease in the accommodative amplitude was thought to be related to the capsular contraction. By readjustment of the IOL position in the eye, using the IOL built-in adjustment mechanism, the IOL performances improved to approximately 50% of the initial design and remained stable at the last check-up (14 months after implantation). We emphasize that the results were obtained in only a few eyes and therefore must be regarded as preliminary.

Pilot Human Study

Due to the high accommodative power observed in the experimental monkey study, the NuLens was proposed as a low-vision aid for age-related macular degeneration patients.

Following the Ethical Board Committee approval of Vissum-Instituto Oftalmologico de Alicante and the Spanish Ministry of Health official approval, 10 patients with stable atrophic forms of age-related macular degeneration were scheduled to be implanted in the worst eye with a NuLens prototype. The age of the patients ranged from 74 to 82 years. Written informed consent following full explanation of the potential of the lens to improve near vision was obtained from all patients. They were all instructed that following implantation, they should be able to experience improved near vision without any specific effort other than to find the adequate focus for near (the prototype to be implanted was going to make them myopic to a calculated magnitude), and that the focus for far should be made on demand. All surgeries were performed by the same surgeon (JLA). There were no complications.

The lens was well tolerated in all cases. There was no inflammatory reaction or subjective symptoms appearing in any case. Following week 1, the patients all exhibited uniformly improved near vision. Far vision was also tested, remaining in most of the cases stable or with slight improvement. The patients' adaptation to this accommodative NuLens model was almost immediate, with no patient requiring specific training. In Figures 8 and 9, we present the preliminary results of this pilot group up to 3 months postoperation. In Figure 8, the average distance visual acuity (Snellen chart) is presented. Note there is only slight improvement shortly after surgery followed by some deterioration over time due to the development of PCO in a few eyes. In Figure 9, near visual acuity is presented measured as the lowest line read in the low vision reading chart. Patients were free to choose the reading distance that they found most suitable. A slight decrease in acuity due to the development of PCO was noted to have negative

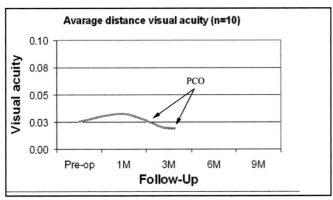

Figure 8. The average distance visual acuity (Snellen chart).

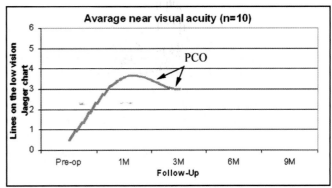

Figure 9. Near visual acuity is presented measured as the lowest line read in the low vision reading chart.

effects on both distance and near visual acuity of the affected eyes. These patients were scheduled for yttrium-aluminum-garnet (YAG) capsulotomy at later time of around 6 months postoperation.

Discussion

Various approaches and designs for accommodating IOLs have been introduced and studied. Although differing in operational concept and design, all of these concepts share 2 principal characteristics. The optical surfaces of these lenses are of fixed power. They are placed next to each other in circles or move along the visual axis as a single lens or dual-optic system.[15-17] These lenses must be accurately centered in the capsular bag for both adequate function and to avoid side effects.

We tried to define the minimal power that an accommodating IOL should generate to avoid any dependence on reading glasses. The accommodative mechanism of young adults can be used as a reference to what nature provides for comfortable accommodation. From studies on this subject[2,3] it seems that this range is between 7 to 10 D. We therefore concluded that an IOL needs to provide approximately 8 D of accommodation to replace the full functional range of distance to near vision. This should minimize side effects such as ocular strain and headache due to fatigue of the ciliary muscle resulting from a lack of accommodative reserve.

We reviewed other accommodating IOL designs and recognized that they would not be able to provide the desired amount of accommodation. It became apparent that the best way to create a dynamic, accommodating IOL was to design one with the ability to change its radius of curvature by applying minimal external force and movement.[18] Utilizing the capsular bag as a component of a moving diaphragm consisting of the collapsed capsular bag, zonules, and ciliary processes, a new mechanical system was developed. In this new design, the dynamic diaphragm could serve to transfer force from the contracting ciliary muscle to any "D generating device" placed near it. The second step was to establish a stable reference plane in front of the dynamic diaphragm to harness these dynamic forces. Once the rigid reference plane is internally fixated by the sclera or the AC angle, a flexible material can be confined between the rigid plane and the capsular diaphragm. The movements of the capsular diaphragm transfer forces that

deform the flexible material through a hole in the rigid anterior reference plane or through the posteriorly pushing piston to create the secondary lens.

It is interesting to note that a similar concept for generating high accommodative forces exists in nature. Water birds such as mergansers, cormorants, penguins, and others are able to compensate for the changes of refractive indexes between air and water. These birds, which possess a very strong sphincter muscle in the iris, have evolved a technique whereby they force the soft crystalline lens to bulge through the rigid iris. The mechanism can dramatically increase the curvature of the crystalline lens. Creating this secondary lens can generate over 70 D of accommodation in certain species.[19]

NuLens Experimental Evidence

Monkeys were selected for the preclinical study because they have an accommodative system that is similar to that of humans. The IOL prototype generated 44 D of accommodative range as documented by UBM imaging between cyclospasm and cycloplegia (see Figure 6) in the study eye. In general, the secondary lens power is related to the refractive index of the flexible material and the radius of curvature of the secondary lens. These parameters can be easily modified to result in double and triple the amount of refractive change. There was a shift in force range seen between the preclinical and clinical model. A lens having the theoretical potential of over 100 D of accommodative range will allow relatively simple adaptation to provide a final add of only 8 D to 10 D of accommodation. We believe this is sufficient to provide comfortable near vision in an emmetropic human eye. The capability of this concept to produce strong refractive power changes has significant design advantages. It enables construction of 6.0-mm lenses with 4.0-mm to 5.0-mm holes for the dynamic lens. Another significant advantage of using the capsular diaphragm as the force-generating element is its internal substructure. The collapsed capsule is expected to scar and contract to an unpredictable extent.

The lenses that were used in this study generated power by direct pressure of the piston on the silicone gel, with maximal power achieved when the ciliary muscle relaxes. It is therefore necessary for the visual system to adapt to operating the focusing mechanism in a different way than was used with the crystalline lens. Clinical evidence from overcorrected myopia supports such a mechanism. Our preliminary results from the monkey preclinical experiments indicate rapid and uncomplicated adjustment to such a reverse mechanism. It is also possible to incorporate a spring-like element into the lens to reverse the mode of the secondary dynamic lens shape so that the lens is operated by the contraction of the ciliary muscle. Currently both models are being studied to learn the advantages and disadvantages of each mode of operation until enough data are accumulated to indicate the preferred alternative.

Future Development of the NuLens True Accommodative IOL

The immediate development of the NuLens project will consist of reducing the incision size to 5 mm. A suitable foldable platform has been designed jointly with an adequate PMMA structure that will allow the mechanism to work without necessitating the large incision performed in the pilot investigation. Neuroadaptation as used in this investigation appears to work in humans and nonhuman primates. A model that approaches the normal mechanism of accommodation has also been designed and is expected to be tested during 2008.

References

1. Ben-nun J, Alio JL. Feasibility and development of a high-power real accommodating intraocular lens. *J Cataract Refract Surg.* 2005;31:1802-1808.

2. Wold JE, Hu A, Chen S, Glasser A. Subjective and objective measurement of human accommodative amplitude. *J Cataract Refract Surg.* 2003;29:1878-1888.

3. Atchison DA, Claydon CA, Irwin SE. Amplitude of accommodation for different head positions and different directions of gaze. *Optom Vis Sci.* 1994;71:339-345.

4. Findl O, Kiss B, Petternel V, Menapace R, Georgopoulos M, Rainer G, Drexler W. Intraocular lens movement caused by ciliary muscle contraction. *J Cataract Refract Surg.* 2003;29:669-676.

5. Lesiewska-Junk H, Kaluzny J. Intraocular lens movement and accommodation in eyes of young patients. *J Cataract Refract Surg.* 2000;26:562-565.

6. Birinci H, Kuruoglu S, Oge I, Oge F, Acar E. Effect of intraocular lens and anterior capsule opening type on posterior capsule opacification. *J Cataract Refract Surg.* 1999;25:1140-1146.

7. Hayashi Y, Kato S, Fukushima H, Numaga J, Kaiya T, Tamaki Y, Oshika T. Relationship between anterior capsule contraction and posterior capsule opacification after cataract surgery in patients with diabetes mellitus. *J Cataract Refract Surg.* 2004;30:1517-1520.

8. Brooks DE, Kallberg ME, Cannon RL, Komaromy AM, Ollivier FJ, Malakhova OE, Dawson WW, Sherwood MB, Kuekuerichkina EE, Lambrou GN. Functional and structural analysis of the visual system in the rhesus monkey model of optic nerve head ischemia. *Invest Ophthalmol Vis Sci.* 2004;45:1830-1840.

9. Cottaris NP, De Valois RL. Temporal dynamics of chromatic tuning in macaque primary visual cortex. *Nature.* 1998;395:896-900.

10. Crawford K, Terasawa E, Kaufman PL. Reproducible stimulation of ciliary muscle contraction in the cynomolgus monkey via a permanent indwelling midbrain electrode. *Brain Res.* 1989;503:265-272.

11. Neider MW, Crawford K, Kaufman PL, Bito LZ. In vivo videography of the rhesus monkey accommodative apparatus. Age-related loss of ciliary muscle response to central stimulation. *Arch Ophthalmol.* 1990;108:69-74.

12. Croft MA, Glasser A, Heatley G, et al. Accommodative ciliary body and lens function in rhesus monkeys: I. Normal lens, zonule and ciliary process configuration in the iridectomized eye. *Invest Ophthalmol Vis Sci.* 2006;47(3):1076-1086.

13. Kaufman LP. Accommodation and presbyopia: neuromuscular and biophysical aspects. In: Kaufman LP, ed, Adler's Physiology of the Eye, ninth edition. St. Louis, Missouri: Mosby-Year Book Inc; 1992:396.

13. Kaufman LP. Accommodation and presbyopia: neuromuscular and biophysical aspects. In: Kaufman LP, ed, *Adler's Physiology of the Eye, ninth edition.* St. Louis, Missouri: Mosby-Year Book Inc; 1992:396.

14. Kaufman PL, Lütjen-Drecoll E. Total iridectomy in the primate in vivo: surgical technique and postoperative anatomy. *Invest Ophthalmol.* 1975;14:766-771.

15. Brydon KW, Tokarewicz AC, Nichols BD. AMO array multifocal lens versus monofocal correction in cataract surgery. *J Cataract Refract Surg.* 2000;26:96-100.

16. Kuchle M, Seitz B, Langenbucher A, Gusek-Schneider GC, Martus P, Nguyen NX; The Erlangen Accommodative Intraocular Lens Study Group. Comparison of 6-month results of implantation of the 1CU accommodative intraocular lens with conventional intraocular lenses. *Ophthalmology.* 2004;111:318-324.

17. Rana A, Miller D, Magnante P. Understanding the accommodating intraocular lens. *J Cataract Refract Surg.* 2003;29:2284-2287.

18. Lesiewska-Junk H, Kaluzny J. Intraocular lens movement and accommodation in eyes of young patients. *J Cataract Refract Surg.* 2000;26:562-565.

19. Sivak JG, Hildebrand T, Lebert C. Magnitude and rate of accommodation in diving and nondiving birds. *Vision Res.* 1985;25:925-933.

CHAPTER 62

CALHOUN LIGHT ADJUSTABLE LENS— PRESBYOPIA CORRECTION

Arturo Chayet, MD; Federico Badala, MD; Christian Sandstedt, PhD;
Shiao Chang, PhD; Paul Rhee, OD; and Daniel M. Schwartz, MD

The multifocal intraocular lenses (IOLs) (refractive, diffractive) that are currently available possess potential drawbacks that prevent them from gaining widespread clinical acceptance. These deficiencies include the unpredictability and inconsistency in achieving emmetropia and perfect IOL centration after surgery. Other problems are variability in patient pupil size and the variability of patients' tolerance of glare, halos, and the loss of contrast. The IOLs themselves do not reverse pre-existing astigmatism, and the procedure is difficult to reverse if the optics are poorly tolerated (ie, explant). In order to address these limitations, Calhoun Vision, Inc (Pasadena, CA) has developed the Light Adjustable Lens (LAL), which enables postoperative, noninvasive adjustment of lens power using ultraviolet (UV) light. The LAL has received CE Mark and is being used in Europe and Latin America to correct postoperative spherical and toric refractive errors. Adjustment of LAL power is performed with a digital light delivery (DLD) device that can be customized to project complex patterns of UV light onto the LAL. The LAL captures these patterns faithfully and this allows surgeons to correct for higher-order aberrations in patients implanted with the LAL. Recently, we have implanted patients with an LAL and postoperatively used the DLD to correct not only defocus but also to "write" a customized multifocal pattern onto the LAL. This approach to creating both emmetropia and a multifocal optic in situ is an appealing alternative to conventional multifocal IOLs.

The LAL consists of photosensitive silicone macromeres embedded in a silicone matrix.[1-3] It has a foldable 6-mm optic and polymethylmethacrylate (PMMA) haptics, similar to conventional silicone IOLs. Spatially modulated polymerization of macromere with the DLD initiates diffusion of unpolymerized macromere into irradiated zones and a change in LAL shape. By projecting appropriate patterns of UV light onto the LAL, precise shape changes are effected. Patients are refracted 1 to 4 weeks after cataract surgery with the LAL and then undergo LAL adjustment with the DLD. Treatment times are between 60 and 120 seconds. The LAL receives a second "lock-in" dose 1 to 4 days after adjustment to polymerize remaining macromere. Following cataract surgery, patients are instructed to wear special UV-blocking spectacles until the LAL is adjusted and locked in. Following lock-in, no protective eyewear is required.

Initial clinical studies with the LAL conducted by the author and Dr. Jose Güell in Barcelona, Spain have confirmed that for spherical refractive errors between +2 and −2 D, adjustments are within 0.25 D of the intended refractive result in more than 90% of cases. Astigmatic adjustment of up to 1.25 D has also been performed in patients implanted with the LAL.

Early in vitro studies conducted at Calhoun Vision, Inc using the DLD demonstrated that the DLD could create a multifocal IOL by projecting the appropriate pattern of light onto a monofocal LAL.[3] Initially, a bulls-eye multifocal optic was written onto the LAL, which could be either near or distance dominant. Furthermore, the optical power and zone size could be readily customized simply by programming the DLD. In Figure 1A and 1B, 2 separate bulls-eye multifocal optics have been written onto a monofocal LAL and are depicted using laser interferometry. In Figure 1C, an annular multifocal pattern has been created. Because in vivo these multifocal patterns would be written postoperatively, it would be easy to customize zone size and power based on each patient's pupillary diameter and visual needs. Furthermore, the ability to correct residual refractive error potentially provides each patient the reassurance that he or she can avoid refractive laser in situ keratomileusis (LASIK) "touch-ups."

Because of recent enthusiasm for the ReSTOR diffractive optic multifocal IOL (Alcon, Fort Worth, TX), Calhoun Vision, Inc tested whether a diffractive optic could also be written onto a monofocal LAL. In vitro experiments showed this was possible. Figure 2 shows a phase contrast image and three-dimensional (3-D) wavefront, respectively, of a diffractive optic written onto a monofocal LAL using the DLD.

Figure 3 shows United States Air Force targets imaged through the diffractive multifocal LAL and compare the resolution to a ReSTOR multifocal IOL. A first iteration of

Figure 1. Laser interferograms.

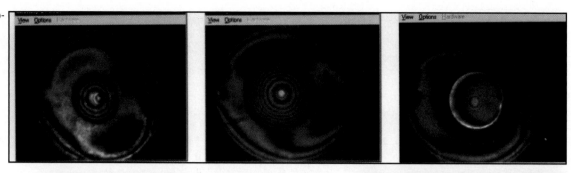

Figure 2. Diffracted LAL.

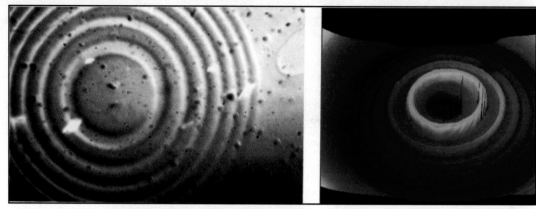

Figure 3. US Air Force target images.

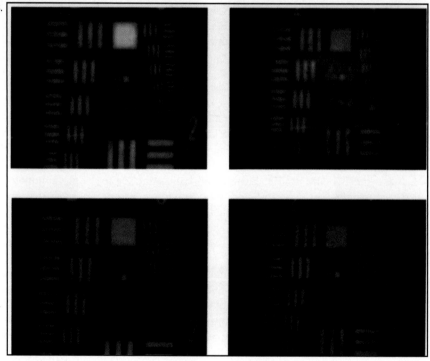

the diffractive multifocal LAL shows that resolution is nearly comparable to the ReSTOR lens.

Based on these in vitro studies, we wished to see whether a multifocal LAL could be written in vivo.

Case Report 1

A 63-year-old male underwent uncomplicated phacoemulsification and implantation of a +19.0-D, monofocal LAL in his right eye. At 2 weeks postimplantation, the patient presented with a manifest refraction of −1.25 D Sph −0.50 D × 7 degrees. The uncorrected visual acuity (UCVA) and best-corrected visual acuity (BCVA) were 20/60- and 20/20-2, respectively. The DLD was employed to correct the myopia and simultaneously write a progressive, multifocal pattern onto the LAL. The 2 day postadjustment refraction was Plano −0.50 D x 5 degrees. UCVA was 20/20-2 and the BCVA was 20/20-1. Near vision without correction was J1. The patient's refraction 9 months postoperatively was stable with a UCVA of 20/20-2 and near vision of J1 without correction. To

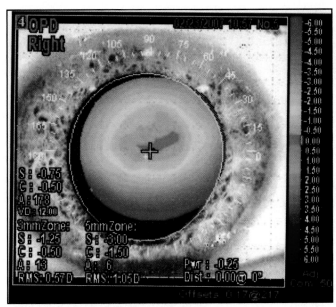

Figure 4. Case 1 wavefront at 9 months postadjustment.

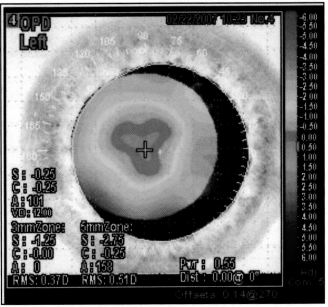

Figure 5. Case 2 wavefront at 9 months postadjustment.

understand the visual mechanism upon which this adjustment is based, it is instructive to view the 9-month post adjustment wavefront of this patient's eye (Figure 4). Inspection of the exit pupil wavefront and comparison with the color-coded dioptric power scale on the right-hand side of the figure indicates that the central part of the wavefront is corrected for distance vision; however, as you move out from the center of the wavefront toward the edges, the power in the periphery becomes progressively more negative, permitting both simultaneous distance and near vision for the patient. Another unique aspect shown in this multifocal wavefront is its gradual, progressive nature. Current diffractive and refractive multifocal IOLs possess sharp discontinuities in the alternating powered zones that produce significant glare and halos to the patient. Inspection of the measured wavefront of the adjusted LAL indicates a gradual increase in power in moving from the periphery to the edge of the pupil and the absence of any sharp demarcation between the different powers.

Case Report 2

A 66-year-old male patient underwent standard cataract surgery with phacoemulsification and implantation of a +19.5-D, monofocal LAL in his left eye. The patient presented with a manifest refraction of -1.50 D Sph −0.50 D × 115 degrees at 2 weeks postimplantation. The UCVA and BCVA were 20/60- and 20/25, respectively. The DLD was again employed to correct the existing myopia and simultaneously write a progressive, multifocal pattern onto the LAL. The 1 day postadjustment refraction was −0.50 −0.25 D x 140 degrees. The UCVA was 20/25-2 and the BCVA was 20/25. The patient's refraction was −0.25 −0.50 D x 100 degrees at 9

months postadjustment and lock-in, with a UCVA of 20/25-1, a BCVA of 20/20-2, and near vision of J1 without correction. As with the first case study, it is instructive to view the 9-month postadjustment wavefront of this patient's eye (Figure 5). Inspection of the exit pupil wavefront and comparison with the color-coded dioptric power scale on the right-hand side of the figure indicates that the central part of the wavefront is again corrected for emmetropia; however, as you move out from the center of the wavefront toward the edges, the power in the periphery becomes progressively more negative, permitting both simultaneous distance and near vision for the patient. This measured wavefront is also absent of any sharp differences in adjacent power zones, indicating that the applied correction minimizes any postadjustment glare and halos.

Conclusion

Adjusting the LAL and creating not only emmetropia, but also a multifocal optic is now being done successfully in patients. The versatility of the DLD enables customization of the multifocal pattern for pupillary size, residual astigmatism, and also the particular visual needs of each patient.

References

1. Schwartz DM. Light-adjustable lens. *Trans Am Ophthalmol Soc.* 2003;101:417-436.
2. Schwartz DM, Sandstedt CA, Chang SH, et al. Light-adjustable lens: development of in vitro nomograms. *Trans Am Ophthalmol Soc.* 2004;102:67-72; discussion 72-74.
3. Sandstedt CA, Chang SH, Grubbs RH, Schwartz DM. Light adjustable lens: customizing correction for multifocality and higher order aberrations. *Trans Am Ophthalmol Soc.* 2006;104:29-39.

CHAPTER 63

CALHOUN LIGHT ADJUSTABLE LENS— PRESBYOPIA CORRECTION

Jose L. Güell, MD; Merce Morral, MD; Felicidad Manero, MD; Maite Sisquella, OPT; and Daniel Schwartz, MD

Despite advances in biometry and the increasingly sophisticated technical aspects of cataract surgery, many patients still require spectacles postoperatively to achieve emmetropia due to an incorrect intraocular lens (IOL) power selection. Specifically, calculations of IOL power are sometimes imprecise because of inaccurate preoperative measurements, postoperative astigmatism, or variability in the final position of the IOL inside the eye.[1] This is especially true in cases of high ametropias or in those patients who have had corneal refractive surgery.[2] As the refractive surgery population ages and begins developing cataracts, appropriate selection of IOL power for these patients will become an increasingly challenging clinical problem.

Previous investigators have recognized the need for an IOL with the capacity of postoperative power adjustment.[3-8] However, these lens designs require invasive adjustment procedures and do not allow correction of astigmatism and higher-order aberrations. Therefore, a means to postoperatively adjust spherical and astigmatic errors after cataract surgery in a noninvasive way would be desirable. In 2000, Dan Schwartz hypothesized that a light-adjustable lens (LAL) could be designed, and a collaboration with scientists at the California Institute of Technology was established. Taking advantage of silicone's low glass transition temperature and resultant facility with which silicone molecules can diffuse in a silicone polymer matrix at body temperature, they developed an adjustable silicone IOL whose power is adjusted noninvasively using low levels of light energy.[9,10] This technology of a silicone lens whose power can be adjusted using light energy may be applied not only in pseudophakic IOLs but also for phakic IOLs, intracorneal lenses, and contact lenses, enabling fine-tuning of our refractive procedures. Moreover, it may be used as part of an injectable lens that refills the capsular bag to restore accommodation.

Basic Science

The currently existing LAL is a 3-piece silicone lens with blue polymethylmethacrylate (PMMA) modified-C haptics, a 6-mm biconvex optic, an overall length of 13 mm, and a dioptric range from 17 to 24 D (Figure 1A).

The silicone formulation is based upon a silicone matrix system composed of polymer, resin, cross-linker, and platinum catalyst. Dispersed within the matrix are low-molecular weight silicone macromer molecules with photoreactive chain ends, benzoin-based photoinitiator with activity at 365 nm, and ultraviolet (UV) absorbers that allow for efficient photoinitiation and adequate UV protection for the retina in the pseudophakic eye.[10,11]

The Light Delivery Device (LDD) consists of a UV light source, projection optics, and control interface installed on a standard slit lamp. The LDD delivers a beam with a center wavelength of 365 nm and a selected spatial intensity profile and diameter to produce a predictable change in the power of the LAL.[11]

The adjustment of the LAL is highly reproducible (within 0.25 D of the desired power). Therefore, appropriate digital irradiation spatial intensity patterns were created to develop nomograms in which adjusted power varies as a function of treatment duration and intensity for correction of myopia, hyperopia, and astigmatism in 0.25-D steps. In vitro studies demonstrated that power changes were reproducible and did not alter optical quality of the LALs. Further, lock-in dosing of the LALs did not alter optical quality nor significantly change LAL power.[12]

Irradiation of the LAL with spatially modulated 365-nm UV light causes the photosensitive macromers to polymerize and form silicone polymers in the irradiated region. For example, if a central zone is irradiated, macromers polymerize in that region alone. Following this polymerization, macromers in the peripheral unirradiated portions of the IOL are highly concentrated relative to the central irradiated zone where they have been depleted by the irradiation. This creates a thermodynamically unstable diffusion gradient that is corrected over 12 to 15 hours as macromers diffuse toward the irradiated region to once again establish a uniform concentration throughout the matrix. As the macromers migrate centrally, this portion

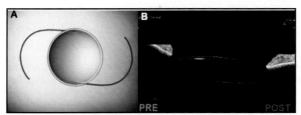

Figure 1. (A) Calhoun LAL. (B) Anterior segment optical coherence tomography (Visante OCT; Carl Zeiss Meditec, Jena, Germany) of the LAL before (green line) and after (blue line) hyperopic adjustment treatment.

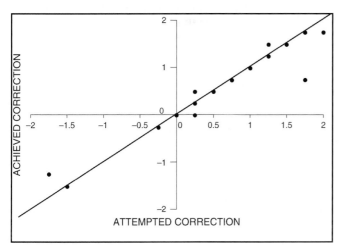

Figure 2. Achieved versus attempted refractive power adjustment of the first 20 LAL implanted by Dr. Güell since June 2006. Three eyes had intended-achieved correction of 0 D, 2 eyes had intended-achieved correction of 0.5 D, and 2 eyes had intended-achieved correction of 1.25 D.

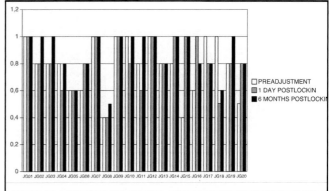

Figure 3. BSCVA before and 6 months after adjustment. None of the eyes lost any line of BSCVA.

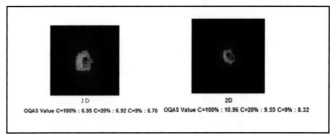

Figure 4. PSF measured by the OQAS of the (A) AcrySof IOL and the (B) Calhoun LAL. Both lenses show excellent optical quality.

of the lens swells and refractive power increases to correct hyperopia (Figure 1B). By irradiating the peripheral portion of the lens, macromer migrates outward, causing a decrease in lens power and producing a myopic correction. The refractive index of the macromer is designed to match the silicone matrix for optimal optical compatibility; therefore, the power change of the LAL upon irradiation is induced primarily by the shape (radius of curvature) change.[11,12]

Once the appropriate power adjustment is achieved, the entire lens is irradiated to polymerize the remaining reactive macromer, thus preventing additional change in lens power. By irradiating the entire lens, macromer diffusion resulting from concentration gradient does not occur, and thus no change in lens power results. This second irradiation procedure is referred to as "lock-in."[11]

In clinical trials, LAL power has effectively been adjusted and locked in over a range of 4 D (–2 to + 2 D) with one light adjustment. Following adjustment, optical quality has been maintained. Astigmatic adjustments have also been introduced, with promising preliminary results. In vitro studies have developed multifocal LAL profiles, and simultaneous correction of defocus and spherical aberration.[13] Finally, new projects in wavefront-guided adjustments are being developed.[12,13]

Clinical Results

The following graphs show the clinical results of the first 20 eyes that underwent LAL implantation since June 2006 by Dr.

Güell at Instituto de Microcirugia Ocular (IMO), Barcelona, Spain. All the patients had LAL implantation in one eye and AcrySof SA60AT IOL (Alcon, Fort Worth, TX) implantation in the fellow eye. Figure 2 shows achieved versus attempted refractive correction in 17 hyperopic and 3 myopic adjustments. Ninety percent (18 of 20) of the eyes achieved ± 0.25 D of the attempted correction. Figure 3 shows best-spectacle corrected visual acuity (BSCVA) before and 6 months after adjustment. None of the eyes lost any line of BSCVA.

All the patients had LAL implantation in one eye and AcrySof SA60AT IOL implantation in the fellow eye. Figure 4 shows the point-spread function (PSF) measured by the Optical Quality Analysis System (OQAS) (Visiometrics SL, Terrassa, Spain) of the (A) AcrySof IOL and (B) the Calhoun LAL. Both lenses show excellent optical quality.

Finally, Figure 5 shows the experience on the LAL for astigmatic treatments.

Pseudoaccommodation

Multifocal IOLs have been designed to respond to patients' increasing demands for spectacle independence. Currently, distance emmetropia is not enough for most patients, as they also desire intermediate distance and near activities without spectacle correction.

Implantation of multifocal IOLs in which patients may be spectacle free for both near and distance has further increased the need for precise IOL power calculation. Moreover, optimization of visual function after implantation of a multifocal IOL is dependent on controlling several variables, including astigmatism,[14] pupil size, and decentration.[15] The capability

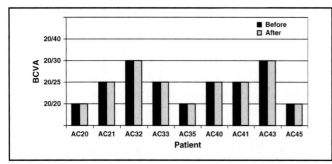

Figure 5. BSCVA before and after test toric treatments.

for in situ creation of a customized multifocal LAL centered on the visual axis and adapted to patient's pupil size in both photopic and scotopic conditions may reduce the undesired adverse events of multifocal IOLs, such as glare and halos. Spatial intensity patterns were designed to create a multifocal optic with customized power and diameter, while simultaneously correcting defocus and spherical aberration. In vitro creation of multifocal patterns demonstrated ability to reproducibly customize zone diameter and power. Both bull's-eye bifocal and annular patterns were successfully created on LAL. Central adds ranging from + 2.0 to + 3.5 D with zone diameters ranging from 1.5 to 2 mm were demonstrated with the bull's-eye pattern. Application of the annular pattern showed that an annular zone ranging from +2.25 to + 2.8 D was written around either an unchanged or −2.5 D-corrected LAL central 2-mm region. Spherical aberration was reduced simultaneously with correction of hyperopia and myopia, both in vitro and in vivo. Additionally, this customized spatial intensity profile can be written onto a LAL that is first adjusted to emmetropia. The ability to readjust the LAL has also been demonstrated.

Despite recently increased interest, multifocal IOLs are not the only way to achieve spectacle independence for both near and distance. Targeting for emmetropia in the dominant eye and leaving the nondominant eye slightly myopic, which is known as monovision, also allows for spectacle independence in more than 90% of the patient's activities. These results are similar to those reported for multifocal IOLs.[16,17]

In our initial study on Calhoun's LAL, 5 patients who underwent bilateral cataract surgery were randomly selected to have Calhoun's LAL implanted in one eye and AcrySof SA60AT IOL implanted in the other. Table 1 shows postoperative refraction and near and far binocular BSCVA and uncorrected visual acuity (UCVA). As it can be seen, all the patients achieved far UCVA greater than 20/27 and near UCVA of at least J2, which allowed them to perform most of their activities without glasses. These excellent results in both far and near binocular UCVA may not only be due to monovision. An additional factor may be the fact that the spatial irradiance profile used for the lens base power adjustments, especially in hyperopic corrections, simultaneously creates a positive aspheric optic that increases the depth of focus in the eye of the LAL. This is similar to what we demonstrated with a special ablation profile with our excimer laser MEL 80 (Carl Zeiss Meditec) in presbyopia corrections (personal communication, American Society of Cataract and Refractive Surgery May 2004 and April 2005; American Academy of Ophthalmology, November

2004; and poster in the Association for Research in Vision and Ophthalmology annual meeting, May 2006) (Table 1).

Conclusion

Our early clinical experience with LAL technology has demonstrated the feasibility to precisely adjust the IOL power to correct postoperative residual refractive errors. All the eyes were within ± 0.5 D of intended correction, and 90% were within ± 0.25 D of intended correction. Although in vitro results have been promising, other possibilities such as creating multifocal patterns or correcting higher-order aberrations need to be validated by clinical trials.

While not addressed in the clinical trials reported above, additional adjustments can be made on the LAL until lock-in. Preliminary studies have indicated that approximately 80% of maximal adjustment can be obtained with a second treatment. Retreatment of the LAL might not only be useful to fine-tune the adjustment but may also allow patients to reversibly try a particular refractive situation, such as monovision or multifocality.

References

1. Narvaez J, Zimmerman G, Stulting RD, Chang DH. Accuracy of intraocular lens power prediction using the Hoffer Q, Holladay 1, Holladay 2, and SRK/T formulas. *J Cataract Refract Surg.* 2006;32(12):2050-2053.

2. Chan CC, Hodge C, Lawless M. Calculation of intraocular lens power after corneal refractive surgery. *Clin Experiment Ophthalmol.* 2006;34(7):640-644.

3. Kraser GN, inventor; CooperVision, Inc, assignee. Small incision intraocular lens with adjustable refractive power. US patent 4,950,289. August 21, 1990.

4. Eggleston HC, Day T, inventors. Adjustable and removable intraocular lens implant. US patent 5,628798. May 13, 1997.

5. Eggleston HC, Day T, inventors. Adjustable intraocular lens implant with magnetic adjustment facilities. US patent 5,800,533. September 1, 1998.

6. O'Donnell FE, inventor. In vivo modification of refractive power of an intraocular lens implant. US patent 5,549,668. August 27, 1996.

7. O'Donnell FE, inventor. In vivo modification of refractive power of an intraocular lens implant. US patent 5,725,575. March 10, 1998.

8. Jahn CE, Jahn MA, Kreiner CF, et al. Intraocular lens with reversibly adjustable optical power: pilot study of concept and safety. *J Cataract Refract Surg.* 2003;29:1795-1799.

9. Jethmalani J, Grubbs RH, Sandstedt CA, Kornfield JA, Schwartz DM, inventors; California Institute of Technology and the Regents of the University of California, assignee. Lenses capable of post-fabrication power modification. US patent 6.450.642 Sept 17, 2002.

10. Schwartz DM, Jethmalani J, Sandstedt CA, et al. Postimplantation adjustable intraocular lenses. *Ophthalmol Clin North Am.* 2001;14(2):339-345.

11. Schwartz DM. Light-adjustable lens. *Trans Am Ophthalmol Soc.* 2003;101:411-430.

12. Schwartz DM, Sandstedt CA, Chang SH, et al. Light-adjustable lens: development of in vitro nomograms. *Trans Am Ophthalmol Soc.* 2004;102:67-74.

13. Sandstedt CA, Chang SH, Grubbs RH, Schwartz DM. Light-adjustable lens: customizing correction for multifocality and higher-order aberrations. *Trans Am Ophthalmol Soc.* 2006;104:29-39.

14. Hayashi K, Hayashi H, Nakao F, Hayashi F. Influence of astigmatism on multifocal and monofocal intraocular lenses. *Am J Ophthalmol.* 2000;13:477-482.

Table 1

BINOCULAR BEST-SPECTACLE CORRECTED AND UNCORRECTED VISUAL ACUITY FOR NEAR AND FAR DISTANCE AFTER BILATERAL CATARACT SURGERY*

Patient	Rx Dominant Eye (D)	Rx Nondominant Eye (D)	UCVA Far	UCVA Near	BSCVA Far	BSCVA Near
1	0.25	-2.25	20/20	J1+ 20/20	20/20	J1+ 20/20
2	0	-0.75	20/20	J1 20/25	20/20	J1+ 20/20
3	85 -1.00	160 -0.50 -0.75	20/25	J2 20/30	20/20	J1+ 20/20
4	140 -0.50 +0.25	-1	20/22	J1 20/25	20/20	J1+ 20/20
5	95 -0.75 +0.25	90 -0.50 – 0.50	20/27	J2 20/30	20/27	J1+ 20/20

* Calhoun's light adjustable lens (LAL) was implanted in one eye and AcrySof SA60AT IOL in the other.

15. Hayashi K, Hayashi H, Nakao F, Hayashi F. Correlation between pupillary size and intraocular lens decentration and visual acuity of a zonal-progressive multifocal lens and a monofocal lens. *Ophthalmology.* 2000;108:2011-2017.

16. Leyland M, Pringle E. Multifocal versus monofocal intraocular lenses after cataract extraction. *Cochrane Database Syst Rev.* 2006;18(4): CD003169.

17. Vingolo EM, Grenga P, Iacobelli L, Grenga R. Visual acuity and contrast sensitivity: AcrySof ReSTOR apodized diffractive versus AcrySof SA60AT monofocal intraocular lenses. *J Cataract Refract Surg.* 2007;33(7):1244-1247.

CHAPTER 64

ACRITEC IOL

José F. Alfonso, MD, PhD and Luis Fernández-Vega, MD, PhD

Current pseudoaccommodative intraocular lens (IOL) implantation may provide good distance and near vision after cataract[1] and presbyopic lens exchange surgery.[2] Differences in visual outcomes achieved with these IOLs come from the optical principle used, such as the shape design of their surfaces, and the role of the patient's pupil size.[3] Refraction and diffraction principles have been used to create multifocality from near to distance. The light distribution between the distance and near foci plays an important role in the final retinal image.[4] Out-of-focus images created by multifocality are responsible for some reduction in contrast sensitivity. Jacobi developed a new concept to overcome some of these limitations.[5] He called this new concept asymmetrical bilateral multifocal IOL implantation. This is the implantation of 2 bifocal diffractive IOLs with different light-distribution between the 2 foci in order to enhance visual performance of the IOL after binocular implantation. A distant-dominant multifocal IOL with a light distribution of 70% for the far and 30% for the near focus is implanted in one eye (model 737D), thus rendering this eye distant dominant. In the contralateral eye, a near dominant multifocal IOL with a light distribution of 30% for the far focus and 70% for the near focus is implanted (model 733D), rendering this eye near dominant. The *Acri. Twin Set, models 737D and 733D (*Acri.Tec, Henningsdorf, Germany) are bifocal diffractive IOLs with different light distributions for distance and near focus (Figure 1).

Asymmetric Implantation

We have recently evaluated 343 consecutive patients who underwent bilateral implantation of the *Acri.Twin IOLs—the distance dominant 737D and near dominant 733D.[6] Monocular and binocular best-corrected distance and near visual acuity and distance contrast sensitivity under photopic (85 cd/m2) and mesopic (5 cd/m2) conditions were determined. Binocularly, the *Acri.Twin system allowed good distance and near vision: 0.031 ± 0.059 and 0.005 ± 0.024 logMAR, respectively. Contrast sensitivity with the *Acri.Twin system was

within normal limits under photopic and mesopic conditions. Binocular implantation of these IOLs should be performed because of the differences in light distribution of the distance dominant and the near dominant IOLs models.

There are 2 drawbacks for the asymmetrical bilateral implantation. First, the evaluation of which eye is dominant in cataract patients is problematic because a denser cataract in the dominant eye could lead to a shift in ocular dominance. Second, the possible binocular intolerance to different light distribution between eyes could lead to dissatisfaction and explantation of the near dominant IOL. We have performed 15 unilateral explantations (3.5%) of the near dominant IOL because of the intolerance to the vision reported by these patients. The near dominant 733D IOL was exchanged for a distance dominant 737D IOL, creating a symmetrical implantation. These patients were questioned about their postoperative vision and reported a significant improvement after IOL exchange to achieve a symmetrical implantation. Thus, bilateral implantation of the distance dominant IOL may solve patient dissatisfaction with vision because there is a symmetric light distribution between eyes, preventing binocular interference. In addition, if both IOLs are distant dominant, ocular dominance is much less important.

Symmetric Implantation

After our experience with the *Acri.Twin system we evaluated 50 patients who underwent bilateral implantation of the distance dominance diffractive bifocal IOL, model 447D (*Acri.Tec, Germany) (Figure 2).[7] Monocular and binocular best-corrected distance and near visual acuities and distance contrast sensitivity under photopic (85 cd/m2) and mesopic (5 cd/m2) conditions were determined. At the 6-month postoperative visit, binocular best-corrected distance acuity and best-corrected distance near acuity were means of 0.02 ± 0.04 logMAR and 0.04 ± 0.03 logMAR, respectively. Postoperatively, 32 patients (64%) reported full independence from spectacle wear at near; 7 patients (14%) said they needed

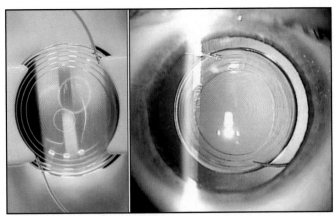

Figure 1. *Acri.Twin 737/733 D IOLs.

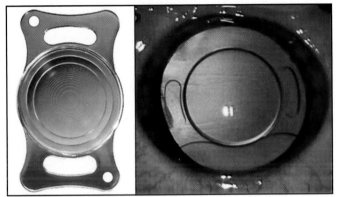

Figure 2. *Acri.Twin 447/433 D IOLs.

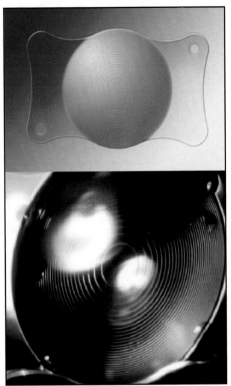

Figure 3. *Acri.LISA 366 D IOL.

glasses all the time. Contrast sensitivity was within normal limits under photopic and mesopic conditions. Binocular implantation of the 447D IOL may overcome binocular interference to different light distributions between eyes, as well as the problem of being unable to determine ocular dominance in cataract patients.

*Acri.LISA Intraocular Lens Implantation

A new optical concept has been recently applied to IOL design—the refractive-diffractive optic. The *Acri.LISA IOL model 366D (*Acri.Tec) uses this hybrid concept to reduce the disadvantages of conventional refractive and diffractive multifocal IOLs (Figure 3). This new IOL, based on symmetrical implantation with a 65/35 ratio of light percentage between distance and near foci, respectively, has been developed to improve on previous outcomes in presbyopia IOL correction. We evaluated 81 patients implanted with the *Acri.LISA 3-months after bilateral implantation.[8] The binocular best-corrected distance acuity and best distance corrected near visual acuity were 0.048 ± 0.111 logMAR and 0.012 ± 0.0084 logMAR, respectively. Contrast sensitivity was within normal limits under photopic and mesopic conditions. Binocular contrast sensitivity was statistically significantly better than monocular contrast sensitivity at all spatial frequencies under photopic and mesopic illumination levels. The *Acri.LISA 366D IOL provides a satisfactory full range of vision. This IOL shows

a high level of uncorrected and corrected distance and near vision with improved contrast sensitivity under photopic and mesopic conditions. Future studies on this IOL should include longer follow-up examinations and comparison with other IOLs based on the same diffractive-refractive concept.

Conclusion

All of the *Acri.Tec multifocal IOLs performed well. Each has predictable characteristics based on its specific optical design. With respect to symmetrical implantation, the *Acri.LISA IOL should be considered in patients with cataracts, high ametropia, and presbyopia. In these cases, our outcomes show that patients achieve good distance, near, and intermediate visual acuity. The model 447 IOL is also indicated for the same patients desiring spectacle freedom for distance and intermediate vision, but patients with this IOL are more likely to use near vision spectacle in some situations. The 737 IOL should be considered for highly hyperopic eyes and as a multifocal piggyback secondarily implanted over a monofocal IOL.[9] The models 447 and 443 IOLs should be used in patients with high myopia and anisometropia, in whom the ocular dominance can be determined.

References

1. Alfonso JF, Fernández-Vega L, Baamonde B, Montés-Micó R. Prospective visual evaluation of apodized diffractive intraocular lenses. *J Cataract Refract Surg.* 2007;33:1235-1243.

2. Fernández-Vega L, Alfonso JF, Rodríguez PP, Montés-Micó R. Clear lens extraction with multifocal apodized diffractive intraocular lens implantation. *Ophthalmology.* 2007;114:1491-1498.

3. Alfonso JF, Fernández-Vega L, Baamonde B, Montés-Micó R. Correlation of pupil size with visual acuity and contrast sensitivity after implantation of an apodized diffractive intraocular lens. *J Cataract Refract Surg.* 2007;33:430-438.

4. Montés-Micó R, España E, Bueno I, et al. Visual performance with multifocal intraocular lenses: mesopic contrast sensitivity under distance and near conditions. *Ophthalmology.* 2004;111:85-96.

5. Jacobi FK, Kammann J, Jacobi WK, et al. Bilateral implantation of asymmetrical diffractive multifocal intraocular lenses. *Arch Ophthalmol.* 1999;117:17-23.

6. Alfonso FJ, Fernández-Vega L, Señaris A, Montés-Micó R. Quality of vision with the *Acri.Twin asymmetric diffractive bifocal intraocular lens system. *J Cataract Refract Surg.* 2007;33:197-202.

7. Fernández-Vega L, Alfonso JA, Baamonde B, Montés-Micó R. Symmetric bilateral implantation of a distance-dominance diffractive bifocal intraocular lens. *J Cataract Refract Surg.* 2007;33:1913-1917.

8. Alfonso JF, Fernández-Vega L, Señaris A, Montés-Micó R. Prospective study of the *Acri.LISA bifocal intraocular lens. *J Cataract Refract Surg.* 2007;33:1930-1935.

9. Alfonso FJ, Fernández-Vega L, Baamonde MB. Secondary diffractive bifocal piggyback intraocular lens implantation. *J Cataract Refract Surg.* 2006;32:1938-1943.

CHAPTER 65

VISION MEMBRANE IOL

Lee T. Nordan, MD and David Castillejos, MD

Cataract extraction has been revolutionized by phacoemulsification, posterior chamber intraocular lenses (PC-IOLs), and the correction of refractive error by laser in situ keratomileusis (LASIK) and photorefractive keratectomy (PRK). Next, the correction of presbyopia will likewise be further advanced by the implantation of phakic multifocal IOLs. This chapter will describe one such IOL—the Vision Membrane (VM) (Vision Membrane Technologies, Inc, Chino Hills, CA). The VM is capable of improving either distance visual acuity alone or correcting distance and near visual function simultaneously.

Optics

The optics created for the VM—multi order optics (MOD)—are a sophisticated form of diffractive optics for both distance and near visual function. Virtually no chromatic aberration is created and a significant area of the central visual axis is free of diffractive elements (Figure 1). It is estimated that 98% of all incoming light is focused at the desired location, which is an astounding percentage for a diffractive optic. This also means that very little glare is created. The impressive depth of focus of a VM multifocal IOL is in the range of 10 cm, thereby allowing for clear reading vision for computer use at 45 cm and routine reading at 35 cm. The VM optic is 600 µm thin for all dioptric powers.

Haptics

Just as challenging as developing an excellent optic is the development of a superior haptic design for an anterior chamber (AC) phakic IOL. This haptic must position and maintain the IOL in the posterior one-third to middle of the AC. The VM haptic is unique in that the haptic flexes in 2 directions: vertically toward the center in order to minimize vaulting of the optic, while the footplates flex horizontally to allow the IOL to conform to the shape and dimension of the angle of the AC.

The VM's contour is convex and thin, thereby increasing endothelial clearance in the mid periphery and allowing the use of a 6.00-mm diameter optic.

Implantation

Accurate implantation of any AC IOL demands the use of optical coherence tomography (OCT) or ultrasound to precisely measure the diameter of the AC. Previous attempts to measure the AC diameter such as with white-to-white or dip stick methods have contributed to the poor sizing of AC lenses in general.

The VM is available in lengths of 13.4 mm, 13.0 mm, and 12.60 mm, and the length to be implanted is always based upon a precise preoperative measurement. In the past, approximately 10% to 15% of pseudophakic AC IOLs have been removed as a result of the IOL being too short (more common) or too long. The new generation of phakic AC IOLs are made of a softer material. The explantation rate has been reduced to less than 1% thanks to their improved design and precise preoperative measurements.

The VM may be implanted by means of an injector through a 2.6-mm corneal limbal incision or a 4.5-mm corneal incision using nonfibrin surgical glue as a sealant. This larger incision induces approximately 1.00 D of astigmatism by flattening the meridian of the wound. By appropriately orienting the wound on the steeper meridian of the cornea, patients with corneal astigmatism in the range of 0.75 D to 1.75 D (90% of all patients) may be treated without the need for a second astigmatic surgery.

Implantation of the VM is performed using topical anesthesia and takes less than 5 minutes. A soft contact lens is placed on the eye without a patch. Visual recovery is noticeable within several hours and a significant improvement in vision is observed by the next morning. Full recovery usually takes 3 to 5 days with a small incision and about 2 weeks with the larger incision (Figure 2).

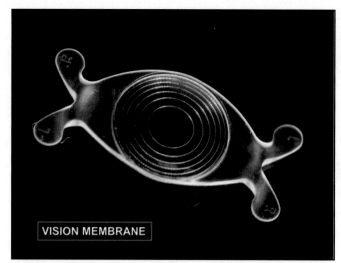

Figure 1. The VM IOL is an AC phakic IOL. The circular diffractive elements may be dedicated to correcting distance or near vision. Notice the convexity of the optic and the compound vertical and horizontal aspects of the haptics.

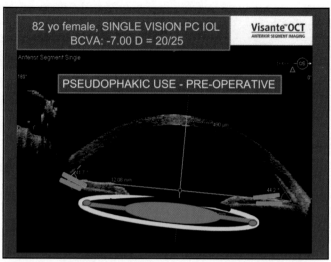

Figure 3. The preoperative Visante OCT of the PC-IOL pseudophakic eye described in the text. Notice the increased depth of the AC.

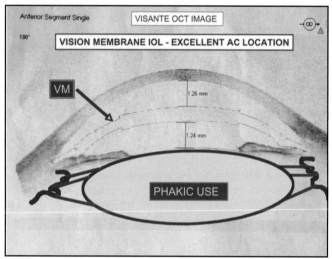

Figure 2. Visante OCT (Carl Zeiss Meditec, Jena, Germany) image of a VM multifocal IOL (arrow) implanted in a phakic eye. The ideal location for the VM in the AC is at the middle to posterior one-third depth.

Philosophy of Use

The correction of ametropia for distance by an IOL is well established. An IOL is superior to keratorefractive surgery for spherical refractive error greater than −6.00 D myopia and +2.00 D of hyperopia. This is because IOLs do not degrade distance vision under night time conditions in the way that midperipheral corneal optical irregularities created by keratorefractive surgery do. Implanting an IOL does not cause corneal irregularity or central corneal scarring.

The correction of presbyopia is the next major challenge to be overcome in anterior segment surgery. Monovision represents a reasonable means to correct presbyopia but leaves 20% to 30% of patients highly dissatisfied and is not nearly as effective as a binocular solution.

The use of a bifocal IOL is a very satisfactory means of correcting presbyopia following cataract surgery, but it certainly should not be the preferred method of presbyopia correc-

tion in a phakic eye that retains useful accommodation. Any residual accommodation from the crystalline lens is totally lost in order to implant the multifocal IOL. On the other hand, adding an AC multifocal IOL to a phakic eye preserves any remaining accommodation and is also completely reversible by removing the AC IOL. The complication rate of a clear lensectomy with implantation of a PC-IOL is about 5%. An elective refractive procedure should not have a long-term complication rate greater than 1%. The VM is unique in its capability to correct distance and near ametropia in phakic and PC-IOL pseudophakic eyes.

Case Report

Although the VM was designed originally for phakic use, interesting clinical situations have arisen. Pseudophakes with a PC IOL cannot accommodate and may have an unexpected refractive error for distance. The following case demonstrates the simultaneous correction of distance and near vision in a pseudophake with a PC-IOL.

An 82-year-old woman underwent uneventful phacoemulsification and PC-IOL implantation in the left eye 9 months ago. Ocular examination revealed the following:

OD: V dis plano = 20/25; V near +3.000 D add = 20/25
OS: V dis: −7.00 D sph = 20/25; V near cc dis = 20/100

Rather than exchange the left IOL, the refractive surprise was managed by implanting a −7.00-D multifocal VM IOL in the AC eye (Figure 3).

At postoperative day 1, her left uncorrected distance acuity was 20/25 and her uncorrected near vision was 20/25 at a distance of 35 to 45 cm. This 10-cm extended depth of field at near is remarkable and allows a patient to use a computer at a convenient distance and to then read comfortably as well (Figures 4 to 6).

If this diffractive optic can reliably provide good far and near vision, it might represent an option as a secondary refractive implant for pseudophakes with monofocal IOLs. For example, a plano VM AC IOL could be placed in an emmetropic monofocal pseudophake to provide the ability to read without glasses as well.

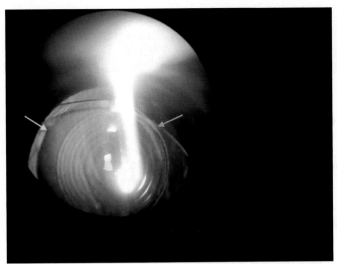

Figure 4. The VM (green arrow) implanted into a PC-IOL (yellow arrow) pseudophakic eye. This VM simultaneously corrected −7.00 D of distance ametropia and provided excellent reading vision at 35 to 45 cm.

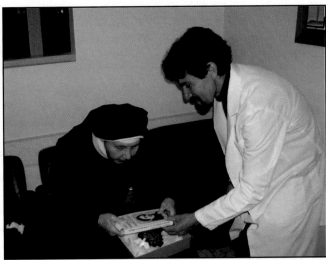

Figure 6. The highly satisfied patient described in Figure 3 demonstrates her newly acquired reading ability as her VM surgeon looks on.

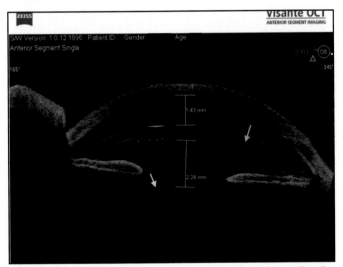

Figure 5. The Visante OCT image of the VM (green arrow) described in Figure 4. The yellow arrow indicates the crystalline lens.

Conclusion

The VM multifocal IOL may represent a major step in our ability to visually rehabilitate phakic and pseudophakic presbyopic eyes while correcting distance ametropia. The correction of presbyopia by means of a diffractive, reversible AC IOL offers significant advantages over performing a clear lensectomy with a bifocal PC-IOL. I predict that newly designed multifocal phakic IOLs will increase in popularity in the future. Anterior segment surgeons will then have an expanded list of refractive IOLs and procedures.

CHAPTER 66

NEW BIOPTICS: REFRACTIVE IOLs COMBINED WITH INTRACORNEAL LENSES

Kevin L. Waltz, OD, MD

The cornea and lens combine to make a dual optic system focusing an image on the retina. It is possible to manipulate the focus of the dual optic system by changing either component. We commonly change the corneal focusing power with laser vision correction and the lens focusing power with cataract surgery. We are now beginning to combine laser vision correction and cataract surgery to achieve results that either procedure alone cannot provide. For instance, it is common to see a 10% or greater incidence of laser vision correction enhancement of presbyopia-correcting intraocular lenses (IOLs) to achieve an optimal result. In the near future, intracorneal lenses will be combined with IOLs to provide benefits that either product alone cannot provide. The combination of an intracorneal implant for presbyopia and an IOL will become the new bioptics.

There are 2 general optical principles guiding the design of intracorneal lenses. They are usually either refractive lenses or lenses that work by the pinhole effect. The ReVision intracorneal lens (ReVision Optics, Lake Forest, CA) is an example of a refractive lens. There are others such as the PermaVision implant by Anamed, Inc (Lake Forest, CA). The ReVision Intracorneal lens is essentially a small, round, clear, thin convex lens with a refractive index identical to the cornea. It works by modifying the cornea shape in an additive manner. The AcuFocus ACI 7000 corneal implant (AcuFocus, Inc, Irvine, CA) is an example of a lens based on the pinhole principle (Figure 1). It is a mostly opaque, donut-shaped disc with many tiny fenestrations and a central 1.6-mm opening and a 3.6-mm outside diameter. It does not modify the corneal shape. It works by limiting the paraxial rays of light entering the eye according to the pinhole effect. Both lenses are placed intrastromally under a corneal flap. They can be placed at the time of a laser in situ keratomileusis (LASIK) procedure or as an enhancement at a later date.[1]

An intracorneal implant for presbyopia is an additive correction versus a subtractive correction like laser vision correction.[2] An additive technology is more readily reversible than a subtractive technology. Intracorneal implants depend less on wound-healing variables than subtractive strategies do. It is also perfectly reasonable to combine a subtractive technology like LASIK and an additive technology like an intracorneal implant.[3] The combination of LASIK and an intracorneal implant can also provide multifocality through a corneal procedure alone.[4] By not requiring an intraocular implant, this presbyopia-correcting strategy could be more easily reversed surgically if the results are not as expected.

It is also possible to consider using an intracorneal implant to minimize the side effects of an IOL implant. Multifocal IOLs are associated with glare and halos, and it is common practice to minimize the unwanted visual sensations of a multifocal IOL by reducing the pupil size with ambient light or with medications such as brimonidine or pilocarpine. An AcuFocus intracorneal implant would also reduce the effective pupil size. It could minimize the negative effects of a multifocal IOL while simultaneously providing improved near vision through the alternative principle of the pinhole effect.

It would be ideal to correct presbyopia once in a lifetime. Conductive keratoplasty is a helpful option for presbyopia, but its effect does not last. It is unlikely that any scleral procedure will permanently correct presbyopia, based on its own theory, even if there were an initial positive effect. It is certainly possible to perform a lens procedure on presbyopic patients, but there are concerns about the safety of refractive lens exchange in myopic patients. When a truly accommodating IOL will become available is also uncertain. An intracorneal corneal inlay may be the best option for a permanent presbyopia correction in all patients and especially myopic patients. It can be combined with laser vision correction. The laser vision correction can correct any ametropia and the corneal implant can correct the presbyopia. This approach would provide good distance and near vision in each eye to maintain binocularity and stereopsis. Certain inlays appear to be well tolerated over the course of many years.[5] It is possible to implant sufficient power in a refractive intracorneal implant to correct

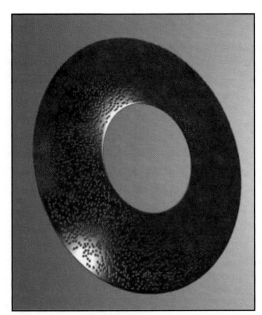

Figure 1. AcuFocus ACI 7000 implant.

presbyopia for many years. The AcuFocus implant should provide about 2.0 D of depth of focus, which should be sufficient for most people for most of their lives.

The great advantage of an intracorneal implant to correct presbyopia is how well it will work with cataract surgery later in life. By whatever principle the intracorneal inlay works, it will still work after cataract surgery. It may even work better with an IOL. The optics of otherwise clear presbyopic crystalline lenses are already beginning to degrade due to excess positive spherical aberration and other higher-order aberrations. Replacing the presbyopic crystalline lens with a manufactured IOL could very well improve the overall vision in someone with a previously placed intracorneal implant. Cataract surgery has already been successfully performed on patients implanted with an AcuFocus inlay. The latter did not make cataract surgery more difficult and the patients maintained good distance and near vision after the procedure.

It is easy to imagine the value of an intracorneal implant that works by improved depth of focus after cataract surgery. Assuming the intracorneal implant could reliably provide 2.0 D of depth of focus, it would make sense to aim for −0.75 D as a refractive endpoint after lens surgery. In this situation, there would be sufficient depth of focus to provide excellent distance and near vision even if the refractive target was missed by a full D in either direction. Likewise, either the ReVision implant or the AcuFocus inlay could be used to enhance the near effect of any accommodating lens. If a patient has an accommodating IOL implanted and is unhappy with the near or distance visual results, the patient could have a LASIK procedure to fine tune the refraction and have a corneal implant placed in the LASIK bed to enhance the presbyopia treatment. Having this kind of a backstop to utilizing an accommodating IOL could greatly enhance the confidence of the surgeon and the patient in the ultimate outcome of the procedure. After a patient has enjoyed an intracorneal implant successfully for many years, they will likely be very motivated to further improve their vision with cataract surgery. It will be a relatively straightforward process to implant an accommodating IOL in a patient with a pre-existing presbyopic intracorneal implant with the expectation of achieving excellent uncorrected distance, intermediate, and near vision.

Combining an intracorneal implant with an IOL to treat presbyopia will become the new refractive bioptics procedure. For the foreseeable future, accommodating lenses will likely be unable to guarantee the distance and near results that our patients desire. Combining intracorneal lenses with accommodating or multifocal IOLs will therefore be a very attractive option. Implanting an intracorneal inlay in an early presbyope will be a very attractive option for the same reason. At some point in the future, the patient will need cataract surgery. By having an intracorneal inlay already placed, any IOL implanted behind it will likely produce better near vision.

References

1. Barragan E. Enhancing the post-LASIK presbyope with additive techniques. Presented at American Society of Cataract and Refractive Surgery; April 27–May 2, 2007; San Diego, CA.

2. Dishler JG. Treating presbyopia: additive versus subtractive techniques. Presented at American Society of Cataract and Refractive Surgery; April 27–May 2, 2007; San Diego, CA.

3. Ismail MM. Correction of hyperopia by intracorneal lenses: Two-year follow-up. *J Cataract Refract Surg.* 2006;32:1657-1660.

4. Chayet A. Creating a multifocal cornea with additive techniques. Presented at American Society of Cataract and Refractive Surgery; April 27–May 2, 2007; San Diego, CA.

5. Doane J. Long-term biocompatibility of intracorneal implants. Presented at American Society of Cataract and Refractive Surgery; April 27–May 2, 2007; San Diego, CA. Available at: ASCRS2007. htm

SECTION VI

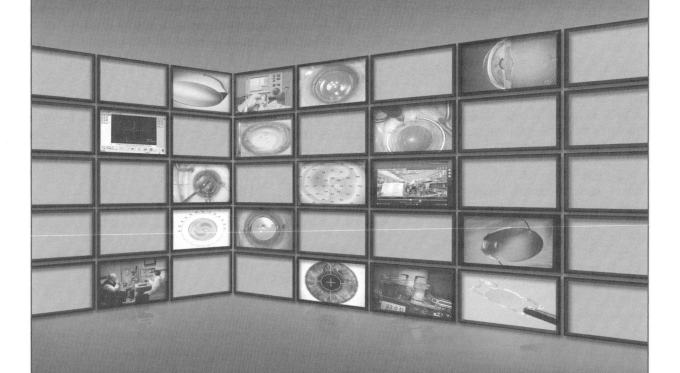

Refractive IOLs—
Quality of Vision

CHAPTER 67

MEASURING OUR IOL OUTCOMES

Pietro Giardini, MD and Nicola Hauranieh, MD

Presbyopia-correcting intraocular lenses (Pr-C IOLs) can provide a full range of visual correction for both far, intermediate, and near vision. It is important to evaluate the outcomes from Pr-C IOLs in order to continually improve our results. Years of experience have taught us to evaluate certain parameters that best correlate with patients' real-life visual performance and satisfaction. We have developed a system to collect important preoperative and postoperative data to accurately access Pr-C IOLs.

The first parameter is the patient's visual acuity. The minimum size letter that a person can resolve at near distance is an important measure of his or her near vision. It is also very important to standardize the measurement. This has been done very well for distance acuity, but not for near acuity. Near acuity is regularly reported in Snellen or Jaeger number formats in the United States, N numbers in the United Kingdom, and Parinaud numbers in France. These differing systems do not lend themselves to comparisons from one study to the next. Our experience has also shown that patients often require print size that is 2 or 3 times larger than their peak near acuity limits before they can achieve their maximum reading speed. It would be very useful to have a standardized method of measuring near vision that was more easily translated into other formats.

Reading speed is an important parameter to consider. In our experience, it is common for a subject not to be able to comfortably read a passage printed in the same size as what vision testing shows their minimum resolvable print size to be. It is common for a patient to desire reading print size that is significantly larger than his or her minimum resolvable letter size. Reading speed is an objective measure of reading performance. Questions regarding how our patients perform in different every day life activities are too subjective for comparison (eg, "…how is your vision during shopping?"). This is simply too general a question, and does not allow a useful comparison between different patients, or between sequential exams of the same patient.

Depth of focus is another important issue. Different IOLs can be expected to perform differently at different distances when reading. A defocus curve is a very useful set of data in order to help us better understand the visual performance of a specific IOL. If a Pr-C IOL is found to have a predictable defocus curve, this information can be valuable for patient selection and counseling.

Another parameter to evaluate is spectacle dependence after surgery. This criterion is not as subjective—if someone does not ever use glasses, this is a very definite endpoint. Likewise, the presence or absence of photic phenomena is important, but it is very helpful to quantify the amount and severity rather than to have the patient respond either yes or no.

We have attempted to estimate patient satisfaction with various IOLs using different kinds of questionnaires that present simple questions regarding quality of life and vision. Unfortunately, these questionnaires are quite boring for our patients, and they do not give us a clear idea about the patients' real visual performance in every day life.

Eyevispod

We have attempted to solve these problems with a new system to measure, collect, record, and analyze near vision data. Early on, we understood the need for an objective measurement system that could also record the information as it was collected. We therefore have developed a diagnostic machine called the "Eyevispod" (PGB srl, Milano, Italy) that can study all of these parameters. In our experience it has proven to be very useful to us and to our patients.

The Eyevispod is a computerized system that allows the convenient measurement, collection, and recording of a detailed assessment of near and intermediate visual performance in patients with or without Pr-C IOLs. It overcomes the limitations of traditional visual acuity charts by presenting the patient with a standardized image and recording the results as soon as they are measured (Figure 1).

Figure 1. The Eyevispod being used by a patient..

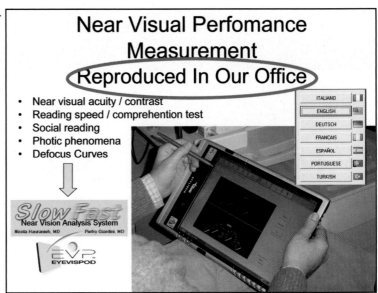

Figure 2. A near vision test with multiple methods used to report the images sizes, such as 20/400 and J19.

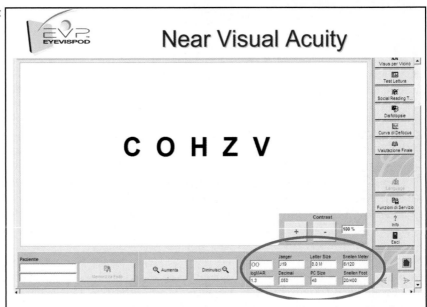

The traditional system of measuring peak near acuity does not correlate well with real-life reading vision. It cannot take into account the variety of every day situations that are normally encountered by our patients, such as shopping, going to restaurants, or driving a car. We also have no way of objectively measuring and documenting common symptoms, such as glare and halos, during our routine examinations. The Eyevispod system performs a comprehensive assessment of near and intermediate visual function, and gives a score (as a percent of normal) of the visual performance of the patient. Through simulation of the most common daily visual tasks and problems on a tablet PC, and by processing the data from a series of subsequent tests, the Eyevispod (previously called SlowFast) creates a functional score of the pre- and postoperative near vision. This score is very useful for practical and medicolegal purposes. It can also be used to compare the outcomes of different surgeries for presbyopia (multifocal IOLs, accommodative IOLs, conductive keratoplasty, scleral bands, or laser keratorefractive surgery).

The system is easy to use, relatively time efficient (a 5-minute time test), and easy to understand. Patients hold the tablet PC in their hands and select the answers with the tip of a pointer on the touch-screen.

The Tests

The different tests are usually administered sequentially. First, near visual acuity is measured with the patient positioned 40 cm away from the screen. A series of progressively smaller letters are shown and the patients stop when they are no longer able to read the letters (Figure 2).

The size of the letters is presented in multiple systems simultaneously. They are shown inside the red ellipse. This value is recorded by the Eyevispod. The next test is reading speed. The program comes with 7 languages. There are reading passages with ratings of low, medium, and high difficulty in each language. Once the patient begins reading the passage a stopwatch on the Eyevispod is started, and then stopped at

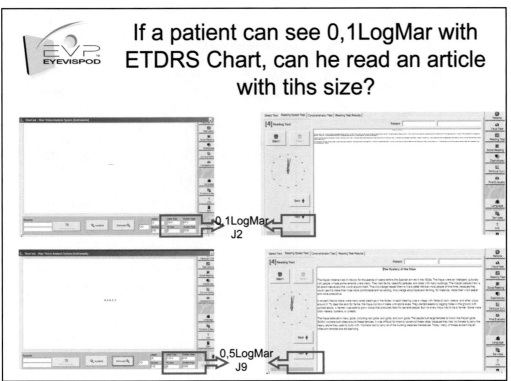

Figure 3. Reading test image sizes compared to the peak near acuity test.

the end of the passage. The reading speed is automatically calculated and recorded. Then the patient is asked a series of questions to estimate his or her comprehension of the passage. We believe that measuring reading speed in this way is the best measure of near vision performance (Figure 3).

Measuring reading speed without testing reading comprehension can also be misleading. Transmitting information to the brain is an essential task of visual function. If we do not test comprehension, we will not know if some patients tended to rush themselves for the test, without allowing enough time to comprehend what they were reading as they would in real life. What we really want to assess is functional every day reading speed, which is a speed that still allows the patient to concentrate enough to understand the text.

The next step is a series of every day visual tasks that are often problematic for presbyopic patients. Standardized images are presented in a reproducible fashion both pre- and postoperatively. Several examples of these commonly problematic objects are reproduced on the screen, and are divided into 3 categories, including near vision (reading newspapers), intermediate vision, and photopic phenomena.

There is an entire set of near images devoted to newspapers. It includes titles, subtitles, articles, different paper colors, and the financial page, where numbers and tables are usually printed in the smallest fonts. Another section contains examples of images from intermediate distance tasks. These include a full-size car dashboard, a door-plate, labels with the price of clothes, ingredients for food products, a road map, and a music score (Figure 4). These are actual size images. They allow us to directly test the every day social visual performance of patients at both near and intermediate distances (Figure 5). Finally, diffractive images and aberrations are simulated with various degrees of severity. Patients select the images that most closely

replicate their own night vision (Figure 6). As these tests are completed, the data is recorded and eventually reported in a numeric scale out of 100.

A final section contains the option of creating a monocular or binocular defocus curve. These curves can be compared to those obtained from other patients using the same standardized testing methodology. Capturing and comparing data in this way allows us to really compare the functional quality of vision after an IOL is implanted (Figure 7).

Toward Standardized Evaluation of Intraocular Performance

In conclusion, the Eyevispod provides us with a complete profile of the patient's visual acuity (including near vision, the quality of their vision, and an assessment of unwanted visual images). With one single testing system, we can measure the overall, real-life visual performance of the patient. Results are then automatically archived in the computer database included in the program. This cumulative database can then characterize a range of typical outcomes for any given IOL. Finally, we can test patients in this way preoperatively, and then obtain a true measure of how much their visual performance improves or how much other visual symptoms worsen after IOL implantation.

Hopefully, this improved way of testing patients' visual outcomes will lead to greater standardization of clinical methods to measure near acuity. Although it has been advocated for many years, standardized outcome testing is becoming increasingly critical as we continue to have many new and different IOLs and procedures to scientifically compare.

Figure 4. There are many different types of images for real world near vision testing.

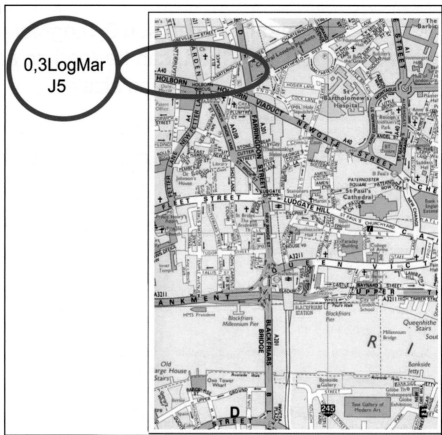

Figure 5. The variety of images used to collect data in the system.

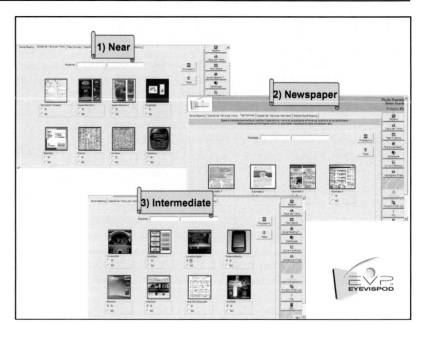

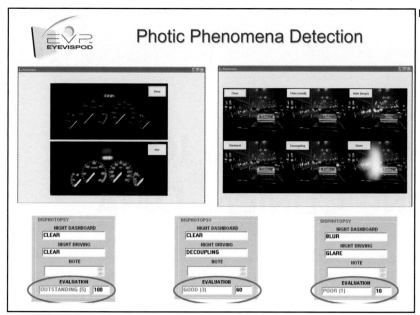

Figure 6. Some of the images used to judge the photic phenomena.

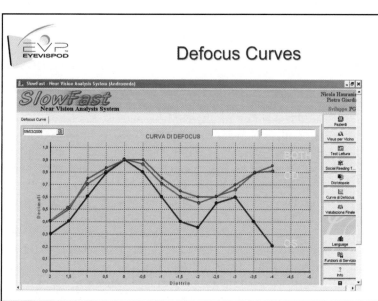

Figure 7. A typical defocus curve for a Pr-C IOL.

PRESBYOPIA-CORRECTING IOLs— INTERPRETING CLINICAL DATA

Kerry D. Solomon, MD; Luis E. Fernández de Castro, MD; Helga P. Sandoval, MD, MSCR; and David T. Vroman, MD

Current tests used to evaluate surgical outcomes include visual acuity measured using the Snellen or the Early Treatment of Diabetic Retinopathy Study (ETDRS) charts that use black letters on an illuminated white background and near vision charts that use individual letters or numbers. Measuring visual acuity by chart testing itself, despite its simplicity and well-established acceptance, still has limitations such as variations in conducting the test and what end point is used, restrictions in the numbers and sizes of optotypes available, and optotype memorization. Moreover, the Snellen chart is optimized for the purpose of refraction, but patients who show no or minimal impairment of Snellen acuity may still have loss of functional vision. Functional vision is what persons use when engaged in any real-world activity, including reading, driving, recreation, or work, and measuring functional vision therefore must go beyond testing with standard visual acuity charts. Reading acuity and reading speed tests have been used as everyday visual function predictors. Given the increasing relevance of reading performance and near-vision function in the clinical setting, there is a tremendous drive to develop standardized tests of reading performance that better replicate real-world visual stimuli. Bailey and Lovie[1] used unrelated words of similar legibility to simultaneously determine visual acuity and reading speed. This method has also been applied to the Minnesota Low-Vision Reading Test (MNREAD) Acuity chart and to the German Radner Reading Charts which use full sentence "optotypes" and variable size. These standardized tests have been used in clinical studies to demonstrate reading performance for patients with a host of ocular conditions, including refractive error, cataract, multifocal intraocular lens (IOL) systems, and maculopathy.[2-6] Similar to visual acuity charts, current reading tests use black letters on a backlit high-contrast background.

Reading is an important skill. It is not only essential to effectively function in society (eg, reading mail, comprehending prescription bottle directions, or keeping-up with current events), but is also a form of recreation.[7] Frequently, return of good reading ability is the principal motivation in a patient's decision to have cataract surgery.[8] Current IOL alternatives include monofocal IOLs, accommodating IOLs, and multifocal IOLs.

Historically, conventional means of evaluating near visual acuity consisted of discerning letters or numbers on a near card. The ability to discern these objects may have no bearing at all on one's functional ability to read. In order to better assess near presbyopia-correcting IOLs, a better reading test needs to be developed that more accurately reflects the functional ability to read. The purpose of the following study was to evaluate a new test (NPReading Test) as a tool to measure near visual function.

A total of 75 patients with a minimum age of 18 years were recruited from the cornea and anterior segment clinic at the Storm Eye Institute and from the staff at MUSC. Exclusion criteria included the inability to read English, previous ocular surgery within the past 3 months or intraocular laser surgery within 1 month of the projected reading test, presence of diabetes mellitus, or an ocular disease or abnormality that would affect visual acuity such as advanced glaucomatous damage, any concurrent infectious/noninfectious conjunctivitis, keratitis or uveitis in either eye, keratoconus, corneal dystrophy, or corneal opacities, to name a few.

Subjects were divided into 4 groups based on lens status and type of IOL. Group 1 (phakic), subjects 35 years old and younger wearing their best distance correction; Group 2 (pseudophakic control), subjects 60 years and older who had undergone cataract extraction and monofocal IOL implantation were evaluated wearing their best distance correction with best near correction; Group 3 (monofocal IOL), subjects 60 years and older who had undergone cataract extraction and monofocal IOL implantation were evaluated wearing their best distance correction without the best near correction; and Group 4 (multifocal IOL), subjects 60 years and older who had undergone cataract extraction and multifocal IOL implantation were evaluated wearing their best distance correction.

Figure 1. The NPReading Test designed for the simultaneous determination of reading acuity, reading speed, and functional vision.

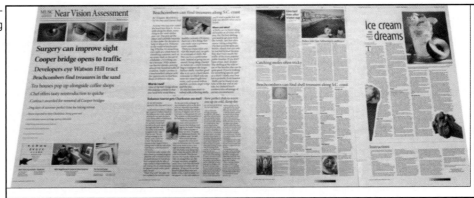

NPReading Test Design

The NPReading test was created and developed by the Magill Research Center for Vision Correction Center at the Storm Eye Institute, MUSC, and was designed and printed by *The Post & Courier*, Charleston, SC (Figure 1). The font type is the one used by the local newspaper (*The Post & Courier*). The character-to-character spacing and line-to-line spacing matched that used in typical everyday print. It is conventional typographical practice for proportionally broader and bolder letters to be used for smaller print sizes. Care was taken so that the smallest letters on the chart were rendered with sufficient resolution so that coarse sampling did not compromise visual acuity assessment. The test was reproduced with a newspaper typesetting method. The ranges of print size were from the American Point-Type 24 through 3 (corresponding to Snellen 20/200 to 20/20 or Jaeger 14 to 1 or logMAR 1.00 to 0). The contrast of the letters and pages are validated for all newspaper print.

All paragraphs were created with the standard 100 words per paragraph, matched for length, and measured by the number of characters. The selection of the number of characters per sentence represented a compromise between 1) enough text to estimate reading performance; and 2) too much text to fit on the newspaper at the large-print end of the scale. To evaluate the formal-linguistic readability we used the tool included in Microsoft Word 2003 (Microsoft Corp, Redmond, WA), which estimates the Flesch Reading Ease score on a scale between 0 (very difficult) and 100 (very easy). Additionally, to evaluate the grade level we used another tool that accompanies Microsoft Word 2003, the Flesch-Kincaid Grade Level score that rates text on a US school-grade level. The paragraphs have a 6 to 8 grade level of education that is the level used by most of the written mass communication media in the United States. Care was taken to avoid use of words with regional spellings or with regional meanings. The paragraphs were taken from actual newspaper articles and as such have been confirmed to be written for a 6th to 8th grade level of education.

Patient Examination

Measurements were performed by only 2 experienced testers who had been trained in this standardized method prior to the study. All tests were performed at a constant chart luminance of 80 to 100 cd/m². Patients were asked to read the paragraph binocularly at a set reading distance of 32 cm. Care was taken to measure the distance to the reading test document, and the seating of the patient prior to the initiation of the exam. Reading distance was repeatedly verified during the procedure. The patients were instructed to read one selected paragraph from each page out loud, without including title, subtitles, and author, starting from the largest font (24 American Point-Type) to the smallest font (3 American Point-Type). Patients were asked to read without correcting any reading error.

Reading speed was measured by recording the reading time for the paragraph at the different print sizes. The reading time was measured with a stopwatch, starting with the first word and stopping with the last word read by the patient. Reading errors were noted by marking the wrong word in the sentence on the study form. If the patient was unable to read a marked paragraph because of decreased font size or if the patient missed ≥20 words, the test was stopped.

Reading acuity was determined as the smallest print size that could be read. Reading speed in words per minute (wpm) was calculated based on the number of words in a paragraph and the time needed to read the paragraph (100 words × 60 seconds/reading time). A training session was not conducted to avoid learning effect over time.

Table 1 summarizes the demographic characteristics of the population evaluated.

The mean reading speed (wpm) and standard deviation for the 8 paragraphs per group are summarized in Table 2 and Figure 2. Patients in Group 1 read in a pattern similar to subjects in Group 2 and 4, that is the "inverted U-shape." Measurements of the 8 paragraphs showed an overall mean reading speed of 218.7 ± 18.2 wpm for patients in Group 1; 178.5 ± 19.3 wpm for patients in Group 4; 157.4 ± 24.5 wpm for patients in Group 2; and 119.2 ± 45.0 wpm for patients in Group 3. The total of patients that were able to read throughout the different paragraphs was constant between the 4 groups (Table 3). The number of subjects that were able to read decreased as the font size decreased.

The distribution of reading errors between the various paragraphs is illustrated in Table 4. In most of the cases just one error was made; the highest number of errors was in patients of Group 3. Overall, the number of errors increased as the font size decreased.

Printed panel charts featuring optotypes (letters or other symbols) of varying sizes are a quick and inexpensive method

Table 1

CHARACTERISTICS OF THE PATIENTS PER GROUP EVALUATED

Results per Group*

Demographics	Group 1 Control <35 years	Group 2 Control >60 years	Group 3 Test >60 years	Group 4 Test >60 years
Age	28.9 ± 6.1	73.2 ± 6.3	62.0 ± 5.3	62.3 ± 6.7
Gender				
Female	21 (70.0%)	7 (58.3%)	7 (63.6%)	11 (50.0%)
Male	9 (30.0%)	5 (41.7%)	4 (36.4%)	11 (50.0%)
Race				
White	23 (76.8%)	11 (91.7%)	8 (72.7%)	22 (100.0%)
Black	3 (10.0%)	0	3 (27.3%)	0
Other	4 (13.2%)	1 (8.3%)	0	0
Highest Level of Education				
High school	0	9 (81.2%)	8 (72.2%)	13 (65.0%)
College or beyond	30 (100.0%)	2 (18.2%)	3 (27.3%)	7 (35.0%)
Sample size	30	12	11	22

*Group 1 (phakic), subjects were wearing the best distance correction; Group 2 (control), subjects who had undergone cataract extraction and monofocal IOL implantation were evaluated wearing the best distance correction with best near correction; Group 3 (monofocal IOL), subjects who had undergone cataract extraction and monofocal IOL implantation were evaluated wearing the best distance correction without near correction; and Group 4 (multifocal IOL), subjects who had undergone cataract extraction and multifocal IOL implantation.

Table 2

READING SPEED OBTAINED PER GROUP AT THE DIFFERENT PARAGRAPHS

Group*	24 American Point-Type	18 American Point-Type	15 American Point-Type	11 American Point-Type	9 American Point-Type	7 American Point-Type	5 American Point-Type	3 American Point-Type
Group 1 Control <35 years	223.8 ± 20.5	215.1 ± 23.2	201.1 ± 17.8	241.8 ± 21.6	244.6 ± 21.2	242.9 ± 23.0	206.1 ± 22.2	174.6 ± 41.9
Group 2 Control >60 years	181.8 ± 37.8	161.1 ± 33.4	156.7 ± 28.4	191.3 ± 43.8	185.6 ± 33.9	170.0 ± 40.9	118.8 ± 44.9	94.1 ± 2.50
Group 3 Monofocal IOL	174.9 ± 32.4	155.0 ± 35.9	132.1 ± 33.2	108.7 ± 44.6	94.4 ± 50.3	49.5 ± 28.0	N/A	N/A
Group 4 Multifocal IOL	199.6 ± 29.6	185.6 ± 32.2	169.7 ± 29.0	198.7 ± 36.5	206.4 ± 34.1	199.9 ± 38.2	153.7 ± 41.3	114.1 ± 38.0
All Groups	202.8 ± 33.7	188.9 ± 37.7	174.6 ± 35.3	201.6 ± 55.4	207.9 ± 53.6	207.1 ± 54.6	171.7 ± 48.5	150.3 ± 50.1

N/A = not available.
*Group 1 (phakic), subjects were wearing the best distance correction; Group 2 (control), subjects who had undergone cataract extraction and monofocal IOL implantation were evaluated wearing the best distance correction with best near correction; Group 3 (monofocal IOL), subjects who had undergone cataract extraction and monofocal IOL implantation were evaluated wearing the best distance correction without near correction; and Group 4 (multifocal IOL), subjects who had undergone cataract extraction and multifocal IOL implantation.

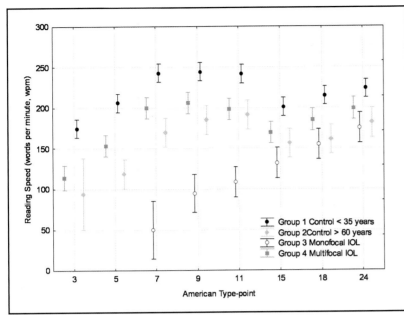

Figure 2. Mean reading speed and standard deviation for the 8 paragraphs read aloud for testing of the 75 participants. Group 1 (phakic), subjects were wearing their best distance correction; Group 2 (pseudophakic control), subjects who had undergone cataract extraction and monofocal IOL implantation were evaluated wearing their best distance correction with best near correction; Group 3 (monofocal IOL), subjects who had undergone cataract extraction and monofocal IOL implantation were evaluated wearing the best distance correction without the near correction; and Group 4 (multifocal IOL), subjects who had undergone cataract extraction and multifocal IOL implantation.

Table 3

TOTAL NUMBER OF SUBJECTS PER GROUP THAT COULD READ EACH PARAGRAPH

Group*	24 American Point-Type	18 American Point-Type	15 American Point-Type	11 American Point-Type	9 American Point-Type	7 American Point-Type	5 American Point-Type	3 American Point-Type
Group 1 Control <35 years	30	30	30	30	30	30	30	30
Group 2 Control >60 years	12	12	12	12	12	12	12	2
Group 3 Monofocal IOL	11	11	11	11	7	3	N/A	N/A
Group 4 Multifocal IOL	22	22	22	22	22	22	22	17
All Groups	75	75	75	75	71	67	65	49

N/A = not available.
*Group 1 (phakic), subjects were wearing the best distance correction; Group 2 (control), subjects who had undergone cataract extraction and monofocal IOL implantation were evaluated wearing the best distance correction with best near correction; Group 3 (monofocal IOL), subjects who had undergone cataract extraction and monofocal IOL implantation were evaluated wearing the best distance correction without near correction; and Group 4 (multifocal IOL), subjects who had undergone cataract extraction and multifocal IOL implantation.

of assessing the spatial resolving capacity of the visual system.[9] As such, they are well suited for use in population-based surveys where visual acuity is often an important outcome measurement, and where time and resources may be limited. Most of these tools have limitations because they use either individual letters or individual words, and they are black-on-white and high contrast, which are not real-world assessments of the patient's visual function. Furthermore, conventional testing methods of reading performance have been developed,[10,11] but

these tests do not relate to actual everyday reading activities (eg, the ability to read magazines, food containers, medicine bottles, newspapers) in a comfortable fashion and reasonable reading speed. In attempting to find a method to evaluate near vision that relates specifically to everyday life, we chose a newspaper. Reading a newspaper is an activity common to most of the population, inexpensive, and easy to administer.

The NPReading Test was developed with the collaboration of a local newspaper. As described previously, the NPReading

Table 4

MEAN NUMBER OF ERRORS PER PARAGRAPH

Group*	24 American Point-Type	18 American Point-Type	15 American Point-Type	11 American Point-Type	9 American Point-Type	7 American Point-Type	5 American Point-Type	3 American Point-Type
Group 1 Control <35 years	0.8 ± 0.9	0.8 ± 1.0	1.1 ± 1.1	0.8 ± 0.8	0.6 ± 0.8	0.9 ± 0.8	1.4 ± 1.7	1.7 ± 1.7
Group 2 Control >60 years	0.2 ± 0.4	0	0.5 ± 0.7	0.6 ± 0.9	0.6 ± 1.2	0.3 ± 0.5	2.1 ± 3.7	4.0 ± 1.4
Group 3 Monofocal IOL	2.2 ± 2.4	3.0 ± 4.6	3.3 ± 2.6	8.8 ± 7.2	5.3 ± 4.9	6.5 ± 2.1	N/A	N/A
Group 4 Multifocal IOL	0.7 ± 1.6	0.4 ± 1.2	1.0 ± 1.2	0.7 ± 1.6	0.6 ± 1.6	1.1 ± 1.9	3.0 ± 3.9	2.5 ± 3.2
All Groups	0.8 ± 1.5	0.9 ± 2.1	1.3 ± 1.6	1.9 ± 4.0	1.0 ± 2.3	1.1 ± 1.6	2.1 ± 3.0	2.1 ± 2.3

N/A, not available.

*Group 1 (phakic), subjects were wearing the best distance correction; Group 2 (control), subjects who had undergone cataract extraction and monofocal IOL implantation were evaluated wearing the best distance correction with best near correction; Group 3 (monofocal IOL), subjects who had undergone cataract extraction and monofocal IOL implantation were evaluated wearing the best distance correction without near correction; and Group 4 (multifocal IOL), subjects who had undergone cataract extraction and multifocal IOL implantation.

Test is comprised of multiple font sizes, with 8 key sizes ranging from 3 to 24 American Point-Type. Only selected paragraphs with these sizes of type were measured. Our results show that subjects older than 60 years of age and wearing the best distance correction with best near correction read in a pattern similar to the patient 35 years old and younger. However, their reading speed was predictably slower (it has been shown that reading speed decreases with age[7]). Patients with multifocal IOLs were able to read faster (178.5 ± 19.3 wpm) than the subjects wearing the best distance correction with best near correction (157.4 ± 24.5 wpm). This was presumably due to improved vision after removal of cataract compared to control population. In all our groups the reading speed versus print size demonstrated an inverted U-shape, in that it decreases from optimum speeds for both small and very large words. This rapid decline in reading rate for letters smaller than 5 American Point-Type is probably related to acuity limitations, whereas the gradual decline for letters larger than 18 American Point-Type may be due to speed limitations in the smooth-pursuit eye-movement system. The number of subjects that were able to read decreased as the font size decreased in all groups.

Although reading is typically done silently, the NPReading test is performed out loud. Legge and colleagues[12] compared oral and silent rates on 5 normal subjects with 3 character sizes on the computer version of the MNREAD. They found that there was no significant difference between oral versus silent reading. Nevertheless, Lovie-Kitchin and coauthors[13] found that silent reading for comprehension was faster than oral reading for comprehension.

For our study we used a stopwatch to measure the reading time in order to calculate the reading speed, a method that is well accepted as reliable for measuring reading speed.[14] However, it is important to know that an acceptable accuracy of stopwatch measurements depends on the examiner's experience and on the procedure. In the validation of the NPReading Test we are seeking to improve our stopwatch measurements and have learned to anticipate the vocal onset of a reader by looking for the initial premovements of the lips.

Our testing population consisted mostly of individuals with above-average education levels. Undoubtedly education plays a role in reading ability, but due to the homogeneity of our sample population this had less of an impact in the current study. In most of the paragraphs only a single error was recorded, with the number of errors seeming to increase as the font size decreased. This could be a result of the patients being forced to read sentences as fast as possible.

In conclusion, these preliminary data demonstrate that the NPReading Test is a practical test because it simulates a normal everyday reading task. Nevertheless, to guarantee accurate, reproducible, and comparable results of the test, an ongoing study is currently underway to validate the testing process. Considering the increasing relevance of functional reading in the real world as well as the clinical setting and research, such validation should be done. An accurate, functional reading test is imperative as newer presbyopia-correcting procedures are developed. Patients and physicians need real life analysis of functional reading vision such as the NPReading test in order to give us a better understanding of what to expect from the technology. Accurate testing will not only be essential for adequate informed consent, but will enable surgeons to better evaluate newer technologies as they are developed.

Acknowledgment

The authors thank Dr. Luanna R. Bartholomew, PhD, Storm Eye Institute, Medical University of South Carolina (Charleston, SC), for her writing assistance.

Financial Disclosure

Supported in part by NIH/NEI EY-014793 (vision core) and an unrestricted grant to MUSC-SEI from Research to Prevent Blindness, New York, NY, USA.

References

1. Richter-Mueksch S, Kaminski S, Kuchar A, Stifter E, Velikay-Parel M, Radner W. Influence of laser in situ keratomileusis and laser epithelial keratectomy on patients' reading performance. *J Cataract Refract Surg.* 2005;31:1544-1548.

2. Rice ML, Birch EE, Holmes JM. An abbreviated reading speed test. *Optom Vis Sci.* 2005;82:128-133.

3. Virgili G, Pierrottet C, Parmeggiani F, Pennino M, Giacomelli G, Steindler P, Menchini U, Orzalesi N. MNREAD charts. Reading performance in patients with retinitis pigmentosa: a study using the MNREAD charts. *Invest Ophthalmol Vis Sci.* 2004;45:3418-3424.

4. Stifter E, Sacu S, Weghaupt H, Konig F, Richter-Muksch S, Thaler A, Velikay-Parel M, Radner W. Reading performance depending on the type of cataract and its predictability on the visual outcome. *J Cataract Refract Surg.* 2004;30:1259-1267.

5. Richter-Mueksch S, Weghaupt H, Skorpik C, Velikay-Parel M, Radner W. Reading performance with a refractive multifocal and a diffractive bifocal intraocular lens. *J Cataract Refract Surg.* 2002;28:1957-1963.

6. Richter-Mueksch S, Stur M, Stifter E, Radner W. Differences in reading performance of patients with Drusen maculopathy and subretinal fibrosis after CNV. *Graefes Arch Clin Exp Ophthalmol.* 2005;27:1-9.

7. Lott LA, Schneck ME, Haegerström-Portnoy G, Brabyn JA, Gildengorin GL, West CG. Reading performance in older adults with good acuity. *Optom Vis Sci.* 2001;78:316-324.

8. Mönestam E, Wachmeister L. The impact of cataract surgery on low vision patients; a population based study. *Acta Ophthalmol Scand.* 1997;75:569-576.

9. Bourne RRA, Rosser DA, Sukudom P, Dineen B, Laidlaw DAH, Johnson GJ, Murdoch IE. Evaluating a new logMAR chart design to improve visual acuity assessment in population-based surveys. *Eye.* 2003;17:754-758.

10. Ahn SJ, Legge GE, Luebker A. Printed cards for measuring low-vision reading speed. *Vision Res.* 1995;35:1939-1944.

11. Rubin GS, Munoz B, Bandeen-Roche K, West SK. Monocular versus binocular visual acuity as measures of vision impairment and predictors of visual disability. *Invest Ophthalmol Vis Sci.* 2000;41:3327-3334.

12. Legge GE, Ross JA, Luebker A, LaMay JM. Psychophysics of reading. VIII. The Minnesota Low-Vision Reading Test. *Optom Vis Sci.* 1989;66:843-853.

13. Lovie-Kitchin JE, Bowers AR, Woods RL. Oral and silent reading performance with macular degeneration. *Ophthalmic Physiol Opt.* 2000;20:360-370.

14. Radner W, Obermayer W, Richter-Mueksch S, Willinger U, Velikay-Parel M, Eisenwort B. The validity and reliability of short German sentences for measuring reading speed. *Graefes Arch Clin Exp Ophthalmol.* 2002;240:461-467.

CHAPTER 69

MULTIFOCAL IOLS: MEASURING ABERRATIONS

W. Andrew Maxwell, MD, PhD and Jim Schwiegerling, PhD

A variety of strategies have been employed to help alleviate pseudophakic presbyopia. The ideal situation would be to implant an intraocular lens (IOL) that had the capability to either change its power as the young crystalline does[1,2] or change its position in response to contraction of the ciliary muscle.[3,4] The latter case provides accommodation by changing the overall power of the eye through a shift in the separation between the cornea and IOL. These strategies and similar variations are being aggressively pursued as "accommodating" IOLs.[5] Results to date though have been somewhat mixed, but improvement is likely as the accommodative mechanism becomes better understood and the lens designs incorporate these actions.

Multifocal IOLs represent a successful bridging technology between conventional IOLs and a true accommodating IOL. Multifocal optics have 2 or more distinct powers within their aperture.[6] These lenses take advantage of simultaneous vision. In other words, both in-focus and out-of-focus images are simultaneously presented to the retina. The role of the brain then is to filter out the blurred component and interpret the sharp component, providing suitable vision for 2 distinct distances. For example, suppose the required monofocal IOL power to correct distance vision in a patient undergoing refractive surgery is 20 D. If a multifocal lens containing dual powers of 20 D and 24 D is implanted instead, the patient will have simultaneous vision following surgery. (Note that a 4-D add power in the IOL plane is approximately equivalent to a 3-D add in the spectacle plane.) If the patient views a distant object, the distance portion of the IOL will form a sharp image on the retina, while the near portion of the lens will create a blurred image of the distant scene on the retina. Similarly, if the patient now views the text of a book, the near portion of the IOL will form a sharp image of the text on the retina, while the distance portion of the IOL will now create a blurred image of the page. In both cases, if the deleterious effects of the blurred portion of the retinal image are sufficiently low, then successful interpretation of the in-focus portion can be made. As a result of simultaneous vision, some contrast is lost in the in-focus image. Multifocal optics, therefore, represent a tradeoff in visual performance. Monofocal lenses provide sharp, high-contrast images for distance and horribly blurred low-contrast images for near objects. Multifocal lenses provide reasonably high-contrast images for both distance and near vision, but there is some loss in contrast compared to monofocal distance vision. When designing multifocal lenses, control of the out-of-focus portion of the retinal image and understanding the conditions under which the lenses are used are important to optimizing the design. Proper understanding of these issues can provide high-quality multifocal images and lead to happy, spectacle-free patients.

Multifocal Technologies

Multifocal IOLs require 2 or more powers to be simultaneously present in the lens. Zonal refractive lenses introduce multiple powers into the lens by having distinct regions or zones that refract light differently.[7-10] The width or area of these zones is large compared to the wavelength of light. As a result of these large zones, the bending of the light rays is determined strictly by refraction. The local surface curvature of the lens determines the local lens power, and different powers can be incorporated simply by having regions with different curvatures. A simple example of a zonal refractive lens would be to bore a 2-mm hole in the center of a 20-D lens and then fill the region with a 2-mm region cookie-cut from a 24-D lens. This resulting lens would act as a 20-D lens with a 4-D add in the center, providing multifocal optics. One clear problem arises in this design. The junction between the 2 lens regions will be abrupt and discontinuous, leading to stray light effects. Zonal refractive lenses blend the transition between regions. This blend can be rapid or the transition can be made slowly to introduce regions of intermediate power. Clearly, this concept can be extended to more than 2 discrete regions so that multiple annular regions of alternating power can be created. Furthermore, the regions do not even need to be concentric circles. Instead, tear-, wedge-, and even swirl-shaped regions have been demonstrated.

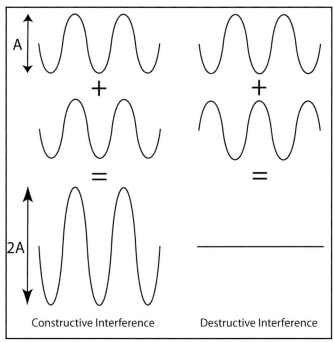

Figure 1. Constructive and destructive interference of waves.

The second optical phenomenon that is exploited to create multifocal optics is diffraction.[11-14] Multifocal optics with diffractive structures are often misunderstood because they move away from the geometrical picture of light rays bending at the surface of the lens. Instead, these lenses take advantage of the wave nature of light. Waves, in general, have the ability to interfere with one another. Consider 2 waves moving toward each other as shown in Figure 1. Each wave is made up of peaks and troughs. The height from the top of the peak to the bottom of the trough is A. When the waves overlap and if the peaks line up, then their amplitudes merge, resulting in a wave with height 2A. This process is called constructive interference. Similarly, if the peaks of one wave line up with the troughs of another wave, then the amplitudes of the waves cancel and the resulting wave has zero height. This process is called destructive interference. In diffractive IOLs, concentric annular zones are created on the face of the lens. At the junction of each zone, an abrupt step appears. Both the height of the step and the dimensions of the zones control the degree of multifocality of the lens. The dimensions of the zones are related to the desired add power and in general, the spacing between zones gets progressively smaller from the lens center to its edge. The height of the step at the boundary of each zone determines how much light is put into the add portion. In typical multifocal diffractive lenses, this step height is chosen so that the peaks of one diffractive zone line up with the troughs of the next larger diffractive zone immediately following the lens. As these waves propagate to the retina, the waves from the various diffractive zones mix and there are 2 distinct regions of constructive interference that correspond to the 2 main foci of the multifocal lens. Roughly 42% of the incident light goes to the add portion, 42% of the incident light contributes to the distance portion, and the remaining light goes into higher diffractive orders. Apodized diffractive lenses modify the step height so that the steps gradually reduce to

zero. This modification has the effect of shifting the energy from the add portion to the distance portion. Consequently, apodized diffractive lenses have nearly equal energy in the near and distance portions for small apertures but become progressively distance biased for larger apertures.

Intraocular Lens Testing Methods

The geometry of how the lens is used within the eye must be taken into account when testing the optical performance of IOLs. Aberrations, which affect the performance, are dependent upon the vergence of light entering the lens. Consequently, a realistic system for testing the IOL must be created. Model eyes are typically used for this testing.[15,16] In general, the model eye consists of a lens that represents an artificial corneal and a wet cell, which is a planar-faced vial containing saline into which the IOL is mounted. The wet cell is placed behind the artificial cornea such that the corneal lens modifies incident planes waves and creates a converging beam onto the IOL. The vergence striking the IOL is meant to be representative of the vergence seen by an implanted IOL. An artificial pupil can also be introduced to simulate performance for different pupil sizes. The performance of the lens can then be evaluated at the image plane of the eye model. Several different types of artificial corneas have been used in eye models. The international standard ISO11979-2 recommends using a model cornea that is virtually free of aberrations in conjunction with the light source used. The standard provides an example model corneal made from a Melles-Griot LAO 034 lens. This lens is a commercially available cemented achromat and consequently is well corrected for both chromatic and spherical aberration. With this model cornea, the aberrations that affect image quality are solely from the IOL. However, the model cornea is not ideal for modern IOLs that incorporate aspheric designs to correct for spherical aberration of the eye or for multifocal designs that intentionally create "aberrations" to give multifocal performance. Model corneas with representative levels of corneal spherical and chromatic dispersion have been proposed and used to test these advanced IOL designs.

Measurement of the modulation transfer function (MTF) is a routine test for measuring the optical quality of IOLs.[17,18] The MTF of an optical system describes the amount of contrast that is passed through the system. If a high-contrast sinusoidal target is imaged by an optical system, then the contrast of the resultant image is reduced. In general, the contrast tends to decrease more severely with higher spatial frequency (ie, finer spacing between the bars of the sinusoidal target). The MTF of a model eye is conveniently calculated by measuring the line spread function (LSF) of the model eye. The LSF, as its name implies, is simply the image of a narrow slit formed by the model eye. The MTF is mathematically calculated from the Fourier transform of the LSF and knowledge of the slit geometry. Figure 2 illustrates some of the properties of the MTF.

In addition to MTF testing, model eyes are useful for qualitatively visualizing the optical performance of different IOLs. A digital camera can be used to capture the "retinal" image formed by the model eye. We have constructed a model eye

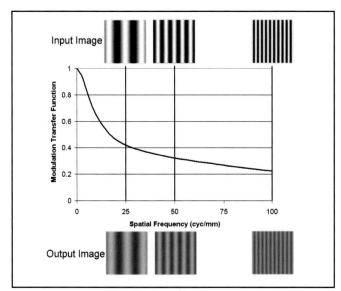

Figure 2. The effects of MTF on sinusoidal targets.

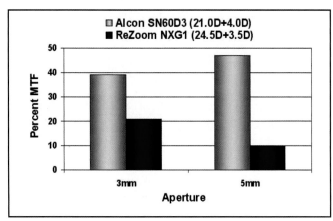

Figure 3. MTF at 100 lp/mm measured with the ISO model eye at 3- and 5-mm aperture distances.

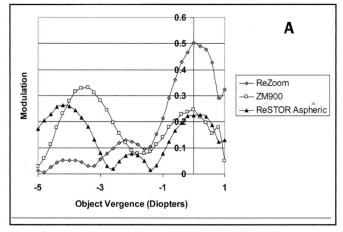

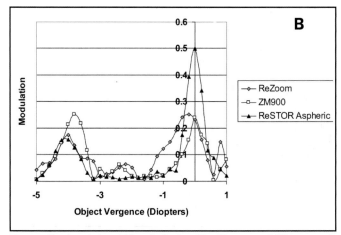

Figure 4. The through-focus MTF results for the 3 IOLs. (A) 3-mm pupil. (B) 6-mm pupil.

that consists of a cornea that contains representative levels of both spherical aberration and chromatic aberration found in the human cornea. We have also constructed a LSF measurement system utilizing the techniques outlined above to measure MTF. The LSF system has also been designed to allow different object vergences, so that we can simulate different target distances and consequently measure through-focus MTFs. This feature allows the IOL performance to be measured for near, intermediate, and distance vision. In addition, the model eye can also be attached to a commercial digital camera to capture arbitrary scenes through a variety of IOL designs. We have explored a night driving scene with this portable system to illustrate the stray light effects introduced by different styles of multifocal IOLs. The multifocal IOLs tested were the ReSTOR aspheric lens (Alcon, Fort Worth, TX), the ReZoom lens (Advanced Medical Optics, Santa Ana, CA), and the Tecnis Multifocal ZM900 (Advanced Medical Optics).

The MTF for the ReSTOR and ReZoom IOLs were measured using an ISO model eye with both a 3- and 5-mm pupil. Comparing the MTF results at 100 lp/mm demonstrates that the apodized diffractive design provides the best MTF values at both pupil sizes (Figure 3).[19]

To compare the MTF results from different IOL styles, we selected MTF value at 50 cycles/mm for each IOL and plotted the through-focus MTF for object vergences of −5 D to +1 D. A spatial frequency of 50 cycles/mm corresponds to the fundamental frequency of the 20/40 line on the Snellen eye chart. Figure 4 shows the results of these measurements. The results for the 3-mm pupil size show that the AMO ReZoom is primarily designed for distance viewing at that pupil size while the other 2 designs balance the performance between distance and near. The 6-mm pupil size shows noticeably different results. At this larger pupil size, the ReSTOR Aspheric shifts its performance toward distance vision, while the other 2 designs continue to balance performance between near and distance vision.

The night driving scene photographs were taken with a 6-mm pupil size to represent the pupil size under dark conditions. The photographs are shown in Figure 5. Inspection of these images shows that the ReSTOR Aspheric IOL has less stray light artifacts compared to the ReZoom and ZM900. The stray light artifacts associated with the diffractive lenses tend to be arcs about light sources. With the zonal refractive lens, the stray light appears as a continuous flare. The continuity of the flare is likely due to the continuous change in power that must occur with zonal refractive lenses in the transition regions between refractive zones. Diffractive lenses, on the other hand, have discrete foci, leading to a more separated

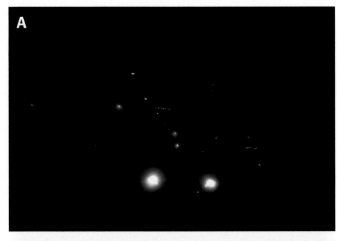

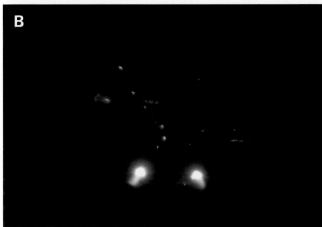

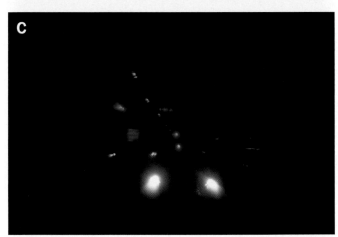

Figure 5. Night driving scene through the different multifocal lenses. (A) ReSTOR aspheric. (B) ReZoom. (C) Tecnis ZM900.

out-of-focus artifact. The reduction of the stray light effects in the ReSTOR Aspheric lens is likely due to the apodized design that only creates the simultaneous vision effect over a small central region of the lens. Consequently, the out-of-focus energy in the apodized diffractive comes from a significantly smaller area of the total aperture than with full-aperture diffractives. This shift to a distance bias in the ReSTOR Aspheric lens is a design strategy, with the thought being that there is a reduced need for near vision under dim lighting.

Conclusion

Advancements in technology and our understanding of visual optics has resulted in the current generation of multifocal intraocular lenses (MFIOL) aimed at restoring vision. The current MFIOLs utilize differing principles of light management to provide recipients a full range of vision. Unfortunately, none of the available lenses are perfect and thus the benefits of a full range of vision are accompanied by a range of potential side effects. Thus a surgeon is left with managing a benefit/risk ratio for each patient. Understanding the light management principles between differing styles of MFIOLs in connection with basic optical bench testing studies, as described in this chapter, should help surgeons better manage the advantages and disadvantages of each MFIOL style and enable them to select the best match for each patient.

References

1. Haefliger E, Parel JM. Accommodation of an endocapsular silicone lens (phaco-ersatz) in the aging rhesus monkey. *J Refract Corneal Surg.* 1994;10:550-555.
2. Nishi O, Nishi K. Accommodation amplitude after lens refilling with injectable silicone by sealing the capsule with a plug in primates. *Arch Ophthalmol.* 1998;116:1358-1361.
3. Mastropasqua L, Toto L, Nubile M, Falconio G, Ballone E. Clinical study of the 1CU accommodating intraocular lens. *J Cataract Refract Surg.* 2003;29:1307-1312.
4. Cumming JS, Colvard DM, Dell SJ, Doane J, et al. Clinical evaluation of the Crystalens AT-45 accommodating intraocular lens: Results of the US Food and Drug Administration clinical trial. *J Cataract Refract Surg.* 2006;32:812-825.
5. Doane JF, Jackson RT. Accommodative intraocular lenses: considerations on use, function and design. *Curr Opin Ophthalmol.* 2007;18:318-324.
6. Avitabile T, Marano F. Multifocal intra-ocular lenses. *Curr Opin Ophthalmol.* 2001;12:12-16.
7. Steinert RF, Aker BL, Trentacost DJ, Smith PJ, Tarantino N. A prospective comparative study of the AMO ARRAY zonal-progressive multifocal silicone intraocular lens and a monofocal intraocular lens. *Ophthalmology.* 1999;106:1243-1255.
8. Steinert RF. Visual outcomes with multifocal intraocular lenses. *Curr Opin Ophthalmol.* 2000;11:12-41.
9. Sen HN, Sarikkola A-U, Uusitalo RJ, Laatikainen L. Quality of vision after AMO Array multifocal intraocular lens implantation. *J Cataract Refract Surg.* 2004;33:2483-2493.
10. Kawamorita T, Uozato H. Modulation transfer function and pupil size in multifocal and monofocal intraocular lenses in vitro. *J Cataract Refract Surg.* 2005;31:2379-2385.
11. Cohen AL. Diffractive bifocal lens designs. *Optom Vis Sci.* 1993;70:461-468.
12. Klein SA. Understanding the diffractive bifocal contact lens. *Optom Vis Sci.* 1993;70:439-460.
13. Schmidinger G, Simader C, Dejaco-Ruhswurm I, Skorpik C, Pieh S. Contrast sensitivity function in eyes with diffractive bifocal intraocular lenses. *J Cataract Refract Surg.* 2005;31:2076-2083.
14. Davison JA, Simpson MJ. History and development of the apodized diffractive intraocular lens. *J Cataract Refract Surg.* 2006;32:849-858.
15. Gobbi PG, Fasce F, Bozza S, Brancato R. Experimental characterization of the imaging properties of multifocal intraocular lenses. *Proc SPIE.* 2003;4951:104-111.

16. Pieh S, Marvan P, Lackner B, et al. Quantitative performance of bifocal and multifocal intraocular lenses in a model eye. *Arch Ophthalmol.* 2002;120:23-28.

17. Portney V. Optical testing and inspection methodology for modern intraocular lenses. *J Cataract Refract Surg.* 1992;18:607-613.

18. Lang AJ, Lakshminarayanan V, Portney V. Phenomenological model for interpreting the clinical significance of the in vitro optical transfer function. *J Opt Soc Am A.* 1993;10:1600-1610.

19. Maxwell A. Modulation transfer function comparison of an apodized diffractive IOL and a zonal refractive IOL. Presented at: ASCRS; April 30, 2007; San Diego, CA.

CHAPTER 70

MULTIFOCAL IOLs: COMPARING ABERRATIONS

Lana J. Nagy, BS; Geunyoung Yoon, PhD; and Scott MacRae, MD

With the recent advent of multifocal intraocular lenses (MF IOLs), the prospect of greater pseudoaccommodation has increased. An understanding of how these IOLs actually affect the optics and visual quality of patients will be helpful in order to maximize patient satisfaction after lens implantation.

Measuring Aberrations in Multifocal Lenses

A high-resolution Shack-Hartmann wavefront sensor was developed in our optics lab and used to measure the 2 most popular MF IOLs, the ReZoom (Advanced Medical Optics, Santa Ana, CA) and the ReSTOR (Alcon, Fort Worth, TX). The ReZoom lens is a distant dominant refractive lens. It consists of 5 concentric refractive zones that correct for distance and near with aspheric transitions between the zones, which help to provide intermediate vision. The ReSTOR lens on the other hand is a near dominant diffractive lens on a refractive base. This lens contains a 3.6-mm central diffractive zone, allowing for 41% of the light energy entering this area to be directed to the near focus with another 41% directed to far, and the remaining 18% is scattered as it is directed into higher diffractive orders.[1] The peripheral portion of the lens beyond the diffractive central zone is a refractive lens designed to maximize light direction to the distant focal point as the pupil size increases.

The Shack-Hartmann wavefront sensor contained a lenslet array with a 133-μm center to center spacing and a focal length of 3.75 mm. This wavefront sensor could record the high spatial frequency information in these IOLs. The wavefront sensor used was a custom design with a much higher resolution (1040 spots for a 5-mm pupil) than the typical commercially available wavefront sensors found in clinical settings. These more commonly used clinical wavefront sensors typically utilize >100 spots,[2] which may represent an insufficient number of lenslets to properly measure high frequency higher-order

aberrations that could be induced by these lenses. Figure 1 illustrates the spot patterns collected with the custom wavefront sensor along with representative images of the ReZoom and ReSTOR lenses. The multiple refractive zones contained within the ReZoom lens can be seen in the spot pattern; the half circles represent the corresponding zones between the representative image and the spot pattern. The first 3 diffractive zones in the spot array of the ReSTOR lens can be visualized, but the spacing between the other diffractive zones are beyond the resolution of the custom-built wavefront sensor.

Higher-Order Spherical Aberrations of Multifocal Lenses

The high-resolution Shack-Hartmann wavefront sensor was able to image the high frequency information with both lenses, which was then converted to Zernike polynomials and yielded the dominant higher-order terms as higher-order spherical aberrations (HOSA). The other higher-order aberrations such as coma, trefoil, and secondary astigmatism were minimal with proper centration. The ReZoom lens had HOSA terms up to the 14th order that were significant, while the ReSTOR lens had them up to the 8th order (Figure 2). The wavefront maps and wavefront profiles for these lenses are illustrated in Figure 2. We also noted that different wavefront reconstruction algorithms such as Fourier and zonal methods provided almost identical wavefront structures.

It has been previously reported that relatively small amounts of primary spherical aberration, when combined appropriately with defocus, can increase retinal image quality and depth of focus.[3,4] In the MF IOLs studied here, the negative primary (4th order) spherical aberration term helps to increase the depth of focus of the lenses into the near dioptric range, allowing for focal points at reading distances. The ReZoom lens also has a significant amount of tertiary or eighth-order spherical

Figure 1. Spot patterns collected with the high-resolution Shack-Hartmann wavefront sensor, in addition to the representative images for both the ReZoom and ReSTOR multifocal IOLs. The half circles represent corresponding zones between the spot pattern (noted with close inspection) and the representative image of the implant shown below. The 3.6-mm zone in the ReSTOR spot pattern is shown in order to provide a sense of where the diffractive zone ends in this lens.

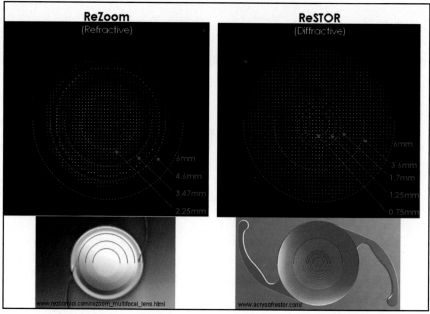

Figure 2. Measured Zernike aberrations for the ReZoom and ReSTOR multifocal IOLs. Both lenses were dominated by HOSAs, the ReZoom lens to the 14th order, and the ReSTOR lens to the 8th order for a 4.6-mm analysis pupil diameter. The representative wavefront maps and their corresponding wavefront side profiles below them clearly illustrate how the HOSA terms affect the wavefront of each lens and how different they are.

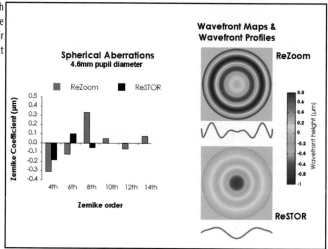

aberration, which may be acting to increase its intermediate focusing abilities, which has been noted with this implant. The dominating negative spherical aberration term in the ReSTOR lens aids in its near focusing abilities while maintaining the distance focus as well. The lack of other HOSA terms though may be why the intermediate focus of this lens is lacking.

Wavefront Interaction Effects on Retinal Image Quality and Depth of Focus

Although the spherical aberrations in the multifocal lenses are acting to increase the depth of focus, they may also be contributing to the diminished retinal image quality that is sometimes reported by patients with these lenses. As you can envisage from the wavefront profiles in Figure 2, light rays entering the eye are being focused by different zones of the optics to create the distant and near focal points but there are aspects of the wavefront that direct light rays away

from the optical axis. It is these scattered light rays that end up creating the halo, glare, or a washed out effect and may reduce the overall contrast around objects of interest. The convolved letters in Figure 3 demonstrate the effect of spherical aberrations and defocus for the ReSTOR and ReZoom multifocal IOLs in white light. Previously reported clinical evaluations of these lenses[5] correspond well to our evaluations for a 4.6-mm pupil. Both the ReZoom and ReSTOR lenses show an increased depth of focus that is accompanied by a diminished retinal image quality at the various dioptric levels of focus. Both ReZoom and ReSTOR yield reasonable near retinal image quality. It is interesting that the image quality for the ReSTOR lens drops off in the intermediate range (~ +1.00 D) and is improved in the near range (~ +2.5D). A trend was found when ReSTOR was tested on the optical bench, which is what is also noted clinically. In addition the ReZoom lens shows good retinal image quality in the hyperopic range. This may mean that undercorrection with this lens could leave the patient with a greater depth of focus. This is not the case with the ReSTOR lens, which has a set depth of

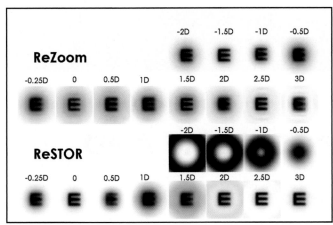

Figure 3. Convolved letter Es, with the aberration information according to our measurements, through focus showing the predicted retinal image quality of the multifocal IOLs with a 4.6-mm pupil. The letters were convolved with white (polychromatic) light. The ReZoom lens has a more even retinal image quality through various levels of focus, which extended into the hyperopic focal range. The ReSTOR lens had definite peaks of retinal image quality for both distance and near focus.

focus. Note that for the focused letters the contrast is slightly degraded and the sharpness of the letters has been compromised, which is an outcome of the multiple spherical aberration terms inherent in these lenses.

Decentration of Spherical Aberrations

As with all IOL implantations, centration of the lens is crucial to the performance of the optics in the eye. We have noted in our model that centration may also play an important role in depth of focus and especially retinal image quality with these MF IOLs. These MFIOLs contain HOSAs that when decentered induce other higher-order aberration terms such as coma and astigmatism, which will also act to degrade the retinal image quality in the eye. In addition, our model resulted in a decrease in depth of focus with decentrations greater than a 200 μm. Thus, moderate levels of decentration with the MF IOL may also contribute to a reduction in image quality compared to a monofocal lens.

Limitations of This Study

Although our measurements correspond to those of recent clinical evaluations for the ReZoom and ReSTOR lenses, there are limitations to our techniques. For instance, the ReSTOR lens is a diffractive lens that has properties that cannot be measured with a Shack-Hartmann–type wavefront sensor. The impact on retinal image quality and depth of focus produced by the diffracted light from the ReSTOR lens was not evaluated with our custom system. However, evaluations of the point spread function (PSF) of this lens measured directly compared to that calculated from our wavefront measurements (data not shown) did show comparable PSFs, indicating that although the wavefront sensor was not measuring the diffraction of the lens, it was accurately characterizing the optical quality of the lens. In addition, the lenslet spacing in the custom wavefront sensor may not be small enough to capture all of the high spatial frequency information contained within these MF IOLs. For a more complete evaluation, bench tests that account for the diffracted light and immeasurable high spatial frequency information will still be important.

Conclusion

MF IOLs are a good step forward in the advancement of presbyopia-correcting lenses. Our evaluations of these lenses showed that HOSAs are acting to improve depth of focus while trying to maintain relatively good retinal image quality for patients. This improved depth of focus, which allows for improved near vision, also reduces retinal image quality at distance, creating the tradeoff that we note clinically. Patients are enthusiastic about being less dependent on spectacles for near, but some individuals note reduced visual quality overall. Further studies demonstrating the role of pupil size, implant decentration tolerances, and other areas may allow us to better predict who is more likely to be successful with multifocal implants.

References

1. Davison JA, Simpson MJ. History and development of the apodized diffractive intraocular lens. *J Cataract Refract Surg.* 2006;32:849-858.
2. Krueger RR. Technology requirements for customized corneal ablation. In: MacRae SM, Krueger RR, Applegate RA, eds. *Customized Corneal Ablation: The Quest for Super Vision.* Thorofare, NJ: SLACK Incorporated; 2001:133-147.
3. Jansonius NM, Kooijman AC. The effect of spherical aberration and other aberrations upon the modulation transfer of the defocused human eye. *Ophthalmic Physiol Opt.* 1998;18:504-513.
4. Nio YK, Jansonius NM, Fidler V, Geraghty E, Norrby S, Kooijman AC. Spherical and irregular aberrations are important for the optimal performance of the human eye. *Ophthalmic Physiol Opt.* 2002;22:103-112.
5. Pepose JS, Qazi MA, Davies J, et al. Visual performance of patients with bilateral vs combination Crystalens, ReZoom and ReSTOR intraocular lens implants. *Am J Ophthalmol.* 2007;144:347-357.

CHAPTER 71

PSEUDOACCOMMODATION AND SPHERICAL ABERRATION

Marc A. Michelson, MD

The treatment of presbyopia is the new paradigm in ophthalmic refractive surgery. Eliminating the need for spectacle correction for both near and distance vision is now an obtainable goal in many patients. First-generation intraocular lenses (IOLs) specifically designed to improve accommodative amplitude are currently divided into 2 categories: accommodating lenses designed to dynamically move in the anterior-posterior visual axis in response to ciliary body contraction and relaxation; and, multifocal static lenses designed to create multiple focal points for near and distance vision. The explanation and functionality of both accommodative and multifocal lenses on the surface appear to be straightforward and simplistic, but a review of our knowledge of accommodation in the pseudophakic eye reveals anything but a simple explanation. A simplistic explanation would account for precise and predictable responses in each and every patient. In fact, patients may have variable responses to these lenses, and our knowledge as to how they work and function is becoming increasingly complex. Understanding interactions of the optical variables in the pseudophakic eye that increase depth of focus will only enhance our ability to improve patients' outcomes for the treatment of presbyopia.

Accommodative potential of either a pseudophakic or aphakic eye resulting in the combination of functional distance and near vision has been described as pseudoaccommodation or apparent accommodation.[1-3] Any degree of accommodative amplitude in the aphakic or pseudophakic state requires the optical system of the eye to overcome the restrictions of an artificial monofocal optical system designed to have a single focal point. Any supra-accommodative potential that an eye possesses with a monofocal implant would be additive, if instead, that same eye were implanted with a lens designed to produce accommodation. This realization alone may help explain why patients with accommodating implants may have variable accommodative responses.

Depth of Field

Apparent accommodation in pseudophakia has been explained by an increase in the depth of field[4] resulting in an expansion of the range of focus around a focal plane that is acceptably sharp. The classic definition of depth of focus is the range of defocus values for which there is a blur of small enough size that it will not adversely affect the performance of the optical system.[4] Depth of field does not produce focal points that change abruptly from sharp to unsharp, but instead occur as a gradual transition. The amplitude of legibility may extend beyond the range of the depth of focus allowing the eye to discern a target even if it is blurred. Therefore depth of focus and amplitude of legibility may be different.

The ability of a spherical monofocal IOL to exhibit pseudo-accommodation has been reported to be 1.27 ± 0.75 D[1] and 2.01 ± 0.95 D.[2] Unaided distance vision of 20/30 and near J5 could be obtained in 80% of pseudophakic eyes with a pupil diameter of 2.2 mm and a refractive error of −0.75 D.[1] An inverse relationship exists between pupillary aperture and depth of field, the smaller the pupil, the greater is the depth of field.[3] In 1984 Nakazawa and Ohtsuki calculated the "anterior" depth of field from near and far focal points in 39 pseudophakic patients with posterior chamber IOLs.[2] The apparent accommodation was significantly correlated to the measured anterior depth of field. The correlation coefficient to anterior depth of field was greater than the correlation coefficient to the reciprocal of the pupillary radius. Depth of field sufficient to produce apparent accommodation in pseudophakia, therefore, is not completely accounted for by pupillary aperture alone. Even though pupillary diameter is significantly correlated to apparent accommodation,[3] additional factors must be concomitantly contributing to the phenomenon of pseudophakic apparent accommodation to increase depth of focus. The emerging application of adaptive optics to the eye may uncover the answers to the mystery of monofocal pseudoaccommodation.

Corneal Factors

The influence of the cornea to enhance depth of field in the pseudophakic patient is beginning to become better elucidated. Corneal multifocality and myopic astigmatism have been identified as factors contributing to pseudophakic apparent accommodation.[5-7] Nanavaty et al showed a positive correlation of pseudoaccommodation in eyes with monofocal lens implants to corneal multifocality.[8] Pseudoaccommodation was present in 9% of patients implanted with the Acrysof SN60AT (Alcon, Fort Worth, TX). These patients had both good near and distance vision. Eyes with uncorrected distance vision of 20/40 or better and near vision on J4 (20/30) were evaluated to determine what influence corneal astigmatism, pupil size, axial IOL movement, age, and axial length had on the amplitude of accommodation. Of all the variables evaluated, against-the-rule astigmatism was found to most positively increase the odds of pseudoaccommodation by a factor of 10.

Corneal-induced Zernike higher-order aberrations may play a significant role in optical performance in pseudophakic apparent accommodation. Oshika et al have demonstrated a positive correlation of corneal multifocality and corneal coma aberrations of the cornea to apparent accommodation in the pseudophakic eye implanted with monofocal posterior chamber IOLs.[9] Third-order coma-like corneal aberrations were associated with greatest amounts of pseudoaccommodation. Corneal trefoil ($Z 3^{-3}$) displayed the highest correlation to apparent accommodation. In contrast, positive corneal spherical aberration had no significant correlation to apparent accommodation. Apparent pseudoaccommodation was found to be 2.08 ± 1.01 D.[9]

Postoperative-induced optical properties of the cornea must also be considered as a variable influencing apparent accommodation. Construction and location of the cataract incision influence the induction of both astigmatism and trefoil, but appear to have little impact on spherical aberration and coma.[10] Negative astigmatism, flattening of the cornea, can occur at the wound site, enhancing corneal multifocality and positively impacting apparent accommodation in pseudophakia.

Lenticular Factors

In the normal lens there is a systematic progression toward negative spherical aberration and an increase in vertical coma with increasing accommodation.[11] Negative spherical aberration from the lens results in paraxial rays focusing anterior to or in front of peripheral rays refracted at the periphery of the lens. Negative spherical aberration acts to manipulate the caustic envelope of light refracted by the curved surfaces of the lens. This increases depth of field by degrading the best focus image to the benefit of out-of-focus imagery.

Newer IOLs have incorporated aspheric designs to compensate for positive corneal spherical aberrations. The intent is to reduce total ocular spherical aberrations in order to improve contrast and retinal imagery.[12] Aspheric IOLs, while designed to improve contrast sensitivity in low light and improve the overall quality of vision, produce an additional benefit: they significantly enhance pseudoaccommodation (Michelson, unpublished data).[13] The relationship between aspheric monofocal IOLs with negative spherical aberration and apparent accommodation in pseudophakic eyes is currently being evaluated. Preliminary observations of eyes implanted with the Acrysof SN60WF (Alcon) aspheric IOL have shown an unusually high degree of pseudoaccommodation as well as an unanticipated greater depth of focus in the clinical setting.

In a review of 42 eyes implanted with the aspheric Acrysof SN60WF, 30 eyes had an uncorrected visual acuity of 20/30 or better. Twenty (20) of the 30 eyes had uncorrected near vision of 20/60 equivalent or better at a range of 12 to 18 inches. Forty-three percent (43%) of eyes with 20/20 uncorrected distance vision could easily read 20/25 or better and a normal reading distance. Eighty-nine percent (89%) of eyes with 20/25 uncorrected distance vision could read 20/60 or better at a normal reading distance. Forty-four percent (44%) of eyes with 20/25 uncorrected distance vision could read 20/30 or better at a comfortable reading distance. Eighty-three percent (83%) of eyes with 20/30 uncorrected distance vision could read at the 20/40 level at a comfortable reading distance. These observations indicate excellent functional pseudoaccommodation in nearly 45% of eyes implanted with an Acrysof aspheric IOL and achieving uncorrected distance vision of 20/30 or better. In addition, these eyes demonstrate an accommodative functionality equal to or better than lenses currently designed for dynamic accommodation or static multifocal pseudoaccommodation. Clinical studies are being designed to establish how corneal wavefront aberrations and aspheric IOLs with negative spherical aberrations can produce enhanced pseudoaccommodation.

There are several references in the ophthalmic literature that support the hypothesis that an IOL with negative spherical aberration would enhance pseudoaccommodation and significantly increase depth of field. Utilizing adaptive optics visual simulation, Artal and Tabernero[13] experimentally demonstrated that correcting an eye with wavefront aberrations simulating an aspheric IOL, neither reduces the depth of field nor renders it more vulnerable to errors of defocus. In fact, they found that, when compared to spherical IOLs, simulated wavefront aberrations from aspheric IOLs generated better retinal image quality for 1) depth of focus, 2) best focus, and 3) different values of defocus. Experimentally removing negative spherically aberrations also reduced depth of focus.

Piers et al[4] utilized an adaptive optics visual simulator to simulate wavefront optics of spherical and aspheric IOLs in normal eyes in order to evaluate the benefits of modified spherical aberration profiles. Simulation of spherical aberration-correcting IOLs outperformed simulations of spherical IOLs. Studies on visual performance also offer a better understanding of the impact of negative spherical aberration on pseudoaccommodation due to depth of focus. Simulation studies have demonstrated that spherical aberration–correcting IOLs functionally improve depth of focus by at least 1 D. Visual performance remained satisfactory for up to 1 D of defocus with aspheric IOL simulation compared to spherical IOL simulation.

Dynamic Properties of the IOL

In addition to static variables of pseudophakic apparent accommodation, there is also controversial evidence that a posterior chamber monofocal lens gains additional accommodative amplitude from anterior axial displacement caused by ciliary body contraction. Vámosi et al[15] have shown anterior axial IOL displacement in both 3-piece MA60BM (Alcon) and single-piece acrylic (Akreos disc) IOLs. IOL displacement was measured when eyes were focused at far points both with and without cycloplegia. Amplitude of accommodation and IOL shift measured approximately 0.2 mm in the early postoperative period and increased to almost 0.50 mm at 6 months postoperatively. Tsorbatzoglou et al[16] however, demonstrated with partial coherence interferometry that implants do not exhibit dynamic changes under physiologic accommodative testing and any pseudoaccommodation of these IOLs is independent of anterior-posterior movement.

Multifactorial Components of Pseudoaccommodation

The phenomenon of pseudophakic accommodation is a function of multiple optical factors involving the cornea, lens implant, and pupil diameter. The sum of static properties from both the lens and the cornea, as well as dynamic properties of the implant caused by ciliary muscle contraction, will determine the total amplitude of apparent accommodation with a monofocal lens. Depth of focus in a monofocal pseudophakic eye is positively influenced by corneal multifocality, against-the-rule astigmatism, and vertical corneal coma. Properties of a lens implant that positively affects apparent accommodation are increasing power of the intraocular lenses[17] and aspheric lenses with negative spherical aberration. Preliminary observations of patients with monofocal aspheric IOLs suggest that negative spherical aberration IOLs may play a significant role in increasing the amplitude of apparent accommodation in pseudophakia.

References

1. Elder M, Murphy C, Sanderson G. Apparent accommodation and depth of field in pseudophakia. *J Cataract Refract Surg.*1996;22:615-619.

2. Nakazawa M, Ohtsuki K. Apparent accommodation in pseudophakic eyes after implantation of posterior chamber intraocular lenses: optical analysis. *Invest Ophth Vis Sci.* 1984;25:1458-1460.

3. Nakazawa M, Ohtsuki K. Apparent accommodation in pseudophakic eyes after implantation of posterior chamber intraocular lenses. *Am J Ophthalmol.* 1983;96:435.

4. Piers P, Fernandez E, Manzanera S. Adaptive optics simulation of intraocular lenses with modified spherical aberration. *Invest Ophth Vis Sci.* 2004;45:4601-4610.

5. Huber C. Myopic Astigmatism as a substitute for accommodation in pseudophakia. *Am Intraocular Implant Soc.* 1981;52(2):123-78.52:123.

6. Trinadade F, Oliveira A, Frasson M. Benefit of against-the-rule astigmatism to uncorrected near vision. *J Cataract Refract Surg.* 1997;23:82-85.

7. Fukuyama M, Oshika T, Amano S, Yoshitomi F. Relationship between apparent accommodation and corneal multifocality in pseudophakic eyes. *Ophthalmology.* 1999; 106:1178-1181.

8. Nanavaty M, Vasavada A, Patel A, Raj S. Analysis of patients with good uncorrected distance and near vision after monofocal lens implantation. *J Cataract Ref Surg.* 2006;32:1091-1097.

9. Oshika T, et al. Apparent accommodation and corneal wavefront aberration in pseudophakic eyes. *Invest Ophth Vis Sci.* 2002;43:2882-2886.

10. Guirao A, Tejedor J, Artal P. Corneal aberrations before and after small-incision cataract surgery. *Investigative Ophth & Vis Sci.* 2004;45:4312-4319.

11. Vilupuru A, Roorda A, Glasser A. Changes in ocular aberrations during accommodation in rhesus monkeys. *J Vis.* 2002;2(10):123.

12. Holladay J, Piers P, Koranyl G, et al. A new intraocular lens design to reduce spherical aberration in the pseudophakic eye. *J Refract Surg.* 2002;18:683-691.

13. Michelson, M.A. 2007: (unpublished data)

14. Artal P, Tabernero J. Do aspheric IOLs worsen pseudoaccommodation? These lenses improve retinal image quality without compromising depth of focus. *Cataract Ref Surg Today.* 2006;6(11):76-77.

15. Vámosi P, Memeth G, Berta A. Pseudophakic accommodation with 2 models of foldable intraocular lenses. *J Cataract Ref Surg.* 2006;32:221-226.

16. Tsorbatzoglou A, Németh G, Berta A. Pseudophakic accommodation and pseudoaccommodation under physiological conditions measured with partial coherence interferometry. *J Cataract Ref Surg.* 2006;32.

17. Hunter J, Campbell M, Geraghty E. Optical analysis of accommodating intraocular lens. *J Cataract Refract Surg.* 2006;32:269-278.

CHAPTER 72

UNDERSTANDING MULTIFOCAL HALOS

Carlos Vergés, MD, PhD

Recently, multifocal intraocular lenses (IOLs) have been developed that offer the pseudophakic patient the possibility of satisfactory vision at both distance and near conditions without the use of spectacles.[1-7] However, the use of multifocal IOLs has been very limited in the past because of several drawbacks and limitations. Surgical techniques were not as refined as they are today, and predictable and accurate biometry to achieve emmetropia was challenging. Finally, the photic side effects, such as glare and halos, were important problems.

Nowadays the newest multifocal IOL designs are engineered to minimize photic phenomena compared with earlier multifocal lenses. However, they are still associated with a higher frequency of halos and glare (20% to 25%)[8,9] when compared to monofocal (3% to 9%)[8] or accommodating lenses (4%).[10] Some, but not all, patients may neurally adapt to these photic phenomena. This may explain why only 16% spontaneously reported glare and halo in one multifocal study, whereas 40% to 50% of these same patients admitted to these side effects upon active questioning (compared with 13% to 20% of patients with a monofocal IOL).[11]

Types of Multifocal Lenses

Three general optical principles have been used in the design of multifocal IOLs: multizone refractive, diffractive, and aspheric lens designs. The multizonal refractive method is defined by 2 different powers that are incorporated into circular or annular (ring-shaped) refractive zones. Some early IOLs had 2 zones (Iolab NuVue), 3 zones (Storz Tru Vista [St. Louis, MO], Alcon AcuraSee [Fort Worth, TX], Ioptex, Morcher, and Pharmacia), 5 zones (Advanced Medical Optics Array [Santa Ana, CA]), and 7 zones (Adatomed). The 5-zone foldable silicone Array IOL (AMO), which was approved by the Food and Drug Administration (FDA) in 1997, is the most common contemporary example of this category.

Each lens zone has a different effective aperture, and this can affect the quality of the image that it provides because the pupil diameter changes in response to different illumination levels as well as with the accommodative reflex. The energy balance between the 2 images and the quality of the images varies with the engineering design and environmental conditions.

The second method to create a lens with 2 powers uses a diffractive surface on a refractive platform.[3,12,13] These designs divide light between 2 images through the use of different diffractive orders, with an equal amount of light directed to the near and distant primary foci for all pupil diameters when the diffractive structure covers the whole lens surface. This design was introduced by 3M (St. Paul, MN) in 1988.

A third design method uses aspheric optic regions that increase the depth of field of the lens. The addition of asphericity in this application does not provide an additional distinct focus but instead aims to expand the range of focus. However, this gain occurs at the expense of image contrast. Lenses that primarily used asphericity as a strategy were the Progress lens from Domilens and the Nordan aspheric. Some zonal lenses also employ a level of asphericity, such as the Ioptex three-zone lens, with distinct aspheric regions between the zones, or the new ReZoom and Tecnis multifocal IOLs, both from AMO.

Why We See Halos With Multifocal Lenses

With multifocal lenses when a distant object is viewed, a sharp retinal image is provided by those parts of the lens within the pupillary area that have the distance correction, and a blurred image is provided by the other parts of the lens. These images are superimposed on the retina (Figure 1). The roles of the corrections change when a near object is observed. In this situation, those regions of the lens occupied by the near correction provide the correctly focused retinal image. In both situations, the unwanted effect of the light from the out-of-focus image reduces the contrast of the in-focus

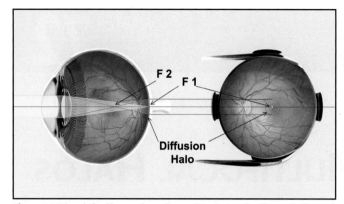

Figure 1. With multifocal lenses when a distant object is viewed, a sharp retinal image is provided by those parts of the lens within the pupillary area that have the distance correction, F1, and a blurred image is provided by the other parts of the lens, F2. These images are superimposed on the retina generating a diffusion halo that impairs visual quality and contrast sensitivity.

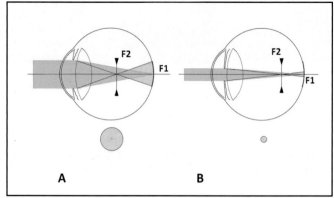

Figure 2. Under scotopic conditions the near focus generates a superimposed image creating a diffusion halo over the principal distance focus (B), larger than a small pupil in photopic conditions when the superimposed image and diffusion halo is at a minimum (A). This explains the increased of depth of field in an eye with a miotic pupil.

Figure 3. Schematic diagram showing the general form of the point images at distance and near conditions for the Array lens (A), The approximations of geometrical optics have been used to show the image blur for ocular entrance pupil diameters of 3.5, and 4.6 mm, as observed at luminance of 85, 5, and 2.5 candelas per square meter (cd/m2), photopic and scotopic conditions, respectively. The images are shown as negatives; the dark spot at the center of each image is the in-focus image formed by the appropriate correction (distance for distance, near for near), and the surrounding circular or annular blur patches are formed by the out of focus images.

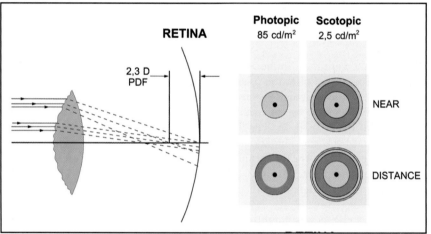

image.[14,15] Visual quality can, however, still be fully acceptable to the patient, and there may be little effect on high-contrast distance and near acuities.

This situation changes depending on the pupillary diameter. When the pupil is small (between 2 and 3.5 mm) as observed under photopic conditions, the diffusion halo generated by the superimposed image of the near focus over the distance focus that converges upon the retina, is at its minimum (Figure 2B). This explains the increase of depth of field in the setting of miotic pupils.

The problem appears when the pupil increases in diameter. The diffusion halo in the retina will now be greater (Figure 2A), and all the exposed rings and zones comprising the multifocal optic will contribute to the retinal image. For example, Figure 3 illustrates how light from the different zones of the lens will strike the retina depending on the pupil size.

Another important fact is related to the additional add for near vision. The higher this is, the greater the distance between the created foci will be (near-distance), and at the same time, the greater the diffusion halo created in the retina will be. This explains why diffractive IOLs with a high add for near vision (eg, 3 D to 3.5 D) produce more halos and glare complications than zone refractive lenses that have a lower add (2.5 D) and devote a lower percentage of light to near vision (20%).

Diffractive Lenses and Halos

Unlike the multizonal refractive optic, with these IOLs, the image quality and energy balance between the images are no longer dependent on pupil diameter. A necessary artifact of any refractive-diffractive optical system is that a portion of the light energy (about 18%) is also directed into higher diffraction orders. This leaves about 82% of the light available to be divided between each of the 2 primary lens foci.

The defocused image of a light at night from the reading add power of any multifocal IOL may sometimes be visible as a halo because it appears against a dark background.

With larger pupils with the ReSTOR IOL, more energy is directed to the distance focus because the outer region of the lens solely provides distance vision. The limited diffractive region limits the size and energy of defocused light under large-pupil conditions. To reduce this side effect a new strategy has been proposed called apodization. This process ensures a gradual redirection of light between the 2 images. This gradual change is optically very important because it avoids sudden optical boundaries, which can create unwanted diffractive effects.[16]

Zonal diffractive lenses can be traced back to the work of Augustin Fresnel, who improved lighthouse optics in the 1820s by segmenting large lenses to reduce their overall weight.

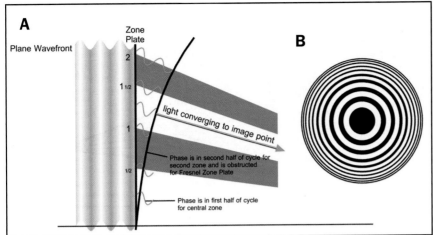

Figure 4. Sketch of Fresnel zone construction. A plane wavefront is divided into zones using circles centered on a distant point P with radius increments of 1/2 wavelength. These divide the wavefront into Fresnel zones (A). Fresnel zone plate that obscures alternate half-period zones (B).

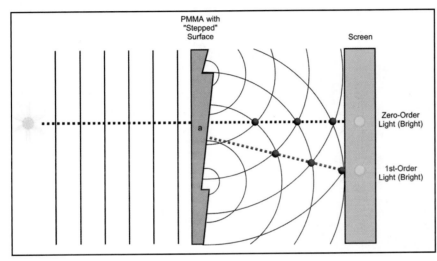

Figure 5. Illustration of a stepped zone plate. The thicker portions of the plate retard the incident light waves as opposed to the thinner portions of the plate, creating an interference pattern of two orders (two foci).

Fresnel's conceptual innovation in 1818 was to incorporate the ideas of amplitude, phase, and interference into the wavelet model of light propagation. This provided the potential for phase manipulations to have a significant effect on final wavefront characteristics. He described what came to be called Fresnel zones in 1818 (Figure 4). Working back from a distant point, the plane wavefront can be divided into zones by placing a zone boundary wherever the optical path increases by half a wavelength. If there is no diffracting obstacle, the light continues to propagate as a plane wave, but the theory indicates that if the central zone is obscured by an opaque object, a bright spot should appear in the shadow. This so-called Arago's spot was found experimentally and helped confirm the significance of Fresnel zones. Fresnel's recognition of the importance of wavelength increments of the optical path distance between 2 points is the fundamental basis for a diffractive lens.

The Fresnel zone plate is not an efficient optical system because it only directs 10% of the light to the point of focus. Lord Rayleigh provided further insight into diffractive lenses by reasoning that the phase of the light could be delayed in alternate zones by a half wavelength, rather than absorbing it using opaque zones. This concept was evaluated experimentally by Wood by bleaching a photographic zone plate of President Wilson in 1898, and demonstrating that it yielded more light at the point of focus. This Wood zone plate, or phase-reversal zone plate, can direct about 40% of the light into each of 2 lens powers, with the remaining light wasted in higher diffractive orders. This is a predecessor to the modern multifocal diffractive lens. Because there are no opaque zones, no light is absorbed.

Multifocal diffractive lenses have an important difference from their monofocal counterparts, namely the phase delay at the step (see Figure 4). For a monofocal lens, the delay is usually 1 wavelength, and for the multifocal lens, it is typically a half wavelength. The zones between steps in a diffractive lens do not refract light so multifocal diffractive lenses cannot be described using a refractive description. If rays were conceptually traced through the zones using the assumption that they were refractive, they would focus halfway between the 2 primary lens powers. In reality, none of the light is concentrated at that location but is directed into the 2 primary lens powers instead.

When light encounters an edge or discontinuity, it slows down and its direction changes slightly. The image quality of the full-optic multifocal diffractive IOL is generally higher than that of a multizonal refractive lens because light from all points in the aperture is directed to both foci. The diffraction that occurs at all the various steps creates the diffractive foci (Figure 5). The optical properties remain relatively constant as the pupil diameter varies with approximately 41% of the light going to each focus at the designated wavelength, whereas the remaining 18% of light is wasted as it is directed into higher diffractive orders (Figure 6).

Figure 6. A diffractive IOL showing the 2 foci for near and distance vision generated for the grooves of the lens.

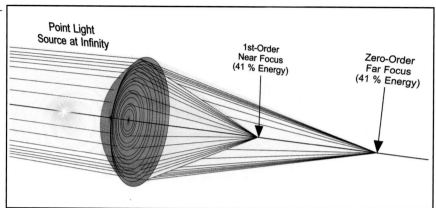

Figure 7. Expanded cross-section of the ReSTOR apodized IOL. The heights of the diffractive steps have been magnified 400 times more than the lens diameter to make them visible on this drawing.

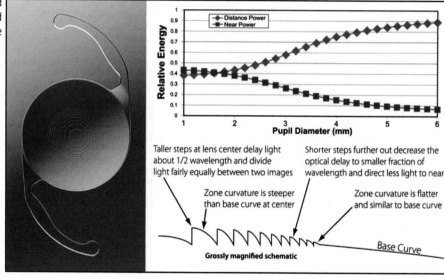

Despite the improvements of new generation diffractive IOLs, there is still a diffusion halo over the retina generated by the superimposed image of one of the two foci. The diffractive designs achieve pupil independence and the balance of energy is the same for the 2 foci (41%). This takes greater advantage of the available light, avoiding any decrease of contrast sensitivity. However, this optical strategy also creates an important negative effect. The secondary focus—the one that is out of focus in the retina—creates higher interference over the primary focus, to a greater degree than would occur with the refractive zone lenses. Because the light balance is 50% for distance vision and 20% for near vision in refractive zone lenses, obviously the close focus induces fewer alterations on top of the distance vision focus. However, this situation reverses when near objects are viewed. The focus for far vision causes a very powerful diffusion halo to be superimposed on the near vision focus, limiting the visual quality of these lenses for near vision as compared to the diffractive lenses.

To resolve this problem the new ReSTOR lens uses apodization and a new diffractive–refractive design concept to provide improved energy distribution. The lens has 2 primary focal points, one at distance and the other at near. The near point is equivalent to approximately a 3.2 D add power in the spectacle plane. The base lens provides the distance power

using its refractive shape and there are 12 diffractive discontinuities, or steps, that have been incorporated in the anterior surface of the cast-molded acrylic optic to provide the diffractive add power (Figure 7).

With respect to a circular lens surface, apodization describes the change in appearance of a plot of the intensity across a point image where the energy in the rings surrounding the central spot is reduced. The apodization property of the ReSTOR lens is radially symmetrical. It is defined by the gradual reduction in diffractive step heights from center to periphery, which results in an energy proportion continuum for light directed to the 2 primary foci.

In the apodized ReSTOR lens, like other diffractive lenses, the radial location of the zone boundaries determines the add power. In full-optic multifocal diffractive lenses, such as the Tecnis multifocal, the step heights are the same, whereas the ReSTOR lens has step heights that decrease with increasing distance from the lens center (it is apodized). This gradually changes the proportion of energy directed to the 2 images as the pupil diameter changes. Apodization provides 2 necessary and complementary improvements to the older design of the 3M diffractive IOL: 1) improved visual quality and 2) fewer unwanted optical phenomena.

Refractive Multizone Lenses and Halos

Once again it is important to remember that any light not contributing to an in-focus retinal image will reduce image quality and image contrast. In practice, the refractive zones used in refractive multifocal lenses mean that the pupil diameter influences the balance of light that contributes to the images formed by the distance and near regions of the lens and, hence, the contrast of the retinal image of any object. In general terms, larger pupils are associated with smaller depth of field because the out-of-focus retinal blur patches are of larger diameter. Consequently visual quality is impaired and contrast sensitivity is reduced.

There have been several previous studies of photic phenomena and contrast sensitivity (CS) after multifocal IOL implantation.[17-21] The most useful were those of Hayashi et al.[18,20] These researchers found that CS with a multifocal IOL was reduced compared with that for a monofocal IOL but was, however, within the normal range. CS with the refractive multifocal correction tended to be slightly lower than with the monofocal correction, but the differences were not significant, and the mean multifocal CS was within normal limits.

Decreased CS in patients with refractive multifocal IOLs, as compared with patients with monofocal IOLs, can be explained by the multifocal IOLs division of the available light energy in the image between 2 or more focal points. Ravalico et al[22,23] by means of a laser optical bench study, found that approximately 50% of the light energy in the full-aperture AMO Array IOL was concentrated at the distance focus and that approximately 20% was concentrated at the near focus. In another study, Montes-Mico et al[21] reported that defocus primarily affects images at higher spatial frequencies. This would imply that, in comparison with an optimal monofocal correction, distance and near CS with the multifocal IOL might be lower at higher spatial frequencies by factors of up to approximately 0.5 (0.3 log units) and 0.2 (0.7 log units), respectively . However, clinical studies (20) show that the loss in photopic CS is somewhat smaller. It may be that the effects of ocular longitudinal chromatic and other types of ocular aberration, together with the blending zones of the IOL tend to mask the differences between the monofocal and multifocal images and hence, the differences in CS.

When evaluating near vision, the CS of the multifocal lenses (both uncorrected and best distance corrected) at the photopic level was worse than that obtained at distance. With real life pupil sizes (probably slightly smaller because of pupillary constriction at near) only approximately one half of the light goes into the full range of near and intermediate foci. As noted previously, Ravalico et al[22,23] found that only approximately 20% of the light contributed to the near focus, in contrast to 50% in the far focus. Thus, the near retinal image is likely to be of reduced contrast in comparison with the distance image. In addition, the in-focus modulation transfer function of a lens with an annular aperture, as in the case of the near add, is depressed at higher spatial frequencies when compared to that with a circular pupil of the same outside diameter.[24] The annular aperture does improve depth of focus, however.[25]

To understand halos and glare with multifocal IOLs, it is necessary to analyze vision under dim lighting conditions. Several previous studies[5,19] have demonstrated that patients with multifocal IOLs show worse CS under dim illumination, particularity at the higher spatial frequencies.[21] This trend agrees with classic data about the effect of luminance level on CS[26,27] and with the values of Montes-Mico and Charman[28] for healthy emmetropic phakic patients.

The pupil diameters are substantially larger under mesopic conditions and it therefore seems reasonable to attribute the observed reduction in multifocal mesopic CS at higher spatial frequencies, relative to the optimal monofocal correction, to the additional blur introduced by the larger-diameter, out-of-focus zones of the multifocal IOL.

Analyzing the AMO Array multizone IOL, only zones 1 and 2 will typically contribute to the retinal images at photopic levels. Under lower light levels, zones 3 and 4 will also become involved with slight mydriasis. For any level of defocus, the size of the annular blur patches will be scaled to the dimensions of the zone of the lens. This indicates that the Array multifocal IOL has a binary refractive profile.[21]

Conclusion

With the refractive multizone IOLs, under photopic conditions, distance CS is only slightly worse than it would be with a monofocal IOL. Near CS, however, is only approximately 30% of that achieved by monofocal patients wearing reading glasses. Under dim mesopic lighting levels, the decrease in relative distance CS with the multifocal at higher frequencies is obvious, whereas near CS with the multifocal correction is much worse than that achievable with a monofocal IOL through reading glasses. Hence, in exchange for the convenience of not using reading spectacles, the multifocal IOL patient may encounter some problems with distance vision at low luminance and with near vision for lower-contrast objects.

References

1. Hansen TE, Corydon L, Krag S, Thim K. New multifocal intraocular lens design. *J Cataract Refract Surg.* 1990;16:38-41.
2. Duffey RJ, Zabel RW, Lindstrom RL. Multifocal intraocular lenses. *J Cataract Refract Surg.* 1990;16:423-429.
3. Lindstrom RL. Food and Drug Administration study update. One-year results from 671 patients with the 3M multifocal intraocular lens. *Ophthalmology.* 1993;100:91-97.
4. Steinert RF, Aker BL, Trentacost DJ, et al. A prospective comparative study of the AMO ARRAY zonal-progressive multifocal silicone intraocular lens and a monofocal intraocular lens. *Ophthalmology.* 1999;106:1243-1255.
5. Sasaki A. Initial experience with a refractive multifocal intraocular lens in a Japanese population. *J Cataract Refract Surg.* 2000;26:1001-1007.
6. Javitt J, Brauweiler HP, Jacobi KW, et al. Cataract extraction with multifocal intraocular lens implantation: clinical, functional, and quality-of-life outcomes. Multicenter clinical trial in Germany and Austria. *J Cataract Refract Surg.* 2000;26: 1356-1366.
7. Javitt JC, Steinert RF. Cataract extraction with multifocal intraocular lens implantation: a multinational clinical trial evaluating clinical, functional, and quality-of-life outcomes. *Ophthalmology.* 2000;107:2040-2048.

8. Solomon R, Donnenfeld ED. Refractive intraocular lenses. Multifocal and Phakic IOLs. *Int Ophthalmol Clin.* 2006;46:123-146.

9. Kohnen T, Allen D, Boureau C, et al. European multicenter study of the AcrySof ReSTOR apodized diffractive intraocular lens. *Ophthalmology.* 2006;113:578-584.

10. Cumming JS, Colvard DM, Dell SJ, et al. Clinical evaluation of the Crystalens AT-45 accommodating intraocular lens. Results of the U.S. Food and Drug Administration Clinical Trial. *J Cataract Refract Surg.* 2006;32:812-825.

11. Souza CE, Muccioli C, Soriano ES, et al. Visual performance of AcrySof ReSTOR apodized diffractive IOL: a prospective comparative trial. *Am J Ophthalmol.* 2006;141:827-832.

12. Simpson MJ. The diffractive multifocal intraocular lens. *Eur J Implant Refract Surg.* 1989;1:115-121.

13. Walkow T, Liekfeld A, Anders N, et al. A prospective evaluation of a diffractive versus a refractive designed multifocal intraocular lens. *Ophthalmology.* 1997;104:1380-1386.

14. Navarro R, Ferro M, Artal P, Miranda I. Modulation transfer functions of eyes implanted with intraocular lenses. *Appl Opt.* 1993;32:6359-6367.

15. Artal P, Marcos S, Navarro R, et al. Through focus image quality of eyes implanted with monofocal and multifocal intraocular lenses. *Opt Eng.* 1995;34:772-779.

16. Davison JA, Simpson, MJ. History and development of the apodized diffractive intraocular lens. *J Cataract Refract Surg.* 2006;32:849-858.

17. Holladay JT, van Dijk H, Lang A, et al. Optical performance of multifocal intraocular lenses. *J Cataract Refract Surg.* 1990;16:413-422.

18. Hayashi K, Hayashi H, Nakao F, Hayashi F. Correlation between pupillary size and intraocular lens decentration and visual acuity of a zonal-progressive multifocal lens and a monofocal lens. *Ophthalmology.* 2001;108:2011-7.

19. Pieh S, Weghaupt H, Skorpik C. Contrast sensitivity and glare disability with diffractive and refractive multifocal intraocular lenses. *J Cataract Refract Surg.* 1998;24:659-662.

20. Hayashi K, Hayashi H, Nakao F, Hayashi F. Influence of astigmatism on multifocal and monofocal intraocular lenses. *Am J Ophthalmol.* 2000;130:477-482.

21. Montes-Mico R, España ED, Bueno I. Visual performance with multifocal intraocular lenses. Mesopic Contrast Sensitivity under Distance and Near Conditions. *Ophthalmology* 2004;111:85-96.

22. Ravalico G, Parentin F, Baccara F. Effect of astigmatism on multifocal intraocular lenses. *J Cataract Refract Surg.* 1999; 25:804-807.

23. Ravalico G, Parentin F, Sirotti P, Baccara F. Analysis of light energy distribution by multifocal intraocular lenses through an experimental optical model. *J Cataract Refract Surg.* 1998;24:647-652.

24. Charman WN, Murray IJ, Nacer M, O'Donoghue EP. Theoretical and practical performance of a concentric bifocal implant lens. *Vision Res.* 1998;38:2841-2853.

25. Welford WT. Use of annular apertures to increase focal depth. *J Opt Soc Am.* 1960;50:749-753.

26. Van Nes FL, Bouman MA. Spatial modulation transfer in the human eye. *J Opt Soc Am.* 1967;57:401-406.

27. Albarran-Diego C, Montes-Mico R, Pons A, Artigas JM. Influence of the luminance level on visual performance with a disposable soft cosmetic tinted contact lens. *Ophthalmic Physiol Opt.* 2001;21:411-419.

28. Montes-Mico R, Charman WN. Mesopic contrast sensitivity function after excimer laser photorefractive keratectomy. *J Refract Surg.* 2002;18:9-13.

CHAPTER 73

UNDERSTANDING MULTIFOCAL HALOS

Kevin L. Waltz, OD, MD

I personally have experienced halos from multifocal intraocular lenses (IOLs) for the last 10 years. I developed cataracts at age 41 and had the Array multifocal IOL (Advanced Medical Optics, Santa Ana, CA) implanted in both eyes in 1998. This chapter is written from my personal experience learning about halos as well as my experience implanting thousands of multifocal IOLs over the last 10 years and learning about them from my patients. Multifocal halos are usually predictable, can be clinically useful, are often distracting, and may even be disturbing. The comments herein are to help you understand them from the patients' perspective.

The eye is but one part of the human visual system. The eye's natural optics—the cornea and the lens—gather and focus light onto the retina. Helmholtz has commented on the relatively poor optical design of the eye. He felt the design of the eye, with its many flaws, left much to be desired. The typical image formed on the retina by the dual lens combination of the cornea and the retina has imperfections that are just now being studied. We have begun to understand how these imperfections we call higher-order aberrations (HOAs) interact to improve or degrade the image focused on the retina. For instance, in the year 2000 almost no eye surgeon was aware of the issue of excess positive spherical aberration caused by standard monofocal IOLs. In the year 2007, standard monofocal IOLs are being phased out and substituted with IOLs that have zero or negative spherical aberration. This is a relatively dramatic change in understanding the optics of IOLs, which have been around for over 50 years. I predict we will make similar changes in our clinical use of multifocal optics as we better understand them in the near future.

Halos are not necessarily abnormal aspects of human vision. They occur naturally in many people. They can be from refractive effects or from diffractive effects (Figure 1). It is common to implant a multifocal IOL in a hyperopic patient who is having refractive lens surgery or presbyopic lens exchange and have that patient comment that the halos with the multifocal IOL are less than with the original natural lens. This almost never happens with a myopic patient. Therein lays an important lesson about the difference between myopic and hyperopic visual systems. Hyperopes commonly have halos as part of their visual experience prior to IOL implantation and are much more forgiving of them after implantation of a multifocal IOL. Myopes rarely have halos as part of their visual experience and are less tolerant of them after implantation of a multifocal IOL.

Because halos are normal after any type of IOL implantation, the important question to ask is not, "Do you have halos?" but rather, "Are the halos bothersome?" Every IOL ever studied has some incidence of halos reported after implantation. Researchers have been known to brag about the IOL they use having a less than 5% incidence of halos. This is largely a matter of definition.

It is very difficult for a doctor and a patient to discuss halos meaningfully. The doctor usually has a preconceived notion of what a halo is and uses the word without really defining it. The patient is seeing something that they assume must be "the halo" the doctor is asking about. Because there is a lot of confusion in this area, it helps to have an image or two to discuss during the patient discussion. How many times have you actually showed the patient an image of what you think the halo looks like, and then asked the patient if that is what he or she sees?

Spherical aberration and other relatively symmetrical HOAs create a glow around a point source of light, especially with a dark background. This can easily be mistaken for a "halo" by a patient. With greater degrees of spherical aberration, it is possible to create a frank halo. A typical amount of spherical aberration from an IOL will only cause a glow around a point source of light and not a frank halo with a clear space between the central image and a surrounding ring of light.

One of the most common causes of a pseudophakic "halo" is unique to an IOL and does not occur in a normal crystalline lens. Approximately 96% of the light striking the cornea in a normal healthy eye is focused on the retina. This is due to the remarkably subtle gradation in the refractive index of the eyes' refracting surfaces. The normal eye effectively has antireflective coatings on its refracting surfaces. The percentage of light

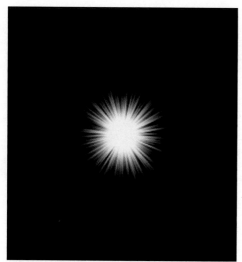

Figure 1. A single point source of light can be diffracted by the crystalline lens fibers to create colored halos or radiating rays of light. (Image courtesy of Val Portney and Advanced Medical Optics.)

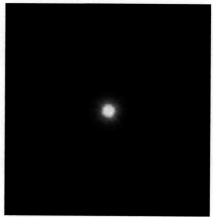

Figure 3. This is a color enhanced image of a point source of light. The central white area is the image of the original point source. The red corona is a combination of spherical aberration creating a blurred image and the reflections of the image as it strikes the surfaces of the IOL. The blue streaks are light diffracted within the lens. The patient will often report this as their "halo." This is the likely source of halos reported in monofocal IOLs. (Image courtesy of Val Portney and Advanced Medical Optics.)

Figure 2. The image is taken from a Tracey wavefront device. The image shows the placement of the red laser test spots for wavefront test. It also shows the relative lack of reflections in the phakic eye and the relatively prominent reflections in the multifocal IOL.

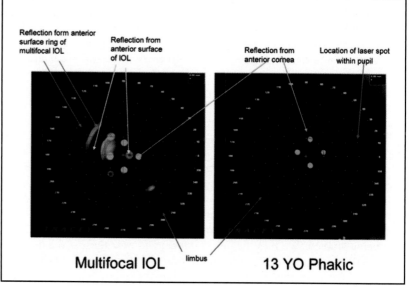

transmission is markedly reduced with an IOL in the eye. The reduction is caused by the accumulated reflections from the surfaces of the IOL creating a glow around a point source of light. All IOLs have reflections at their surfaces. The reflections from the surface of a normal lens are minimal (Figure 2), and this is related to their index of refraction. As the index of refraction of the IOL increases, the reflections from the IOL surfaces increase. The reflected light from the posterior surface of an IOL will in turn strike the anterior surface and be redirected toward the retina. The reflected light will be out-of-focus and will cause a glow of decreasing intensity around the point source of light (Figure 3).

A true halo has a central image, a surrounding ring of light of the same color, and an intervening clear zone (Figure 4). This is the typical image caused by a multifocal IOL. It is caused by the out-of-focus near image being superimposed on the in-focus distance image on the retina. There should be a complete ring of light around the central image. This information can be diagnostically useful. If a part of the halo is missing, something is blocking the light rays entering the eye. The most common situation causing this problem is blepharoptosis. After cataract surgery, a patient may describe an incomplete halo with a portion of the upper half missing, and this is virtually diagnostic of clinically significant blepharoptosis. Another useful characteristic is the shape of the halo. A halo that is not circular indicates the presence of additional HOAs that might be potentially treated to reduce clinical symptoms. For example, an oblong halo usually indicates coma.

Myopes tend to not have halos in their normal phakic state, and generally like to be slightly over-minused in their

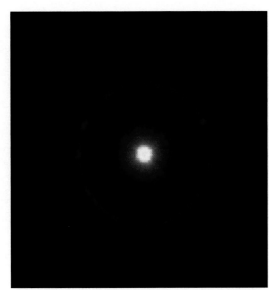

Figure 4. This is the same image as Figure 3 with an added, surrounding halo and an intervening clear zone that is typical of a multifocal IOL. This image is color enhanced; the halo is almost always the same color as the central image in real life. (Image courtesy of Val Portney and Advanced Medical Optics.)

refraction to create an artificial, hyperopic state. This allows the myope to accommodate slightly and fine tune the focus of their retinal image. Hyperopes, on the other hand, generally like to be slightly undercorrected in their refractions. This causes a significant amount of light to be focused behind the retina, creating a corona around the central image. The light focused behind the retina can make either a glow or a frank halo around a point image of light. For this reason, myopes tend to be relatively intolerant of the halos associated with multifocal IOLs and, all other things being equal, will comment about their halos more persistently and vociferously than hyperopes. Most people in developed countries are hyperopic so they are less likely to be bothered by halos after implantation with a multifocal IOL. Most ophthalmologists in developed countries are myopic so they are less likely to experience halos themselves. Because of lack of personal experience, ophthalmologists are more likely to be bothered by their patients' subjective reports of halos.

Halos are optical phenomena, but the patient's perception of them is a mental one. Our ability to perceive what is and what is not important is remarkable. This is similar to floaters, which most patients over 40 years of age experience to some degree, and especially following a posterior vitreous detachment. Most patients are reassured that floaters are normal and that they will get used to them. Most people who experience floaters are usually much more bothered by them in the first several months. After some time, most people get used to their floaters and notice them much less. Some will complain bitterly about them for months, and may even have their floaters surgically removed. The same could be true when considering patients with halos after multifocal IOL implantation. The halos always improve over time, but faster in some individuals than in others. The patient would likely adapt to halos better if their ophthalmologist reassured them they were normal and would improve with time, just like floaters. One important dif-

ference is that most ophthalmologists over 40 years of age have floaters and have had to learn to adapt to them, but most have not had to adapt to multifocal halos.

Halos are also a part of our artistic culture. We have all heard of a "moon glow" in music and film, which is a collection of halos or corona. Older eyes see moon glows due to the imperfections of their visual systems and we immortalize them in song. A single star or point source of light imaged through a multifocal IOL makes a single halo. The moon is an infinite number of point sources of light that are overlapping. The infinite point sources of light create an infinite number of overlapping halos that collectively appear as a "moon glow."

A point source of light imaged through a multifocal IOL creates a halo that is not absolute, even in the same eye. The true size of the halo does not vary by much after the point source of light is about 100 feet away from the eye with a multifocal IOL. However, the perceived size of the halo is dependent on its surroundings. The apparent size of the halo will vary dramatically with its surroundings. The most common and dramatic example of this is the halo around a car headlight.

The apparent magnification of the headlights of cars is one of the most troubling experiences for a multifocal IOL patient in the early stages of adaptation. It is very helpful for the patient to understand this is an illusion. When the car is close to the observer, the headlight will not be a point source of light. It will become an infinite number of point sources like the moon. The overlapping halos will fuse and become a glow around the headlight. As the car is farther away, the headlight becomes a point source again and there is a single halo. As the car moves even further away, the size of the car seems to shrink while the halo seems to enlarge. In reality, the apparent size of the car decreases with distance and the halo is stable in size. Therefore, the halo appears to enlarge as the car decreases in size with further distance from the observer. Now reverse this and imagine what the patient sees. At a distance of a mile, the car is very small and the halo is relatively huge. It appears larger than the car. As the car approaches, the halo appears to decrease in size, even though we know the car is really increasing in size. Ultimately, the car is so close there is a glow around the headlight and the halo is gone. Now imagine this sequence happening in real time as a line of traffic approaches the driver with a multifocal IOL. It takes some time to adapt to this.

Every ophthalmologist I know who has been implanted with a multifocal IOL counsels their own patients about halos in a manner similar to how they counsel their patients about floaters. "Don't worry. They will get better." The best images of this process come from Michael Woodcock, MD and an artist he implanted with multifocal IOLs several years ago (Figures 5, 6, and 7). The first image (see Figure 5) is the artist's impression of her halos when she was first implanted with a multifocal IOL. Even the trees have a glow or halo. After 3 months the subjective effects are much less (see Figure 6). The lens has not changed in the eye, but the mind has started to adjust. In the final images created approximately 3 years later (see Figure 7), the extra glow previously seen around objects is gone. Only the halos around the headlights and streetlights remain and they are much less. In 3 years, the brain adjusted to its new circumstances and is doing quite well. This sequence of initial strong reaction followed by adjustment is the norm with floaters, and with halos associated with multifocal IOLs.

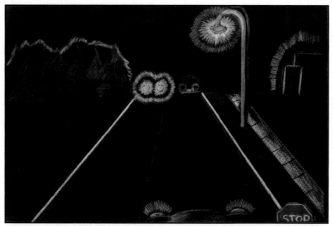

Figure 5. This is the initial image created by an artist implanted with multifocal IOLs. Her visual and mental reaction to the multifocal halos is significant. (Image courtesy of Michael Woodcock, MD.)

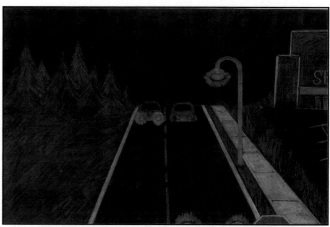

Figure 7. This is the same image by the same artist 3 years later. She demonstrates continued neural adaptation to the multifocal images. (Image courtesy of Michael Woodcock, MD.)

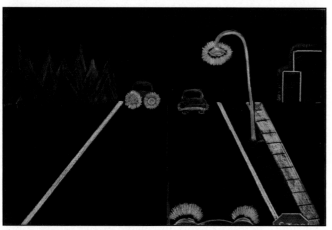

Figure 6. This is the same image by the same artist patient 3 months later. The multifocal IOL has not changed. She has mentally adapted to the multifocal images much like she would to floaters. (Image courtesy of Michael Woodcock, MD.)

Multifocal halos are real. They can cause significant problems, which are often made much worse by our reaction to them. It is important to listen to our patients and acknowledge their concerns, but not to over react to them. Halos will sometimes offer diagnostic clues to other sources of visual complaints. It is safe to tell and practically promise our patients that their perception of halos will decrease over time, usually below a clinically relevant level.

PEARLS FOR MANAGING HALOS

Dwayne Logan, MD

The ReZoom intraocular lens (IOL) (Advanced Medical Optics, Santa Ana, CA) has emerged as the primary presbyopia-correcting IOL in my practice due to its outstanding distance vision in daylight and excellent near and intermediate vision in dim light. It offers the best opportunity to simulate a natural vision lifestyle; however, patients with moderately dilated pupils due mostly to night time conditions can complain of visual aberrations often described as halos and/or starbursts. This phenomenon is caused largely by the near dominant zone of the ReZoom optic.

I explain the concept of neuroadaptation to all of my symptomatic patients with the theory that the halos may dissipate with time. I do not believe the process of neuro-adaptation can begin until I have eliminated all other postoperative variables that may potentially be contributing factors for visual aberrations. These include an inadequate tear film, corneal epithelial and stromal haze, residual spherocylinder refractive errors, IOL decentration,

capsular fibrosis, vitreous opacities, and cystoid macular edema (CME).

Tear film insufficiency can result in decreased visual acuity, excessive glare, and halos at night. All of my ReZoom patients are placed on artificial tears and Restasis (Allergan, Irvine, CA) for 3 to 6 months following surgery. Silicone punctal plugs are also used if needed.

Spherocylinder residual refractive errors greater than +0.50 D of sphere and 0.50 D of cylinder increase the perception of halos at night. Astigmatism should be treated intraoperatively with limbal and/or corneal relaxing incisions based on the corneal topography. I believe cylindrical refractive error can play the most significant role in halo severity; hence, controlling it at the time of surgery is important. At 12 weeks postoperatively, residual refractive cylinder can be treated with repeat limbal relaxing incisions and spherical refractive errors can be treated with excimer laser surface ablation.

IOL Centration: It is not uncommon for patients to complain of a coma or a crescent in their visual field secondary to nasal decentration of the central optic. This phenomenon is more aggravating than the 360-degree halo found in a perfectly centered ReZoom IOL.

The first step is to determine if the lens is centered on the optical center. This can easily be established by having the patient look into the center of the 2 half-moon lights from the microscope and adjusting the IOL position so the light reflex is directly in the center of the ReZoom IOL.

Second step: If the pupil is not symmetrical around the central optic, an iridoplasty can be performed with the argon laser. This procedure not only decreases visual aberrations, but also improves near vision.

Capsular Fibrosis: Within the first postoperative month, early capsular fibrotic changes can occur giving the appearance of an orange peel on the capsule. At night this can result in a starburst-like halo. I typically wait 3 months with monofocal IOLs before considering a yttrium-aluminum-garnet (YAG) capsulotomy. I have found that by performing this procedure at 4 to 6 weeks with multifocal IOL patients, it is effective in reducing visual aberrations and halos, thereby decreasing the timeline for the neuro-adaptation process.

Vitreous Opacities: They are very annoying with or without halos. I am now breaking up the vitreous opacities with the YAG laser in order to decrease complaints of visual aberrations.

Cystoid Macular Edema: I have found that patients with decreased visual acuity secondary to CME feel that halos are more symptomatic. I believe that excellent residual cortical clean up along with using pre- and postoperative topical non-steroidal anti-inflammatories is mandatory.

Once these aforementioned variables are eliminated or stabilized, and I am satisfied with the outcome, I can confidently tell my patients that they are doing great. When I am happy they are too. The process of neuroadaptation will begin once the patient is confident you have a roadmap to success. If night time halos continue to be moderately to severely problematic, I will ask my patients to use topical Alphagan P (Allergan) 5 minutes prior to driving at night.

CHAPTER 74

ASPHERIC IOLs—MATCHING CORNEAL AND IOL WAVEFRONT

George Beiko, BM, BCh, FRCS(C)

Until recently, the goal of cataract surgery has been to restore a patient's Snellen visual acuity to its greatest potential. Much emphasis was placed on minimizing sphere and cylinder, and obtaining emmetropic results for these patients. The goal of cataract surgery now has become the rejuvenation of vision by the restoration of youthful contrast sensitivity and by restoring accommodative potential. In this chapter, I would like to address contrast sensitivity in pseudophakic patients.

Wavefront analysis of the ocular optical system has increased our knowledge of the aberrations, other than sphere and cylinder, in the eye, which impact significantly on visual function. Using Zernike polynomials, the aberrations of the ocular system can be characterized. The Zernike coefficient for spherical aberration (SA) has been found to be linked to contrast visual acuity; as this value increases, contrast sensitivity has been found to decrease.[1-4] The best contrast sensitivity has been measured in young patients, aged 20 to 30 years.

The total higher-order aberrations of the phakic eye are composed of aberrations arising from the anterior corneal surface, the posterior corneal surface, the crystalline lens, and the retina; however, in the aphakic eye, 98.2% of the aberrations arise from the anterior corneal surface.[5,6] As this discussion is about pseudophakia, then necessarily the corneal aberrations are of importance, and for our purposes, can be thought of being representative of the whole aphakic eye.

Zernike coefficients of the higher-order aberrations can be derived from corneal topographic data.[1,6-9] With current small-incision cataract surgery, it has been reported that the average postoperative corneal topography does not differ significantly from average preoperative corneal topography.[5,10] Thus, for cataract patients, it is possible to measure their corneal SAs using corneal topography preoperatively and then use these data to manipulate the outcome of cataract surgery by implantation of aspheric intraocular lenses, with the goal of achieving an optimum SA for the eye and maximum contrast sensitivity. A reduction of higher-order wavefront aberrations in the eye results in improved contrast vision.[11-13]

The cornea has positive SA, which does not vary significantly with aging. The corneal SA has been reported to be approximately +0.27 μm[14-16] for a diameter of 6.0 mm. By implanting an aspheric intraocular lens, such as the Tecnis Z9000 (Advanced Medical Optics, Santa Ana, CA), with a SA of −0.27 μm, it has been reported that the image quality and contrast sensitivity under mesopic and photopic conditions can be improved as compared to patients who receive a standard intraocular lens, which, contrary to the Tecnis lens, have positive SA that increase with lens power (Figure 1).[17-19]

In Figure 1, it may seem that different powers of the Tecnis lens have different SA values. This study measured the SA in isolation. Two factors contribute to the differing SA of the Tecnis lenses of different powers when measured in isolation. The first of these factors is caused by the fact that the radii and thickness change with lens power, therefore you must compensate for different amounts of aberration per lens power to have the same compensation in the eye. All Tecnis lens powers compensate for the same amount of corneal SA, the difference in the isolated lenses arises due to the different amount that different power lenses must compensate for because of their different curvatures and power. The second factor is the convergence angle of incident light (ie, the angle of the light approaching the lens). The value of SA of a lens varies with this convergence angle. Because the radii and thickness of the Tecnis lens change with lens power, the convergence angle of the light approaching the posterior surface changes for each lens power in isolation. In the eye model with an average cornea, the lens is designed to compensate for this. (The explanation in the preceding paragraph was kindly provided by Patricia Piers, PhD.)

In simulated night driving tests, it has been shown that patients with the Tecnis lens were able to identify a pedestrian 45 feet or 0.5 seconds sooner at 55 miles per hour than patients with a spheric intraocular lens.[20] Thus not only does correction of SA improve vision, but it also increases patient safety.

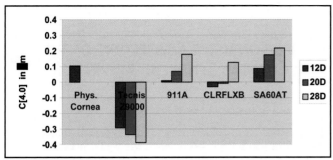

Figure 1. Spherical aberrations of isolated lenses. (Reprinted with permission from Terwee T. The correcting effect of the Tecnis IOL on corneal spherical wavefront aberration and its influence on optical performance. Presented at the XX Congress of the ESCRS, September 7 to 11, 2002; Nice, France.)

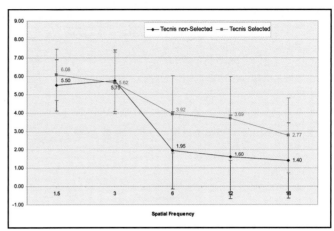

Figure 2. Postoperative photopic (85 cpd/mm) contrast sensitivity.

However, what must be borne in mind is that these studies were comparing patients whose mean postoperative SA was zero in the Tecnis group, and in the order of 0.30 to 0.40 μm in the comparative group.

Currently, there are 3 lens approved by the Food and Drug Administration (FDA) for correction of SA. In addition to the Tecnis, there are the SofPort AO (Bausch & Lomb, Rochester, NY) and the AcrySof IQ (Alcon, Fort Worth, TX). The 3 lenses have different strategies for correction of SA. The SofPort AO lens has an effective SA of almost zero and produces minimal change in the SA of the eye. (In fact, the Sofport AO is designed to correct the SA of the isolated lens, as such when it is inserted into the eye, it contributes small amounts of positive SA due to the converging incident light from the cornea.) The AcrySof IQ has a negative SA of –0.20 μm. Thus, if one considers the average corneal SA of +0.27 μm, the SofPort AO does not change this value significantly, whereas the Tecnis corrects this SA fully and the AcrySof IQ compensates to a lesser degree.

Different studies have demonstrated that there may be a correlation between SA and natural supervision (defined as vision of 6/4.5 or better). Levy and colleagues quantified the total SA across a naturally dilated pupil with a diameter equal or superior to 6 mm, in 70 eyes of 35 subjects with a mean age of 24.3 ± 7.7 years and natural supervision, using the Nidek OPD scan wavefront aberrometer (Nidek Co, Ltd, Gamagori, Japan). Mean total root-mean-square SA in this population was found to be +0.110 ± 0.077 μm.[21] Similarly, in a study by Grimson and colleagues, student naval pilots showed better-than-average visual acuity associated with better-than-average contrast sensitivity, which was correlated with more SA in this population.[22]

Therefore, considering an average corneal SA of +0.27 μm, I hypothesized that contrast sensitivity would be better in patients with a residual mean SA of approximately +0.10 μm after cataract surgery with implantation of the Tecnis lens. Thus, I compared 13 patients with average preoperative SA of +0.37 μm, with 20 patients with average preoperative SA close to that found in the studies by Holladay and colleagues[15] and Beiko and Haigis.[23] Considering that the Tecnis lens has a fixed negative SA of –0.27 μm, in theory, the patients in the first group would have a residual average SA of +0.10 μm, whereas those in the second group would have a mean SA of zero.

My results confirmed that 13 patients in the group who had a corneal SA of +0.37 μm (this group was called "Tecnis-selected") showed better contrast sensitivity than those who had an average corneal SA of +0.27 μm (this group was called "Tecnis-nonselected"), after Tecnis implantation. Statistically significant differences were detected for spatial frequencies of 12 cpd, under photopic conditions, and for 6.0, 12, and 18 cpd, under mesopic conditions. Also, the differences were barely nonsignificant for spatial frequencies of 6.0 and 18 cpd, under photopic conditions (P = .0570 and P = .0585, respectively). Contrary to other studies comparing the Tecnis lens with hydrophobic acrylic lenses, the differences in contrast sensitivity between the 2 groups of patients in this present study cannot at any rate be related to differences in intraocular lens material and optic characteristics[24] (Figures 2 and 3).

This was then followed up with studies looking at unselected groups of patients, whose average corneal SA was similar to that of the general population, namely 0.27 μm, and who were implanted with the AcrySof IQ lens or the Sofport AO lens. The Acrysof IQ lens performed almost identically to the previous Tecnis-selected group, which was targeted for 0.10 μm of SA postoperatively, whereas the Sofport AO group performed similarly to the Tecnis-nonselected group; the test conditions were photopic and mesopic contrast sensitivity testing. In terms of vision testing, targeting a mean SA of 0.00 (which was the case with the Tecnis-nonselected group) or 0.27 μm (as in the Sofport AO group) was inferior to targeting 0.10 μm.[25]

It has been proposed by each of the manufacturers that implantation of one of their lens and its targeted strategy will result in superior vision for all patients. For this premise to be true, it presupposes that the corneal SA of all patients lies in a tight distribution about the mean, and that the value targeted by each strategy is the optimum one. In order to be able to adequately investigate the proposals of the manufacturers, it is essential to know the distribution in the population of the corneal SA. A small standard deviation relative to the value of the mean would support the premise and a large value would not, as this would necessarily support the need for a range of intraocular lenses correcting for different values of SA.

In a study of 696 eyes, we found that the corneal SA was 0.274 ± 0.095 μm in a normal Gaussian distribution[23] (Figure

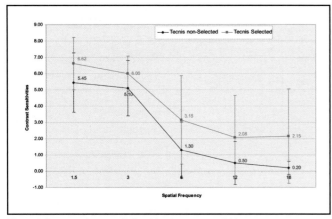

Figure 3. Postoperative mesopic (3 cpd/mm) contrast sensitivity.

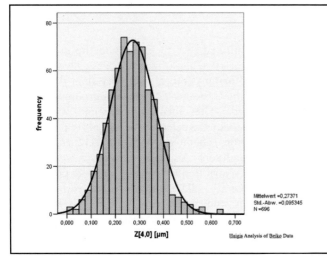

Figure 4. Corneal SA.

Table 1

PERSONALIZED CORRECTION OF THE CORNEAL SPHERICAL ABERRATION

Corneal Spherical Aberration	Lens Implanted
–0.15 to +0.15 μm	Advanced Medical Optics Clariflex, Bausch & Lomb Sofport AO, or Bausch & Lomb Akreos AO
+0.16 to +0.33 μm	Alcon IQ (SN60WF)
>+0.33 μm	AMO Tecnis
<–0.15 μm	Nonwavefront intraocular lens

This area is constantly evolving. The previous discussion does not take into account that higher-order and lower-order aberrations may interact to impact on contrast sensitivity, and that the target SA may need to be revised. A recent finding certainly confirms this: MacRae and Yoon[28] have reported that in laser refractive cases, patients with 0.10 μm of SA prefer to have a manifest refraction of –0.25 D. Although not confirmed in cataract patients, this would necessarily imply that these patients should be targeted not only for a SA of 0.10 μm, but also for a sphere of –0.25 D.

4). Thus, this large standard deviation of the distribution does not support the assertions of the manufacturers.

Based on performance on contrast sensitivity testing, I am currently advocating a personalized correction of the corneal SA and targeting 0.10 μm for cataract patients. The ideal situation would be to have a range of powers of SA available on different lens platforms. However, in the current market, only a small number of aspheric lenses are available. Thus, this is my current practice. I measure preoperative corneal SA, and then select the lens, as outlined in Table 1.

After corneal refractive surgery, some generalizations can be made if one cannot directly measure the SA. Myopic laser ablation tends to increase the SA, so a high negative SA lens, such as the Tecnis, is probably appropriate. Conversely, hyperopic ablation tends to decrease the SA, and possibly make it negative, so a standard lens with positive SA should be considered.

Although I advocate a target of 0.10 μm, recent studies by R. Chu[26] and by M. Packer and colleagues[27] have suggested that targeting 0 μm is superior to not targeting any value. The study that needs to be done is a comparison of targeting different values, prospectively. Thus, the only statement that can be made at present is that targeting is better than not.

References

1. Guirao A, Artal P. Corneal wave aberration from videokeratography: accuracy and limitations of the procedure. *J Optom Soc Am A Opt Image Sci Vis.* 2000;17:955-965.

2. Glasser A, Campbell MC. Biometric, optical and physical changes in the isolated human crystalline lens with age in relation to presbyopia. *Vision Res.* 1999;39:1991-2015.

3. Glasser A, Campbell MC. Presbyopia and the optical changes in the human crystalline lens with age. *Vision Res.* 1998;38:209-229

4. DeValois RL, DeValois KK. *Spatial Vision.* Oxford, UK: Oxford University Press; 1988.

5. Bellucci R. *Eurotimes.* 2002;June.

6. Barbero S, Marcos S, Merayo-Lloves L, Moreno-Barriuso E. Validation of the estimation of corneal aberrations from videokeratography in keratoconus. *J Refract Surg.* 2002;18:263-270.

7. Rubinowitz YS, McDonnell PJ. Computer assisted corneal topography in keratoconus. *Refract Corneal Surg.* 1989;5(6):400-8.

8. Schweigerling J, Greivenkamp JE. Using corneal height maps and polynomial decompensation to determine corneal aberration. *Optom Vis Sci.* 1997;74:906-916.

9. Gobbe M, Guillan M, Marissa C. Measurement repeatability of corneal aberration. *J Refract Surg.* 2002;18:S567-S571.

10. Guirao A, Tejedor J, Artal P. Corneal aberrations before and after small-incision cataract surgery. *Invest Ophthalmol Vis Sci.* 2004;45:4312-4319.

11. Liang J, Williams DR, Miller DT. Supernormal vision and high-resolution retinal imaging through adaptive optics. *J Optom Soc Am A.* 1997;14:2884.

12. Williams DR, Yoon GY, Guirao A, Hofer H, Porter J. How far can we extend the limits of human vision. In: MacRae SM, Kreuger RR, Applegate RA, eds. *Customized Corneal Ablation: The Quest for SuperVision.* Thorofare, NJ: SLACK Incorporated; 2001:11.

13. Marcos S. Aberrations and visual performance following standard laser vision correction. *J Refract Surg.* 2001;17:596.

14. Wang I, Dai E, Koch D, Nathoo A. Optical aberrations of the human anterior cornea. *J Cataract Refract Surg.* 2003;29:1514-1521.

15. Holladay JT, Piers PA, Koranyi G, van der Mooren M, Norrby S. A new intraocular lens design to reduce spherical aberration of pseudophakic eyes. *J Refract Surg.* 2002;18:683-691.

16. Beiko G. Measurement of the wavefront aberrations using the Oculus Easygraph Topographic System. Lecture presented at the American Society of Cataract and Refractive Surgery Annual Meeting; May 1-5, 2004; San Diego, CA.

17. Kershner RM. Retinal image contrast and functional visual performance with aspheric, silicone, and acrylic intraocular lenses: prospective evaluation. *J Cataract Refract Surg.* 2003;29:1684-1694.

18. Packer M, Fine IH, Hoffman RS, Piers PA. Initial clinical experience with an anterior surface modified prolate intraocular lens. *J Refract Surg.* 2002;18:692-696.

19. Barbero S, Marcos S, Jimenez-Alfaro I. Optical aberrations of intraocular lenses measured in vivo and in vitro. *J Optom Soc Am A Opt Image Sci Vis.* 2003;20:1841-1851.

20. Data on file. Tecnis package insert. April 2004. New York: Pfizer Inc.

21. Levy Y, Segal O, Avni I, Zadok D. Ocular higher-order aberrations in eyes with supernormal vision. *Am J Ophthalmol.* 2005;139:225-228.

22. Grimson JM, Schallhorn SC, Kaupp SE. Contrast sensitivity: establishing normative data for use in screening prospective naval pilots. *Aviat Space Environ Med.* 2002;73:28-35.

23. Beiko GHH, Haigis W, Steinmueller A. Distribution of the corneal spherical aberration in a comprehensive ophthalmology practice, and can keratometry be predictive of the value of the corneal spherical aberration? *J Cataract Refract Surg.* 2007;33(5):848-858.

24. Beiko GHH. Personalized correction of spherical aberration in cataract surgery. *J Cataract Refract Surg.* 2007;33(8):1455-1460..

25. Beiko GHH. Correction of spherical aberration in cataract surgery: where should we be? Presented at the Annual Meeting of Canadian Ophthalmological Society; June 2005; Edmonton, Canada.

26. Chu R. Clinical comparison of the Tecnis Z9000, the Acrysof IQ and the Sofport AO IOLs. Presented at the XXV Congress of the ESCRS; September 8-12, 2007; Stockholm, Sweden..

27. Packer M, Fine IH and Hoffman R. Customizing selection of aspheric intraocular lenses. Presented at the XXV Congress of the ESCRS, September 8-12, 2007; Stockholm, Sweden.

28. Guttman C. Balancing lower and higher order aberrations enables fine-tuning of customized ablation algorithm. *Eurotimes.* 2006;August:13.

CHAPTER 75

Aspheric IOLs—Matching Corneal and IOL Wavefront

Mark Packer, MD, FACS; I. Howard Fine, MD; and Richard S. Hoffman, MD

In the current era of presbyopia-correcting intraocular lenses (IOLs), toric IOLs, and aspheric IOL technology, the practice milieu is changing. Informed consent takes on new meaning when the surgeon and the patient decide together which IOL technology represents the best fit for a particular lifestyle and its visual demands. Customizing IOL choice is no longer optional; it is essential to the practice of refractive lens surgery.

Because the positive spherical aberration of a spherical pseudophakic IOL tends to increase total optical aberrations, attention has turned to the development of aspheric IOLs.[1] These designs are intended to reduce or eliminate the spherical aberration of the eye and improve functional vision as compared with a spherical pseudophakic implant. Three aspheric IOL designs are currently marketed in the United States: the Tecnis Z9000/2/3 IOLs (Advanced Medical Optics, Santa Ana, CA), the AcrySof IQ IOL (Alcon, Fort Worth, TX), and the SofPort AO IOL (Bausch & Lomb, Rochester, NY). Other aspheric IOL designs not yet available in the United States also show promise for the reduction of spherical aberration.[2]

The Tecnis IOL was designed with a modified prolate anterior surface to compensate for the average corneal spherical aberration found in the adult eye. It introduces (–)0.27 μ of spherical aberration to the eye measured at the 6-mm optical zone. The clinical investigation of the Tecnis IOL submitted to the US Food and Drug Administration (FDA) demonstrated elimination of mean spherical aberration as well as significant improvement in functional vision when compared to a standard spherical IOL.[3]

The AcrySof IQ shares the ultraviolet (UV) and blue light-filtering chromophores found in the single-piece acrylic AcrySof Natural IOL. The special feature of the IQ IOL is the posterior aspheric surface designed to reduce spherical aberration by addressing the effects of over-refraction at the periphery. It adds (–)0.20 μ of spherical aberration to the eye at the 6-mm optical zone. The SofPort Advanced Optics (LI61AO) IOL is an aspheric IOL that has been specifically designed with zero spherical aberration so that it will not contribute to any pre-existing higher-order aberrations.

Multiple peer-reviewed, prospective, randomized scientific publications have demonstrated reduction or elimination of spherical aberration with the Tecnis modified prolate IOL when compared to a variety of spherical IOLs.[4-13] Data show that the mean spherical aberration in the eyes implanted with the Tecnis IOL is, in the words approved by the FDA, "not different from zero." Studies have also documented superior functional vision with the Tecnis IOL. Subjects in the FDA-monitored randomized double-masked night driving simulation study of the Tecnis IOL performed functionally better in 20 of 24 driving conditions (and statistically better in 10 conditions) when using best-spectacle correction with the eye implanted with the Tecnis IOL, as compared to best-spectacle correction with the eye implanted with the AcrySof spherical IOL.[2] Data from the night driving simulation showed a significant correlation between reduction of spherical aberration and detection distance for the pedestrian target under rural conditions with glare (the most difficult target to discern).

More recently, peer-reviewed published clinical studies have also supported reduction of spherical aberration and superior functional vision with the AcrySof IQ when compared with spherical IOLs.[14-17] In fact, the optical advantages of aspheric IOL technology have become fairly well accepted, although some controversy remains in the areas of functional benefit as it relates to pupil size, IOL decentration, depth of focus, and customization.[18] Some studies have shown little or no benefit of aspheric IOLs with smaller pupils[12,13] whereas one laboratory study showed that the SofPort AO provides better optical quality than either a negatively aspheric or a spherical IOL under conditions of significant decentration.[19] One study has shown diminished distance-corrected near-visual acuity, a surrogate measure for depth of focus, with the AcrySof IQ aspheric IOL as compared to the AcrySof SN60AT spherical IOL.[17]

Regarding customization of the aspheric correction, it has been suggested that achieving zero total spherical aberration postoperatively provides the best quality of vision. Piers and coauthors utilized an adaptive optics simulator to assess letter acuity and contrast sensitivity for 2 different values of spherical aberration. The first condition was the average amount of spherical aberration measured in pseudophakic patients with spherical IOLs. The second condition represented the complete correction of the individual's spherical aberration (Z [4,0] = 0). The researchers found an average improvement in visual acuity associated with the correction of spherical aberration of 10% and 38% measured in white and green light, respectively. Similarly, average contrast sensitivity measurements improved 32% and 57% in white and green light. When spherical aberration was corrected, visual performance was as good as or better than for the normal spherical aberration case for defocus as large as ±1 D. Therefore, these researchers concluded that completely correcting ocular spherical aberration improves spatial vision in the best-focus position without compromising the subjective tolerance to defocus.[20]

On the other hand, it has alternatively been suggested that providing Z [4,0] = +0.1 μ of postoperative spherical aberration represents a better choice.[21] This line of reasoning originated from a study demonstrating that 35 young subjects with uncorrected visual acuity of 20/15 or better had a mean total spherical aberration of Z [4,0] = +0.110 ± 0.077 μ.[22] However, there is no logical basis to infer that the spherical aberration is responsible for the supernormal visual acuity. In fact, the authors of this study concluded that "The amount of ocular HOAs in eyes with natural supernormal vision is not negligible, and is comparable to the reported amount of HOAs in myopic eyes."[22] This conclusion is born out by a study performed by Wang and Koch demonstrating a mean total spherical aberration of Z [4,0] = +0.128 ± 0.074 μ in a series of 532 eyes of 306 subjects presenting for refractive surgery.[23] Nevertheless, Beiko[21] used the Easygraph corneal topographer (Oculus, Lynwood, WA) to select patients with corneal spherical aberration of +0.37 μ, thus targeting a postoperative total ocular spherical aberration of +0.10 μ following implantation of the Tecnis IOL with −0.27 μ (the Easygraph includes an optional software package that provides Zernike analysis). The selected patient group demonstrated significantly better contrast sensitivity than an unselected group of control patients under both mesopic and photopic conditions.

Recently, Beiko, Haigis, and Steinmueller presented data from a series of 696 eyes confirming the mean corneal spherical aberration of +0.27 μ used in the design of the Tecnis IOL.[24] They found a wide standard deviation of 0.089 μ, with a range from +0.041 to +0.632 μ, and significantly different corneal spherical aberration means in men and women. In some cases the corneal spherical aberration differed significantly between fellow eyes. The authors concluded that "individuals should be measured to determine their unique value when considering correction of this aberration."[24] In addition, they noted that keratometry and the corneal Q value do not correlate well with spherical aberration, and that therefore corneal spherical aberration must be measured directly with a topographer.

One method of proceeding with customized selection of aspheric IOLs involves the following protocol:

∗ Preoperative testing to include corneal topography as well as axial length determination, anterior chamber depth, phakic lens thickness, and corneal white-to-white diameter.

∗ Application of a software package such as VOL-CT (Sarver and Associates, Carbondale, IL) to transform the topography elevation data into preoperative corneal Zernike coefficients, with special attention to Z [4,0], fourth-order spherical aberration at the 6-mm optical zone.

∗ Application of an IOL calculation formula, such as the Holladay 2 (available as part of the Holladay IOL Consultant & Surgical Outcomes Assessment Program, Jack T. Holladay, Houston, TX) to determine correct IOL power for desired postoperative spherical equivalent.

∗ Determination of desired postoperative total ocular spherical aberration and selection of IOL type.

For example, if the desired postoperative total ocular spherical aberration is zero and the preoperative corneal spherical aberration measures about +0.27 μ, the Tecnis with −0.27 μ would be selected. In general, the aspheric IOL that comes closest to providing the desired correction should be selected (Figure 1).

Initial results of customizing the selection of aspheric IOLs have shown promise. In a series of 18 eyes of 12 patients with a mean preoperative corneal spherical aberration of + 0.24 ± 0.075 μ and a targeted postoperative total spherical aberration of Z [4,0] = 0, the Tecnis IOL was selected for 10 eyes, the AcrySof IQ for 7 eyes, and the SofPort AO for 1 eye. The overall mean postoperative total spherical aberration measured −0.0065 ± 0.060 μ, which is statistically not different from zero (p = 0.65). For the Tecnis group, mean Z [4,0] = -0.019 ± 0.061 μ; for the AcrySof group mean Z [4,0] = 0.0073 ± 0.063 μ; for the SofPort eye Z [4,0] = 0.025 μ.

In order to determine the feasibility of correcting preoperative corneal spherical aberration, we calculated the mean absolute error for each type of IOL. The mean absolute error is equal to the absolute value of the difference between the predicted total postoperative spherical aberration and the measured postoperative spherical aberration. The predicted postoperative spherical aberration is simply the preoperative corneal spherical aberration at the 6-mm zone plus the spherical aberration of the IOL implanted. In evaluating the results, allowance should be made for surgically induced spherical aberration; an accepted value for this quantity is 0.03 ± 0.17 μ.[25] The surgically induced spherical aberration represents an estimate of the degree of variation one should expect in the postoperative Z [4,0] wavefront.

In the Tecnis group, the calculated mean absolute error was 0.052 ± 0.044 μ; in the AcrySof group the mean absolute error was 0.052 ± 0.033 μ; for the SofPort AO eye the absolute error was 0.040 μ. The overall mean absolute error for all IOLs was 0.052 ± 0.038 μ. There were no statistically significant differences in the mean absolute error among the different groups or between any group and the entire group.

Our results indicate that targeted postoperative spherical aberration can be achieved within a range very close to the

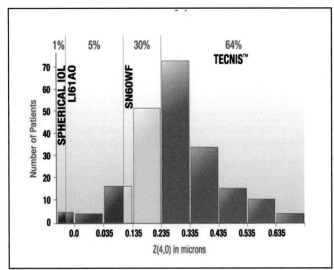

Figure 1. Aspheric IOL selection chart based on the frequency distribution of corneal spherical aberration in the population (for background information, see Holladay JT, Piers PA, Koranyi G, van der Mooren M, Norrby S. A new intraocular lens design to reduce spherical aberration of pseudophakic eyes. *J Refract Surg.* 2002; 18: 683-691; and, Beiko GH, Haigis W, Steinmueller A. Distribution of corneal spherical aberration in a comprehensive ophthalmology practice and whether keratometry can predict aberration values. *J Cataract Refract Surg.* 2007 May;33(5):848-858.)

limits of surgically induced spherical aberration. Future directions for research include expansion of this initial study and consideration of psychophysical measures such as contrast sensitivity to elucidate the real value of eliminating spherical aberration. It is important to realize that these psychophysical tests of functional vision are generally performed with best spectacle correction in order to exclude the effects of blur from test results. The ability to achieve superior functional vision with best spectacle correction reflects both the strength and weakness of wavefront-corrected IOLs. Given the state of the art of biometry and IOL power calculation it is not possible to achieve precise emmetropia in all eyes. Many pseudophakic patients find that their uncorrected vision is adequate for most tasks of daily living and therefore do not wear spectacles. The amount of defocus and astigmatism they accept may negate the pseudophakic correction of their spherical aberration. Nio and colleagues noted in 2002, "Both spherical and irregular aberrations increase the depth of focus, but decrease the modulation transfer (MT) at high spatial frequencies at optimum focus. These aberrations, therefore, play an important role in the balance between acuity and depth of focus."[26] For some patients with adequate uncorrected distance acuity, the advantages of a bit more depth of focus may be worth a little loss of contrast. The ultimate expression of this trend is embodied in the multifocal IOL, which by its design reduces optical quality in order to enhance spectacle independence. The Tecnis Multifocal IOL, now in FDA-monitored clinical trials, represents a conscious compromise between optical efficiency and functional vision on the one hand, and quality of life on the other.

References

1. Holladay JT, Piers PA, Koranyi G, van der Mooren M, Norrby S. A new intraocular lens design to reduce spherical aberration of pseudophakic eyes. *J Refract Surg.* 2002;18:683-691

2. Kurz S, Krummenauer F, Thieme H, Dick HB. Contrast sensitivity after implantation of a spherical versus an aspherical intraocular lens in biaxial microincision cataract surgery. *J Cataract Refract Surg.* 2007;33(3):393-400.

3. Tecnis Foldable Ultraviolet Light-Absorbing Posterior Chamber IOL [package insert]. Santa Ana, CA. Advanced Medical Optics, Inc.; 2005.

4. Packer M, Fine IH, Hoffman RS, Piers PA. Initial clinical experience with an anterior surface modified prolate intraocular lens. *J Refract Surg.* 2002;18:692-696.

5. Mester U, Dillinger P, Anterist N. Impact of a modified optic design on visual function: clinical comparative study. *J Cataract Refract Surg.* 2003;29(4):652-660.

6. Packer M, Fine IH, Hoffman RS, Piers PA. Improved functional vision with a modified prolate intraocular lens. *J Cataract Refract Surg.* 2004;30:986-992.

7. Bellucci R, Scialdone A, Buratto L, et al. Visual acuity and contrast sensitivity comparison between Tecnis and AcrySof SA60AT intraocular lenses: a multicenter randomized study. *J Cataract Refract Surg.* 2005;31(4):712-717.

8. Kennis H, Huygens M, Callebaut F. Comparing the contrast sensitivity of a modified prolate anterior surface IOL and of two spherical IOLs. *Bull Soc Belge Ophtalmol.* 2004;294:49-58.

9. Kershner RM. Retinal image contrast and functional visual performance with aspheric, silicone, and acrylic intraocular lenses: prospective evaluation. *J Cataract Refract Surg.* 2003;29:1684-1694.

10. Ricci F, Scuderi G, Missiroli F, Regine F, Cerulli A. Low contrast visual acuity in pseudophakic patients implanted with an anterior surface modified prolate intraocular lens. *Acta Ophthalmol Scand.* 2004;82(6):718-722.

11. Martinez Palmer A, Palacin Miranda B, Castilla Cespedes M, Comas Serrano M, Punti Badosa A. Spherical aberration influence in visual function after cataract surgery: prospective randomized trial [in Spanish]. *Arch Soc Esp Oftalmol.* 2005;80(2):71-77.

12. Munoz G, Albarran-Diego C, Montes-Mico R, Rodriguez-Galietero A, Alio JL. Spherical aberration and contrast sensitivity after cataract surgery with the Tecnis Z9000 intraocular lens. *J Cataract Refract Surg.* 2006;32(8):1320-1327.

13. Kasper T, Buhren J, Kohnen T. Visual performance of aspherical and spherical intraocular lenses: intraindividual comparison of visual acuity, contrast sensitivity, and higher-order aberrations. *J Cataract Refract Surg.* 2006;32(12):2022-2029.

14. Awwad ST, Lehmann JD, McCulley JP, Bowman RW. A comparison of higher order aberrations in eyes implanted with AcrySof IQ SN60WF and AcrySof SN60AT intraocular lenses. *Eur J Ophthalmol.* 2007;17(3):320-326.

15. Sandoval HP, Fernandez de Castro LE, Vroman DT, Solomon KD. Comparison of visual outcomes, photopic contrast sensitivity, wavefront analysis, and patient satisfaction following cataract extraction and IOL implantation: aspheric vs spherical acrylic lenses. *Eye.* 2007 Jul 6; [Epub ahead of print]

16. Rocha KM, Soriano ES, Chalita MR, et al. Wavefront analysis and contrast sensitivity of aspheric and spherical intraocular lenses: a randomized prospective study. *Am J Ophthalmol.* 2006;142(5):750-756.

17. Rocha KM, Soriano ES, Chamon W, Chalita MR, Nose W. Spherical aberration and depth of focus in eyes implanted with aspheric and spherical intraocular lenses: a prospective randomized study. *Ophthalmology.* 2007;114(11):2050-2054.

18. Werner L, Olson RJ, Mamalis N. New technology IOL optics. *Ophthalmol Clin North Am.* 2006;19(4):469-483.

19. Altmann GE, Nichamin LD, Lane SS, Pepose JS. Optical performance of 3 intraocular lens designs in the presence of decentration. *J Cataract Refract Surg.* 2005;31(3):574-585.

20. Piers PA, Fernandez EJ, Manzanera S, Norrby S, Artal P. Adaptive optics simulation of intraocular lenses with modified spherical aberration. *Invest Ophthalmol Vis Sci.* 2004;45(12):4601-4610.

21. Beiko G. Personalized Correction of Spherical Aberration in Cataract Surgery. Presented at the Annual Meeting of the American Academy of Ophthalmology, 18 October 2006, Chicago, IL.

22. Levy Y, Segal O, Avni I, Zadok D. Ocular higher-order aberrations in eyes with supernormal vision. *Am J Ophthalmol.* 2005;139(2):225-228.

23. Wang L, Koch DD. Ocular higher-order aberrations in individuals screened for refractive surgery. *J Cataract Refract Surg.* 2003;29(10):1896-1903.

24. Beiko GH, Haigis W, Steinmueller A. Distribution of corneal spherical aberration in a comprehensive ophthalmology practice and whether keratometry can predict aberration values. *J Cataract Refract Surg.* 2007;33(5):848-858.

25. Guirao A, Tejedor J, Artal P. Corneal aberrations before and after small-incision cataract surgery. *Invest Ophthalmol Vis Sci.* 2004;45:4312-4319.

26. Nio YK, Jansonius NM, Fidler V, Geraghty E, Norrby S, Kooijman AC. Spherical and irregular aberrations are important for the optimal performance of the human eye. *Ophthalmic Physiol Opt.* 2002;22(2):103-112.

ASPHERIC IOLS—MATCHING CORNEAL AND IOL WAVEFRONT

Roberto Bellucci, MD

The discussion about the advantages and drawbacks of aspheric intraocular lenses (IOLs) has been long-standing, with some agreement that their practical use should be postponed until decentration problems had been solved.[1] It was the availability of IOLs that remained centered within the capsular bag, when implanted after uneventful lens surgery, that renewed interest in this area. At the moment, several IOLs with different asphericity are available, making it somewhat cumbersome for those not deeply interested in optics to select the best IOL for a specific patient.

Optical Aberrations of Interest in Cataract Surgery

Positive spherical lenses refract parallel rays differently according to their distance from the optical center. Paraxial, or central, rays are refracted onto the main focus of the lens, while more peripheral rays are refracted onto points that are closer to the back lens surface. This disparity in the focus of central and marginal rays is termed *spherical aberration* (Figure 1A). Spherical aberration may be described as either positive or negative. If the marginal rays are focused behind the central rays, it is termed positive and if they are focused behind the central rays it is termed negative.[2] A second important aberration is "coma." Coma occurs when refracted rays are deviated toward one side of the main focus of the lens, adding a comet-like distortion to the image (Figure 1B). Coma can be positive or negative, according to the shifting direction. Coma is produced when the elements of an optical system are decentered.[2]

Optical aberrations affect the quality of the image by decreasing both the resolution and contrast transmitted to the retina. Such a decrease in contrast and resolution results in a reduced modulation transfer function and point spread function.[3] Spherical aberration is the most important of the optical aberrations of lenses—and of the eye as an optical system. It can be reduced by progressively decreasing the lens power toward the periphery. However, coma can only be corrected by perfecting centration of the various refractive surfaces.

Determining the Corneal Wavefront

Almost all of the refractive power of the cornea is provided by its anterior surface. The difference in the refractive indexes between the corneal stroma and the aqueous humor is too small for the posterior corneal surface to exert a significant influence, thus simplifying evaluations and calculations.[4] For this reason, corneal aberrations can be studied from corneal topography, which measures the amount and differences in anterior corneal surface elevation. Topographers with special software are now able to generate a Zernike tree that contains information regarding the amount of anterior corneal spherical aberration, as well as other higher-order aberrations (Figure 2).

One characteristic of the anterior surface of the human cornea is positive spherical aberration that does not generally change with increasing age (Figure 3).[5,6] Larger variations occur after corneal refractive surgery. There is typically an increase in positive spherical aberration with myopic ablations (Figure 4), and an increase in negative spherical aberration with hyperopic ablations.

It has been demonstrated that the youthful crystalline lens compensates for the amount of positive spherical aberration of the normal anterior corneal surface by adding a lesser amount of negative spherical aberration to the human eye. But unlike the spherical aberration of the anterior cornea, the amount of negative spherical aberration of the crystalline lens decreases over time, leading to an overall increase in the amount of positive spherical aberration.[7]

When we perform cataract surgery in a previously unoperated eye, the positive spherical aberration of the IOL will add to that of the cornea, reducing the optical quality of the eye and the overall quality of vision.[8,9]

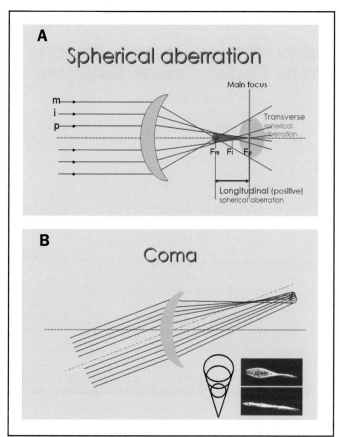

Figure 1. (A) Spherical aberration of a positive spherical lens is *positive* (ie, eccentric rays are refracted closer to the lens). (B) Coma occurs when the images—or the refracting lenses—are decentered.

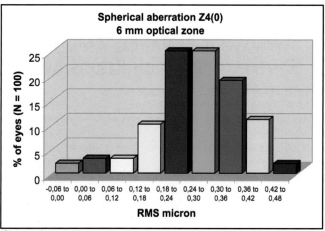

Figure 3. Corneal spherical aberration Z4 (0) for 6-mm optical zone, calculated from 100 unoperated corneas.

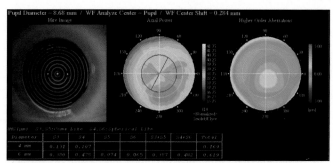

Figure 4. Corneal spherical aberration is double than usual in this cornea operated for 7-D myopia.

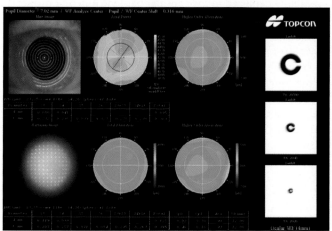

Figure 2. Corneal topography and simultaneous ocular aberrometry allow direct comparison between corneal and ocular wavefront.

The amount of coma of the corneal surface is similar as the amount of spherical aberration, but vision is less affected for optical reasons. After refractive corneal surgery, coma increases in the presence of a decentered ablation. IOL decentration also produces coma, which can either add to the corneal coma or subtract from it, thus worsening or improving the overall optical quality of the eye.

Aspheric IOLs

Aspheric IOLs were designed to overcome the problem of adding additional positive spherical aberration to the pseudophakic eye. Different aspheric IOLs contain different amounts of asphericity according to different theoretical approaches. The first approach aims at correcting all the positive spherical aberration of the cornea, with an IOL providing −0.27 µm of negative spherical aberration (Tecnis IOL; Advanced Medical Optics, Santa Ana, CA).[10] A second approach takes into account the variability of the corneal asphericity among different subjects, and the possible induction of coma with IOL decentration. This type of aspheric lens corrects only its own positive spherical aberration (Advanced Optics IOL; Bausch & Lomb, Rochester, NY).[11] A third approach is only designed to correct for a part of the positive spherical aberration of the anterior cornea, with the overall objective being the preservation of a small amount of positive spherical aberration as found in eyes with "supernormal" vision (Acrysof IQ; Alcon, Forth Worth, TX).[12]

From an optical point of view, only the so-called "neutral" lenses should be labeled "aspheric," whereas the other lenses should be called "hyperaspheric." Aspheric IOLs with negative spherical aberration in reality have poor optical quality. Such lenses represent compensating, or correcting optics, rather than a stand-alone optic device.

Table 1

HYPERASPHERIC, NEUTRAL ASPHERIC, AND SPHERICAL INTRAOCULAR LENSES PRODUCE DIFFERENT ABERRATION RESULTS ACCORDING TO THE EXISTING CORNEAL ASPHERICITY

# of Patients	Corneal SA μm	IOL SA μm	Ocular SA μm	Result
18%	-0.06 to +0.18	-0.27	-0.33 to -0.09	◐
		0	-0.06 to +0.18	●
		+0.20	+0.14 to +0.38	◐
69%	+0.18 to +0.36	-0.27	-0.09 to +0.09	●
		0	+0.18 to +0.36	◐
		+0.20	+0.38 to +0.56	●
13%	+0.36 to +0.48	-0.27	+0.09 to +0.21	◐
		0	+0.36 to +0.48	●
		+0.20	+0.56 to +0.68	●

Result: (●) Good; (◐) Acceptable; (●) Poor

Regardless of the amount of asphericity, it is helpful to keep some fundamental principles in mind. The aspheric surface can be either anterior or posterior without affecting the basic properties of an IOL[1]; as the power of the eye is changed by the implant, no IOL can actually behave as truly "neutral"[1]; the SRK/T A-constant for IOL power calculations, compared to a regular spherical IOL of the same design, should be increased approximately by 0.25 for an aspheric IOL and by 0.50 for an aspheric IOL that adds negative spherical aberration[13]; hyperaspheric IOLs will not induce coma in the presence of "physiological" decentration[14]; in eyes with the compensation of the anterior corneal spherical aberration, both an increase in image quality and a decrease in depth of focus occur.[15] In the presence of a small pupil diameter, the advantage of an aspheric IOL, with or without the addition of negative spherical aberration, becomes imperceptible.[1]

Wavefront Matching

To compensate for the positive spherical aberration of the anterior cornea with an IOL, we must start with a value as obtained from corneal topography. Practically speaking, several conditions can arise (Table 1), and the surgeon can generally predict the amount of postoperative spherical aberration of the pseudophakic eye, although not precisely. In the pseudophakic state, spherical aberration close to zero will increase the sharpness of the perceived image.[16] Residual amounts of spherical aberration will increase depth of focus while decreasing image quality. The increase in depth of focus due to large amounts of spherical aberration is probably the reason for the reduced near add required after implantation of high-power spherical lenses.

When matching the corneal asphericity with a hyperaspheric IOL, the optical center of the cornea and the IOL should be coincident so as not to induce coma. However, the eye is not a centered optical system due to the fact that the optical axis and the visual axis are slightly different. Thus even if the IOL is perfectly centered in the capsular bag, the inherent property of the human eye will result in some degree of decentration. As a result, some coma will be induced by any IOL with positive or negative spherical aberration. This coma will combine with the coma already present from the corneal surface, sometimes adding to or subtracting from it. As a result, it has been found that hyperaspheric IOLs induce as much coma as a spherical IOL, when clinically centered.[14] With gross decentration, the aberrations induced by a hyperaspheric IOL will outweigh those induced by a spherical IOL, which themselves are still greater as compared with those induced by a neutral aspheric IOL. For this reason, neutral lenses should be preferred when IOL decentration can be anticipated, such as in eyes with weak zonules or previous trauma.

By personalizing the IOL profile according to measured Zernike coefficients for each individual eye, it could be possible to correct the whole spherical aberration in any particular eye. This expensive approach is offered in Europe by *Acri.tec (Hennigsdorf, Germany), and is suggested for selected cases of unusual spherical aberration of the cornea. This approach can be useful in eyes with previous corneal refractive surgery, but the attempt to counteract high corneal spherical aberration with excessive IOL asphericity will probably induce too much coma even with good IOL centration. In this regard, the desire to correct every amount of corneal spherical aberration with the IOL will probably not be satisfied.

Another possible problem with aspheric IOLs is the amount of flattening required by the aspheric design. This could produce an anterior surface much flatter than that of a spherical IOL, especially with high refractive index material and low-power lenses. Anterior flattening is known to produce positive and negative dysphotopsias,[17] which therefore could be more frequent with aspheric IOLs.

Clinical Results

The first clinical studies conducted on aspheric IOLs demonstrated that the reduction of spherical aberration, as compared to conventional IOLs, leads to improved contrast sensitivity (Figure 5).[18-20] Current attention is more devoted to aberration measurements in implanted eyes, and to their relation with functional vision. In a theoretical setting, Wang and Koch[21] calculated the residual aberrations after implantation simulation of centered and decentered IOLs correcting either corneal spherical aberration or corneal total wavefront error. They concluded that hyperaspheric IOLs can improve the corneal higher-order aberrations in approximately 45% of eyes, when clinically centered. Marcos and colleagues found the spherical aberration of the entire eye to be lower in the eyes with the Tecnis lens than in the eyes with spherical IOLs, with better optical quality as measured by modulation transfer function (MTF) and point spread function (PSF) (Strehl ratio).[22] Interestingly, they also found some changes in the corneal surface aberrations after surgery with 4.1-mm incisions, suggesting that the smallest possible incision be used when planning postoperative aberration control. Similar results about the efficacy of hyperaspheric lenses in matching corneal spherical aberration were obtained by other investigators.[23-25] We could demonstrate good compensation of the corneal spherical aberration with no increase in the coma of the entire eye with the Tecnis lens, as compared with the parent spherical IOL.[14] Our recent investigations comparing 3 aspheric IOLs confirm those previous results both for spherical aberration (Figure 6A) and for coma (Figure 6B).

The usefulness of patient selection according to their corneal asphericity has been underscored by Beiko, who demonstrated lower aberrations and better contrast sensitivity when hyperaspheric lenses had been implanted in eyes with high positive spherical aberration, as compared to an unselected group of eyes receiving the same IOL.[26]

Conclusion

Earlier and recent studies indicate that aspheric IOLs effectively reduce spherical aberration in implanted eyes, with the possible exception of those patients who prior to surgery have close to zero, or negative, spherical aberration. The clinical advantage of matching corneal aberrations with IOL technology has been demonstrated, and in the future new lenses with different amounts of asphericity will appear. On a theoretical basis, the advantages of using various types of aspheric IOLs could be limited by decentration, dysphotopsias, and small pupil diameters, and by any problems with optical clarity.

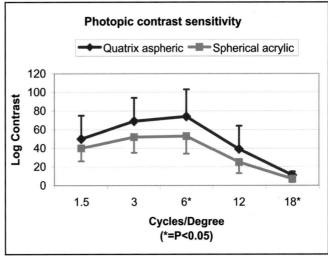

Figure 5. Contrast sensitivity comparison between the 2 eyes of 20 patients implanted in one eye with a hyperaspheric IOL and in the contralateral eye with a spherical IOL.

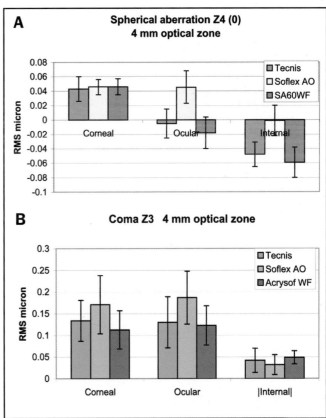

Figure 6. (A) Corneal, ocular, and internal (IOL-related) spherical aberration with 2 hyperaspheric IOLs and 1 aspheric neutral IOL. (B) Corneal, ocular, and internal (IOL-related) coma with 2 hyperaspheric IOLs and 1 aspheric neutral IOL.

Although not yet clearly demonstrated, these drawbacks suggest that when anticipating any amount of IOL decentration, the implantation of a neutral aspheric lens may be advantageous. Also, the correction of excessive amounts of negative and positive asphericity with an IOL should be avoided.

References

1. Atchison DA. Design of aspheric intraocular lenses. *Ophthalm Physiol Opt.* 1991;11:137-146.

2. Atchison DA, Smith G. *Optics of the Human Eye.* Edinburgh: Butterworth; 2000

3. Charman WN. The Charles W Prentice Award Lecture 2005. Optics of the human eye: progress and problems. *Optom Vis Sci.* 2006;83:335-345.

4. Dubbelman M, Sicam VADP, Van der Heijde GL. The shape of the anterior and posterior surface of the aging human cornea. *Vis Res.* 2006;46:993-1001.

5. Navarro R, Gonzalez L, Hernandez JL. Optics of the average normal cornea from general and canonical representations of its surface topography. *J Opt Soc Am A.* 2006;23:219-232.

6. Vinciguerra P, Camesasca FI, Calossi A. Statistical analysis of physiological aberrations of the cornea. *J Refract Surg.* 2003;19:S265-S269.

7. Alio JL, Schimchak P, Negri HP, Montes-Mico R. Crystalline lens optical dysfunction through aging. *Ophthalmology.* 2005;112:2022-2029.

8. Guirao A, Redondo M, Geraghty E, et al. Corneal optical aberrations and retinal image quality in patients in whom monofocal intraocular lenses were implanted. *Arch Ophthalmol.* 2002;120:1143-1151.

9. Bellucci R, Morselli S, Piers P. Comparison of wavefront aberrations and optical quality of eyes implanted with five intraocular lenses. *J Refract Surg.* 2004;20:297-306.

10. Holladay JT, Piers PA, Koranyi G, van der Mooren M, Norrby S. A new intraocular lens design to reduce spherical aberration of pseudophakic eyes. *J Refract Surg.* 2002;18:683-691.

11. Altmann GE, Nichamin LD, Lane SS, Pepose JS. Optical performance of 3 intraocular lens designs in the presence of decentration. *J Cataract Refract Surg.* 2005;31:574-585.

12. Awwad ST, Lehmann JD, McCulley JP, Bowman RW. A comparison of higher order aberrations in eyes implanted with AcrySof IQ SN60WF and AcrySof SN60AT intraocular lenses. *Eur J Ophthalmol.* 2007;17:320-326.

13. Becker KA, Holzer MP, Reuland AJ, Auffarth GU. [Accuracy of lens power calculation and centration of an aspheric intraocular lens]. *Ophthalmologe.* 2006;103:873-876.

14. Bellucci R, Morselli S, Pucci V. Spherical aberration and coma with an aspherical and a spherical intraocular lens in normal age-matched eyes. *J Cataract Refract Surg.* 2007;33:203-209.

15. Rocha KM, Soriano ES, Chamon W, Chalita MR, Nose W. Spherical aberration and depth of focus in eyes implanted with aspheric and spherical intraocular lenses: a prospective randomized study. *Ophthalmology.* 2007;114:2050-2054.

16. Levy Y, Segal O, Avni I, Zadok D. Ocular higher-order aberrations in eyes with supernormal vision. *Am J Ophthalmol.* 2005;139:225-228.

17. Shambhu S, Shanmuganathan VA, Charles SJ. The effect of lens design on dysphotopsia in different acrylic IOLs. *Eye.* 2005;19:567-570.

18. Packer M, Fine IH, Hoffman RS, Piers PA. Prospective randomized trial of an anterior surface modified prolate intraocular lens. *J Refract Surg.* 2002;18:692-696.

19. Mester U, Dillinger P, Anterist N. Impact of a modified optic design on visual function: clinical comparative study. *J Cataract Refract Surg.* 2003;29:652-660.

20. Bellucci R, Scialdone A, Buratto L, et al. Visual acuity and contrast sensitivity comparison between Tecnis and AcrySof SA60AT intraocular lenses: a multicenter randomized study. *J Cataract Refract Surg.* 2005;31:712-717.

21. Wang L, Koch DD. Effect of decentration of wavefront-corrected intraocular lenses on the higher-order aberrations of the eye. *Arch Ophthalmol.* 2005;123:1226-1230.

22. Marcos S, Barbero S, Jimenez-Alfaro I. Optical quality and depth of field of eyes implanted with spherical and aspheric intraocular lenses. *J Refract Surg.* 2005;21:223-235.

23. Kasper T, Buhren J, Kohnen T. Intraindividual comparison of higher-order aberrations after implantation of aspherical and spherical intraocular lenses as a function of pupil diameter. *J Cataract Refract Surg.* 2006;32:78-84.

24. Denoyer A, Roger F, Majzoub S, Pisella PJ. [Quality of vision after cataract surgery in patients with prolate aspheric lens.] *J Fr Ophtalmol.* 2006;29:157-163.

25. Padmanabhan P, Rao SK, Jayasree R, Chowdhry M, Roy J. Monochromatic aberrations in eyes with different intraocular lens optic designs. *J Refract Surg.* 2006;22:172-177.

26. Beiko GH. Personalized correction of spherical aberration in cataract surgery. *J Cataract Refract Surg.* 2007;33:1455-1460.

CHAPTER 77

MONOVISION WITH ASPHERIC IOLS

J. E. "Jay" McDonald II, MD and David J. Deitz, MPhil

Patients increasingly demand spectacle independence as the goal for intraocular lens (IOL) surgery. Surgeons have responded by mixing and matching IOLs in order to achieve better results through more successful combinations. Multifocal and accommodating IOL strategies have realized significant gains over standard monofocal implementation, yet the ability to restore or imitate accommodation remains elusive.

This chapter presents a new look at an old technique: monovision. We have found that new generation monofocal IOLs in conjunction with monovision produces superior results and patient satisfaction. This chapter will explain the clinical success we have had with the monovision technique in tandem with aspheric monofocal lenses and accommodative IOLs. Then in Chapter 78, we will further explore the reasons for this success, examining the neurocognitive correlates of both monovision and multifocal IOLs. We believe that the reason why monovision trumps a multifocal approach can be explained when the processes involved in visual processing are fully understood.

The Monofocal Approach Revisited

Standard bilateral lens replacement with distance monofocal IOLs typically leads to a deficit in near vision for presbyopic patients, which normally results in a need for reading glasses.[1,2] However, utilizing monovision can overcome this difficulty while maintaining excellent contrast sensitivity.

In monovision, a slight defocus is applied to one of the two eyes while the other is corrected for normal distance. Although this only produces slight losses in distance vision, the technique greatly improves the patient's ability to see objects at close range. The monovision technique has been popular with contact lenses, successful in laser in situ keratomileusis (LASIK), and successfully employed with IOLs.[3-6] Combining new generation monofocal IOLs with a monovision technique is an excellent strategy for achieving spectacle independence, although patients with weaker or mixed dominance tend to fair better in monovision than those with strong dominance.[7] Figure 1 demonstrates the range of visual acuity possible with monovision in a patient with an eye corrected to −1.5 D for near vision and an eye corrected for distance vision (plano). One eye is targeted for distance, whereas the other produces high-contrast images when used for near vision.

Our Results

In our practice, we have had considerable success with the monovision technique in conjunction with aspheric IOLs. Our practice conducted a formalized study measuring the visual outcomes of 40 patients (80 eyes) who underwent uneventful bilateral cataract surgery. After determining dominance between the 2 eyes, the dominant eye was corrected for distance vision (goal between plano and −0.50 D) whereas the nondominant eye was corrected for near vision (goal between −0.75 D and −2.00 D).

Following lens replacement with the SofPort AO lens (Bausch & Lomb, Rochester, NY) and subsequent incisional enhancement, the 40 distance eyes (goal 0 to −0.50) had a mean spherical equivalent (SE) of −0.21 (sd 0.39), whereas the 40 eyes corrected with a myopic goal (−0.75 to −2.00) had a mean SE of −1.42 (sd = 0.71). Eleven of the 40 patients (28%) underwent postoperative astigmatic keratotomy (AK) or limbal relaxing incisions (LRI) touch-ups. Among the 40 patients for distance vision, 100% achieved binocular uncorrected visual acuity of 20/30 or better, and 73% achieved 20/20 or better (Figure 2). For binocular near vision, 88% achieved J2 uncorrected visual acuity (UCVA) or better, and 48% achieved J1 or better (Figure 3). Binocularly, patients had an average distance logMAR UCVA of 0.036 (20/20-2 Snellen equivalent) and an average near logMAR UCVA of 0.077 (J2+ Jaeger equivalent).

A spectacle dependence survey was conducted with all patients approximately 1 year postoperatively with 37 out of

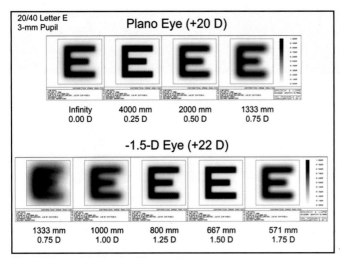

Figure 1. Range of visual acuity with monovision.

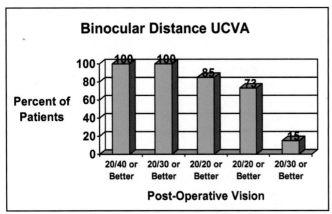

Figure 2. Binocular distance UCVA for patients with aspheric IOLs with monovision (n = 40).

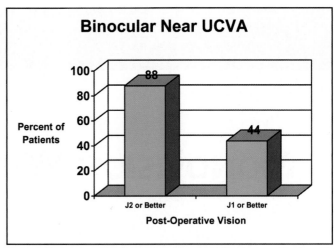

Figure 3. Binocular near UCVA for patients with aspheric IOLs with monovision (n = 40).

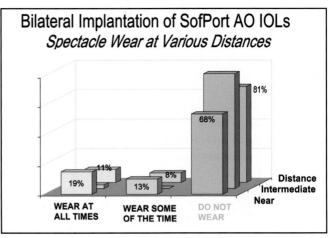

Figure 4. Spectacle Independence Survey of patients at 6 months postoperative (n = 37).

40 patients responding. This survey showed that 97% of these patients were free from glasses for intermediate vision, 81% were spectacle free at distance, and 68% were completely spectacle free at near (Figure 4). Only 3% of patients required glasses at all times for intermediate vision, whereas 11% required glasses for distance, and 19% required glasses for near vision at all times.

The Triumph of Aspheric and Accommodative IOLs

The newest generation aspheric monofocal lenses have improved contrast sensitivity over their spherical counterparts. An aspheric aberration-free IOL removes the additional spherical aberration seen with conventional IOLs, preserving the natural spherical dimensions of the cornea. The aspheric lens normally preserves a small amount of naturally occurring positive spherical aberration, which has been shown to be beneficial in compensating for higher-order aberrations, such as coma and foil.[8,9] An aberration-free aspheric is also more forgiving of IOL decentration, and thus helps to ensure excellent visual outcomes.[10,11] Additionally, studies have demonstrated that aspheric lenses produce better best-corrected

visual acuity (BCVA) and contrast sensitivity than conventional IOLs.[12,13]

Furthermore, spherical aberration increases an eye's depth of field. When the object distance is infinity, image clarity is sharpest in an eye with no spherical aberration (the IOL with negative spherical aberration produces this). However, as vergence increases, image quality degrades with an IOL that has negative spherical aberration. Although other monofocal IOLs work well, we believe a patient is better suited with an aberration-free IOL. By delivering a better image at the focused distance, the aspheric IOL overcomes the depth of field advantage of conventional IOLs. We hypothesize that the inherent image degradation caused by the conventional IOL creates a less advantageous position. The higher contrasted images of the aspheric optic provide stronger drive for visual cortical contrast gain enhancement of the regarded eye thus a better form of monovision. This is not to say that a spherical IOL is wholly inappropriate—we believe that successful monovision can certainly be achieved with spherical IOLs.

Figure 5 (from Holladay) shows the modulation transfer function versus defocus.[14] In the graph, higher modulation corresponds with higher contrast sensitivity. For both the aspheric (diagramed here as "MP") and spherical lenses,

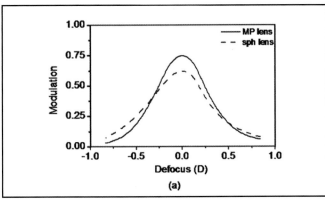

Figure 5. Modulation curves for aspheric and spherical IOLs.

contrast sensitivity (or modulation) is greatest when defocus is at a minimum. As the amount of defocus increases, the contrast sensitivity decreases similarly to a normal curve. This diagram illustrates the superiority of the aspheric IOL over spherical models by achieving a higher modulation at its focal point.

Another recent study has confirmed this finding, demonstrating that on average contrast sensitivity is best when the amount of spherical aberration contributed by the IOL is zero.[15] Due to the cerebral cortex's ability to invoke contrast gain for reading, the aspheric lens delivers better function (J1) but at a farther distance away (28 inches), even with only a −1.25-D defocus. We have found this to be clinically manifest as well.

Our practice has had great success with aspheric IOLs and monovision, but we believe that the future of this technique will involve accommodating IOLs. If accommodating IOLs were combined with a monovision technique in the same fashion, a patient who received an IOL with the distance eye corrected to plano and the near eye corrected to −1.50 D would exhibit a near perfect and extended range of visual acuity. Assuming that the accommodative lens provided an additional −0.75 D of accommodation, the near eye would have an effective range of accommodation from −1.50 to −2.25. If the eye corrected for distance vision also has −0.75 to −1.00 D of accommodation, the 2 eyes stay within 0.75 D of spatial frequency separation at all distances. Spatial frequency degradation should be minimal in this range and fusion would occur at all distances.

Surgeon's Perspective

There are many practical reasons to employ monovision:

* It always leaves the surgeon and patient with a readily available temporary and permanent fall back position. The optical effects can be intermittently reversed with spectacles or contacts. This is great comfort to the doctor and the patient when deciding to embark on the journey of spectacle independence. As well, it is surgically reversible or alterable by a refractive procedure.
* It provides the highest quality of vision.
* The patient maintains their eligibility for currently unavailable downstream technology.

* The procedure allows for the largest margin of surgical latitude. A poor capsulorrhexis, need for sulcus placement, or decentration of IOL do not necessarily compromise the plan.

When surgical outcomes are not ideal, there are many options available for the monovision IOL patient. Most commonly, we use a 2-incision radial keratotomy (RK) to decrease the near eye from a −2.25 to −1.50, for instance. Clinically, we find the most common issue is residual astigmatic or myopic correction, as we always err in our calculations on the myopic side to account for our bell curve of refractive predictions. Those not comfortable with using incisional surgery can certainly use laser vision correction for this need.

Every refractive IOL surgeon must have at his or her disposal a comfortable course of astigmatic management, refractive tune ups, accurate biometry, and a staff and doctor that understands the refractive patient, as well as how to set and manage expectations. We will touch only on a few of these issues, as they pertain directly to monovision with IOLs.

Indications for Aspheric Monovision

* Desire for spectacle independence
* 20/20 expected visual acuity result in each eye
* Willingness to understand the process of vision is binocular
* Patient understands that spectacles will always be a fall back for full distance and near

Blur Tolerance

We like to hold a +1.50-D lens over the distance correction of the non-dominant eye to "illustrate" the principle. If the patient strongly objects or reacts to this situation, we will eliminate him or her. We encourage them that this is better tolerated when the difference is inside the eye, but we also eliminate those patients who have questionable adaptability at this trial.

The surgeons fall-back position is that if the patient does not tolerate monovision, it is easily fixed with a refractive procedure. Usually this amounts to taking a D at most out of the cornea, which we do with a mini RK. This can certainly be done with laser vision correction as well if one chooses.

Contact Lens or Not

We do not do a contact lens trial. The contact lens trial will eliminate some patients who would otherwise do well with pseudophakic monovision. Because the IOL is closer to the nodal point of the eye than a contact lens, the resultant difference in size of the 2 images is smaller than with contact lenses and thus less objectionable to the brain in terms of the ability to fuse. Just as a trial of spectacles employing monovision is not a good indicator of contact lens success with monovision, a contact lens trial is not a good indicator for success with pseudophakic monovision.

Near Eye Focal Distance

Because of a growing dependence on computer use, many of today's patients are more appreciative of excellent intermediate vision than a closer focal distance. We have thus moved more toward a lower dioptric power in the near eye, which gives great vision at "computer" distance and better fusion overall.

Special Preoperative Testing

EYE DOMINANCE

The standard test is a card with a hole in it held at arms length. We have moved to handing the patient a camera and asking them to "take my picture." The eye the patient uses for sighting is recorded as the dominant eye. We ask men if they shoot rifles or pistols. If they answer yes, we usually use the eye they aim with as the dominant eye. Ocular dominance plays a major role in ease of adaptation to monovision.[7] We are in the process of developing an easily administered quantitative test that will allow us to determine the strength of eye dominance within the patient.

PHORIAS

We utilize a Maddox rod test. Patients who have 12 or more degrees of esophoria are eliminated from monovision.

CORNEAL TOPOGRAPHY

Abnormal corneal topography should be identified as patients with this condition may not have 20/20 visual potential. As for any presbyopia-correcting IOL, astigmatism should be dealt with preferably at the time of cataract surgery. We treat 0.75 D or more with astigmatic keratotomy unless the axis of refractive versus topographic astigmatism differs significantly. In this case, we inform the patient of the astigmatism but explain that we will wait until after cataract surgery to perform astigmatic keratotomy at 6 weeks postoperatively if it is manifest. Patients appreciate hearing this information up front.

All of these aforementioned diagnostic and treatment processes are noncovered and may be considered to be added on services and charges.

Conclusion

Monofocal IOLs present an option for spectacle independence that offers the best quality of vision. We have had great clinical success with aspheric IOLs, which deliver a high contrast percept across a range of distances. When the monofocal strategy is used with an accommodating IOL, this range of vision as well as fusion can be extended. Our optimum separation is 1.50 D with the aspheric monofocal and 1.00 D with the accommodating Crystalens (Eyeonics, Inc, Aliso Viejo, CA). Accurate biometry, astigmatism reduction to 0.50 D or less, and the capability to make small corrections of residual spherical error with incisional or laser vision correction are necessary tools for the successful implementation of this strategy. An understanding of all these issues is mandatory for the entire staff from front office to back. The process begins with the initial phone call and ends only when the patient's expectations have been met or exceeded.

References

1. Nijkamp MD, Dolders MGT, de Brabander J, et al. Effectiveness of multifocal intraocular lenses to correct presbyopia after cataract surgery; a randomized controlled trial. *Ophthalmology.* 2004;111:1832-1839.

2. Leyland MD, Langan L, Goolfee F, Lee N, Bloom PA. Prospective randomised double-masked trial of bilateral multifocal, bifocal or monofocal intraocular lenses. *Eye.* 2002;16:481-490.

3. Jain S, Arora I, Azar DT. Success of monovision in presbyopes: review of the literature and potential applications to refractive surgery. *Surv Ophthalmol.* 1996;40:491-499.

4. Goldberg DB. Laser in situ keratomileusis monovision. *J Cataract Refract Surg.* 2001;27:1449-1455.

5. Boerner CF, Thrasher BH. Results of monovision correction in bilateral pseudophakes. *J Am Intraocul Implant Soc.* 1984;10:49-50.

6. Greenbaum S. Monovision pseudophakia. *J Cataract Refract Surg.* 2002;28:1439-1443.

7. Handa T, Mukuno K, Uozato H, et al. Ocular dominance and patient satisfaction after monovision induced by intraocular lens implantation. *J Cataract Refract Surg.* 2004;30:769-774.

8. Artal P, Berrio E, Guirao A, Piers P. Contribution of the cornea and internal surfaces to the change of ocular aberrations with age. *J Opt Soc Am A Opt Image Sci Vis.* 2002;19:137-143.

9. Applegate RA, Marsack JD, Ramos R, Sarver EJ. Interaction between aberrations to improve or reduce visual performance. *J Cataract Refract Surg.* 2003;29:1487-1495.

10. Altmann GE, Nichamin LD, Lane SS, Pepose JS. Optical performance of 3 intraocular lens designs in the presence of decentration. *J Cataract Refract Surg.* 2005;31:574-585.

11. Hayashi K, Hayashi H, Nakao F, Hayashi F. Correlation between pupillary size and intraocular lens decentration and visual acuity of a zonal-progressive multifocal lens and a monofocal lens. *Ophthalmology.* 2001;108:2011-2017.

12. Belucci R, Scialdone A, Buratto L. Visual acuity and contrast sensitivity comparison between Tecnis and AcrySof SA60AT intraocular lenses: a multicenter randomized study. *J Cataract Refract Surg.* 2005;31:712-717.

13. Marcos S, Barbero S, Jimenez-Alfaro I. Optical quality and depth-of-field of eyes implanted with spherical and aspheric intraocular lenses. *J Refract Surg.* 2005;21:223-235.

14. Holladay JT, Piers PA, Koranyi G, van der Mooren M, Norrby NE. A new intraocular lens design to reduce spherical aberration of pseudophakic eyes. *J Refract Surg.* 2002;18:683-691.

15. Piers PA, Manzanera S, Prieto PM, Gorceix N, Artal P. Use of adaptive optics to determine the optimal ocular spherical aberration. *J Cataract Refract Surg.* 2007; 33:1721-1726.

CHAPTER 78

NEUROADAPTATION TO MONOVISION

J. E. "Jay" McDonald II, MD and David J. Deitz, MPhil

Starkly absent from many intraocular lens (IOL) discussions is informed consideration of the consequences of IOLs on the neural machinery underlying vision. In other words, what is happening in the precortical and cortical visual areas as images are filtered through IOLs? The dialogue between ophthalmologists and neuroscientists has not been as strong as it could be, especially considering that the 2 disciplines share much of the same subject matter. This chapter attempts to reconcile this shortcoming by providing an overview of developing literature in neuroscience as it may pertain to the consequences of different IOL choices.

We will attempt to illuminate the neurological processes impacted by both monovision and multifocal IOLs, providing a possible theoretical explanation of the clinical results reported in the literature. We believe monovision is a more effective solution that preserves good contrast sensitivity and visual acuity by capitalizing on the ways in which the eye and visual cortex process optical information specifying form and contrast. Our reasoning may also explain why multifocal solutions can result in decreased contrast, halos at night, and why some patients complain of blurry images despite having 20/20 vision.[1-4]

Intraocular Lenses and the Brain

The eye and brain contain neural elements that behave somewhat like complex integrated circuits comprising an incredibly powerful computer. Those neural circuits are capable of translating the patterns of light that fall on the photoreceptors into meaningful visual impressions of the objects and events in our field of view. Despite the computational power of the retina and brain, the performance of that neural circuitry is limited by the quality of the images triggering sensory signals. Good vision is impossible without good optics, which is why disturbances in the quality of the eye's refractive components can have devastating consequences on vision. In the case of

patients with cataracts, surgical replacement of a clouded lens with a high quality intraocular lens implant can provide what seems like a visual miracle from the patient's perspective. For the IOL to be successful over the long term, the decision about which implant to use must be informed by the consequences of the IOL on the neural operations performed by the eye and brain. These neural elements will be operating on images formed and altered by that newly introduced refractive component. Therefore, we should prefer IOLs that best cooperate with the normal image processing operations of the brain.

We can think of the visual nervous system as comprising multiple stages distributed from the retina to a rich network of brain areas stretching from the occipital cortex into the temporal, parietal and frontal lobes of the brain. This network continues from the retina into the thalamus and the primary visual cortex, which in turn channels visual information to higher areas of the brain. Figure 1 summarizes one conceptualization of this complex, richly interconnected network of processing stages.[5] Located at the gateway to this network, at the bottom of this diagram, are the RGCs (RGC) whose axons form the optic nerve that projects from the eye to the brain. The human eye contains, on average, just over 100 million photoreceptors (rods and cones) but only about 1 million ganglion cells. This 100/1 disparity in numbers tells us that already, within the retina, information contained in the light imaged on the photoreceptors is being significantly transformed. Specifically, this neural transformation condenses and collates the point-like sensory data registered by the 100 million photoreceptors into one million neural signals that specify the spatial structure contained in the image.

What do we mean by spatial structure? In the context of image formation, spatial structure refers to regions in the image where there exist differences in the intensity distribution ("lightness contrast") and, often, wavelength distribution ("color contrast") of light. Spatial structure corresponds to the presence of contours and edges within local regions of an image; those contours and edges define the sizes, shapes, and surface characteristics of the objects we are looking at. Among

Figure 1. A conceptualization of neural networks involved in vision. This diagram does not include subcortical structures involved in oculomotor function, such as control of the pupil and the eye muscles. (Reprinted with permission from Felleman DJ, Van Essen DC. Distributed hierarchical processing in the primate cerebral cortex. *Cereb Cortex.* 1991;1:1-47.)

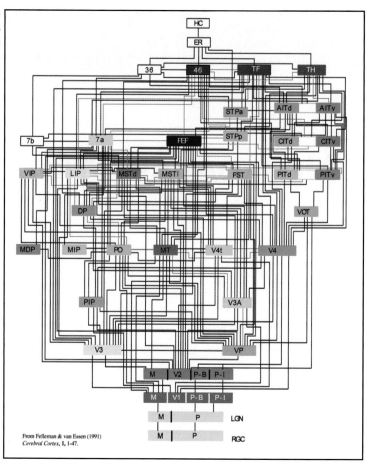

From Felleman & van Essen (1991)
Cerebral Cortex, **1,** 1-47.

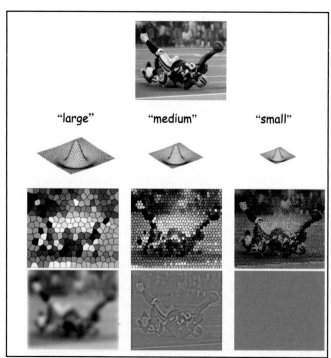

Figure 2. A demonstration showing how vision is dependent on the summation of different levels of contrast perception. (Images and arrangement courtesy Randolph Blake.)

trast) over relatively broad areas of space whereas others are representing light distributions within relatively small areas of space. Neuroscientists characterize these different ganglion cells as registering image information at different spatial scales, where scale is roughly synonymous with size.

The concept of spatial scale is illustrated in Figure 2, where we see a visual scene—a football player attempting to make a difficult catch—portrayed at 3 different spatial scales (governed by the sizes of the receptive fields of 3 hypothetical ganglion cells). In fact, spatial information is represented at more than just 3 scales, but this simplified picture nonetheless portrays how a complex visual image can be construed as multiple neural images represented simultaneously at different scales.

Note that the broadest spatial scale represents what we would term a blurred depiction of the scene and the finest spatial scale portrays just the outline-like details in the scene. No single spatial scale provides all the information needed for good object recognition; that requires collating information across spatial scales, which in turn means combining information contained in the different ganglion cells. We are not perceptually aware of these neural operations underlying multiscale representation: we cannot visually sort out the different levels of spatial scale comprising a scene. But the RGC can, and do, sort out those spatial scales and convey that multiplexed pattern of data to the brain via the 1 million ganglion cell axons comprising the optic nerve. The brain ordinarily receives 2 highly correlated streams of data from the 2 optic nerves; these signals are correlated because the 2 eyes are

the approximately 1 million retinal ganglion cells (RGCs) within each eye, some are registering light distributions (con-

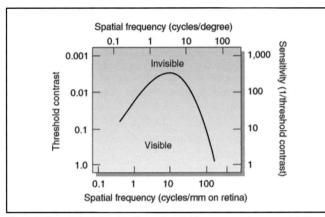

Figure 3. A graph depicting the effects of spatial frequency on the range of visible and invisible light at differing levels of sensitivity. (Courtesy Randolph Blake.)

viewing the same objects from slightly different perspectives.

Turning to the next stage shown in Figure 1, we encounter the lateral geniculate nucleus (LGN), a layered structure within the subcortical thalamus that contains roughly the same number of neurons as the retina. The LGN, besides preserving the spatial scale information conveyed by the RGCs, is also the first stage where information from the 2 eyes comes in very close proximity within the LGN's adjacent layers. Thus within the LGN, neural activity evoked by the stimulation of one eye can impact the neural activity evoked by stimulation of the other eye. These between-layer interactions can play an important role in setting the balance of influence exerted by the 2 eyes on visual perception.

From the LGN, visual information is channeled to the primary visual cortex, labeled V1 in the diagram in Figure 1. Located in the very back of the brain within the occipital lobe, V1 is a large brain area that comprises an estimated 1 billion neurons. This is a remarkably large number in relation to the 1 million RGCs from each eye feeding V1 via the LGN. Obviously, the multiplexed information contained in the RGCs is being demultiplexed within V1; in other words, signals from individual ganglion cells are feeding multiple neurons in V1. Neurons in V1, like their retinal counterparts, are responsive to contrasts within the visual image conveyed at different spatial scales. In addition to this, V1 neurons also signal the orientation of the contours and edges portrayed by those image contrasts. In effect, the one billion V1 neurons provide a complete description of the locations of contours located throughout the visible visual field, with those descriptions portrayed at multiple spatial scales. We can begin to understand why V1 contains so many neurons: these neurons must be capable of representing the countless different images of objects we encounter in our complex visual environments.

From area V1, these neural image descriptions are channeled to multiple visual areas within the hierarchy shown in Figure 1, consisting of an estimated 30 distinct brain areas each specialized for analysis of a particular aspect of visual processing. Within Figure 1 the flow of information within the visual areas is designated by the connecting black lines, and for every visual area connected with another there are reciprocal feedforward and feedback connections.

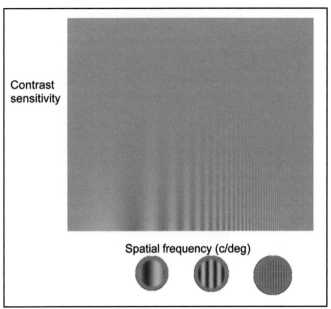

Figure 4. A graph demonstrating contrast sensitivity over a range of spatial frequencies. As spatial frequency increases, the bands alternate more quickly. Maximum perceived contrast sensitivity occurs in the medium range spatial frequency bands. (Courtesy Randolph Blake.)

This complex diagram begins to articulate the absolute processing power of the visual cortex in terms of its image processing capabilities. It is courtesy of this complexity that we are able to effortlessly and automatically recognize objects within our environment: this network allows us to drive an automobile, to read text, to discern the ripeness of fruit, to pick out the clothes to be worn that day, to recognize the face of a loved one, or to discern the angry expression of a stranger. But for this network to work efficiently, these visual areas must have at their disposal high-quality data provided by the RGCs. Optical technologies that prohibit or alter information in the early stages of neural transmission can seriously limit neural image processing, which brings us back to the image characteristics of IOLs.

To appreciate the information ordinarily available to human vision, we need to consider our sensitivity to contrast patterns depicted at different spatial frequencies. Vision scientists have measured the contrast sensitivity of human vision by asking people to adjust the contrast of oriented contours of different sizes (different spatial frequencies) until those contours are barely visible. Figure 3 shows how these contrast sensitivity measures vary with spatial frequency, and Figure 4 allows you to see the consequences of your own contrast sensitivity.

In these figures, spatial frequency (a measurement quantifying the regular alternation of contrasting bands of lightness and darkness) increases from relatively few cycles per degree of visual angle to many cycles per degree of visual angle. Notice that contrast sensitivity increases up to an intermediate value after which sensitivity steadily decreases to zero as the bands of lightness and darkness become too thin to be resolved. What these figures do not convey is that your perception of the different spatial frequencies is registered by neurons responsive to these different sized contours; looking at different regions of Figure 4 activates different neurons responsive to these different spatial frequencies.

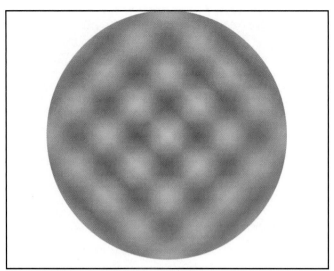

Figure 5. An image that may trigger monocular suppression. (Reprinted with permission from Blake and Logothetis, 2002.)

Armed with this overview of neural processing of spatial forms and contrast, we are now prepared to consider the effects of different IOLs on contrast sensitivity.

Why Multifocals Fail to Produce Optimum Contrast Sensitivity

IOLs can significantly affect contrast sensitivity. Monofocal IOLs can provide excellent near, intermediate, and distance vision when implanted in conjunction with the monovision technique. Monofocal IOLs are superior to multifocal IOLs in that they do not suffer from a high proportion of glare, halo, and lowered contrast sensitivity, all of which can be problems with multifocal IOLs.[1-4] It can be difficult to perceive sharp contrasts with multifocal lenses over a wide range of light conditions. The following 2 sections will clarify why we believe monofocal IOLs with monovision produce superior gains as compared to multifocal IOLs; our thinking is guided by some of the neuroscience concepts outlined earlier.

Multifocal IOLs employ one of several different techniques to divide the artificial lens into different zones intended to provide simultaneous distance, intermediate, and near vision to each eye.[6] These lenses produce multiple overlapping images each refracted to produce clear vision for different viewing distances. In principle, the combined optical image contains image information appropriate for viewing objects at the desired distance (eg, close-up focus for words on a page versus distance focus for a pedestrian crossing an intersection several car lengths ahead of a driver). However, the challenge with multifocal IOLs is that this mixture of images requires the brain to deal with spatial frequency components associated with the out of focus objects located at distances other than the currently desired viewing distance. Because these multiple image components appear superimposed within a single eye's image, the brain has no effective way to segregate the desired from the undesired components. Consequently, these conflicting signals are effectively blended in a way that reduces image contrast and compromises contour visibility. With diffractive

IOLs, up to half of contrast in the image can be defocused by 3.50 D depending on pupil size.[7] This defocused, nonregarded image still activates RGCs, thereby creating unwanted "noise" incorporated into the neural signals transmitted from those RGCs to the visual cortex. With refractive IOLs the same degradation occurs for all but the smallest optical zone whereby only one focal distance is refracted. In the ReZoom IOL (Advanced Medical Optics, Santa Ana, CA), this monofocality happens at the 2.3 pupil diameter at distance.

How does the visual system react to the distorted images resulting from multifocal IOLs? One possible reaction is to reduce the effective contrast of all image components owing to the neural process called monocular suppression.[8-10] This type of suppression refers to the reduced neural responsiveness of visual neurons when they are stimulated simultaneously by their preferred visual stimulus and a nonpreferred stimulus. In effect, the neuron reduces its contrast gain in response to the added, but nonpreferred, visual signals, effectively reducing the neuron's contrast sensitivity. This is ordinarily an adaptive function that operates under ordinary viewing conditions where multiple images are not superimposed. Figure 5 shows an example of an image that is thought by some to engage monocular suppression and produce fluctuations in visibility.[11] While viewing this figure, notice how the 2 superimposed features appear to wax and wane in visibility, as if the neural signals associated with one and then the other are rising and falling in strength. The picture itself remains unchanged; however, the fluctuations in apparent clarity of the 2 images occur because of neural events in your visual system.

Monocular suppression can be likened to the visual effect that can occur within multifocal IOLs. In these IOLs, near, intermediate, and distance visual information is presented to both eyes simultaneously. Each eye must individually suppress extraneous visual information in order to promote clarity of vision. We believe that the suppression within multifocal IOLs may stem from the same neural processes thought to underlie monocular suppression. Thus, as contrast sensitivity is reduced, patients experience reduced ability to see objects clearly under low contrast conditions. This monocular suppression could begin in the retina, continue through the LGN, and build up to full strength in the visual cortex.[8] According to this view, the quality of visual information is stifled at the entry point of the neural pathways, compromising the information reaching higher areas within the visual hierarchy (see Figure 1). This occurs because our visual system is not designed to distinguish overlapping images of confusing spatial frequencies simultaneously.[9,10]

To reiterate, monocular suppression means that significantly stronger contrast would be needed within the retinal image for that image to evoke the same level of responses within neurons subjected to monocular suppression. Because the object relative to its background does not itself produce an increase in image contrast, contrast sensitivity will inevitably be compromised owing to monocular suppression; this is an inevitable, undesirable consequence of multifocal IOLs. For inherently high contrast objects such as black letters appearing on a white page, the loss in effective image contrast may be minimal, but for many natural scenes this loss in contrast response could be noticeable. Figure 6 provides a simulation of one such situation. The picture on the left represents what

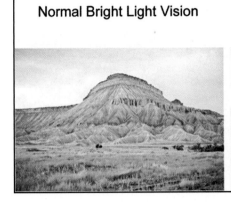
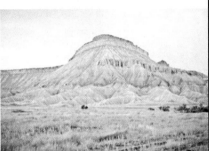

Normal Bright Light Vision   Bright Light with Multifocal IOL

Figure 6. Demonstration of the contrast that is lost with a multifocal IOL in bright light conditions inducing "waxy vision." The image on the left is normal illumination.

one might see when viewing through the eye's natural optics in bright light conditions; the picture on the right depicts the contrast sensitivity lost in bright light conditions with multifocal IOLs. Contrast orientation, when the edges are more closely related in contrast, challenges the suppression of the out of focus, low spatial frequencies. This then results in "bleed" over into the properly mixed low, mid, and high spatial frequencies. As such, the edges and textures are blurred under the higher luminance simulation.

There could also be a secondary effect of the image components associated with the temporarily undesired viewing distance, as these components are not selectively suppressed from the image. If both eyes are outfitted with multifocal IOLs, the effective contrast of these components could be boosted owing to binocular contrast summation.[12] The neural consequence of this could be stronger than desired contrast responses that accentuate lower spatial frequency components in the image. The perceptual consequence could be distortions in the appearance of objects, distortions that may be what patients describe as "waxy vision" and haloes.

Why Monofocals With Monovision Preserve Contrast Sensitivity and Promote Spectacle Independence

In contrast to the potentially degraded visual quality produced by multifocal IOLs, we believe that monofocal IOLs with monovision may preserve the full neural integrity of high contrast images. Applying monovision with the aid of monofocal IOLs can induce binocular fusion and promote clear contrast vision, thereby producing desired clinical outcomes.[13,14] The following reasoning supports these suppositions.

Binocular fusion occurs when the retinal images formed in the 2 eyes are sufficiently similar to allow the brain to establish interocular correspondence. The brain can tolerate small differences in the spatial frequency content of the images in the 2 eyes without disruption to binocular fusion. Moreover, binocular fusion can occur even when left and right eye images differ in contrast. Under these conditions, the brain averages the 2 overall contrast levels to produce an intermediate perceived contrast. When the contrast differences between the eyes is large, the eye exposed to the higher contrast dominates

perception while the contribution from the eye receiving the weaker contrast is suppressed from vision.[13,14] Thus, at the focal point of the monofocal IOL, the visual cortex has the complete, nondistorted signal of the regarded eye and can complement the image from the alternate eye depending on the spatial frequency compatibility of the alternate eye.

However, left- and right-eye images that differ greatly in spatial frequency and/or orientation cannot be combined by the brain; in such cases, binocular fusion gives way to interocular suppression.[15,16] In this situation, the temporarily dominant eye suppresses the contrast gain of the other eye, the result being that the dominant eye has the same contrast sensitivity as if monocular viewing was occurring. In our experience in the clinic, binocular fusion is maintained so long as the refractive difference between the 2 eyes does not exceed 1.5 D; this value promotes sufficient overlap in spatial frequency content in the 2 eyes to support binocular fusion. Using monofocal IOLs that differ by greater amounts than this tends to undermine binocular fusion and interfere with binocular depth perception.

The pairs of images in Figures 7A, 7B, and 7C illustrate the points just made. These pairs of images were created to be viewed by crossing the eyes, so that the left eye views the right-hand image and vice versa. In Figure 7A, the left eye and right eye images simulate what one would experience when viewing a natural scene through lenses differing in refractive power by approximately 1 D. You can see the visual differences between the images because the spatial frequency content of the 2 images is not identical. The clearer image contains high spatial frequency information not contained in the other, less clear image. However, when viewed dichoptically (one image to each eye) the 2 images blend into a single binocular impression that is stable and clear. This occurs because the spatial frequency information in the "blurred" image is also contained in the "clear" image and there is sufficient overlap in those spatial frequencies to promote binocular combination.

In Figure 7B, the spatial frequency content in the 2 views differs by an amount corresponding to a refractive difference between the 2 eyes of about 2.5 D. Consequently, the region of overlap in spatial frequency content is reduced in the 2 images, creating a more challenging matching problem for the brain and compromising binocular fusion. Finally, Figure 7C illustrates what happens when the 2 eyes receive radically different views in which spatial frequency, color, and orientation information is uncorrelated. Here binocular fusion is impossible. Fortunately, neither monofocal nor multifocal

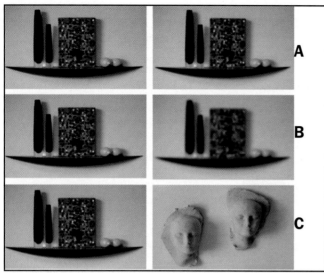

Figure 7. (A) When viewed with crossed eyes, these two pictures simulate the effects of a 1 D difference between the eyes (images courtesy Randolph Blake). (B) When viewed with crossed eyes, these two figures demonstrate the effects of a 2.5 D difference between the eyes. (C) When viewed with crossed eyes, these two figures demonstrate the effects of two completely disparate images presented to the eyes, making binocular fusion impossible (all images in Figure 7 courtesy Randolph Blake).

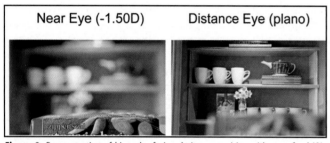

Figure 8. Demonstration of binocular fusion during monovision with monofocal IOLs (cross eyes to experience).

IOLs produce the confusing situation simulated in Figure 7c. However, this confusion can occur when a patient has eye misalignment causing the foveae of the two eyes to view different objects within of the visual field. As such, patients with strabismus are guarded candidates for monovision or multifocal IOLs. We usually try and correct these patients' eyes to the same dioptric power.

In summary, vision provided by a monofocal IOL is supported by the full range of spatial frequencies associated with viewing at a given distance. In the case of bilateral, monofocal IOLs, one eye can be provided with a lens whose dioptric power is appropriate for near vision while the other eye's lens is tailored for distance vision. In practice, this can be accomplished with a pair of IOLs that differ by no more than 1.5 D of refractive power (this is possible because the depth of field associated with the 2 IOLs expands their ranges of imaged spatial frequencies). Even for spatial frequencies contained only in one eye's image, this information can be attenuated within the visual cortex, thereby effectively lowering the contrast amplitude of those unmatched spatial frequencies.[14] This reduced contrast gain permits the partner eye to enjoy full contrast sensitivity and good visual acuity.[13] For these reasons,

2 Multifocal IOLs

Figure 9. Demonstration of binocular fusion with multifocal IOLs (cross eyes to experience).

we believe monofocal IOLs promote superior contrast sensitivity owing to the ability of the brain to fully utilize natural discriminatory channels within the visual cortex and maximize the amount of information available for object and grouping perception.[17] Unlike multifocal IOLs, monofocal IOLs with the monovision technique can generate clearer images with minimal distortion for objects appearing at all viewing distances. The visual cortex—and the specialized cortical areas within higher stages of the visual hierarchy—receives visual data more nearly matching that experienced prior to development of cataracts.

Figures 8 and 9 provide a visual demonstration of why we think the monofocal approach is superior to multifocal IOLs. Figure 8 simulates 2 images of a group of household objects located at different distances from the eye. The left image simulates the image quality experienced by the near eye (−1.50 D) and the right image simulates the quality experienced by the more distant eye (plano). Compare this pair of pictures to the ones shown in Figure 9, which depicts an example of the perceived images of 2 eyes with multifocal IOLs. In this latter pair of pictures, both the near and far images are in focus, yet both suffer reductions in image contrast.

By crossing your eyes to view each pair of images, you can experience the binocular consequence produced by these 2 distinct lens types. Notice that with the monofocal simulation, the contrasts of the objects experienced with binocular viewing of the visual scene are as clear as those associated with monocular viewing of that scene. There is no compromise in contrast sensitivity, and the binocular view is stable and clear. On the other hand, when the right and the left eye with multifocal IOLs view this scene, the images are in focus at all distances but the contrasts of those objects are reduced. This reduced contrast sensitivity results from the inevitable compromise in image contrast produced by the multiple optical zones with different focal lengths. Objects located at the correct viewing distance for one of the zones results in a retinal image that is the sum of an in-focus image plus all the out-of-focus images for the other zones. No matter what the viewing distance, these out-of-focus images will always attenuate the overall image quality.

In our view, this represents the crucial reason why monovision trumps multifocal vision. The brain is able to use its normal contrast gain control mechanisms while adjusting sensitivity to optimize the spatial frequency content of the best focused image. If necessary, the brain will also attenuate the weaker spatial frequency components in the nondominant eye's view. But with multifocal IOLs, the selective attenuation of contrast information associated with particular spatial frequencies also drags down the effective contrast of the spatial frequencies associated with the objects of regard. Monocular suppression, in other words, impairs contrast sensitivity in the case of multifocal IOLs but not monofocal IOLs.

Conclusion

We have tried to describe the neurophysiological consequences associated with different solutions commonly utilized to achieve spectacle independence with IOLs. We argue that monovision, in conjunction with an aspheric monofocal IOL, leverages the power of the visual nervous system to provide high-quality image contrasts of objects viewed at near, intermediate, and far distances. When lower amounts of focal distance separation are employed within IOLs in the 2 eyes, binocular fusion and stereopsis can be supported at all distances. The patient is more likely to experience a full range of near to far continuous vision. In contrast, multifocal IOLs produce optical images that are degraded by the out-of-focus optical zones. These degraded images cannot then be adequately demodulated by the visual nervous system. Instead, contrast gain control is compromised, as is the quality of the signals channeled to higher visual areas associated with object recognition. We acknowledge that parts of this neurophysiologically grounded account of IOLs remain to be confirmed, but we hope that future research guided by neurophysiology will produce more principled, successful decisions about compensatory optical prosthetics employed following cataract surgery.

Acknowledgment

We acknowledge the assistance and insight into the neurocognitive processes involved and outlined in this chapter to Dr. Randolph Blake, professor of psychology and founding member of the Vanderbilt Vision Research Center.

References

1. Chiam PJ, Chan JH, Aggarwal RK, et al. ReSTOR intraocular lens implantation in cataract surgery: quality of vision. *J Cataract Refract Surg.* 2006;32:1459-1463.

2. Souza CE, Muccioli C, Soriano ES, et al. Visual performance of AcrySof ReSTOR apodized diffractive IOL: a prospective comparative trial. *Am J Ophthalmol.* 2006;141:827-832.

3. Rocha KM, Chalita MR, Souza CE, et al. Postoperative wavefront analysis and contrast sensitivity of a multifocal apodized diffractive IOL (ReSTOR) and three monofocal IOLs. *J Refract Surg.* 2005;21: S808-S812.

4. Javitt JC, Steinert RF. Cataract extraction with multifocal intraocular lens implantation: a multinational clinical trial evaluation clinical, functional, and quality-of-life outcomes. *Ophthalmology.* 2000;107:2040-2048.

5. Felleman DJ, Van Essen DC. Distributed hierarchical processing in the primate cerebral cortex. *Cereb Cortex.* 1991;1:1-47.

6. Bellucci R. Multifocal intraocular lenses. *Curr Opin Ophthalmol.* 2005;16:33-37.

7. Claoue C, Parmar D. Multifocal intraocular lenses. *Dev Ophthalmol.* 2002;34:217-237.

8. Tse PU, Martinez-Conde S, Schlegel AA, Macknik SL. Visibility, visual awareness, and visual masking of simple unattended targets are confined to areas in the occipital cortex beyond human V1/V2. *Proc Nat Acad Sci USA.* 2005;102:17178-17183.

9. Sengpiel F, Baddeley RJ, Freeman TCB, Harrad R, Blakemore C. Different mechanisms underlie three inhibitory phenomena in cat area 17. *Vision Res.* 1998;38:2067-2080.

10. Sengpiel F, Vorobyov V. Intracortical origins of interocular suppression in the visual cortex. *J Neurosci.* 2005;25:6394-6400.

11. Blake R, Logothetis NK. Visual competition. *Nat Rev Neurosci.* 2002;3:13-21.

12. Rose D, Blake R, Halpern DL. Disparity range for binocular suppression. *Invest Ophthalmol Vis Sci.* 1988;29:283-290.

13. Schor C, Heckmann T. Interocular differences in contrast and spatial frequency: effects on stereopsis and fusion. *Vision Res.* 1989;29:837-847.

14. Abadi R. Induction masking—a study of some inhibitory interactions during dichoptic viewing. *Vision Res.* 1967;16:269-275.

15. Schor C, Heckmann T, Tyler CW. Binocular fusion limits are independent of contrast, luminance gradient and component phases. *Vision Res.* 1989;29:821-835.

16. Liu L, Tyler CW, Schor CM. Failure of rivalry at low contrast: evidence of a suprathreshold binocular summation process. *Vision Res.* 1992;32:1471-1479.

17. Roelfsema PR. Cortical algorithms for perceptual grouping. *Annu Rev Neurosci.* 2006;29:203-227.

CHAPTER 79

NEUROADAPTATION AND MULTIFOCAL IOLS

Robert M. Kershner, MD, MS, FACS

Neuroadaptation is the process by which the brain modifies its sensory input, in response to touch, heat, cold, pain, sight, sounds, or smell. Nervous system adaptation enables us to cope with a constantly changing environment.

The adult nervous system is remarkably plastic. Numerous studies have shed light on the molecular basis for this fascinating process from the regulation of stem cell function to how neurotransmitters influence behaviors. In the adult, neurogenesis, including adaptive roles in learning and memory, changing environments, depression and moods, and responses to injury including neuropathic pain, are all linked to the hippocampal region of the brain. The hippocampus is responsible for consolidation of memory, emotion, navigation, and of importance to ophthalmologists, spatial orientation. Research has revealed an intimate relationship in this area between neuroadaptive mechanisms and addictive behavior.

Our need to understand the underlying mechanisms of neuroadaptation, as it relates to visual function, has once again taken center stage. It has become a poignant topic of conversation between physicians who must treat patients who, as a result of an alteration in their visual system, are struggling to adapt. Patients who undergo a modification in the visual system, whether induced by the wearing of a new pair of eyeglasses or bifocals, or by having undergone a corneal ablative procedure or lens implantation with the novel optics of multifocal intraocular lenses (IOLs),[1] will undoubtedly be challenged by the newly created perceptive change. How quickly and how well they adapt to this will ultimately determine whether they become evangelistic believers in this new technology, or whether they will disparage it and their physicians for the rest of their lives. Although many patients adapt quickly and successfully to a surgical procedure, some adapt slowly, if at all. As ophthalmologists, we can be stymied by the dissatisfaction of an unhappy patient, especially in the face of a successful visual outcome from a surgical procedure. What factors are at play that can allow one individual to embrace refractive revision and another to reject it? The answer to these questions remains within the realm of this rich and elusive process called neuroadaptation.

Neuroadaptation can occur within the visual system in response to either a monocular or binocular visual disturbance. Visual adaptation depends to a great extent on visual awareness. In the case of a monocular visual disturbance, the brain learns to compensate by altering its perception. It has been shown that even in cases where a clear image is focused onto the retina, that neuroadaptation may still be required if there are inherent optical aberrations within the visual system that the brain cannot accept.[2] Given time, the mind applies its negating effect to the undesirable pattern. Should the aberrations be eliminated (as in wave-front enhanced, custom, excimer-laser ablation), then the brain will, at least for a period of time, apply the negating effect that it has previously learned to this new clearer image, thus degrading it. Ultimately, if age and time work in the patient's favor, then the final image quality becomes acceptable.[3,4] Both patient and physician must be cognizant of the nuances of this process. It is not acceptable to simply tell a patient to "give it some time."

To better understand this phenomenon of neuroadaptation, let us use *meridional aniseikonia* as an example. Meridional aniseikonia is a binocular phenomenon that occurs when there is a difference in the astigmatic refractive error between the 2 eyes. It can occur in either eye and can result in amblyopia if it appears early in life. Strabismic amblyopes who do not have significant astigmatism often exhibit a decrease in contrast sensitivity measurements when tested with vertical rather than with horizontal gratings. This is believed to be the result of horizontal image displacement in the deviating eye. The more ametropic meridian in highly astigmatic individuals can be associated with a marked reduction in acuity despite optical correction. What is going on? A defocused image in one meridian can actually prevent the establishment of normal neural pathways from the eye to the occipital cortex. What happens if a previously nonexistent astigmatic error is inadvertently introduced? The postoperative patient, with an increase in magnitude or change in direction of an astigmatic refractive error, must adapt to the visual perceptive change. First, the brain becomes confused with the new imagery. The conflict must be resolved if the patient is to accept the refractive change. The ability of an individual to resolve such conflict may rest more with his or her chronological age than with the degree or magnitude of the refractive error. What we know is that the "plasticity" of this neuroadaptive process is a function of age. The younger the patient is, the more likely he or she is to accept this newfound perceptive alteration. Time in this case, is not on our side. If the patient is fortunate, then the neuroadaptive process will take over and the final image quality will be perceived as satisfactory. This is precisely how, when confronted with the first pair of bifocal glasses that cause an intolerable blurring at first, the new presbyope develops a level of acceptable visual function within a matter of days. Remember when we used to frequently hear from our patients their postoperative complaint of *erythropsia* prior to the advent of ultraviolet-blocking IOLs? By the second postoperative visit, the complaint was gone, when obviously the altered visual perception was still present. The brain had adapted.

Stereopsis, or 3D vision, provides an enhanced perception of depth; it is the ability of the binocular optical system to merge 2 images, one from each of the slightly disparate parallax points of view from each eye. When we as surgeons intentionally disrupt the "one-eye, one-image" perception that is required for successful merging of the images from 2 eyes, we can create a perceptive paradox that the brain simply cannot undo. An example of this chicanery is the newly embraced portfolio of multifocal IOLs. By requiring the simultaneous perception of multiple images, in focus only at the differing focal lengths created by these optical marvels, we undermine the ability of the optical system to adapt.

Some can ignore the perceptive annoyances, others cannot, and the success of these IOLs depends entirely on the brain's ability to act on the disturbance.

The study of neuroadaptation is based primarily in psychophysics. Two extensively studied phenomena are known as *binocular rivalry* and *visual crowding*.[5,6] These visual phenomena are capable of erasing visual stimuli from conscious awareness. Unlike factors that lead to visual processing early in the system, processing of these phenomena occurs within the primary visual cortex (V1) and the middle-temporal visual areas. Brain imaging and EEG studies have demonstrated that suppression of unwanted images during retinal rivalry reduces the visual stimuli perceived in the monocular regions of V1 and keeps them from conscious awareness. Randolph Blake and colleagues at the Department of Psychology of the Vanderbilt Vision Research Center at Vanderbilt University have extensively researched this area and suggest that suppression of vision rivalry and crowding involves a *reduction* of neural activity, and not an increase or elimination of it.

Just how the brain recruits the neurons to make this happen is a scientific fascination in itself. Just as every processing point along the visual pathway contributes to the final, clearly perceived optical image, an interruption in the smooth flow of information can become problematic. Until the image signal hits the sixth-order neurons, both images are monocular. It is here where ocular dominance and retinal rivalry exists. From the lateral geniculate bodies, the images begin to fuse. If we flood these centers with retinal signals from multiple images, then the deep centers of the brain that need to make sense of the chaos begin to fail. Neural adaptation associated with both retinal rivalry and image crowding occur at the earliest stages of visual processing. The fact that neuroadaptation to this visual disparity can happen at all is testimony to the amazing plasticity of the system. For it to occur over a period of weeks to months and even years signifies that complex neurogenesis is at work. It takes time to make new neural connections or suppress old ones.

Neuroadaptation begins at the beginning of life and remains an encompassing, ongoing phenomenon, unless something intervenes to disrupt it.[7] When light first strikes a baby's retina at birth, the startled look in the baby's opened eyes reflects a dramatic flood of information to the occipital cortex. The hardware is there, but the software has not yet been developed. The earliest images that reach the occipital cortex will be inverted. Neuroadaptation flips them cortically so that up is down and down is up. The brain continues to process visual stimuli throughout life and make sense of the images the retina receives. When reading, our eyes move in spurts across the page. To meld the saccadic movement of our eyes into a smooth perception of letters and words requires higher cortical processing. The brain adapts to the information from these images and combines them across glances.[8] When an individual with a vertical hemianopia is presented with a triangle or a square, he or she perceives the images as a rectangle and a spear. The brain has filled in the blanks. If, during the course of our lives, we lose the ability to modulate visual information, then retraining the brain to perceive visual stimuli differently is required. That is precisely what is done for vision rehabilitation in cases of injury or disease, such as in stroke patients and those with age-related macular degeneration. Permanent damage to the processing areas in the primary visual cortex may unfortunately render neuroadaptation useless.

What should our patients expect when we, as surgeons, modify a lifetime of visual perception with one quick stroke of a diamond blade or a laser beam? It is certainly intriguing to postulate a pivotal role for the neuroadaptive mechanisms, which can act as friend or foe, in predicting which patients will accept visual perceptive change and which will not. The psychological implications of neuroadaptation, which have been well studied in addictive behaviors such as drug dependence and excessive gambling tendencies, may provide some insight. If the same regions of the brain are involved, and they are, can there be a potential link between addictive personalities and failure to accept and adapt to refractive change? Should we be avoiding risk-taking personalities as poor candidates for cataract and refractive surgery? Certainly more work is needed in this area. What is certain, however, is that our assessment of our patients behavioral, social, and psychological needs are at least as important as the analysis of their A-scans and wavefront maps.

References

1. Javitt JC, Steinert RF. Cataract extraction with multifocal intraocular lens implantation: a multinational clinical trial evaluating clinical, functional, and quality-of-life outcomes. *Ophthalmology*. 2000; 107(11):2040-2048.

2. Artal P, Guirao A, Berrio E, Williams DR. Compensation of corneal aberrations by the internal optics in the human eye. *J Vis.* 2001;1:1-8.

3. Webster MA, Georgeson MA, Webster SM. Neural adjustments to image blur. *Nat Neurosci.* 2002;5:839-849.

4. Artal P, Chen L, Fernández EJ, et al. Neural compensation for the eye's optical aberrations. *J Vis.* 2004;4:281-287.

5. Kim CY, Blake R. Psychophysical strategies for rendering the normally visible "invisible". *Trends Cognit Sci.* 2005;9:381-388.

6. Tong F, Engel SA. Interocular rivalry revealed in the human cortical blind-spot representation. *Nature.* 2001;411:195-199.

7. Blake R, Tadin D, Sobel KV, et al. Strength of early visual adaptation depends on visual awareness. *Proc Natl Acad Sci USA.* 2006; 103(12):4783-4788.

8. Melcher, D. Predictive transfer of visual adaptation before saccadic eye movements [Abstract]. *J Vis.* 2007;7(9):1003, 1003a.

CHAPTER 80

NEUROADAPTATION AND MULTIFOCAL IOLS

Pablo Artal

The visual system in normal eyes provides a clear image of the objects in the scene despite the aberrations caused by the eye's optics.[1,2] It is well known that every eye is affected by specific optical aberrations that produce a particular light pattern in the retina of an object point; the image caused by the aberrations is represented by the point-spread function (PSF). If the brain has adjusted for the individual eye's optical aberrations, vision should be clearest when looking through the familiar aberrations of that eye. Replacing these with different and unfamiliar optical aberrations may actually cause the vision to be "worse." If this is true, this has important implications for any surgical procedure that modifies the eye's optical properties and aberrations.

Adaptation and plasticity in the visual system are known to play major roles in many important visual tasks. For centuries, clinicians have recognized the benefit of neural adaptation. Many patients' complaints disappear without any apparent reason simply by waiting long enough. Perhaps one of the most dramatic examples of adaptation in the visual system was an experiment performed in the 1950s. Several subjects were fitted with goggles having prisms that inverted the image. Initially, the subject saw the visual scene inverted; however after a period of anywhere from a few days to a few weeks the subjects found that the image of the world became spontaneously normal again. This was despite the fact that the actual image projected onto the retina remained inverted. The "surprise" for the subject was when the goggles were removed and the world again became inverted! The brain would again correctly orient the image after a few days to weeks without the prism. I confess that I am not sure I would have volunteered to be a subject in this simple, but "scary" experiment.

There are many more common examples of how the visual system adapts. The mechanisms of blur adaptation,[3] the adaptation to color perception, and the adaptation to distortions in the visual field are an important part of many patients' adjustment to their treatment. In clinical practice, patients commonly adapt to progressive addition lenses (PALs). Initially, most patients notice the evident distortions in the retinal image caused by the optical surfaces in the PALs.[4] However, these problems tend to disappear after some time as patients adapt. When PALs were first introduced, it was common for lens companies to guarantee the adaptation by promising to replace any PAL with a standard bifocal if the patient could not adapt. The reported success rate with the first generation of PALs was over 90%.

Following this reasoning, we were interested in demonstrating if the individual visual system was also particularly adapted to its own unique optical aberrations. To do this, we performed an experiment in collaboration with Prof. David Williams at the University of Rochester using adaptive optics.[5] This technology has proved quite useful for obtaining high-resolution retinal images. Another important research application of adaptive optics, however, is the ability to produce controlled aberration patterns in the eye of a subject. This is what we called an adaptive optics visual simulator.[6] This permitted us to determine if each individual visual system is adapted to the unique optical aberrations of its own eye. We performed a controlled experiment of subjective blur matching with the normal and rotated aberrations. The adaptive optics system consisted of a real time wavefront sensor[7] to measure the eye's aberrations and a deformable mirror to modify the aberrations. A visual channel presented the stimulus to the subject. By using this instrument (see reference 5 for additional technical details), we were able to rotate the aberrations (and the PSFs) of the subject while maintaining the same magnitude of the aberration. Figure 1 shows an example of this procedure. Subjects were asked to view a binary noise stimulus through the system with their own aberrations or with a rotated version of their aberrations. The stimulus was seen alternatively for 500 msec with both the normal and the rotated PSF. The subject's task was to adjust the magnitude of the aberrations to match the subjective blur of the stimulus to that seen when the wave aberration was in the normal orientation. In all subjects tested, the wavefront error of the rotated wave aberration required to match the blur with the normal wave aberration was found to be less than in the normally oriented aberration

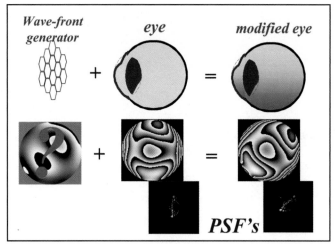

Figure 1. Schematic example of how aberrations and the PSF are rotated using adaptive optics.

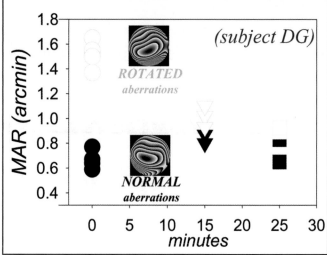

Figure 3. Visual acuity (expressed in MAR) measured for the normal aberrations (dark circles) and rotated aberrations (white circles) as a function of adaptation time for the rotated aberrations.

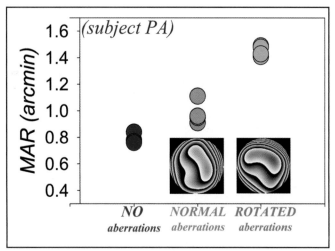

Figure 2. Visual acuity (expressed in MAR) measured in the right eye of the author for corrected aberrations (brown), normal aberrations (orange), and rotated aberrations (green).

case. This indicates that the subjective blur for the stimulus increased significantly when the PSF was rotated. We also measured visual acuity for different aberration profiles. Figure 2 shows visual acuity in one subject (the author) expressed as minimum angle of resolution in minutes of arc without any aberration, with the normal aberrations, and with the rotated aberrations. The performance was lowest with the rotated version of the aberrations.

More recently, the same instrument was used to evaluate how neural adaptation effect might affect the best subjective image quality.[8] In all tested subjects, the best subjective visual quality occurred when some small amount of higher-order aberrations were left uncorrected. This result may have some practical implications for any type of customized vision correction.

A very important issue relating to neural adaptation is the temporal characteristics of the process. The clinical implications will be very different if the adaptation last seconds, hours, or months. Adaptation to blur or contrast seems to take a few seconds, while for other effects it may take minutes

or weeks. We measured high contrast visual acuity with the normal and rotated aberrations after asking the subject to see through the unfamiliar rotated aberrations. After some minutes of adaptation to the abnormal aberrations, visual acuity improved, nearly reaching the level for the normal aberrations (Figure 3).

Although it is obvious that the visual system cannot deal with very large amount of aberrations, it is also important to understand the amount of aberration that is required to induce the adaptation. The impact of the age of the subjects could also be studied in the future.

Aberrations in the eye are dynamic by nature.[9] They change with varying pupil diameter and accommodation during normal viewing. This creates an apparent paradox. If those changes prevent the eye from producing a PSF that is stable over time, how can optimal neural adaptation be achieved? A possible explanation is that the PSF preserves most of its characteristic shape features during normal viewing. We tested this hypothesis by using a real-time Hartmann-Shack wavefront sensor to measure the PSF for a combination of varying pupil diameters (3 to 7 mm) and accommodation (0 to 3 D) that simulate real life. Figure 4 shows a collection of those images for the author's right eye. We computed a parameter, the maximum of the cross-correlation function, which provided information on the shape differences among PSFs. In the subjects tested, despite scale changes, shape features in the PSFs remained stable under most normal conditions. This may allow the brain to achieve a coarse adaptation to an average aberration pattern, which somewhat explains this phenomenon.

Finally, I will elaborate on the possible impact of this adaptation mechanism in different clinical situations. In the area of wavefront-guided customized refractive surgery, this adaptation effect will reduce the immediate benefit of attempts to surgically produce diffraction-limited eyes. This is because if the brain is already adapted to a particular familiar aberration pattern, when this is permanently altered by surgery, the neural compensation mechanism will still be adjusted for the previous aberration pattern. Figure 5 shows a "cartoon-like"

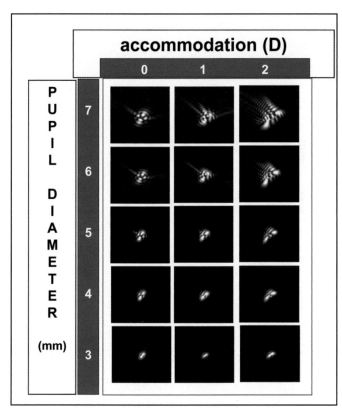

Figure 4. PSFs for the author's right eye measured for different common situations of pupil diameter and accommodation. This series of PSFs reproduces the typical variations of image quality during normal viewing. Despite changes in scale, they seem to keep some shape feature. This could favor a neural adaptation to the overall aberrations.

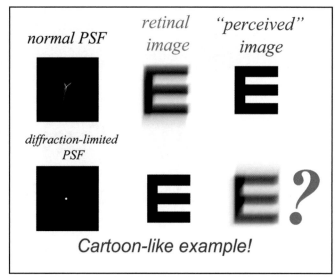

Figure 5. Schematic example of the possible effect of neural adaptation in the retinal images before and after an ideal correction of the aberrations.

simulation of this possible effect. If the brain normally attempts to restore a degraded retinal image, it would also initially degrade a perfect retinal image that has been suddenly produced by refractive surgery. Of course, the clinical relevance of this depends on the time required to reverse the previous compensatory adaptation and for the visual system to readapt to the new induced aberrations.

There is tremendous interest in mixing different multifocal IOLs in each eye to increase the overall depth of focus. This technique is often called mix and match. The role of neural adaptation in this approach is probably very important but related to binocular vision. This is likely a complex scenario in which both monocular aberrations and binocular interactions should be considered. For better clinical understanding of these IOL mixing methods, more research is needed. For instance, a better understanding of binocular performance as a function of individual or binocular aberrations is required. Applying

adaptive optics to binocular vision may help to answer some of these questions. Future experiments in this exciting area of research will help clinicians to ultimately provide patients with superior quality of vision.

References

1. Artal P, Guirao A, Berrio E, Williams DR. Compensation of corneal aberrations by the internal optics in the human eye. *J Vis.* 2001;1:1-8.
2. Artal P, Benito A, Tabernero J. The human eye is an example of robust optical design. *J Vis.* 2006;6(1):1-7.
3. Webster MA, Georgeson MA, Webster SM. Neural adjustments to image blur. *Nature Neuroscience.* 2002;5:839-849.
4. Villegas EA, Artal P. Comparison of aberrations in different types of progressive power lenses. *Ophthalmic Physiol Opt.* 2004;24:419-426.
5. Artal P, Chen L, Fernández EJ, Singer B, Manzanera S, Williams DR. Neural compensation for the eye's optical aberrations. *J Vis.* 2004;4:281-287.
6. Fernández EJ, Manzanera S, Piers P, Artal P. Adaptive optics visual simulator. *J Refract Surg.* 2002;18:S634-S638.
7. Prieto PM, Vargas-Martín F, Goelz S, Artal P. Analysis of the performance of the Hartmann-Shack sensor in the human eye. *J Opt Soc Am A.* 2000;17:1388-1398.
8. Chen L, Artal P, Hartnell DG, Williams DR, Neural compensation for the best aberration correction. *J Vis.* 2007;7:1-9.
9. Hofer H, Artal P, Singer B, Aragón JL, Williams DR. Dynamics of the eye's wave aberration. *J Opt Soc Am A.* 2001;18:497-506.

VISUAL FUNCTION TRAINING FOR MULTIFOCAL PATIENTS

Hakan Kaymak, MD and Ulrich Mester, MD

Multifocal IOLs (MIOLs) are a powerful tool to help patients become less dependent on glasses after cataract surgery and refractive surgery. The latest generation of MIOLs have produced a higher percentage of patients who are independent of glasses after surgery. For this reason, MIOLs are an interesting option for patients considering cataract surgery and refractive surgery.[1,2] MIOLs have been shown to require a significant learning curve in several studies.[1,3,4] We have demonstrated a computer-based visual training method of accelerating this learning process with MIOLs.

MIOLs work by the simultaneous presentation of 2 images. A learning period is required for patients to fully adapt to these simultaneous images with their reduced contrast and decreased edge distinction.[5] Psychophysical experiments have taught us that neural plasticity is present even in adults. Visual learning can lead to faster and more dramatic improvement of performance in perceptual tasks.[6,7] The recognition that these functions improve over time motivated us to develop a method to train the visual system.

"Perceptual learning" of visual tasks is a well-recognized subject in the neurobiological literature. Perceptual learning is defined as any relatively permanent change of perception as a result of experience.[7] One of the tasks employed most often to test perceptual learning is visual hyperacuity. Several hyperacuity tasks such as vernier discriminations have been shown to improve with practice in both adults with normal vision[6,8] and adult amblyopic patients.[9,10] It has been shown that visual acuity could be improved while practicing a very different and functionally more basic task using stimuli different from those used for the acuity tests. Improving the early processing in the visual system resulted in an improvement of all higher levels of processing that depend on the quality of the low-level visual representation.[8] Such a low-level feature of the stimulus could be the orientation discrimination of tilted bars, which we used in our study.[7]

To evaluate our method of visual training, we tested 16 patients who had bilateral phacoemulsification with MIOL implantation both eyes. Eight patients had bilateral AcrySof ReSTOR (Alcon, Fort Worth, TX) IOLs implanted and 8 patients had bilateral Tecnis (Advanced Medical Optics, Santa Ana, CA) MIOLs implanted. All patients received computer-based visual training beginning 6 weeks postoperatively. The functional outcome of the eyes with the ReSTOR MIOL was not significantly different from the eyes with the Tecnis MIOL.

The training is based on the concept of perceptual learning of discrimination line orientations. The training was performed in 6 sessions over 2 weeks on the nondominant eye of each patient. The untrained, fellow eye served as the control. The patients were fully evaluated prior to the training period, immediately after the training period, and 6 months after the training period. We noted a significant improvement in orientation visual acuity (OVA) (Parameter Estimation by Sequential Testing, PEST) after 2 weeks of training. The mean improvement in OVA in the trained eyes was 82% whereas the mean improvement in control eyes was 9% (p < .001). Contrast sensitivity and near vision under different contrast levels also showed a significant benefit of training. The superior function of the trained eyes relative to the untrained eyes persisted after 6 months of follow-up.

The training procedure is based on the orientation discrimination of tilted bars, which are presented on a computer monitor. The patients sat at a fixed distance of 1 m from a Samsung LCD 19" Monitor (1280 × 1024 resolution, 75 hertz) that was controlled by a personal computer.

The test stimuli consisted of thin (1 arc min wide) bright lines, presented on a dark surround. The length of the test stimulus was 50 arc min and presentation time was 500 ms. After a 300 ms pause, the patient was asked to respond to the stimulus by pushing a button. After the response, the next stimulus was presented. The patients had to indicate in a binary, forced-choice test without time pressure whether the stimulus was slightly inclined to the left or to the right for vertical stimuli. The decision was indicated by pushing either the left or right of 2 buttons. The training consisted of 6 sessions

Table 1

PATIENTS' DEMOGRAPHICS

	Tecnis	ReSTOR
Age (years)	69±3	71. ±9
Lens power (diopters)	21.8±1.7	22.3±3.9
Sphere (diopters)	0.2±0.3	0.0±0.1
Cylinder (diopters)	0.3±0.3	0.24±0.3
Spherical equivalent (diopters)	0.0±0.3	-0.1±0.2

Figure 1. OVA for horizontal bars had improved in the trained eyes but not in the untrained eyes, also OVA for horizontal bars showed in the trained eyes no improvement after training end. Means and SDs of 16 eyes. (***= p<0.001; *= p<0.05; n.s.= not significant)

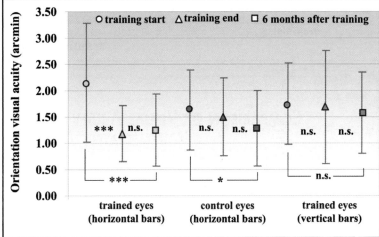

Figure 2. Scatter plot of the relation of individual OVA improvement and pretraining OVA including r value of correlation (Pearson correlation).

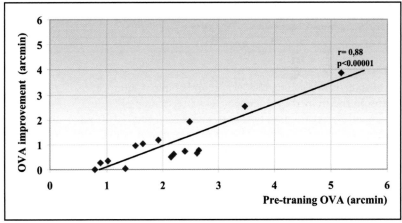

over 2 weeks. A total of 7 sets with 50 stimulus presentations each had to be completed in each session. The mean time of each session was 30 min ± 5 min. There was a maximum of one session per observer per day. Subsequent sessions were completed in no more than 3 subsequent days. The individual OVA was measured in arc min, which defines the minimum angle of the inclined stimulus the patient was able to discriminate, relative to a fully vertical or horizontal line.

All patients completed the training protocol. All eyes of all patients were normal postoperatively. The mean capsulorrhexis size was 5.3 mm with circular overlap of the optic rim. The patient demographics and postoperative refraction are summarized in Table 1.

The functional tests were performed immediately (1 day) after finishing the training program.

They showed a highly significant improvement of OVA for the trained eyes for bars presented in the trained or vertical orientations (p = .001). The fellow eyes showed only a slight, insignificant improvement. We then tested OVA with bars in the nontrained horizontal axis and found only a slight improvement without statistical significance. This situation was nearly unchanged at the 6-month follow-up (Figure 1). We found the eyes with the lowest OVA benefited the most from the training (Figure 2) and the greatest improvement occurred after the first 3 sessions (Figure 3).

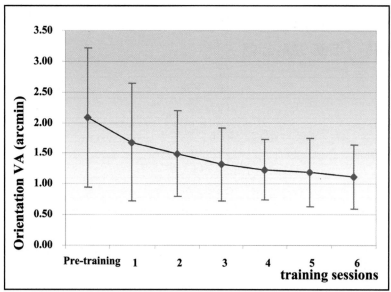

Figure 3. Orientation VA (arcmin) versus number of 6 sessions within 2 weeks. Means and SDs of 16 eyes.

Table 2

COMPARISON OF VISUAL ACUITY BETWEEN TRAINED AND CONTROL EYES IMMEDIATELY AFTER TRAINING END

	Training end		
	Trained eyes (reading letters)	*Control eyes (reading letters)*	*Significance level*
100% contrast Distance VA	50±8	48±8	p=0.06
100% contrast Near VA	65±8	60±6	p<0.05
25% contrast Near VA	44±6	40±5	p=0.07
12.5% contrast Near VA	42±5	39±7	p<0.01

Distance visual acuity (VA) was slightly but not significantly better in the trained eyes immediately after training (Table 2). Six months after training best-corrected visual acuity (BCVA) had improved in both eyes. This improvement was statistically significant (p < .05) for both eyes (Figure 4). The difference between the distance VA in trained and untrained eyes was significantly (p < .01) in favor of the trained eyes (Table 3). Near VA was significantly better immediately after training (Figures 5, 6, and 7). The control eyes showed a significant improvement only for the lowest contrast level. These results were stable after 6 months (see Table 3). The improvement in contrast sensitivity under different conditions (photopic, mesopic, and mesopic with glare) was only significant in the trained eyes, and not in the untrained eyes (Figures 8, 9, and 10). This improvement persisted for 6 months (Table 4).

Our results confirm the findings of previous studies that OVA can be improved by training using orientation discrimination without interocular transfer.[7,10,11] The improvement did not transfer to another task. For example, there was no significant change in the trained eyes for the horizontal stimulus orientation. Another interesting finding is the correlation of OVA improvement with the pre-training OVA. The lower the OVA before the training program the greater the gain in visual performance after the training program. Although this was statistically

significant, there was a high inter-individual variability of OVA (see Figure 2). Distance VA showed a slight, nonsignificant improvement immediately after training, but there was a significant difference at the 6-month follow-up (see Figure 4). The near vision was significantly better compared to the control eyes at all visits.

One major drawback of MIOLs is impaired contrast sensitivity.[12,13] We paid particular attention to the impact of our training method of orientation discrimination on contrast sensitivity.

The influence of training with orientation discrimination seems to be stronger on contrast sensitivity than on Snellen visual acuity. The gain in acuity by training became more evident with decreasing contrast immediately after the training. These findings are in agreement with results published by Matthews et al.[13] Examining normal adult humans they found that contrast sensitivity improved significantly after observers demonstrated practice-based increases in orientation discrimination. Several other investigators demonstrated a significant impact particularly on contrast sensitivity after vernier task training in amblyopic eyes.[9,10] Polat et al[8] documented a 2-fold improvement in contrast sensitivity in adult amblyopes following training of Gabor detection (bars with blurred edges). Training of basic psychophysical tasks improves

Figure 4. Change of mean BCVA measured using high contrast ETDRS charts in trained eyes (yellow) and control eyes (red). Means and SDs of 16 eyes. (***= p<0.001; **= p<0.01 *= p<0.05; n.s.= not significant)

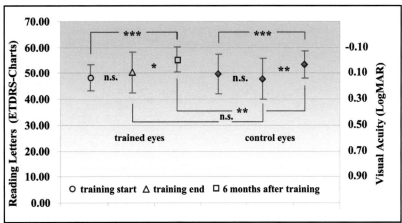

Table 3

COMPARISON OF VISUAL ACUITY
BETWEEN TRAINED AND CONTROL EYES 6 MONTHS AFTER TRAINING

	6 months after training		
	Trained eyes (reading letters)	Control eyes (reading letters)	Significance level
100% contrast Distance VA	56±5	53±5	p<0.01
100% contrast Near VA	67±6	63±8	p<0.01
25% contrast Near VA	43±6	39±7	p<0.01
12.5% contrast Near VA	40±6	37±6	p<0.01

Figure 5. Change in mean distance-corrected near contrast visual acuity in trained (yellow) and control eyes (red). Means and SDs of 16 eyes. (****= p<0.00001;*** p<0.001; **= p<0.01; *= p< 0.05; n.s.= not significant)

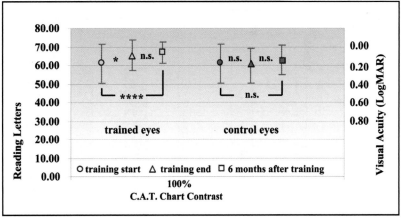

processing/coding of basic visual features that in turn facilitate performance in the high level visual acuity task, while training of visual acuity may not have allowed direct access to some of the basic visual features.[14,15]

The functional results were not significantly different for the 2 MIOLs investigated. The 2 lenses were not equal in optic design. This finding supports our assumption that the effect of perceptual learning is not due to a specific design of MIOLs, but is due to 2 simultaneous images the MIOL creates on the retina. A fundamental question concerns the persistence of the training effect found immediately after the training period. The evaluation after 6 months showed almost unchanged OVA

and near VA for different contrast levels. Distance BCVA was significantly improved in both the trained and the untrained eyes, but the trained eye was even better than the untrained eye. Interestingly, contrast sensitivity showed the greatest impact of training under all lighting conditions whereas the untrained eyes showed only a slight improvement. Contrast sensitivity in the fellow eyes was almost unchanged from the pre-training values after 6 months under photopic conditions and slightly improved under mesopic conditions with or without glare. These data support the findings of Zhou et al[11] and Polat et al[8] who found an excellent retention of the training benefit up to 1 year post-training.

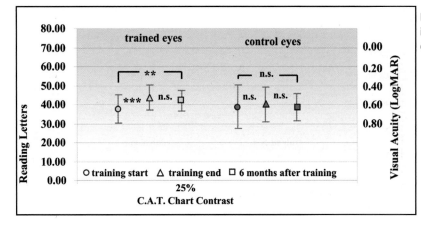

Figure 6. Change in mean distance-corrected near contrast visual acuity (25%) in trained (yellow) and control eyes (red). Means and SDs of 16 eyes. (*** p<0.001; **= p<0.01; n.s.= not significant)

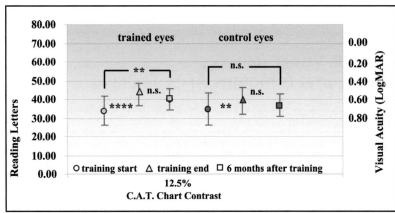

Figure 7. Change in mean uncorrected near contrast visual acuity (12.5%) in trained (yellow) and control eyes (red). Means and SDs of 16 eyes. (****= p<0.00001; **= p<0.01; n.s.= not significant)

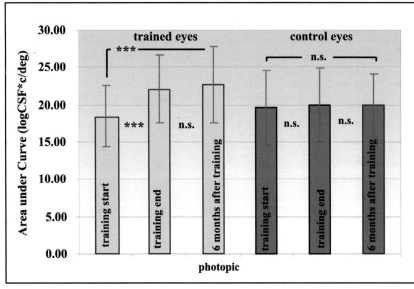

Figure 8. Change in contrast sensitivity under photopic conditions calculated as mean of the area under curve (AUC). Means and SDs of 16 eyes. (***= p<0.001; n.s.= not significant)

We still do not know how much training is needed to improve visual function. Our training program consisted of 6 sessions within 2 weeks. The assessment of OVA at each session revealed the greatest gain after the first 3 sessions (see Figure 3). From a practical point of view, it might be possible to shorten the training program. The ideal training method and time is not known. It is also possible that visual perception training could be suitable to diminish the perception of halos by improved suppression of the second, out-of-focus image.

References

1. Mester U, Hunold W, Wesendahl T, Kaymak H. Functional outcome after implantation of the Tecnis multifocal intraocular lens ZM900 compared to the Array SA40. *J Cataract Refract Surg.* 2007;33:1033-1040.

2. Kohnen T, Allen D, Boureau C, Dublineau P, Hartmann C, Mehdorn E, Rozot P, Tassinari G. European multicenter study of the AcrySof Restor apodized diffractive intraocular lens. *Ophthalmology.* 2006;113:578-584.

Figure 9. Change in contrast sensitivity under mesopic conditions calculated as mean of area under curve (AUC). Means and SDs of 16 eyes. (***= p<0.001; *= p<0.05; n.s.= not significant).

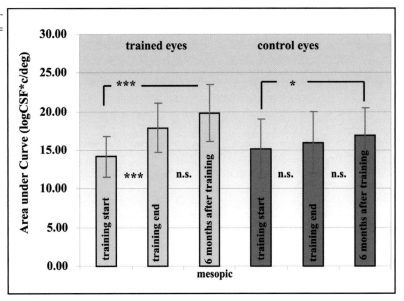

Figure 10. Change in contrast sensitivity under mesopic with glare conditions calculated as mean of the area under curve (AUC). Means and SDs of 16 eyes. (***= p<0.001; **= p<0.01 *= p<0.05; n.s.= not significant).

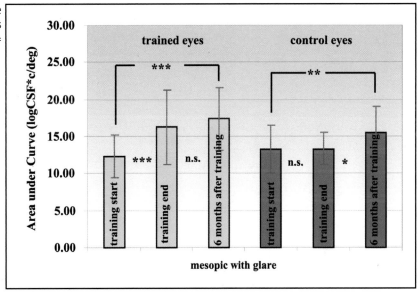

Table 4

COMPARISON OF CONTRAST SENSITIVITY CALCULATED AS AREA UNDER CURVE (AUC) BETWEEN TRAINED AND CONTROL EYES AFTER TRAINING END AND 6 MONTHS

	Trained eyes Area under curve (logCSF*c/deg)	Control eyes Area under curve (logCSF*c/deg)	Significance level
Training end			
Photopic	22.1±4.5	20.0±5.0	p<0.005
Mesopic	17.9±3.2	15.7±4.0	p<0.050
Mesopic with glare	16.2±5.0	13.3±2.1	p<0.006
6 months after training			
Photopic	22.7±5.0	19.9±4.0	p<0.05
Mesopic	19.8±3.7	17±3.4	p<0.02
Mesopic with glare	17.3 ±4.2	15.4 ±3.5	p<0.05

3. Montés-Micó R, Alio JL. Distance and near contrast sensitivity function after multifocal intraocular lens implantation. *J Cataract Refract Surg.* 2003;29:703-711.

4. Petermeier K, Szurman P. Subjecitve and objective outcomes following implantation of the apodized diffractive AcrySof Restor. *Ophthalmologe.* 2007;48:399-404.

5. Steinert RF. ASCRS Binkhorst lecture 2004: the search for perfect vision: ophthalmology's Holy Grail? *J Cataract Refract Surg.* 2005;31:2405-2412.

6. Fahle M, Edelman S, Poggio T. Fast perceptual learning in visual hyperacuity. *Vision Res.* 1995;35:3003-3013.

7. Fahle M. Perceptual learning: a case for early selection. *J Vision.* 2004;10:879-890.

8. Polat U, Ma-Naim T, Belkin M, Sagi D. Improving vision in adult amblyopia by perceptual learning. *Proc Natl Acad Sci USA.* 2004;101:6692-6697.

9. Levi DM, Polat U. Neural plasticity in adults with amblyopia. *Proc Natl Acad Sci USA.* 1996;93:6830-6834.

10. Levi DM, Polat U, Hu YS. Improvement in vernier acuity in adults with amblyopia. Practice makes better. *Invest Ophthalmol Vis Sci.* 1997;38:1493-1510.

11. Zhou Y, Huang C, Xu P, Tao L, Quiu Z, Li X, Lu ZL. Perceptual learning improves contrast sensitivity and visual acuity in adults with anisometropic amblyopia. *Vis Res.* 2006;46:739-750.

12. Jacobi FK, Kessler W, Held S. Abbildungseigenschaften multifokalerIntraokularlinsen. *Ophthalmologe.* 2007;104:236-242.

13. Matthews N, Liu Z, Qian N. The effect of orientation learning on contrast sensitivity. *Vis Res.* 2001;41:463-471.

14. Ahissar M, Hochstein S. Learning pop-out detection: specificities to stimulus characteristics. *Vis Res.* 1996;36:3487-3500.

15. Dosher BA, Zu ZL. Perceptual learning reflects external noise filtering and internal noise reduction through channel reweighting. *Proc Natl Acad Sci USA.* 1998;95:13988-13993.

CHAPTER 82

ADAPTING TO MY OWN MULTIFOCAL HALOS

Guy E. Knolle, MD, FACS

I began using the Advanced Medical Optics' (AMO) Array multifocal (MF) intraocular lens in my cataract patients in 2000. I had the advantage of previous experience in 1989 with the Wright Medical MF lens (California), which offered a varying radius of curvature on the anterior surface rather than concentric circles of varying power. This Wright lens worked well in the few patients that I implanted, and I followed 2 of them for over 10 years. The lens was removed from the market in the early 1990s because of the lack of Food and Drug Administration approval.

After AMO sales representative, Vicki Williams, encouraged me several times to consider using the Array, I went to visit Andy Watkins, MD in Houston, TX. Andy was using the Array lens frequently in his cataract patients. I examined and questioned Andy's patients and because of my previous experience in 1989, I was convinced the Array lens worked. I returned to Austin, TX and educated my staff. I then began using the lens in all of my patients who understood the concept. I educated patients by talking to them face to face about the lens and what it could do to enhance their postoperative visual function. I told them about the circles the lens would put around a point of light at night and that the lens would not make them "glasses free," but it would give them more freedom from wearing glasses. I explained that their vision could be clear at all distances and that they could have increased depth of field as compared to a monofocal lens implant. I talked to them about neutralizing their corneal astigmatism with "limbal" relaxing incisions (LRIs). I showed them surgical videos and Kevin Waltz, MD's video "Halos and the Good Life 2." I used the illustrations that Michael Woodcock, MD's patient Thelma McGugan created for him illustrating headlights at night immediately after surgery and then again some months later. Since Robert Watson had not developed the IOL Counselor (Patient Education Concepts, Houston, TX) at the time, preoperative counseling was fairly extensive and demanding of my personal time. Although in those years there was no additional financial reimbursement for MF lenses, I found the time spent was very gratifying. I was truly rehabili-

tating these patients and the "wow" factor was reward enough. I was convinced that it was patient education and not patient selection that led to success. I believed from the beginning that the informed patient would select the proper lens choice for his or her needs if given the opportunity.

In any event, I used the Array lens in 95.2% of my cataract patients beginning in 2000. I used it in conjunction with both a monofocal and MF lens in the fellow eye. The MF lens filled in the gaps left by the monofocal intraocular lens and was most commonly the patient's lens of choice. The first observation most patients expressed postoperatively was that their distance vision was better than ever before. I questioned them about the circles around lights at night and got variable responses. Most patients had adapted to the sight of these halos within the first few months after surgery and felt the advantages in depth of field and good vision at all distances without glasses was worth the small trade off. Occasionally, I used Alphagan P (Allergan, Irvine, CA) 3 times a day to reduce pupillary dilation and help patients with night driving, but this was only during the early adaptation period. Before using the Array MF lens, I had never had a patient sit up on the operating table and exclaim, "I can see." I believe this was because of the overall operating room environment being simultaneously in focus in spite of the immediate postoperative haze that was present.

After 3 years of examining and listening to my patients tell me about their visual abilities and observing them reading in our dimly lighted waiting room without glasses, I decided to have the lenses implanted in my own eyes. I simply did not want to continue wearing hyperopic trifocals. My corrected vision was 20/15 with no glare disability, but I disliked being dependent on eyeglasses for good vision. On Wednesday May 21, 2003, I flew my airplane from Austin to Alexandria, Louisiana. Bruce Wallace, MD and I compared the measurements my staff had made earlier to those of his office staff, and we selected a lens power. That afternoon Bruce did my surgery. The next day I was 20/20 both at distance and near without correction. Bruce said, "You are good to fly," and I flew my airplane home and went to work in my office the following day. The second eye was a repeat performance. It has now been over 4 years since my surgery, and I am still excited about how well I see without glasses.

I have been using the ReZoom MF lens (Advanced Medical Optics, Santa Ana, CA) since it came on the market 2 years ago. Because added cost to the patient has become a factor, I am implanting currently 60.47% of my cataract patients with the ReZoom. My clinical impression is that patients adapt more quickly to the circles around lights at night and their reading ability is better in a shorter period of time. This is purely a subjective impression on my part, and it may be that MF lenses are now regarded as an accepted way of visual rehabilitation.

How do I see and how do my patients see? It is pretty simple—we just open our eyes and look at any object of regard. The ReZoom lens, like the Array, has 5 concentric circles of varying power. Rings 1 (the center), 3, and 5 are for distance and rings 2 and 4 are for near. This is straight forward, but I think that the transition between the center and second ring and between the second and third rings is the reason for truly flawless, blended vision at all distances. The lens is 6 mm in diameter, so surely the outer rings add little to enhance vision regardless of pupil size or ambient lighting. The lens is weighted for distance, so for prolonged reading or to increase the speed of performing near work, a +1.50 half glass helps some patients. The distance vision is never an issue if the power calculation, LRIs, and healing are appropriate.

There are occasional individuals that never adapt to the lens and cannot use it well. In my experience, they are maybe 5 in 1000, but I cannot tell you how to find them. They find themselves after the fact. The more intelligent the patient and the more compulsive he or she is, the better he or she does in my experience. I have 16-cut radial keratotomy (RK) patients that are delighted with their distance, intermediate, and near vision and say their night vision is no worse than before implantation of the MF lens. I have seen only a single unhappy post-laser in situ keratomileusis patient with these lenses while many patients are very happy that they can now see at all distances without correction.

There is no "trick" that I can find to seeing with these 2 lenses. Just open your eyes and engage your brain. Those individuals who "doubt" will take longer to adapt to the circles at night and to reading. A −12 myope with cataracts that I recently operated on is still nervous in spite of 20/25 vision distance and near without correction. However, she no longer sleeps in her glasses at night, no longer has to sleep with light in the room, and can see a white bar of soap in the bottom of the bathtub. She bought only colored soap bars before her surgery. Her office staff cannot believe she works all day long at her computer without glasses. Her husband is delighted because he no longer has to drive her to work. Since she was afraid to drive using her eyeglasses, he was her chauffeur for months while her corneal topography stabilized after discontinuing her hard contact lenses.

Driving at night is not a problem with these MF lenses. Even when driving in the rain for hours on the highway, I have not found my vision limited. The road marking, signs, parked vehicles, and bicycles are clearly visible. I can say the same for flying an airplane at night in and out of clouds and rain. Instrument approaches are made easy by my ability to effortlessly scan the instrument panel. Multifocal lenses truly enhance cockpit management.

I have been asked if I see halos through the operating microscope while performing surgery. The answer is no because, as Kevin L. Waltz, OD, MD has pointed out, the microscope forms a second entrance pupil before light reaches the surgeon's eyes. This is similar to the effect produced by using a pair of binoculars to remove the ring of light created by the MF lens around a full moon. In fact, my depth of field at the microscope is so enhanced that the entire view is generally in focus from the cornea to the posterior capsule. I change the focus only occasionally during surgery to be sure that I have the best possible clarity.

Who may not be a good candidate for these MF lenses? I think from a functional standpoint the patient with early macular degeneration (AMD) may not adapt well if annoyed by having to use extra light in dimly lighted areas. Except for increased lighting requirements to enhance definition and contrast sensitivity, the MF intraocular lens may offer depth of field benefits to these patients that again are difficult to objectively quantify. This subject is controversial at this point in time to say the least, but as a rule the AMD patients I have implanted with MF lenses are generally pleased with their outcome. Irregular central corneal astigmatism can be another concern against using these lenses. However, as previously mentioned, I have had good success with radial keratotomy patients with up to sixteen incisions.

The Array/ReZoom MF intraocular lens can truly enhance one's visual lifestyle, whether operating, flying an airplane, fly fishing, walking on uneven ground while hunting game, golfing, water skiing, or just watching the sunset as the moon rises.

CHAPTER 83

How I See With the ReZoom

Tom M. Coffman, MD

After having dealt with hard contact lenses and the gas permeable contacts for 47 years and after implanting almost 10,000 multifocal lenses I was ready for my own relief from glasses or contacts. Choosing the lens was easy, because all the presbyopia-correcting lenses work and I have implanted the Crystalens (Eyeonics, Inc, Aliso Viejo, CA), the Array lens (Advanced Medical Optics, Santa Ana, CA), and the ReZoom lenses (Advanced Medical Optics). I felt that in my case, as with most of my patients, the ReZoom would offer me the best result.

My right eye is my dominant eye, and my refractions were −1.75 OD and −1.12 OS. When I became presbyopic, I achieved monovision by not wearing any correction for my left eye. However, after my left contact lens had been out for 3 years the −1.12 monovision had become inadequate for reading. Having observed Dr. Gayle Martin in surgery and having shared ideas with him for over 20 years, I picked him to perform my refractive lens exchange starting in my non-dominant left eye. I had my technicians measure me for the implant power and made my own calculations. Then this was repeated at Carolina Eye in Southern Pines, NC. We picked a lens and Dr. Martin opted to add a limbal relaxing incision (LRI) for .75 D of astigmatism.

That afternoon the surgery was performed through a smallish pupil without complications. I must have talked too much under the influences of Versed (Hoffman-LaRoche, Inc, Nutley, NJ) so they gave me more. As a result I missed the procedure and it took me 45 minutes in recovery before I could even walk awkwardly out to my ride back to the motel. A 2-hour nap seemed appropriate at that point. Upon awakening I was significantly improved but my vision was smoky from corneal edema or just epithelial edema from the drops. It was amazing that I did not feel like the Versed had totally worn off until the third day postoperative. At the 1 day postoperative visit I was 20/20 at a distance and 20/40 at 18 inches. If I looked at reading material for 30 seconds it would slowly become sharper. Over the first week I improved to 20/15 at distance and 20/25 at near. I could read the newspaper from 10

to 30 inches, but it was somewhat difficult due to ghosting. At 2 weeks postoperative and through 4 months postoperatively I was 20/15 +2 at distance and 20/20 at near. My refractive error is +.25 and with a +.50 lens the near 20/20 line was easily read and with minimal ghosting. Also, by month 4 the reading vision did improve after about 2 seconds of concentration, when I used the operative eye.

After the first week postoperative, I left out my gas permeable lens in the second (right) eye to allow the corneal molding to dissipate. This took 4.5 months to stabilize. This complicated matters some because I was −1.75 in the dominant unoperated right eye and it constantly competed with the left ReZoom eye for near vision. As a result, my brain did not accept the near image until 3 days after the second eye received its ReZoom. At that point, it suddenly became easy to read newsprint.

I must share an important event at week 6 in the first eye. Having finished my Pred Forte (Allergan, Irvine, CA) 3 days prior, I awakened to a 20/30 blur in the left eye at distance. I also noticed a crinkled cellophane appearance in the center 5 degrees of field. I had an optical coherence tomography (OCT) performed and documented the cystoid macular edema (CME). I started Pred Forte and Acular (Allergan) both hourly and within 3 hours my vision had returned to 20/15 +2! I used these drops for a few weeks longer and have had no further CME.

By 14 weeks after discontinuing my second eye's contact lens the keratometry readings were still steepening .25 D every few weeks. By 4 and 1/2 months after the first operation, the refraction in my unoperated right eye finally stabilized and I was ready for surgery. I looked forward to the second refractive lens exchange and having a matched set of eyes.

My goal for the right eye was to have a target refraction of −0.37 in order to boost the near vision. I aimed at −0.50 and at 5 weeks postoperative, I was −0.50, −0.25 × 25 and 20/15 at near. I also had fantastic computer distance vision, without correction. Amazingly, I developed CME in the second eye at day 14. I increased my Pred Forte and Acular LS to every

2 hours, but no change in my vision or OCT occurred. At week 4, a retro bulbar Kenalog injection hastened my improvement back to 20/20 near and distance. However, I still had enough CME adjacent to the fovea to cause some blur.

Halos are always the big concern about multifocal IOLs among ophthalmologists. In my series of multifocal IOLs (mostly Array and ReZoom) 4% of the patients needed Alphagan or pilocarpine 0.5% at sundown to palliate them. Less than 0.5% of my patients stop driving due to halos and I have only removed four multifocal IOLs from 2 patients due to halos. This is out of almost 10,000 multifocal implantations by me. With my left eye I am able to see a crescent of halo adjacent to street lights. It is about the size of the street light and 40% of a circle. With my right eye this is similar on the right of the light. This is an observation but certainly in no way is it a nuisance. I believe it is similar to what I observed with my contacts for decades. I do not know why a few patients are bothered by the halos but astigmatism correction or a yttrium-aluminum-garnet (YAG) capsulotomy helps some. I have never found any correlation between any preoperative complaint or personality leading to postoperative complaints of halos. Hyperopes have more halos and glare with glasses than patients with multifocal lenses.

Basically, in the past 6 months my halos have not changed. Importantly, they are so insignificant that I only study them for my interest. A significant number of patients have noticed their disappearance by 1 year. Occasionally, this occurs the day after the second eye surgery.

I had my second contact lens out for 5 months before the second eye surgery. This was a nuisance as mentioned earlier, with the distant blur and competition for near. In my experience the happiest patients have the second eye done in 1 to 3 weeks.

I have never had an unhappy patient in the years between eyes, if the second eye is emmetropic and without a significant cataract,. Also, I have put a multifocal lens in the second eye in about 60 patients that had a monofocal in the first eye in the past. One hundred percent have been very happy with the result. Of course, the first eye has to be close to emmetropia.

Conclusion

I am ecstatic with my crystal clear 20/15 distance vision. My near vision is acceptable with some posterior capsular haze and after a posterior capsulotomy should approach 20/15 as well. It certainly is a pleasure to not be frustrated by the need for glasses for distance, near, or in between.

CHAPTER 84

HOW I SEE WITH THE ReSTOR

Daniel Vos, MD

Laser in situ keratomileusis (LASIK) is a great operation but as a –2.50 presbyope it would just be trading distance glasses for reading glasses. Besides, bifocal contact lenses preserved my stereopsis and were tolerated well until the last few years. At 53, a combination of a 1 D myopic shift and progressively dryer eyes diminished the quality of vision with the contacts. In addition to being an ophthalmologist, I am into model railroading and water skiing. All of these require excellent depth perception up close and at distance, so monovision is out. After doing about 90 ReSTOR (Alcon, Fort Worth, TX) patients I was impressed with their spectacle independence. I was aware of the night glare issue and a little puzzled that some of them had to be shown how to hold what they want to read. I decided that I would like to do it but the hard part was getting my partners past their wariness about the lens.

My dominant eye was implanted on a Monday, the left eye on Wednesday, and I made good time operating on 15 cataracts on Friday with better vision than the week before. I dialed +0.25 and +0.50 into the scope. No correction is required for minor surgeries, punctal plugs, or reading micrometers.

The first day was a little "edgy" because of the Cyclogyl (Alcon, Fort Worth, TX). Distance vision was color desaturated like being dilated plus a little worse and reading was frightful. If I really stared at the "water colors" where the print should be, I could gradually make out the letters at 15 inches; but they were low contrast and one-fourth thickness at full height. The background had grey water color brush strokes 3 times the height of the letters and overlapping the next line. The degree of monocular diplopia surprised me because almost all of my ReSTOR patients can read their appointment card at the 1 hour postoperative, if I push it up to 13 inches for them. Maybe that is because I use nonsteroidal anti-inflammatory drugs (NSAIDs), neosynephrine, and mydriacyl but no cyclogyl. It was possible to read with a +2.50 reader but I fear that it delays adaptation.

Postoperative day 1 the reading was improved but the depth of field was shallow and there was still a faint "ghost image." Distance appeared clear, but oddly letters were dyslexic and I could only see 20/40. That improved to a crystal 20/15 with +0.75. I thought my bifocal contact lens experience would have made the adaptation better than it did. I did try the contact lens in the nonoperated eye postoperative day one and it did help the operated eye significantly.

Monocular implantation was not an option for me because of my critical need for stereopsis. Also, summation seemed to be a great advantage with the second eye. Normally I do not operate on the second eye sooner than a week, but I was anxious to get back to work and patients definitely do better the closer their surgeries are. The second eye had exactly the same recovery but the clarity was slightly worse and indeed it took a +1.00 to get to 20/15 on post-op day one. By postoperative day 2, I was 20/15 OD and 20/25 OS. Both could be corrected to 20/15 with +0.25 OD and +0.50 OS. Reading was comfortable at 15 inches with a little more depth of field but "arms length" was hit and miss and often plagued with a blurred ghost image.

Night glare on day one looked like someone twirled a Fourth of July sparkler at arms length around head lights. There were discrete micro strokes within the ring at 3x the width of oncoming cars while the pupil was dilated. With normal pupil size the rings reduced to one-fourth the width of the car immediately. Over the last 3 weeks the halos are only present for some lights with high contrast backgrounds. They are distance dependant—absent beyond a mile, most prominent at a half mile, and absent again within 1/4 mile. Curiously, if I concentrate on seeing the circles they are more prominent. In fact, a point source of light in the dark can have a placido disk appearance at 0.5 mile, if I admire it. If I concentrate on the shape of the bulb itself, the halos lose "awareness" rapidly. That makes me worry that the patients who concentrate on the glare will not adapt as fast. Glare is getting better steadily, but it is worse with high contrast and less if I know the shape of what I am trying to see. By 3 weeks I said, "Even if it does not get better than this, I would still be happy with the lens." And by 2 months glare around lights at night is really no issue.

Lighting and background make a difference, especially at arm's length. More light usually helps, but if I solder wires with a bright light I have to move a light-colored background behind the wires to decrease the reflections or decrease the light to a moderate level.

Many cataract patients talk about how much brighter colors are after surgery, especially blues and greens. The SN6AD3 is yellow and maybe it matched my preoperative nuclear sclerosis exactly but I did not notice any color change. Relative hues are unchanged and distance color intensity may be about 5% improved overall. No colors are different than what I thought and near colors are no worse.

As a pseudophake I am not supposed to have accommodation, but my near point moves out a couple of inches when I am tired and arm's length reading gets worse. If I try to read something in "the circle of most confusion," 18 to 30 inches, it works better if I start close and move toward the dreaded arm's length or start out beyond and move the object into the "circle" to avoid monocular diplopia. Part of the neural adaptation is suppressing the blurred image, so if you start at the shift point between the distant and near focal lengths they are equally blurred and the brain does not know which to choose. Accommodation also works against you if you are at the distal part of your near range so it takes practice to relax accommodation. That only happens if you mentally lock onto the image and push away the image repeatedly. Conversely, accommodation can help if you can stay locked onto the distance focal image as your image approaches the "circle." All of that takes practice and coaching. I wonder how to motivate patients who expected it to be instant and automatic. In case of emergency, you can use a +1.50 reader for the computer. It works, but I prefer to lean in a little and eventually the other patients will too. I agree with one of my patients who wrote on his satisfaction survey, "Distance and close up are great, but I think I'll get a bigger computer monitor."

I started with the bias that a low hyperopic result would be better than a low myopic result but it really depends on the distance with which that the patient is working. Fortunately my surgeon, Jim Davison, delivered just what I desired; +0.25 Sph OD and +0.50 Sph OS. I simulated various refractions and used trial frames with reading fine print, computers at arm's length, and driving. Of course the best distance vision was with −0.25 to +0.25. All 3 were 20/15. The myopic tests actually improved reading and the distant edge of the "circle of most confusion" (18 to 30 inches). So a −0.25 or −0.50 result helped with the dash instruments while driving and the computer distance. Here are some of my simulated postoperative refractions and observations:

* +0.50 Sph distance 20/25+, near Jaeger 1 @ 16"
* +0.25 Sph distance 20/15, near Jaeger 1 @ 15"
* Plano Sph distance 20/15, near Jaeger 1 @ 13"
* −0.25 Sph distance 20/15, near Jaeger1+ @ 11"
* −0.50 Sph distance 20/20, near Jaeger 1+ @ 10"

Arm's length tasks surprised me the most. The dash and the computer were significantly clearer at 27 to 30 inches with the −0.25 and −0.50. That reminded me of a patient of mine that ended up Plano in one eye and −0.75 in the other. She was very happy but admitted to some night glare when pressed. I have offered her a laser in situ keratomileusis (LASIK) enhancement several times, but she refused. I simulated it and have 20/15—with OU @ distance, and it does work better with the computer. In fact there is a seamless transition from 9 inches through distance. A Plano/−0.50 is a little blurred with small print from 14" to 22" but does improve 22 to 30 inches significantly. Less than 1.00 D of anisometropia does not affect threading a needle for me.

A Plano result in one eye and −0.75 in the other eye eliminated "the circle of most confusion" at arm's length without sacrificing needle threading or creating night glare in my simulation.

I am really fortunate to not have astigmatism, but wondered how much is tolerable. Here is my simulation for distance:

Plano Sph	20/15
+0.25 to 0.50 @ 90	20/20+2
+0.37 to 0.75 @ 90	20/25+
+0.50 to 1.00 @ 90	20/25−
+0.62 to 1.25 @ 90	20/40−
+0.75 to 1.50 @ 90	20/60−

Switching the axis to 180 had no effect on the results. There is a dramatic drop off in acuity above a D of astigmatism. This was at least as bad for intermediate or near.

More than a D of residual astigmatism would certainly explain the "waxy vision" reported by some. More than 0.75 D of anisometropia may be another explanation. I cannot rule out a failure to adequately suppress the out of focus image for those who concentrate on it instead of the intended image. Keep in mind that we have created monocular diplopia and we are depending on neural adaptation to suppress one image. I noticed that for me that was prominent the first day and even a week later would occasionally be seen as a "cartoon thought bubble" surrounding a line of white print on a black background. This was more noticeable in low light conditions, but always improved with moving the paper closer.

Another of my patients, despite 20/20 at distance and the witnessed ability to read a magazine without glasses, asked one of my colleagues for bifocals. It turns out that preoperatively he was a −5.50 and would take off his glasses to read blueprints. All of his co-workers used a magnifier to do that task. He was disappointed that he could not do that with the ReSTOR alone. The +2.25 add made him able to work at 7" because the ReSTOR's 3.2 plus the bifocal's + 2.25 equals a 5.45 D add. In fact, that combination gave him a high-powered "quadrifocal" with focals at distance, +2.25, +3.25, and +5.45. A more practical combination for the "watchmakers" in your practice might be a +1.50 reader. That would give a good mid range, and combined with the ReSTOR near focal, an effective +4.70 add. Yes, I would do it again, and no it is not for everyone. Patience and optimism are rewarded with spectacle independence. LASIK enhancement may be needed to fine tune the results.

CHAPTER 85

HOW I SEE WITH THE ReSTOR

Jess C. Lester, MD, FACS

In March 2006, I noticed that I had difficulty reading with my right eye. An exam by a retina specialist confirmed a normal macula, but a posterior subcapsular cataract (PSC) was found. By August 2006, the visual disturbance was bothersome. Cataract surgery with a ReSTOR intraocular lens (IOL) (Alcon, Fort Worth, TX) was performed in September. The postoperative vision in my left eye was crystal clear, and I was able to read an entire newspaper without reading glasses on postoperative day 1. All 3 ranges of vision were so incredibly clear that I had the same procedure performed on my right eye even though the vision was relatively clear and the PSC was small. Since then I have been 100% glasses free for distance, intermediate, and near vision. I do not have "20-year-old eyes" because I do not have 20-year-old maculas (I am in my mid-70s). I do enjoy 20/15 vision in my left eye and 20/20 vision in my right eye. I am able to see to do anything I need to do or want to see without glasses. This includes seeing through an operating microscope, slit lamp, or indirect scope; driving at night even in heavy rain; woodworking; flying; shooting; performing all intermediate tasks; and reading from a variety of ranges, whether close to reading in my lap. My best intermediate distance is 23 to 24 inches. My reading range is 9 to 20 inches. I have been presbyopic for 25 years, and the ability to perform all my visual tasks without glasses is quite a luxury.

I chose to have a ReSTOR IOL implanted because I wanted the best opportunity to be glasses free. That implant also had the fewest side effects. I had been implanting that implant in my patients for 1 year and was very impressed with the number of patients who presented with excellent postoperative results. Nearly 90% of those patients were glasses free. Intermediate distance problems were very rare, and their reading vision was outstanding. Glare and halos were extremely rare as well as symptoms of negative dysphotopsia. Excellent near vision was another finding in our patients that helped me decide on the ReSTOR lens. This was enhanced in dim or poor lighting and in situations of low contrast by increasing the light at near. Increasing the light, even though it caused miosis dramatically improved near vision.

When I began implanting the Array Multifocal IOL (Advanced Medical Optics, Santa Ana, CA) when it became available about 8 or 9 years ago, I was initially enthusiastic. After 2 or 3 years, my enthusiasm diminished because 50% of those patients need reading glasses. Some patients complained of very bothersome night time glare and halos. A few were so unhappy with this symptom that they asked to have their lenses removed. We still offered the lens to patients but our office staff was very careful to explain to patients about the potential need for glasses for near and the nighttime glare and halos. Even though the percentage of patients with this complaint was small we felt that preoperative counseling was extremely important. Another problem that was encountered was the finding that increasing the light for near caused the reading to be worse because of the miosis and the relationship of small pupil to the add in the IOL. This was very disturbing and is in direct contrast to the improvement in near vision when light was introduced at near in a ReSTOR patient.

My eyes adapted rapidly to the ReSTOR IOLS. I did not need to hold reading material close for 1 to 2 weeks as some patients have reported. My intermediate distance was 23 inches immediately after surgery. My distance vision is crisp and clear in both eyes.

At night I do see the rings in the IOL centered around lights, such as headlights, tail lights, traffic signal lights, and parking lot lights. These rings do not interfere with driving at night even in the rain. These rings are diminishing in number and distinctness and are now picked up much further in the distance and disappear much further in the distance than in the immediate postoperative time frame. They are totally different than glare and halos .

I am very pleased with the decision to have bilateral ReSTOR implantations in my own eyes. My wife also has bilateral ReSTOR implantations and her results are also excellent.

I took a medical retirement in September 2006 at the advice of a neurosurgeon who found some "serious neurological problems" in my lower back. My refraction in my OD is +0.75 and OS is +0.50. Since all of my preoperative Ks and axial lengths were confirmed by measurements at 2 different locations, I am assuming that when the capsule contracted in my OD, the IOL was "pushed" posteriorly causing the plus increase. (Sometimes the refraction in my OD is closer to +1.00.) I am totally unaware of any loss of contrast. I am extremely pleased at how well I can read in dim light such as during concerts and plays or reading a road map in a dimly auto at night. I have always been emmetropic with no refractive error for distance, myopic or hyperopic. I did develop about 1.25 to 1.50 D of cylinder in my OS probably due to wearing a monovision SCTL for about 25 years. That is why I had an "on axis" incision with 2 small limbal relaxing incisions. I have no cylinder in my refraction now. I would not have had surgery prior to the availability of the ReSTOR IOL because of the disappointing reading results with the only other multifocal IOL available at the time, the Array. If surgery had been necessary, I would have had an Array since that would have been my best opportunity to be glasses free. However, my need for surgery came after the availability of the ReSTOR IOL. Knowing what I now know, I would definitely have considered refractive lens exchange with the ReSTOR IOL, but not any other lens.

CHAPTER 86

How I See With the Crystalens

Harvey Zalaznick, MD

As an ophthalmologist, it was awkward needing help following my golf ball. My wife had to read the hockey scores to me from the television. Office examinations presented difficulties with indirect ophthalmoscopy. Memorizing the Snellen chart was a definite help. I was diagnosed with bilateral cataracts with a reduction in vision to 20/60+. I was a bit surprised just how intolerable that vision was. It did not take long to decide on surgery or my surgeon, Dr. Alan Aker.

The preoperative evaluation was routine with the discussion mostly centering around the choice of implant. As a mild myope, I had worn glasses my whole life and did not mind the likelihood of requiring postoperative correction, although the less the better. Monovision, for me, was not an option. At the American Academy of Ophthalmology meeting 1 month prior, I had attended lectures on the different available implants. While the lectures were informative, I found them confusing, imprecise, and contradictory. What I wanted was to see well without any side effects. The Crystalens 4.5 (Eyeonics, Inc, Aliso Viejo, CA) was my choice of implant since it offered the best chance of spectacle-free distance and computer vision over most lighting situations. I was prepared for the likelihood of requiring readers, but I preferred that to the likelihood of glare and contrast issues with other implants.

Although my surgery went well technically, one eye developed cystoid macular edema that cleared quickly with steroids and nonsteroidal anti-inflammatory drops. My postoperative refraction is −0.50 in both eyes. My distance and computer vision are excellent without correction. My binocular vision improved after the second operation but not as dramatically as after the first procedure. Although I can read Jaeger-2 without correction in good lighting, I much prefer my +1.50 readers. I did notice that a +2.00 reader felt much too strong. My guess is that the implant is actually accommodating but no more than +1.00 D to +1.25 D. I have no problems with glare or night vision.

My personal experience has impressed upon me just how individualized cataract surgery has become. It is anything but routine. Success no longer depends solely on the surgeon's technical skill. The patient's expectations and the limitations of any of these implants must be clearly defined preoperatively.

Basically, I have been thrilled with my surgical outcome. At a distance, I can see my golf ball enter the water and at near, read the 8 on my scorecard.

CHAPTER 87

How I See With the Crystalens

Brian D. Lueth, MD

When I saw flickering lights in my peripheral vision that Saturday morning, my heart sank. As a 49-year-old ophthalmologist with an ambulatory surgery center (ASC) and an active cataract and refractive practice, I was virtually certain that I was developing a retinal tear and quite possibly a detachment. Later that day my suspicions were confirmed, and I underwent repair of a localized detachment with intraocular injection of SF6 and cryopexy. The details of that experience are another story, but let me tell you—cryopexy is COLD!

Fortunately, the repair was very successful. Other than a week spent with my head tipped at an odd angle, (which limited my ability to see patients and do surgery), I was none the worse for wear… for the time being.

I then began to notice a gradually progressive decline in my acuity that I could not correct as I dialed the various lenses through the phoropter. Point sources of light had triangular radiations that looked like the Mitsubishi emblem. I realized that the intraocular gas had caused one of its well-known adverse effects and that I had better start thinking about my preferred options for an intraocular lens implant.

I spoke with a colleague who did a lot of Food and Drug Administration (FDA) studies on intraocular lenses (IOLs) about his opinion about my various choices. I was pretty well acquainted with my current options and wanted to know what he saw coming down the pipeline—soon. He mentioned a promising new lens implant called the Crystalens (Eyeonics, Inc, Aliso Viejo, CA) with which he had favorable experience. He thought FDA approval for this lens was only a short time off and that it had the ability to give me what I was looking for in the way of spectacle independence. After years of hearing about the need to select patients carefully for multifocal lens implantation, I was pretty sure I valued quality distance acuity and the possible need for occasional use of readers for near vision over the type of vision I could expect with multifocal lens implants available at the time. Not long afterwards, FDA approval was granted, and my decision was confirmed.

The surgery experience itself was pretty easy. I was able to provide my surgeon with all the necessary parameters to order the implant using our own facilities. I chose to leave my family (and moral support network) at home and travel to his office on my own. I have big, myopic eyes with wide corneas and deep chambers. My preoperative refraction measured about −6.50 D of myopia and 1.5 D of myopic astigmatism with gross inferior steepening both eyes (OU). This finding, along with the fact that my brother has frank keratoconus, prevented me from considering keratorefractive surgery for myself. My Ks are median and corneal thickness is normal. My 6.5-mm pupils with a 4.5-mm diameter optic were a bit of a concern, so I anticipated some halos around lights at night with the Crystalens. We decided to correct the astigmatism as much as possible with limbal relaxing incisions placed a little asymmetrically to better account for the inferior steepening. We also discussed the possibility of an endocyclophotocoagulation (ECP) treatment for pigment dispersion, elevated intraocular pressures, and tilted myopic discs suspicious for cupping (with normal visual fields). My surgeon recommended that he defer the ECP because of the possibility that it might have an adverse effect on the ability to accommodate with the Crystalens.

I flew down to the surgeon's office on a Tuesday and had him confirm the biometry and finalize his surgical plan, and on Wednesday he placed a Crystalens implant in my right eye, targeting −0.75. The next day I was able to read 20/20- with my right eye and it had a satisfactory postoperative appearance, so later that day he placed a second Crystalens in my left eye. Things looked fine for both eyes on Friday, and I was able to read 20/15 with my left eye, so I flew home. The following Monday I was seeing patients of my own in my office, and on Tuesday I was performing cataract surgery in my ASC with a spectacularly clear view through the operating microscope. Atropine was used postoperatively in both eyes, so there was quite a pronounced glare and the near vision was very poor without correction for the first week.

What is my vision like with the Crystalens? Uncorrected distance acuity is much sharper than I expected. After a lifetime of significant myopia, I rejoice every day in my crystal clear distance vision. Although my first eye was able to read 20/20- without correction, it did in fact measure −0.75 spherical as planned. My right eye refracted to +0.25 −0.50 × 165 and maintained 20/15 uncorrected distance vision. My near vision varies tremendously depending upon lighting conditions. Ocular surface disease (dry eye/blepharitis) and floaters degrade the near vision on occasion. I generally read J3 OD, J5 OS, and J3 OU in average light. I can easily read the small print on a medicine bottle or on a business card with bright light. The near vision occurs automatically and without conscious effort, but I can perceive accommodative effort when present, and this guides my focusing through the operating microscope. The near vision function seems to defy conventional teaching about optics. Rather than behaving like a near lens, it behaves more like an expanded range of focus. Where one might expect a relatively sharp focus at arm's reach, especially for the −0.75 right eye, the image appears readable but a bit fuzzy even at that distance. Bringing the object of regard closer does not make it less legible as expected; it is still fuzzy but closer, therefore larger, and thus still legible. I can read nearly as well at 10 inches as I can at 24 inches if there is very good light. The near vision is poor in very dim lighting conditions, and no amount of accommodative effort seems to make much difference. I am not sure that the near function is achieved entirely by a shift in the lens position, the mechanism of action proposed by Eyeonics, or I would expect better reading vision even in reduced light. I suspect at least part of the effect is provided by the posterior vault of this lens, which places it closer to the nodal point of the eye, and the pinhole effect that is provided by both bright lighting and the miosis of accommodation. I did have ultrasound biometry that indicated about 1.5 mm of anterior shift with accommodation, so we do know that the lens changes position during accommodation.

Shortly after the surgery, I was very sensitive to glare and experienced considerable halos around lights. There was a very sharply focused point of light surrounded by a well-defined halo a considerable distance away from the light source in a fairly narrow ring. A bit further out there was a pair of parallel lines of light that originated from the hinges. I could tell exactly the orientation of both lens implants, based upon these lines of light. The effect was a bit disconcerting, but faded progressively at about 6 months after the surgery and now has completely resolved. I have little doubt that my perception of these lines occurred because of my large pupils, and that effect has resolved with peripheral capsule opacification. The central capsule has remained clear in both eyes, and I have not required a YAG capsulotomy in either eye to date some 3.5 years after my surgery. You might expect poor night vision, with these rings or halos, but oddly enough I am very comfortable and confident in my night driving vision, in large part due to the sharpness of my focus. The instrument panel is crisp and clear, even at night (although it is a bit farther away than arm's reach for me).

I do notice some sensitivity to glare and reduced contrast sensitivity in the presence of intense backlighting conditions. If I face the sun and talk with someone, I can see him or her clearly, but if I hold up my hand to shield my eyes from the glare, I notice an increase in the contrast and density of colors and the vision becomes noticeably more comfortable. Oddly, I cannot remember for certain if I noticed this even before the surgery, but I believe it is more apparent now. Maybe a YAG would reduce that effect somewhat. Shortly after the surgery we had a power outage at our house, and I was going to use a candle to light my way downstairs to retrieve a flashlight. I was startled to notice that due to the glare, the only thing I could see was the candle light itself, with its rings and parallel lines of light. Only when I held the light behind me to the side did it illuminate the stairs enough for me to see where I was going. I have not repeated this experiment since then, but it is my perception that the effect would not be quite as troublesome now.

I function in the office without glasses almost completely. I can read the patient's chart with moderate room light and read the numbers off the phoropter with only modest effort. I need glasses only to read the faded print-out of correspondence produced at the end of the useful life of the ink cartridge. Certainly, bold contrast greatly improves my near ability. I use loupes routinely for minor office surgery. I use +2.00 readers and sit fairly close for lid plastics cases. Otherwise, I enjoy spectacle independence for the most part. I usually bring readers with me and find that even when I can read something without glasses I will sometimes use the readers anyway. The print is bolder and better focused, and I can expend less concentration and effort. As an added bonus, my intraocular pressure dropped into the low teens after the cataract surgery, the pigment dispersion has stopped, and I have much less concern about the possibility of pigmentary glaucoma.

After being highly myopic since the age of 7 or so, I am now enjoying all the delights that your patients have been telling you about. It is not perfect vision; I wish I could read even better without the "fuzzy" appearance to the print, and I would prefer not as much glare with backlighting conditions. All in all, I am very happy with my decision and implant the Crystalens myself as a result of my own personal experience. Having your vision corrected like this is a life-changing experience for which I am truly grateful. It gives me even greater satisfaction to do my job with the knowledge that we can affect such a profound improvement in the vision and the lifestyle of our patients. We are truly fortunate.

CHAPTER 88

HOW I SEE WITH THE TECNIS MF AND REZOOM

R. Lee Harman, MD, FACS

The Conquering of Presbyopia

It has been stated many times over that the last refractive frontier was the conquering of presbyopia. "Was" is the appropriate word because options available to the presbyope of 2007 have dramatically improved with the recent marriage of corneal laser surgery with multifocal lens technology. As a practicing refractive and anterior segment surgeon of some 29 years, I know; in January of 2007 I opted for refractive lens exchange utilizing the latest in mixed-lens, multifocal technology. My story follows.

Scleral Expansion Bands

I have often said that I would not do any "cutting edge" procedure that I did not believe in enough to have done for myself, my friends, and family. As a manifest hyperope, I tried monovision with contact lenses. In the lanes, monovision worked fine but I discovered that my right eye was so fiercely dominant that the reading lens had to be worn in my right eye. By the end of clinic, I was ready to shed the contact and return to spectacle correction. Dozens of reading glasses were stashed hither and yonder but I finally graduated to bifocals, followed by trifocals as my hyperopia and presbyopia progressed.

An early adopter of new technologies, I embraced scleral expansion band surgery. I traveled to Mexico to do 4 carefully selected patients from my practice. Holding true to my word, I had the bands inserted in my own eyes, becoming 1 of 3 US ophthalmologists who can personally relate their experiences with this technology. Obviously, surgery on one's own eyes is not taken lightly and my decision followed extensive study of and belief in Dr. Schachar's revised theory of accommodation. I personally received the benefit predicted by the surgery but the positive effects of improved reading were short lived. By about 18 months, the improved accommodative amplitudes waned in myself and my patients. I removed the bands from my patients without untoward effect and had them removed from my own eyes. My refractive error and presbyopic status was unchanged by the experience once the bands were removed.

Multifocal Lens Implants: Zonular Refractive, Diffractive, and Pseudoaccommodating

Five years after my experience with scleral expansion band technology and 12 after my initial use of the Array multifocal lens (Advanced Medical Optics, Santa Ana, CA), I first seriously considered multifocal lens implants for my own eyes. The lens types had evolved into basically three: zonal refractive, diffractive, and pseudoaccommodating. An active aviator, having excellent vision is everything (but no less so for all patients). The Dell Survey that matches patient needs and desires to one multifocal lens or another, suggested that I was NOT a good candidate for ANY multifocal lens because I fell into the "precision-oriented," "high-maintenance," "approach with great caution" category of the chart. (My practice partners would agree.)

From an optical standpoint my aviator's bilateral 20/15 – J1 vision was achieved with +1.75 −0.50 × 090 OD and +1.50 − 0.25 × 120 OS refractions and +2.25 reading adds. This made me an ideal multifocal implant patient because I could neither see near or far without spectacle correction. My ocular and general health exam was otherwise normal notwithstanding scleral expansion band surgical scars. My corneas, Ks, retina, and so on, were all normal. Minimal 1 to 2+ nuclear sclerosis of the lens had not yet affected my vision but was present despite years of using UV 400 filters and anti-oxidant vitamins. With the exception of my expectations I was a decent candidate for the refractive lens exchange.

The question was—which lens? Rick Milne, MD, of Columbia, SC was among the first to address the mix or match question and convinced me of the technical rationale of mixing implants even though it went against my own practice of recommending symmetrical IOLs for my own patients. I was finally swayed by the happiness quotient of our own mixed IOL patients, who typically received the zonal refractive ReZoom lens (Advanced Medical Optics) in their dominant eye as the first surgery, followed by the diffractive ReSTOR lens (Alcon, Fort Worth, TX) in the nondominant eye 2 weeks later. We offer bilateral ReZoom IOLs for those with appropriate pupil sizes, but we use bilateral ReSTOR IOLs less often owing to markedly reduced intermediate vision. When we do, it is after a thorough discussion about limited intermediate vision. With my own needs as a pilot, I therefore opted for mixed IOL surgery. The excellent intermediate vision of the ReZoom would permit me to see instruments and gauges essentially at arm's length (also considered to be computer vision) and a diffractive lens, such as the ReSTOR or Tecnis multifocal (Advanced Medical Optics), would work well for the small print and low contrast of the cockpit charts, particularly under the variety of lighting conditions encountered. My "small beady" hyperopic eyes with 2.5 to 3.0 mm pupils also influenced the decision because I would be unlikely to achieve the precision that I needed to read with the ReZoom. Therefore, despite my experience(s) with monovision, I opted for a mixed IOL strategy, placing the ReZoom in my very dominant right eye and an AMO Tecnis multifocal in my left eye.

Surgeon as Patient Sheds Light on Multifocal Lens Outcome

I am now 10 months postoperative and extremely pleased with my new vision. I gloat and generally make a nuisance of myself to my friends and colleagues, telling them about my new vision with multifocals (watching them in their spectacle corrections while I enjoy the vision of a 20-year-old emmetrope!). I have not worn glasses of any type since my first surgery and I would never opt to go back to them. I have passed my aviation flight physical for the first time in nearly 20 years with the "glasses required for distance and near" limitation removed. I have lived my life with all the usual daily tasks performed without glasses and without the need to look for brighter light. I read menus for my friends in any lighting situation. I point out airplanes in the sky at great distances. I can jog or walk down stairs without worrying about foot falls or missing a step. In short, I see with precision and facility like I used to. I really have turned back the clock.

Now, as Mr. Paul Harvey would say, "The Rest of the Story." Right eye: 20/15, J3 at 40 centimeters, J5 at 20 centimeters. Refraction OD: +0.25 −0.50 × 170 (spherical equivalent plano.). Left eye: 20/15, J5 at 40 centimeters, J1+ in a band at 20 to 30 centimeters. Refraction OS: plano −0.50 × 119 (spherical equivalent −0.25 D). To the victor goes the spoils!

Now the price: Live by the Sword, Die by the Sword! Eight procedures (if you count 2 punctal plug procedures) over a 3-month period as follows: Despite extremely careful preoperative biometry my lens implants like to reside 600 µm posterior to the intended intraocular position (small, beady eyes). This led to a TWO (count them) TWO D hyperopic surprise in my dominant right eye (20/50, J 10 vision postoperative day 1). At 72 and 96 hours the vision and refraction remained essentially unchanged. At week 1, the lens was removed and exchanged with a power-adjusted ReZoom lens, obtaining a 20/25, J3

postoperative day one result. One week later, my left eye was implanted with a power adjustment based on nearly identical biometries and the unplanned hyperopic outcome experienced in my right eye. Postoperative day one OS: 20/20, J1 with a final and persistent refraction at 10 months of plano −0.50 × 119. At 8 weeks, a yttrium-aluminum-garnet (YAG) capsulotomy was performed for my left due to glare vision OS under certain lighting conditions. This was not relieved by the YAG (more about that in a moment under diffractive lens "waxy" or "gauze-like" vision). Vision and refraction OD at 3 months: 20/25−, J5 with -0.25 - 0.75 x 090 (spherical equivalent −0.62 D). At 4 months, PRK right eye for final vision at 10 months of 20/15, J3 with +0.25 −0.50 ×170 (spherical equivalent plano). Two incidental punctal occlusion procedures with plugs, inferior canaliculi.

Binocular vision at 10 months 20/15+, J1 at 20 to 30 centimeters primarily left eye; J5 at 40 centimeters primarily right eye. The reading differences between my 2 eyes at near improves in dim illumination as my right pupil enlarges to uncover the near reading add of the ReZoom lens. I can also achieve this by pharmacologically dilating my right eye. I am considering a laser pupilloplasty in the future (if I can talk my surgeon(s) into it). My subjective reading speed and comfort is better than experienced preoperatively as a former +2.00 hyperope using a monovision contact in my non-dominant left eye. My overall subjective reading speed is not as fast as it was in trifocals or wearing a monofocal contact lens in my dominant right eye but is improving with practice. This is because my very dominant right eye interferes with reading, particularly if I am tired, less attentive, or trying to read in dim or less than high-contrast lighting conditions. My best (J1+) reading is in a 10-cm band starting at about 20 centimeters and is independent of lighting, which is to say, if a presbyope wearing spectacles can read in the available light, so can I. The same is true for pre-presbyopes. If they can function or read in the available light, so can I. My cockpit and computer vision is excellent and I am usually word processing with #12 font size.

At about 6 weeks, I noticed an unusual glare from my diffractive Tecnis multifocal IOL in the left eye. This only occurred (then) and occurs now when the object of regard is back-lit by a large luminous source such as bright sky or sunshine through a picture window. It is not point source glare but large-scale background luminance that "softens" the view. It is only noticeable when covering and comparing eyes, right to left and it is definitely associated with the diffractive lens in my left eye. Some have referred to this as a waxy or gauze-like quality to the vision; it is not debilitating or a problem of any kind, but it is a difference between the 2 lenses. It proved unrelated to the posterior capsule and did not improve subsequently with a YAG capsulotomy. Place a single drop of Pred Forte in one of your eyes, blink a dozen times, wait 5 minutes and compare eyes: the sheen caused by the diluted prednisolone acetate suspension in your tear film will approximate the qualitative difference between the Tecnis diffractive lens and the ReZoom refractive lens when a large-area of background luminance overpowers a proximal object of regard.

Glare: I do not experience any except as noted earlier. Halos! A different story entirely and present for both eyes from day one. As advertised, the process of neuroadaptation reduced the phenomenon for me on about a weekly basis. Driving prior to the lens exchange for my right eye was very exciting and improved markedly when the lens of a more appropriate power was implanted a week later. With the implantation of my second eye, the halos intensified. Being a "cup half full" kind of guy, I knew to expect them, knew they would improve with time and hence, was not in the least concerned about them. Nevertheless, patient informed consent and prior discussions about the halo phenomenon are essential. If the halos are encountered without prior explanation (and/or warning) they would be indeed worrisome, even debilitating beyond distraction. Knowing to expect them really allowed a measure of enjoyment to their presence, because they are indeed quite beautiful. After careful analysis, I noted that the quality of the halos varied with residual refractive error and the light source. Halos were most prominent in my right eye when I became an unexpected (surprise!) 2-D hyperope. When the lens was exchanged a week later, the halos dramatically improved. They improved even further when (3 months later) my −0.62 residual spherical equivalent refractive error was converted by photorefractive keratectomy (PRK) to plano. So, the visual disturbances are affected by residual refractive error. As to light sources, point sources, like the popular white Christmas lights, were surrounded by a faint globe of light, not unlike placing a candle in a small fish bowl. Brighter, more intense lights were surrounded by true halos, which varied with the time of day (most prominent at dusk/twilight). They also varied with the distance I was from the source: the further away, the larger the halo; the closer to the source, the smaller the halo until at some variable distance (closer), the halo disappears altogether into the source of bright light. By way of example, headlight halos at three-quarters of a mile distance combined to encircle the entire car in a single ring about twice the width of the car. At a half-mile distance, the large single halo diverged into 2 separate halos centered around each headlight and overlapped in the middle of the car or truck's hood. The closer the light source approached, the halo reduced in diameter until at some closer distance (about 100 feet), the halos converged with the light source and essentially went away. The quality of each halo stayed the same during the approach to the light source but the width of the halo reduced in a constant relationship to the overall diameter. In other words, the "doughnut" of light surrounding each central light source reduced in both diameter and width until it finally disappeared within the light source. It also appeared that the point of halo-collapse into the approaching light source occurred further and further away from my eyes with the passage of time. Similarly, the intensity of the halo diminished with time so that at 10 months postoperative, I do not notice the halos except when looking for them (neuroadaptation?). The halos are still there but I have to look for them.

The quality of the individual halo produced by the ReZoom refractive lens is that of a halo or ring you might see around a light source in thick fog. The halo ring appears like interrupted, overlapping soft radial lines or spokes, which are too numerous to count. There is no other "fog" in the vicinity, just the darkness of night or the illumination by the light. Except for the halo, the rest of the scotopic scene is "normal" with no discernible missing information. The halo is added information, not subtractive.

The quality of the individual halo produced by the Tecnis diffractive lens is different. The "doughnut" of light is the same width as that from the refractive lens but the lighted area is made up of closely packed radial lines of sparkling, tiny diamonds. They, too, diminish with proximity to my eyes and eventually coalesce within the originating light source just as occurs in the ReZoom refractive eye. Similarly, the diffractive halos are additive and the surrounding scotopic scene is "normal."

The Importance of Patient Counseling and Informed Consent

If one is properly prepared in advance, both halo types can best be described as entertaining. If not properly forewarned and especially in the early adaptive phase, the halos could be problematic. Because they are so interesting and pretty to see, they are quite distracting, to the point that driving might be challenging. Recall that I went without spectacle correction from postoperative day 1 of my first surgery and drove on postoperative day 2. I also flew my plane early in the postoperative period and because I was interested in the visual phenomena, I actually flew at night with my instructor pilot in the fourth week. (The Federal Aviation Administration restricts commercial pilots for 90 days to allow for neuroadaptation to occur.) The cockpit and chart environment presented no problems; the landing environment, particularly taxing, was distracting due to the beauty of each blue taxi light surrounded by a blue globe-like glow. Finding the parking spot on a blackened, moonless night was inconsequential.

Halos are a distinct part of this generation of multifocal lenses. They are beautiful to see but in the early adaptation period, could be dangerous due to the visual distraction they present. As advertised, the halos have greatly diminished for me with time but at 10 months are still present if I look for them. For me they have been inconsequential and I will miss them should they eventually disappear entirely.

Conclusion

I could have traveled anywhere in the world to have my surgery done. I selected my 2 partners, however, inviting each to do an eye. I am not foolish; I have participated with them in the clinic and mentored them in surgery. They are truly gifted and talented practitioners. We practice in the small, provincial town of Arlington, WA, located between Seattle and the Canadian border. If my partners were not good enough to do the eyes of "the boss," why did I invite them to join me in Arlington? Thus, the story of my experience has been a "work in progress" but at this point I see with the vision of a 20 year old, or nearly so. Certainly there is not anything as good as 20-year-old standard equipment vision but multifocal lens implants certainly come close. I am thrilled with my new multifocal vision and I would never go back to spectacle correction. I owe a debt of thanks to my partners and staff, who have made multifocals a reality for me and the people of our community.

How I See with Mixed Multifocals

Anonymous

David F. Chang, MD posed several questions to a cataract and refractive surgeon who had undergone refractive lens exchange with mixing of ReSTOR and ReZoom. The surgeon wished to remain anonymous.

Describe Why You Underwent Mixed ReSTOR (RS)/ReZoom (RZ) Implantation

I had bilateral radial keratotomy (RK) in the early 1990s, and then had laser in situ keratomileusis (LASIK) 10 years ago for residual myopia and astigmatism. The onset of presbyopia symptoms occurred later than one might have expected. I suppose this might have been due to some asphericity of my corneas. By the age of 48, however, I needed readers all the time and in March 2006, at the age of 52, I decided to have a refractive lens exchange with a ReSTOR intraocular lens (IOL) in my left eye. I had kept all my medical records including the pre-RK refraction and K readings for each eye. I calculated my own IOL power using the Holladay IOL Consultant using the "K bypass method."

Initially, I had a large experience implanting only ReSTOR/ReSTOR in my own patients. I subsequently gained some experience with implanting the ReZoom IOL as well. I have observed that ReZoom/ReZoom patients are often not happy with their reading vision. On the other hand, ReSTOR/ReSTOR patients often complain of poor reading ability in dim illumination and either difficult or absent intermediate vision. I was a late adopter to mixing multifocal IOLs, but this approach has turned out to be very successful in my own patients. During the past 6 months virtually all of my patients have received ReSTOR/ReZoom! Once I noticed that my right eye had became presbyopic it was therefore an easy decision to choose a ReZoom IOL for my dominant right eye, which underwent a refractive lens exchange in September 2007.

At the time of this writing (December 2007) my manifest refraction is +0.50 − 1.50 × 57 (OD) and +0.25-0.75 × 116 (OS). I am now 20/20 uncorrected in both eyes at distance and near, and can sit as far away from my desktop computer as I need to read. Actually, in the exam room I am usually behind the scribe reading the chart over her shoulder with no problem, and can read a drug insert. I really am not at all bothered by glare and halos. My pupil diameters as measured by the Procyon are:

- Scotopic (0.04 lux) 6.8 mm (R); 7.28 mm (L)
- Mesopic low (0.40 lux) 3.85 mm (R); 4.20 mm (L)
- Mesopic high (4.0 lux) 3.02 mm (R); 3.10 mm (L)

I do have a little astigmatism, which can be tweaked in a couple months, but it does not really prevent me from reading or operating. I did require a yttrium-aluminum-garnet (YAG) capsulotomy in the ReSTOR eye at 3 months (the haze came on very quickly) and within several months following the ReZoom eye implantation as well.

Describe Your Uncorrected Vision

With both eyes open, I see just fine at distance, near (even reading in dim illumination) and can read the fine print of the Vigamox (Alcon) drug insert. If I close my left (ReSTOR) eye I can notice a slight ghosting of letters at near, which is probably my astigmatism, but I am not really symptomatic and I function just fine for surgery, and so on. I will probably have a LASIK or photorefractive keratectomy (PRK) touch up in the next 6 months when my schedule allows it.

The binocular reading vision is many times better than monocular reading, and it gets better month by month. There is truly something to the neural processing that we hear about in lectures. I have no problem reading in a dimly lit restaurant, but of course read better with more light. I can read printed material in the dimly lit exam lane. The only time I will pick up a pair of readers is to remove a chalazion or lid lesion, or in the operating room when I perform an eyelid procedure. I can perform the entire Intralasik procedure without spectacles. Overall, I consider my vision to be quite remarkable, and am spectacle independent.

Describe the Difference in Intermediate Vision Between the Two Eyes

After the left ReSTOR implant, and before the right ReZoom IOL, I had to hold reading material close and I had to get pretty close to the computer to read it. For example, I could not sit behind my scribe and see the computer monitor in the exam room. She had to move aside for me to get close enough to read the computer screen. Since the right ReZoom was implanted, I can sit with my nose 6 inches from the screen and read it, and move slowly away and still read everything until I am 3 feet from the computer screen.

Describe Any Difference in Visual Quality between the Two Eyes

I have a ReSTOR Natural (yellow tint) in the left eye and clear ReZoom in the right eye. I have absolutely no difference in color perception between the eyes. I have heard a few patients with RS/RZ comment about seeing "yellow" in one eye for a few weeks, but I did not experience this. With my astigmatic correction in my right eye the quality of vision is the same. The intermediate vision is better with both eyes open and not as good with either eye alone, and this is also noticed with near reading. The quality of the distance vision is the same with either the ReSTOR or ReZoom.

Compare the Kinds of Halos That Are Seen at Night Between the ReSTOR and ReZoom Eyes

I had halos around lights at night for about a month in each eye. My night vision has been excellent after 1 month from either IOL, and I currently have absolutely no halos around lights at night. The ReSTOR caused several thin circles of light around a headlight or streetlight. The ReZoom just produced more of a glare around a headlight. Neither has persisted in my case, which is interesting because I have had prior corneal refractive surgery (RK and LASIK). As I recall, the night vision was worse for a few months with RK than with either IOL. It is difficult for me to understand why an occasional patient really complains about halos—their pupils or eye optics must be different.

Are There Patients in Whom You Would Not Implant or Mix ReSTOR/ReZoom?

The patient's personality is important. If he or she appears clinically depressed, have many somatic complaints, take more than one antidepressant—watch out. At every visit this patient will have a new complaint. If a patient is taking an antidepressant but appears otherwise healthy and well treated, he or she is a good patient postoperatively. I avoid implanting multifocal IOLs in commercial truck drivers who drive at night or commercial airline pilots. I have corrected many private pilots and they love being able to read charts, see their instruments, and see well in the distance.

What Insights Does Your Personal ReSTOR/ReZoom Experience Offer About Complaints That Some Patients Have?

Visual imbalance—I was one of those patients! Yes, I had visual imbalance, which I understood and just put up with

until I had my second eye performed. I waited until I saw many happy postoperative patients with the RS/RZ combination before making my decision. Hardly any patient has postoperative complaints unless they have early posterior capsule opacification (PCO) or residual refractive error. I developed early PCO within 1 to 2 months of surgery and had a YAG capsulotomy in both eyes. Even a small amount of PCO significantly impairs the reading vision in both eyes, so I am very liberal in performing YAG procedures after multifocal IOL implantation.

If you see a patient with postoperative fluctuation of vision/refraction, or who is unhappy with their vision in the absence of posterior capsule opacification or macula disease, it is usually a dry eye. One should perform a Schirmer's test to document the dry eye, insert punctal plugs, and prescribe ReStasis, viscous artificial tears, and fish oil capsules. Treat any blepharitis/meibomian gland dysfunction that may be affecting tear stability. It is best to perform a Schirmer's test preoperatively on all patients over age 40.

Please Describe Your Own Refractive IOL Practice and Your Current Thinking About Mixing Multifocal IOLs

About half of my patients are cataract patients having multifocal IOLs, and the other half are refractive lensectomy patients who want to be rid of reading glasses or bifocals. Many of the latter patients have had prior RK, LASIK, PRK, conductive keratoplasty (CK), and they seem to do just fine. One must be willing and capable of performing a LASIK or PRK enhancement 6 weeks after implanting multifocal IOLs, or at 3 months if prior refractive surgery has been performed. Patients must expect to need temporary astigmatic correction following multifocal IOL implantation until the laser touch up is performed.

I have converted many patients from monovision with contact lenses or prior LASIK to ReZoom/ReSTOR, and all of them like it better. There are only 2 types of patients who may tend to be unhappy with mixing ReSTOR/ReZoom. Mild myopes in their mid-forties who never wore bifocals and instead removed their glasses to read may complain that the quality of reading vision was better before surgery when he or she took off the distance glasses. The second type of unhappy patient is the one that performs a visual task further away than the normal desk top computer distance. Be sure to take a work/hobby history at the time of the consultation.

SECTION VII

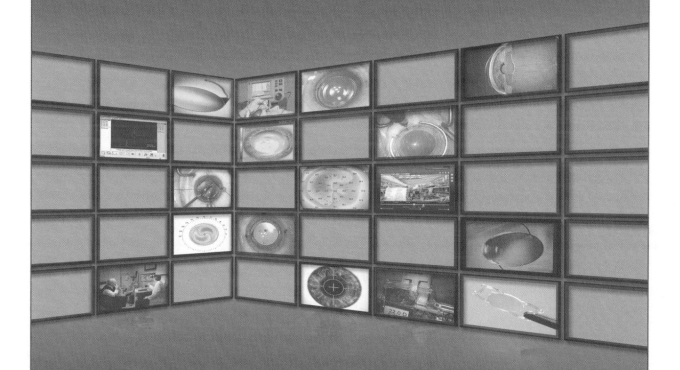

Patient Selection and Education

CHAPTER 89

THE MINDSET OF THE REFRACTIVE **IOL** PATIENT

Kerry K. Assil, MD and William K. Christian, MD

To improve results with multifocals and achieve success, surgeons should listen closely to their patients' needs and desires.

Surgeons should consider the mindsets of their staff as well as the prospective refractive intraocular lens (IOL) patient in order to achieve a successful multifocal IOL experience for everyone involved. These dual mindsets in addition to other factors, such as proper preoperative patient selection, discussions with patients, and proper surgical planning, are integral parts of optimal outcomes with multifocal lenses (Figure 1).

Talking to Patients

The biggest disconnect between the doctor's office and the patient is that often the doctors and their office staff believe that the patients are paying this premium (or surcharge) for receiving a multifocal lens or some other premium IOL. However, that is not the case. In actuality, the patients are paying a premium to be able to see without glasses. They are paying a surcharge for the lifestyle liberation.

Therefore, the first thing that needs to come into play is the discussion with a patient about lifestyle liberation. The wording we use to talk with patients is critical. It is important for the surgeon and office staff to make sure that they are not overly technical early on by explaining the different lens types and different types of options.

Instead, after it has been established that a patient will have cataract surgery we should simply ask the question:

"Would you like to see everything without glasses?"

Not: "Would you like to receive a multifocal intraocular lens?"

Not: "Would you like to see up close and far away better?"

Not: "Would you like to be less dependent on glasses?"

Instead just simply ask "Would you like to see everything without glasses?" Then wait and let the patient drive the desirability portion of the discussion.

The key words in that phrase are *everything* and *without glasses* because on average I do not find that patients who have a reduction in their dependency on their glasses end up highly satisfied.

Once the common goal is understood, the practice needs to do an internal assessment to determine what systems need to be set up in order to be able to deliver on that expectation. Just implanting the multifocal lens is not enough to ensure spectacle independence and when these patients require glasses afterward they will not be very happy with their surgeon. Unfortunately, this type of experience has led many surgeons to be discouraged to the point of deciding to stop providing this service.

Of course, it should also be very clear at the end of the discussion that no promises can be made to the patient. Instead the surgeon and patient can talk about reasonable expectations and have a discussion of the percentages with regard to likely outcomes.

A Successful System

Surgeons must first select an appropriate patient, who meets the medical criteria (see later). This ideal patient is also someone who is motivated and excited about the idea of seeing without glasses, and who understands the procedure and has realistic expectations.

Next, very precise biometry is needed to determine the appropriate lens power for each eye. Then, an assessment for lens selection is needed. For example, would this particular patient be best suited for a diffractive multifocal, a refractive multifocal, a pseudoaccommodating lens or is custom matching (in which two different types of multifocal IOLS are used) the best option?

In our practice, we only consider the pseudoaccommodating lenses in a setting in which a patient is highly glare phobic and who has specifically requested such a lens. The lay public is not sophisticated enough to recognize that as the lens capsule fibroses the accommodation that comes with this lens type will be lost over time.

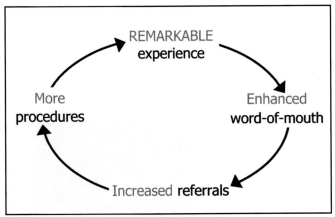

Figure 1. The Cycle of Great Patient Experience. Happy 1st and 2nd generation multifocal IOL patients will in turn educate others, saving you time on the education process and allowing you to spend more quality time with your patients. This is how we expect to grow our practice over time.

Table 1

PATIENT INCLUSION
IDEAL CANDIDATES FOR PCIOL

- Medicare age group
- Presbyopic hyperopes and high myopes
- Not big night drivers
- No retinal pathology
- Avoid pessimists

The vast majority of our patients are going to get a diffractive or a refractive multifocal lens or a combination of these lenses because they are designed to ensure multifocality and the results are therefore more predictable and reproducible.

Which Lens or Combination Is Best?

In general, if the patient has medium-sized pupils, the patient can receive a refractive IOL in both eyes aiming for Plano in the distance dominant eye and about a −0.5 or −0.75 D in the near dominant eye. For example, this would be true with a photopic pupil that measures 3.2 mm to 4.0 mm (as the photopic pupil diameter is similar to the miotic pupil diameter in the reading state). If the patient has either very small pupils or very large pupils then implanting a refractive lens in both eyes would not likely achieve satisfactory results. Patients with very large pupils might potentially be bothered by significant halos or glare (at night) with bilaterally implanted refractive lenses. Patients with small pupils (under most lighting conditions) will not be able to enjoy reading as the near add portion of the refractive IOL will be covered by the iris.

In our own clinical experience, we have found that there are very few settings in which a diffractive IOL in both eyes will result in optimally satisfied patients. One of the challenges with these lenses is that if the pupils are very small the distance acuity becomes less crisp. For example, when driving in the day-

---

Table 2

DOS AND DON'TS: RESULTS

"Rolls Royce" expectations
- Must achieve excellent results. Period.
- Use tight inclusion parameters:
  - No ocular pathology
  - Lens available in their dioptric range
  - Residual error manageable
  - Patient not prone to "underachieving"
  - Aware of glare

---

time far away road signs will not appear very clear. Conversely, when the pupils are very large, such as when trying to read a menu in a dimly lit restaurant, then the vast majority of light rays are committed to distance and they blur out the near image. Thus these patients get frustrated and have a hard time reading a menu no matter how close or far away they hold it. Working at computer distance can also be problematic. (This reflects my experience with currently approved multifocal IOLS in the United States. The Tecnis MF [Advanced Medical Optics, Santa Ana, CA], with which we have conducted clinical trials and which is currently available in Europe, might over come some [but not all] of the deficits.)

Custom Matching, or Custom Lens Selection, is a process of evaluating a patient's lifestyle and visual needs and then matching the best lenses accordingly. This approach provides the optimal functional vision for most patients. For example, for patients who receive custom matching in my clinic, the refractive lens is placed in the distance dominant eye (aiming for Plano to −0.25 D), and the diffractive lens in the near dominant eye (aiming for Plano to +0.25).

Patient Inclusion/Exclusion

In the multifocal lens setting, it is best to steer clear of unrealistic patients or patients with a skewed sense of entitlement (Table 1). These are not necessarily pessimistic patients or underachievers. In my experience, it is the patients with a skewed sense of entitlement who are unhappy no matter what service you are performing.

In addition, other patients to avoid in this setting are those who have significant pathology in their visual pathway that would inherently handicap their contrast acuity. These include patients with an extremely dry ocular surface, severe map dot finger print dystrophy of the corneal epithelium or other corneal epitheliopathies, opacities in the corneal stroma, advanced corneal endothelial dystrophy, significant vitreous opacities, such as large and highly symptomatic vitreous floaters, maculopathy (hypertensive retinopathy, diabetic retinopathy, and macular degeneration that is manifesting itself in some compromise of potential 20/20 best corrected acuity). Patients with very advanced glaucoma (although not moderate or medically controlled glaucoma) should also be excluded. These patients may experience critical loss of contrast acuity and potentially some best corrected acuity as well (Table 2).

Table 3

DOS AND DON'TS: SURGEON

Do it yourself
- Surgeon should be active in patient exams
- 60 year old versus 30 year old or nursing home patient
- Accustomed to doctor relationship

Table 4

ASTIGMATISM CONTROL

- Astigmatic Keratotomy (AK)
- Limbal Relaxing Incisions (LRI)
  - 550 µ extension
  - Genesis Diamond Blade
  - Nomograms

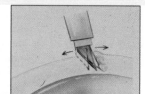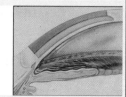

Postoperative Procedures and Follow-Up

Another important component of a successful multifocal IOL practice is the surgeon's personalized follow-up with the patient and also the capability to perform subsequent proce-

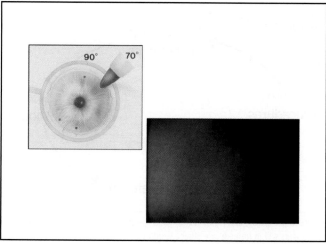

Figure 2. Astigmatism control.

dures, such as limbal relaxing incisions, laser enhancement, IOL exchange, a piggyback lens procedure, YAG capsulotomies, and/or pupilloplasty (Table 3).

For example, performing limbal relaxing incisions at the time of surgery to sufficiently debulk the astigmatism allows for patients to have reasonably good uncorrected vision in the immediate postoperative period (Table 4 and Figure 2). Surgeons should also have the capability of doing laser enhancement—either laser in situ keratomileusis (LASIK) or Epi-LASIK or photorefractive keratectomy—to treat any residual refractive error. The surgeon should be ready to perform a YAG capsulotomy at a relatively early stage postoperatively to treat early capsular opacity.

These are some of the main objectives that the clinic needs to commit to in order to live up to our patients' expectations of visual quality from multifocal refractive IOLs.

CHAPTER 90

THE MINDSET OF THE REFRACTIVE IOL PATIENT

Alan B. Aker, MD

It is important to realize that each patient is different, so it might be better to consider, not the mindset, but rather, the various mindsets of our patients. When considering implanting a premium intraocular lens (IOL), we must recognize a number of basic truths about patients. The first of these is that patients represent a host of personalities, and some have personality disorders as well. Some people are easy to please whereas others are obsessive in nature and extremely difficult to please. Some patients are like land mines—the danger they pose is hidden from view. And here we are simply considering the various personality types—we have not even begun to consider multiple other factors such as preoperative refractive error, prior eye history, financial means, age, occupation, and hobbies, just to name a few.

So how can we accurately assess the mindset of that patient sitting before us? Communication is one of our key tools. It may be a challenge, but there are ways to ensure that you effectively communicate with each patient before surgery. Communicating clearly and concisely with each patient before surgery must be a priority!

Communication must be a dialogue. For this to be effective, we must take control of the discussion and use it to educate the patient on what their vision will be like with a premium IOL. It is important to gain an understanding of your patient's expectations and you must be certain that both you and the patient have the same understanding regarding what their postoperative vision will be. We must also be able to discern what the patient is saying in both words and body language.

What Does the Patient Want?

Almost all of our patients want "perfect vision" following "perfect surgery" performed by a compassionate and "perfect surgeon." The patient also would like the surgery to painless, without any bruising or other postoperative "complications." The patient wants the vision to be outstanding as soon as pos-

sible. And, of course, it would also help if the surgery could be free or at minimal cost. This description is perhaps a bit severe, but it probably fits a great number, if not all, of our patients.

Truly the mindset of the each premium IOL patient is unique. Typically, their expectations are a function of a number of variables such as their refractive error, their age, and even external factors such as advertising of premium IOLs.

Preoperative Refraction

It is important to recognize that the preoperative refraction of our patients has a great deal to do with how happy they might be following surgery. Patients with significant myopia or hyperopia will typically be "wowed" by being brought to emmetropia with any IOL.

Hyperopic patients are the easiest to please. These are patients who have been living with a refractive error that has made them dependent upon glasses or contacts for virtually all tasks. Their uncorrected acuity makes them vulnerable in many settings. My hyperopic patients are quick to tell me they cannot differentiate between their shampoo and their conditioner in the shower. These patients are usually thrilled with postoperative emmetropia. And yet, these same patients will have high expectations for uncorrected intermediate and near vision because of the price tag associated with a premium IOL.

Myopic patients pose a greater challenge in terms of their near vision with a premium IOL. Their expectation is often influenced by the excellent uncorrected near acuity they experienced prior to developing cataracts. Because of this, it is very important to specifically address this subject with your myopic patients prior to surgery. They should be told upfront that their near vision will most likely not be as good as it was if they were a −3 myope. Your discussion should focus on your ability to provide great functional vision following surgery.

A Word of Caution Regarding Emmetropic Patients

Prior to the availability of premium IOLs, most of us have experienced the disappointment of emmetropes who suddenly found they needed a spectacle correction following cataract surgery. These patients are quick to educate us that, prior to the removal of their cataract, they never needed any correction for distance vision. They typically do not expect less than emmetropia following our surgery. For this reason, it is extremely important for us to be able to target and achieve emmetropia routinely in our patients.

Astigmatism is another challenge that must be recognized and discussed. Patients with astigmatism need to be educated regarding how this can impact their final outcome. It is important to discuss the amount of astigmatism and the various surgical remedies available. You must be comfortable performing limbal relaxing incisions (LRIs) or clear cornea relaxing incisions (CCRIs) as you move into premiums IOLs. Many surgeons have refined these techniques anticipating presbyopia-correcting (Pr-C) IOLs. It is important to know how much cylinder you can eliminate with your incisions. Patients with higher amounts of regular astigmatism should be counseled about the possibility of a bioptic procedure.

External Factors

Beyond preoperative refractive errors, there are a number of external factors that impact the mindset of our premium IOL patients. Encounters with friends who are either satisfied or dissatisfied with their Pr-C IOLs will have a significant impact. In addition, unrealistic promises made in the media by colleagues offering these IOLs will most certainly raise patient expectations. Whether through a discussion with a friend or viewing an advertisement on cable TV, our patients often come in with a bias about these lenses. Having said this, it should be obvious that we can help promote and protect this exciting aspect of ophthalmic surgery by exercising discretion in any advertising. Later in this chapter I will describe the steps we take to ensure that our patients leave feeling they have received good value for the fees charged for these premium IOLs.

The Whole Concept of Premium Products

One of the points we consistently stress with our patients is that "premium" does not imply "perfect." We explain the significant advantage these lenses have in being able to provide much more functional vision. However, we also explain that they should not expect perfect vision in every setting. This is a most important aspect of our patient education package. Once we have established this point, we go on to let the patient know that we will do everything possible to help them achieve the best possible results.

So it should be now be obvious that there are many factors that influence our patients' thinking about premium IOLs. Your role as the surgeon in dealing with these different mind-

sets is to level the playing field, establish reasonable expectations, and ensure the patient has heard and understood the information being conveyed by you and your staff.

I'd like to offer some important rules and measures we take to help ensure our success.

DON'T "SELL" PREMIUM IOLS

Your results and your happy premium IOL patients will do the selling for you. You and your staff members should be certain to explain this new capability of achieving great functional vision with each and every patient. As this is shared with patients, most will be curious about these Pr-C IOLs.

SET REALISTIC EXPECTATIONS

This is perhaps one of the most important aspects of dealing with premium IOL patients. Regardless of the many previously discussed variables there is one common expectation—the average patient wants their surgery to be perfect! To them, this means no discomfort or pain, no red lids or red eyes postoperatively, good vision on that first day following surgery, and no excuses from the surgeon in whom they have placed their trust. In light of this common mindset, what we tell our patients is most important. We must prepare them by setting realistic, achievable expectations, and then be sure they have heard and understood our discussion.

DON'T OVER PROMISE!!!

Regarding our premium IOL patients, it is absolutely imperative that we don't over promise. The clear road to success with these patients is to underpromise and over deliver. This can be achieved if you and your staff commit to a consistent and positive approach in all your discussions with your premium IOL patients. You and your staff must seize the initiative and proactively set patient expectations. Because this can be an excellent way of avoiding patients with unrealistic expectations, it is extremely important that this process is consistent with every patient. You must ensure that each and every patient accepts and embraces what they can realistically expect following surgery.

OUR DISCUSSION BEFORE SURGERY

Because of the patient education materials placed throughout our center as well as the inevitable interactions with our many postoperative premium IOL patients, our preoperative patients usually broach the subject of Pr-C IOLs. If a patient does not ask about these lenses, they are always discussed with our cataract patients. Failure to discuss these new IOLs is a mistake. You do not want to have one of your postoperative patients upset with you because you failed to offer them the option of a Pr-C IOL.

Prior to my preoperative evaluation, each patient has been made aware of the various IOL options by both a workup technician and one of our clinical optometrists. What I would like to stress here is that a consistent message is presented. As our technicians discuss the premium IOLs, they use a reading card provided by Eyeonics, Inc (Aliso Viejo, CA). They point out that with a standard IOL correcting their vision for distance, they will most likely need reading glasses to read everything on the card. They then explain that with the Crystalens (Eyeonics, Inc), all our patients achieve 10-point near vision without glasses. The technicians emphasize that this means they will be able to read magazines, hardcover books, and menus in restaurants without using glasses. In addition, they are told they can anticipate being able to see their cell phones and have excellent vision when using their computers.

Following the workup technician, one of our clinical optometrists examines the patient. At this point the various options are again discussed and the Eyeonics reading card is once again used. The patient's level of interest in the Crystalens is indicated on the chart to help make my evaluation more efficient.

My evaluation is a very forthright discussion of the Crystalens. Some of our patients ask about problems their friends have experienced with premium IOLs. These are almost always related to either quality of vision or glare and halo issues. At this point I will explain the difference between the multifocal IOLs (Array [Advanced Medical Optics, Santa Ana, CA], ReZoom [Advanced Medical Optics], and ReSTOR [Alcon, Fort Worth, TX]) and the Crystalens accommodating IOL. I discuss my experience with all these different IOLs as well as the earlier 3M diffractive multifocal IOL (St. Paul, MN).

I believe this is also an important part of our patient education package on these premium IOLs. Patients need to sense our comfort and confidence with the lens we will be implanting. An honest discussion of the history of this technology seems to put their minds at ease. Often a patient will ask me what I think they should do. I tell them that the choice has to be their own. I then mention that I have implanted the Crystalens in my family members and friends. I also tell them that if I were having surgery myself, the only lens I would have implanted would be the Crystalens. As I do this, I take this opportunity to once again explain what we describe as excellent functional vision—being able to read magazines, books, and menus, as well as use their computer and cell phone, all without glasses.

They are told that for tiny print like the phone book or stock quotes they might still need glasses, but in most settings they will be able to function very well spectacle free.

OUR EVALUATION AND DISCUSSION FOLLOWING SURGERY

We feel that it is extremely important to demonstrate the consistency of our message in the postoperative visits with our patients. To do this we fall back on the Eyeonics reading card, which is used at each visit. On their first postoperative visit, we usually can demonstrate 20/30 or better distance acuity and at least 10-point near vision. By their 1-week visit, they are usually in the 20/20 range and reading 8 points. The bottom line is that we have promised 10 points and our patients are typically achieving 8, 6, or even 4 points. This is demonstrated by our staff at each visit to ensure that our patients realize they have achieved what was promised—and more!

DEMONSTRATE THE VALUE OF THE PREMIUM IOL

To quickly and easily demonstrate that the premium IOL was worth the additional cost, simply have a few –2.00-D glasses in each examination room. Have the patient look at your reading card or a magazine and read. As they do this, slip on these glasses. We tell the patient that this is what their near vision would be like without the Pr-C IOL. The effect is dramatic and provides an excellent way of demonstrating the value of these IOLs.

In closing, we need to recognize that the mindset of the premium IOL patient is such that they typically expect more than we can deliver. To ensure your patients are satisfied, you and your staff must seize the initiative and proactively set patient expectations. It is essential that you communicate this effectively with each of your patients.

CHAPTER 91

THE MINDSET OF THE REFRACTIVE IOL SURGEON

Alan B. Aker, MD

I feel I would be remiss and the material presented in the preceding chapter would be incomplete without this discussion on the mindset of the surgeon. By this, I am referring to how we feel about our surgical abilities and our surgical outcomes with premium intraocular lenses (IOLs).

Your Abilities as a Surgeon

If you are going to participate in the presbyopia-correcting (Pr-C) IOL market, it is imperative that you have a clear and honest understanding of your capabilities as a surgeon. Are you able to consistently perform excellent surgery? What are your typical 1-day postoperative acuities? Can you effectively correct astigmatism with either limbal relaxing incisions (LRIs), clear cornea relaxing incisions (CCRIs), or combined with laser in situ keratomileusis (LASIK) or other excimer procedures? If you have a postoperative refractive surprise, are you comfortable performing lens exchanges?

What is your track record in achieving emmetropia? How are IOL power calculations performed? Do you have a team in place conducting ongoing outcomes analysis? Do you and your measurement team counsel patients who present greater challenges such as those who have had prior refractive surgery, those with high astigmatism, or patients with dense nuclear or PSC cataracts.

Your ability to perform will determine your ability to deliver. You have to be able to produce consistent, excellent, uncomplicated emmetropic results if you are going to successfully participate in the premium IOL market.

You must be able to do this if you are going to deliver what the premium IOL patient expects and deserves.

Your comfort level with your premium IOL results will be evident to your patients and will impact your staff as well.

So this actually has to do with the mindset of the patient, the surgeon, and his staff. The patient needs to sense the confidence the surgeon and his staff have in these new IOLs.

A Brief History of Our Experience With Premium IOLs

Years ago, my wife, Ann Kasten Aker, MD, and I were invited to participate in the 3M (St. Paul, MN) Vision Care Food and Drug Administration (FDA) study of the diffractive multifocal IOL. This was the first FDA study of a Pr-C IOL. Together we had the largest series of patients implanted with this lens and were encouraged by the study results. Though disappointed that 3M never got to market this lens, we did implant the Array IOL (Advanced Medical Optics, Santa Ana, CA) when it became available. Unfortunately, we felt we should discontinue using the Array lens because of patient complaints of halos and difficulty with lights while driving at night.

When the Crystalens (Eyeonics, Inc, Aliso Viejo, CA) became available, we quickly embraced this technology and were quite pleased with our results. Then we began to see patients returning with refractive shifts, which were usually myopic, despite near emmetropic early postoperative refractions. This was about the same time the troublesome "Z syndrome" presented in a number of our patients. Though we were able to correct these Z syndromes using the YAG laser, their occurrence combined with what we described as refractive instability caused us to cease using the Eyeonics Crystalens AT-45 and AT-45SE. Our reasons for discontinuing use of these IOLs was discussed with both Stuart Cumming, MD, the developer of the accommodating Crystalens, and Andy Corley, CEO of Eyeonics.

At about the same time, the multifocal IOLs became available following FDA approval. I initially implanted the Alcon (Fort Worth, TX) ReSTOR IOL, which was based on the 3M diffractive technology. This lens was, in fact, an improved diffractive IOL and provided very good near vision. Unfortunately, a number of our patients were bothered by quality-of-vision issues and the loss of their intermediate vision.

Still seeking a premium IOL that would provide consistent results and satisfy the demands of patients in the premium

IOL market, we decided to try the ReZoom IOL (Advanced Medical Optics, Santa Ana, CA). Our initial reaction to this lens was extremely positive. Once again, however, as the number of our patients implanted with this IOL increased, we had to deal with patient complaints.

These typically centered on problems with glare and halos. We encouraged our patients to "hang in there" and see if their difficulty would resolve over time. Unfortunately, I found myself performing IOL exchanges on patients after 6 to 18 months, despite excellent distance and very good near vision without correction.

As we continued to spend considerable chair time with these patients, our frustration mounted with these Pr-C IOLs. Our patients who had paid for a premium product were also challenged and frustrated in the face of these difficulties.

I am including this discussion in an attempt to be completely forthright in presenting my own experience. Our experience impacts our mindset as we present the option of a Pr-C IOL to our patients. In the midst of dealing with our unhappy patients with the multifocal IOLs, Eyeonics introduced the third version of their accommodating IOL, the Crystalens AT-50.

My principle desire at this point was to have an IOL I could feel confident about implanting in all my patients. I did not want to deal with refractive instability, quality of vision issues, or complaints of glare and halos.

After discussions with my staff, we decided to revisit the accommodating IOL and began implanting the Crystalens AT-50. Because of patient complaints and challenges seen with the other premium IOLs, our staff was hesitant and doubtful about this new IOL.

Staff and surgeon confidence in the technology is essential if your presentation is going to motivate a patient to request and pay for a premium IOL. They can sense our lack of confidence. I knew we had to overcome the concerns of our technicians and optometrists. They see themselves as patient advocates rather than a premium IOL sales force. I would have it no other way. Because of this, our early use of the Crystalens AT-50 was cautious and our results and patients' responses were carefully monitored.

Fortunately, we have been extremely pleased with the outcome. The Crystalens AT-50 is a consistent performer. We have not had to deal with any patient issues either early on or more than 1 year after implantation. Our patients interested in presbyopia correction usually come in asking for the Crystalens by name.

Having said all this, I would like to state that we do have a fair number of patients quite pleased with either ReSTOR or ReZoom IOLs. However, I do believe the accommodating technology has a significant advantage. Rather than splitting light or seeking to create two focal points, the Crystalens provides intermediate and near vision through anterior arching during accommodation. It basically seeks to copy God's design. John Sheets, MD, was one of the early proponents of "in the bag" placement of IOLs. When explaining the Sheets lens produced by 3M, he said it is best not to argue with God in terms of lens design and placement. For the same reason, I would go on record stating that I believe the future for correction of presbyopia will be in accommodating IOLs.

I have many friends using multifocals. The key thing is that you and your staff must be comfortable with your results and the level of satisfaction you are achieving with your patients.

Your Confidence in Premium IOLs

Beyond the comfort level you and your staff have regarding your surgical abilities, it is extremely important that you share a great deal of confidence in the premium IOLs you are implanting.

As discussed earlier, when we were dealing with "issues" at my eye center regarding our early premium IOL results, these concerns impacted our entire staff. It was not a question of my surgical ability, but rather issues relating to the premium IOLs we were using. We were concerned about our ability to deliver a consistent good result without postoperative issues, which patients quickly described as "complications." This loss of confidence resulted in our technicians and optometrists being reluctant to offer these new refractive IOLs. This reluctance persisted until the introduction of the Crystalens Five-0.

Your staff has to "buy in" to whatever technology you embrace. The degree to which they are able to do this will be a function of your surgical skill and the consistency of your patients' satisfaction. If you and your staff hear ongoing complaints from your patients regarding the quality of their vision or difficulty with halos and glare, you will find this will "spill over" into your discussion regarding these IOLs. As a result, patients will be aware that your premium IOL presentation lacks confidence. As surgeons we want a premium IOL that will enable us to consistently deliver great functional vision without any time-consuming postoperative concerns. Regardless of the type of Pr-C IOL you are using (accommodating or multifocal), you must have a high level of comfort with your ability to produce consistent good results if your presentation is to be convincing.

Great Wisdom Comes With Great Age

Finally, we need to recognize that we certainly have our own bias as we view our patients. We subconsciously make judgments based on their dress, their appearance, and their age.

I vividly recall a most instructive encounter with one of my elderly patients. As I entered the examination room, I noted from the chart that she was 94 years old. Because of her age, I did not even bring up the availability of premium IOLs. Finishing my evaluation, I told her that following her surgery, we anticipated that her uncorrected distance vision would be excellent and we would fit her with glasses for reading. She then told me she was hoping to get "that new lens" that would eliminate the need for reading glasses. My quick response in light of her age (my age bias) was that neither Medicare nor her insurance would pay for this special new lens. She said she was aware of this. I then informed her that the lens was quite expensive. At this, she smiled and gently admonished me saying, "I know Doctor, but we are talking about my eyesight which is a most precious gift." As I then explained the Crystalens to this patient, I also reflected on how great age is sometimes accompanied by great wisdom.

CHAPTER 92

SCREENING AND COUNSELING REFRACTIVE IOL PATIENTS

Steven J. Dell, MD

A few short years ago, it was not unusual for some surgeons to implant the same intraocular lens (IOL) in 95% of their patients. The decision of which IOL to use was only an issue in unusual cases or in those cases with inadequate capsular support. The available spectrum of presbyopia-correcting IOLs (Pr-C IOLs), aspheric, and spherical IOLs has completely changed this. Preoperative counseling has become infinitely more complex, and IOL inventory management has become a new challenge for ambulatory surgery centers and hospitals. In addition, the possibility of mistakenly inserting an unintended IOL has become much, much more likely.

With the anticipated arrival of the Tecnis multifocal, we will soon offer 4 completely different Pr-C IOL platforms to our patients. There are subsets of different styles of these IOLs within these platforms. For example, the AcrySof ReSTOR (Alcon, Fort Worth, TX) is available in tinted and nontinted versions, as a single-piece or 3-piece lens, and in spherical and aspheric configurations, with various combinations of these options. Soon there will also be differing AcrySof near powers from which to choose. The Eyeonics Crystalens (Aliso Viejo, CA) comes in both 4.5-mm and 5.0-mm versions with varying overall lengths. The ReZoom and Tecnis Multifocal from Advanced Medical Optics (Santa Ana, CA) round out this stable of lenses. There is no reason to think that the dizzying spectrum of available lenses will get any smaller in the future.

Since the optical characteristics of these lenses vary considerably, the patient's visual needs factor significantly in the decision tree of which lens to offer each patient. Each lens has its own unique constellation of advantages and disadvantages that is complicated even further by the fact that these lenses are often mixed with each other in the same patient. I quickly found that there was no practical way to discuss every possible permutation of lens choice with my patients in a timely fashion without a radical change to my patient work-up regimen. Endless discussions of all these lens choices left the patients bewildered and frozen with indecision. Other patients degenerated into an information-seeking spiral, resulting in several follow-up consultations that could only be described as highly reiterative.

I recognized that patients were much more interested in a visual outcome than a particular technology, so I began to focus on what they really wanted to achieve after surgery. A brief questionnaire was developed to asses these needs (Figure 1). In essence, it forces the patient to make some difficult choices regarding his or her visual priorities. This provides me with invaluable information, while simultaneously conveying the subtle message to the patient that all these IOL choices involve compromise.

After the patient watches a video introducing the concept of Pr-C IOLs, he or she is asked to fill out the questionnaire. A tremendous amount of information can be obtained by putting hundreds of patients through this stereotyped process. For example, when we perform applanation tonometry on our patients, we observe a spectrum of physical and psychological reactions from them during the testing process. These can range from nonchalance to abject horror. By providing this single largely uniform stimulus, we can observe the response and learn a great deal about our patients. By the same token, the ways in which patients fill out the questionnaire provide precious insights into their visual needs as well as their personalities. Some patients mark the form up in a fit of indecision, while others give outright contradictory responses. However, most will logically and thoughtfully outline what they would like to achieve postoperatively.

With the questionnaire completed, I perform my examination and consultation. The process has become relatively simple and quick. By the time the patient sees me, he or she generally has a very thorough understanding of the available options and, most importantly, he or she understands the concept of presbyopia. This allows us to converse fluently without having to establish a common vocabulary first. Some patients indicate that they have no desire to correct their presbyopia surgically. Others choose to remain nearsighted postoperatively and use distance correction. Many are not candidates

Figure 1. Cataract and refractive lens exchange questionnaire.

Date_____   Name_____

Cataract and Refractive Lens Exchange Questionnaire

The term "cataract" refers to a cloudy lens within the eye. When a cataract is removed, an artificial lens is placed inside the eye to take the place of the human lens that has become the cataract. Occasionally, clear lenses that have not yet developed cataracts are also removed to reduce or eliminate the need for glasses or contacts. If it is determined that surgery is appropriate for you, this questionnaire will help us provide the best treatment for your visual needs. It is important that you understand that many patients still need to wear glasses for some activities after surgery. Please fill this form out completely and give it to the doctor. If you have questions, please let us know and we will assist you with this form.

1. After surgery, would you be interested in seeing well **without glasses** in the following situations?
    Distance vision (driving, golf, tennis, other sports, watching TV)
    ___Prefer no **Distance** glasses.   ___ I wouldn't mind wearing **Distance** glasses.

    Mid-range vision. (computer, menus, price tags, cooking, board games, items on a shelf)
    ___Prefer no **Mid-range** glasses.   ___ I wouldn't mind wearing **Mid-range** glasses.

    Near vision (reading books, newspapers, magazines, detailed handwork)
    ___Prefer no **Near** glasses.   ___ I wouldn't mind wearing **Near** glasses.

2. Please check the **single** statement that best describes you in terms of **night vision:**
    ___ a. Night vision is extremely important to me, and I require the best possible quality night vision.
    ___ b. I want to be able to drive comfortably at night, but I would tolerate some slight imperfections.
    ___ c. Night vision is not particularly important to me.

3. If you **had** to wear glasses after surgery for one activity, for which activity would you be **most** willing to use glasses?   ____**Distance Vision.**   ____**Mid-range Vision.**   ____**Near Vision.**

4. If you could have good **Distance Vision during the day without glasses**, and good **Near Vision for reading without glasses**, but the compromise was that you might see some **halos or rings** around lights at night, would you like that option?   ____Yes   ____No

5. If you could have good **Distance vision during the day and night** without glasses, and good **Mid-range Vision** without glasses, but the compromise was that you might need glasses for reading the finest print at near, would you like that option?   ____Yes   ____No

6. Surgery to reduce or eliminate your dependence upon glasses for **Distance, Mid-range and Near Vision** may be partially covered by insurance if you have a cataract that is covered by insurance. Would you be interested in learning more about this option?
    ____Yes   ____No   ____Maybe, it depends on how much is covered by insurance.

7. Please place an "X" on the following scale to describe your personality as best you can:
    [--I--]
    Easy going   Perfectionist

Please Sign Here_____

for anything but a monofocal lens due to ocular pathology. After digesting the historical and physical information, I make a very definitive recommendation of which IOL technology I believe is best for the patient. It is very important that this recommendation be definitive. If you provide the patient with a multitude of choices and place the decision in his or her lap, he or she will come away confused and worried that he or she will make the wrong choice. It really is the surgeon's responsibility to provide a recommendation based upon the available information.

Some surgeons might disagree, but I tell patients receiving Pr-C IOLs that they will all need glasses postoperatively for some visual tasks. It is impossible to tell them for which tasks they will need these glasses in advance, but my goal is to reduce their need for these glasses to a bare minimum. Patients are generally very tolerant of this message. If they are not, I prefer to know this in advance so I can address this misconception or decline to perform their surgery and refer them elsewhere. In reality, the vast majority of patients do not use glasses postoperatively, and they are happily surprised to have beaten our expectations.

Perhaps one of the more interesting facets of the questionnaire is the final question, which asks the patient to rate his or her own personality on a scale from "easy going" to "perfectionist." I looked at the correlation of this response to the overall satisfaction of the patient postoperatively. In 43 patients, I implanted 1 of 5 possible IOL combinations: bilateral Crystalens, bilateral ReZoom, bilateral ReSTOR (spherical version), ReZoom mixed with ReSTOR, and Crystalens mixed with ReSTOR. All patients in the study had to achieve a "perfect" result to be included in the study. They had to be within 0.25 D of their refractive target with no enhancements or postoperative complications. In essence, the study examines what happens if everything turns out exactly as planned (Figure 2).

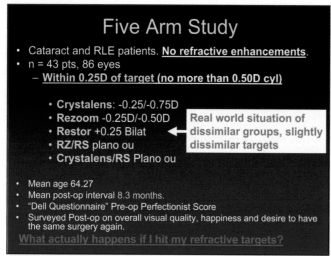

Figure 2. Five arm study.

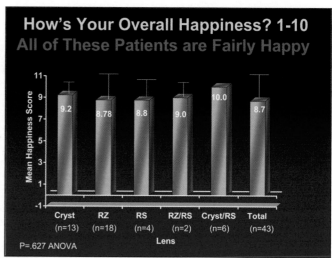

Figure 5. Patients' overall happiness rated on a scale of 1 to 10.

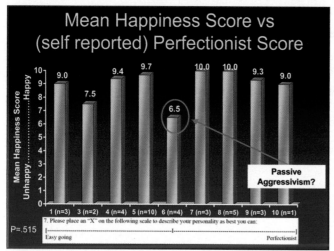

Figure 3. Mean happiness score versus (self-reported) perfectionist score.

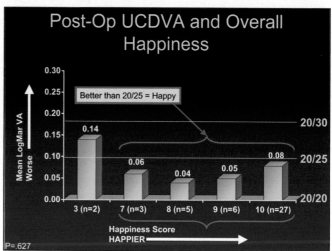

Figure 6. Postoperative uncorrected distance visual acuity and overall happiness.

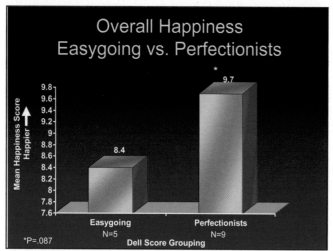

Figure 4. Overall happiness: easygoing versus perfectionist.

One interesting finding (Figure 3) was that patients were generally quite happy no matter how they rated their personality preoperatively, but those who marked their personality as falling in the exact middle of the spectrum were less happy than others. This might represent a passive-aggressive dislike

for the questionnaire or for the process in general. I am speculating that such patients might have a tendency to arbitrarily mark the form right in the middle. I also found that contrary to my assumptions, patients ranking themselves as extreme perfectionists turned out happier postoperatively than those who ranked themselves as extremely easy going (Figure 4). This may represent selection bias on my part, since I tended to very thoroughly counsel a self-described perfectionist. I have learned that all personality types require vigorous counseling.

There is no easy answer to which IOL combination(s) proved the "best." However, some very important conclusions can be drawn from the study. As might be expected in a cohort achieving refractive perfection, all of these patients were generally quite happy, regardless of IOL type (Figure 5). There were nuanced differences in IOL performance that are generally well known and have been thoroughly described elsewhere. The real key to happiness seemed to be uncorrected distance vision that was better than 20/25 (Figure 6). Importantly, those patients who saw the very best at near were no happier than those whose near vision was slightly less clear (Figure 7). The bottom line is that in this small study, slight near trouble was much better tolerated than any distance trouble.

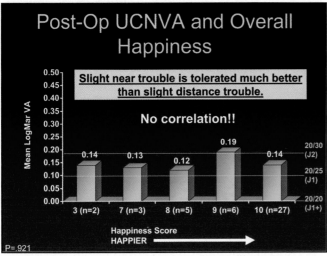

Figure 7. Postoperative uncorrected near visual acuity and overall happiness.

This study suggests that it is possible to identify a patient's preoperative visual desires using a questionnaire and translate those desires into a logical surgical plan with a high degree of success. Obviously, no single IOL technology is suitable for all patients, and as our options multiply, these decisions will grow in complexity. It is very likely that excimer laser enhancement is needed to achieve high levels of satisfaction in a larger cohort of patients since in this study patient happiness was so closely tied to emmetropia. While other modalities such as piggyback IOLs, limbal relaxing incisions, and IOL exchange might be suitable for some postoperative ametropias, it seems likely that excimer laser enhancement will be needed in some patients. For those surgeons who do not perform keratorefractive surgery, comanagement with a refractive surgeon will be important.

CHAPTER 93

SCREENING AND COUNSELING REFRACTIVE IOL PATIENTS

David F. Chang, MD

Since the Centers for Medicare & Medicaid Services' 2005 ruling made presbyopia-correcting intraocular lenses (Pr-C IOLs) available to every cataract patient, each new Pr-C IOL has been greeted with great interest and excitement. For experienced IOL surgeons, the technical transition was easy. What we were not prepared for was the unpredictable and substantial increase in chair time that offering these premium IOLs would entail.

Does this sound familiar? Drawn-out explanations are met with confusion, blank stares, or even a postponement of surgery. Indecision results in repeated telephone calls and requests to speak to other patients. You fall so far behind schedule from an endless consultation that you pray that the next patient wants a standard IOL. I offer all 3 Pr-C IOLs and an accommodating IOL in clinical trial, but too many choices will overwhelm most patients and can result in what Steven Dell, MD calls an "information-seeking spiral."

It is all too easy for patients to develop unrealistic expectations about eliminating glasses and about perfect "20/20" vision. Indeed, the greater the emotional and financial investment in the refractive outcome, the higher the expectations will be. Postoperative dissatisfaction is excruciating to both the patient and the surgeon for this reason. Residual astigmatism, myopia or hyperopia, or macular pathology that may have been missed preoperatively are much more disappointing for a refractive cataract patient. Despite flawless surgery, emmetropia, and a healthy eye, dissatisfaction may still arise because of halos, glare, waxy vision, and other imperfections that may correctly or incorrectly be attributed to the "special" IOL.

To Promote or Not?

For appropriate candidates, toric IOLs or astigmatic keratotomy have no major downside aside from their additional cost. Compared to the alternative of postoperative laser vision correction, they represent a good value and I am comfortable encouraging a patient to have them if they are desirable and affordable for that individual. How strongly we should promote the option of Pr-C IOLs, however, is controversial and is more a matter of the surgeon's personal style, opinion, and philosophy.

Our current Pr-C IOL technologies are not without tradeoffs, and knowing that we do not have a powerful accommodating IOL, I am uncomfortable with promoting these options too strongly. I believe that they are a great solution for many patients but not for everyone . Realizing the power of my influence, I therefore strive to educate patients about these options in a neutral way. For this reason, I avoid the term *deluxe lenses* and I avoid third-party promotional brochures and displays. I do not advertise, nor do I enlist my staff to market these products internally. I am collaborating with Eyemaginations (Towson, MD) to script a Pr-C IOL education video that is more neutral and less promotional than some that I have seen. Such decisions will depend upon your personal style and your own assessment of and experience with the technologies. It is important to note that I do not perform laser vision correction and that mine is primarily a cataract referral practice.

Undecided cataract patients often ask whether I would recommend that they choose the Pr-C IOL option. I explain that I would recommend that anyone living in California should buy a car. In doing so, they will be given options such as leather seats, a GPS tracking system, or a sunroof. Whether or not they want or value these add-on luxury options is a very personal choice. Once they decide to have a Pr-C IOL, however, I will make a recommendation as to which option I believe will best match their priorities.

Educating Patients Efficiently and Effectively

Most patients understandably need a lot of time to make this complex decision. It is therefore far more efficient and effective to initiate Pr-C IOL education in advance of their office visit. My staff now sends a packet of handouts that I personally wrote to every patient who is referred (or self-referred) with a diagnosis of cataract. Besides a basic brochure on cataract surgery, they receive a general handout describing the option of Pr-C IOLs (Appendix D). This handout attempts to explain presbyopia, and the concept of paying extra to upgrade to a Pr-C IOL that reduces but does not eliminate the need to wear spectacles.

Patients also receive and are asked to complete the Dell questionnaire at home (my modification is in Appendix C). In addition to eliciting personal preferences and goals, the process of completing this survey makes it clear to the patient that 1) they utilize and require multiple different working distances, and that 2) there are tradeoffs with these lenses that require each patient to establish certain priorities. When they come in, interested patients are prepared to hear whether they are a good candidate for these IOLs and to discuss their cost. Some immediately volunteer that they do or do not want these IOLs. The Dell questionnaire gives me an instant indication of their interest and functional profile.

Presbyopia-Correcting IOL Handouts

During their visit, interested patients without medical or refractive contraindications are given a longer 4-page handout that I wrote about multifocal IOLs (Appendix E). I first introduce the multifocal option to most patients who desire spectacle independence because it is the technology most likely to meet this specific goal. My handout covers must-read information about adapting to halos, the possible need for a laser enhancement, and unpredictable results due to variable macular function. It is also provides formal informed consent and includes far more detail than I would want to give cataract patients who do not express a strong interest in the subject. I do not mention or compare different multifocal IOL designs, but rather discuss the generic product.

Because manufacturer-supplied brochures optimistically promote a single product, I also wrote this handout in order to temper expectations (it stresses a reduction rather than an elimination of spectacle use). Although they are asked to read it while they are dilating, this take-home handout allows patients to review the important points at home with their family. After the examination, most undecided patients can make up their minds by reviewing the handout at home without any further input from me. If patients are dissatisfied about something postoperatively, this handout provides a clear reminder that we did present certain pros and cons in advance.

If the patient is interested in reducing spectacle dependence, but either they or I have reservations about using a multifocal IOL, I explain the option of an accommodating IOL (Crystalens; Eyeonics, Inc, Aliso Viejo, CA). I find that the pros and cons of this option are easier to understand once the patient is already familiar with how multifocal IOLs work. Again, I have prepared a take-home handout to explain certain pros and cons about the Crystalens (Appendix F).

Who Does the Patient Counseling?

By saving me from having to repeat the basics every time, these handouts allow me to personally do the patient counseling, as opposed to entrusting this to a staff member. In many refractive practices staff counselors educate patients about how laser vision correction works and how much it will cost. This makes sense if most patients want to hear about and are presented with the same options. It is tempting to delegate the lengthy patient education process about Pr-C IOL options as well. I view this decision, however, as being much more complex than deciding to have laser in situ keratomileusis (LASIK).

Most of my Pr-C IOL candidates with cataracts did not come to me seeking refractive surgery. There is no consensus as to the best technology. None of the choices is without significant tradeoffs, and satisfaction will depend upon realistic and informed expectations. Because of this, I may determine that many motivated patients are not ideal candidates despite their being able to afford the procedure and having a healthy eye. Patients who are willing to invest thousands of extra dollars in this technology deserve my expertise in patient selection, and I get subtle clues regarding their personality and priorities as we discuss the option and the costs together. We will both be happier if I am able to determine if, because of their personality, their glass will be half full or half empty postoperatively, and I can factor this information into steering their expectations and decision. This approach has definitely lengthened the average preoperative chair time for my cataract patients. However, that is the essence of why this service commands a premium. Just a few unhappy postoperative Pr-C IOL patients can easily offset the preoperative time savings of having your staff do the majority of patient counseling.

After taking the history, we perform automated keratometry and IOL Master (Carl Zeiss Meditec, Jena, Germany) biometry as part of every cataract patient's pretesting. My optometrist refracts the patient and determines his or her best-corrected distance and near acuity. If indicated, Amsler Grid and BAT glare testing is performed. As determined by the optometrist, interested patients who appear to be appropriate candidates are given handouts or shown videos (astigmatic keratotomy, Pr-C or toric IOLs) while they dilate.

In addition to the history, I review the refraction, current eyeglasses, and visual acuity. I check the biometry and keratometry readings and read the patient's responses to the Dell survey. After performing the dilated slit lamp and ophthalmoscopic exams, I generally know whether or not we will be discussing refractive IOLs at length. I mention the option to everyone as it is better to address this preoperatively than to have the patient wonder later why they were not told about this choice. I therefore explain to patients with ocular pathology or high astigmatism why they are poor candidates for Pr-C IOLs.

The Concept of Convenience

I first explain to my cataract patients that they would be happy with a standard IOL following surgery. Realizing that the majority of my cataract patients will receive a monofocal IOL, I do not want the process of refractive IOL education to send subliminal messages that monofocal IOLs are an inferior technology. In next explaining the advantages of Pr-C IOLs, I emphasize the concept of convenience. This properly defines what is at stake—namely, that these IOLs are not "better" for their eye or of "better" quality. Nor is this a life-or-death decision to agonize over. Finally, for Pr-C IOL patients, having emphasized the concept of "convenience" will help them to better accept that having to wear glasses postoperatively may be disappointing but is not a disability.

Many consultants and practitioners prefer to have staff members discuss pricing with the patient. For my own practice, I disagree. I mention the additional cost early in the discussion and explain that the convenience of reduced spectacle dependence is not covered by insurance because it is not "medically necessary." Upon hearing what the premium cost is, some previously interested patients immediately volunteer that they have been wearing eyeglasses all along and that they really do not mind them. This is their way of saying "I can't or don't want to spend that kind of money for this convenience." At this point I take the hint, and we can now skip the lengthier explanation of multifocal IOL pros, cons, and expectations. I like to have them feel positive about their surgery, so I confirm that they will "do great" with the standard IOL. I have my own bias about the financial value of these Pr-C IOLs and it is hard not to be influenced by the fact some patients must struggle to afford the premium, while other patients dismiss cost as a "non-issue." I was ready to implant a multifocal IOL in one patient until I learned that he was going to take out a home equity loan to afford it. After I clarified once more that the advantage was one of convenience and not what was "better" for his eyesight, he opted for a monofocal IOL instead.

The Process of Resetting Expectations

Most patients want and will tend to believe that refractive IOLs will eliminate glasses. This idea may have first been planted in their mind by LASIK advertising, by third-party brochures depicting a smiling spectacle-free patient, or by hearing a contemporary brag that they "no longer wear glasses" after surgery. An important goal of patient counseling, therefore, is to reset and manage these expectations. The oft stated dictum of "under-promising and over-delivering" is another way of saying that we want to be confident that we can meet or exceed the patients' expectations. This is certainly easier to do if they have a dense cataract or are completely spectacle dependent from high myopia or hyperopia to begin with.

Optical concepts such as focus, depth of field, contrast sensitivity, astigmatism, and refractive error are difficult for many patients to grasp. How effectively you are able to explain these concepts is just as important as how much time you spend doing so. It is best to honestly emphasize that these IOLs do not reliably eliminate glasses. A frequent response is, "If I still need to buy reading glasses, then what is the advantage?" I use the analogy that our winter weather is so much better here in California than in Minnesota, but it is not perfect and we still own a coat. We just own a lighter weight coat that we wear much less frequently. In other words, "better" is a good result, even if it is not "perfect."

Conclusion

Besides the advanced IOL technology, the "premium" part of the refractive IOL channel is not necessarily the way we perform surgery or the extra preoperative testing that we perform. Rather, it is our judgment, experience, and expertise in both patient and IOL selection that defines ours to be a premium service. The critical elements of patient selection and education are as much art as science. With so many IOL options, each with different pros and cons, and with the wide range of individual personalities and lifestyles, this art is not easily mastered.

CHAPTER 94

SCREENING AND COUNSELING REFRACTIVE IOL PATIENTS

Mark Packer, MD, FACS

In general, there are 2 situations in which new patients need counseling on refractive intraocular lens (IOL) selection. First, there are patients who present for a refractive screening. We offer a free screening that includes a history; autorefraction; autokeratometry; pachymetry; and discussion of alternatives, risks, and questions. These people are looking forward to freedom from glasses or contact lenses and want to know their options. Generally, if they are in the presbyopic age range, I will discuss refractive lens exchange (RLE). Second, there are patients presenting for cataract surgery who may not be aware of astigmatism and presbyopia. They want to see better but may not yet have given much consideration to spectacle independence. I pose the question to this second group, "After your surgery, would you like to be able to read and drive without glasses?"

I do not have a preconceived notion of what goals a particular person may have for his or her vision. I consider it my role to create solutions for each individual. Many people like the idea of freedom from glasses; however some, prefer to wear glasses, and others may not know what they want. The high myope or hyperope who has worn spectacles from a young age may have a significant shift in self-image that occurs with spectacle independence. The ease with which they adapt to life without glasses may reflect their degree of self-confidence. On the other hand, the emmetropic presbyope who never wore glasses until age 45 may see nothing but good in getting rid of the specs. The surgeon, however, may be less comfortable operating on a patient with uncorrected distance acuity approximating 20/20.

Screening and counseling patients is really about communicating realistic expectations. Everyone needs to be prepared for imperfect outcomes. I like to discuss my approach to residual spherical refractive error (which is usually due to the limitations of biometry and IOL power calculation) and my

treatment of residual astigmatism (which is often due to the variability of response to limbal relaxing incisions). I also stress the limitations of the IOL technology itself, best analyzed by Food and Drug Administration (FDA)-monitored clinical trial results. I provide percentages from these studies, relating, for example, how many subjects experience halos after multifocal IOL implantation and how many can use the computer without glasses after accommodative IOL implantation. These data give prospective patients a realistic idea of what to expect following surgery and set the stage for enhancement procedures if they prove necessary.

My enthusiasm for RLE and presbyopia-correcting IOLs comes straight from my patients; they are among the very happiest postoperative patients in my practice. Ironically, it is sometimes patients who require an enhancement procedure who seem most grateful. I recall one hyperopic presbyope whose astigmatism regressed 6 weeks after RLE; her binocular uncorrected acuity slipped from 20/20 and J2 to 20/60 and J7. She was upset and crying when I walked in the room to see her, but she recovered her calm once she understood the problem and its solution. Later she told me it had been incredibly frightening because she thought she was going blind. she reported that she was seeing better after bilateral laser in situ keratomileusis than she ever had in her life.

One of the critical decisions that refractive lens surgeons must make relates to enhancement strategies. Traditionally, LASIK enhancements have been included in the initial price. However, enhancements after RLE may take the form of LASIK, piggyback IOLs, limbal relaxing incisions, photomydriasis, or other procedures. These techniques have widely varying costs, so applying a blanket percentage fee across the board seems unrealistic. Instead, I have generally charged the patient my cost for doing the enhancement. I explain this policy during the preoperative counseling; I think it helps

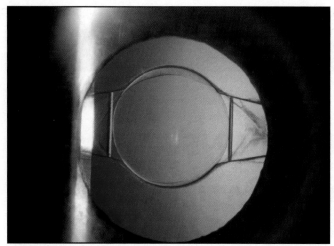

Figure 1. Slit lamp retroillumination image of the Crystalens AT-45 (Eyeonics, Inc, Aliso Viejo, CA) 1 year after surgery demonstrates how 360 degree overlap of the capsulorhexis on the optic in combination with thorough capsule polishing and meticulous cortical clean up enables maintenance of extraordinary capsule clarity.

patients remember that they may in fact need an enhancement if they also are told they will be paying for it. Additionally, this policy underlines the fact that enhancements may be necessary despite flawless procedures. That is the state of the art.

CHAPTER 95

Screening and Counseling Refractive IOL Patients

Robert J. Cionni, MD

The 3 most important factors in ensuring a successful refractive intraocular lens (IOL) outcome are proper patient selection, proper patient selection, and proper patient selection. Those who are experienced in laser refractive surgery have come to understand this concept very well, whereas those who are not laser refractive surgeons must come to understand the importance of patient selection or they will fail miserably. Many cataract surgeons learned the importance of patient selection for multifocal IOLs (MFIOL) years ago when the Array IOL (Advanced Medical Optics, Santa Ana, CA) was introduced. Surgeons who did not carefully screen their patients to determine the best candidates and cull out those who were not, found themselves with many unhappy patients. This led many surgeons to abandon the Array IOL for fear of a high percentage of unhappy patients.

Although presbyopia-correcting IOL (Pr-C IOL) technology has improved tremendously over the last 2 decades, the importance of selecting the proper patients for these IOLs has not changed. The next few pages will outline some of the important factors in determining who might be a good candidate for a Pr-C IOL. Notice that I did not say, "will" be a good candidate, but instead, "might" be a good candidate. Despite our best efforts, even the most selective surgeons will occasionally have unhappy patients. Therefore, what may be even more important than determining who is likely to do well is determining who will likely NOT do well with a Pr-C IOL.

Although toric IOLs are certainly considered refractive IOLs, the only real determining factor for implanting a toric IOL is whether or not the patient has corneal astigmatism. Therefore, this chapter will focus on Pr-C IOLs.

It is probably best to separate selection criteria into objective criteria and subjective criteria. Some of the important objective criteria are listed below with explanations as to why each criterion is important.

* Best-corrected preoperative vision: The quality of preoperative best-corrected vision affects the likelihood that we will be able to make the patient happy postoperatively. A patient who has poor vision that limits his or her quality of life will be far easier to please than someone who can be corrected with glasses or contact lenses to an acceptable level.

* Preoperative refractive state: Patients who need corrective lenses at all distances are easiest to please. Patients who can see fine in the distance and only require reading glasses will likely not end up happy if their distance vision is decreased at all. Likewise, patients who can take off their glasses and read perfectly fine are going to be harder to please with regard to their reading vision.

* Bilateral versus unilateral implantation: We have found that bilateral implantation of Pr-C IOLs results in significant improvement in vision at all distances (bilateral summation reference needed) (Figure 1). Therefore, patients who are prepared to have surgery on both eyes within a short period of time are generally going to fare better than patients who only want surgery on one eye. Still, for those patients who already have a near plano result in one eye with a monofocal IOL from previous surgery, and are desirous of better reading vision without glasses, we can offer a Pr-C IOL in the second eye. However, it is important to inform this patient preoperatively that the result will likely not be as good as if the Pr-C IOL were implanted in both eyes.

* Surface pathology: The tear film and corneal surface are extremely important elements in creating an acceptable image through a Pr-C IOL. This is more important for multifocal IOLs than for pseudoaccommodating IOLs. Therefore, patients with a poor tear, or an irregular corneal surface from basement membrane disease or other such corneal abnormalities are not the best candidates for these IOLs. This includes patients who have had prior radial keratotomy surgery.

* Pupil size in light and dark: Pupil size leads me to favor one style of Pr-C IOL over another. For instance, the ReSTOR IOL (Alcon, Fort Worth, TX) performs

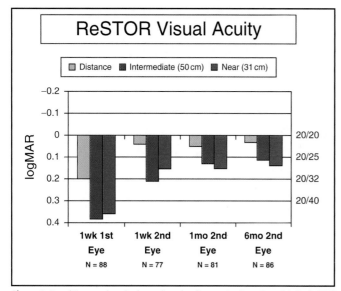

Figure 1. A multicentered study shows that after first eye implantation with the ReSTOR IOL, vision at distance is acceptable but near and intermediate is not very good. After second eye implantation of the same style IOL, vision improves at all distances and continues to improve with time.

very well at all distances in patients with small pupils. However, patients with large pupils under normal lighting conditions are not as likely to reach excellent reading and intermediate vision with the ReSTOR IOL. These patients may do better with a ReZoom (Advanced Medical Optics) or Crystalens Pr-C IOL (Eyeonics, Inc, Aliso Viejo, CA). The aspheric ReSTOR may perform better for those with large pupils but I do not have enough experience with this IOL to come to a conclusion yet.

 * Other ocular pathology: Any ocular pathology that would preclude good postoperative vision such as diabetic macular edema, macular degeneration, epiretinal membrane, or significant glaucoma places the patient at a higher risk for dissatisfaction with a Pr-C IOL.

 * Age: In general, the older the patient, the easier to please. Younger patients tend to be more active with more rigorous vision requirements. Additionally, younger patients may have not yet experienced presbyopia and therefore do not fully understand the benefits of a Pr-C IOL over a monofocal IOL.

 * Ability to attain a near-plano result with less than 0.5 D of cylinder: Patients with more than 0.5 D of residual astigmatism will be less likely to be happy with their uncorrected vision and less likely to gain spectacle freedom. Either select patients with little pre-op astigmatism, or be certain that you can reduce their astigmatism with limbal relaxing incisions (LRIs) or laser refractive surgery.

Subjective criteria are not as "black and white" but can yield clues as to the best choice for each patient.

 * Occupation/hobbies/life activities: Knowledge of a patient's daily activities will help the surgeon determine the patient's distance, intermediate, and near vision

requirements. This may affect the decision to suggest a Pr-C IOL and may move the surgeon to suggest one particular Pr-C IOL over another.

 * Tolerance to halos: Although most patients feel that these visual disturbances are mild to moderate and a fair tradeoff for increased spectacle freedom, a small percentage feels that these disturbances are quite significant. If patients are light sensitive or concerned about the likelihood of halos around lights while driving at night, they may be more likely to be unhappy with a MFIOL. In this instance a pseudoaccommodating IOL may be a better choice.

 * Adaptable personality: Although this is a quality that is hard to measure, suffice it to say that patients who can "go with the flow" will adapt more easily to Pr-C IOLs.

 * Realistic expectations: Patients need to realize that every style of Pr-C IOL has compromises and that none are as good as the natural crystalline lenses with which we were born. A patient who expects perfect uncorrected vision at all distances and lighting conditions will very likely be disappointed after surgery. Likewise, a patient who believes that anything other than complete spectacle freedom means failure is a very poor candidate for a Pr-C IOL. It is better to tell patients preoperatively that they will likely be free from glasses for 90% of everything they do rather than quote them a chance for complete spectacle freedom.

The aforementioned selection criteria represent a guide to selecting the best candidates for consideration of refractive IOL surgery. As with everything in life, there will be exceptions to the rules but your odds of achieving patient and practice success with refractive IOLs are best if you follow these guidelines. For those just venturing into the refractive IOL market, begin with those patients most likely to do well. The ideal patient to begin with would be a 70-year-old hyperope with bilateral cataract, no other ocular pathology, normal axial lengths, and keratometric cylinder of 0.50 D or less who drives only during the day. Only after tackling a few patients like this one should the surgeon consider moving on to those that need a little more finesse, such as the post-LASIK patient.

Almost as important as patient selection for refractive IOLs is how your patients are presented with these options. Experience has taught us that if the patient does not know about these options until he or she is in your exam chair, he or she is much less likely to choose a refractive IOL. Therefore, pre-consultation education is hugely important! If you work with referring doctors, ideally the referring doctor has brought up and discussed these options with the patient. Additionally, mailing an informational brochure to the patient before the consult helps to educate your patient about the availability of these new options. Many patients go on to investigate refractive IOLs in more depth through the Internet before they come to see you. Many already know whether or not they want a toric IOL or a Pr-C IOL and some even come in requesting a specific Pr-C IOL.

The in-office experience with all cataract patients has changed dramatically since the introduction of the new refractive IOLs. Each patient regardless of whether or not they are a refractive IOL candidate now requires more chair time with the technician, the surgeon, and the surgery scheduler or surgery counselor. As the technician is bringing the patient into the exam room, the patient is asked if they have any questions about the information they received preoperatively and the technician begins to answer those questions. While the patient is dilating they watch a DVD concerning cataract surgery and the new refractive IOL options.

Prior to seeing the surgeon it is helpful to have the patient complete a Vision Preference Questionnaire and have keratometric and axial length testing completed so the surgeon will know whether or not they are a candidate for a refractive IOL and with which type they may do best.

It is of paramount importance to have a family member join the patient in the exam room for the consult as the patient may not understand the options well enough to relay this information correctly to the spouse or other family member. Additionally, it is not uncommon for the patient to say, "Well, I'd like to get rid of these glasses but I don't think we can afford it." If the spouse is not in the room with the patient, the chance that the patient will convert to a refractive IOL is almost zero. However, if the spouse is in the room it is common to hear the spouse say, "Honey, you are worth it. I want you to have the best."

The surgeon needs to spend enough time with each patient to fully explain the options available to the patient and to discuss advantages and limitations of each design. Consequently, the surgeon should consider changing his or her appointment scheduling to allow more time with each consult. Surgeons who spend 20 minutes with each patient tend to have better informed patients and consequently, higher conversion rates than those who run through a cataract evaluation every 5 minutes. The extra time allotted allows the surgeon to fully discuss realistic expectations with the patient and their family member. Some key points that should be stressed are reading distance, likelihood of halos, and the importance of bilateral implantation. In fact, it is far better to under-promise and over-deliver rather than to over-promise and under-deliver. With that in mind, I tell all patients that they will see halos with MFIOLs, and about 4% of patients feel the halos are quite bothersome, but they do diminish with time. Patients are also told that they are likely to be under-whelmed after the first eye is implanted but that their vision at all distances should be significantly better after the second eye surgery has been completed (see Figure 1). Taking the time with each patient preoperatively not only increases the chance for a happy postoperative patient, but also enriches the doctor/patient relationship. I encourage surgeons to try this approach and I trust you will enjoy the nature of your practice far more than you have in years.

Conclusion

Without a doubt, the happiest patients in our practices today are those who gain a high level of spectacle freedom following cataract surgery. The surgeon who spends enough time and energy to select the right patients, put them with the best IOL to suit their needs, and educate these patients completely about refractive IOLs will be rewarded with the highest percentage of happy patients.

CHAPTER 96

MANAGING PATIENT EXPECTATIONS

David F. Chang, MD

Patient satisfaction with their uncorrected vision following a refractive IOL reflects success in 4 separate areas. There must be 1) uncomplicated surgery, 2) avoidance or reduction of astigmatism, 3) selection of the optimal intraocular lens (IOL) power, and 4) reasonable expectations on the part of the patient. The first 3 prerequisites have long been the goal of every cataract surgeon. It is in this fourth area of patient selection where the availability of presbyopia-correcting IOLs (Pr-C IOLs) has required us to develop and refine our skills.

Choosing to implant a Pr-C IOL certainly increases the demands placed on the cataract surgeon. The patient has agreed to pay extra for and accept the possible optical disadvantages of this lens because of the expectation of reduced spectacle dependence. Contrast these expectations with those of a patient whose procedure is entirely covered by insurance, and who anticipates wearing bifocals following bilateral cataract surgery. If we miss the spherical target by +1 D, the correction simply ends up in the eyeglasses. This is also true for 1 to 2 D of surgically induced astigmatism or 1 to 2 D of unintended anisometropia. The patient will likely be unaware of 0.5 to 1 mm of optic decentration and, barring late complications, the patient will probably be just as happy with an anterior chamber (AC) IOL in the event of posterior capsule rupture.

Unfortunately, all of these scenarios compromise the uncorrected visual function of the bilateral multifocal IOL patient, particularly if the 2 eyes are compared. The expectation of good vision without glasses reduces our margin for error, and increases the potential for patients to become dissatisfied. The results of the various clinical studies of these lenses, however, indicate that skilled IOL surgeons are indeed able to meet this challenge.

With respect to our outcomes, we can readily measure objective parameters such as uncorrected Snellen and Jaeger acuity, and spherical or cylindrical refractive error. Nevertheless, we must remember that patient satisfaction and the perceived benefits and drawbacks of these lenses are largely subjective.

For example, 2 bilateral multifocal IOL patients with identical refractive and anatomical results may differ greatly in their frequency of using reading glasses. This is influenced by the individual's lifestyle and vocation, expectations, comparative preoperative function, and the motivation or determination to function without glasses.

We know from keratorefractive surgery that there is great variability in just how much patients value having good uncorrected vision. For some individuals, the motivation to see without glasses was so strong that even the tremendous glare and fluctuating vision characteristic of a 16-incision radial keratotomy (RK) was a very acceptable tradeoff. Individuals with such strong motivation are also more likely to accept and adapt to the optical aberrations of a multifocal IOL. These are the patients who, after hearing about the potential for night time aberrations with a multifocal lens, start trying to convince me why they should not have any problems. "Oh, I already have plenty of halos now anyway." "Well, I really don't do that much night driving."

Although we certainly leave the final decision up to the patient, refractive error, pseudoaccommodation, contrast sensitivity, and optical aberrations are confusing topics for most patients to comprehend. Appropriately, they depend on our experience and understanding of the available options for guidance. With the heightened financial and emotional investment in the refractive outcome, it is the potential intensity of patient dissatisfaction that truly frightens us. Clearly, not every refractive IOL patient will achieve a superb functional result. If that patient, however, is still able to understand the advantages of their Pr-C IOL compared to a standard monofocal lens, they may be disappointed but will usually not regret their decision. Preoperatively, a "good candidate," therefore, is a patient who understands this concept and has reasonable expectations that we are confident can be met.

Besides what patients tell us during our discussion, are there other clues that predict their likelihood for satisfaction with a Pr-C IOL? To get a sense of their motivation to avoid glasses, I usually ask prospective candidates how often they wear their bifocals during the average day. As we know, there are a number of people with significant refractive error who do not wear their glasses that often. These individuals are apparently willing to tolerate the extra blur rather than be inconvenienced with wearing spectacles. On the other hand, a nearly emmetropic patient who wears bifocals all day long because he or she is too blurred without that $-0.50 + 0.50 \times 90$ correction may be equally intolerant of multifocal IOL ghost images.

We also know from our general ophthalmology practices that individual patients vary greatly in their ability to adapt to distracting imperfections in their vision. Whether it be a floater, an oily contact lens, monovision, or the distortions of progressive add bifocals, patients who are highly intolerant of such flaws might be at higher risk of dissatisfaction with the unwanted images from a multifocal IOL. The degree of cataract and visual complaint is also telling in this regard. A patient with advanced brunescent lenses, 20/80 acuity, and yet relatively understated complaints is telling you that they are not a very "picky" person. This is in contrast to the 20/25 patient with minor lens opacities who, despite being reassured 3 months ago, is already back again feeling utterly disabled by his or her deteriorating vision. Obviously, this person may be equally intolerant of the glare and halos from a multifocal IOL.

Pupil size is important with respect to both night vision and near acuity. A patient with small pupils will enjoy greater depth of field and will experience less optical aberration at night. A patient with large pupils will more likely experience halos with the ReZoom (Advanced Medical Optics, Santa Ana, CA) or Crystalens (Eyeonics, Inc, Aliso Viejo CA), and it is important to inquire about that patient's night time lifestyle. Finally, expect patients to compare their postoperative uncorrected visual function to their preoperative state. For example, uncorrected J5 vision will seem miraculous to someone who was +3.00 preoperatively, but will be disappointing to someone who was formerly −3.00. Likewise, it is hard to imagine a patient starting with a 20/400 PSC cataract not being ecstatic with or without glasses postoperatively.

We cataract surgeons are accustomed to routinely exceeding our patients' expectations. Our patients are typically surprised and unexpectedly pleased with the lack of pain during and after surgery, the speed of the surgery and their visual recovery, the unanticipated clarity and enhanced color vision, the improvement in refractive error (in highly ametropic individuals), and so on. Contrast this with the frustrating prospect that flawless surgery may still disappoint a refractive IOL patient with unrealistic expectations.

Because expectations are such a critical determinant of patient satisfaction, all refractive surgeons have no doubt mastered the art of understating the anticipated results. Who should we be particularly cautious about? Be careful with patients who are depressed, obsessive compulsive, passive-aggressive, or manipulative (patients with a so-called borderline personality). Some of these patients will be unhappy no matter what the outcome, and if they perceive that you promoted a more expensive option, they may unfairly blame all of their woes on this decision, which you "pressured" them into making. Patients with a strong sense of "entitlement" may

also be hard to please. Examples would be patients who are uncooperative with your staff, or who tend to feel that every problem or inconvenience is someone else's fault. These may be hints that they will hold you responsible for providing a perfect refractive result.

What makes some engineers so difficult? Their livelihood depends on precision and they are conditioned to detect and uncover imperfection and subtle "bugs" that, if undiscovered, might undermine performance. Some engineers are so accustomed to solving problems with precise technical solutions that they have difficulty accepting that we do not have a perfect answer for refractive error and presbyopia. The process of adaptation will be stalled if an obsessive individual cannot accept any imperfection, distraction, or inconvenience, and in fact dwells on these problems. This is not to say that these patients should not be given the same options as everyone else. Rather, we should emphasize the risk of dissatisfaction due to any number of potential scenarios when we counsel that particular patient. I may diplomatically point out that they seem to be a very "precise" individual who may be more bothered by certain optical characteristics of a multifocal IOL that otherwise go unnoticed by the general patient population.

Particularly when getting started with multifocal and refractive IOLs, it is important to select patients who will be among the easiest to satisfy. I liken this to taking high percentage shots in basketball. Easy going patients with advanced cataracts, minimal astigmatism, and significant preoperative myopia or hyperopia will have the most to gain and will be the easiest to please. Performing cataract surgery with Pr-C IOLs in these patients is like shooting layups. On the other hand, obsessive or perfectionist patients with minor lens opacities will be more difficult to impress. This is particularly true if they have significant astigmatism, low myopia, or are already achieving monovision with contact lenses, and satisfying these patients is the basketball equivalent of an off balanced 3-point shot. In my basketball analogy, the inexperienced surgeon is better off sticking to short shots from the lane, rather than attempting low percentage long-range bombs. As more and more success begets confidence, one can start to think about moving further away from the basket.

Overall, electing to implant a premium refractive IOL is analogous to other nonmedical decisions that we make with our patients every day. Examples would be the decision to pursue refractive surgery, cosmetic surgery, monovision contact lenses, progressive bifocals, and so on. Each of these options has pros and cons that are time consuming to discuss, but which prevent them from being the universal best solution for everyone. However, just as it would be inappropriate to push these options on every patient, it would be just as wrong to conceal or routinely discourage these options because of potential drawbacks or because some patients are dissatisfied. In each of these instances, there is a subset of informed patients who are delighted to have had these options, and grateful to the physician who explained and provided them. For this reason, I believe we all owe it to our cataract patients to acquire the skills needed to offer Pr-C IOLs, and to spend the necessary time discussing and considering these options with them.

CHAPTER 97

MANAGING PATIENT EXPECTATIONS

Jay S. Pepose, MD, PhD

In general, the key to a successful premium intraocular lens (IOL) practice is appropriately managing patient's expectations. Tom Peters' advice, "Formula for success: under promise and over deliver," emphatically applies to the premium IOL experience. In our practice, we have taken the following approach to patient education about premium channel IOLs.

Preoperative Assessment

The preoperative assessment begins with the patient filling out the Dell questionnaire (Appendix A). This gives us the first clues about the patient's expectations in considering surgery. Demands of perfection in all 5 ranges of vision constitute obvious warning signs of a patient with unachievable goals. Special attention should be paid to patients with a history of rigid gas permeable (RGP) contact lens use who may expect the same level of high-quality vision without correction postoperatively than they achieved with RGP correction in the past (perhaps 35 years ago prior to the onset of presbyopia). Patients with refractive errors between –1.5 D and –2.5 D will have higher anticipation of good uncorrected near vision since they are already used to clear close vision and will require extensive counseling regarding realistic achievable expectations. Patients with irregular corneal astigmatism or those presenting with numerous pairs of glasses, none of which has ever been satisfactory, are not good premium IOL candidates.

In assessing the patient's expectations preoperatively and in educating him or her as to what can be likely delivered, it is unwise to recommend a premium IOL to a patient whose only satisfactory outcome is perfect uncorrected vision at all distances, in all lighting conditions, all of the time. Since a satisfied patient will recommend the surgery to 10 friends and a dissatisfied patient will tell 100 people, it is the better part of valor to counsel a patient with unrealistic expectations appropriately and explain that it is not possible for you to provide what he or she is seeking. Since no IOL or IOL combination

has been shown to allow 100% of patients to be completely free of glasses under all conditions all of the time, the very nature of patient counseling must focus on accepting some degree of compromise and it is best to deal with this issue openly up front.

If the patient says, "Why would I be willing to pay extra out of pocket costs if I may still need to use glasses?" the ophthalmologist should emphasize that the goal of premium IOLs is to reduce one's dependence on glasses. Studies have shown that premium IOL patients are glasses free a much higher percentage of the time as compared to monofocal lenses, but it may not eliminate the need for glasses in all cases. I tell the patient that these deluxe lenses have many features that are superior to monofocal IOLs of the past. However, these are still all man-made lenses and our Creator continues to hold the patent on the "perfect" lens.

Use of Educational Materials

Some people are primarily auditory learners, some visual learners, and some are both. The availability of brochures, posters, models, and illustrations of the various premium IOLs are useful ancillary tools. However, we have found that the use of customized computer software, such as the IOL Counselor (Patient Education Concepts, Houston, TX) (available free to American Society of Cataract and Refractive Surgeons [ASCRS] members) and other software programs available from Eyeonics, Inc (Aliso Viejo, CA), greatly facilitate patients' understanding the differences between monofocal and premium IOLs by allowing the patients to picture themselves in common situations such as driving or shopping. In addition, patients can better visualize and understand the risks and benefits of the cataract surgery and accompanying limbal relaxing incisions (LRIs), as well as possible side effects of multifocal IOLs such as photic phenomenon along with postoperative neural adaptation (Figure 1).

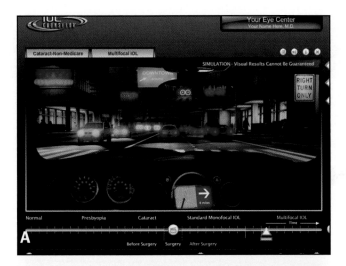

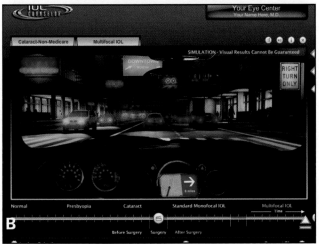

Figure 1. The IOL Counselor is a useful adjunct that can be used to prepare the patient for potential side effects of multifocal IOLS, such as dysphotopsia (A), as well as the process of neural adaptation (B).

Explain the Premium IOL Process From Start to Finish

Many people enjoy surprise birthday parties, but no one enjoys unanticipated postoperative surprises. While it may seem like an information overload to the patient, it is very important to explain that there is a series of sequential steps that may be necessary for some patients to achieve a satisfactory visual outcome and to emphasize that some period of healing will be required before all of these steps can be completed. It behooves the ophthalmologist to discuss the more common possible events that may occur and procedures that may be necessary to complete the entire premium IOL process. This discussion does not necessarily have to happen during the initial visit, which may be already lengthy and a bit overwhelming for the patient, but it must be accomplished at some time prior to surgery.

The ophthalmologist may not view these common occurrences as complications, but the uninformed patient may view them as a failure of the surgery. For example, patients must be told that they can develop secondary cataract and require a neodymium:yttrium-aluminum-garnet (Nd:YAG) laser capsulotomy postoperatively. They need to know that this can happen following any IOL implantation, is not peculiar to a premium IOL, and that this office-based surgery is generally covered by insurance. They also must be told that while every effort is made to pick the appropriate lens power, there is some uncertainty to this determination (especially in the setting of prior keratorefractive surgery) and that, in addition, IOLs are only manufactured in given steps or powers. I explain that just as a man may go to a store to buy a suit and a woman a dress, if they fall between the sizes hanging on the rack, then a tailor must alter the suite or dress to better fit them. I draw the same analogy to postoperative laser vision correction, which may be necessary to "fine tune" the power to customize the patient's needs more exactly.

All fees for premium IOL surgery as well as potential postoperative procedures that are not bundled should be discussed with the patient before scheduling surgery. This task is not handled by any of the doctors in my office, but by other staff members. In addition, I do mention that glasses may be required at times following surgery and that there can be no way to guarantee a specific outcome. If I am considering implanting a multifocal IOL in one or both eyes, I inform the patient that he or she will initially experience some night glare or halos when he or she drives in the dark, which in most cases diminishes with time but may not be totally eliminated in all patients. I explain that this is one of the tradeoffs in exchange for the benefit of better near vision that comes with the multifocal technology. I also inform them that certain intraoperative events or findings could preclude the intended implantation of a premium IOL and that we will have a backup monofocal IOL available in the operating room if needed.

It is useful to provide the patient with additional written material at various stages following the surgery that emphasizes and reiterates the need for binocular IOL implantation to achieve maximum results, to allow time for improved function and adaptation with both accommodating and multifocal IOLs, and the potential need for YAG capsulotomy or laser vision correction over the ensuing months.

Start at the End

The premium IOL experience begins with managing the patient's expectations and then carefully guiding him or her through the entire process, which may require a number of steps beyond lens implantation. If the ophthalmologist can visualize this entire process from beginning to end from the patient's perspective, starting with an anxious patient's first reaction to the news that he or she has a cataract, often knowing little about cataract surgery or IOL options, this will help you create the premium IOL experience. Like any premium service, this highly proactive and interactive patient-centered process entails much more than implanting the deluxe IOL itself.

CHAPTER 98

MANAGING PATIENT EXPECTATIONS

Richard S. Hoffman, MD

Success with refractive intraocular lenses (IOLs) is a function of accuracy and includes accuracy in biometry, lens power calculation, surgical technique, and addressing preoperative astigmatism. In addition, one must choose the right lens model for the right patient. Perhaps most important to a successful outcome is accuracy in patient selection and managing patient expectations (Table 1). A +6.00-D presbyope who presents wanting refractive surgery and states, "I do not mind wearing reading glasses after the procedure," is easy to please, but most patients requesting refractive lens exchange are not this cut and dry. Selecting your refractive patients appropriately and managing their expectations properly will go a long way toward creating a happy and satisfied patient.

When counseling patients for refractive lens exchange, it is important to evaluate their occupation, expectations, motivations, and refractive error. With the various choices of refractive IOLs available, each with their particular strengths and weaknesses, the lens must be customized to the individual.

An individual who spends much of their day working in front of a computer would be a better candidate for a ReZoom (Advanced Medical Optics, Santa Ana, CA) or Crystalens IOL (Eyeonics, Inc, Aliso Viejo, CA) rather than a ReSTOR IOL (Alcon, Fort Worth, TX) due to the current weakness in intermediate vision inherent in the latter's design. Similarly, a watchmaker or seamstress might make a better ReSTOR candidate due to the excellent near vision delivered from this IOL compared to the other refractive IOLs. Is the patient a truck driver or does he or she have an occupation that involves frequent night driving? This individual would need to be counseled extensively regarding the potential drawbacks of halos from multifocal IOLs and perhaps steered toward an accommodating IOL if halos or poor night vision could be an issue. Every patient implanted with a multifocal IOL must be made aware that although halos tend to improve several months after surgery, they may be a permanent consequence of these lenses.

Additionally, the ophthalmic examination might suggest implantation of one lens model over another. Corneal guttatae, macular drusen, or faint epiretinal membranes can all affect the efficiency of multifocal IOLs. Patients with these pathologies might be better served with an accommodating IOL as long as they are aware of the near limitations and lower likelihood for spectacle independence with currently available accommodating IOL technology. Pupil size can also be an issue. Small pupils during reading will occlude the near-dominant rings of a ReZoom IOL and diminish near acuity. Similarly, pupils that do not dilate adequately for distance will occlude the outer refractive portion of the ReSTOR IOL and may affect the quality of distance vision. Large pupils that do not react adequately are cause for concern with any multifocal IOL, but less so for an accommodating IOL.

Highly motivated, laid-back individuals with large refractive errors are the easiest patients to please. Fussy, introspective, obsessive, type-A individuals should be avoided. When presented with patients who have unreasonable expectations, it is essential that their expectations are brought into reasonable alignment with the projected outcomes. It is best to undersell and over deliver than to oversell and have an unhappy patient who was expecting 20/20 and J1 vision and only achieved a 20/25 and J2 outcome. If a patient's preoperative expectations cannot be made reasonable, he or she should be discouraged from proceeding with surgery.

Part of managing expectations is making each patient aware of the possibility that he or she may not achieve adequate near vision or may need an enhancement procedure to achieve emmetropia. The strengths and benefits of each IOL model open up the possibility of mixing and matching various IOLs to maximize depth of focus. The potential for placing a different IOL that gives better near vision in the second eye after the first surgical eye delivered unacceptable near acuity should be discussed with the patient. Discussing the benefits and limitations of each IOL model preoperatively will help the patient participate in the IOL choice and make him or her

Table 1
CRITERIA FOR MANAGING PATIENT EXPECTATIONS
• Occupation and hobbies
• Preoperative refractive error
• Ophthalmic pathology
• Pupil size
• Motivation

more responsive and accepting of changes in IOL models for the second eye if this is desired.

Enhancement procedures are inevitable in a certain percentage of refractive lens exchange patients. Each patient should be made aware of this possibility and of the options for refinement, including corneal refractive surgery or a piggyback IOL. The costs of these enhancement procedures should also be discussed preoperatively but the patient can be reassured that if they are required, these procedures are relatively safe and effective in improving the final result.

Presbyopic hyperopes are great candidates for refractive lens exchange. If they do not achieve good uncorrected near vision, they are usually still thrilled with their uncorrected distance vision. Low myopes, however, are the most difficult patients to please because their preoperative near acuity is many times better than their likely postoperative near acuity. It is for this reason that I tend to dissuade low myopes from refractive lens exchange unless they are extremely motivated and willing to accept reading glasses for near tasks.

The lure of refractive lens exchange for both the surgeon and the patient require us to screen patients adequately and to manage their expectations appropriately. I tend to be very conservative with refractive IOLs and I try to lower patients' expectations so that I can exceed them postoperatively. I would rather turn away 10 patients from refractive lens exchange than deal with a single unhappy patient. Customizing the IOL to the patient and preparing the patient for all possible scenarios will help increase patient satisfaction and prevent us from creating a patient who is unhappy despite a good surgical and refractive result.

CHAPTER 99

MANAGING PATIENT EXPECTATIONS

Richard Tipperman, MD

Managing patient expectations is one of the most critical processes for success with presbyopia-correcting intraocular lenses (Pr-C IOLs). This is accomplished in most cases through an interactive counseling process.

One of the most oft-quoted lines on the subject of counseling patients for Pr-C IOL surgery is to "under sell and over deliver." While the logic behind this aphorism is clear, it can unfortunately lead to difficulties for the surgeon just beginning to utilize Pr-C IOLs.

The problem with "under sell and over deliver" is that it can create a confusing situation in which the surgeon is trying to convey 2 disparate and conflicting messages to his or her patients: 1) This lens has problems and things you will not like about it and 2) we should use this lens because it will work well for you and you will like it. If this approach is taken, the patient will often sense "uncertainty" either in his or her surgeon or at the very least in the support staff of the office.

The easiest way to resolve this paradox is to counsel the patient from a different perspective. One approach that can be helpful is the concept of "educate and manage expectations" rather than "under sell and over deliver."

With the focus on educating the patient, the first step is to advise the patient with regard to what his or her visual function would be like if he or she chose a conventional monofocal IOL. If the patient understands the absolute presbyopia that accompanies emmetropia with a monofocal IOL and does not desire this situation, then he or she can at least be considered as a candidate for a Pr-C IOL.

There is no "underselling or overselling" in this approach but instead the patient is counseled or "educated" regarding first the potential benefits (as well as drawbacks) of Pr-C IOLs versus monofocal IOLs. A basic approach to this is outlined below:

Physician: "Well, I understand that you have decided to proceed with cataract surgery. You need to realize that with standard cataract surgery with a conventional lens you will see well in the distance without glasses but you will need *spectacles* for all visual activities from arms length on in.

If you do not want to have to wear *spectacles* for all visual tasks from arms length on in, there is a *better* surgical option. It is called (insert the name of the particular lens platform you would use) cataract surgery."*

The cornerstone in managing expectations and educating patients about Pr-C IOLs is really to educate them about what their other option would be like if they chose a monofocal IOL. We have all had the experience of operating on a patient for conventional cataract surgery who is perplexed as to why he or she needs reading glasses after surgery despite having been informed preoperatively "you will see well in the distance without glasses but will need them for reading." This is because none of these concepts are instinctive or intuitive for our patients. It is our goal as surgeons to educate the patient preoperatively so he or she can understand the poor functional near vision that accompanies bilateral emmetropia with monofocal IOLs. The entire process becomes easier once patients understand that this is what things would be like if they do not choose a Pr-C IOL. Their expectation for Pr-C IOL surgery is that you will make them better than they would be if they chose a monofocal IOL.

In +95% of cases you will dramatically "over deliver" beyond this mark and the patients will be extremely pleased. In the small number of cases where this is not the case, you at least will not have "over promised." As a result with the approach of "educate and manage expectations," you can deliver a coherent unified message to the patient, and yet still be able to "under promise and over deliver." This frees the surgeon from

*I have italicized the words *spectacles* and *better* in the above discussion because I believe they are important specific terms to use. Using the word *spectacles* in the discussion fixes the patient's attention on the need for continued optical correction in the way that the more commonplace term *glasses* cannot. I have italicized the term *better* because many surgeons utilizing this template have a tendency to say "I have something 'newer.'" Many patients will be hesitant about considering a technology that is newer but will be able to understand the advantages of a technology that is "better."

having to "under sell" the Pr-C IOL because he or she can appropriately educate his or her patients that the functional near vision will be better than that with a monofocal IOL. Yet at the same time he or she can inform the patient of any potential concerns that might exist regarding the specific presbyopic platform he or she is utilizing.

The discussion can progress as follows:

"With Pr-C IOL cataract surgery, you will have much more functional vision for near than what you would have with conventional cataract surgery. Approximately 95% of my patients are extremely *pleased with their functional vision and overall results,** and are thrilled that they chose this option. Of the remainder, almost all of them can still tell they are better off than they would have been with a conventional monofocal IOL. However, they may not think they are "perfect" and may wish their vision function was even better. A small percentage of patients may notice issues with _____ (here is where you would include any potential issues with your lens platform of choice [eg, difficulty reading in certain lighting situations, dysphotopsia]).

What if a patient asks you, "What is the biggest risk?"

I answer, "In some way, shape, or form, you may not be happy with how you are seeing with the presbyopic lens in place. Conceivably if you are frustrated enough with the vision, the procedure is reversible and the Pr-C IOL can be removed and a conventional lens put in its place. This would obviously require more surgery but is fortunately a rare event."

Preoperative education and counseling are critical for success with any Pr-C IOL platform. The time commitment necessary to accomplish this becomes less as surgeons gain familiarity with their overall spectrum of clinical results. In addition, education and counseling ,when performed appropriately, also make the entire process easier for both the patient and the surgeon. Ultimately, this saves significant time, as happy and satisfied patients are easier and less stressful to care for. Investing the time preoperatively and postoperatively to manage your patient's expectations is extremely valuable, as it will allow you to achieve the highest rate of clinical success with your chosen platform.

---

*In discussing satisfaction with multifocal lenses and managing patient expectations, it is much better to discuss "overall satisfaction and improvement in functional vision" as a measure of success rather than spectacle independence. If the preoperative counseling stresses spectacle independence as a measure of success, then any patient who wears spectacles occasionally may consider his or her surgery a "failure." Dr. Stephen Dell has described a great phrase he tells patients interested in presbyopic lenses: "You will still wear some type of glasses, some of the time, for some activities." This is a very succinct way to set and manage reasonable expectations.

CHAPTER 100

MANAGING PATIENT EXPECTATIONS

Frank A. Bucci, Jr, MD

The typical large volume cataract practice efficiently "moves information" about the surgical experience from the practice (doctor) to the patients. Brochures, videos, and surgical counselors educate patients about their upcoming surgery in an effort to decrease patient anxiety and decrease the doctor's chair time. Combining high-quality cataract surgery with efficient patient flow in both the clinic and ASC usually results in excellent outcomes, high patient satisfaction, and economic prosperity.

The Centers for Medicare & Medicaid Services (CMS) ruling in 2005 introduced a new option for cataract surgeons—multifocal or presbyopia-correcting intraocular lenses (Pr-C IOLs). Each cataract patient (by paying an additional fee) now has the option to upgrade to a premium IOL that can reduce or eliminate his or her need for reading glasses. In recent surveys, high-volume cataract surgeons have reported increased chair time with cataract patients (discussing premium IOLs), which has resulted in disappointing conversion rates. The typical response of these efficient successful cataract practices is to do more of what they do well. Based on the assumption that their patients need more and higher quality information to make quicker definitive decisions, the practice drives new and greater quantities of presbyopic IOL information from the practice (doctor) to the patient— "so the patient can decide."

What results from intensifying the transfer of information from the practice to the patient? The result has been frustration. The conversion rates to premium IOLs are still poor. The increased information only serves to increase patient inquiries, resulting in further increases to the doctor's chair time. In addition, surgeons are also surprised to encounter excessive complaining by patients postoperatively even after, for example, "telling the patient there would be halos."

What accounts for these observations? The premium IOL component of the doctor/patient relationship introduces a new paradigm—elective surgery. In this new elective surgery paradigm, the pathology/cataract model will fail. In the new paradigm of elective IOL surgery, the quality of the preoperative decision making is directly related to, and dependent upon, the amount of information moving not from the practice to the patient, but on the amount of valuable information moving from the patient to the doctor.

This can only occur if the doctor improves the quality of the doctor/patient relationship. The surgeon must educate him- or herself as to who the patient really is and what he or she actually wants to achieve. Open-ended questions that elicit spontaneous patient responses, in combination with improved listening and observational skills, is a first step in acquiring this necessary information needed to engage in proper patient selection. The patient will give you all the information you need to know—if you will let him- or herself. Combine this information with a thorough exam and then make a definite recommendation to the patient based on your professional opinion about what course will lead to the highest levels of success. Do not ask the patient to decide; lead him or her to the best alternatives based on what he or she has revealed about him- or herself in the preoperative consultation and exam.

Some of the obvious patient characteristics that we learn about in the preoperative interview include patient expectations (personality), visual function and demands, economic status, and refractive status. However, the 2 most interesting and revealing characteristics are the patient's lens status (cataract versus clear lens) and the patient's "purpose for the consultation."

The lens status will frequently divide potential patients into subcategories based on age and culture (Figure 1). Lensectomy and younger cataract patients (baby boomers) are generally more demanding. They will compare their postimplant vision with their excellent preoperative corrected vision. The inherent visual improvement that comes with all cataract surgery makes the entire process more forgiving when cataracts are removed in more senior individuals. These older patients are more accepting by culture, have paid less, perform less demanding visual tasks, and—in general—are less demanding and less litigious.

The "patient's purpose for the consultation" may be the most revealing characteristic of a surgical candidate. We need

Figure 1. The lens status will frequently divide potential patients into subcategories based on age and culture

Age & Culture

Cataract	Lensectomy
• late 60's, 70's, 80's	• 40's, 50's, early 60's
• "Brokaw cataract" WW II	• "Boomer cataract" & clear lens
• Accepting by culture	• Demanding by culture
• Poor corrected pre op VA	• Excellent corrected pre op VA
• Reasonable expectations	• High expectations
• Pay less – expect less	• Pay more – expect more
• Less litigious	• More litigious
• Less computer	• More computer

to just ask the question, "Why is the patient seeking an evaluation?" Is he or she pursuing the diagnosis and treatment for pathology (cataract) or is he or she seeking spectacle independence? Even if the prospective patients were identical twins with identical exams upon presentation, the distinctly different intent or "purpose for the consultation" causes a significant divergence in the course of the preoperative consultation.

Those seeking treatment for a possible cataract have little or no awareness of refractive options. Those seeking spectacle independence are usually very educated by the media, seminars, Internet, word of mouth, or optometry consults regarding their refractive options. If the patient who is concerned about having a (cataract) is told that no cataract is present, he or she is delighted and returns home, telling his or her family that he or she does not need "that growth" removed from his or her eye. If the patient seeking spectacle independence is told he or she does not have a cataract, he or she is extremely upset that he or she has "missed out" on the potential large discount for his or her Pr-C IOL.

If the pathology-minded patient is told that he or she does have a cataract, it may be initially difficult to efficiently present all the refractive options and economic realities. I implement what I call "the three core questions." The answers to the following 3 questions quickly elevate you to a new level of awareness about the patient:

1. Do you have any interest in achieving spectacle independence? Yes or no?

2. Would you be willing to tolerate some light phenomena while driving at night to achieve this freedom? Yes or no?

3. Would you be willing to pay something out of pocket to achieve this increased freedom from glasses? Yes or no?

If the answer to the first question is no, the patient will likely receive an insurance covered monofocal IOL (with or without monovision) at the time of surgery. If the sequence of answers is yes, yes, no, we than offer what I call "the opportunity." We

inform the patient that many presbyopes with bifocals that do not have cataracts pay in excess of $4000.00 per eye to be free of their glasses. However, because he or she has cataracts, he or she will pay less than $2000.00 per eye to achieve the same thing. Do not directly compare the cost of upgrading to a premium IOL to the "free" IOL that comes with his or her health insurance. If his or her sequence of answers is yes, yes, yes, he or she will eventually choose an aspheric or Pr-C IOL.

If the patient seeking spectacle independence does not have a cataract, we then need to distinguish the emmetropes from the nonemmetropes. If the patient is a non-emmetrope, will he or she have laser in situ keratomileusis (LASIK) or a refractive lensectomy? I start the differentiating process with the "one fundamental question": "If we use custom LASIK to give you excellent distance vision and all you need is reading glasses after surgery, will that make you happy?" If you receive a strong yes, do LASIK. If you receive a strong no, discuss the essential aspects of refractive lensectomy with the patient and you will likely end up performing that procedure. If you hear a weak "yes" or a weak "no," begin to discuss the pros and cons of each procedure in a balanced fashion. Watch and listen to his or her responses. The patient will lead you to an awareness or an understanding as to which procedure is best for him or her. Do not quickly manipulate the patient into having a particular procedure because you will get burned. Through a respectful exchange with the patient, offering information and listening to his or her responses, seek and perceive the "truth" about the patient. Who is he or she and what does he or she really want to achieve? The quality of your decision making will escalate. When you decide that you have enough valuable information and you are aware of what is best for the patient, then proceed to lead him or her in a nonbalanced manner to the procedure that you have determined will make him or her most satisfied.

The approach changes significantly if the patient is an emmetropic presbyope. Since these patients already have relatively good uncorrected distance acuity, they are more difficult to please. I strongly "counsel down" their expectations. I tell them that I am very respectful and cautious about performing intraocular surgery in patients with 20/20 uncorrected distance vision. I tell the patient that if he or she can fully grasp the high-risk profile of this surgery, I might offer them a Pr-C IOL in the nondominant eye, and I will likely require a significant period (months) of neuroadaptation after the first eye surgery before ever considering surgery in his or her second eye. I discuss every possible complication. After offering him or her the procedure in one eye, I then begin to withdraw this offer. I closely observe the patient's reaction because it will reveal his or her true demand for spectacle independence. In my opinion, a strong sincere desire for spectacle independence, as compared to any other patient characteristic, has the greatest correlation with postoperative success when implanting multifocal IOLs.

Conclusion

The new paradigm of elective implant surgery demands that you facilitate a genuine doctor/patient relationship. The "3 core questions," "the opportunity," and "the one fundamental question" are only tools for stimulating the patient so you can then observe, listen to, and learn from the elicited response. The basic underlying principle of this approach is that if you choose to listen to your patients, they will give you the answers.

CHAPTER 101

MANAGING PATIENT EXPECTATIONS

Kenneth J. Rosenthal, MD, FACS

General Principles: A Balanced Approach

The patient who has been diagnosed with visually significant cataracts requiring surgery poses a special challenge to the physician who must outline the available options for vision correction. Unlike the (usually) younger laser in situ keratomileusis (LASIK) candidate, whose only goal is independence from spectacles, the cataract patient's primary goal is the removal of the impediment to clear vision, and he or she is likely to be completely unaware that an option for spectacle independence even exists. At the time of this writing, multifocal intraocular lenses (IOLs) have been available in the United States for approximately 10 years, but they have not enjoyed the widespread acceptance that laser vision correction has achieved in a similar time span. As a result, a patient who is diagnosed with a cataract is not likely to have heard about presbyopia-correcting (Pr-C) IOLs, and it is most likely that the experience of his or her acquaintances did not include such choices. Furthermore, patients have become accustomed to the idea, in most instances, that their medical care will be a "covered" service under their health insurance policy.

Managing patient expectations therefore involves a multistep process that must proceed in a progression that is logical to the patient and that apprises him or her not only of the options and their costs, but of what he or she may derive from such options. The process should help the patient decide if the cost of multifocal IOLs represents a good value for his or her money as well.

A carefully balanced approach should be followed for informing the patient not only of the benefits but also of the limitations and possible downside of multifocal lenses. I rely on my strong positive experience of 10 years with respect to patient satisfaction in recommending this option to patients, emphasizing that they will likely be relatively but not completely free of spectacles. It is important to discuss possible limitations of the technology, such as the possibility of needing reading glasses for intensive near vision tasks, in poor lighting, or for reading small print (what I call "stress reading conditions"), and that each patient has a different endpoint in his or her ability to be spectacle independent. I also point out that the patient is almost never completely free of spectacles but that a small (and especially happy!) number of patients actually achieve the goal of complete freedom from glasses. In having this discussion, one must be careful to emphasize the most likely outcome while discussing but not emphasizing the downside. We must tell patients that they may experience night time starbursts around light, but at the same time emphasize that such visual phenomena tend to fade with time and are almost never vision impairing. I may recommend the accommodating IOL (ie, Crystalens [Eyeonics, Inc, Santa Ana, CA]) over the multifocal IOL (ReZoom [Advanced Medical Optics, Santa Ana, CA] or ReSTOR [Alcon, Fort Worth, TX]) to those patients who are unduly concerned about this issue. We must also tell patients that while they are most likely to be pleased with their choice of IOL, there is the unlikely possibility that the multifocal IOL may need to be exchanged for a monofocal lens and that there are risks involved in this process (Table 1).

This is really the same informed consent discussion we have with "standard" surgical procedures: we discuss the risks in the context of how often they occur and how severe they may be, but emphasize the positive features when the risk benefit ratio is legitimately favorable to having surgery. All too often I hear of surgeons who offer multifocal IOLs but with a weak-hearted approach. Telling a patient, "Well, there are the multifocal lenses, and maybe you'll see better up close but you will still need glasses and a lot of patients are uncomfortable at night with glare and halos," does not give the patient encouragement and may provide fertile ground for ultimate patient discontent postoperatively as he or she dwells on these negative aspects. Furthermore, such an approach may discourage a legitimately excellent candidate from choosing Pr-C IOLs.

Table 1

A BALANCED COUNSELING APPROACH

- Unlike LASIK patient, cataract surgical patients are not expecting to have options.
- Prepare them thoroughly and in a way that they can understand.
- Explain choices in a way that realistically represents the risk/benefit ratio.
  - Positives:
    - Relative but not absolute spectacle independence
  - Negatives:
    - May still need spectacles for some tasks
    - May experience visual side effects, but usually dissipate in time
    - Unlikely possibility (and risks) of IOL exchange

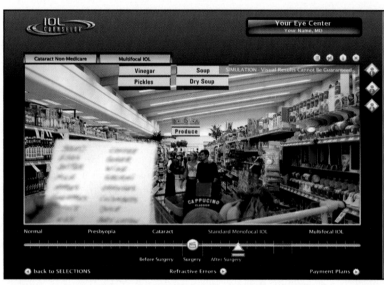

Figure 1. The IOL Counselor illustrates to patients the difference between multi- and monofocality.

Use of Examples From Life Activities

Discussion of the multifocal choices should emphasize the "experience" rather than the "science" of multifocal vision. We use visual aids such as the Eyemaginations (Towson, MD) video clips and the IOL Counselor (Patient Education Concepts, Houston, TX) (Figures 1 and 2) to illustrate to patients the difference between multi- and monofocality. Equally important is helping the patient to imagine life without depending on spectacles: arising from bed in the morning, seeing the time on the alarm clock, preparing breakfast and reading the morning newspaper, then seeing the grandchildren off to school, making a shopping list and then driving to the grocery store, all without putting on glasses. This approach, rather than a dry discussion of "near, intermediate and distance" vision, helps the patient to understand what he or she may expect as it relates to the real world (Table 2). When appropriate, we offer the opportunity to speak with patients who have previously undergone this surgery.

Discuss Bilateral Sequential Implantation

Bilateral implantation of the lens, in most cases, will result in the best multifocality and the best results in terms of quality of vision, and minimizing unwanted visual side effects such as starbursts. Because of this, in cases in which bilateral surgery is anticipated to be needed, a tentative date for the second eye surgery is established prior to the initial surgery. The patient is made to understand that he or she may not be fully satisfied and, in fact, may be unhappy with the initial unilateral result until the second eye is operated upon. I counsel patients that they may need to take a "leap of faith" in having the surgery for the second eye, even in face of their uncertainty after first eye surgery but that this is most likely to lead to the best result.

As a corollary to this principle, Pr-C IOLs can be implanted unilaterally (eg, in the case of a unilateral cataract or in a patient with a pre-existing monofocal IOL in one eye). However, it is essential to educate patients about the limitations of such an approach. They will achieve better distance and near uncorrected vision than with a multifocal IOL but not as good vision as if the same lens is implanted bilaterally.

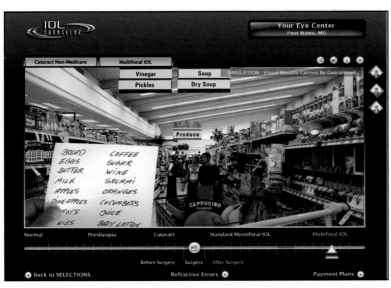

Figure 2. The IOL Counselor illustrates to patients the difference between multi- and monofocality.

Table 2

DISCUSS DETAILS

- Use examples from life activities
  - * Outline "a day in the life" and how spectacle independence may positively affect the average day.
- Use visual aids:
  - * Eyemaginations Videos
  - * IOL Counselor
- Explain need for second eye surgery soon after first, when indicated.

Provide an Assertive Recommendation

My approach to the prospective refractive surgical patient thwarts the conventional practice that separates potential candidates into "good" and "bad" prospective candidates based on their "motivation" to be spectacle independent (Table 3). While it has become commonplace to provide a patient with a "lifestyle" questionnaire assessing his or her motivation to be spectacle independent, my recommendation is based solely on whether the physical state of the patient's eyes supports the decision for a Pr-C IOL. My experience in implanting multifocal IOLs is that patients cannot intuit the value of being free of spectacles. Even the patient who, before surgery, was guarded or skeptical about being spectacle independent ("I've worn them all my life, so I'm happy to continue to do so") is usually pleased beyond his or her expectations afterwards.

A positive, assertive recommendation to the patient helps to guide him or her in his or her decision and creates the atmosphere for success after surgery. Therefore, if the patient's eyes are essentially healthy, I do not ask the patient whether or not he or she would like to be free from spectacles; I tell him or her that he or she is a good candidate for multifocal or accommodating IOLs and that I would recommend them.

Postoperative Adaptation

Managing the visual expectations of a patient about to receive multifocal IOLs comprises preoperative counseling as well as postoperative guidance and training.

Preoperatively I explain to the patient that I will be revamping his or her visual system and that the eyes will see well almost from the beginning but that the brain has to slowly adapt to the new visual system. The process of "neuroadaptation" (and I use that word) will allow the patient to gradually become used to seeing things differently than before surgery (Table 4). A good analogy that helps patients understand this is that of adapting to a new spectacle correction they may have received when they were younger. Many people can remember that they put on the new spectacles and instantly saw more clearly than before but that they were uncomfortable for a while until they "broke in" the new glasses.

This "breaking in" period of neuroadaptation is a poorly understood process and it occurs with wide variations in time for different patients. While it is not at all uncommon for patients to note clear vision at all distances even on the first post operative day (following the second eye surgery), this may take up to a year for some patients. I tell patients to expect that it will take at least 6 months and as much as a year to achieve the optimal results, citing our "no complaint" policy (Kevin L. Waltz, OD, MD): we will not heed complaints of near vision

---

Table 3

HELP PATIENT TO CHOOSE

- Provide an assertive recommendation based on surgeon's understanding of previous patients' experiences.
- Do not rely on assessment of patients "motivation" and "lifestyle" needs
- **Recommend multifocal to all patients who are suitable candidates based primarily on physical health of the eyes, regardless of perceived "motivation."**
- **"Buyers remorse" is primarily from the patient who chooses the monofocal IOL!**
- **Ask patient to sign off on choice of IOL.**

Table 4

EXPLAIN POSTOPERATIVE ADAPTATION

- Discuss the process of "neuroadaptation."
- Explain the expected time course of full adaptation:
  * Some have immediate improvement in near vision
  * Expect about 6 months but may take up to 1 year for optimal result
  * May need more frequent visits to achieve goals.
- "No complaint" time out = 6 months (Kevin L. Waltz, OD, MD)
- Possibility that they may need spectacles early on, and possibly in future.
- Encourage non-use of spectacles during the adaptation period.

---

deficiencies for at least 6 months postoperatively. I also advise them that they may need to participate in the adaptive process by refraining from wearing glasses unless absolutely necessary, or by performing eye exercises to improve their near vision, and by additional office visits to aid in the process. I also add that a minority of patients will not achieve near vision good enough to do ordinary reading. This type of result is most likely to be seen in patients who were nearsighted preoperatively, those who have demanding near vision needs, those who are perfectionists, or those who have skeptical or demanding personalities. We have adopted Steven J. Dell, MD's approach in which he advises the patient that "the IOL does not care if you are a perfectionist."

Counsel the Monofocal Patient Too

It is also important to point out that we need to manage the expectations of the patient who chooses a monofocal IOL. Because they have options, patients who did not choose one of the multifocal options often experience "buyer's remorse," particularly when they are in the company (usually in my reception area as they await their post operative office visit!) of patients who have had multifocal IOLs who are reading comfortably without spectacles. These patients should be counseled about the possibility that they may actually regret their decision, and if they express such a regret post operatively, they are reminded of the initial discussion. As a corollary to this approach, I discuss multifocal IOLs with all patients even if they are not candidates, so that they will not be upset after surgery if they learn such an option was available.

In order to codify the patient's final decision, and to ensure that there are no misunderstandings afterwards, we have the patient choose and sign off on his or her choice of lens from a written menu of lens options, and we provide him or her with a copy.

In the end, the success of Pr-C IOL implantation is contingent not only on careful preoperative testing, impeccable biometry, and meticulous surgical technique, but also on the proper counseling of patients as to the choices they have, to the array of potential outcomes, and to the expected time course necessary for optimal visual rehabilitation. A presentation that is positive, yet incorporates realistic goals, will result in the most satisfactory outcomes.

CHAPTER 102

THE ROLE OF THE REFRACTIVE IOL COUNSELOR

James D. Dawes, MHA, CMPE, COE

Most traditional cataract practices have struggled with how to incorporate the best practices of the laser vision correction industry to develop a refractive intraocular lens (IOL) patient flow model. Surgeons throughout the country have experimented with various staffing and patient flow models to optimize the conversion of traditional IOL patients to a refractive IOL procedure. Below, I have outlined the key elements of the refractive IOL consultation and evaluation as developed by our practice. I do not attempt to discuss the actual surgical procedure or follow-up care and have intentionally limited my discussion to the consultation and evaluation of the refractive IOL patient. In this chapter, I routinely reference accommodating and multifocal IOLs as premium lenses and refractive IOLs.

Phones/Reception

The patient's first contact with the practice must create a first impression that is courteous, professional, and inviting. It is important to identify patients who are potentially seeking a refractive procedure and to schedule them for the appropriate consultation and evaluation. Some patients are reluctant to schedule a consultation immediately. These patients must have the option to ask questions prior to the consultation if they so desire. Speaking to a counselor prior to the consultation allows the patient to be educated and comfortable with the surgeon prior to actually coming to the office. Some practices have chosen to outsource these refractive consumer calls whereas others choose to handle them in-house. The important factors are to ensure that a patient can access a well-informed counselor without waiting on hold or going to voice mail, and to ensure a consistent tracking mechanism for call volumes, referral sources, and follow-up contacts.

Prior to the actual visit, the patient should receive educational information related to refractive procedures and IOLs either via mail, referring doctor, or the practice Web site. As demonstrated by recent Internet studies, many Americans over 50 years of age rely on the Internet for medical informa-tion. An informative and easy to navigate Web site can reduce expenses associated with mailing and will allow patients to learn the basics about the refractive IOL procedure prior to the visit. This is the key to increasing efficiency and effectiveness of the consultation and evaluation.

Office Reception and Greeting

Once the patient arrives at the practice for a consultation, they are well on their way to making the decision to have a premium lens procedure. Even patients who are coming in for a routine eye examination are potential refractive IOL patients; therefore, the initial greeting must differentiate your practice from others. Professional and polite front office staff with inviting smiles are surprisingly rare in today's medical practices. Much like the telephone interaction, this first personal contact will set the tone for the entire patient experience. At this point in the visit, if the patient has not received educational information about the premium lens procedure, every effort must be made to put this in his or her hands. The lobby area where the patient may wait should contain educational information and patient testimonials while creating a relaxing environment.

Technician Work Up

In addition to the technician's clinical function, this is the point at which the patient should be told what exactly will transpire during that day's office visit. The technician must set the tone of excitement about the latest technological advancements in refractive IOLs and cataract surgery. Often patients are not only unaware of refractive IOLs but are surprised to learn that they have a cataract. In our experience, it is best for the technician to confirm the existence of a cataract and the presence of any astigmatism with the goal of reducing the patient's potential anxiety and answering any questions that may arise.

The technician also has an opportunity to confirm the patient's desire for the premium lens procedure based on lifestyle information obtained earlier in the scheduling process. For example, a technician may say to the patient, "Yes, Mr. Smith, it does appear that you have a cataract, but with today's premium lens technology you may have the opportunity to experience life without glasses. Imagine being able to see the golf ball on the tee, see the ball in the fairway, and write down your score all without glasses. Mr. Smith, you are now going to talk with one of our counselors about your lens options. The counselor will discuss the details related to your insurance coverage, potential costs, and review the benefits of the various lenses with you."

With clearly defined parameters developed by the surgeon, a technician can deselect any patients who do not meet the clinical criteria for a refractive IOL and move the patient out of the refractive IOL patient flow to a traditional cataract patient flow. This would eliminate the need for a nonqualifying patient to meet with a counselor. This is also a great time for the technician to credential the surgeon by referencing training, experience, and other factors that reaffirm the patient's selection.

Refractive IOL Counselor

At this point in the visit, the patient should be well aware of refractive IOL technology. The counselor now has the opportunity to work through detailed information and answer questions prior to the patient seeing the surgeon. Although the surgeon has not yet recommended a specific lens or finalized the decision that the patient will qualify for the premium lens procedure, the benefits, risks, price, and insurance coverage can all be discussed with the patient. Again, like the technician, the counselor is using the patient's lifestyle questionnaire responses to associate an emotional connection to the lifestyle benefit of a refractive IOL procedure. This entire conversation with the patient can be completed in less than 10 minutes while the patient is dilating prior to the consultation with the surgeon. It is important that the counselor complete a summary of the patient's lifestyle-based vision needs, desire for the procedure, and any concerns or questions that need to be addressed by the surgeon.

Surgeon

Prior to sitting down with the patient, the surgeon should have had the opportunity to review the summary provided by the counselor and be prepared to answer any questions or address any concerns the patient may have. Assuming the patient meets the surgeon's clinical criteria, it is imperative that the surgeon makes a specific and definitive lens recommendation. The surgeon now has an opportunity to talk about his or her experience with refractive IOLs and discuss historic patient outcomes. At this point, price has been discussed by the counselor, so there should be no need for the surgeon to discuss price. Due to the complications related to coverage by Medicare and private insurance, as well as copayments and deductibles, specific pricing discussions should be conducted by the counselors. Once the patient indicates a preference to proceed with a premium lens procedure or traditional cataract surgery, the appropriate consents and authorizations must be handled. In order to maximize the efficiency of the surgeon and to allow time to review all of the information, a clinical assistant can typically handle this part of the consultation.

Refractive IOL Counselor

Once the patient has made the decision to have a premium lens procedure, the visit is not complete. The counselor must "close the deal"; that is, schedule the procedure and postoperative follow-up, finalize all consents and forms, receive payment, and/or arrange any financing necessary. At this point, surgical preoperative testing may have already been performed; however, discussions regarding covered and non-covered tests, and the signing of Advanced Beneficiary Notices (ABNs) and the Notice of Exclusion of Medicare Benefits (NEMB) form must be carefully coordinated by the counselors to ensure that the patient fully understands the out of pocket costs. By now the patient has been in the practice for well over an hour and has been bombarded with information, tests, clinical staff, and forms. The counselor must work to ensure that all of the patient's questions have been sufficiently answered, that the chart forms are in order, and that the patient is excited about the benefits of the premium lens procedure. The patient should leave the practice with a complete preoperative packet, appointment reminder cards, contact information for the counselor, and most importantly a feeling of confidence in the surgeon, the practice, and the lens technology.

Conclusion

I have only discussed the consultation and evaluation portion of the refractive IOL patient experience. The patient must still have the surgical procedure and required follow-up examinations. The patient's excitement and emotional connection about the lifestyle benefits of the procedure must be continually reaffirmed throughout the process. However, the same principles and commitment to exceeding the patient's expectations and creating a premium experience must be applied to the remaining components of the premium lens procedure and follow-up care. Achieving the best visual outcome for the patient through diagnostic and surgical excellence can never be replaced by counseling and sales techniques. These techniques only allow the patient to make an informed decision so that they might have the opportunity to enjoy the benefits of all distance vision provided by today's refractive IOLs. All patients who meet the surgeon's criteria for a refractive IOL should have the opportunity to experience life without glasses.

CHAPTER 103

WHO IS A PREMIUM IOL CANDIDATE?

Alan Shiller, MD

We ophthalmic surgeons live in an incredibly exciting time because we have more choices than ever before to obtain the best possible outcomes for our patients. This is true whether they are primarily refractive patients or whether they are cataract patients who are wanting to achieve a greater level of spectacle independence. Our practice has had a good deal of experience when it comes to refractive lensectomy as well as cataract patients who are opting for a presbyopia-correcting premium intraocular lens (IOL), and my primary choice has landed squarely on the Crystalens IOL (Eyeonics, Inc, Aliso Viejo, CA). There are several reasons for this choice, not the least of which is that the Crystalens is the only Food and Drug Administration (FDA)-approved accommodating IOL.

Patient Selection

The issue of patient selection has become a big topic in regard to presbyopia-correcting IOL. Certainly, patient selection is an important process, but I believe we make it much more complicated than it really should be. We all pretty much agree that if we perform a cataract procedure or clear lensectomy on a patient, then we are almost always going to place an IOL in that eye. Well, if you stop and think about it in its most basic terms, the main difference between a traditional monofocal IOL and the Crystalens IOL is that one of them flexes and accommodates. At its very core, that is the main difference. Therefore, it is my very strong belief that if we agree that a patient is a candidate for a traditional monofocal IOL, then that same patient is certainly a candidate for a Crystalens accommodating monofocal IOL, assuming that there is an intact capsular bag with intact zonules. The only difference is that the Crystalens IOL will provide a larger range of vision than the traditional lens. There are certainly some patients who simply are not good candidates for a multifocal ReZoom (Advanced Medical Optics, Santa Ana, CA) or ReSTOR (Alcon, Fort Worth, TX) IOL because of the induced aberrations that are inherent with their design. Such patients could include those with prior radial keratotomy (RK), laser

in situ keratomileusis (LASIK), or even corneal scars. So far, I have implanted a Crystalens IOL in several patients after previous LASIK and RK as well as one patient that had an old hexagonal keratotomy without fear of inducing more aberrations over what they already had. These patients have so far been extremely happy.

Even in light of macular pathology when there is potential improvement of vision with a cataract procedure, certainly it would be a benefit to have a broader range of vision than not. There is obviously a spectrum of achievable vision that some patients can obtain, and it is my strong belief that it should be the patient's decision if a broader visual range at their expected acuity level warrants the extra cost of this premium IOL. I find that if we educate our patients on what to expect and then deliver the highest quality results, then the Crystalens is a fantastic choice for the majority of our patients.

I believe that it is important not to prejudge whether or not a patient can afford a premium IOL. Let me emphasize that it is not my job to prejudge whether a patient wants or can afford a premium IOL. It absolutely is my job to let patients know what technology is available, so that they can make an informed decision.

I will give several examples from my own experience as to why I believe this is of utmost importance. About a year ago I performed cataract surgery on a very nice lady and implanted a traditional monofocal IOL. She did very well and was very happy with her improved vision. However, at her one month visit she was a little miffed at me. Upon questioning her, she let me know that I had implanted a Crystalens IOL in a good friend of hers, and this friend was enjoying more spectacle independence than she was. This nice lady also let me know that I had not offered her the same. After I reviewed my traditional monofocal patient's records, it was very clear to me that I had prejudged her ability to pay for the Crystalens upgrade even though later she informed me that money was not an issue. Did she forgive me? Yes. Did I learn a lesson? Absolutely!

A second example of my potential misjudgment occurred about 2 months ago. I was seeing an active 87-year-old man who lives a lifestyle that I hope I am blessed with when I am that age. He needed cataract surgery and I was not even going to offer the Crystalens option to him based on his age. However, during his examination the thought came to me that my very own father is almost 86 years old and is active, and if I were about to do cataract surgery on him, he would definitely get a Crystalens. I thought how beneficial it would be to someone like my very own father to be less dependent on glasses. Then the humbling thought occurred to me that this nice, active 87-year-old man's lifestyle is no less valuable than my very own dad's. I offered the Crystalens upgrade to him, thinking that he surely would not opt for it because, after all, he is too old. Right? Wrong. He is now enjoying spectacle independence because he chose the Crystalens upgrade and is not regretting it one bit.

Therefore, my belief is that we should NEVER prejudge a patient's desire for a premium IOL or his or her willingness to pay for it. Simply give the patient the option and let him or her decide. The primary reason I would not offer the option of a Crystalens is when a patient has preoperative evidence of abnormal zonulae.

Finally, never underestimate the importance of a superb refractive coordinator. Our refractive coordinator treats all of our refractive lensectomy patients and cataract patients with the same importance that she does our LASIK patients. After all, our cataract patients have now become potential refractive patients. She counsels the patient by discussing options, expectations, and costs. A patient does not leave our office without being offered financing and going through the approval process if financing is chosen. I know that I am blessed to have one of the best refractive coordinators in the industry, and because of this my extra chair time with these patients is minimal. When I consider the added profit that these lenses provide to our practice, it's easy for me to see that the economics are clearly on my side.

Surgical Technique

My surgical technique is fairly straightforward, as I perform routine phaco through a 2.75-mm incision. I will do limbal relaxing incisions (LRI) on patients with >1.00 D of astigmatism, which I believe decreases the need for enhancements postoperatively. I rotate the lens with a cystotome so that the haptics are oriented along the 90 degree axis. This is so that the haptics will not be affected by any potential subincisional cortex that could be left behind. Furthermore, hydration of the incision, as well as the paracentesis, is always done. We should never underestimate the paracentesis as a possible site of wound leak after the patient leaves the facility. Any momentary wound leak can shallow the anterior chamber and cause the Crystalens to vault forward. To date we have not had anterior vaulting of the Crystalens, and I credit this to the

hydration of both the primary incision as well as the paracentesis.

Postoperative Targets

Getting good outcomes requires very accurate preoperative K readings and axial length measurements. I am very blessed to have a staff that understands the importance of these measurements. We ALWAYS obtain 3 sets of manual K readings and select the best one for our IOL calculation. We also use the IOL Master (Carl Zeiss Meditec, Jena, Germany) for our biometry, but we never use the K readings that the IOL Master provides. We use immersion A-scan axial lengths if an IOL Master reading cannot be done. We never, ever stray from this methodology.

I prefer to operate on the non dominant eye first with a postoperative target of −0.37 D to −0.62 D with the Crystalens. The dominant eye is typically done 2 weeks later with a postoperative target of Plano to −0.25 D. These targets give us slightly overlapping visual ranges, which is different from the monovision achieved with monofocal IOLs. These slightly overlapping visual ranges give a binocular functional range of around plano to −2.00 D. This refractive range gives patients the ability to do most of their activities without spectacles.

Postoperative Counseling

Our patients are told during their preoperative consultation that it is okay to use weak readers of about +1.00 D as a crutch for reading the smallest print. We encourage our patients to avoid using the readers as much as possible, and we definitely see their reading ability improve over time. I believe this improvement is due to the strengthening of the ciliary muscles as well as the fact that patients have the ability to neuroadapt to the new visual system they now have.

To maximize patient satisfaction, we must be able to perform enhancements after the Crystalens implantation for any residual refractive error. For pure mixed astigmatism, I tend to do astigmatic conductive keratoplasty (CK) as early as 3 weeks postoperatively. If a patient needs spherical correction, I typically choose to use LASIK. So far, using these adjunctive refractive procedures has not caused any problems and has satisfied the patients that needed it. Our enhancement rate after Crystalens implantation is about 6%. I credit this low rate to my staff because of the accuracy of the preoperative measurements.

Finally, we must remember that each of our patients has unique vocational demands as well as lifestyle desires. It is our job as physicians to provide our patients with the technology that will give them the greatest chance of meeting these needs and desires. In my experience, the Crystalens fits the bill.

CHAPTER 104

REFRACTIVE CANDIDATES— WHO IS GOOD? WHO IS NOT?

Stephen G. Slade, MD, FACS

In the past, corneal refractive surgery was for our younger patients, and our cataract surgery patients were a separate group where less attention was paid to the final refractive outcome. Today we offer more choices than ever to all our patients. With the current advanced intraocular lens (IOL) options for presbyopia, cataract surgery is as much refractive as corneal based refractive surgery.

The Advanced "Presbyopia"— Correcting IOL Population

All we have to do to identify our presbyopia-correcting Pr-C) IOL population is to follow the baby boomer generation through time. The post–WWII baby boom today, in 2007, is centered on those of us who are close to 50 years of age. Ten years ago these patients were 40 and produced the record numbers of laser in situ keratomileusis (LASIK) we were doing at that time. Now boomers are at the age where they will begin to seek cataract surgery and solutions for presbyopia. Indeed, by 2020 the US population over 65 will double from current levels. This patient group will need high-quality care from today's ophthalmologists and the next generation of ophthalmologists.

Baby boomers are of a different mind set. They are unwilling to drift quietly into senescence. They have more wealth than any other group in history and are willing to spend their money on themselves. They attach significant value to cosmetic procedures and view aging as a weakness. As such they do not want to be identified as "aged" by virtue of wearing bifocals or reading spectacles (Figure 1).

Benefits of Presbyopia-Correcting IOLs

Specifically, who can benefit from these advanced lenses? The traditional cataract patient has the most to gain as they are visually disabled with no refractive fix. A patient with presbyopia can also benefit from the ability of these lenses to decrease dependence on glasses for near and intermediate vision. A patient with large amounts of myopia or significant hyperopia will also gain better uncorrected distance vision. In our practice, we are more conservative for clear lens extraction and reserve this for larger amounts of hyperopia (>4.00 D). A patient without a cataract and a large amount of myopia would likely receive a phakic IOL. A good rule of thumb is to treat the patients with significant cataracts, and be more aggressive with presbyopic refractive patients and high hyperopes. Finally, patients often perceive one further benefit of having refractive lens exchange and IOL surgery, which is not something that we traditionally discuss as ophthalmologists. This benefit is that we are removing the early cataract before it can ever become a problematic cataract. This patient population does not want to live their life incubating a visually significant cataract in their eye until they have become disabled from doing certain daily activities, such as driving (Figure 2).

Value Versus Cost of the Presbyopia Lenses

Most patients realize that the choice of a premium IOL is a decision of cost versus value. This is a common dilemma with which we are all familiar. Patients need information and time to make decisions such as whether to take a vacation, cover other personal needs, make financial investments, remodel their home, or invest in their future eyesight. They will seek the surgeon's recommendation and reassurance. Remind them that they are spending money on their most important sense and one that they use every waking moment of every day. In fact, many of them have spent more money on their dental work than on their vision. It is better to present the cost of an advanced lens as being "discounted" by the insurance payment rather than as an "added" price over traditional Medicare- or insurance-covered cataract surgery. To be able to be successful with this technology the physician has to recognize the great value that modern Pr-C IOL surgery can provide. You must

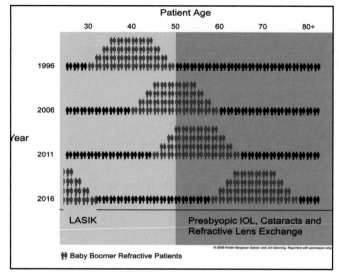

Figure 1. A demographic chart which demonstrates the baby boomer generation in red moving through time. The new group of red figures at the far left in 2016 represents "Gen Y" by some accounts, larger than the baby boomer generation.

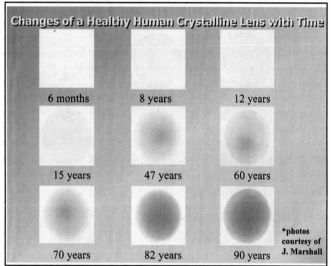

Figure 2. A comparison of human lenses at different points in time. Even at an earlier age than traditional cataract surgery, the lens has lost clarity, gained color, and lost accommodation.

believe in your price and that yes, this is a reversal of the trend of declining fees for cataract surgery over the last 20 years.

Lens Selection and Patient Selection

There are 3 main choices for Pr-C IOLs today; ReSTOR (Alcon, Fort Worth, TX), ReZoom (Advanced Medical Optics, Santa Ana, CA), and the Crystalens (Eyeonics, Inc, Aliso Viejo, CA). Their characteristics are well documented elsewhere in this book. Importantly, none of them are perfect and this forms a critical concept for patient education. These lenses cannot assure glasses-free vision at all distances. The old refractive surgery adage "under promise and over deliver" is the right one for these patients. The surgeon must ensure that the patient understands the different ranges of vision and the choices. Of

particular importance is intermediate vision. Many patients use their intermediate vision much more than near vision compared to how other generations did in the past. We simply view cell phones, PDAs, and computer screens more frequently than we read novels with small print. Of course, each patient will have different needs and wishes. Again, stress the potential for complications such as dysphotopsias and the need for glasses and/or refractive enhancement procedures after surgery.

For lenticular refractive surgery, like corneal refractive surgery, about 10% of our effort is in performing the surgery and 90% of our effort is in providing the rest of the services. These include selecting the procedure and lens, selecting and counseling the patient, and performing the preoperative workup and postoperative care. Patient selection is a major component of presurgical planning, where the patient's personality is a huge consideration. A patient that understands risk and imprecision often is better suited for our IOL options today. Typically professionals such as lawyers or doctors are better candidates than architects or engineers. Lawyers are less exact and more flexible, in my experience. Always listen to your staff's impressions of a patient's personality. Usually they spend more time with the patient than you, and in a more relaxed, "real life" atmosphere than the physician. Try to identify patients with unrealistic expectations, those who demand perfect vision, and those who have a poor understanding of cataract surgery risks. These individuals should either be disqualified for the refractive IOL or counseled further.

A main goal for patient selection is to avoid the patient that would eventually become so unhappy as to require IOL explantation (Table 1). A successful refractive lens practice should be judged not only by the number of excellent outcomes, but also by how small the number of bad results is. The optical qualities of the different IOL choices must also be specifically weighed for more complex eyes such as those with retinal abnormalities, or those having previously undergone corneal surgery. Whereas monofocal lenses are most often explanted for power errors, decentration, and dysphotopsias, in that order, multifocal lenses are explanted for (in order of frequency), dysphotopsias, power errors, and lens decentration. A final crucial point is to make sure that the patient understands that they might not get the planned lens if there were unexpected intraoperative problems. If they are aware of this possibility, they certainly will be more accepting if such an occasion arises

Ocular factors can influence a patient's suitability as well. Examples include diabetes, macular degeneration, uveitis, glaucoma, previous retinal detachment, irregular astigmatism, pseudoexfoliation, zonular weakness, posterior polar cataracts, and surgical complications such as capsular tears at surgery. Refractive surgeons have learned the importance of identifying patients with corneal dystrophies who may be compromised in terms of laser vision refinement after lens surgery. Whereas keratoconus can occur in 1 in 2000 patients in the general population the incidence of ectasia after laser vision correction is unknown. It is associated with eye rubbing, family history, genetic predisposition, Down's syndrome, ocular allergy, and contact lens wear. For these patients, lens exchange for spherical errors and other options for astigmatism may be better choices. The diagnosis is aided by observing the presence of local areas of ectasia and steepening, noting differing states

Table 1

MOST COMMON REASONS FOR IOL EXPLANTATION

Monofocal IOL

1. Power error
2. > Lens decentration
3. > Unwanted visual phenomenon
   Total < 1%

Multifocal IOL

1. Unwanted visual phenomenon
2. > Power error
3. > Lens decentration
   Total: > 2%

ASCRS Surveys

of progression, mirror image symmetry, folds in Descemet's membrane, spectacle blur, and an abnormal retinoscopy reflex. Review the patient's old records for refractive stability, family history, and their age.

Although there are no blood tests or magic numbers that provide a definitive diagnosis,[1] a typical pattern on topography of asymmetric bowties with skewed radial axis is very helpful in the diagnosis.[2] We attempt to avoid ectasia after laser vision correction by recognizing forme fruste keratoconus preoperatively, fully informing the patient of any additional, unique risks they may have, and being able to offer different options for such patients.

Patient Counseling

Let the patient become educated about you and your expertise as well. Just as you need to learn about your patients, they need to learn about you. Of course, explain what the best possible outcome could be—glasses-free vision—but also mention the worst case scenario including, but not limited to, vitreous loss, retinal detachment, and infection. The surgeon should give the patient some idea about his or her level of experience, especially early on in the surgeon's learning process. Often it is better for the surgeon to introduce the costs, in a positive manner, as described earlier, before leaving a discussion of details to the staff.

Try to ensure that the patient has realistic expectations. Remember "better" is the enemy of "good." This holds true for Pr-C IOL surgery. The need for surgery on one eye, or both and the timing between the 2 eye operations must be fully explained to the patient. The predictability of the initial and final result after any enhancement should be reviewed in terms of the patient's pre-existing astigmatism, ease of lens calculations, and so on. Tell the patient about the potential need for refractive corneal surgery postoperatively as well as the possible need for a ytrrium-aluminum-garnet (YAG) laser procedure. Ask the patient about any night vision complaints they currently have and document them. This can prove to be invaluable postoperatively if the patient starts to express such complaints at that time. A good tip is to record the patient's uncorrected near vision for the chart by having them circle the smallest line they can read uncorrected preoperatively so that it can be referenced postoperatively. The more you can learn about the patient's lifestyle and daily activities, whether they like monovision, and their expectations for "glasses free" vision, the easier the choice of IOL will be.

Conclusion

Among all refractive procedures, lenticular surgery has become just as important as corneal surgery. Lenticular refractive surgery is done on relatively healthy eyes, the patients are paying for all or part of the costs out of pocket, and they are expecting a "perfect" result. We find that these patients are all best treated together as refractive surgery patients.

References

1. Binder P. Risk factors in post LASIK ectasia. *J Cataract Refract Surg.* 2007;33:1530-1537.
2. Rabinowitz YS, Rasheed K. KISA index: a quantitative videokeratography algorithm embodying topographic criteria for diagnosing keratoconus. *J Cataract Refract Surg.* 1999;25:1327-1335.

CHAPTER 105

REFRACTIVE CANDIDATES—
WHO IS GOOD? WHO IS NOT?

Weldon W. Haw, MD and Edward E. Manche, MD

The development of presbyopia-correcting intraocular lenses (Pr-C IOLs) has expanded the options available to refractive cataract surgeons and patients alike. However, the merging of the cataract patient's problem with the refractive surgery patient's expectations for "20/20" or "perfect vision" outcomes creates challenges. Many patients now expect excellent uncorrected visual acuity at far, intermediate, and near distances under all ambient lighting conditions. In addition, they may also expect no glare/halos, no contrast sensitivity loss, no residual astigmatism, emmetropia, and more than 3.0 D of accommodative amplitude. Unfortunately, current generation Pr-C IOLs may fall short of the patient's elevated and often unrealistic expectations. The refractive cataract patient is in many ways similar to the refractive/laser in situ keratomileusis (LASIK) patient. From this standpoint, we can learn a great deal from the experience of our refractive surgeon colleagues.

The Pr-C IOLs available in the United States can be divided into 2 categories: 1) multifocal IOLs and 2) Accommodating IOLs (Figure 1). The currently available multifocal IOLs include ReSTOR (Alcon, Fort Worth, TX) and ReZoom (Advanced Medical Optics, Santa Ana, CA). At the time of the writing, the anticipated launch of the Tecnis multifocal IOLs (Advanced Medical Optics) in the United States has been delayed by the Food and Drug Administration (FDA)'s request for additional follow-up data. The Crystalens (Eyeonics) is currently the only available accommodating IOL on the US market and is available with a 4.5-mm optic and 5.0-mm optic. Understanding the current generation of each of these Pr-C IOLs and their respective strengths and weakness may assist us with selecting the optimal IOL for each patient. Appropriate candidate selection and accurate, predictable IOL calculation are, however, the most essential aspects in transitioning to a successful refractive cataract practice.

Candidate Selection

PREOPERATIVE REFRACTIVE ERROR

The best results are obtained in hyperopic presbyopic cataract patients because preoperatively they are already dependant on spectacle correction for all distances (Table 1). These patients usually have reasonable expectations and are therefore quite accepting of uncorrected distance visual acuity of 20/40 or better (DMV requirement for driving without corrective wear) and with uncorrected near visual acuity of J3 or better (reading the newspaper in sufficient light without requiring corrective wear). Patients with high myopia (>–6.0 D) may also be reasonable candidates because, preoperatively, they are spectacle dependent for distance as well as for a comfortable reading distance. Less optimal candidates are emmetropic patients with presbyopia although they also tend to have realistic expectations for functional uncorrected near vision. Low myopic (<–3.0 D) patients with presbyopia (ie, those who enjoy reading without their spectacles) may be particularly difficult to please given their expectation of improved postoperative near uncorrected visual acuity. Regardless of their preoperative refractive error, patients should be aware of the possibility of requiring corrective lenses, especially for prolonged near activities or activities that are particularly visually demanding such as driving in a scotopic/nocturnal environment. Patients should also be counseled regarding the possible need for keratorefractive surgical enhancement such as photorefractive keratectomy (PRK) or LASIK to treat any residual refractive error or astigmatism.

LIMITED POSTOPERATIVE VISUAL POTENTIAL

Patients with obvious and significant pre-existing morbidity (ie, macular degeneration, cellophane maculopathy, macular scar, cystoid macular edema, ischemic maculopathy)

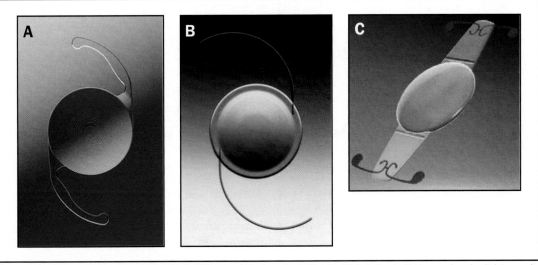

Figure 1. The FDA-approved Pr-C IOLs: (A) ReSTOR. ReSTOR is a multifocal apodized diffractive IOL that allocates light energy based on lighting conditions and activity. There are 12 concentric steps (1.3 to 0.2 µm) providing a range of vision. The reading add of +3.2 D in the spectacle plane is the strongest of the currently available presbyopia multifocal IOLs. (B) ReZOOM. ReZOOM is a second generation refractive multifocal IOL with 5 optical zones including a central distance dominated area. It provides excellent distance and intermediate vision. (C) Crystalens. The Crystalens is a nonpupil dependent accommodating lens that uses 100% of the available light rays all of the time. By changing position, the lens allows accommodation and provides excellent distance and intermediate vision. The lens is not a multifocal IOL and therefore avoids many of the reported side effects of a multifocal optical system.

Table 1
PRESBYOPIA-CORRECTING IOL CANDIDATES
1. Hyperopic presbyopes (best candidates)
2. High myopia
3. Emmetropic presbyopes
4. Low myopic presbyopes (worst candidates)

are unlikely to fully benefit from the technology offered by the premium Pr-C IOLs. Less obvious, but nonetheless, poor candidates are those patients with an eccentric pupil, high myopia and stretched photoreceptors from a posterior staphyloma, slight amblyopia, minimal macular drusen or retinal pigment epithelial changes, chronic dry eye or ocular surface disease, uncorrected corneal astigmatism >1.0 D, and the unilateral monofocal pseudophakic. The potential loss of contrast sensitivity and degradation of the quality of vision from a multifocal IOL may be additive to the patient's pre-existing eye disease in adversely impacting the patient's vision to a significant degree. In addition, patients with central nervous system (CNS) issues may be at risk for an inability to neurally adapt to multifocal IOLs.

POSTKERATOREFRACTIVE SURGERY

The normal physiologic cornea retains a prolate shape, such that it is steeper in the center and flatter in the periphery. Eyes that have undergone previous keratorefractive surgery no longer have a physiologic prolate shape. In addition eyes that have had radial keratotomy, PRK, or LASIK may have irregular central corneal astigmatism resulting in a reduction of best spectacle correction to less than 20/20. Any visual symptoms resulting from an opacity (ie, posterior capsular opacity) or optical abnormality (ie, irregular astigmatism) along the visual

axis can be dramatically accentuated or exaggerated in an eye with a multifocal optical system (ReSTOR, ReZoom). Thus, eyes that have undergone previous keratorefractive surgery with a decrease in best spectacle-corrected visual acuity out of proportion to what would be expected from the cataract should be evaluated with manual keratometry or videokeratography to determine whether there is irregular astigmatism. This must be done before a multifocal IOL is implanted. In addition, a greater improvement in best corrected visual acuity with a rigid gas permeable contact lens compared to a soft contact lens or spectacle lens may also be consistent with irregular corneal astigmatism.

PUPIL SIZE

In refractive surgery, it is important to carefully measure and document scotopic pupil size preoperatively. Patients with larger pupil size need to be counseled that they may be at increased risk of developing unwanted scotopic symptoms of glare, halos, starbursts, and night vision phenomena. The pupil size in the refractive cataract patient is also important. ReZoom is a distance dominated IOLs in which the central zone (<2.1 mm) provides distance only correction. Thus, patients with small pupils are unlikely to benefit fully from the multifocal design of the IOLs. Patients with miotic pupils are more likely to have poor uncorrected near and intermediate vision. The apodized diffractive design of ReSTOR is less pupil size dependent and allows a near 50:50 distance:near split from the incoming light. It therefore provides reasonable near and distance vision regardless of the pupil size. Patients with larger pupils are subjected to the possibility of developing glare and halos. The large pupil effect is mitigated in ReZoom due to its Opti-Edge design. Nevertheless, in most instances, glare and halos resulting from a multifocal IOL subside over 6 months.

Table 2

TRANSITIONING TO A REFRACTIVE CATARACT PRACTICE: PEARLS AND PITFALLS

- Preprinted literature given to patients about their IOL options before their appointment (minimizes "chair" time discussion).
- Assess the visual needs and expectations before surgery.
- Manage the patient's expectations **before** surgery. Exclude patients with unrealistic expectations.
- Preprinted survey/questionnaire assessing and ranking the patient's visual demands may also be useful.
- Demonstrate to patients undergoing a multifocal IOL that they have glare/halos preoperatively with a light source.
- Place −3.0 D lens over each eye to duplicate the difficulty with reading with a monofocal distance-corrected eye.
- Customize the IOL selection based on the patient's visual demands (may consider mix/match with ReSTOR/Crystalens/ReZoom, etc).
- Optimize the IOL Calculation (see Tables 3 and 4).

UNREALISTIC EXPECTATIONS

A refractive cataract surgeon will inevitably be faced with a patient with unrealistic expectations. Obtaining a detailed perspective on a patient's expectations is essential as all current generation Pr-C IOLs have shortcomings that may result in an outcome that falls short of a patient's high expectations. By listening to the patient's expectations, spending the necessary "chair" time with the patient *before* surgery, and educating the patient on what the different Pr-C IOLs can and cannot achieve, the refractive cataract surgeon can improve the probability of having a 20/"happy" patient (Table 2). For example, a rigid gas permeable contact lens wearer who was unhappy with his or her contact lens vision before the cataract developed may not be the best candidate for a multifocal IOL. A patient who would not be satisfied with anything but complete independence from spectacles in all ambient settings is also not an optimal candidate for the current generation Pr-C IOLs.

PATIENT PERSONALITY

We have all experienced patients whose personality makes us uneasy or uncomfortable. Typically, these are the patients that we dread seeing on our schedule and might hope to avoid seeing at all costs. Many of these patients are driven by the need to achieve perfection in every aspect of their lives, including vision correction. Unfortunately, these are typically the same patients requesting vision correction surgery from our refractive surgeon colleagues and now, presbyopia-correcting cataract surgery from refractive cataract surgeons.

These patients with difficult personalities may have trouble understanding that the outcomes of current generation Pr-C IOLs are by no means perfect. The situation is exacerbated by the patient's perception of entitlement to "perfect" vision after incurring additional out of pocket expense for the Pr-C IOL technology. Despite a comprehensive discussion, consent, and documentation of the consent process, these patients may be significantly disappointed with their visual outcome. Additionally, they may not recall the limitations that were discussed during the preoperative visit.

PATIENT WITH A DIFFERENT SPECTACLE FOR EVERY DIFFERENT ACTIVITY ("100 DIFFERENT GLASSES")

Patients with a different spectacle correction for every different activity (ie, reading in dim light, reading in bright light, computer, knitting, cooking, driving in bright light, driving at night) are a well-known personality type to the refractive surgeon. A classic sign is a patient that brings in more spectacles than he or she can carry in his or her 2 hands (ie, requires a bag to carry all of the different spectacles that are used throughout the day). These patients typically express general dissatisfaction and frustration with their vision in any setting and are therefore, by nature, difficult to please.

EXCESSIVE VISUAL DEMANDS (WORK OR HOBBY)

Patients with extraordinary visual demands that are unlikely to be satisfied with a Pr-C IOL should be educated about the consequences of proceeding with surgery. In particular, patients whose vision may adversely be impacted by the contrast sensitivity loss or additional glare/halos during scotopic circumstances are not ideal candidates for multifocal IOLs. For example, a professional truck driver or commercial airline pilot needing 20/15 scotopic vision are not optimal candidates for a multifocal IOLs.

UNWILLING TO ACCEPT THE DOWNSIDE RISK

A patient's acceptance of both the surgical risk and Pr-C IOL limitation is a prerequisite for proceeding with refractive cataract surgery. Current generation Pr-C IOLs are not perfect optical systems. Multifocal IOLs may result in glare/halos, contrast sensitivity loss, and difficulty seeing in all ambient lighting conditions.[1-5] The Crystalens is a monofocal accommodative IOL and therefore minimizes many of the adverse events ascribed to a multifocal IOL.[6] However, uncorrected near vision may not be as comparable to the ReSTOR IOL. In addition, patients must be willing to accept the possibility of requiring subsequent enhancement surgery with keratorefractive surgery to manage any residual refractive error or astigmatism. Patients should also be accepting of the possibility of requiring spectacle correction for visually demanding activities such as driving at night or reading fine print for an extensive duration.

IOL Calculation

As in refractive surgery, poor preoperative measurements result in unacceptably unpredictable postoperative results and ultimately, an extremely vocal unsatisfied patient. In refractive surgery manifest and cycloplegic refraction, corneal pachymetry, and topography are essential tools in evaluating a prospective candidate for LASIK. Similarly, the refractive cataract surgeon needs to be able to accurately and

---

Table 3

MAXIMIZING KERATOMETRY AND AXIAL LENGTH MEASUREMENTS

Keratometry	*Axial Length Measurement*
Avoid taking measurements immediately after contact (ie, tonometer)	Noncontact methods (Immersion or IOL Master [Carl Zeiss Meditec, Jena, Germany]) are preferred
Discontinue contact lens 2 to 4 weeks prior to ensure stable K reading	Use the average of multiple consistent measurements
Use one dedicated keratometer and technician for all measurements	Reconcile with bilateral axial length measurements
Manual keratometer is the preferred technique	A difference >0.33 mm between eyes requires independent confirmation from another technician
Use topography to confirm Ks for irregular mires or astigmatism >4.0 D	If the axial length is <22 mm or >26 mm, a second person independently confirms the measurements
RECHECK if a) K <40 D or >47 D; b) corneal astigmatism by K does not correlate with refraction	Review the actual A-scan (and repeat if necessary) for measurements that do not make sense

---

Table 4

RECOMMENDED IOL CALCULATION FORMULA ACCORDING TO AXIAL LENGTH

Prevalence of Eyes With the Noted Axial Length Measurement (%)	*Axial Length (mm)*	*Recommended IOL Calculation Formula*
8%	Short eyes (<22 mm)	Hoffer Q
72	Average eyes (22 to 24.5 mm)	Holladay 1, Hoffer, SRK-T
15	Slightly long eyes (24.5 to 26.0 mm)	Holladay 1
5	Long eyes (>26.0 mm)	SRK-T

Consider using Holladay 1 for flat K readings and using Holladay 1 or Hoffer Q for steep K readings. If the IOL power difference between eyes is greater than 1.0 D or there is any question about the accuracy of the axial length or keratometry, repeat the measurements. It should be the goal of every practice to eventually transition to the Haigis or Holladay 2 formulas. These newer generation formulas are highly accurate and can be applied to most axial lengths.

---

reproducibly perform keratometry and axial length measurements in a patient undergoing cataract surgery with a Pr-C IOLs implantation (Table 3).

The inability to obtain reliable or reproducible preoperative readings results in inaccurate IOL calculations that can be devastating for a physician's reputation among his or her patients. In particular, refractive cataract patients who pay an out of pocket premium for the Pr-C IOLs may be particularly vociferous about outcomes that fall short of their elevated expectations.

Noncontact methods of measuring the axial length (ie, immersion ultrasonography or IOL Master) and manual keratometry are recommended techniques for patients undergoing a refractive cataract procedure. The IOL Master is a noncontact, optical device that uses partial coherence interferometry to obtain the necessary measurements for prediction IOL power for patients that are undergoing cataract surgery. This technology was approved by the FDA in March 2000 and has been found to be accurate, reproducible, and easy to use. It is

also can be particularly useful in eyes with posterior staphylomas, extreme hyperopia or myopia, or eyes with silicone oil. It may not be effective in eyes with certain media opacities in the optical axis (corneal scar, dense cataract, vitreous hemorrhage).

Choosing an appropriate IOL calculation formula is critical for optimizing postoperative refractive results (Table 4). Several third-generation IOL calculation formulas must be tailored according to the axial length measurements: Hoffer Q is accurate for short axial lengths (<22 mm), Holladay 1 is accurate for normal to slightly long axial lengths (23 to 26 mm), and the SRK/T is accurate for long axial lengths (>26 mm).

However, it should be the goal of every surgical practice to incorporate the more modern and sophisticated formulas such as the Holladay 2 and Haigis formulas. These newer generation IOL calculation formulas can offer increased predictability and accuracy. The Holladay 2 was developed in 1998 by Jack Holladay, MD and utilizes 7 variables including the axial length, white to white, corneal diameter, anterior chamber depth, lens thickness, patient's age, and preoperative prescription. This stand- alone software can be purchased as an IOL package (ie, IOL Consultant). The Haigis formula was developed by Wolfgang Haigis, PhD in 1991 uses the true anterior chamber depth and 3 constants: a0, a1, and a3. It is available through the Web site of Warren Hill, MD at www. doctor-hill.com. In addition, determining the true central keratometry reading in post-keratorefractive eyes must also be performed. A full discussion of this topic is beyond the scope of this chapter.

Conclusion

The Pr-C IOLs represent one of the most innovative technological advancements in the IOL market in recent history. However, with the evolution of new technology comes the responsibility of determining the appropriate candidacy of patients that are likely and unlikely to benefit from the potential advantages that Pr-C IOLs offer. Indeed, identifying patients that may potentially experience adverse consequences from this technology may be similarly important. Appropriate candidate selection and accurate IOL measurements are integral in maximizing the patient's visual outcome. As in refractive surgery, the "chair time" spent with these patients discussing their options may be lengthier, the informed consent may be more complicated, and the documentation process may be more involved. Nevertheless, when the technology is appropriately integrated into the refractive cataract surgeon's practice, it is a considerably valuable option that results in a more satisfied patient with functional "20/happy" vision.

References

1. Vingolo EM, Grenga P, Iacaobelli L, Grenga R. Visual acuity and contrast sensitivity: AcrySof ReSTOR apodized diffractive versus Acrysof SA60AT monofocal intraocular lenses. *J Cataract Refract Surg.* 2007;33(7):1244-1247.
2. Zeng M, Liu Y, Liu X, Yuan Z, Luo L, Xia Y, Zeng Y. Aberration and contrast sensitivity comparison of aspherical and monofocal and multifocal intraocular lens eyes. *Clin Experiment Ophthalmol.* 2007;35(4):355-360.
3. Leyland M, Pringle E. Multifocal versus monofocal intraocular lenses after cataract extraction. *Cochrane Database Syst Rev.* 2006;18(4): CD003169.
4. Chiam PJ, Chan JH, Aggarwal RK, Kasaby S. ReSTOR intraocular lens implantation in cataract surgery: quality of vision. *J Cataract Refract Surg.* 2006;32(9):1459-1463.
5. Leccisotti A. Secondary procedures after presbyopic lens exchange. *J Cataract Refract Surg.* 2004;30(7):1461-1465.
6. Pepose JS, Qazi MA, Davies J, Doane JF, Loden JC, Sivalingham V, Mahmoud AM. Visual performance of patients with bilateral vs combination Crystalens, ReZoom, and ReSTOR intraocular lens implants. *Am J Ophthalmol.* 2007;144(3):347-357.

CHAPTER 106

REFINING MY INDICATIONS FOR MULTIFOCAL IOLs

James A. Davison, MD, FACS

Food and Drug Administration Studies

Food and Drug Administration (FDA) studies for new surgical devices are performed to establish that products are safe and effective. They are scientifically specific and rigid in their definition, patient inclusion criteria, surgical execution, and performance measurement. Follow-up and reporting are rigorous even to the point of specifying that only black-ink pens can be used for signatures. Because of the validity of this process, once a device has been approved surgeons should be confident in their expectations of achieving FDA-study performance levels if they perform their surgery in the same way on similar patients. However, we should also understand that results may vary if even one of the components of the FDA study routine is not followed. As I have strayed from strict FDA patient inclusion criteria, that variation in performance is exactly what I have experienced as I have used the Alcon ReSTOR (Fort Worth, TX) diffractive intraocular lens (IOL).

I was one of the clinical investigators for the ReSTOR and was therefore well aware of the key components of the FDA study: patient inclusion criteria, preoperative patient counseling, preoperative biometry, surgical technique, and postoperative care and performance assessments. All of the patients I operated on in the study had excellent results and were very happy with their visual performance. Now that I am using the IOL following FDA approval, there are 3 key differences that have made things slightly different for me. First, there are some patients who want the technology even though they do not conform to the FDA patient inclusion criteria. This might be because of either major or minor pathologies in their eyes or visual systems. FDA study patients were basically normal. Second, patients with healthy eyes but who have regular keratometric astigmatism of greater than 1 D want the diffractive IOL. These patients would not have been candidates in the FDA study. Finally, all patients are expected to pay an out-

of-pocket "upgrade" fee as part of their surgical fee. The FDA study patients did not.

What follows are my impressions of the impact of these 3 key differences on my clinical results. They are based on my personal anecdotal experience and are not the result of a formal controlled study. I have the most experience with the Alcon ReSTOR IOL. I also have some experience with the Crystalens by Eyeonics, Inc (Aliso Viejo, CA), and minimal experience with the ReZoom by Advanced Medical Optics (Santa Ana, CA). I have not mixed multifocal technologies.

Normal Patients

We mail out a 1-page information brochure that describes monofocal, toric, and multifocal IOLs along with an appointment card to new patients so they can start thinking about options and choices before their office visit. A new patient will receive a technical evaluation by one of our technicians before I see him or her. A biometry determination by IOL Master (Carl Zeiss Meditec, Jena, Germany) is part of that initial work-up. That, along with the refraction and history, are displayed on the computer screen for my nurse to review prior to my arrival in the exam room. The nurse will make an assessment of the technical work-up and the patient's interest in reducing spectacle dependence. She will then initiate an introduction of IOL options based upon this information. If patients have employed a monovision contact lens strategy, we usually encourage them to consider continuing with pseudophakic monovision after cataract surgery. Nine times out of 10, my staff can determine the patient's interest and candidacy for a premium IOL before I enter the room. They will include this part of their assessment in their introductory summary to me in the hall before I enter the exam room.

If a patient is interested in multifocal or toric IOL options and they have a healthy ocular examination, I review the highlights of the FDA data on the IOL that they are qualified for and are likely to be happy with. A reasonable ReSTOR candidate wants to be able to read small print or read for extended periods of time without glasses but does not mind having to wear intermediate glasses for computer use. They should also be able to tolerate the risk of some halos and glare or the risk that their visual system may not completely satisfactorily adapt to the ReSTOR technology. I tell them that I have only had to exchange 3 ReSTOR IOLs because of idiosyncratic poor visual adaptation and that those patients all ultimately did well with their monofocal IOLs. If patients prefer good uncorrected distance and intermediate vision and would not mind wearing glasses for reading small print in most situations, I would consider them to be a reasonable candidate for the Crystalens. This is also a good option for someone who might be at increased risk for pseudophakic dysphotopsia or is afraid of being intolerant of multifocal glare and halos or incomplete cortical adaptation. I tell patients that we may yet determine that they are not good multifocal IOL candidates if other subsequent tests are found to be abnormal. In particular, we look for abnormalities on computerized video keratography and Orbscan (Bausch & Lomb, Rochester, NY), which might make them ineligible for potential laser in situ keratomileusis (LASIK) enhancement.

Pathology of the Visual System

Before I knew better, I used the ReSTOR in patients with other significant compromises in their visual system and found that the results in those patients were not what they had hoped for or what I would been happy to accept. I have had to exchange only 3 ReSTOR IOLs (<1% incidence for me), but I would not implant these 3 patients today knowing what I know now. The first patient was a prominent businessman who had an epimacular membrane after a scleral buckle and pars plana vitrectomy for a macula off retinal detachment. He only had a 20/30 potential and developed low-grade cystoid macular edema (CME) after surgery. Even after resolution of the CME with medical treatment, he still had a very poor subjective quality distance and near vision (but did measure 20/40 uncorrected distance and near equivalent) after surgery. He really pushed for the ReSTOR during his preoperative exam, in fact that is why he had come to me specifically, but I should have just said no. He was quite dissatisfied with his vision with the ReSTOR IOL but was very happy after I exchanged the multifocal IOL for a monofocal distance focused AcrySof IOL (Alcon).

The second patient was a woman who had a very minimal cataract but lots of glare complaints, including a lifelong history of glare with night driving. She experienced immediate positive dysphotopsias and glare with her ReSTOR, which partially persisted even after exchange with an Advanced Medical Optic SI40 silicone IOL. She was a poor candidate for ReSTOR or even a monofocal high refractive index square-edge acrylic optic. She never returned to get her second eye done. The third patient was a woman with a history of possible mild amblyopia. After uneventful ReSTOR implantation, her vision was "hazy" and she had "spots missing" when she looked at objects or print. Interestingly, she had normal pseudophakic vision and was very happy after exchanging the ReSTOR for an AcrySof monofocal IOL focused for distance.

Most ReSTOR patients do well and are happiest if they have a perfect plano result and if they have no other pathology in their visual system. Some patients have had acceptable results with mild degrees of other ocular pathologies. Examples of such mild abnormalities would include grade 1 corneal anterior basement dystrophy, grade 1 corneal endothelial guttata, a few small macular drusen or extremely minimal central macular pigmentary changes, or a grade 1 epimacular membrane with no macular thickening. In my experience, if patients have more advanced degrees of these types of abnormalities, they are very likely to underperform objectively and subjectively and not be happy with their results. The same is true if they have combinations of such low-grade problems, even though each abnormality is individually mild. If I do not expect at least a solid crisp 20/25 visual result, I usually do not think about offering ReSTOR technology.

While there is nothing more satisfying than having a perfect bilateral ReSTOR patient, the performance of the ReSTOR-enabled visual system depends upon everything being perfect or near perfect. In other words, when the demanding requirements of this system are met, it performs at a very high level. All patients who elect a multifocal IOL receive a refractive surgery evaluation as well so that we can be sure that we can apply LASIK technology to enhance clinically significant residual refractive error after the primary surgery. The correction of very small residual refractive errors can make a huge improvement in the performance of ReSTOR patients. These patients will experience decreased performance with small amounts of posterior capsule opacification and will need Nd:YAG laser treatment earlier than monofocal IOL patients.

Patients who have some low to intermediate degree of ocular pathology and would still like good uncorrected distance and intermediate vision may be good candidates for the Crystalens technology. The Crystalens-enabled visual system is less demanding in terms of perfect emmetropia and perfect ocular health. However, Crystalens patients usually require reading glasses for extended or fine near work or small print.

Multifocal IOL implantation does not always have to be bilateral as unilateral ReSTOR or Crystalens patients do very well. I have implanted quite a few monocular ReSTOR IOLs in young patients in their teens, 20s, and 30s, and they have all done very well.

Regular Keratometric Astigmatism

In order to be included in the FDA ReSTOR study, patients could not have more than 1.0 D of regular keratometric astigmatism. Since its introduction, I offer the AcrySof toric IOL rather than the ReSTOR or Crystalens IOL to patients with greater than 1.0 D of keratometric astigmatism. If they insist that they really want multifocal technology, then I have to plan for LASIK after their lensectomy. Limbal relaxing incisions can be done, but in my hands they are notoriously imprecise, especially when compared to contemporary LASIK performance. Residual refractive error is better tolerated in Crystalens patients than in those implanted with the ReSTOR.

Planned LASIK bioptics patients should understand that they will need to wear some temporary spectacle correction (at their own expense) following lensectomy but before his or her laser enhancement procedure. In my practice, LASIK enhancement following a multifocal IOL is included in the premium charge. It can usually be done about 1 month after cataract surgery.

The "Upgrade" Fee

I do not use this term because it implies a different level of service than monofocal patients receive. We try to provide each and every one of our patients with only the highest level of service possible. We simply introduce the multifocal or toric IOL as "premium" IOL options for them to consider and tell them that these options have different costs associated with them. We tell patients that the "standard" monofocal IOL has many high technology features already built into it and that 80% of our patients select that technology. If being less spectacle dependent is not that important to them or the increased cost of a premium option bothers them, then they should not consider the option.

One of the reasons the ReSTOR FDA study patients were happy is that they did not have to pay extra for their access to the new technology. There can be a considerable difference in expectation and attitude in patients who have their costs covered by insurance or Medicare and those who pay a surgeon extra out-of-pocket money for a technology "upgrade." The latter group of patients have different expectations, a different appreciation of the value of the service, and a greater potential for dissatisfaction and frustration. When using a multifocal IOL, I feel that I have taken on a refractive surgery patient and I will have to be committed to making him or her happy no matter what. This may include frequent no-charge postoperative appointments for reassurance and LASIK for even small amounts of residual refractive error if necessary.

Conclusion

There is nothing more spectacular than hearing the comments and witnessing the performance of patients who have received multifocal IOLs. Patients consider this a truly miraculous experience. And while the multifocal visual system can be life changing for patients, we must constantly resist the temptation to try to "sell" it. The patients most likely to be happy are those who truly want to achieve some significant level of spectacle independence and will be able to fully appreciate the true and enduring increased value that a premium IOL will add to their lives For many, it may be something that they have always dreamed of. Let the patients and their families make their own determination and assessment of the options. The added cost and the increased risk of dissatisfaction or additional adjunctive surgery must be offset by the potential value. Listen to the patients and their families and try to offer multifocal technology to highly motivated healthy people with healthy eyes and you will have good results.

CHAPTER 107

REFRACTIVE IOLS AND PATIENT OFFICE FLOW

William D. Gaskins, MD, FACS

Planning for patient flow in the ophthalmic practice, large or small, is essential for maintaining patient satisfaction. Patients are informed about new lens technology from traditional sources such as advertisements, and they will present with questions that must be answered to their satisfaction. Preparation for timely, accurate, and factual presentations to your patients serves as an indicator of your capability to provide them with the latest technology available. Patient flow in the era of noncovered refractive intraocular lenses (IOLs) used in cataract surgery is important due to the time constraints of both the ophthalmologist and the patient. Refractive IOL discussions and evaluations add significantly to the time necessary to educate patients.

Preparation includes providing helpful sources of information to patients. Informational pamphlets may be included with correspondence to the patient for their initial visit or with bills. Brochures or video technology such as DVDs can educate patients while they are in your reception area (Figure 1). Waiting time can be effectively used to assist the patient in making the decision of whether or not to receive a refractive lens. This information may be useful for the patient or his or her family and friends.

These informational sources serve as a stimulus for discussion and can be addressed by appropriate members of your staff. When trusted and well-trained staff members display a positive attitude toward new lens technology this will break down barriers and reduce concerns about whether these new implants are appropriate for the patient's lifestyle. Staff enthusiasm, or the lack of it, will definitely influence patients' perception of any new technology.

Enthusiasm must be tempered with the realization that new technology lenses are not the correct choice for every patient. Patients need to know that each individual must be separately evaluated for their candidacy for the new technology lenses, and that every effort will be made to make the extra time and cost of the evaluation worthwhile. Even if the patient is not a candidate for the new refractive IOL, he or she will appreciate the knowledge gained and will understand the logic behind your decision not to use the new lens technology.

Dr. Mark Gorovoy of Fort Myers, FL recommends introducing the patient to the refractive lens option as early in the cataract evaluation as possible to eliminate those who are not able or willing to spend out of pocket money. He has patients fill out a visual task sheet to indicate where their preference for best uncorrected vision is for near, intermediate, or distance. Patients interested in the refractive lenses are asked to view a video while he sees another patient before returning for further discussion. The amount of astigmatism directs his recommendations for a toric lens with astigmatism of greater than one D. With less than one D of astigmatism he considers using the multifocal lens, and he discusses drawbacks of the lens with the patient.[1]

For patients who are interested, hands-on demonstration of the implant shape, flexibility, and design may be easily shown with the props such as an IOL model or pictures of the implant (Figure 2).

By the time the patient sees the ophthalmologist, a baseline level of knowledge and reassurance should have been obtained so that more time can be devoted to answering specific "nongeneric" questions. A discussion of multifocal and toric lenses with every patient allows them to understand that new lens technology is available and helps them understand your perspective. William W. Culbertson, MD, professor of ophthalmology at Bascom Palmer Eye Institute and member of the American Academy of Ophthalmology Ethics Committee, feels that the decision to use these lenses is best made when the patient has a complete understanding of the advantages and disadvantages of the procedure. "You can partially off-load it to brochures and videos and patient counselors. In the end, however, it comes down to the doctor helping the patient make the best choice and answering all the patient's questions"[2]

Richard J. Mackool, MD recommends 4 principal preoperative steps to ensure the highest level of success when implanting premium lenses. "Seek motivated patients and inform them

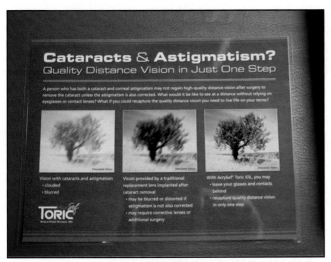

Figure 1. Brochures or laminated teaching aids may enable the patient to visualize the effects of cataracts or astigmatism, and the benefit of correction with the appropriate intraocular lens. (Reprinted with permission of Alcon.)

well, evaluate pupil diameter, evaluate keratometry readings, and customize the incision sizes to treat astigmatism."[3]

Preoperative evaluation in these patients requires attention to the accommodative pupil diameter. It is desirable to have an accommodative pupil diameter of 2.5 mm or less to avoid ghost images. Postoperative astigmatism of 0.5 D or less will optimize refractive outcomes. Residual postoperative astigmatism can be modified by the size and positioning of the phaco incision, adding limbal relaxing incisions or performing laser in situ keratomileusis (LASIK). Use of devices such as the IOL Master (Carl Zeiss Meditec, Jena, Germany) can simplify the measurement of axial length and keratometry and expedite calculations for premium lenses with the ability to personalize your surgeon's factor for each implant model.

Even though added paperwork that informs patients about their out of pocket costs adds to the time involved in getting these patient through your office, it needs to be integrated into your routine. Appropriate documentation with forms such as the "Notice of Exclusion from Medicare Benefits" are signed and understood by each patient. If there are extra costs for additional procedures such as limbal relaxing incisions, LASIK, or other procedures, the patient needs to be informed of these costs and risks before surgery.

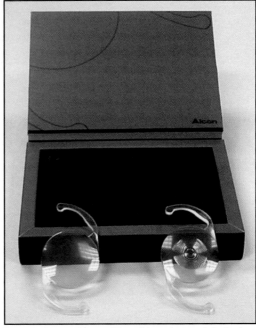

Figure 2. Props such as an IOL model or pictures of the implant. (Reprinted with permission of Alcon.)

Patients are more receptive to the additional cost of the procedure when they understand the extra testing, planning, and premium expense of the implant. Avoid unrealistic patient expectations by discussing likely outcomes of the procedure and by selecting appropriate candidates. One of the most rewarding aspects of working with refractive IOLs, even with the extra time, effort, and paperwork involved, is to see the smile on the face of the "20/happy" patient. Patient satisfaction may be one of the best forms of advertisement.

References

1. Mark Gorovoy, MD, personal discussion, September 18, 2007.
2. Miriam Karmel, High road ethics for a high-tech era. *Eye Net.* 2007;11(8):53-57.
3. Richard J. Mackool, MD, Customizing surgery for premium IOL success. *Eyeworld Suppl.* 2007;July 10;8-10.

CHAPTER 108

MULTIFOCAL IOLS AND GLAUCOMA— HOW MUCH IS TOO MUCH?

Iqbal Ike K. Ahmed, MD and Joshua Teichman, MD

With the emergence of multifocal intraocular lenses (IOLs) and increasing patient expectations, their use in patients with concomitant diseases such as glaucoma raises both opportunity and questions. The impact of glaucoma on the visual system, and the potential alterations created by a multifocal IOL, obviously raises concerns. Relevant questions include the effect of these IOLs on visual function, and their impact on glaucoma screening and monitoring in this population. Unfortunately, there is a paucity of data in this area, leaving clinicians with only theoretical and anecdotal evidence to guide their decision making. The severity and stability of glaucoma must be factored into this. Consideration of the potential risk-to-benefit ratio for an individual glaucoma patient will assist in determining the appropriateness of a multifocal IOL, and perhaps a specific multifocal technology.

Concerns with the use of multifocal IOLs in glaucoma and their effect on visual function center on 2 main issues: the reduction of contrast sensitivity (CS) and the effect on mesopic and scotopic vision. It is known than CS is reduced in glaucoma, even in mild disease prior to discernible perimetric defects, and is correlated to the degree of visual field (VF) loss. Evidence suggests a greater impairment of mesopic visual quality and slower dark adaptation in the glaucoma patient, which is also correlated with the degree of VF loss.

Some overall reduction of CS to some degree has been found with all currently available multifocal IOLs. These IOLs use optical splitting technologies, either primarily diffractive or zonal refractive, thus producing 2 or more simultaneous foci. For a specific focal point of interest, there is a defocused veil of light that is directed to the second image, and reduction of light intensity at a specific focal point. Compared to monofocal IOLs, there is a mild reduction of CS with multifocal technology. This reduction is more evident at near than at distance, and is greater under mesopic than photopic conditions (in glaucoma, there is a comparatively greater loss of mesopic CS as well). Higher spatial frequencies are also more likely to be impacted with multifocality, although in glaucoma, there is a greater loss of CS at lower spatial frequencies. Although for most patients without concurrent eye disease this is not a significant issue, this has implications for CS and mesopic/scotopic vision in the glaucoma population.

High-pass-resolution central perimetry has shown a loss of sensitivity for eyes implanted with multifocal IOLs when compared to phakic or monofocal IOL eyes in patients without glaucoma. Diffractive multifocal IOLs were found to perform better than refractive designs. However, it is unknown whether one multifocal design is more optimal for a glaucoma patient versus another.

With a reduction in higher-order aberrations and the expected benefit for CS, the addition of asphericity to multifocal IOL technology should help to offset some of the CS and mesopic functional loss.

It is important to note the both diffractive and refractive multifocal IOL designs impact the amount of light available for a particular focus. In a diffractive design, light energy is divided between 2 foci, with some lost within the system, whereas in a refractive design, light energy is scattered over a large number of foci.

The impact of multifocal IOLs on perimetric testing in the glaucoma patient is also debatable, with little data available to provide firm conclusions. These IOLs have the potential to have an impact on overall threshold values, with a possible mild reduction. Clinicians should consider a possible depression (ie, 1 to 2 dB) in grey scale, raw values, total deviation, and mean deviation values in standard automated perimetry. However, anecdotal reports in glaucoma patients with mild to moderate VF defects have found minimal effect on these values. Threshold perimetry should be performed using an optical add for near despite the presence of a multifocal IOL. Indices that are less likely to be affected by focus/multifocality issues include pattern deviation plots, pattern standard deviation, and the glaucoma hemifield test. Frequency-doubling technology (FDT), which utilizes a larger target and is less dependent on refraction, is less likely to be affected by the presence of a multifocal IOL.

Table 1

PATIENT SELECTION: PATIENTS WITH GLAUCOMA WHO MAY BE CANDIDATES FOR MULTIFOCAL IOL IMPLANTATION

- Glaucoma suspects and ocular hypertension with no disc or VF damage who have been stable.
- Glaucoma with early or mild VF damage that has been controlled and stable.
- Level of glaucoma in fellow eye is similar, and not severe, advanced or progressive.

Despite the potential impact on some perimetric values, clinicians can use early postoperative VF testing to establish a new baseline for these patients, as should be done for any glaucoma patient undergoing cataract extraction. This can then be used to monitor for future progression. Furthermore, the use of disc and retinal nerve fiber layer (RNFL) imaging, such as scanning laser tomography, optical coherence tomography, and scanning laser polarimetry, should be considered. The impact of multifocality upon these modalities appears to be minimal to none.

A valid concern for any patient with a chronic, potentially progressive disease, such as glaucoma, is his or her unknown future visual function. For example, although it may be reasonable to implant a multifocal IOL in a patient with ocular hypertension or mild glaucoma, what if that patient progresses to more advanced glaucoma, and thus may be more negatively impacted by the choice of IOL? For this reason, it is advisable to determine a patient's risk for glaucoma progression to guide IOL decision making (Table 1). Glaucoma patients who have been stable for a period of time (ie, >1 year) with adequate follow-up are potential candidates. On the other hand, patients with advanced VF damage, unstable or progressive disease, substantial visual loss in one eye, and possibly pseudoexfoliative glaucoma with moderate-advanced disease are not ideal candidates.

Multifocal IOL performance is felt to be dependent on pupil size and dynamic characteristics of the pupil. As an excessively miotic or mydriatic pupil may affect performance, the presence of posterior synechiae, or pseudoexfoliation, in the glaucoma patient may be an issue and should be factored into the decision to proceed with a multifocal IOL.

The only published data on the use of multifocal IOLs in glaucoma found an improvement in near visual acuity with no reported subjective issues, and "management was not compromised." However this study had a small number of glaucoma patients (n = 11), and did not use objective assessment of CS or perimetry.

One must temper the IOL selection issues with the fact that cataract extraction alone in all glaucoma patients will improve visual quality, CS, and have an impact on perimetric testing. Clinicians should therefore expect that even in those patients with more advanced glaucomatous damage, a significant visual improvement will be found with monofocal and multifocal IOLs. The question here is one of maximizing visual function

in these patients. Certainly in early glaucoma, although there is some loss of CS, it is mild and likely insignificant for most patients. As in the patient without concurrent disease, some may be willing to comprise some loss of CS and/or mesopic visual function for the benefit of reduced spectacle dependence. An accommodating IOL, which should have less impact on these visual function issues, should be considered as well.

The risk-to-benefit ratio of using a multifocal IOL in the glaucoma patient remains debatable and uncertain. To deny all patients with glaucoma or glaucoma suspicion of the potential benefit of multifocal technology may be excessive. Many clinicians have achieved success in patients with ocular hypertension and "preperimetric" glaucoma, and those with mild VF damage, and this appears reasonable. Aspheric IOL designs, which are likely to benefit all patients, should particularly be considered for the glaucoma patient. Caution must be exercised in patients with moderate to advanced VF damage, and in unstable and progressive disease. As always, appropriate preoperative discussion and patient selection are critical to success in the use of these advanced IOL technologies.

Key Points

* Patients with glaucoma have a degree of CS and mesopic visual function loss, which correlates with disease severity, and which may occur prior to documented VF damage.

* Multifocal IOLs have been found to result in a reduction of CS and mesopic visual function when compared to monofocal IOLs.

* There are limited data on the use of multifocal IOLs in glaucoma patients, although a number of anecdotal have reported safety and success.

* An aspheric multifocal IOL design is preferred if there is optic neuropathy.

* The stability and severity of glaucomatous disease, and the fellow-eye status should be considered.

* Appropriate preoperative assessment, counseling, and patient selection are critical when considering implantation of a multifocal IOL in the glaucoma patient.

* Certain values in threshold VF testing may be affected in the glaucoma patient with a multifocal IOL.

Bibliography

Hawkins AS, Szlyk JP, Ardickas Z, et al. Comparison of contrast sensitivity, visual acuity, and Humphrey visual field testing in patients with glaucoma. *J Glaucoma.* 2003;12:134-138.

Kameth GG, Prasad S, Danson A, Phillips RP. Visual outcome with the Array multifocal intraocular lens in patients with concurrent eye disease. *J Cataract Refract Surg.* 2000;26:576-581.

Kumar BV, Phillips RP, Prasad S. Multifocal intraocular lenses in the setting of glaucoma. *Curr Opin Ophthalmol.* 2007;18:62-66.

Ravalico G, et al. Spatial resolution threshold in pseudophakic patients with monofocal and multifocal IOLs. *J Cataract Refract Surg.* 1998;24:244-248.

CHAPTER 109

MULTIFOCAL IOLS AND GLAUCOMA— HOW MUCH IS TOO MUCH?

Parag D. Parekh, MD, MPA and Thomas W. Samuelson, MD

The use of multifocal intraocular lenses (IOLs) in patients with glaucoma is a topic with little direct research upon which to form evidence-based guidelines. A significant amount of indirect evidence exists, however, to suggest the use of aspheric IOLs and to approach the use of multifocal IOLs in glaucoma patients with caution.

Contrast Sensitivity, Multifocal IOLs, and Aspheric IOLs

The cornea has positive spherical aberration that is relatively stable throughout life. The crystalline lens in a younger patient has a negative spherical aberration that offsets this, rendering the youthful eye relatively aspheric. With aging and cataract formation, the crystalline lens increases in positive sphericity, leaving the eye with a greater amount of positive total spherical aberration and further deteriorating the quality of vision (Figure 1).

Traditional IOLs have positive sphericity, which, when added to the positive sphericity of the cornea, gives the pseudophakic eye an even larger amount of positive spherical aberration. Currently, several aspheric IOLs are available (Table 1), with different amounts of negative sphericity: Advanced Medical Optics Tecnis ZA9002 (Santa Ana, CA) and ZA9003 (approximately −0.27 µm), Alcon SN60WF (Fort Worth, TX) (approximately −0.17 µm), or Bausch & Lomb SofPort LI61AO (Rochester, NY) (zero sphericity). Therefore, the use of "aspheric" IOLs can offset the corneal positive sphericity and simulate the youthful eye's vision more closely.

Packer et al compared the aspheric Tecnis Z9000 to the spherical Advanced Medical Optics AR40e, in a randomized, prospective study of 30 patients with 3 months follow-up.[1] They compared sine-wave grating contrast sensitivity testing under mesopic and photopic conditions. In all eyes, patients with the aspheric IOL demonstrated statistically significant better contrast sensitivity at 3 and 6 cycles per degree (cpd) under photopic conditions and at 1.5, 3, and 6 cpd under mesopic conditions (Figure 2).

Belluci et al compared the aspheric Tecnis Z9000 to the spherical Alcon AcrySof SA60AT, in a randomized, prospective study of 30 patients. Again, the aspheric IOL demonstrated statistically significant better contrast sensitivity at spatial frequencies of 3, 6, 12, and 18 cpd in photopic and mesopic conditions.[2]

The Tecnis ZA9003 and the Alcon SN60WF, having negative spherical aberration, must be very precisely positioned in the eye. For example, the Tecnis lens must be centered within 0.4 mm of the visual axis and tilted less than 7 degrees from the visual axis to provide better optical quality than a spherical IOL.[1] In an IOL with zero sphericity, such as the Bausch & Lomb lens, the precise centration of the lens is less important. Thus, in situations of uncertain capsular stability or integrity such as combined phacoemulsification and trabeculectomy in exfoliative glaucoma, the more forgiving IOL could represent a better choice. In the case of a straightforward phacoemulsification/IOL placement procedure, there is typically less than 0.3-mm decentration and less than 3 degrees of tilt[3]; thus any of the aspheric IOLs could be a fine choice.

Multifocal IOLs, whether based on a diffractive or refractive mechanism, reduce contrast sensitivity. Several studies have directly compared aspheric IOLs and multifocal IOLs in terms of contrast sensitivity. Zeng et al studied the Tecnis Z9001 (aspheric), the Alcon SA60AT (spherical), and the Advanced Medical Optics SA40N (multifocal) in a prospective, randomized trial with 124 eyes of 124 patients. Spherical aberration was highest in the multifocal and lowest in the aspheric, with the traditional monofocal spherical IOL in the mid-range. Accordingly, contrast sensitivity was best in the aspheric lens and lowest in the multifocal in all spatial frequencies tested—3, 6, 12, and 18 cpd.[4]

Montes-Mico et al published a prospective, nonrandomized series of 64 patients followed for 18 months, comparing the Advanced Medical Optics Array SA-40N multifocal IOL

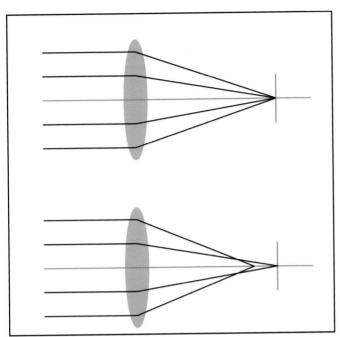

Figure 1. Positive spherical aberration caused by peripheral light rays being bent more by the optical system than the para-axial rays.

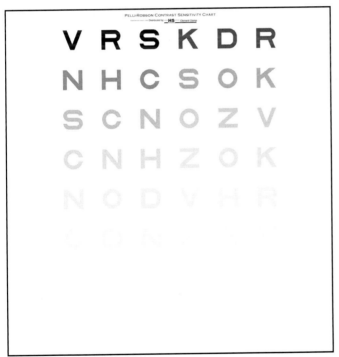

Figure 2. Pelli-Robson Contrast Sensitivity Chart commonly used to test contrast sensitivity. (Reprinted with permission of Haag-Streit UK Ltd.)

Table 1			
ASPHERIC INTRAOCULAR LENSES			
Intraocular Lens	*Design*	*Material*	*Spherical Aberration*
AMO Tecnis Z9002 and Z9003	3 piece; 6-mm optic	Silicone	Approximately −0.27 um
Alcon AcrySof SN60WF	1 piece, 6-mm optic	Acrylic	Approximately −0.17 um
Bausch & Lomb SofPort LI61AO	3 piece; 6-mm optic	Silicone	Approximately 0.0 um

Although an aspheric multifocal IOL is upcoming from both Advanced Medical Optics and Alcon, the contrast sensitivity data are not currently available.

Contrast Sensitivity in Glaucoma

The disease process of glaucoma preferentially damages contrast sensitivity before visual acuity. Snellen visual acuities measure high-contrast central vision, often remaining near-normal until late in the disease process and not necessarily simulating low contrast situations. Glaucoma patients can have contrast sensitivity losses at spatial frequencies between 0.25 and 8 cpd.[7] Contrast sensitivity is one of the earliest functions damaged by glaucoma, and it correlates with glaucoma progression. In fact, several authors have tried to use the loss of contrast sensitivity as an early glaucoma-detection test.[8] Hawkins et al studied 250 eyes of 144 patients with glaucoma, suspected glaucoma, or ocular hypertension with better than 20/40 vision and found that reduced contrast sensitivity was significantly correlated to visual field loss in patients with glaucoma.[9] Regan et al also demonstrated decreased contrast sensitivity in patients with glaucoma and ocular hypertension.[10]

The loss of contrast sensitivity has very practical applications far beyond academic or theoretic interest. Owsley and McGwin correlated the loss of contrast sensitivity, visual acuity, and horizontal visual field with increased accident incidence in drivers over the age of 65.[11] In a prospective study of 25 glaucoma patients with age-matched controls, Szlyk et al compared driving skills using a computer simulator. As expected, the glaucoma patients had similar visual acuities compared with the control group but had diminished contrast sensitivity. These glaucoma patients with diminished contrast sensitivity in their better eye demonstrated slower driving speeds, more lane boundary crossings, and longer braking response times.[12]

to the spherical monofocal Advanced Medical Optics SI-40NB. Under bright conditions, contrast sensitivity was not statistically different in either group at any of the spatial frequencies. However, at low luminance, the contrast sensitivity was worse in the multifocal group at the highest spatial frequencies (12 and 18 cpd) at distance and near.[5]

Leyland confirmed the loss of contrast sensitivity in multifocal patients in a meta-analysis of 8 randomized controlled trials.[6]

Accommodating IOL

Pepose et al examined bilateral and combination Crystalens (Eyeonics, Inc, Aliso Viejo, CA) (accommodating IOL), ReZoom (Advanced Medical Optics), and ReSTOR (Alcon) multifocal IOLs. The Crystalens fared statistically significantly better than both of the multifocal IOLs at all spatial frequencies in a monocular comparison. In a binocular comparison under mesopic conditions, patients with the Crystalens in one or both eyes had better scores than patients with bilateral multifocal IOLs, although the difference was only statistically significant in comparison to the bilateral ReZoom group.[13] Contrast sensitivity was comparable to a standard monofocal IOLs in the Food and Drug Administration clinical trial of the Crystalens.[14]

Conclusion

In the absence of studies directly investigating the use of multifocal and aspheric IOLs in patients with glaucoma, the concept of contrast sensitivity may drive selection of the appropriate IOL. Multifocal IOLs should be used with caution in patients with glaucoma, given that both the IOL and the disease can decrease contrast sensitivity. Crystalens use could be considered in patients who are highly motivated to decrease their spectacle dependence, as the evidence demonstrates its comparability to a traditional IOL in terms of contrast sensitivity. On the other hand, an aspheric IOL can enhance contrast sensitivity, thereby potentially offsetting some of the contrast sensitivity loss in glaucoma and maintaining a better quality of vision. Positioning of the Alcon or Tecnis aspheric IOL must be precise because they both have negative spherical aberration; the Bausch & Lomb aspheric lens has zero sphericity. In cases of questionable zonular integrity, this may represent a more forgiving lens. Finally, monovision achieved with bilateral aspheric IOL implantation remains a very effective option in patients with glaucoma in whom spectacle independence is desired. With this strategy, patients may enjoy effective vision at both distance and near, and yet their best-corrected acuity can be maximized by spectacle correction when most needed.

References

1. Packer M, Fine IH, Hoffman RS, et al. Improved functional vision with a modified prolate intraocular lens. *J Cataract Refract Surg.* 2004;30:986-992.

2. Bellucci R, Scialdone A, Buratto L, et al. Visual acuity and contrast sensitivity comparison between Tecnis and AcrySof SA60AT intraocular lenses: A multicenter randomized study. *J Cataract Refract Surg.* 2005;31:712-717.

3. Holladay JT, Piers PA, Koranyi G, et al. A new intraocular lens design to reduce spherical aberration of pseudophakic eyes. *J Refract Surg.* 2002;18:683-691.

4. Zeng M, Liu Y, Liu X, et al. Aberration and contrast sensitivity comparison of aspherical and monofocal and multifocal intraocular lens eyes. *Clinical and Experimental Ophthalmology.* 2007;35:355-360.

5. Montes-Mico R, Espana E, Bueno I, et al. Visual performance with multifocal intraocular lenses. *Ophthalmology.* 2004;111:85-96.

6. Leyland M, Zinicola E. Multifocal versus monofocal intraocular lenses in cataract surgery. *Ophthalmology.* 2003;110:1789-1798.

7. Seiple WH. The clinical utility of spatial contrast sensitivity testing. *Duane's Foundation of Clinical Ophthalmology.* 1991;114:1-13.

8. Wood JM, Lovie-Kitchin JE. Evaluation of the efficacy of contrast sensitivity measures for the detection of early primary open angle glaucoma. *Optom Vis Sci.* 1992;69:175-181.

9. Hawkins AS, Sylyk JP, Ardickas Z, et al. Comparison of contrast sensitivity, visual acuity and Humphrey visual field testing in patients with glaucoma. *J Glaucoma.* 2003;12:134-138.

10. Regan D, Neima D. Low-contrast letter charts in early diabetic retinopathy, ocular hypertension, glaucoma, and Parkinson's disease. *Br J Ophthalmol.* 1984;68:885-889.

11. Owsley C, McGwin G. Vision impairment and driving. *Surv Ophthalmol.* 1999;43(6):535-550.

12. Szlyk JP, Taglia DP, Paliga J, et al. Driving performance in patients wit mild to moderate glaucomatous clinical vision changes. *J Rehabil Res Dev.* 2002;39(4):467-482.

13. Pepose JS, Qazi MA, Davies J, et al. Visual performance of patients with bilateral vs. combination Crystalens, ReZoom, and ReSTOR intraocular lens implants. *Am J Ophthalmol.* 2006;144:347-357.e1

14. Cumming JS, Colvard DM, Dell SJ, et al. Clinical evaluation of the Crystalens AT-45 accommodating intraocular lens: Results of the U.S. Food and Drug Administration clinical trial. *J Cataract Refract Surg.* 2006;32:812-825.

CHAPTER 110

MULTIFOCAL IOLS AND MACULOPATHY— HOW MUCH IS TOO MUCH?

Martin A. Mainster, PhD, MD, FRCOphth and Patricia L. Turner, MD

The global population grows and ages.[1,2] The percentage of individuals over 60 years of age in developed countries will increase from 20% of the population at present to 33% by 2050.[2] People survive to older ages and live longer.[1] Amongst the rising number of individuals with presbyopia and cataract formation will be people who develop macular abnormalities (maculopathy) from aging (age-related macular degeneration) or diabetes (diabetic retinopathy). Multifocal intraocular lenses (IOLs) can reduce the spectacle dependence of people with normal maculas. Are they potentially helpful or ill-advised for individuals with macular abnormalities or at risk for developing them? This chapter identifies and analyzes relevant issues, but significant scientific and clinical questions remain unanswered.

Multifocal IOLs

Monofocal IOLs efficiently transfer optical information from an object (target) to an image (retina) plane. Depth of field is the distance proximal and distal to a visual target over which the target appears in focus. Depth of field in object space has a corresponding depth of focus in image space. Depth of focus can be described as the maximum defocus in diopters that an observer can tolerate without detecting blur in an optimally focused target. Many factors affect depth of focus, including pupil diameter; ocular aberrations; retinal eccentricity; and target size, brightness, and contrast.[3,4] Pseudoaccommodation provides a depth of field large enough for useful distance thru near vision in some monofocal pseudophakes.[5,6] Mean pseudophakic pseudoaccommodation is roughly 2 D.[7] Factors that can enhance it include myopic astigmatism, pupillary miosis, and corneal multifocality, although each has its own disadvantages.[5,7-9]

Multifocal IOLs use diffractive or refractive optics to produce 2 or more optical foci and their corresponding superimposed retinal images.[10-13] When a distant object is perceived through a multifocal IOL, enlarged defocused secondary retinal images from near or intermediate components are combined with the primary, well-focused distance image. Similarly, a near object's primary retinal image is overlain by enlarged defocused secondary images from the IOL's intermediate and distance components. Enlarged, blurred secondary images produce haloes and decrease primary image contrast. The fraction of incident light energy distributed to near, intermediate, and distance foci varies with pupil diameter and IOL design.

The human visual system exhibits remarkable plasticity at the retinal and cortical levels, changing adaptively to alterations in sensory input or anatomy.[14] Adaptation at or above the level of the primary visual cortex (V1) affects summation[15] and other binocular processes involved in postoperative adaptation to multifocal IOLs. Contrast sensitivity improves in the first 6 months after implantation,[16,17] a poorly-understood slow neural adjustment that also occurs after corneal refractive surgery.[18] Additionally, contrast sensitivity is better in bilateral than unilateral multifocal pseudophakes,[19,20] orientational visual acuity in multifocal pseudophakes is improved after visual training (perceptual learning),[21] neural processing by the retina and brain may compensate for ocular optical aberrations,[22] perceptual adaptation to sustained blur occurs in myopia,[23-25] and defocus blur is an important accommodative stimulus.[26-28]

Multifocal IOLs reduce retinal image contrast to improve unaided near vision.[12] Numerous studies have compared the contrast sensitivity provided by different multifocal and monofocal IOLs using a variety of protocols.[16,29-33] Systematic literature reviews[20,34] estimate that a 2- to 3-fold increase in depth of field is achieved typically at the expense of a 50% loss in contrast sensitivity. That trade-off is quite satisfactory for many people with normal retinas. Its impact on people with maculopathy is best examined in terms of pseudophakic visual, optical, and retinal-cortical sensitivity.

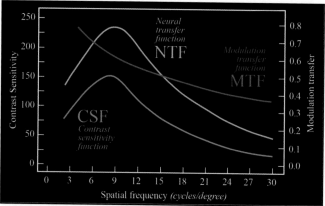

Figure 1. The overall contrast sensitivity of the human eye is described by a contrast sensitivity function (CSF) that shows how sensitive it is to sine-wave gratings of different spatial frequency (fineness). Coarse and fine grating targets have low and high spatial frequencies, respectively. Spatial frequency is measured in cycles per degree (cpd) of visual angle. Six, 15, and 30 cpd gratings correspond to 20/100, 20/40, and 20/20 visual acuity targets, respectively. It takes more contrast to see fine detail than coarse detail, so contrast sensitivity decreases with increasing spatial frequency from its peak around 3 to 6 cpd. The neural transfer function (NTF) describes the visual sensitivity of the retina and brain independent of the eye's optics. The modulation transfer function (MTF) describes how the transfer of contrast information by ocular optics decreases with increasing spatial frequency. The CSF (overall contrast sensitivity) decreases with increasing spatial frequency (target fineness) because the retina and brain are less sensitive to higher spatial frequencies (NTF) and the cornea, lens, and other ocular media transfer less contrast information to the retina at higher than lower spatial frequencies (MTF). Curves are adapted from data in the classic study of Campbell and Green.[63]

Maculopathy

EPIDEMIOLOGY

Age-related macular degeneration (AMD) and diabetic maculopathy are the most common maculopathies. AMD is the leading cause of severe, irreversible visual impairment in developed countries.[35] Its prevalence varies from 8.5% in 43- to 54-year-old adults to 37% in people 75 years of age or older.[36] The only risk factors consistently identified in epidemiological studies of AMD are aging, smoking, and ethnicity.[35] Nine of the 11 major epidemiological studies showed no correlation between environmental light exposure and AMD.[37,38] Patients with numerous medium-sized drusen and one or more large drusen in one eye (intermediate AMD) have an 18% chance of progressing to advanced AMD in 5 years, which increases to a 26% chance if large drusen are present in both eyes.[35]

Treatment for diabetic retinopathy can reduce the risk of severe vision loss by 90%, but diabetic retinopathy remains a leading cause of new blindness in developed countries. The duration of diabetes and severity of hyperglycemia are important risk factors for diabetic retinopathy.[39] Retinopathy affects 40% of people who have had type 2 diabetes for less than 5 years if they are taking insulin and 24% if they are not taking insulin.[39] It affects 25% of people with type 1 diabetes for more than 5 years.[39] Rates for the progression or development of diabetic retinopathy over a period of 1 year are 5% to 10%.[39]

VISION

Loss of visual acuity and contrast sensitivity can impair the performance of routine daily tasks.[40-44] Decreased contrast sensitivity is associated independently with difficulties in mobility, face recognition, reading, driving, and overall quality of life.[40,41,45,46] A 25% reduction in contrast sensitivity can produce functionally significant loss in night driving visibility distances and reaction times.[42] A 50% loss in contrast sensitivity or visual acuity in phakic adults over 65 is associated with a 3- to 5-fold odds of reporting difficulty in performing routine daily tasks independent of visual acuity loss.[43] A 90% reduction in contrast sensitivity is one criterion for visual impairment.[47] Conversely, with normal vision, a 10-fold contrast sensitivity loss has been reported to produce only a 2-fold reduction in reading rate[48] and ambulation involves low spatial frequencies relatively unaffected by multifocal optics.[49]

Contrast sensitivity testing can detect functional vision losses in retinal disease that are not demonstrated by visual acuity measurements.[46,50,51] Several studies have shown that AMD even in its earliest stages impairs contrast sensitivity.[46,50-57] Contrast sensitivity worsens as AMD progresses. Findings are similar in diabetic retinopathy.[46,58-61] Contrast sensitivity is reduced in diabetics versus nondiabetics as well as in diabetics with retinopathy versus those without retinopathy.[58,59,61,62] A variety of contrast sensitivity measurement techniques have been used to study the visual effects of macular disease so numerical results are not directly comparable.

OPTICS

The contrast sensitivity function (CSF) describes overall visual function (functional vision).[41,63-67] It specifies how much contrast a patient needs to detect a sine-wave grating of a particular fineness (spatial frequency). Coarse and fine grating targets have low and high spatial frequencies, respectively. Spatial frequency is measured in cycles per degree (cpd) of visual angle. Six, 15, and 30 cpd gratings correspond to the detail in 20/100, 20/40, and 20/20 visual acuity targets, respectively. Spatial frequencies most important for detecting simple edges and newspaper letters are 3 and 12 cpd, respectively[68] (corresponding to 20/200 and 20/50 visual acuity targets, respectively). It takes more contrast to see fine detail than coarse detail, so contrast sensitivity decreases with increasing spatial frequency from its peak around 3 to 6 cpd as shown in Figure 1.[63] Contrast sensitivity also decreases with increasing distance from the fovea (retinal eccentricity).[69]

The visual sensitivity of the retina and brain, independent of the eye's optics, can be described by the neural transfer function (NTF).[63,64,70-72] The NTF and CSF have similar forms, as shown in Figure 1.[63] The sine-wave grating targets used to measure NTFs are produced directly on a patient's retina using interference fringes largely unaffected by ocular aberrations.

The CSF (overall contrast sensitivity) decreases with increasing spatial frequency (target fineness) for 2 reasons. First, the retina and brain are less sensitive to high spatial frequencies, as shown by the NTF in Figure 1. Second, the cornea, lens, and other ocular media transfer less contrast information to the retina at higher than lower spatial frequencies, as shown by the MTF in Figure 1.

The modulation transfer function (MTF) describes how the transfer of contrast information by ocular optics decreases with increasing spatial frequency.[63,64,73-77] In essence, the eye's optics act as filters for contrast information, transferring (transmitting) lower spatial frequencies more efficiently than higher ones (see Figure 1). This situation is analogous to the transfer of color information by aging, yellowish crystalline lenses, which transmit lower optical frequencies (longer, redder wavelengths) more effectively than higher ones (shorter, bluer wavelengths).[78]

The following simple transfer equation describes how overall contrast sensitivity (CSF) depends on ocular optics (MTF) and retinal-brain function (NTF)[63,64,74]:

$$CSF = MTF \times NTF$$

Clinical applications are straightforward. If retinal-brain function (NTF) does not change after implant surgery, then postoperative functional vision (CSF) improvement is proportional to the improvement in ocular optics (MTF) after surgery. If ocular optics (MTF) do not change after multifocal IOL implantation, then improvements in functional vision (CSF) in the months that follow surgery are proportional to increases in retinal-brain function (NTF) due to neural adaptation. The equation therefore provides a formalism for quantifying postoperative neural adaptation. If ocular optics (MTF) do not change in the process of macular scarring, then loss of functional vision (CSF) after scarring is proportional to decreased retinal-brain function (NTF).

Multifocals and Maculopathy

Visual acuities were similar in groups of monofocal and multifocal pseudophakes with concurrent retinal disease in one study, but patients were not stratified by their disease severity.[79] There are no reported clinical trials of the relative performance of monofocal and multifocal pseudophakes with maculopathy regarding their postoperative contrast sensitivity, quality of life, or effectiveness of low-vision aid usage.

Tasks requiring lower spatial frequencies (coarser details) are more tolerant to defocus than those involving higher frequencies (finer details), so low vision patients with decreased visual acuity have greater tolerance to defocus than people with normal vision.[80] Conversely, loss of contrast sensitivity is an important correlate and predictor of problems that maculopathy patients experience in reading, mobility, and other important daily living tasks.[48,56,81-85] Patients with vision loss from maculopathy often benefit from devices such as hand-held and stand magnifiers or closed circuit television reading machines.[85] There are no published studies on how multifocal IOLs affect optimal low-vision aid usage.

The transfer equation discussed previously provides a convenient way of understanding the combined effects of concurrent contrast sensitivity loss from multifocal IOLs and maculopathy. Contrast sensitivity decrements can be expressed as percentage or logarithmic losses. For example, a 2-fold (50%), 4-fold (75%), or 10-fold (90%) loss is a 6, 12, or 20 decibel (dB) loss, respectively (an alternative definition halves dB losses to 3, 6, and 10 dBs, respectively).[46,50]

The transfer equation shows that CSF losses are additive when expressed in logarithmic units. For example, uniform 6 dB (50%) optical sensitivity losses from multifocality that might be quite acceptable to normally sighted patients and 6 dB retinal-brain sensitivity losses from maculopathy that might be well tolerated by AMD patients would be combined theoretically into 12 dB contrast sensitivity losses (4-fold, 75% losses). There are no reported clinical trials to validate this type of analysis or to reveal whether patients with maculopathy would find hypothetically reduced spectacle independence to be a satisfactory trade-off for any additional contrast sensitivity loss.

Maculopathy patients may benefit from cataract surgery even when visual acuity is not improved. Contrast sensitivity loss from lens opacities[86,87] and macular abnormalities are also additive, so implant surgery may improve medium spatial frequency performance even when macular scarring has permanently impaired a patient's high spatial frequency (fine detail) performance. Aspheric IOLs with their higher MTFs should potentially provide the best improvement,[88-90] particularly when low chromatic dispersion optic materials are used as in Tecnis ZA9003 monofocal or ZMA00 multifocal IOLs (Advanced Medical Optics, Santa Ana, CA).[91] Wavelengths in the center of the visible spectrum determine pseudophakic performance at medium and high spatial frequencies, explaining why blue-blocking chromophores fail to improve contrast sensitivity clinically.[91]

Rod photoreceptor sensitivity is decreased in people with AMD and diabetic retinopathy, making it more difficult for them to perform important daily tasks such as ambulation and night driving.[92-96] Circadian dysfunction increases with aging, a loss linked to insomnia, depression, numerous systemic disorders, and shortened longevity.[37,38,97] Cataract surgery can improve rod and circadian photoreception and reduce insomnia.[37,38,97-99] Multifocal IOLs without blue-blocking filters would preserve this gain. Blue-blocking filters decrease rod and circadian photoreception by 14% to 21% and 27% to 38%, respectively, reducing important potential benefits from cataract surgery.[37,38,100,101] Recent Swiss and Chinese studies support Age-Related Eye Disease Study conclusions that cataract surgery is not a significant risk factor for advanced AMD.[102-104]

Ophthalmoscopy and vitreoretinal surgery may be more difficult in some multifocal patients than monofocal patients,[105,106] although these procedures can usually be performed successfully, as can fluorescein angiography and optical coherence tomography. The power of the near component of a multifocal IOL is small in comparison to overall pseudophakic ocular power, so laser spot size differences in retinal photocoagulation due to multifocality are less than 5%, insignificant for clinical procedures.[107] Such small power differences should not increase the risk of operating microscope phototoxicity (photic retinopathy).[108,109] There is a case report of photic retinopathy after multifocal implant surgery,[110] but photic retinopathy has been reported after most forms of anterior and posterior segment surgery.[109]

Neuroplasticity accommodates traumatic and other changes in the structure of and neural input to the brain's visual centers. The brain creates visual images by sampling small portions of retinal images and processing this local data in relatively narrow spatial frequency channels.[111] Monocular data are initially segregated by eye in the visual cortex and subsequently transferred to higher order neurons, which extract binocular and other complex information. There is currently only rudimentary knowledge of how the brain selects between completing images in multifocal pseudophakes with or without maculopathy, but clinical data show that neural adaptation occurs and may be hastened by perceptual learning.[16,17,21]

Conclusion

Most multifocal pseudophakes without retinal problems who are properly selected preoperatively are satisfied with trading some contrast sensitivity for the convenience of spectacle independence. Multifocal blur adaptation and image selection remain poorly understood. Patients with vision loss are more tolerant to image defocus, but their contrast sensitivity is an important measure of their ability to read and perform important daily tasks. Contrast sensitivity loss from multifocal pseudophakia and maculopathy are additive. It is possible that these combined losses could be visually significant for some patients or that multifocal IOLs could interfere with low-vision aid usage, but only controlled clinical trials can determine the potential advantages or disadvantages of multifocal IOLs for patients with or at risk for maculopathy.

Acknowledgment

This research was supported in part by the Kansas Lions Sight Foundation, Inc, Manhattan, KS.

References

1. United-Nations-Population-Division. World Population Ageing: 1950-2050, ST/ESA/SER.A/207. New York: United Nations; 2001.

2. United-Nations-Population-Division. *The World at Six Billion, ESA/P/WP.154.* New York: United Nations; 1999.

3. Freeman MH, Hull CC, Charman WN. *Optics.* 11th ed. London: Butterworth and Heineman; 2003.

4. Wang B, Ciuffreda KJ. Depth-of-focus of the human eye: theory and clinical implications. *Surv Ophthalmol.* 2006;51:75-85.

5. Nanavaty MA, Vasavada AR, Patel AS, Raj SM, Desai TH. Analysis of patients with good uncorrected distance and near vision after monofocal intraocular lens implantation. *J Cataract Refract Surg.* 2006;32:1091-1097.

6. Koch DD. Revisiting the conoid of sturm. *J Cataract Refract Surg.* 2006;32:1071-1072.

7. Menapace R, Findl O, Kriechbaum K, Leydolt-Koeppl C. Accommodating intraocular lenses: a critical review of present and future concepts. *Graefes Arch Clin Exp Ophthalmol.* 2007;245:473-489.

8. Oshika T, Mimura T, Tanaka S, et al. Apparent accommodation and corneal wavefront aberration in pseudophakic eyes. *Invest Ophthalmol Vis Sci.* 2002;43:2882-2886.

9. Fukuyama M, Oshika T, Amano S, Yoshitomi F. Relationship between apparent accommodation and corneal multifocality in pseudophakic eyes. *Ophthalmology.* 1999;106:1178-1181.

10. Charman WN, Murray IJ, Nacer M, O'Donoghue EP. Theoretical and practical performance of a concentric bifocal intraocular implant lens. *Vision Res.* 1998;38:2841-2853.

11. Pieh S, Marvan P, Lackner B, et al. Quantitative performance of bifocal and multifocal intraocular lenses in a model eye: point spread function in multifocal intraocular lenses. *Arch Ophthalmol.* 2002;120:23-28.

12. Bellucci R. Multifocal intraocular lenses. *Curr Opin Ophthalmol.* 2005;16:33-37.

13. Lane SS, Morris M, Nordan L, Packer M, Tarantino N, Wallace RB, 3rd. Multifocal intraocular lenses. *Ophthalmol Clin North Am.* 2006;19:vi, 89-105.

14. Tremere LA, De Weerd P, Pinaud R. A unified theoretical framework for plasticity in visual circuitry. In: Pinaud R, Tremere LA, De Weerd P, eds. *Plasticity in the Visual System: From Genes to Circuits.* New York: Springer; 2006.

15. Steinman SB, Steinman BA, Garzia RP. *Foundations of Binocular Vision: A Clinical Perspective.* New York: The McGraw-Hill Companies; 2000.

16. Montes-Mico R, Alio JL. Distance and near contrast sensitivity function after multifocal intraocular lens implantation. *J Cataract Refract Surg.* 2003;29:703-711.

17. Mester U, Hunold W, Wesendahl T, Kaymak H. Functional outcomes after implantation of Tecnis ZM900 and Array SA40 multifocal intraocular lenses. *J Cataract Refract Surg.* 2007;33:1033-1040.

18. Pesudovs K. Involvement of neural adaptation in the recovery of vision after laser refractive surgery. *J Refract Surg.* 2005;21:144-147.

19. Arens B, Freudenthaler N, Quentin CD. Binocular function after bilateral implantation of monofocal and refractive multifocal intraocular lenses. *J Cataract Refract Surg.* 1999;25:399-404.

20. Leyland M, Pringle E. Multifocal versus monofocal intraocular lenses after cataract extraction. *Cochrane Database Syst Rev.* 2006: CD003169.

21. Kaymak H, Ott G, Mester U. Training visual quality after implantation of multifocal IOLs. Paper presented at: American Society of Cataract and Refractive Surgery, 2007 Annual Meeting; April 27 to May 2, 2007; San Diego, CA.

22. Artal P, Chen L, Fernandez EJ, Singer B, Manzanera S, Williams DR. Neural compensation for the eye's optical aberrations. *J Vis.* 2004;4:281-287.

23. Mon-Williams M, Tresilian JR, Strang NC, Kochhar P, Wann JP. Improving vision: neural compensation for optical defocus. *Proc Biol Sci.* 1998;265:71-77.

24. George S, Rosenfield M. Blur adaptation and myopia. *Optom Vis Sci.* 2004;81:543-547.

25. Rosenfield M, Hong SE, George S. Blur adaptation in myopes. *Optom Vis Sci.* 2004;81:657-662.

26. Fernandez EJ, Artal P. Study on the effects of monochromatic aberrations in the accommodation response by using adaptive optics. *J Opt Soc Am A Opt Image Sci Vis.* 2005;22:1732-1738.

27. Chen AH. Is there any difference in using blur as a stimulus for accommodation between emmetropes and myopes? *Doc Ophthalmol.* 2002;105:33-39.

28. Kruger PB, Pola J. Stimuli for accommodation: blur, chromatic aberration and size. *Vision Res.* 1986;26:957-971.

29. Zeng M, Liu Y, Liu X et al. Aberration and contrast sensitivity comparison of aspherical and monofocal and multifocal intraocular lens eyes. *Clin Experiment Ophthalmol.* 2007;35:355-360.

30. Alfonso JF, Fernandez-Vega L, Baamonde MB, Montes-Mico R. Prospective visual evaluation of apodized diffractive intraocular lenses. *J Cataract Refract Surg.* 2007;33:1235-1243.

31. Vingolo EM, Grenga P, Iacobelli L, Grenga R. Visual acuity and contrast sensitivity: AcrySof ReSTOR apodized diffractive versus AcrySof SA60AT monofocal intraocular lenses. *J Cataract Refract Surg.* 2007;33:1244-1247.

32. Haaskjold E, Allen ED, Burton RL, et al. Contrast sensitivity after implantation of diffractive bifocal and monofocal intraocular lenses. *J Cataract Refract Surg.* 1998;24:653-658.

33. Allen ED, Burton RL, Webber SK, et al. Comparison of a diffractive bifocal and a monofocal intraocular lens. *J Cataract Refract Surg.* 1996;22:446-451.

34. Leyland M, Zinicola E. Multifocal versus monofocal intraocular lenses in cataract surgery: a systematic review. *Ophthalmology.* 2003;110:1789-1798.

35. American Academy of Ophthalmology. *Age-Related Macular Degeneration, Preferred Practice Pattern.* San Francisco, CA: American Academy of Ophthalmology; 2006.

36. Klein R, Klein BE, Linton KL. Prevalence of Age-Related Maculopathy. The Beaver Dam Eye Study. *Ophthalmology.* 1992;99:933-943.

37. Mainster MA, Turner PL. Blue light: to block or not to block. Cataract & Refractive Surgery Today Europe. 2007;2:64-68. (Can be found at www.crstodayeurope.com/Html%20pages/0507/f4_mainster.pdf).

38. Mainster MA. Violet and blue light blocking intraocular lenses: photoprotection versus photoreception. *Br J Ophthalmol.* 2006;90:784-792.

39. American Academy of Ophthalmology. *Diabetic Retinopathy, Preferred Practice Pattern.* San Francisco, CA: American Academy of Ophthalmology; 2003.

40. West SK, Rubin GS, Broman AT, Munoz B, Bandeen-Roche K, Turano K. How does visual impairment affect performance on tasks of everyday life? The SEE Project. Salisbury Eye Evaluation. *Arch Ophthalmol.* 2002;120:774-780.

41. Owsley C. Contrast sensitivity. *Ophthalmol Clin North Am.* 2003;16:171-177.

42. Ginsburg AP. Contrast sensitivity and functional vision. *Int Ophthalmol Clin.* 2003;43:5-15.

43. Rubin GS, Bandeen-Roche K, Huang GH, et al. The association of multiple visual impairments with self-reported visual disability: SEE project. *Invest Ophthalmol Vis Sci.* 2001;42:64-72.

44. Mones J, Rubin GS. Contrast sensitivity as an outcome measure in patients with subfoveal choroidal neovascularization due to age-related macular degeneration. *Eye.* 2005;19:1142-1150.

45. Wolffsohn JS, Cochrane AL. Design of the low vision quality-of-life questionnaire (LVQOL) and measuring the outcome of low-vision rehabilitation. *Am J Ophthalmol.* 2000;130:793-802.

46. Eperjesi F, Wolffsohn J, Bowden J, Napper G, Rubinstein M. Normative contrast sensitivity values for the back-lit Melbourne Edge Test and the effect of visual impairment. *Ophthalmic Physiol Opt.* 2004;24:600-606.

47. Leat SJ, Legge GE, Bullimore MA. What is low vision? A re-evaluation of definitions. *Optom Vis Sci.* 1999;76:198-211.

48. Legge GE, Rubin GS, Luebker A. Psychophysics of reading—V. The role of contrast in normal vision. *Vision Res.* 1987;27:1165-1177.

49. Akutsu H, Legge GE, Showalter M, Lindstrom RL, Zabel RW, Kirby VM. Contrast sensitivity and reading through multifocal intraocular lenses. *Arch Ophthalmol.* 1992;110:1076-1080.

50. Wolkstein M, Atkin A, Bodis-Wollner I. Contrast sensitivity in retinal disease. *Ophthalmology.* 1980;87:1140-1149.

51. Marmor MF. Contrast sensitivity versus visual acuity in retinal disease. *Br J Ophthalmol.* 1986;70:553-559.

52. Sjostrand J, Frisen L. Contrast sensitivity in macular disease: A preliminary report. *Acta Ophthalmol (Copenh).* 1977;55:507-514.

53. Kleiner RC, Enger C, Alexander MF, Fine SL. Contrast sensitivity in age-related macular degeneration. *Arch Ophthalmol.* 1988;106:55-57.

54. Collins M, Brown B. Glare recovery and age related maculopathy. *Clin Vision Sci.* 1989;4:145-153.

55. Midena E, Degli Angeli C, Blarzino MC, Valenti M, Segato T. Macular function impairment in eyes with early age-related macular degeneration. *Invest Ophthalmol Vis Sci.* 1997;38:469-477.

56. Kuyk T, Elliott JL. Visual factors and mobility in persons with age-related macular degeneration. *J Rehabil Res Dev.* 1999;36:303-312.

57. Bellmann C, Unnebrink K, Rubin GS, Miller D, Holz FG. Visual acuity and contrast sensitivity in patients with neovascular age-related macular degeneration: Results from the Radiation Therapy for Age-Related Macular Degeneration (RAD-) Study. *Graefes Arch Clin Exp Ophthalmol.* 2003;241:968-974.

58. Arend O, Remky A, Evans D, Stuber R, Harris A. Contrast sensitivity loss is coupled with capillary dropout in patients with diabetes. *Invest Ophthalmol Vis Sci.* 1997;38:1819-124.

59. Ismail GM, Whitaker D. Early detection of changes in visual function in diabetes mellitus. *Ophthalmic Physiol Opt.* 1998;18:3-12.

60. Sokol S, Moskowitz A, Skarf B, Evans R, Molitch M, Senior B. Contrast sensitivity in diabetics with and without background retinopathy. *Arch Ophthalmol.* 1985;103:51-54.

61. Stavrou EP, Wood JM. Letter contrast sensitivity changes in early diabetic retinopathy. *Clin Exp Optom.* 2003;86:152-156.

62. Krasny J, Vyplasilova E, Brunnerova R, et al. [The human lens' transparence changes in children, adolescents, and young adults with diabetes mellitus type I]. *Cesk Slov Oftalmol.* 2006;62:304-314.

63. Campbell FW, Green DG. Optical and retinal factors affecting visual resolution. *J Physiol.* 1965;181:576-593.

64. Mainster MA. Contemporary optics and ocular pathology. *Surv Ophthalmol.* 1978;23:135-142.

65. Barten PGJ. *Contrast sensitivity of the human eye and its effects on image quality.* Bellingham, WA: SPIE Optical Engineering Press; 1999.

66. Amesbury EC, Schallhorn SC. Contrast sensitivity and limits of vision. *Int Ophthalmol Clin.* 2003;43:31-42.

67. Ginsburg AP. Contrast sensitivity: determining the visual quality and function of cataract, intraocular lenses and refractive surgery. *Curr Opin Ophthalmol.* 2006;17:19-26.

68. Nio YK, Jansonius NM, Wijdh RH et al. Effect of methods of myopia correction on visual acuity, contrast sensitivity, and depth of focus. *J Cataract Refract Surg.* 2003;29:2082-2095.

69. Frisen L, Glansholm A. Optical and neural resolution in peripheral vision. *Invest Ophthalmol.* 1975;14:528-536.

70. Thibos LN, Bradley A. New methods for discriminating neural and optical losses of vision. *Optom Vis Sci.* 1993;70:279-287.

71. Sekiguchi N, Williams DR, Brainard DH. Aberration-free measurements of the visibility of isoluminant gratings. *J Opt Soc Am A Opt Image Sci Vis.* 1993;10:2105-2117.

72. Charman WN, Simonet P. Yves Le Grand and the assessment of retinal acuity using interference fringes. *Ophthalmic Physiol Opt.* 1997;17:164-168.

73. Kingslake R. *Optical System Design.* New York: Academic Press; 1983.

74. Lang A, Portney V. Interpreting multifocal intraocular lens modulation transfer functions. *J Cataract Refract Surg.* 1993;19:505-512.

75. Mouroulis P. Aberration and image quality representation for visual optical systems. In: Mouroulis P, ed. *Visual Instrumentation: Optical Design and Engineering Principles.* New York: McGraw-Hill; 1999:27-68.

76. Atchison DA, Smith G. *Optics of the Human Eye.* Oxford, UK: Butterworth-Heinemann; 2000.

77. Guirao A, Porter J, Williams DR, Cox IG. Calculated impact of higher-order monochromatic aberrations on retinal image quality in a population of human eyes. *J Opt Soc Am A Opt Image Sci Vis.* 2002;19:1-9.

78. Boettner EA, Wolter JR. Transmission of the ocular media. *Invest Ophthalmol.* 1962;1:776-783.

79. Kamath GG, Prasad S, Danson A, Phillips RP. Visual outcome with the array multifocal intraocular lens in patients with concurrent eye disease. *J Cataract Refract Surg.* 2000;26:576-581.

80. Legge GE, Mullen KT, Woo GC, Campbell FW. Tolerance to visual defocus. *J Opt Soc Am A.* 1987;4:851-863.

81. Loshin DS, White J. Contrast sensitivity: the visual rehabilitation of the patient with macular degeneration. *Arch Ophthalmol.* 1984;102:1303-1306.

82. Rubin GS, Legge GE. Psychophysics of reading—VI: The role of contrast in low vision. *Vision Res.* 1989;29:79-91.

83. Leat SJ, Woodhouse JM. Reading performance with low vision aids: relationship with contrast sensitivity. *Ophthalmic Physiol Opt.* 1993;13:9-16.

84. Crossland MD, Culham LE, Rubin GS. Predicting reading fluency in patients with macular disease. *Optom Vis Sci.* 2005;82:11-17.

85. Fletcher DC, Schuchard RA. Visual function in patients with choroidal neovascularization resulting from age-related macular degeneration: the importance of looking beyond visual acuity. *Optom Vis Sci.* 2006;83:178-189.

86. Adamsons I, Rubin GS, Vitale S, Taylor HR, Stark WJ. The effect of early cataracts on glare and contrast sensitivity: a pilot study. *Arch Ophthalmol.* 1992;110:1081-1086.

87. Elliott DB, Situ P. Visual acuity versus letter contrast sensitivity in early cataract. *Vision Res.* 1998;38:2047-2052.

88. Holladay JT, Piers PA, Koranyi G, van der Mooren M, Norrby NE. A new intraocular lens design to reduce spherical aberration of pseudophakic eyes. *J Refract Surg.* 2002;18:683-691.

89. Piers PA, Fernandez EJ, Manzanera S, Norrby S, Artal P. Adaptive optics simulation of intraocular lenses with modified spherical aberration. *Invest Ophthalmol Vis Sci.* 2004;45:4601-4610.

90. Piers PA, Norrby NE, Mester U. Eye models for the prediction of contrast vision in patients with new intraocular lens designs. *Opt Lett.* 2004;29:733-735.

91. Zhao H, Mainster MA. The effect of chromatic dispersion on pseudophakic optical performance. *Br J Ophthalmol.* 2007;91:1225-1229.

92. Brown B, Brabyn L, Welch L, Haegerstrom-Portnoy G, Colenbrander A. Contribution of vision variables to mobility in age-related maculopathy patients. *Am J Optom Physiol Opt.* 1986;63:733-739.

93. Sunness JS, Rubin GS, Applegate CA, et al. Visual function abnormalities and prognosis in eyes with age-related geographic atrophy of the macula and good visual acuity. *Ophthalmology.* 1997;104:1677-1691.

94. Owsley C, Jackson GR, Cideciyan AV, et al. Psychophysical evidence for rod vulnerability in age-related macular degeneration. *Invest Ophthalmol Vis Sci.* 2000;41:267-273.

95. Owsley C, Jackson GR, White M, Feist R, Edwards D. Delays in rod-mediated dark adaptation in early age-related maculopathy. *Ophthalmology.* 2001;108:1196-1202.

96. Greenstein VC, Thomas SR, Blaustein H, Koenig K, Carr RE. Effects of early diabetic retinopathy on rod system sensitivity. *Optom Vis Sci.* 1993;70:18-23.

97. Mainster MA, Turner PL. Intraocular lens spectral filtering. In: Steinert RF, ed. *Cataract Surgery.* 3rd ed. London: Elsevier Ltd.; 2007.

98. Asplund R, Lindblad BE. Sleep and sleepiness 1 and 9 months after cataract surgery. *Arch Gerontol Geriatr.* 2004;38:69-75.

99. Asplund R, Ejdervik Lindblad B. The development of sleep in persons undergoing cataract surgery. *Arch Gerontol Geriatr.* 2002;35:179-187.

100. Mainster MA. Intraocular lenses should block UV radiation and violet but not blue light. *Arch Ophthalmol.* 2005;123:550-555.

101. Mainster MA, Sparrow JR. How much blue light should an IOL transmit? *Br J Ophthalmol.* 2003;87:1523-1529.

102. Ferris FL, 3rd. Discussion of a model of spectral filtering to reduce photochemical damage in age-related macular degeneration. *Trans Am Ophthalmol Soc.* 2004;102:95.

103. Sutter FK, Menghini M, Barthelmes D, et al. Is pseudophakia a risk factor for neovascular age-related macular degeneration? *Invest Ophthalmol Vis Sci.* 2007;48:1472-1475.

104. Xu L, Li Y, Zheng Y, Jonas JB. Associated factors for age related maculopathy in the adult population in China: the Beijing eye study. *Br J Ophthalmol.* 2006;90:1087-1090.

105. Vanderschueren I, Zeyen T, D'Heer B. Multifocal IOL implantation: 16 cases. *Br J Ophthalmol.* 1991;75:88-91.

106. Mainster MA, Reichel E, Warren KA, Harrington PG. Ophthalmoscopy and vitreoretinal surgery in patients with an ARRAY refractive multifocal intraocular lens implant. *Ophthalmic Surg Lasers.* 2002;33:74-76.

107. Mainster MA. Decreasing retinal photocoagulation damage: principles and techniques. *Semin Ophthalmol.* 1999;14:200-209.

108. Mainster MA, Boulton M. Retinal phototoxicity. In: Albert DM, Miller JW, Blodi BA, Azar DT, eds. *Principles and Practice of Ophthalmology.* 3rd ed. London, UK: Elsevier; 2007.

109. Mainster MA, Turner PL. Retinal injuries from light: mechanisms, hazards and prevention. In: Ryan SJ, Hinton DR, Schachat AP, Wilkinson P, eds. *Retina.* 4th ed. London: Elsevier Publishers; 2006:1857-1870.

110. Menezo JL, Peris-Martinez C, Taboada Esteve J. Macular phototrauma after cataract extraction and multifocal lens implantation: case report. *Eur J Ophthalmol.* 2002;12:247-249.

111. Hess RF. Spatial scale in visual processing. In: Chalupa LM, Werner JS, eds. *The Visual Neurosciences.* 2 vol. Cambridge, MA: The MIT Press; 2004:1043-1059.

CHAPTER III

WHAT IF MULTIFOCAL IOL PATIENTS DEVELOP ARMD?

Johnny L. Gayton, MD

The most common cause of Caucasian seniors losing their ability to read and drive is age-related macular degeneration (ARMD). Today we have an unprecedented number of presbyopic patients having accommodative and multifocal implants in the hopes of reading and driving without the need for glasses or contacts. It is obvious that these 2 situations are going to coexist more and more in the future. There are 3 main questions:

1. Should I implant this lens in someone who may develop macular degeneration?

2. What should I do if an implanted patient develops macular degeneration?

3. Should these lenses be implanted in individuals with macular degeneration?

Addressing the first question is critical because even though we now may know who is at higher risk for ARMD, we do not know who will develop ARMD. There is an old southern saying that applies here, "If you hang 'em all you get the guilty." By refusing to put these lenses in anyone who is at risk for ARMD, we deprive a significant number of people of receiving the life-enhancing qualities of presbyopia-correcting lenses. Because of our work with ARMD and the ReSTOR lens (Alcon, Fort Worth, TX), I do not believe it is a catastrophe when a person develops ARMD in the presence of a premium lens. Therefore, I maintain that patients without ARMD but who are at higher risk for ARMD should be considered as candidates for these lenses. They should be encouraged to make appropriate lifestyle changes that lessen the risk of ARMD. Some of these changes are avoidance of tobacco, weight control, exercise, and nutritional supplementation. If they develop ARMD, do not hesitate to take advantage of optical correction, CPF lenses, and/or magnification. If they develop severe ARMD, I have some ideas that I will share at the end of this chapter.

For many years, we have frequently induced pseudophakic myopia of approximately 5.0 D in our ARMD patients. This aided in near vision recovery and allowed patients to resume some activities. It also avoided spectacle-induced loss of contrast sensitivity when performing near tasks. The patients were pleased with their near acuity; however, they were frequently displeased with their high myopic correction for distance.

The myopic target refraction was based on the premise of relative distance magnification (RDM).[1] The premise of RDM is that materials appear larger when they are held closer to the eye.[1] For example, depending on the distance, your finger can appear larger than the Empire State Building. The accommodative/reading correction needed increases from 2.5 D for the 40-cm working distance to 5.0 D for the 20-cm working distance. Thus, the material being read will appear 2 times larger than material at 40 cm. Remember, it is not the size of the object that is important, it is the size of the object's image on the retina.

We have been using the ReSTOR lens as an intraocular low vision aid to enhance the quality of life in patients with significant ARMD. The AcrySof ReSTOR apodized diffractive IOL provides high-quality distance vision. Its step heights decrease peripherally from 1.3 to 0.2 μm. This lens has a +4.0 add at the lens plane that equals a +3.2 add at the spectacle plane. We decided to take advantage of this characteristic by making macular degeneration patients 2.0 D myopic with the ReSTOR lens.

Under photopic conditions, a –2.00 distance refraction provides a near equivalent of +5.20 D with a best focus of 20 cm. The ReSTOR lens technique does not reduce uncorrected distance acuity nearly as much as a –5.0-D myopia-inducing monofocal lens. The patients were much happier now that they only needed a –2.0-D distance correction.

The first 2 ARMD patients implanted with the ReSTOR lens were absolutely ecstatic, so we started a pilot study. This study was a prospective series of cataract patients with vision loss from ARMD who received an off-label AcrySof ReSTOR IOL following phacoemulsification. Surgery was planned for a desired postoperative refraction of –2.00 to –3.00. This study also indicated that many patients' quality of life was improved; therefore, a multicenter study was started.

The 6-month study included 43 eyes of 32 patients with moderate to severe ARMD. All patients had best-corrected

Figure 1. ReSTOR ARMD uncorrected near visual acuity.

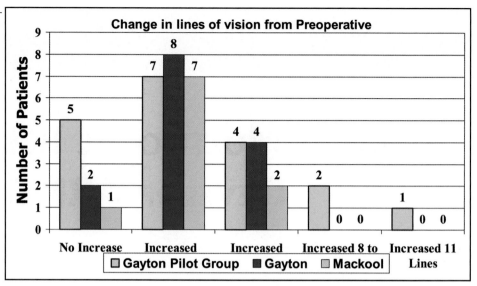

Figure 2. ReSTOR ARMD best-corrected near visual acuity.

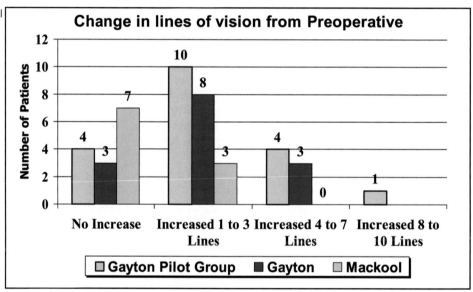

visual acuity between 20/50 and 20/400, and they had stable dry or disciform scarring.

Near and distance Snellen visual acuities with and without correction were collected both pre- and postoperatively, and subjective quality of life statements were collected both pre- and postoperatively. The National Eye Institute Visual Function Questionnaire (VFQ-25 Version 2000) was administered both pre- and postoperatively.[2]

Improvement in Uncorrected Near Visual Acuity

Of the 43 eyes included in the study, 8 had no increase in uncorrected near visual acuity, 22 had an increase of 1 to 3 lines, 10 had an increase of 4 to 7 lines, 2 had an increase of 8 to 10 lines, and 1 patient had an increase of 11 lines (Figure 1). Additionally, 14 had no increase in best-corrected near visual acuity, 21 had an increase of 1 to 2 lines, 7 had an increase of 4 to 7 lines, and 1 had an increase of 8 to 10 lines (Figure 2).

With regard to uncorrected distance visual acuity, 14 had a decrease in distance vision, 18 had no increase, 8 had an increase of 1 to 3 lines, and 3 had an increase of 4 to 7 lines. No eyes had a decrease in best-corrected distance visual acuity, while 18 had no increase, 19 had an increase of 1 to 3 lines, and 6 had an increase of 4 to 7 lines. This is to be expected since the patients are purposefully made myopic (Figure 3).

Increasing Quality of Life

Quality of life is multidimensional and includes physical, function, social, and psychological factors.[3] The National Eye Institute Visual Function Questionnaire (VFQ-25 Version 2000) is designed to measure vision-specific, health-related quality of life and it consists of a base set of 25 vision-targeted questions and a supplement of 14 additional questions addressing general health, general vision, ocular pain, near activities, distance activities, as well as vision-specific social functioning, mental health, role difficulties, dependency, driving, color vision, and peripheral vision.[2]

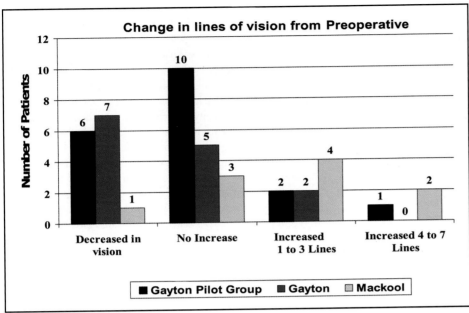

Figure 3. ReSTOR ARMD uncorrected distance visual acuity.

According to the questionnaire, patients' general vision increased, near vision activities increased, distance vision activities increased, social functioning limitations decreased, mental health increased, role limitations due to vision decreased, dependency on others due to vision decreased, driving difficulties decreased, and peripheral vision limitations decreased.

However, the measurements of success may not be in lines of vision or other objective findings. Subjective observations may tell us more. The following are patient comments:

* ✳ "I have not used glasses to read since surgery."
* ✳ "I can read the newspaper and the phonebook now."
* ✳ "I finished reading a book that was started 5 years ago."
* ✳ "I can see the steps and sidewalk."
* ✳ "I can see to pick out clothes that match."
* ✳ "I can see the faces of others."
* ✳ "I can see my watch."
* ✳ "I can see the labels on spices for the first time in years."
* ✳ "I can see the microwave numbers."
* ✳ "I can see to thread a fish hook."
* ✳ "I can see to comb my hair."
* ✳ "You gave me my life back."

Telescopic Implant

Another option for these patients is the Implantable Miniature Telescope (VisionCare Ophthalmic Technologies, Saratoga, CA). However, according to the 1-year efficacy data, while patients' best-corrected visual acuity and best-corrected near visual acuity improved 3 lines on the ETDRS, patients experienced a 25% loss of endothelial cell density, which was assumed to be a result of the surgical procedure. Additionally, patients experienced a limited distance vision increase with a marked loss of peripheral visual field. Longer-term follow-up is ongoing.[4] While the ReSTOR lens does not increase central vision as much as the telescopic lens, it is definitely much

better when is comes to peripheral vision. It is also technically an easier operation, resulting in less trauma to the eye.

Conclusion

Macular degeneration is one of the most serious health issues facing our country. Its incidence is expected to double over the next few years primarily because of the aging of our population. Because of this increased incidence of ARMD and the desire for an enhanced quality of life in our senior population, the modern lens surgeon is going to be frequently faced with the dilemmas presented in this chapter. The ReSTOR IOL is a promising option for these patients, and its use is appropriate in relatively young patients who may develop ARMD in the future. Should an implanted patient develop ARMD, the lens can be converted to a low vision aid using a laser vision correction procedure or a piggyback IOL to make the patient 2.0 D myopic. I hope the information that I have presented here helps in deciding how to handle these situations. I believe that the presbyopia-correcting lens patient with ARMD may face some extra challenges, but just like the monofocal patient he or she can usually be kept functional. Any improvement in the ARMD patient's quality of life is worthwhile. If the ARMD becomes more severe, they may have the advantage of having a built in potential low vision aid.

References

1. Wilkinson ME. *Essential Optics Review for the Boards*. Iowa City, IA: MedRounds Publications; 2006.
2. Rand Corporation. National Eye Institute Visual Function Questionnaire (VFQ-25), Interviewer Administered Format, Self-Administered Format. , Santa Monica, CA: Author; 1996.
3. Stelmack JA, Stelmack TR, Massof RW. Measuring low-vision rehabilitation outcomes with the NEI VFQ-25. *IOVS*. 2002;43:2859-2868.
4. Lipshitz I. Miniature telescope improves vision at 12 months. VisionCare Ophthalmic Technologies, Implantable Miniature Telescope (IMT™ by Dr. Isaac Lipshitz).

WHAT IF MULTIFOCAL IOL PATIENTS DEVELOP ARMD?

Richard J. Mackool, MD

I would not expect this to be problematic because of the following.

I have implanted the ReSTOR lens (Alcon, Fort Worth, TX) in approximately 30 monocular patients with macular degeneration in whom the postoperative best-corrected visual acuity (BCVA) was expected to be somewhere between 20/50 and 20/200. In these individuals, intentional myopia of −2.00 to −7.00 D was targeted (the higher levels of myopia were targeted for those patients whose postoperative BCVA was anticipated to be the worst). This in effect provided the patients with myopia between −5.00 and −10.00 D for reading. It has been my experience that these and other myopic individuals are able to read much better than emmetropic patients of similar best-corrected distance acuity who wear a strong near add. The reasons for this are probably 2-fold. First, inherent myopia provides better contrast sensitivity for reading than does emmetropia aided by a reading spectacle. Second, the smaller, brighter image present in the myopic eye "fits better" on the best functioning macular region in these individuals who have relative or absolute macular scotomas as a result of the degenerative process. Reading speed is therefore dramatically improved in the myopic eye, as compared to the emmetropic or hyperopic eye, with macular degeneration.

CHAPTER 112

PREMIUM **IOLS** IN POST-**LASIK** EYES

Uday Devgan, MD, FACS

Patients who undergo refractive surgery have a desire to improve their unaided vision and decrease their dependence on glasses. This personality trait remains throughout their life and when they develop cataracts in the future, they will still want to maintain a large degree of freedom from spectacles. Performing cataract surgery in these patients is more complex due to the difficulty in intraocular lens (IOL) calculations, the issues of visual quality and higher-order aberrations, and the high level of patient expectations.

IOL Selection

Patients who have undergone prior corneal refractive surgery often have induced higher-order aberrations in their corneas as well as a degree of irregularity. This is particularly true in patients with prior radial keratotomy and those who have undergone high degrees of excimer-based laser correction. For this reason it is imperative to perform corneal topography to determine the amount of corneal irregularity. Wavefront aberrometers are helpful in determining the degree of higher-order aberrations.

Use of a multifocal IOL, either refractive or diffractive, involves intentionally creating aberrations in order to provide a greater range of uncorrected vision via multifocality. In normal virgin eyes multifocal IOLs reduce contrast sensitivity. Combining a multifocal IOL with an irregular or highly aberrated cornea can create an excessive loss of image quality. Patients who have undergone mild to moderate degrees of excimer-based laser correction, typically in the form of laser in situ keratomileusis (LASIK) or photorefractive keratectomy (PRK), tend to have relatively regular corneas with reasonable degrees of higher order aberration. These patients are suitable candidates for a multifocal IOL.

Patients who had undergone prior radial keratotomy (RK), particularly those with hexagonal cuts, more than 8 radial cuts, and small optical zones, tend to have high degrees of corneal irregularity. Patients who previously had aggressive excimer corneal ablations to treat high degrees of ametropia usually have excessive levels of higher-order aberrations and may even have early corneal ectasia and thinning. These patients are not good candidates for multifocal IOLs. Instead, an accommodating IOL or even a monofocal IOL may be a better choice.

One advantage of an accommodating IOL is that the accommodative amplitude can allow for more variance in the accuracy of the lens calculations. For example, should the patient end up somewhat hyperopic after surgery, they are able to use some of his or her accommodative amplitude to focus at distance. This is similar to performing LASIK surgery in a 25-year-old patient—a slight over-correction resulting in mild hyperopia is of little concern because these patients can accommodate in order to achieve a plano refractive result.

Aspheric IOLs may be a particularly good choice for post-myopic LASIK patients due to their significant corneal aberrations. Implanting a negative spherical aberration aspheric IOL can help to off-set the large amount of positive spherical aberration often seen in RK corneas. When the corneal aberrations are not known and a degree of irregularity and other higher order aberrations are suspected, I prefer an IOL with zero spherical aberration because it will not confound the aberrations.

IOL Power Calculation

In this subset of patients who desire the most accurate postoperative results, the lens calculations are the least predictable. This is due to the corneal changes induced by the prior corneal refractive surgery.

Many formulas and techniques have been described for calculating IOL power in post-RK patients—this tells me that there is no single method that yields great results. The principal error in calculation in previously myopic patients is overestimation of the corneal power, which results in implantation of a lower power IOL, with a resultant postoperative hyperopia. Because these patients have typically been myopic their entire life, leaving them with residual hyperopia is particularly uncomfortable and bothersome. To help prevent postopera-

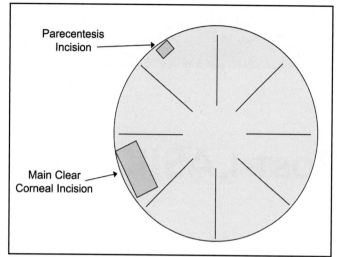

Figure 1. Cataract incisions in 8-cut RK patients. Clear corneal incisions can be used as long as they are placed between the existing RK incisions without intersecting them.

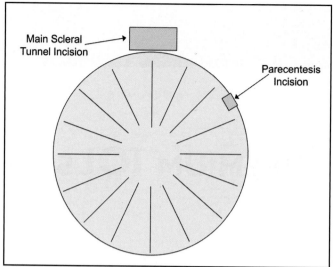

Figure 2. Cataract incisions in 16-cut RK patients. A scleral tunnel incision should be used for the cataract surgery since it will not intersect any of the many existing RK incisions.

tive hyperopia, a more myopic result can be targeted such as −0.75 D instead of the typical −0.25 D.

In patients with no old records, the method that I use most often to calculate corneal power was initially proposed by Robert Maloney, MD and later revised by Doug Koch, MD and Li Wang, MD.[1] It uses the central corneal power as measured by topography and therefore does not depend on prior history or records. The power of the cornea is a combination of the anterior corneal power and the posterior corneal power. By converting the overall central corneal power from topography back to the anterior corneal power, then subtracting the expected posterior corneal power, we can achieve a fairly accurate estimation for our IOL calculations. This formula is as follows:

Estimated K power = (Central K power on topo × 376/337.5) − 6.1

Intraoperative Considerations

When creating the clear corneal incision during the cataract surgery it is important not to damage the LASIK flap. Care should be taken to initiate the incision closer to the limbus so that it avoids contacting the corneal flap.

In patients with prior RK, the old incisions are weak and are prone to opening during surgery. Any incisions made during cataract surgery must avoid intersecting the pre-existing RK incisions, lest they unzip and cause excessive fluid leakage during surgery. In patients with previous 8-cut RK (Figure 1), clear corneal incisions can be made between the existing RK incisions. In patients with 16-cut or more RK (Figure 2), it becomes very difficult to avoid the existing RK incisions unless a scleral tunnel cataract incision is used.

To be gentle on the weakened cornea, I prefer using a lower aspiration flow rate and a lower bottle height, with a smaller phaco needle to ensure that fluid inflow remains greater than fluid outflow. If the RK incisions open during surgery, be aware that there could be sudden instability and shallowing of anterior segment and the chance for posterior capsule rup-

ture is increased. At the end of these surgeries, I like to paint the entire cornea with fluorescein dye to check for any leaks, which can easily be sutured while the patient is in the operating room.

In patients with prior phakic IOL surgery, this lens implant must be removed prior to starting the cataract surgery. I strongly recommend using two separate incisions, both of which are placed on the steep axis. The first incision is to remove the phakic IOL and the second incision is to perform the cataract surgery (Figure 3). The first incision should be sutured to ensure a water-tight anterior chamber during phacoemulsification. The second incision should be placed in the meridian that allows for the greatest ease of performing the cataract surgery (Figure 4).

Postoperative Management

The LASIK flap can swell during the postoperative period, causing some refractive instability. RK incisions swell during even the gentlest cataract operation and this swelling can induce central corneal flattening, which results in excessive hyperopia immediately postoperatively. These RK patients will experience fluctuations in their refractive state for many weeks after their cataract surgery, so a mild amount of initial hyperopia should not be a cause of concern. After waiting at least 6 weeks for the keratometry readings to return to their preoperative level, if the patient is still significantly hyperopic, a second procedure can be performed. Note that the corneas in RK patients will continue to become progressively flatter in the years to come, with a slow shift toward hyperopia.

The primary determinant of the patient's postoperative refractive spherical state is the effective lens position of the IOL after surgery. This is complex because the patient's healing response and level of fibrosis and capsular contraction after surgery are largely unknown. I explain to patients that my calculations and my surgery assume that they will have an average healing response, but if they heal more or less aggressively than normal, I may need to perform a second

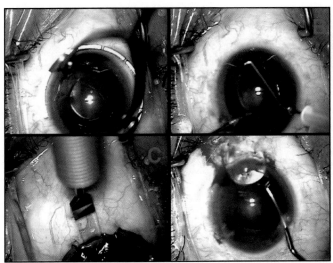

Figure 3. (A) Preoperative configuration showing the phakic IOL and the cataract. (B) De-enclavating the phakic IOL from the iris. (C) Making a nasal clear corneal incision at the steep axis. (D) Removal of the phakic IOL via the nasal incision.

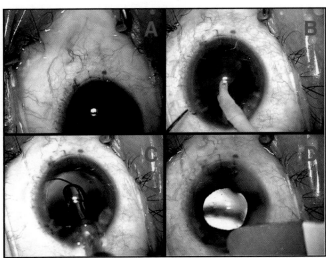

Figure 4. (A) The nasal incision is sutured closed. (B) Phacoemulsification of the cataract via a temporal clear corneal incision at the steep axis. (C) Insertion of the posterior chamber IOL. (D) Checking all incisions with fluorescein dye.

touch-up procedure to help them. They understand this and they appreciate that the surgeon is willing to do whatever it takes. In our practice, this is included at no additional cost to the patient, so it gives the practice an incentive to be as accurate as possible in IOL calculations. Because enhancements are necessary in only a small percentage of patients, this has a mild impact on the practice finances.

In post-LASIK eyes, where the IOL selection is more estimation than calculation, doing an enhancement after IOL surgery is not difficult because the prior corneal flap can be lifted. In other patients, I prefer to wait at least a couple of months until the cataract incisions have fully healed before performing LASIK to fine tune their refractive status. In cases where there is a very high likelihood of needing to perform LASIK enhancement following the IOL surgery, a corneal flap can be created prior to the intraocular surgery. In post-RK eyes, performing a piggy-back IOL may be a better choice in order to avoid inducing any further corneal irregularities or weakening.

Perhaps the most important issues in refractive surgery patients with cataracts are explaining to them that their IOL calculations are, at best, estimations, and that their surgery and postoperative recovery will likely be more challenging for both the surgeon and the patient.

Reference

1. Wang L, Booth MA, Koch DD. Comparison of intraocular lens power calculation methods in eyes that have undergone LASIK. *Ophthalmology.* 2004;111(10):1825-1831.

CHAPTER 113

PREMIUM IOLS IN POST–LASIK EYES

Jeffrey D. Horn, MD

Laser vision correction surgery has become one of the most popular elective surgeries, with approximately 1.4 million laser in situ keratomileusis (LASIK)/photorefractive keratectomy (PRK) procedures performed annually in the United States. However, cataract surgery is still the most commonly performed vision corrective procedure in the United States, with approximately 2.5 million procedures performed per year. This is projected to increase to 3.5 million per year in the next 5 to 10 years, as the baby boomers age. It is evident, therefore, that many of the patients that will undergo cataract with intraocular lens (IOL) surgery will have had prior corneal laser surgery. Fueled by LASIK marketing, advances in technology and IOL design, and increased needs and demands by this aging baby boomer population, patient expectations for spectacle independence following cataract surgery are ever increasing.

However, it is well known that the alteration in corneal curvature achieved with LASIK makes calculating IOL power more complicated and therefore less accurate. Specifically, LASIK modifies the anterior corneal curvature with minimal effect on the posterior cornea (in the absence of ectasia), altering the normal anterior/posterior ratio of approximately 82%. Because traditional keratometry (manual, automated, and placido disc based corneal topography) measures only the anterior cornea and assumes a normal ratio, the change in this ratio following LASIK results in an inaccurate measurement of corneal power. Typically, with previous myopic LASIK, for example, the measured corneal curvature overestimates the true value, resulting in under powering of the IOL leading to a hyperopic outcome. There have been at least 10 different methods designed to calculate (and therefore estimate) corneal power. Most rely on historical information, such as pre-LASIK keratometry and/or manifest refraction (which may not be available), whereas some others do not. Although a discussion of all the published and proposed methods is beyond the scope of this chapter, I would direct the reader to the Web site of Dr. Warren Hill (www.doctor-hill.com) as an excellent resource. In addition, the American Society of Cataract and Refractive Surgery (www.ASCRS.org) provides a free online calculator. My personal preference is to use the Holladay Report provided by the Pentacam (Oculus Inc, Lynwood, WA). This calculates corneal power by measuring both the anterior and posterior corneal curvatures. I then use the equivalent K provided by the report and input that into the previous refractive surgery screen of the Holladay II formula provided with the Holladay Consultant. This formula also uses a double-K calculation to take into account effective lens position, which would be erroneously predicted using post LASIK keratometry only. With this method, my mean deviation from desired refractive aim has been within ± 0.50 D (unpublished data).

It is imperative, therefore, that any patient who presents to you with cataracts and who has had previous LASIK must understand the potential for a refractive surprise despite your best efforts and intentions. They must be made aware, without confusing them, that there is a good chance they will require some surgical enhancement, be it IOL exchange, piggyback lens, or LASIK, or that they may need eyeglasses after cataract surgery. However, I let my patients know that although I may not get it right the first time, there should be no reason why I cannot ultimately achieve the desired refractive outcome. In addition, they should know that there may additional costs associated with these enhancing procedures, especially if you were not the original LASIK surgeon. Properly managing their expectations preoperatively is mandatory.

Once patients understand the ramifications that their previous laser surgery will have on their cataract surgery, we must select the lens implant. Because corneal asphericity may change secondary to laser ablation, especially with increased treatment powers and older generation laser technology, some IOL types may be more appropriate than others. For instance, in a postmyopic LASIK patient, the typical prolate corneal curvature (steeper centrally than peripherally) may become more oblate. Negative aspheric lens implants, such as the SN60WF (Alcon, Fort Worth, TX) and the Tecnis (Advanced Medical Optics, Santa Ana, CA) may be good choices as they will help offset the prolate spherical aberrations. In a patient status posthyperopic LASIK, however, the increased curvature results in a more prolate cornea, and would therefore do better if matched with a spherical lens implant. This assumes that the patient desires a monofocal implant without addressing presbyopia (unless he or she chooses monovision). Remember, the most common side effect of any cataract procedure is presbyopia.

It has been my experience that these patients want to reduce their dependence on glasses as much as possible. After all, this is the reason they underwent LASIK in the first place. All of my patients are counseled as to their lens implant options, including monofocal (with or without monovision), toric monofocal (in the case of pre-existing corneal astigmatism), and multifocal or accommodating. In fact, in the last 2 years, every one of those patients presenting to me who had previous LASIK and requiring cataract extraction opted for a presbyopia-correcting solution. The vast majority of these chose multifocal or accommodating implants.

How do you, as the surgeon, determine if a patient who has had LASIK is a candidate for a presbyopia-correcting lens implant? First, the same prerequisites for a good outcome as for any other patient receiving a presbyopia-correcting (Pr-C) IOL (especially a multifocal) apply. These include a good tear film and normal corneal surface, minimal astigmatism (or regular astigmatism that can be reduced to less than 0.75 D with limbal relaxing incisions (LRIs) and/or LASIK or surface ablation enhancement), and the absence of pathology that may contribute to decreased contrast sensitivity (macular disease, glaucoma, significant corneal guttata or edema, etc). This is in addition to having reasonable and appropriate expectations. In addition, corneal topography to evaluate centration of the ablation is important because a decentered ablation will create irregular astigmatism, which can degrade vision quality, especially with a multifocal implant. The LASIK flap itself should be evaluated, as even small microstriae within the visual axis may result in a degradation of visual quality if combined with a multifocal implant. Tear film issues need to be addressed aggressively. I have heard that any one who has had prior LASIK should be excluded from receiving anything other than a monofocal implant. This does not make sense to me, as we teach that many patients who receive multifocal implants may require a LASIK enhancement, so it should not matter whether the LASIK came before or after the cataract surgery. Granted, the amount of ablation will be greater in the patient who had LASIK surgery first, but as long as the aforementioned issues are addressed and evaluated, excellent outcomes can be achieved.

My personal algorithm for determining the appropriate lens implant is as follows. For those patients who choose monovision (or monofocal distance IOL with reading glasses), I will implant an aspheric lens in patients who had previous myopic LASIK, and a spherical lens in those who had previous hyperopic LASIK. However, for those patients who have pre-existing regular corneal astigmatism, I prefer the Alcon Acrysof Toric IOL (with or without monovision). This is especially true for posthyperopic LASIK eyes, but also for postmyopic LASIK eyes as well. An argument can be made for placing an aspheric lens combined with an LRI in these patients. For those patients who choose a Pr-C IOL to address their near vision tasks (the majority of these patients in my experience) and are otherwise

good candidates as described previously, I first determine what their visual requirements and needs are. For instance, is reading the most important near task? Do they do other near tasks like sewing, and so on? Do they spend much time on the computer? If so, is it a stationary desktop computer, or do they travel with a laptop? We question our patients extensively in this regard, in addition to utilizing a vision preferences survey form that the patient completes. Because no single Pr-C IOL necessarily corrects all distances equally well, we use this information to determine which implant to give them, and whether to mix the technologies. Next, I determine whether they have had myopic or hyperopic LASIK. This, of course will be known to you if you did the original LASIK, but many times this is not the case. You may be surprised at how many patients do not know whether they were near or far sighted prior to LASIK, whether they were given monovision, and if so, which eye was set for reading. Once the patient presents to us we request their previous LASIK records, but often they are incomplete or nonexistent. Frequently, the patient must be questioned as to when hr or she began wearing spectacles or contacts, if hr or she wore distant or reading glasses as his or her first pair, and so on. Although not everyone has a Pentacam, I find it extremely useful in this regard, because it shows the relative anterior/posterior corneal curvature in percent. Previous myopes should have a ratio less than 82% (hyperopes greater than 82%), and the difference between measured and normal can be a fairly good indication of the magnitude of the original treatment. In the case of patients who are status postmyopic LASIK, I prefer the Alcon ReSTOR SN6AD3, which is a ReSTOR lens on the aspheric platform. For those patients who require excellent intermediate vision, and who are postmyopic LASIK with monovision, I will consider a monovision type approach, where the nondominant eye is implanted with the ReSTOR Aspheric with a target of −1.00. In the dominant eye, I will use the same lens aiming for emmetropia. This will allow the non-dominant eye to provide intermediate vision, while also providing a higher add for such close up tasks such as threading a needle. Binocularly these patients will have a tremendous overall range of vision, and usually do extremely well. However, they may require greater hand holding and reassurance during the postoperative period, because neuroadaptation often takes longer. Again, the key to success with any premium IOL is to manage the patient's expectations preoperatively. If the patients have not had monovision before, then I will implant the SN6AD3 in the nondominant eye first, and then decide on whether to implant the lens bilaterally, or to use a different lens in the fellow eye, which may provide better intermediate vision. This determination is based on the patient's satisfaction with their vision after the first surgery is performed. If mixing lenses is indicated, then I will either implant a Crystalens (Eyeonics, Inc, Aliso Viejo, CA), or an Advanced Medical Optics ReZoom in the second eye. Just as for any eye receiving a multifocal implant, pupil size, and tolerance for possible night vision issues (greatest with ReZoom), and so on must be taken into account. In my experience, the Crystalens provides excellent intermediate vision but is less predictable because of its axial instability. This results in a slightly greater need for enhancement, especially in these post LASIK eyes. For eyes that have undergone hyperopic LASIK, I prefer the original nonaspheric ReSTOR, and then follow a similar protocol to determine whether it should be implanted bilaterally. If a multifocal lens is otherwise contraindicated, but the patient still desires presbyopia correction bilaterally, then I will implant the Crystalens, aiming for −0.25 D in one eye and −0.75 in the other.

My need for laser enhancements using this technique and methodology has been less than 5% in these patients. For those who may need an enhancement, especially for a spherical refractive error, my preference is to perform a surface ablation enhancement with mitomycin C over the flap. I wait several months, as I prefer to perform a yttrium-aluminum-garnet (YAG) capsulotomy first, as this may affect the ultimate refractive error requiring treatment. Alternatively, one can do an IOL exchange or piggyback sooner. There is a possibility of iris chafing, pigment dispersion, and possible chronic iritis and or cystoid macular edema with a piggyback lens. The choice of procedure ultimately will be determined by relative cost, access to a laser, feasibility of further corneal laser ablation (corneal pachymetry needs to be performed prior to cataract surgery), and the comfort level of both the surgeon and patient. As far as cost to the patient, the surgeon can either implement a "pay as you go" model, in which the patient pays extra for the enhancement, or utilize an all inclusive approach, in which enhancements costs are covered by the original payment. I prefer the latter.

Conclusion

There will be a growing number of patients requiring cataract surgery who have undergone previous laser refractive surgery. This population of patients has essentially been self-selected as requiring (if not demanding) as good a refractive outcome, if not better, from their cataract surgery as they achieved from LASIK. Therefore, it may be necessary to give them as much spectacle independence as possible, including correcting their presbyopia with multifocal and/or accommodating lens implants. This in turn requires meticulous attention to detail to determine who is a good candidate, and then performing excellent biometry and surgery with appropriate lens selection for the individual patient. Management of patient expectations long before the patient is taken to the operating room is vital. With that said, in my experience, these patients are some of the happiest people in my practice, and although it takes extra work and effort on my part, it is one the most gratifying things I can do.

CHAPTER 114

PREMIUM IOLs IN POST-LASIK EYES

Renée Solomon, MD and Eric Donnenfeld, MD

Over 8 million refractive procedures have been performed in the United States over the last decade. As these postlaser in situ keratomileusis (LASIK) patients have aged, there has been an increased incidence of cataract surgery in this population. Significant breakthroughs in intraocular lens (IOL) technology now allow clinicians an alternative to monofocal IOLs. With dramatic improvement in IOL technology, multifocal IOLs including the multifocal diffractive posterior chamber IOLs (PCIOL), the ReSTOR lens (Alcon, Fort Worth, TX), and the Tecnis multifocal lens (Advanced Medical Optics, Santa Ana, CA) (available in Europe), the multifocal refractive PCIOL, the ReZoom lens (Advanced Medical Optics), the accommodative IOL, the Crystalens (Eyeonics, Inc, Aliso Viejo, CA), and toric IOLs by STAAR Surgical (Monrovia, CA) and Alcon are assuming an increasing role in the refractive armamentarium. These premium IOLs have revolutionized the rehabilitation of the post-LASIK cataract patient.[1-11] However, reduced contrast sensitivity and symptoms of glare and halos following implantation of multifocal IOLs have been reported and are more significant in patients who have undergone prior refractive surgery.[11] For a few patients, these symptoms are so debilitating that they have required explantation of these IOLs. Toric IOLs may be indicated in patients with residual cylinder or in patients with lenticular astigmatism who will manifest astigmatism following cataract extraction.

Post-LASIK patients often have a relative intolerance for diminished vision and often request early cataract surgery. Many LASIK patients with cataracts desire spectacle independence and are interested in presbyopia-correcting (Pr-C) IOLs. When the cataract surgery is done early and before their vision has deteriorated badly, these patients will still have high expectations. If the postoperative refraction is not close to Plano or if there is residual cylinder, then these post-refractive surgery patients tend to be unhappy. Following prior refractive surgery, it is particularly important to carefully select appropriate patients for multifocal IOLs. A sample screening questionnaire for multifocal IOLs developed by Steven J. Dell, MD,

(Appendix A) is available on the internet at www.crstoday.com under the header "Dell Questionnaire." This questionnaire is not specific to post-LASIK patients but is extremely useful as a screening guide.

The more "chair time" a surgeon spends with the patients before the surgery, the less time will be needed after surgery. A significant discussion prior to surgery eases the patient's expectations. Patients receiving a Pr-C IOL after prior keratorefractive surgery tend to be the most demanding and the most challenging patients seen in cataract and refractive practices. It is important to extensively discuss the added risk of glare and halos when the premium lenses are inserted in eyes that have undergone prior laser vision correction (LVC). In addition, patients must be made aware of the increased need for refractive enhancement after prior refractive surgery and the difficulty in perfectly achieving the target refraction in eyes that have undergone prior LVC. The greater the original ametropia, the more difficult it will be to predict the proper IOL power. Patients need to be informed that as many as 10% of multifocal IOL patients will require an excimer laser enhancement postoperatively. Following LASIK the inherent refractive uncertainly and the high patient expectations may significantly increase the need for additional refractive enhancements.[12] In addition, patients need to be aware that best-corrected visual acuity (BCVA) immediately after surgery may not be as good as multifocal and accommodative IOLs placed in eyes without previous refractive surgery but with a refractive enhancement patient satisfaction is usually excellent.[12]

Patients presenting for premium IOLs in post-refractive eyes require an extensive informed consent of the risks and benefits of these lenses. The informed consent should include the normal information important to all patients and should specifically address the added risks of glare and halo and the need for additional refractive enhancements that are inherent with using these IOLs in a post-LASIK eye. Multifocal IOLs have the greatest risk of additional glare and halo, whereas accommodating IOLs and toric IOLs have less additional risk.

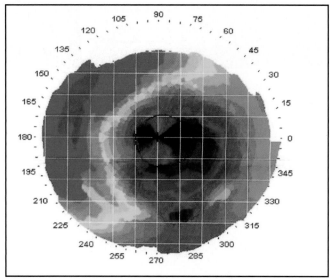

Figure 1. Image of corneal topography after decentered excimer ablation in an eye that had previously undergone LASIK. A patient with this topography would not be a candidate for a multifocal IOL.

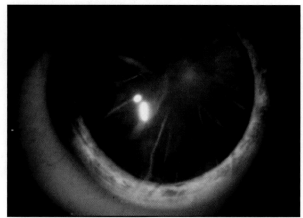

Figure 2. Cataract in a patient who has had a prior RK. The decentered nature of the RK incisions would make this patient a poor candidate for a multifocal IOL.

In addition, following LVC, patients need to understand that they will most likely be dissatisfied with their overall vision after having only one eye operated on. The importance of having both eyes implanted is critical for the success of the procedure as is an adequate adaptation period. Patients who have had prior radial keratotomy (RK) need to understand that insertion of a multifocal IOL will not eliminate the refractive fluctuations that are common after RK. Cataract surgeons who do not perform laser refractive surgery need to work with a laser refractive surgeon with whom they are comfortable comanaging their patients for postmultifocal IOL enhancements.

IOL power calculations are less precise in eyes following previous refractive surgery. Although there are a variety of different techniques to calculate the IOL power, it is important to remember that the refractive goal following elective IOL implantation varies based on the IOL implanted. ReZoom lenses are generally most effective with a postoperative refraction of Plano. For ReSTOR lenses the postoperative goal is usually Plano to +0.25 D and for the Crystalens the postoperative goal is usually −0.25 D. Toric IOLs may be indicated in patients with residual cylinder or in patients with lenticular astigmatism who will manifest astigmatism following cataract extraction and for whom the target postoperative refraction is Plano.

The optics of multifocal IOLs make IOL centration extremely important for improved patient outcomes.[13] Multifocal lenses should not be inserted in cases of zonular dehiscence or capsular rupture. The size of the anterior capsulorrhexis is critical in these patients and should be close to 6 mm in diameter. After implantation of a multifocal IOL, a lens that is centered within the capsular bag may not be aligned with the center of the pupil. This decentration of the IOL with respect to the pupil occurs because the anatomical pupillary axis of the eye, the visual axis, and the optical axis are not aligned.[14]

Misalignment of a multifocal IOL with the pupil may compromise the optical outcome, resulting in a decrease in the quality of vision. Clinically it has been noted that patients who had decentration of the multifocal IOL relative to the pupil had more complaints of glare and halo than patients with the IOL well aligned with the pupil.

Prior to considering multifocal IOLs in patients who have undergone prior refractive surgery, patients must have an assessment of their post-LASIK topography, pachymetry, and keratometry values. Patients need to have well-centered ablations (Figure 1), sufficient stromal depth, and appropriate corneal steepness to undergo an enhancement. If the ablation is decentered and the multifocal IOL is decentered by a different amount than the ablation, then the deleterious effect of the decentration will be compounded and the patient will not achieve a good visual result. If the peripheral cornea is very flat (oblate), the patient may not tolerate a multifocal IOL because of compounded spherical aberration. Similarly, if the patient has had prior photorefractive keratectomy (PRK) or a variant, such as LASIK or Epi-LASIK, the postrefractive topographies must be reviewed to confirm that the treatments were well centered. If the patient has had prior RK, it is very important for the RK incisions to be well-centered as confirmed by corneal topography before inserting a multifocal IOL (Figure 2). Patients who have a multifocal IOL implanted after a decentered ablation or decentered RK surgical incisions are at greater risk of increased glare, halos, and poor quality of vision even though they may see a Snellen visual acuity of 20/20.

Before considering laser vision enhancement for postoperative complaints of glare and halos, it is important to be sure that all other potential causes of these complaints have been addressed or ruled out. The 5 Cs designate potential problems that must be sought or addressed: cylinder and residual refractive error, capsular opacities, cornea and ocular surface disease, cystoid macular edema (CME),[15] and centration of the IOL with the pupil.

For patients whose IOL is not well centered with the pupil (Figure 3) an argon laser iridoplasty can be performed.[16,17] Four 500-milliwatt, 500-µm diameter spots of 0.5 second duration are placed in the iris mid-periphery in the area in which the pupil margin is impinging on the center of the multifocal IOL. If there are still complaints of glare and halo and the patient is emmetropic then Alphagan P (Allergan, Irvine, CA) can be prescribed to treat the glare and halo complaints.

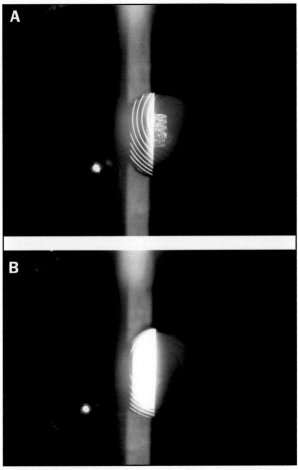

Figure 3. Slit lamp biomicroscopy of ReSTOR multifocal IOL before (A) and after (B) treatment with argon laser iridoplasty.

Patients presenting for cataract surgery after prior LASIK are usually older individuals, who have less adherent epithelium and are better PRK candidates. In addition, a LASIK enhancement performed years later in older individuals is more likely to result in epithelial ingrowth. Unlike LASIK, PRK does not exacerbate dry eye or pose the risk of epithelial ingrowth beneath a flap. A conventional ablation will often give better results after multifocal IOL implantation than a wavefront ablation because current aberrometers may not accurately measure through multifocal IOLs. Patients undergoing cataract surgery following LASIK should be told they may require a conventional PRK rather than the custom wavefront treatment, which they may have previously underwent. In conclusion, we recommend a conventional PRK enhancement in older patients who need a refractive enhancement following insertion of a multifocal IOL.

Refractive IOL explantations are uncommon. However, patients and physicians need to understand prior to the insertion of Pr-C IOLs that additional touch-ups may be needed including additional laser vision correction, treatment of dry eye disease, limbal relaxing incisions, yttrium-aluminum-garnet (YAG) capsulotomy, treatment of any macular pathology, and argon laser iridoplasty to improve centration of the IOL with the pupil. When all possible causes of decreased visual acuity have been addressed the majority of patients should

enjoy their spectacle independence with Pr-C IOLs.

In addition, it is important to remember that older myopic excimer laser ablation profiles were oblate with minimal blend zones. These ablation profiles are associated with a greater positive spherical aberration, which, when coupled with the intrinsic loss of contrast and glare seen in multifocal IOLs, may result in dissatisfied patients. In general, patients with minimal ablations, which are well centered, and have a prolate architecture are good candidates for multifocal IOLs. Conversely, patients with deeper ablations, which are oblate and decentered have an increased risk of a poor visual outcome with a multifocal IOL. Patients who are not good candidates for multifocal IOLs may be acceptable candidates for an accommodating IOL. With a thorough preoperative workup, an extensive informed consent, and, finally, excellent surgical and postoperative care, premium IOLs offer enhanced visual rehabilitation of the cataract patient following previous refractive surgery.

References

1. Solomon R, Donnenfeld ED. Refractive intraocular lenses multifocal and phakic IOLs. In: Friedlaender MB ed. *Int Ophthalmol Clin.* Vol. 46. Philadelphia, Pa: Lippincott Williams and Wilkins, 2006:123-143.

2. Bellucci R. Multifocal intraocular lenses. *Curr Opin Ophthalmol.* 2005;16:33-37.

3. Dick HB. Accommodative intraocular lenses: current status. *Curr Opin Ophthalmol.* 2005;16:8-26.

4. Rocha KM, Chalita MR, Souza CE, Soriano ES, Freitas LL, Muccioli C, Belfort R Jr. Postoperative wavefront analysis and contrast sensitivity of a multifocal apodized diffractive IOL (ReSTOR) and three monofocal IOLs. *J Refract Surg.* 2005;21:S808-812.

5. Mamalis N. Accommodating intraocular lenses. *J Cataract Refract Surg.* 2004;30:2455-2456.

6. Rana A, Miller D, Magnante P. Understanding the accommodating intraocular lens. *J Cataract Refract Surg.* 2003;29:2284-2287.

7. Versteeg FF. Multifocal IOLs for presbyopia. *J Cataract Refract Surg.* 2005;31:1266.

8. Olson RJ, Werner L, Mamalis N, Cionni R. New intraocular lens technology. *Am J Ophthalmol.* 2005;140:709-716.

9. Nijkamp MD, Dolders MG, de Brabander J, van den Borne B, Hendrikse F, Nuijts RM. Effectiveness of multifocal intraocular lenses to correct presbyopia after cataract surgery: a randomized controlled trial. *Ophthalmology.* 2004;111:1832-1839. Erratum in: *Ophthalmology.* 2004;111:2022.

10. Pineda-Fernandez A, Jaramillo J, Celis V, Vargas J, DiStacio M, Galindez A, Del Valle M. Refractive outcomes after bilateral multifocal intraocular lens implantation. *J Cataract Refract Surg.* 2004;30:685-688.

11. Leyland M, Zinicola E. Multifocal versus monofocal intraocular lenses in cataract surgery: a systematic review. *Ophthalmology.* 2003;110:1789-1798.

12. Solomon R, Donnenfeld E, Perry H, Palmer C. Multifocal, Accommodative, and Aspheric Lenses in Patients Who Have Undergone Prior Refractive Surgery. Presented at the ASCRS Symposium on Cataract, IOL, and Refractive Surgery, San Diego, California, April 2007.

13. Wang L, Koch DD. Effect of decentration of wavefront-corrected intraocular lenses on the higher-order aberrations of the eye. *Arch Ophthalmol.* 2005;123:1226-1230.

14. Holladay JT, ed. Understanding optics. In: *Quality of Vision.* Ch 1. Thorofare, NJ. Slack Incorporated; 2005:3-5.

15. Donnenfeld E, Roberts CW, Perry HD, Solomon R, Wittpenn JR, McDonald MB. The Effect of the Topical Nonsteroidal Anti-inflammatory Drug, Ketorolac Tromethamine 0.4%, on Quality of Vision with a Multifocal Intraocular Lens. Presented at American Society of Cataract and Refractive Surgery Annual Meeting 2006.

16. Solomon R, Donnenfeld ED, Perry HD, et al. Argon Laser Iridoplasty to Improve Visual Function Following Multifocal IOL Implantation. Presented at the American Academy of Ophthalmology Annual Meeting, New Orleans, Louisiana, November 2007.

17. Donnenfeld ED, Solomon R, Perry HD, et al. Argon Laser Iridoplasty to Improve Visual Function Following Multifocal IOL Implantation. Presented at the Refractive Surgery Subspecialty Day, New Orleans, Louisiana, November 2007.

CHAPTER 115

PATIENT EDUCATION— USING THE IOL COUNSELOR

Robert D. Watson

Let us be honest. If given a choice between "restricted near vision" after cataract surgery with a monofocal intraocular lens (IOL) or a "full range of vision" with a refractive IOL, the vast majority of us would prefer a full range of vision with little or no dependence on corrective eyewear. Then why did only 4.6% of all cataract procedures in 2006 involve refractive IOLs?

If you think cost is the reason, you are only partly correct. The real culprit is lack of proper education. Unless you educate patients in a manner that raises the perceived value of refractive IOLs, your conversion percentage will not rise. Fortunately, the IOL Counselor (Patient Education Concepts, [PEC] Houston, TX) patient education software program is now available to help you raise the perceived value of refractive IOLs, with some of our beta test practices now averaging over 70% conversion!

Most doctors are not good at selling their services, and many do not have patient counselors trained in sales and closing techniques. Year after year of reduced Medicare reimbursements have ingrained in their minds that they have to see more cataract patients just to break even. Getting doctors to consider the fact that they could actually make more money seeing fewer patients if they take the time to educate patients about refractive IOLs is not an easy assignment for any practice development manager or lens representative.

The IOL Counselor patient education program was introduced in March 2007 and delivered to approximately 5000 US-based American Society of Cataract and Refractive Surgery (ASCRS) members through an educational grant from Alcon and Advanced Medical Optics,. It was created to accomplish one primary objective—increase the number of patients electing a refractive IOL versus a standard IOL.

In order to accomplish this goal, the program had to make the educational process quick and simple. Most patients do not even know what a cataract is, much less how they would see with a monofocal or refractive IOL. So the cataract surgeon is right… it does take too much of his or her time to educate patients, but he or she probably should not be the ones doing it anyway.

When doctors take on the task of explaining IOL options to patients in the exam room, the odds of conversion are against them. First, some patients cannot focus on the conversation after hearing the doctor say "surgery." While the doctor is explaining IOL options, patients are often in a mild state of shock, thinking they might go blind if there are complications or wondering who will take care of them while they are recovering.

Second, the doctor is putting a lot of pressure on the patient to make an immediate decision that will affect the quality of his or her vision for the rest of his or her life. Patients simply do not have time in the exam room to fully reflect on the importance of this decision and often utter a defensive, "No thanks."

Third, doctors just want to be doctors, so they tend to give patients too much information, which often confuses them. Imagine someone who thought a cataract was something that grows over the cornea trying to make a decision about the pros and cons of a refractive, diffractive, or accommodating IOL. When it comes to the difficulty of describing the benefits of a refractive IOL along with the cost, it is no wonder doctors were not successful in converting patients.

Frustrated with both the lack of time and tools to educate patients properly and lack of success in up-selling, many doctors would either just briefly mention refractive IOLs with little effort to up-sell or they would delegate the educational duty to their surgical counselors. If a practice was already performing corneal refractive surgery, their surgical counselor usually had some experience in sales and closing techniques. If a cataract practice did not have a skilled surgical counselor, the job was passed on to the surgery scheduler or ophthalmic technician who often had no sales training or counseling skills.

With the table set on why conversions were so low, PEC began working with Eyeland Design Network (Germany) on the IOL Counselor. We needed to develop a multifaceted approach to this educational problem that would enhance the counseling skills of both surgical counselors and doctors, regardless of their sales and counseling skills.

Figure 1. The IOL Acceptance Form documents each patient's final choice of IOLs and that the simulations were not shown as a guarantee.

Patient's Name _____ Date of Consultation: _____

IOL Acceptance Form

Because you will only have cataract surgery one time, it is very important to understand how the Intra-ocular Lens (IOL) you choose to have during surgery can affect the quality of your vision for the rest of your life. Please indicate your choice of IOL below and sign at the bottom. Your signature verifies that you have been made aware of your IOL options and you understand the importance of choosing the right IOL to meet your visual and lifestyle needs. DO NOT SIGN BELOW IF YOU ARE STILL IN DOUBT ABOUT WHICH IOL YOU WOULD LIKE TO HAVE IMPLANTED DURING YOUR PROCEDURE.

__ I have decided to have the _____ presbyopia correcting IOL, designed to provide a full range of vision and reduce my need for bifocals or reading glasses.

__ I have decided to have the ___Standard or ___Aspheric Monofocal, designed to provide good distance vision and I understand that I will most likely need to wear corrective lenses for my intermediate and near vision.

I also understand that the simulations presented to me on the IOL Counselor™ were not presented as a guarantee of how I will see with the lens selection I made. I understand that it is impossible to simulate how anyone will see with any IOL due to a variety of optical, surgical, and individual healing factors.

_____   _____
Signature of Patient   Date

_____   _____
Witness   Date

The IOL Counselor ultimately developed into a set of tools that, when used together, provided the practice with a beginning, middle, and ending to the educational process. These tools include the following:

* Dr. Steven Dell's Vision Assessment Questionnaire (VAQ)
* A patient education video
* The IOL simulation module
* The IOL acceptance form (Figure 1)
* A "How to Use the IOL Counselor" tutorial

Dr. Dell's VAQ is given to the patient to complete prior to the exam. It provides the doctor with an easy to interpret, analytical tool to assess the patient's vision needs based on his or her responses about his or her lifestyle preferences. The doctor reviews the VAQ and recommends a specific IOL by circling the type of lens at the bottom of the form. This provides the patient with a positive directive, "Based on your vision lifestyle needs, I think you would do best with the ___ refractive IOL." The patient then takes the VAQ with him or her to the surgical counselor who immediately identifies which IOL simulation the doctor wants shown to the patient (Figure 2).

The 8-minute "presbyopia-correcting IOLs" video can be shown to patients waiting for the doctor in the exam room or the counselor and incorporates the same animations they will see during the interactive presentation (Figure 3). This generic video can also be shown in DVD format in the reception room to pre-educate patients.

Counseling patients within the IOL simulation module is where the magic of the IOL Counselor begins to work. Using a slider bar, the surgical counselor guides the patient through a visual presentation depicting normal vision, presbyopic vision, and progressive cataract vision. Next, it shows vision with a monofocal IOL, corrected for distance and then vision with a multifocal IOL, showing a full range of vision (Figure 4).

The differences between "restricted near vision" and a "full range of vision" are very obvious. Even if the patient has bilateral cataracts and cannot see well, the IOL Counselor simulations usually encourage the codecision maker, who came to the exam with the cataract patient, to strongly recommend the refractive IOL option.

The surgical counselor can choose from a number of real life scenes to match the personality and lifestyle of each patient. They can show the baseball park scene, a grocery store scene, or a city driving scene. If the doctor recommended a multifocal IOL, the driving scene has a night time companion scene that allows the counselor to show how multifocal IOLs create rings and halos around lights (Figures 5 and 6).

Moving the pointer down the timeline within the multifocal IOL's night time simulation shows patients what the rings and halos might look like immediately after surgery and how they might appear during and after the neuroadaptation process. Although the characteristics of these artifacts vary between refractive and diffractive optics, showing the night time simulation prepares the patient for the inevitable while assuring

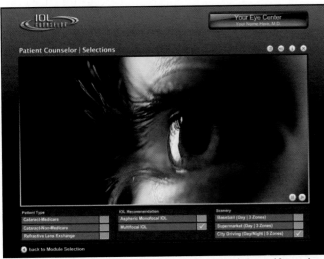

Figure 2. The counselor selects the Patient Type, IOL Recommendation, and Scenery based on Medicare coverage, the doctor's IOL recommendation, and the patient's lifestyle.

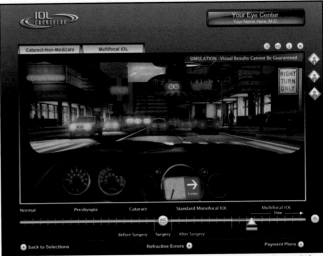

Figure 5. Night time simulation showing rings and halos immediately after multifocal IOL implantation.

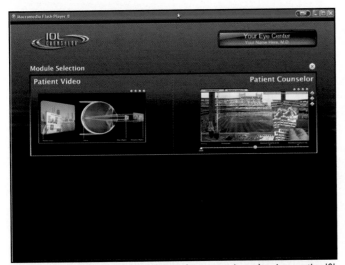

Figure 3. The surgical counselor can elect to show a generic presbyopic-correcting IOL video or enter the interactive patient counseling pages from the Module Selection page.

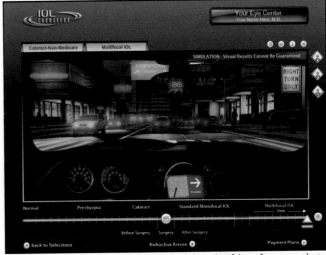

Figure 6. Night time simulation shows reduction in intensity of rings after neuro-adaptation.

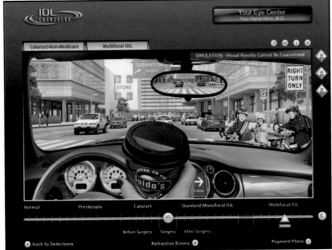

Figure 4. The city driving day scene showing full range of vision with a multifocal IOL.

him or her that, in spite of their presence, they are not debilitating and for most patients diminish over time.

Without the pressure of the doctor's presence in the exam room, after the patient has had time to absorb the fact that he or she will have cataract surgery and after he or she realizes that the chances of going blind are extremely rare, it is much easier for a patient to focus on how the decision he or she is being asked to make will affect the quality of his or her vision for the rest of his or her life. Some patients actually prefer wearing glasses, but for the vast majority, the decision to wear or not wear "granny glasses" or "readers" after cataract surgery comes down to the "How much?" question.

If the patient says, "Fine, let's do it" after you tell him or her how much the surgery costs, the counseling session is over. If the patient shows any hesitation at all, the counselor clicks on the "Payment Plans" button (Figure 7). This takes the patient to a side-by-side comparison showing vision through the "government-issued" IOL covered by Medicare and the multifocal IOL available for a low monthly payment through CareCredit. Just like with other refractive procedures or any kind of luxury

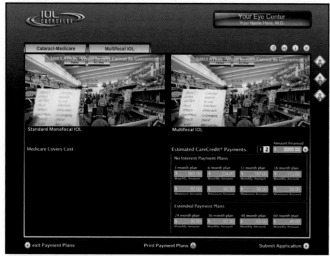

Figure 7. If patients hesitate about procedure costs, the counselor uses the Payments Page to show how affordable the procedure can be using CareCredit.

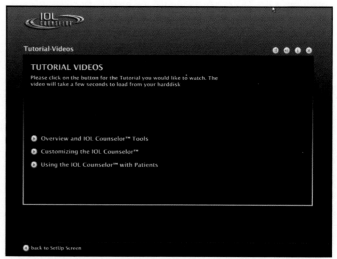

Figure 9. The IOL Counselor makes it easy to train counselors with a number of video tutorials on the CD.

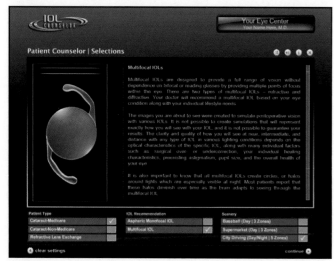

Figure 8. Counselors are encouraged to read the disclaimer page prior to showing IOL simulations.

item, you want to show its affordability along with the benefits of owning the product. If the counselor's computer is connected to the Internet, one more click takes them to CareCredit's "apply online" Web site where the patient can be approved for credit within minutes.

The IOL Counselor is first and foremost an educational tool to help patients understand their IOL options and excite them about the possibility of being lens free after cataract surgery. It is not an informed consent tool. However, the software was designed so that before each patient can view the IOL simulations, a disclaimer page appears (Figure 8). The surgical counselor reads the disclaimer to the patient, informing him or her that it is impossible to simulate exactly how he or she will see with any IOL and that what he or she is about to see is not being presented as a guarantee. PEC also advocates using a presbyopia-correcting IOL informed consent video to help create more realistic expectations about these IOLs that covers potential risks, side effects, and complications of the procedure.

After the counseling session, the patient is presented with the IOL Acceptance Form regardless of his or her choice (see

Figure 1). This form documents that the patient understood that the simulations were not presented as a guarantee and asks him or her to put his or her initials next to the final choice of a monofocal or refractive IOL. If the patient chooses a monofocal, he or she is reminded again that with this choice he or she is going to need reading glasses for most of his or her close activities. This moment can be a turning point in the patient's decision process as he or she thinks one more time about being dependent on reading glasses or imagines living a lens-free lifestyle after cataract surgery.

Before using the IOL Counselor, practices are encouraged to view the "How to Use the IOL Counselor" tutorial (Figure 9). Ideally, both the surgical counselor and the doctor should watch it together. Then, they should take turns role playing to fine tune their presentation and to ensure the doctor that the counselor is proficient in its use.

The IOL Counselor has 2 additional sections that can be used when the patient has further questions. Since refractive IOLs do not correct astigmatism, there is a "surgery" section that has brief animations of limbal relaxing incisions along with photorefractive keratectomy and laser in situ keratomileusis. There is also a brief animation showing small incision cataract surgery (phacoemulsification) with IOL implantation (Figure 10). Additionally, if a patient does not understand the differences between nearsightedness, farsightedness, and astigmatism, the counselor can access the "refractive errors" animations page (Figure 11).

The IOL Counselor, when used as it was intended, does not have to add time to the surgeon's schedule. If the rest of the staff is on board, patients will learn about refractive IOLs through collateral materials such as videos and brochures while in the reception room. Then, technicians usually have 1 hour or more to talk to patients during their work-ups about how their surgeon is making their patients happy with refractive IOLs. The surgeon, using the VAQ, needs only a minute or two more to make his IOL recommendation before sending the patient on to the surgical counselor who uses the IOL Counselor to close the sale.

The IOL Counselor requires a PC computer and looks best when shown on a flat screen monitor. Once a practice recog-

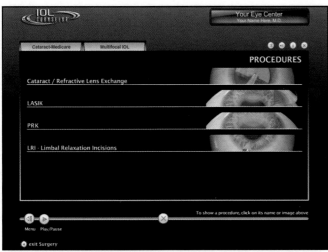

Figure 10. A short animated segments show cataract surgery while other animations are helpful and showing other enhancement procedures.

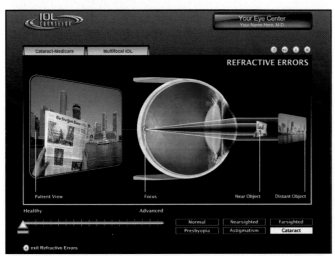

Figure 11. The counselor can explain refractive errors including astigmatism from the Refractive Errors animations.

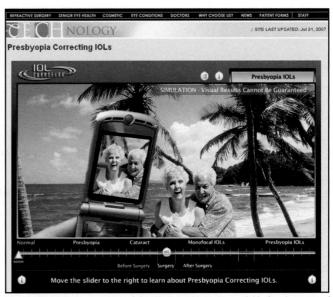

Figure 12. An Internet version of the IOL Counselor is also available for placement of individual Web sites.

nizes its value, it must decide the best way to incorporate it into its patient flow. In a recent survey of IOL Counselor users, 78% had a surgical counselor presenting it in a counseling room, while 7% of the presentations were being done by doctors in the exam room and 14% indicated both the doctor and the surgical counselor showed patients the program. Fifty-five percent showed it on a desktop computer and 30% used laptop computers, while 15% used a combination of laptop, tablet PC, and desktop computers. Seventy-nine percent showed the IOL Counselor only to patients whom the doctor wanted to see it, while 21% showed it to every cataract patient.

Thirty-seven percent of the responders indicated they used the IOL Counselor to train their staff with an additional 20% planning to train their staff in the future. Sixty-three percent indicated the IOL Counselor was very helpful in converting patients. The number one obstacle to getting started with the IOL Counselor was determining how to incorporate it into the existing patient flow.

In our beta practice sites, those doctors showing the IOL Counselor to patients in the exam room increased their con-

versions from 5% to 15%, while other beta sites that used surgical counselors after the doctor recommended a specific IOL increased their conversions from 15% to a high of 80%.

The IOL Counselor software is sold with a single-user license that can only be activated on one computer or with a multi-user license that can be activated on as many as 8 different computers within a practice. The program can be purchased from PEC directly, or while supplies last, CareCredit will provide CDs to their existing practices or any new practice willing to open an account with them.

There is also an IOL Counselor Web Tool available to install on individual practice Web sites (Figure 12), and PEC has introduced several alternative language versions for the international market. In addition to the 3 scenes on the initial version, additional scenes and ancillary IOL Counselor products can be purchased from their Web site at www.iolcounselor.com.

Success in increasing the percentage of patients converting to refractive IOLs at any practice depends on the degree to which both the surgeon and the staff form a collective mindset about performing refractive cataract surgery and how and when to counsel patients using the IOL Counselor. Hesitation or lack of enthusiasm or confidence on the part of any one staff member will induce doubt and skepticism in the patient and undermine all other efforts to grow the refractive cataract business. That is why role playing and educating the entire staff about the benefits and affordability of refractive IOLs are so important.

It has been speculated that if only 20% of cataract patients elect refractive IOLs by the year 2010, ophthalmology will own the number one (laser vision correction) and the number two (refractive IOLs) elective procedures in medicine. Almost all of our beta sites found the 20% conversion mark easy to achieve. 2010 should be an excellent year for all of us in the ophthalmic community.

CHAPTER 116

PATIENT EDUCATION— USING EYEMAGINATIONS

Michael Sopher

The focus of this chapter is to introduce cataract surgeons to a suite of products and how these products may help to improve the patient education process for presbyopia-correcting intraocular lens (IOL) surgery.

Patient Education

What do patients want to know? This question was asked by Eyemaginations (Towson, MD) almost 10 years ago—before the development of its 3D-Eye Office patient software system. Although it is not an easy question to answer, Eyemaginations found that most patients were concerned with answers to 4 very important questions:

1. What problem(s) will the doctor find?

2. What treatment options are available for the problem(s)?

3. What is the cost of treating the problem(s)?

4. Is there a correlation between the premium options and the surgical outcome?

Ask yourself as a cataract surgeon, how do you handle these questions in your clinic? What do you do to help your patients understand what they might be at risk of? How do you help them to understand the treatment options available? How do you help them to deal with the financial realities of costly treatment plans? How do you manage their expectations and make sure that they understand that each option has pros, cons, risks, and benefits? Importantly—how do we underscore that nothing happens in a vacuum and that many other factors beyond their optical system can impact the perceived outcome of the surgery? Such factors include, but are not limited to, their profession, personality, lifestyle, etc.

Patient education is the process used to help patients understand the answers to these questions. As mentioned at the outset, this chapter seeks to answer the question of how to improve the patient education process for presbyopia-correcting IOL surgery using the technologies developed by Eyemaginations.

Why Three-Dimensional Animation?

We experience the world in 3 dimensions so why educate patients in any other way. Written text and 2-dimensional images are less effective than 3-dimensional (3D) animation in improving a patients understanding of a subject. In fact, Dr. Michael Hermann from the University of Vienna published a study in 2002 proving this very point. His analysis focused on a prospective randomized study of 3D animations versus text in terms of both patient acceptance and assessment. The following is his conclusion from the study:

"Understanding of and subjective knowledge about the surgical procedure and possible complications, the degree of trust in professional treatment, the reduction in anxiety and readiness for the operation were significantly better after watching... computer animation than after reading...text."[1]

His study found that 3D animation was a new medium for supporting patient education before surgery (Figures 1 and 2). In 2006, a similar study was performed by Drs. Carl Glittenberg and Susanne Binder on the "advantages of interactive 3D computer animation technology in the demonstration of complex ophthalmological subjects." They found that ophthalmology students who were taught using 3D animation understood complex subject matter better than via conventional lecture text. "We conclude that 3D computer animation technology can significantly increase the quality and efficiency of the education and demonstration of complex topics in ophthalmology."[2]

Eyemaginations has built its business and reputation on providing cataract surgeons with educational and marketing tools using the highest quality 3D animation design. Our belief is that the most effective way to communicate refractive IOL surgery options is through 3D computer simulation.

There are other medical specialties (eg, dentistry, plastic surgery) that have relied on commercial forms of education and marketing. Dentistry and plastic surgery are examples of fields where television and other forms of media have offered

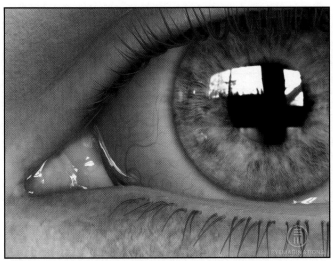

Figure 1. 3D images from Eyemaginations. (Courtesy of Eyemaginations.)

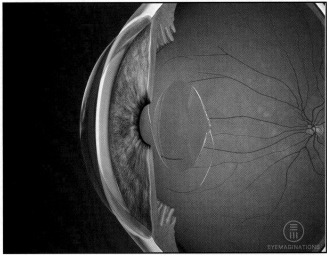

Figure 3. 3D image of the eye with cataract and the affect on vision. (Courtesy of Eyemaginations.)

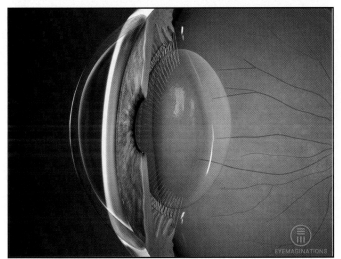

Figure 2. 3D images from Eyemaginations. (Courtesy of Eyemaginations.)

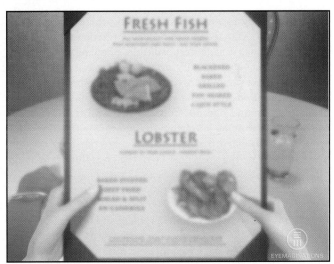

Figure 4. 3D image of the eye with cataract and the affect on vision. (Courtesy of Eyemaginations.)

a large variety of educational and explanatory modules. With eye care in general and cataracts in particular, there are not commercial and mainstream forms of education. Accordingly, a 3D animated software program represents a powerful tool to explain and educate.

The 3D-Eye Office Program

The 3D-Eye Office program enables a practice to preset a number of critical topics that the doctors and staff can access through the push of a single button. The technology enables the practice to customize the program and save the presentations to the "F" keys that reside at the top of any keyboard. Practices should consider having preset explanations on topics such as anatomy of the eye, refractive errors, cataracts, what the opacification or cloudiness may look like from a patient point of view, how a cataract can impact your lifestyle, phacoemulsification, and the various IOL options (Figures 3 and 4).

Patients who visit the reception area of the clinic should be presented with information that creates general awareness of various refractive procedures and products available. For example, having a loop running on toric IOLs or astigmatic keratotomy will help patients to understand new developments in the field of cataract surgery, and to be better prepared for their discussion with the physician. The idea is not necessarily to promote any product or specific procedure, but rather to introduce concepts, create awareness, and debunk the myths. When the information is delivered using 3D animation, patients are likely to find the subject matter more entertaining and easy to understand.

Some clinics will look to use DVD technology to play the 3D animation information in their reception area. However, DVD technology is considered "static" technology and does not allow the information to be readily updated, personalized and customized to each individual practice. This is only achievable using "dynamic" technology such as computer software. The 3D-Eye Office system will allow the clinic to achieve this dynamic approach in the reception area.

A visit to the examination room should allow the patients to receive animated information in a more personalized way from the physician. Animation software enables the physician

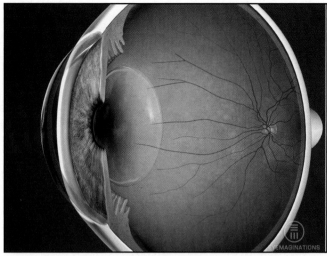

Figure 5. The aging lens. (Courtesy of Eyemaginations.)

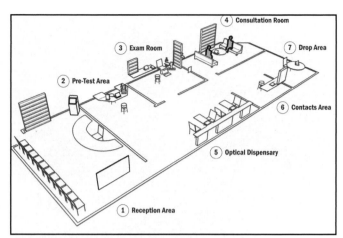

Figure 6. The virtual office. (Courtesy of Eyemaginations.)

to simulate progression of disease. Using the 3D-Eye Office "sketch mode" can reduce the video presentation time significantly as chair-time is very valuable. Showing how the lens hardens or loses its flexibility over time does not need to take more than a few seconds. For example, you can begin by rotating the head 90 degrees and explaining how the lens becomes presbyopic around age 40. You can draw on the image and explain how the aging lens begins to interfere with close vision around age 40 when the patient's arms are not long enough. You can simulate the opacification of the crystalline lens at age 60 explaining that the cataract begins to develop. This type of presentation should take the physician no more than 20 to 30 seconds (Figure 5).

Patients will see their specific problem and the treatment for the problem in a few seconds under the watchful eye of their attending physician. Having a presentation that is fast, effective, and efficient in its playback is almost as important as the content itself. In addition, 3D-Eye Office offers the doctor the capability of drawing on top of the moving animation, adding a "wow" factor to the presentation. Helping the doctor represent him- or herself in the best possible light makes the strongest impact on the patient during the education process.

Although chair-side consultation is always a great idea to optimize the patient education process, there is not always enough time to attend to each and every patient in this manner. For this reason, 3D-Eye Office offers the flexibility of running the animation in "video mode." Similar to a screensaver, patients can review information before or after the doctor leaves the room. This option is ideal for practices with multiple examination lanes.

The Importance of Managing Expectations

When the patient sits with a counselor in the consultation lane, animation becomes the vehicle to explain all the details of surgery, including risks associated with the procedure. Using 3D-Eye Office in the consultation lane will help patients to

understand the simplicity of cataract surgery and the risks versus benefits of different IOL options. For example, you can simulate the effects of a multifocal IOL by showing the patient the ability to have focus at both near and distance at the same time. You can segue to a simulation of a car driving at night to illustrate how postoperative glare can be one of the effects of the multifocal lens with the concentric ring technology. You can also show how the brain begins to compensate for this glare by demonstrating what neuroadaptation might achieve. Patients who need a deeper knowledge of refractive errors such as astigmatism can receive this information during the consultation session. When showing the premium lens options, it is important for the doctor or technician to indicate that spectacle independence is possible but not guaranteed.

Patient Administration Using Software Technology

Although we believe 3D animation to be the most powerful way for a cataract physician to express his or her ideas, concepts, and information, we have found that simply creating content alone is not sufficient for optimal patient education. Our findings show that the most successful refractive IOL practices present animation to their patients in a style similar to how data administration is performed.[3] Data administration is performed through the use of practice management software (PMS) and/or electronic medical record (EMR) technology. These systems require computer terminals in strategic areas of the clinic to ensure efficient data entry and information recall. In the best PMS/EMR models, information efficiently moves through the clinic along with the patient. This process allows for instantaneous electronic health record access. By using the same PC terminals or adding additional terminals, 3D animation can be made available to the patient as they are matriculated through the clinic. As patients move from room to room, they would observe different animations in different ways depending on where they are in their healthcare process. The office diagram in Figure 6 demonstrates areas in a clinic that are considered ideal for patient education.

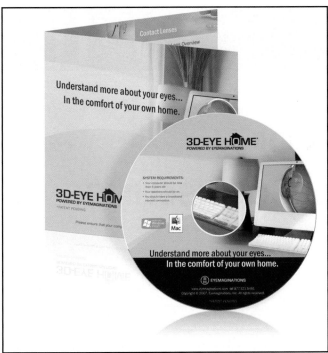

Figure 7. The new 3D-Eye Home platform. (Courtesy of Eyemaginations.)

3D-Eye Home

According to David F. Chang, MD, "…it is… far more efficient and effective to initiate presbyopia IOL education in advance of [the patients] office visit."[4]

With Eyemaginations' latest technology, 3D-Eye Home, patients can have education delivered to them prior to their visit or after leaving the practice. This technology allows the doctor to provide detailed information specific to the patient on topics such as cataracts, phacoemulsification, presbyopic IOL technology, and much more (Figure 7).

3D-Eye Counselor

With the assistance of David F. Chang, MD, and other prominent ophthalmic thought leaders, Eyemaginations will be developing a new presbyopia-correcting IOL counselor technology to compliment the practicing style of different surgeons. With customizable content, the doctor may select how neutral or promotional they want to be.

How to Learn More

Those who wish to learn more about Eyemaginations' products and services may contact Eyemaginations directly at 877-321-5481 or visit their Web site at www.eyemaginations.com.

References

1. Hermann M. 3-Dimensional computer animation—a new medium for supporting patient education before surgery. *Chirurgica.* 2002;73:500-507.
2. Binder S, Glittenberg C. Computer simulations in ophthalmic training. The College of Optometrists. *Ophthal Physiol Opt.* 2006;26:40-49.
3. According to Wikipedia, "data administration" is the administration of the organization of data, usually as stored in databases under some database management system or alternative systems such as electronic spreadsheets.
4. David F. Chang, personal communication.

CHAPTER 117

ETHICS OF REFRACTIVE IOL COUNSELING

Charles M. Zacks, MD

Since intraocular lenses (IOLs) were first introduced in the 1970s, we have witnessed a progression from rudimentary designs to a highly refined technology, guided by formal clinical research and individual surgeons' experience. Until recently, however, the entire evolution of IOLs was directed toward essentially the same goal—optimizing the monofocal implant. These lenses now deliver remarkable and predictable outcomes for the cataract patient, with a very low risk of complications. With the recent introduction of multifocal and accommodative IOLs, however, options for pseudophakic vision have expanded significantly, creating new challenges for the surgeon in recommending the appropriate lens design for a particular patient. Because of these new dimensions, detailed patient education, accurate clinical assessment, and truly informed consent are even more critical aspects to preoperative management. Some modifications and additions to our preoperative evaluation of cataract patients have therefore become necessary to maximize patient satisfaction with lens implant procedures, and to maximally respect the ethical principles that govern surgical care.

Cataract Surgery as Refractive Surgery

With improvements in technique and instrumentation, it is generally recognized that the risk/benefit profile for cataract surgery has improved substantially. Correspondingly, the criteria for diagnosis of cataract itself has evolved from a disabling disease for which any visual improvement was hailed as a success, toward earlier diagnosis based on lesser degrees of visual disability. This evolution has apparently lowered the threshold for considering cataract procedures compared to decades ago. Until recently, when only spherical monofocal IOLs were available, it was relatively easy to inform a cataract surgery patient about the nature of the expected pseudophakic vision. A patient's "options" for pseudophakia were generally limited to choice of the target refraction. With the advent of

aspheric, multifocal, and accommodative lenses, there are new options to discuss. With wider choices, a particular lens, with its attendant advantages and disadvantages, has greater potential to significantly affect the patient's satisfaction with the procedure. In this way, cataract surgery more closely resembles refractive surgery than ever before. These trends toward earlier surgery, and recent developments in lens designs, place additional responsibility on the surgeon to be certain that the individual patient is truly informed, that their expectations for outcomes are realistic, and that their exposure to surgical risk is appropriate to the anticipated benefit.

Preoperative Evaluation and the Process of Informed Consent

It is the responsibility of the ophthalmologist to act in the best interest of the patent.[1] Treatment should be recommended only after a careful consideration of the patient's physical and other associated needs,[2] and must be preceded by appropriate informed consent.[3] Given these ethical obligations, the informed consent process for cataract surgery actually begins with a discussion about whether it should be done at all, or whether further observation and non-surgical approaches could mitigate the patient's symptoms until the cataracts progress.[4] After this preliminary discussion of patient needs, if the patient concludes that surgery is appropriate, the discussion can then include available options for pseudophakic vision.

It is generally understood among surgeons offering multifocal and accommodative lenses that they must assess the lifestyle and occupational needs of the patient in greater detail than they did before the wider lens choice was available. Correspondingly, patient education about the new lens technology has required additional attention to discussion of the characteristics of individual lens designs. With more options, the informed consent discussion should not only include an assessment of a given patient's preference for attributes of available technologies, but also their anticipated tolerance of undesired visual phenomena intrinsic to each, such as halos, glare, and loss of contrast sensitivity.[5,6] Every optical system has inherent compromises that will affect lens choice, such that the desired attributes and the shortcomings of each lens option should be presented together. The less desirable optical characteristics of some lenses are best represented not as uncommon complications that could occur, but as potentially objectionable features of an otherwise technically normal procedure that will occur, but may be variably objectionable to individual patients. This emphasis offsets the patient's natural inclination to assume that if the surgery goes well, these adverse effects will not occur in their case. Although carefully selected staff could be entrusted to convey some of this information, this discussion may be sufficiently nuanced that the discussion is most effective when conducted between surgeon and patient and adjusted to the patient's responses, rather than delegated to others or by excessive reliance on printed materials and audio-visual presentations.

The use of accommodative and multifocal lenses has also required a change in discussion of the possibility of ancillary or additional surgery. Following successful conventional IOL surgery in a healthy eye, the need for additional procedures (with the exception of ytrrium-aluminum-garnet (YAG) laser capsulotomy) is generally very low. For multifocal and accommodative IOLs, however, successful surgical outcomes are much more likely to involve other procedures, including relaxing incisions for astigmatism, or corrections for residual refractive errors using laser refractive techniques. In both cases, the informed consent process must include a discussion of the likelihood that additional procedures will be needed, and their associated risks.

Although legal standards of informed consent vary with jurisdiction, the ethical imperative for any preoperative discussion is to provide sufficient information so that a reasonable patient may make well-informed decisions about treatment.[7] Especially for new technology lens surgery, preoperative assessment and informed consent are complex elements of this process. If this discussion is reduced inappropriately to an expedient effort to obtain a signature on a prepared form, these ethical obligations are not met and the stage is set for conflict after surgery—even after a technically "perfect" procedure.

Informed Consent and Discussion of Fees

Ethical billing for surgical services depends in large measure on preoperative disclosure of fees, including additional charges for noncovered devices and procedures,[8] the finances of comanagement arrangements,[9] and ideally some disclosure of covered or noncovered services that reasonably might be anticipated.

There is some divergence of opinion about how and when the additional "out of pocket" cost of accommodative and multifocal lenses should be disclosed. It might seem logical that when cost appears likely to be a barrier, the price should be disclosed "up front" to satisfy full disclosure before an extended discussion. However, it is also unethical to prejudge a patient's ability to pay additional fees based on subjective or incomplete information, and this argument omits the relationship of the patient's perception of cost to benefit ratio, which is the value of the premium device. Instead, the cost of the surgery should be considered as but one aspect of balancing the advantages and disadvantages of all medically reasonable options for the patient.

If postoperative comanagement is part of a fee arrangement with other practitioners, ethical care requires preoperative consent to have some aspects of care delegated, and disclosure of the financial relationship.[10] Documentation of patient consent for delegated services may also be a regulatory or legal requirement depending on the situation.

If additional procedures, either anticipated or unanticipated, are to be included or excluded in the surgical fee, the specifics should be disclosed. This might include intraoperative corneal relaxing incisions, or corneal refractive procedures that could become necessary postoperatively. In the event that the patient is unable to adapt to the multifocal optic, removal of the IOL may become necessary. The patient's discovery that this is not a covered service after the fact has been known to further anger a dissatisfied patient, causing misery for both the patient and surgeon.

Informed Consent and the Learning Curve

When a surgeon assimilates new technology into his or her practice, there is an inevitable learning curve that affects the outcomes of early cases. After completion of formal residency training, surgeons are largely responsible for their own education. Fortunately, the use of new technology IOLs requires incremental steps, rather than sweeping changes, but some technical aspects may be entirely new, such as enhanced biometry or astigmatic procedures. Ethical patient care requires that the surgeon become competent with new techniques, which can be gained with an incremental educational approach. This can range from instruction courses and didactic materials, to mentored surgery, with eventual assimilation of the new procedure. Because a reasonable patient will be interested to know if a surgeon has ever performed a given procedure before, it is ethically imperative to disclose aspects of one's early experience. This topic is discussed in detail in the Academy's Advisory Opinion "Learning New Techniques after Residency."[11]

Conflicts of Interest and Disclosure

The intrinsic conflict of interest arising from remuneration for physicians' services is nothing new. Traditions in professional ethics dating back to antiquity require that, despite the expectation of a fee for service, decisions are made in the best interest of the patient, and not the doctor. Today, an ophthalmologist's enthusiasm for using these new lenses, however well intended, should never interfere with one's clinical judgment that deferring surgery, or using a conventional monofocal

IOL, may be appropriate management for a particular patient despite less remuneration for the surgeon.[7]

Other, more specific conflicts of interest may arise when the surgeon is a consultant for a device manufacturer, or is conducting clinical research on outcomes of the proposed surgery. In the former case, full disclosure of the relationship with industry is mandatory,[12] and professional restraint may be required to put the patient's interests first and to avoid clouding judgment with other incentives.[13] In the latter case, the fact that a patient is participating in clinical research must be specifically disclosed.[14,15] In conducting research, the surgeon's desire to obtain data on outcomes for reasons of advancing one's academic or professional stature are also potential conflicts of interest that must be acknowledged, and managed with professional restraint.

Conclusion

Newer intraocular lens designs offer expanded options for patients, but also pose new challenges for the surgeon, both technically and professionally. Needless to say, the trends toward innovation and greater complexity in surgical care are expected to continue. Although these new technologies will place additional demands on us in the future, they will improve outcomes for the patient, and reward us for our expertise. In this environment we must continue to maintain competence in a rapidly changing field, and challenge ourselves to learn and offer new technology. In doing so, it is critical to remain objective in how we offer these new products to patients. No one can predict whether today's "miracle" will be superseded by new innovations, or if it will prove to be tomorrow's mistake.

As we offer the benefits of new technology to patients, failure to respect basic precepts of professional ethics will compromise the trust that patients have in us— namely, that we are working with their best interest in mind, rather than for ourselves or for industry. This trust will always be a better guarantor of our success than the short- term benefits of merely "selling" the newest device or procedure. At the very least, careful attention to ethical requirements reduces the risk of being confronted by disappointed patients, either in the exam room or the court room. More importantly, adherence to ethical principles distinguishes us as physicians, to the credit of the profession and the benefit of society.

References

1. The Academy's Code of Ethics, Principle 1, available at http://www.aao.org/about/ethics/code_ethics.cfm
2. Ibid., Rule 6.
3. Ibid., Rule 2.
4. Advisory Opinion: Unnecessary Surgery and Related Procedures, available at http://www.aao.org/about/ethics/upload/Unnecessary_Surgery_12.pdf
5. Restor manufacturer product information, available at http://www.acrysofrestor.com/cataract-surgery/iol-choices.asp
6. Rezoom manufacturer product information, available at http://www.rezoomiol.com/faqs.html
7. Advisory Opinion: Informed Consent, available at http://www.aao.org/about/ethics/informed_consent.cfm
8. Code of Ethics, Rule 9.
9. Advisory Opinion: Employment and Referral Relationships Between Ophthalmologists and Other Health Care Providers, available at http://www.aao.org/about/ethics/employment_referral.cfm
10. Advisory Opinion: Postoperative Care, available at http://www.aao.org/about/ethics/employment_referral.cfm
11. Advisory Opinion: Learning New Techniques Following Residency, available at http://www.aao.org/about/ethics/upload/Learning_New_Techniques_5-4-07.pdf
12. Advisory Opinion: Disclosures of Professionally Related Commercial Interests, available at http://www.aao.org/about/ethics/disclosure.cfm
13. Code of Ethics, Rule 11.
14. Code of Ethics, Rule 3.
15. Advisory Opinion: Clinical Trials and Investigative Procedures, available at http://www.aao.org/about/ethics/clinical.cfm

CHAPTER 118

ETHICS OF REFRACTIVE IOL COUNSELING

David F. Chang, MD

The availability of new presbyopia-correcting (Pr-C) intraocular lenses (IOLs), and the Centers for Medicaid & Medicare Services (CMS) ruling allowing patients to pay for them as noncovered refractive services, has dramatically altered the practice of every cataract and refractive surgeon. Ready or not, the availability of these options has made every cataract patient a potential refractive patient. Furthermore, presbyopic refractive patients who believed laser vision correction to be the only refractive procedure available now have entirely different surgical alternatives to consider. These myriad new options, and the premium remuneration that they command, create a number of ethical issues for ophthalmologists. In a profession where the IOL industry spends a great deal of money to market products to us, we have the challenge and the important responsibility to educate patients as objectively as possible.

Offering and explaining the option of reduced spectacle dependence would be far easier if we had an accommodating IOL that consistently and permanently provided 3 to 5 D of accommodation in every patient. The benefit would be easy to understand, and qualified candidates would decide what they wanted based upon the affordability of this option. Lacking such an elegant solution, we and our patients must analyze and understand the potential benefits and tradeoffs of current Pr-C IOLs, knowing that the results will vary from one individual to the next.

Patients consulting a plastic surgeon already understand that their interest in elective cosmetic surgery is not because of a health need or recommendation. This concept may not be clear, however, to patients hearing about Pr-C IOLs for the first time prior to scheduling cataract surgery. Already somewhat confused about cataracts and IOLs, many patients will not understand the distinction between what is the refractive treatment and what is the cataract treatment. They may not understand that the financial decision they are being asked to make concerns lifestyle benefits, such as convenience, rather than what is "best" for their eyes.

The nature of medical ethics is such that reasonable minds may have differing opinions and philosophies about a particular question. I am certainly not an expert. However, we probably all agree that the essence of ethical practice means treating our patients in the same way that we and our families would want to be treated in an identical situation. With that in mind, what are some common ethical issues that cataract and refractive surgeons now face with respect to refractive IOLs?

Should Every Patient Undergoing Cataract Surgery Be Informed of These Options?

I believe that most patients want to hear about all of their options prior to cataract surgery. Even if they are not a good multifocal IOL candidate, they would prefer to have the surgeon explain why, rather than to learn about this option later from a boastful friend. The question of "Why wasn't I told about this option?" may arise long after the patient was discharged from the surgeon's care. If left unanswered, this doubt may be a nagging source of disappointment and resentment. What if the surgeon does not offer these IOLs? If you are worried about the drawbacks of these implants, you can share your concerns with your patients. However, you should then be willing to refer that patient if, after your discussion, you determine that he or she is an excellent candidate who wants a Pr-C IOL.

Another issue might be one that I call "financial profiling." Based upon their attire or their home address, it is tempting to assume that certain individuals would not be able to afford a premium IOL. Such assumptions are often, but not always, accurate. I believe that patients would be disappointed to learn that certain options were not explained to them because it was assumed that they could not afford them. Instead, we should still explain the choices, but in a way that is sensitive to their needs and means.

What About New Technology in the Pipeline?

This is an important question, as we have all read about improved IOL technologies being developed for the future. I remember hearing a practice consultant in the early 1990s recommending that with the anticipated approval of the excimer laser and the ensuing competitive free-for-all, now was the time to establish one's reputation as a refractive surgeon by learning to perform radial keratotomy (RK). Was I the only one wondering how a patient would feel seeing all of the ads touting the new laser's advantages less than a year after he or she had had bilateral RK?

For cataract patients, the decision is often simple. Unless I felt that a better technology would be imminently available, I would want my own family member to enjoy the benefits of cataract surgery now rather than later. Some of our current refractive IOLs took between 10 to 12 years following initial human implantation to gain Food and Drug Administration (FDA) approval. Even after it was finally approved, it took widespread clinical use of the Allergan Array IOL (Irvine, CA) to truly understand its capabilities and limitations. Meanwhile, postponing cataract surgery that is otherwise functionally indicated may increase the risk of falls or traffic accidents.

Refractive lens exchange (RLE) patients are a different story. We all acknowledge that current refractive IOL technology is not perfect, and this is why we are reluctant to perform RLE for a presbyopic emmetrope. RLE is a legitimate option for hyperopes and higher myopes that are presbyopic. However, if I were myopic, I would want to be told about the uncertain but higher risk of retinal detachment in pseudophakes. I would also want to know whether there was a better technology on the foreseeable horizon worth waiting for. This might not influence a frustrated high hyperope who has become contact lens intolerant and increasingly presbyopic. On the other hand, consider a presbyopic myope who is reasonably happy with contact lenses but came in for a laser in situ keratomileusis (LASIK) consultation only to learn that this will not eliminate reading glasses. Although he or she may be a multifocal IOL-RLE candidate, this patient might prefer to wait for better IOL technology if this possibility was explained.

How Aggressively Should Our Practice Promote This Option to Patients?

Compared to radial keratotomy, LASIK is a great procedure. In appropriate candidates, there are very few risks and downsides, the benefit is stable, and the satisfaction rate is extremely high. Marketing not only spreads the word about this exciting procedure but can help to justify the significant cost by pointing out the benefits. In my opinion, Pr-C IOLs are not yet on par with laser vision correction in terms of patient satisfaction. Costs aside, there are inherent optical drawbacks with multifocal IOLs that must be counterbalanced by that patient's strong motivation to see without glasses. In a significant percentage of patients, the upside potential to multifocal IOLs outweighs the downside; in many other patients, it does not.

The manner by which patients are informed about these options is therefore very important. In most cataract practices, the majority of patients will still receive a monofocal IOL. Over-touting Pr-C IOLs through internal marketing may leave those who cannot have or afford them feeling shortchanged. It is also very easy for patients to misunderstand that the more expensive lens is "better" for their eyes. Could they afford to, most patients would pay extra for a technology that benefitted their ocular health—particularly if they perceive that the doctor favors it. "My eyes are important to me," we so often hear. Historically, this was the concern that CMS had with allowing surgeons to balance bill patients for noncovered services. Would some surgeons take advantage of elderly patients by selling them on costly upgrades that they did not need? It is important that patients who choose these premium technologies understand the real nature of the benefits.

Can I Maintain Objectivity Despite Strong Financial Incentives?

The higher the reimbursement, the more important this question becomes. As physicians, we have enormous power to influence elective decisions that our patients make. This is only true because patients trust us to make treatment recommendations without regard to which choice is more profitable to us. The tradition of implicit patient trust in this fundamental responsibility has been forged throughout the long course of modern medical history. Putting ourselves in our patient's shoes should guide each of us with respect to issues such as comanagement, specialist referrals, and recommendations for testing and procedures.

In the end, being constantly mindful of this sacred responsibility will provide us with good guidance. Patients can accept that you tried your best on their behalf, even if they are disappointed with their postoperative vision. However, by virtue of the high out-of-pocket premium that they paid, unhappy refractive IOL patients may look back and view what they perceive to have been promotion or sales pressure with suspicion. Your unhappiest refractive IOL patients will be those who are dissatisfied and believe that someone in your practice talked them into choosing the more expensive IOL.

Should Surgical Fees Be Billed to the Insurance Company?

For insurance purposes, if the decision to have lens replacement surgery is because of visually significant cataract symptoms, then it should be billed as cataract surgery. On the other hand, if the patient's primary motivation for surgery is the correction of refractive error, then it should be billed as a refractive lens exchange, which is not medically necessary. Insurance companies rely upon the surgeon to ethically make this distinction. The reason why the operation is or is not covered by insurance should also be explained to the patient. This decision is similar to other elective surgeries, such as for ptosis in which the functional indications must be distinguished from the cosmetic motivation.

What Is a Fair Price for a Noncovered Service?

Are patients being gouged by current prices? Unlike prescription medications and gasoline, refractive surgery and refractive IOLs are luxury items. I believe that as long as patients understand the optional and elective nature of this service, then they can ultimately judge the value of the service and whether the cost is fair. I certainly do not profess to know what the correct premium charge should be. I do know what it should be based upon, and additional surgical time is not the deciding factor. I charge for elective astigmatic keratotomy because many years of surgical experience with thousands of cases have made me very skilled at knowing when and how to correct astigmatism at the time of cataract surgery. The primary determinant of the charge is not the additional operative time. Refractive IOL surgery undeniably raises the bar, both in terms of patient expectations and necessary surgical precision. Offering these IOLs requires an entirely different level of preoperative evaluation, counseling, and education. The necessary commitment to excellence is not insignificant. I do not believe that the value of the professional component of reducing spectacle dependence should be calculated based on the additional surgical time or preoperative testing necessary to implant these IOLs. As a patient, it is what lies in between the surgeon's 2 ears that matters most to me—knowledge, experience, preparation, clinical judgment, compassion, and the ethical commitment to do what is best for me.

CHAPTER 119

ETHICS OF
REFRACTIVE IOL COUNSELING

Lisa Brothers Arbisser, MD

"Do unto others as you would have done to yourself" expresses the distillation of ethical patient care. The challenge of having the wisdom to glean what is best for another, let alone oneself, further complicates our task. I do not claim to provide answers but rather offer my reflections on the subject of integrating premium intraocular lenses into our ethical practice of ophthalmology. Most of us are comfortable with charging what the market will bear for laser in situ keratomileusis (LASIK) but let us consider the unique position of the cataract patient as opposed to the refractive patient. I believe the ethics are very different as the former has no alternative to surgery in order to function in his or her daily activities whereas the latter is electively choosing an alternative to glasses or contacts. The cataract patient cannot wait to save up money over time or wait for better technology development without compromising his or her lifestyle in the interim. He or she looks to us, his or her physicians, for honest counsel. Do we offer only the tried and true despite its significant limitations to restoring the function of a 70-year-old eye when we have the opportunity to mimic a 40-year-old one? Do we encourage the choice of the premium lenses despite their risks and cost? Can we avoid bias? We must strive to.

This is the first time in my career that I have been unable to offer all my patients the same access to technology based on their needs and wants alone. Decisions must now also be based on what they can afford. This makes me uncomfortable. I have often heard the argument that not everyone in our society is entitled to drive a Cadillac; some will drive a Yugo. Because we accept this as fair and just, the analogy does not hold with implants. Why? Because the Yugo owner can always hope to improve his situation in the future while the cataract patient will, for all practical purposes, never be able to upgrade his or her implant without major risk. I think it is very important to avoid the tendency to give a pejorative connotation to the use of a standard implant that is subtly implied by the jargon or rhetoric sometimes used to promote premium lenses. I make it clear to patients that there is no inferior or superior choice. There are potential benefits and risks to every choice. I learned to use the word *convenience* from David Chang when describing the benefits of independence from glasses. To "sell up" to someone who is comfortable wearing glasses is not my goal. Neither do I want to disappoint a patient who would prefer to be independent of them but cannot afford the premium lens. I always offer blended vision to mimic the advantages of the premium lens as one of the alternatives and stress the low-risk nature of this choice.

Part of the dilemma is that today's technology is not flawless. Most patients are thrilled with their outcomes. Unfortunately neuroadaptation to the noise of multifocal simultaneous vision is so variable and hard to predict we actually cause some people harm. We need to be very candid and detailed about the challenges involved and, in the end, the patient must evaluate whether they believe they are adaptable. Decreased contrast means that these lenses are virtually contraindicated for patients lacking a normal visual system. We must ruthlessly exclude inappropriate or borderline patients. Accommodative technology is still in its infancy and is variable in its ability to deliver true spectacle independence. The current silicone implants remain inappropriate in eyes at significant risk for retinal detachment. The toric lens is nearly a "free lunch"; however, there is the potential to create an uncomfortable new meridian of astigmatism that may result in the need for a second surgery unique to this technology.

The privilege to charge out of pocket in a world where previously all choices were covered by third-party payers is a significant paradigm shift for ophthalmology and, indeed, for medicine in the United States. In principle I do believe that we as a society cannot afford to pay for everything. If we did we would lack the ability to cover the necessities. Psychologically the entitlement attitude that patients have adopted is deleterious to our recognition of the value of what we receive. It is also necessary that there be a stream of income that is not legislated by fiat to maintain the health and quality of medical practice. We cannot afford to live in a socialist environment on the income side when expenses are determined by capitalist market forces. I am grateful to the ophthalmic industry for this new opportunity, and I am glad that in this respect our incentives align.

If we are to adopt this technology, the financial gain goes hand in hand with the need to commit to excellence. These lenses are not forgiving, demand attention to minute detail, and sometimes require further intervention. Today more than ever the bottom line for most practices is sufficiently slim that investment in new technology and in time for training and advancement is limited. We, however, are ethically obliged to diligently progress through a learning curve when adopting new techniques and technology to avoid exposing the patient to unnecessary risk. It is not enough to be a good surgical technician. It is essential to critically assess the literature to know what we are comfortable to adopt and when. We must partner with industry but not allow ourselves to be pressured by it against our better judgment.

Being the patient's advocate means being a communicator. This skill has never been more in demand now that we have such a rich panoply of choices to offer our patients. Full disclosure of significant options to all patients regardless of their apparent ability to pay and regardless of the surgeon's willingness to adopt the various technologies is becoming a medical–legal as well as an ethical imperative. The value of informed consent is closely related to the values of autonomy and truth telling and the concept that an uninformed agent is at risk of mistakenly making a choice not reflective of his or her values. If we do not choose to implement these changes in our own practice, we must be willing to refer patients to those who have. Our Hippocratic oath states that "I will not be ashamed to say "I know not," nor will I fail to call in my colleagues when the skills of another are needed for a patient's recovery."

All this said, I have enjoyed being challenged and delight in this new dimension in the quality of life that I can offer patients as well as the opportunity to improve my productivity. I have embraced refractive cataract surgery for years working with blended vision, astigmatic keratotomy, and multifocals since their Food and Drug Administration approval. I waited until the latest iterations to adopt toric implants and accommodative lenses. About 30% of my surgery is done with premium implants at the time of this writing. This has required that I strive always to perfect my techniques, upgrade my equipment and my technical staff, and stay on top of an ongoing learning curve. I invest far more chair time than before, and I still seek strategies to delegate and improve my efficiency while keeping the good of the patient as the highest priority.

Incredibly, Maimonides' oath from centuries ago is apropos to our current situation: "The eternal providence has appointed me to watch over the life and health of Thy creatures. May the love for my art actuate me at all times; may neither avarice nor miserliness, nor thirst for glory or for a great reputation engage my mind; for the enemies of truth and philanthropy could easily deceive me and make me forgetful of my lofty aim of doing good to Thy children."

CHAPTER 120

RISK MANAGEMENT AND INFORMED CONSENT

Richard L. Abbott, MD

A number of new intraocular lenses (IOLs) have been introduced into the US ophthalmology market over the past several years with technological features described as accommodating, apodized diffractive, or presbyopia correcting. These lenses correct for all ranges of vision—near, intermediate, and distance. The new IOL options for correcting both near and distant vision via cataract or refractive lens exchange surgery raise important risk management and informed consent issues for the ophthalmologist.

Informed Consent

The distinction between a refractive and cataract surgeon has become blurred with the advent of these new lenses. Every patient requiring cataract surgery is now a potential refractive surgery patient. Furthermore, cataract surgeons are ethically obligated to inform their cataract patients about the pros and cons of these new lenses, including what patients can and cannot expect from them in terms of postoperative vision, and other options that may be available. Patients must be informed that they will not have clear uncorrected vision at all distances with these lenses. This translates into more one-on-one counseling of patients, requiring significantly more "chair" time than with the more routine cataract patients of the past.

There are several principles of informed consent for patients seeking refractive IOLs that are similar to the principles recommended for patients undergoing elective refractive surgery. Most importantly, these lenses may not be appropriate for patients with unrealistic personal expectations or strict professional visual acuity requirements (ie, commercial airline pilots) as even the most accurate biometry and uncomplicated surgery in the hands of the most experienced surgeon may not guarantee a perfect visual outcome. Since multifocal lens surgery typically costs the patient more out-of-pocket money, such inflexible expectations can lead to dissatisfaction and ultimately litigation in the event of a suboptimal visual outcome. Certainly more questions need to be asked of and by

the patient, as the informed consent process does not simply consist of signing a preprinted standardized consent form. Adequate information has to be provided to the patient, ideally well in advance of surgery, with the opportunity to be able to ask questions of the surgeon face to face.

The whole process of informed consent for refractive lens exchange surgery should be similar to that of a refractive surgeon performing laser in situ keratomileusis (LASIK). Many ophthalmologists do not realize that if they are performing a refractive lens exchange in a younger patient or offering an older cataractous patient a multifocal or accommodating IOL, the patient's expectations are high for both excellent near and distant vision. In addition, multifocal IOLs are not typically covered by health insurance if there is no cataract present, so patients are paying out of pocket for the benefits of the lenses and have come to expect near perfection in the surgical outcome.

Risk Management

The following risk management recommendations are intended to promote the patient's safety and reduce liability exposure when performing cataract or refractive lens exchange surgery.

PREOPERATIVE COUNSELING OF PATIENTS

It is important to discuss with patients what it means for an IOL to be Food and Drug Administration (FDA) approved and how it is intended to be used. If the lens was recently approved, surgeons need to inform patients about the lack of long-term outcomes and experience with the lens and advise them that unanticipated problems may possibly occur. Surgeons should advise patients that refractive lens exchange procedures are considered off-label and a full explanation of what "off-label" means should be discussed with the patient. This discussion should be documented in the patient's medical record.

The informed consent should include a detailed description of alternatives to refractive lens exchange. A dialogue with patients about presbyopia and the options for near and/or distance vision correction should occur. Patients should not feel they are under any pressure to choose one option over another. Furthermore, patients appreciate the additional explanation regarding the rationale for your recommendation. Options that patients should be made aware of include monofocal IOLs, reading glasses, monovision, and multifocal IOLs.

Disclose and document the option of monovision, and demonstrate what a patient's postoperative vision may be like using a contact lens or glasses. If the patient refuses a short-term trial of monovision, document this in the medical record. If the patient agrees to pursue monovision, explain the possible difficulties with depth perception. This is the value of having the patient wear a contact lens in one eye for a short period of time to simulate the monovision condition. Although popular with many patients, there are others who simply cannot tolerate monovision.

One should explain that the goal with multifocal IOLs is to reduce the patient's dependency on glasses or contact lenses for both distance and near vision but that there is no guarantee that this goal can be fully achieved. The objective of a multifocal IOL is to restore some or all of the near (and intermediate, depending upon the IOL) focusing ability, but other factors may affect postoperative outcomes (eg, IOL power, IOL position, wound healing, functioning of the ciliary muscle).

Side effects associated with multifocal IOLs may include less sharp vision, worse vision in dim light, halos around lights, decreased contrast sensitivity, and difficulty driving at night. Patients need to be informed of all these possibilities. Furthermore, one must explain that if an intraoperative complication occurs, a monofocal IOL may have to be implanted instead of the scheduled multifocal lens.

Patients also need to know whether LASIK and/or photorefractive keratectomy (PRK) are available in the same office if additional correction is required following refractive lens exchange. If the surgery center does not offer these procedures, the surgeon should be ready to provide the patient with a list of refractive surgeons in the area. Also, patients must be told whether refractive surgery, spectacles, or other forms of correction, if required, are included in the global fee for the cataract surgery with a multifocal IOL.

Another important clinical issue to discuss is the risks of retinal detachment in high myopes. There is a greater risk for retinal detachment, especially in a younger patient with high myopia undergoing a clear lens extraction or a refractive lens exchange. The peripheral retina should be examined very carefully, and if the surgeon is not comfortable in doing scleral depression of the peripheral retina, these patients should be referred to a retinal specialist for a careful examination preoperatively.

During the informed consent process, verbally emphasize to patients that they may not achieve a specific postoperative visual acuity with refractive lens exchange. The selection of a proper implant for a specific patient is based upon sophisticated equipment and a computer formulae, but it is not an exact science. Let patients know that eyeglasses, refractive surgery, or repositioning or replacement of the IOL may be required if a postoperative refractive result is considerably different than planned. Discussion of the costs related to these procedures should also be clearly explained both verbally and in writing so that there is no misunderstanding if these are required.

Sometimes during surgery, the refractive lens chosen for insertion cannot be placed due to unexpected intraoperative complications. This risk needs to be discussed prior to surgery, especially in those patients at increased risk for such complications (eg, diabetics). Document in the patient's medical record that this topic was addressed during preoperative counseling.

PAY ATTENTION TO YOUR STAFF

Oftentimes, the staff will screen or spend more time with a patient than the surgeon. If the staff reports that a patient is acting inappropriately, this should convey an important message to the surgeon. The true colors of a patient often are displayed in front of the staff and are not obvious to the physician when he or she first meets the patient. If anything should go wrong in surgery, these "hidden" personality traits frequently manifest themselves and one is left dealing with a very difficult and sometimes unreasonable patient. It is recommended to pay close attention to one's staff and their insights and avoid operating on these patients if at all possible.

IDENTIFY INAPPROPRIATE PATIENTS FOR MULTIFOCALS

Communicate to patients that although surgery may eliminate a cataract, and/or refractive error and presbyopia, it will not correct any potentially sight-threatening condition of the eye (ie, peripheral retinal degeneration) that may be found in a high myope. Furthermore, the surgery cannot guarantee to make a patient happy, more popular, or improve his or her life if he or she is inherently unhappy. It is true that satisfaction with a successful postoperative outcome can result in short-term happiness, but it will often not cure longstanding issues of depression or dissatisfaction in one's life situation.

It is strongly recommended to use a questionnaire to identify inappropriate patients. Talk to patients about their responses and ask them what they expect to obtain while assessing their emotional stability and reasonableness. Some patients to look out for are those on antidepressant medications. Others are engineers, pilots, doctors, and lawyers because of their high and often unrealistic expectations. Other poor candidates for multifocal IOLs are those who drive long distances at night and/or perform detailed work that requires closer focus than just reading. Often, a monofocal IOL with reading glasses may be a better option for these patients.

FINANCIAL IMPLICATIONS

Patients

For refractive lens exchange, the beneficiary is responsible for the charge that exceeds that of a conventional IOL. Patients should be given the Notice of Exclusion from Medicare Benefits[1] and should know that the Centers for Medicare & Medicaid Services (CMS) will only pay for one pair of glasses or contact lenses if needed after the implantation of a presbyopia-correcting IOL. If the lens needs to be removed due to medical complications, CMS will cover the insertion of a conventional IOL as a replacement. Also, make it known that private insurance may or may not pay for a multifocal IOL.

Insurance generally does not cover costs of a refractive lens exchange (RLE) procedure.

Surgeons

The American Academy of Ophthalmology (AAO) Code of Ethics advises surgeons against providing inducements that could encourage the use of services. An example would be offering incentives such as free rides to and from the surgery center.

Implanting refractive IOLs as an elective procedure for patients will demand more of one's time due to the informed consent process and may impact the total number of patients seen in one's practice. This may require more staff, the use of audio/visual aids, and possibly the need to conduct evening seminars where an exchange of information outside of patient hours can take place.

ADVERTISING

Marketing and advertising include any promotional or informational activity used by an ophthalmic practice. With the addition of intraocular refractive surgery as a surgical alternative to vision correction with laser, spectacles, or contact lenses, marketing efforts have increased as ophthalmic surgeons promote their new services. While advertising by physicians remains an acceptable way to market one's practice, it is required by the Federal Trade Commission, many state laws, and the AAO Code of Ethics that all material must not be false or deceptive in the way it is presented to the public. Even advertising that states true facts, but conveys a misleading impression to reasonable consumers may be considered illegal. Ophthalmologists must be able to substantiate all claims made in their advertising. From a risk management perspective, any deviation from appropriate marketing and advertising principles could weaken the defensibility of a claim or lawsuit since

this information is often considered to be part of the initial informed consent process.

Conclusion

The risk management recommendations discussed in this chapter highlight the actions ophthalmologists can take to reduce the likelihood of a legal claim or suit. Cataract surgery is the most frequently performed ophthalmic procedure in the United States and the source of the majority of medical malpractice claims reported to Ophthalmic Mutual Insurance Company (OMIC). The addition of multifocal IOLs and the refractive lens exchange procedure has raised the bar for potential increased medicolegal risk for the surgeon and requires careful attention to the informed consent process. A comprehensive informed consent process, as well as careful chart documentation helps to protect the surgeon against unforeseeable risks.

A sample informed consent form containing the minimum information that the surgeon should personally disclose to the patient has been developed by OMIC and is available for anyone to use by accessing the OMIC Web site at www.omic. com.[2]

References

1. Centers for Medicare & Medicaid Services. Notice of Exclusion from Medicare Benefits. http://www.cms.hhs.gov. Accessed January 15, 2007.
2. Ophthalmic Mutual Insurance Company. Informed consent for refractive lens exchange (RLE) for the correction of hyperopia (farsightedness) or myopia (nearsightedness). http://www.omic.com/resources/risk_man/forms.cfm. Accessed October 3, 2007.

CHAPTER 121

RISK MANAGEMENT AND INFORMED CONSENT

James J. Salz, MD

This chapter is a revision of an article originally published in the October 2006 issue of *Refractive Eyecare* titled "Informed consent for intraocular refractive surgery" and is published with permission.

The risk/benefit ratio for a presbyopia-correcting intraocular lens (Pr-C IOL) as part of a cataract operation is similar to the risks of a standard monofocal implant. Potential complications such as endophthalmitis, cystoid macular edema (CME), retinal detachment, implant malposition, and improper implant power are possible with any IOL surgery. The unique additional complications of a Pr-C IOL may be considered expected side effects related to the design of the implant itself and include increased risk of halos, glare, ghost images (usually more noticeable at night), and "waxy" vision that may result in loss of best spectacle-corrected vision not related to eye pathology such as CME. Although it is true that most patients eventually adapt to the night halos and glare, some do not and in rare cases the only solution may be explantation of the IOL. A thorough discussion of these side effects with estimates of their frequency with the particular implant selected for the patient should be covered both orally and with an addendum to the written informed consent.

The informed consent process in patients who are considering refractive lensectomy simply to eliminate their need for glasses presents a very different risk/benefit ratio compared to traditional cataract surgery. Because intraocular refractive surgery can be thought of as a surgical alternative to extraocular laser vision correction (laser in situ keratomileusis [LASIK] or photorefractive keratectomy [PRK]) or nonsurgical correction with glasses or contact lenses, the risk to both surgeon and patient is high. This makes the informed consent process particularly important in these cases.

Although there is a tendency to think of "informed consent" as the general surgical informed consent document and any procedure-specific addenda that the patient signs once a decision to proceed with surgery has been made, these are but links in the chain of events that constitute the informed consent process.

Informed Consent Starts Before You See the Patient

The informed consent process begins with a prospective patient's first contact with a surgeon's office. That initial contact could include information relayed by a technician during the patient screening process, a glowing description of the doctor's surgical skills by a receptionist, or claims made on a Web site or in advertising. If the practice Web site says that 99% of Dr. Smith's cataract patients no longer require glasses after Pr-C IOLs, that information is part of Dr. Smith's informed consent process.

Regardless of what is written in the signed informed consent documents or what is said during the patient's evaluation, an advertising claim such a "99% no longer require glasses" can lead patients to assume that they too will achieve that outcome. Thus, it is vital that any outcomes claims are both true and documented.

It is important to realize that all of the materials and activities that make up one's marketing effort such as seminars, brochures, advertising, etc constitute a critical component of informed consent. If a complication arises and a lawsuit ensues, any of these marketing claims can be introduced in court.

The Value of Informed Consent Documents

While some might suggest that the signed informed consent documents carry more weight than these other modes of sharing information, I disagree. To appreciate how much credence patients put into the informed consent documents, think about how often you have signed documents full of legalese that have been handed to you in the midst of complex transaction, such a buying a car. Do you read every word? Do you ask multiple clarifying questions and get written answers? Most people consider such documents merely a formality and give them only a cursory review.

While oral communication between physician and patient may eclipse the informed consent documents, the forms are by no means superfluous, and their value can be increased. We provide our patients with the informed consent forms on the day of their consultation, so that they can take them home, review the information, call with questions, and return with a signed form on the day of surgery. There is nothing worse than having the patient sign the informed consent on the day of the surgery. Sitting in the doctor's office with staff rushing to get the patient ready for surgery can be considered a coercive setting. If the patient can reasonably claim to have signed under pressure, the value of the document is compromised.

The protection such a document offers the practice plummets once a patient has been given a sedative. The same is true if the patient has been dilated and cannot read easily. On the other hand, if the patient has been given adequate time to review the document in a relaxed setting away from the physician's office, a judge or jury could reasonably infer that the patient made an informed decision of his or her own free will.

While there is no sure way to know whether a patient truly understands what he or she is agreeing to, one way to improve the odds is to use plain language. For instance, describing swelling of the center of your retina that can cause distorted reading and distance vision is far more meaningful than listing CME.

The Risk/Benefit Ratio and Refractive Lensectomy

Justifying a procedure based on a reasonable risk/benefit ratio is a key element of the informed consent process. If a complication arises and the informed consent is called into question, the physician must be able to justify the risk taken by the patient in relationship to the desired outcome.

There are numerous additional risks inherent in refractive lenticular surgery over and above the inherent risks of cataract surgery. For instance, in clear lens exchange the patient assumes all of the risk of cataract surgery without the same potential benefits as a patient with a cataract. That is, if the refractive IOL candidate were to decide against surgery, he or she could still see well with glasses or contact lenses. By contrast, a cataract patient would experience continued vision loss and eventual blindness without surgery. The surgical benefit for the clear lens exchange patient is a preferred mode of vision correction; the benefit for the cataract patient is prevention of blindness.

In fact, because of this skewed risk/benefit ratio, I personally will not implant a refractive IOL in a patient just to correct presbyopia in an emmetropic patient. This is also an Ophthalmic Mutual Insurance Company (OMIC) requirement for coverage for refractive lensectomy (Appendix H). The patient has to, at the very least, have a refractive error and not be a good candidate for corneal refractive surgery. Otherwise the degree of benefit is too small to expose the patient to the risks of intraocular surgery, which include endophthalmitis, CME, and retinal detachment. An emmetropic patient should not bear the risk of losing an eye simply to eliminate having to wear a $10 pair of glasses for reading.

On the other hand, consider a high hyperope. The patient cannot see well at either distance or near without glasses or contact lenses, and LASIK has traditionally been a poor solution for high hyperopia. In this case, refractive lens exchange may offer enough benefit to justify the risk. The same is true of a patient with early signs of cataract.

Multifocal and Accommodating IOLs

The availability of multifocal or accommodating IOLs further complicates the informed consent process. Patients have to understand that there is a possibility that they will not have clear uncorrected vision at all distances with these lenses. They may well require glasses for specific tasks such as reading very small print or looking at a computer monitor. None of us can guarantee that we will nail the biometry and get the power exactly right every time. Patients need to understand this clearly, and they need to be informed of their options should they be dissatisfied with their uncorrected vision. These options include IOL explantation, glasses, contact lenses, or laser refractive surgery to correct residual refractive errors. They also need to have been clearly informed of the additional costs if they opt to have their outcome enhanced with LASIK for example.

I recently had a patient come to me looking for a second opinion after having had a Pr-C IOL implanted. It turned out that he had not been clearly informed that this particular implant required that reading material be held at 14 inches for clear focus rather than at 18 inches, which is what he was used to. Patients cannot be expected to know this in advance, nor are they likely to be capable of intuitively figuring it out. It is critical that the informed consent process include device nuances such as this.

Astigmatism

A similar situation occurs when the patient is an astigmat. Astigmatism in a pseudophakic patient can mean that the patient will have to wear glasses after surgery or have the astigmatism corrected by surgical means such as limbal relaxing incisions (LRIs) or LASIK. A diopter of astigmatism in the cataract patient with a monofocal IOL might not be terribly significant (and it is correctable), but it can be the difference between perceived success and failure in the multifocal IOL patient because he or she expected nearly perfect vision without glasses.

Patients need to understand that 1 D of astigmatism is the equivalent of blurry vision and that it has to be corrected with either LRIs at the time of surgery or with glasses or laser surgery postoperatively. I also review the monovision option with patients preoperatively because I still think monovision is a perfectly reasonable alternative to multifocal IOLs.

Specific Risks

Providing patients with as much information as possible in both verbal and written form is the best defense against a patient's claim of being uninformed or underinformed. If this belt-and-suspenders approach seems like information overload, it is possible to streamline the approach. However, for each refractive lenticular procedure there are certain things that absolutely must be addressed in the informed consent process. For instance, the risk of a retinal detachment must be emphasized when performing clear lensectomy in a highly myopic eye.

Patient selection is also important. Because of the very different risk/benefit ratios, performing clear lens extraction on a 45-year-old emmetrope creates far more risk for the surgeon than operating on a high myope with early cataracts. That being said, I still would not perform clear lens exchange on a 30-year-old who is –14 D, because I think the increased risk of a retinal detachment over that patient's lifetime is unacceptably high. I would inform the patient of this.

The issue that needs to be emphasized with multifocal IOLs is the increased risk of night vision problems. Clouding of the capsule is a common complication that must be mentioned in the informed consent process as well. For all intraocular procedures, patients should be aware of the risk of CME, retinal detachment, and infection. It is equally important to make sure the patients are aware of unusual risks. For instance, before implanting a Pr-C IOL, the patient should be told that if during surgery the anterior capsulorrhexis extends and the capsule breaks, a different type of IOL will have to be used. This is typically a sulcus-supported monofocal lens, so the patient will not get the benefit of the Pr-C IOL. Patients need to be told ahead of time that even though this complication is unusual, should it happen they will have a standard implant and they will have to wear glasses.

Documentation

The importance of documentation to the informed consent process cannot be overstated. If a patient experiences a serious complication and a lawsuit results and goes to trial, a jury tends to believe the plaintiff unless the possibility of that complication had been discussed and that discussion was clearly documented in the patient's chart.

Any off-label usage, such as wavefront surgery for PRK (wavefront is so far only approved for LASIK), needs to be spelled out clearly in the informed consent. The use of wavefront software in PRK may be considered the standard of care. However, if a patient gets a poor result and says that he or she was not told that the wavefront was not approved for his or her surgery, there may then be an issue. The attorney could argue that the patient had not been properly informed because that seemingly innocuous piece of information was missing.

The Bottom Line

With respect to refractive intraocular surgery, as long as the patient is willing to accept the risks of an intraocular procedure (ie, endophthalmitis, CME, and retinal detachment), the risk/benefit ratio of the specific procedure is favorable, all of these risks have been disclosed to patient, and that disclosure has been documented, then the informed consent process should be considered sound.

Download Ophthalmic Mutual Insurance Company Consent Forms From the Web Site

The OMIC Informed Consent for Refractive Lensectomy is included in Appendix H and can also be downloaded along with the cataract consent form and modified even by non-OMIC insureds. To download a copy in Word format, go to www.omic.com. Click on Informed Consent Documents on the home page, then scroll down to the cataract consent form or click on Refractive Surgery Consent Forms and scroll down to Refractive Lens Exchange Consent Form.

INFORMED CONSENT

Dos
- Realize that informed consent is an educational process rather than a legal document.
- Know that advertising and Web site information are part of the process.
- Make patients aware of the risk/benefit ratio.
- Discuss alternative treatment options.
- Be truthful about your outcomes.
- Be able to back-up your outcomes claims.
- Document everything that is discussed with the patient.

Don'ts
- Assume that the patient understands.
- Think you are covered because the patient signed a form.
- Have the patient sign on the day of surgery (or after taking a sedative or while dilated).
- Use a drug/device off label without telling the patient.
- Implant a Pr-C IOL without stressing the unique side effects such as increased glare, halos, ghost images, and near focusing distance that are uncommon issues with monofocal implants.

POTENTIAL COMPLICATIONS OF WHICH PATIENTS MUST BE INFORMED

- Poor vision, total loss of vision, or loss of eye
- Bleeding in eye
- Loss of corneal clarity
- Chronic inflammation
- Infection
- Temporary or permanent blurring of vision because of retinal swelling
- Detachment of the retina
- Glaucoma
- Double vision
- Night vision problems, glare, halos, ghost images
- Best focusing distance, reading or intermediate

SECTION VIII

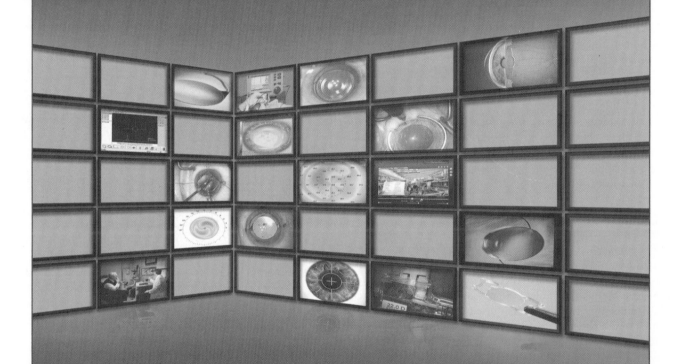

Presbyopia-Correcting IOL Selection

CHAPTER 122

WHY OFFER MULTIPLE PREMIUM IOLs?

David F. Chang, MD

The goal of having a sufficiently powerful accommodating intraocular lens (IOL) continues to elude us.[1] Compared to multifocal IOLs, the optical quality of such a lens would not be compromised by night time haloes or reduced contrast sensitivity.[2] Patients could dynamically shift their focus along a continuous range of distances from far to intermediate to near. With no major drawbacks, the choice of IOL would simply depend on the patient's desire and willingness to pay for this technology.

Despite significant improvements in current designs, multifocal IOLs will always fall short of these lofty goals. Image splitting designs require an inherent compromise in both optical quality and pseudoaccommodative performance. Because of these necessary tradeoffs, proper patient selection is especially critical.

The optical differences in the design of current diffractive multifocal IOLs and refractive multifocal IOLs should be well understood by all refractive IOL surgeons.[3] Eyes with high or irregular astigmatism, with maculopathy or reduced vision potential, and with zonular problems predisposing to IOL decentration are poor candidates. However, assuming that an interested patient is a good multifocal candidate, each design has different pros and cons. It is the job of the ophthalmologist to determine the best match for each individual patient.

ReZoom

The central distance-only zone of the ReZoom (Advanced Medical Optics, Santa Ana, CA) makes this multifocal "distance-dominant" with normal pupil sizes.[3] This means that uncorrected reading vision is poor through small pupils, and patients may read better if ambient light is reduced enough to avoid miosis. Halos, although less severe than with the Array (Advanced Medical Optics), are still quite noticeable to patients whenever the pupil dilates widely, such as in younger patients at night. ReZoom has a lower effective near add (+2.6 D) than ReSTOR (Alcon, Fort Worth, TX) (+3.2 D). In addition, the blending of ReZoom's refractive zones creates a progressive add, which devotes some focus to intermediate distances. However, having more light emanating from distance and intermediate points reduces the near vision performance of ReZoom, compared to ReSTOR.

The zonal refractive design seems to make this technology slightly more forgiving of being +0.5 D hyperopic or myopic. Distance contrast sensitivity should be superior to that with ReSTOR, because the central 2-mm zone essentially functions like a monofocal distance lens. In addition, there is no loss of incoming light with the zonal refractive optic.

ReSTOR

The apodized diffractive design of ReSTOR provides excellent near and distance function despite the loss of some incoming light due to diffractive scattering.[3,4] The 50:50 distance/near split throughout the center of the lens provides good reading ability even with small pupil sizes. The higher near add allows a closer reading distance, which is the habitual preference of many myopes. A closer reading distance also increases the magnification of smaller print, but the tradeoff is having less light coming from intermediate distances. When they become available, lower add models of ReSTOR should improve intermediate function much as a lower add bifocal does.

With increasing dilation, the incoming distance/near light ratio increases dramatically due to the ReSTOR design (no peripheral diffractive optic). This significantly reduces the severity of night time halos, compared to the ReZoom. Although ReSTOR patients still notice halos and rings around lights, the severity is much less compared to Array and ReZoom.

Pupil centration is very important with a diffractive optic in order to avoid coma and other aberrations. Because the pupil is usually decentered nasally, I have found that orienting the ReSTOR haptics from 6:00 to 12:00 and slightly nudging the IOL nasally improves the centration of the diffractive pattern. Paulo Vinciguerra, MD has suggested this strategy based on improved wavefront scans and decreased patient complaints in

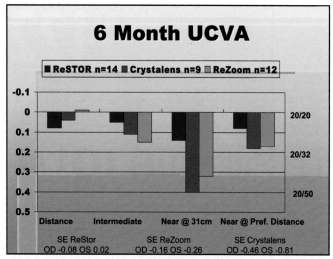

Figure 1. Comparative performance of bilateral IOLs showing uncorrected visual acuity in logMAR scale. Preferred reading distance means that the patient can hold the test card at any distance to maximize reading ability.

eyes in which he re-positioned the ReSTOR because of symptomatic decentration with the pupil.

Aspheric Multifocal IOLs

Both the AcrySof aspheric ReSTOR (Alcon) and the Tecnis multifocal IOL (Advanced Medical Optics) are diffractive lenses with aspheric optics that provide a high effective add power. The aspheric design better compensates for contrast sensitivity loss compared to spherical diffractive multifocal IOLs. Theoretically, aspheric multifocal IOLs should provide better visual quality at distance compared to spherical counterparts with larger pupil diameters. This difference might be particularly important for driving under dimmer illumination.[5] It is important to realize that the aspheric surface does not affect the very center of the IOL, and should not impact IOL spherical aberration when the pupil is small. The concentrated near focus of these diffractive optics results in excellent close reading ability that comes at the expense of decreased focus at intermediate distances.

Crystalens 5.0

The Crystalens (Eyeonics, Inc, Aliso Viejo, CA) has an entirely different set of pros and cons compared to multifocal IOLs. With emmetropia, near performance is reduced and is more variable compared to both ReSTOR and ReZoom. However, particularly if the eye is slightly myopic, uncorrected intermediate focus is generally good without the tradeoff of halos and reduced contrast sensitivity.[6] The ability to hit emmetropia with the Crystalens 4.5 model was less consistent because of an added variable—the effective lens position of a hinged IOL will vary according to bag and capsulorrhexis size. However, refractive accuracy has been improved with the broader haptics, larger optic diameter, and greater overall length of the 5.0 model. This technology is an excellent alternative for those patients who desire and are accustomed to monovision, and are concerned about the risk of bothersome

halos or diminished quality of vision at night. I also favor this choice if there is a possibility of decreased macular function (eg, a patient following macular hole repair who nevertheless has a strong desire to try to reduce spectacle dependence).

The Crystalens mechanism of action remains controversial, as the results are simply not explained by the proposed mechanism of forward optic movement.[1] Whether it is through some combination of pseudoaccommodation and lens arching or movement, the accommodative results can vary significantly from one individual to the next. Individual variability is less with multifocal IOLs, where a defined focus shift is built into the optic. If the first eye is emmetropic but provides disappointing accommodation, one can aim for slight myopia (eg, −0.50 sphere) in the second eye to provide a slight monovision boost to reading function. Generally, night time halos are of minimal severity with the Crystalens, and contrast sensitivity should be comparable to that of a spherical monofocal IOL.

Prospective Comparison of Bilateral ReSTOR and ReZoom in Younger Patients

When ReSTOR and ReZoom both became available in late 2005, I undertook a prospective study to evaluate and better understand their comparative performance characteristics.[7] After informed consent, I prospectively enrolled 30 patients: my first 15 consecutive bilateral ReSTOR and my first 15 consecutive bilateral ReZoom patients that were younger than age 70. Multifocal IOL selection was not randomized, but was determined based on what I thought would best match that individual patient's needs. I chose this arbitrary age cutoff in order to evaluate IOL performance in younger patients who, as a whole, could be expected to be more demanding. I reasoned that these patients would be more likely to use computers, to drive at night, and to perform more visually demanding tasks. Furthermore, testing was performed at 6 months postoperatively to allow for adaptation to night time optical aberrations and to the new visual system. For further comparison, 9 patients under the age of 70 implanted with bilateral Crystalens 4.5 IOLs were also tested at 6 months postoperatively.

After 6 months, we evaluated uncorrected distance, intermediate (50 cm), and near acuity using standard ETDRS charts. In order to understand the intrinsic near and intermediate properties of an IOL, however, you must correct for any residual refractive error so that testing is conducted in an eye that is functionally emmetropic. We therefore also tested distance-corrected near and intermediate vision. We recorded pupil size and tested contrast sensitivity. Patients were asked to complete a standardized quality of life questionnaire, and we attempted to correlate this with a functional vision evaluation using standardized real-life props such as newspapers, magazines, medicine bottles, and a laptop computer.

Bilateral uncorrected visual acuity is represented with a logMAR scale in Figure 1. The last column (preferred reading distance) measures near vision when the patient is allowed to hold the reading card at any distance they want. The mean spherical equivalent for right and left eyes is listed at the bottom of

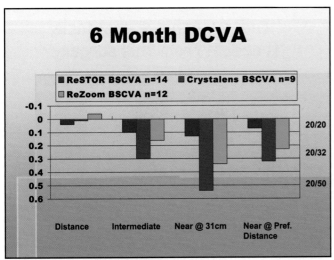

Figure 2. Same test criteria as Figure 1, except all testing is done while wearing best distance correction, to simulate emmetropia.

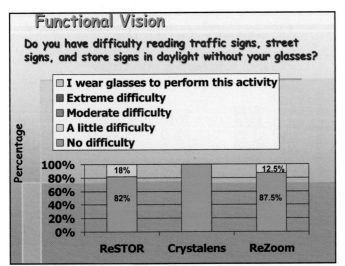

Figure 3. Results of questionnaire asking patients to rate their difficulty seeing distance objects without glasses.

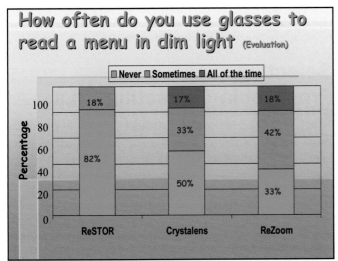

Figure 4. Results of questionnaire asking patients to rate how often they wear glasses to read a menu in dim light.

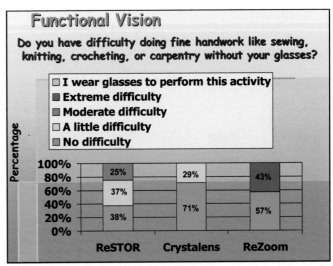

Figure 5. Results of questionnaire asking patients to rate their difficulty doing detailed near tasks without glasses.

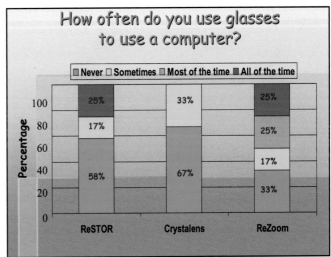

Figure 6. Results of questionnaire asking patients how often they wear glasses to use a computer.

the chart, and shows that the Crystalens patients tended to be slightly myopic. Figure 2 shows the results of bestdistance-corrected visual acuity. As expected, all 3 IOLs show excellent distance acuity. However, the Crystalens performance at near and intermediate was decreased when these eyes were made emmetropic. This demonstrates that the Crystalens had less intrinsic near function when compared to a multifocal IOL. ReSTOR clearly performed the best at near. Both multifocal IOLs were comparable at an intermediate distance of 50 cm.

According to a standardized lifestyle questionnaire, patients in all 3 groups had excellent uncorrected vision for driving, store signs, television, and cooking. All patients reported excellent spectacle free distance vision (Figure 3). Most patients could read a menu without glasses, although ReSTOR was the best for this task (Figure 4). More patients struggled with fine handwork (Figure 5). ReSTOR performed the best for these near tasks. One-fourth of both ReSTOR and ReZoom patients needed glasses all the time to view the computer, whereas Crystalens patients enjoyed the most spectacle independence for this activity (Figure 6).

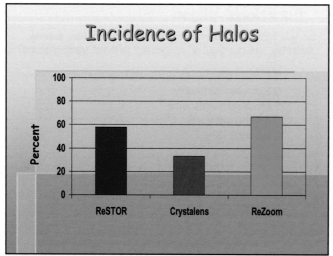

Figure 7A. Incidence of those patients responding yes to the question, "Do you see halos at night?"

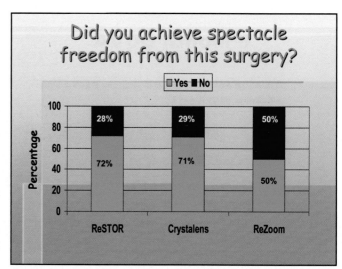

Figure 8. Percentages of each group who reported spectacle freedom at 6 months after surgery.

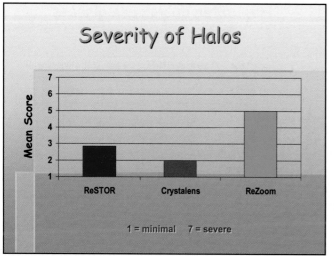

Figure 7B. Mean halo severity score, with patients asked to rate their halos on a scale from 1-7.

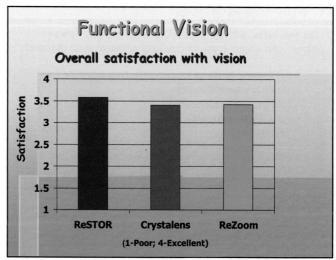

Figure 9. Mean satisfaction scores, based on a 1 to 4 scale.

Approximately 60% of subjects in each multifocal IOL group reported halos, which was roughly double the incidence of halos in Crystalens patients (Figure 7A). However, halo severity was rated much higher by ReZoom patients (Figure 7B). In fact, 2 patients in the ReZoom group refused to have their second eye implanted following their first surgery. Although both patients achieved uncorrected monocular 20/20 and J1, they had great difficulty adapting to halos. One patient had the ReZoom IOL explanted, and the other eventually chose a monofocal IOL for the second eye.

As shown in Figure 8, roughly 70% of bilateral ReSTOR and Crystalens patients achieved spectacle freedom in this study, compared to only 50% of bilateral ReZoom patients. Although these percentages are lower than in other studies, this was a selective population of younger patients all under the age of 70. This may reflect a greater range of demanding visual requirements in the study group compared to an older pseudophakic population. Given these results, it might seem surprising that overall satisfaction with all 3 IOLs was extremely high (Figure 9). Clearly, this would not have occurred if patients had expected never to need glasses. Having realistic expectations clearly impacts patient satisfaction.

Selecting Presbyopia-Correcting IOLs

Based on these observations, I tend to favor ReSTOR for patients with smaller or larger pupils, or if the patient frequently drives at night. ReSTOR is more likely to satisfy the reading expectations of myopes, who tend to hold reading material fairly close without glasses and are unaccustomed to having good uncorrected intermediate vision. ReZoom works very well for hyperopes and taller patients with longer arms and for whom intermediate vision is important. Hyperopes usually do not hold reading material very close and have lower expectations for uncorrected reading ability. Emmetropia is less consistently attained in higher hyperopes with short axial lengths, and ReZoom is more forgiving of slight ametropia. Finally, only ReZoom is available in low diopter powers at present.

Patients with possible mild macular degeneration are not good multifocal candidates because they would be less likely to reap the benefits and may be impacted by reduced contrast sensitivity. However, when using reading glasses, there should be less contrast sensitivity loss with ReZoom compared to ReSTOR should a patient later develop macular degeneration.

Based on these guidelines, bilateral ReSTOR matches the profile for more of my refractive IOL patients than bilateral ReZoom. Both groups performed well without glasses and had high satisfaction scores in my own small study. ReZoom gave slightly better distance performance, and ReSTOR was superior at near. Although the incidence of halos was similar in both groups, they were more severe in the ReZoom group. It should be mentioned that at the time of this writing, the Tecnis multifocal IOL is not available in the United States.

Mixing Presbyopia-Correcting IOLs

As pointed out by Frank A. Bucci, Jr, MD, Dick Lindstrom MD, John Doane MD, and others, the strengths and weaknesses of different presbyopia IOL designs are complimentary in many respects. The growing interest in a mixing approach affirms that no available IOL is perfect, and we are learning that many patients tolerate and achieve functional advantages with these combinations.[7] With respect to mixing different multifocal IOLs ReZoom can potentially fill the intermediate gap found with ReSTOR. ReSTOR or the Tecnis multifocal provide a stronger reading add, and allow patients to read even when their pupils constrict under brighter illumination. ReZoom should provide better contrast sensitivity in the distance, whereas ReSTOR can make it easier to suppress the night time halos from the ReZoom eye. Pairing a Crystalens in the dominant eye with a diffractive multifocal IOL in the non-dominant eye is another excellent mixing strategy. ReSTOR and the Tecnis multifocal offer much better near reading ability. The Crystalens provides better intermediate function, however, and should provide better quality of vision at distance, particularly at night.

Presently, the biggest impetus for mixing IOLs seems to be refractive lens exchange (RLE) patients, who certainly have much higher refractive expectations than senior citizens with cataracts. The latter group is usually thrilled with any IOL, and attaining good pseudoaccommodation is a surprising bonus for someone who lost accommodation two decades ago. My older cataract patients are usually so happy after their first surgery that they would question the notion of doing anything different for their second eye. Most of my cataract patients have the same multifocal IOL in both eyes for this reason.

In contrast, the presbyopic refractive lens exchange patient already has excellent spectacle corrected vision and will be less forgiving of new optical aberrations and halos. They would not be considering expensive refractive surgery if they did not expect to be spectacle free for most activities afterwards. Younger cataract surgery patients also have a different concept of presbyopia than 75 year olds, and their refractive expectations are more similar to those of RLE patients. Baby boomers are accustomed to having technology solve most problems and like to research which technology is the best. Those who spend many hours on the Internet researching which cell phone to buy will feel that their IOL decision deserves the same careful analysis. They are more open to a mixing strategy in order to attain the complementary benefits which no single lens can provide.

Staging the IOL decision also makes sense if there is any question as to which IOL to choose. Both the patient and the surgeon can assess the result of the first eye implantation, before deciding which IOL to implant in the second eye. For example, implanting a monofocal or accommodating IOL in the second eye can be an excellent fall-back strategy for patients having trouble adapting to multifocal IOL halos or aberrations in their first eye. Such a contingency plan helps reassure patients preoperatively who are worried about being "locked in" to a multifocal that they may not tolerate well. Likewise, if a patient was disappointed with their reading ability following implantation of a Crystalens or ReZoom in one eye, the ReSTOR IOL can be implanted in the second eye.

Conclusion

The premium IOL channel appropriately allows surgeons and patients to differentiate between cataract treatment and optional refractive surgical goals. That we have no universally perfect solution increases the importance of careful patient selection. Understanding the differences between the available presbyopia correcting IOL designs permits us to individualize our approach, which for some patients may include mixing different lenses.

References

1. Findl O, Leydolt C. Meta-analysis of accommodating intraocular lenses. *J Cataract Refract Surg.* 2007;33:522-527.
2. Vingolo EM, Grenga P, Iacobelli L, Grenga R. Visual acuity and contrast sensitivity: AcrySof ReSTOR apodized diffractive versus AcrySof SA60AT monofocal intraocular lenses. *J Cataract Refract Surg.* 2007;33:1244-1247.
3. Lane SS, Morris M, Nordan L, et al. Multifocal intraocular lenses. *Ophthalmol Clin North Am.* 2006;19:89-105, vi. Review.
4. Alfonso JF, Fernández-Vega L, Baamonde MB, Montés-Micó R. Prospective visual evaluation of apodized diffractive intraocular lenses. *J Cataract Refract Surg.* 2007;33:1235-1243.
5. Hütz WW, Eckhardt HB, Röhrig B, Grolmus R. Reading ability with 3 multifocal intraocular lens models. *J Cataract Refract Surg.* 2006;32:2015-2021.
6. Cumming JS, Colvard DM, Dell SJ, et al. Clinical evaluation of the Crystalens AT-45 accommodating intraocular lens: results of the U.S. Food and Drug Administration clinical trial. *J Cataract Refract Surg.* 2006;32:812-825.
7. Chang DF. Prospective functional and clinical comparison of bilateral ReZoom and ReSTOR IOLs in patients under age 70. *J Cataract Refract Surg.* In press.
8. Pepose JS, Qazi MA, Davies J, et al. Visual performance of patients with bilateral vs combination Crystalens, ReZoom, and ReSTOR intraocular lens implants. *Am J Ophthalmol.* 2007;144:347-357. Epub 2007 Jul 25.

CHAPTER 123

WHY OFFER
MULTIPLE PREMIUM IOLS?

Joel K. Shugar, MD, MSEE

At the time of this writing, there are 3 presbyopia-correcting IOLs (Pr-C IOLs) that have been approved by the Food and Drug Administration (FDA) for implantation in the United States: Crystalens (Eyeonics, Inc, Aliso Viejo, CA), ReSTOR (Alcon, Fort Worth, TX), and ReZoom (Advanced Medical Optics, Santa Ana, CA). Crystalens is designed to function as a true accommodative IOL whereas ReSTOR and ReZoom are multifocal IOLs that provide multiple, simultaneous distance and near foci. In my opinion, it is imperative for any surgeon who wishes to maximize success with premium IOLs to gain experience with all 3 Pr-C IOLs and be able to offer each of these lenses to the most appropriate candidates. The other key technical pieces to the puzzle for maximizing success with these lenses are highly accurate biometry, precise astigmatism reduction, seamless laser vision correction (LVC) capability, and, most importantly, impeccable surgical technique. Of at least equal importance is the necessity for thorough preoperative counseling including the determination and management of both clinical and financial patient expectations—the latter being a skill set generally much more familiar to surgeons with significant experience in refractive surgery relative to those whose practices have focused mainly on cataract and anterior segment surgery and/or comprehensive ophthalmology.

Each Pr-C IOL has relative strengths, weaknesses, and nuances related to its use.

Of the 3 Pr-C IOLs, Crystalens provides the best distance and intermediate vision and is more forgiving of residual ametropia than either of the multifocal IOLs. Quality of vision is highest with Crystalens, which offers the same crispness and contrast sensitivity as monofocal IOLs. This is particularly important in patients in whom any compromise in macular function is present or likely to occur in the future, particularly patients with drusen or a strong family history of age-related macular degeneration (ARMD). One drawback of Crystalens in this cohort is that the optic currently has no ultraviolet blocker, and patients who receive Crystalens must be counseled to wear sun-protective eyewear whenever exposed to sunlight. On average Crystalens typically provides about 1.5 D of accommodative amplitude, so either a mini-monovision or a mix-and-match strategy is imperative if the patient is to be able to read fine print postoperatively. Patients receiving this IOL bilaterally must be willing to accept the possibility of needing reading glasses for finest print. Optimal surgical technique with Crystalens, which is of modified plate haptic design and therefore requires an intact posterior capsule and capsulorrhexis, involves creation of a capsulorrhexis of at least 6 mm in diameter such that the capsulorrhexis margin is peripheral to the 5-mm diameter IOL optic. Creation of such a capsulorrhexis increases the surgical complexity in using this lens and its presence precludes the use of capsulorrhexis capture in the event a three-piece IOL must be implanted in the ciliary sulcus. Best practice includes polishing of not only the posterior capsule but also the undersurface of the anterior capsule to remove A-type lens epithelial cells in order to avoid postoperative capsular phimosis as well as seeding of the posterior capsule once capsular fusion has occurred. Following IOL placement, avoidance of intra- or postoperative anterior chamber shallowing is critical. For this reason Langerman-groove-style incision architecture is strongly recommended, as is pre-hydrating the stroma of the sideport and possibly also the main incision. The Crystalens is more difficult to exchange after about 4 weeks postoperatively because the haptics become fibrosed into the equator of the capsular bag and attempts at simple extraction can cause zonular dehiscence. In the event late IOL exchange becomes necessary, haptic amputation or preplacement of a capsular tension ring prior to attempting to explant the haptics are recommended. Accommodative amplitudes increase postoperatively and accommodative exercises are recommended starting several weeks postoperatively. A final advantage of this IOL model is that wavefront-guided LVC is both possible and predictable (provided pupil size permits), which is of particular importance in cases in which a bioptics approach is planned ahead of time. PCO tends to occur earlier and more vigorously with this IOL than with either multifocal IOL, and in many circumstances my preference with Crystalens is to defer LVC until after yttrium-aluminum-garnet (YAG) capsulotomy has been performed.

The ReSTOR offers the best uncorrected near vision but the worst uncorrected intermediate vision of the three approved Pr-C IOLs. At the time of this writing, the only available ReSTOR model has a near add of +3.5 D in the spectacle plane. Bilateral ReSTOR implantation can be a delight to those with high near and low intermediate vision need, such as avid readers who eschew computer use. One of my happiest Pr-C IOL patients is a middle-aged jeweler with bilateral ReSTOR lenses (who had undergone a relatively large optical zone radial keratotomy by another surgeon many years previously). Because of this high add power, ReSTOR outcomes should be targeted at between Plano and +0.25 D; even a small amount of postoperative myopia can markedly reduce patient satisfaction. I cannot overemphasize the disappointment with intermediate vision expressed by prolific computer users or other individuals with other significant visual needs at intermediate distance and I recommend avoiding placing a ReSTOR lens in at least the dominant eye of such an individual. These IOLs are available in one- and 3-piece models, the latter of which is suitable for sulcus implantation in the event of posterior capsular rupture (in which case I strongly suggest capsulorrhexis capture of the optic). A significant percentage of patients implanted with ReSTOR complain about a waxy quality to their vision, which is the other major area of complaint with this design apart from complaints about intermediate vision. Complaints about waxy vision often resolve after implantation of the second eye, even if the second eye is implanted with a different model of Pr-C IOL. Aspheric optics have recently become available, thus offering the potential to reduce postoperative spherical aberration and perhaps addressing the waxy vision complaint. Although patients receiving either multifocal IOL should be counseled preoperatively about halos with night driving, such complaints are typically rare with ReSTOR and usually resolve within several months.

The ReZoom offers better uncorrected intermediate vision than ReSTOR but worse uncorrected near vision. Distance vision with ReZoom is typically quite good although Crystalens usually provides even better distance and intermediate vision. ReZoom provides better near vision in dim illumination whereas ReSTOR provides better near vision in bright illumination. The biggest drawback to the ReZoom is halos, with some patients complaining about halos and glare with different types of artificial lights as well as with night driving. Neuroadaptation can continue for up to 2 years, and I have heard patients comment on significant improvement in visual artifacts occurring well into the second year following implantation. The 3-piece design of this IOL renders it suitable for sulcus implantation, and my sole case to date of sulcus implantation of a Pr-C IOL (with capsulorrhexis capture, following posterior capsular rupture) of a multifocal IOL involves a ReZoom and an excellent long-term outcome. Other than halos and suboptimal near vision, the other major drawback to this IOL is a poor injector design with a propensity to gouge the optic surface (which in my experience has not yet required exchange nor produced any symptoms postoperatively).

Possible strategies to improve outcomes with these IOLs are as follows:

* Mini-monovision with Crystalens, targeting dominant eye at −0.25 D and nondominant eye at −0.75 D.
* Mix-and-match with ReSTOR in nondominant eye and ReZoom or Crystalens in the dominant eye.
* Bilateral ReSTOR implantation in individuals with strong near vision needs and limited intermediate needs.
* Bilateral ReZoom implantation in easy-going individuals who do not mind halos at night and do not have strong near vision needs.

I have personal experience with strategies 1 through 3.

So how is one to match the right strategy to the right patient? Both patient preferences and comorbid pathology come into play. I have found Steve Dell's questionnaire invaluable in determining the former. I pay particular attention to whether a patient is willing to accept good intermediate vision with limited ability to read fine print, if a patient is willing to accept night glare/halo, and how a patient rates him- or herself on a scale from easy-going to perfectionist. I also ask patients about occupation and avocations. The most commonly encountered comorbid pathologies are ARMD, diabetic retinopathy, glaucoma, and Fuchs dystrophy.

Rule number one is *primum non nocerum*—first do no harm. I currently consider significant retinal pathology a contraindication to multifocal IOL implantation, although I am often willing to consider Crystalens placement in patients with ARMD or well-controlled diabetic retinopathy. Such patients must be educated about the need for close follow-up and treatment of comorbid pathology. All Crystalens patients and particularly those with ARMD must commit to wearing good UV400 protection whenever exposed to sunlight. Fuchs dystrophy presents a conundrum, because guttatate can reduce contrast sensitivity, but Crystalens might make Descemet's stripping automated endothelial keratoplasty (DSAEK) more difficult, particularly if YAG capsulotomy has already been performed. I have performed both bilateral Crystalens and ReSTOR/ReZoom mix-and-match both with excellent short-term results in Fuchs patients; in such a scenario detailed informed consent and involvement of the patient in the decision making are imperative.

Patients unwilling to risk night halos/glare are obvious candidates for bilateral Crystalens implantation. In such a scenario, extra discussion should focus on the fact that the Crystalens cannot provide the full range of accommodation. Would the patient prefer a thin pair of glasses for night driving to eliminate halos from mini-monovision or would the patient prefer to forgo the likelihood of such glasses at the expense of virtually guaranteeing the need for reading glasses for small print? Patients who are equally and totally unwilling to risk night glare/halos or the need for reading glasses for fine print, and particularly those who classify themselves as "perfectionists" are best served by a frank discussion that their expectations exceed the limits of current technology. If they are unwilling to compromise on one area or the other they would not be suitable candidates for available premium lens technology. Once they learn there is no simple panacea many patients will prove less dogmatic and ask the surgeon to simply "do the best you can" to minimize both night halos as well as the need for any reading glasses. In such a scenario, after exhaustive consent I will either implant a ReSTOR in the nondominant eye and a Crystalens in the dominant eye or use bilateral Crystalenses with a more aggressive monovision target.

Patients unwilling to risk the need for reading glasses for fine print but who do not mind night glare/halos are obvious candidates for either ReSTOR in the nondominant eye or Crystalens with a refractive target between −1.0 D and −1.25 D, depending on comorbid pathology and patient willingness to accept perceptibly lower uncorrected visual acuity (UCVA) in the nondominant eye. Patients implanted with a Crystalens in the nondominant eye are always implanted with a Crystalens in the dominant eye, whereas those with a ReSTOR in the nondominant eye are implanted with either a Crystalens or a ReZoom in the dominant eye depending on a number of factors. Avid computer users will receive a Crystalens in the dominant eye, whereas outdoorsmen who may not reliably wear sunglasses or those with large pupils and/or those who specifically wish to be able to read in dim illumination are more likely to receive a ReZoom in the dominant eye.

Very easy-going patients who do not mind glasses for fine print or halos at night are good candidates for either bilateral Crystalens with mini-monovision or mix-and-match ReZoom/ReSTOR in the dominant/nondominant eyes, respectively. I find myself gravitating more and more to bilateral Crystalens as my "fastball" option. This is because I would rather deal with 10 patients complaining about still needing reading glasses for fine print than one multifocal IOL patient complaining about intractable halos or "waxy" vision or suffering from decreased best-corrected visual acuity (BCVA) that is either idiopathic or follows worsening of comorbid pathology such as ARMD. A small percentage (<5%) of mix-and-match ReZoom/ReSTOR patients will complain that most of the time either one eye or the other is doing the work at near and the eyes just will not work simultaneously at near in many situations. Most of these complaints will diminish with passage of time, correction of dry eye and residual ametropia, and YAG capsulotomy for posterior capsular opacification that can cause symptoms seemingly disproportionate to the degree of posterior capsule opacification (PCO).

Although many surgeons suggest waiting to perform surgery on the second eye until the patient is happy with the first eye, in my experience such a strategy can set the patient and surgeon up for "refractive purgatory" in which the patient is unhappy with the result in the first eye, which paradoxically would be resolved once surgery is performed on the second eye. For patients receiving a multifocal implant in the first eye I prepare them for the possibility that they will be unhappy with their vision until the second eye has been operated on, which will be scheduled as soon as is medically prudent following surgery on the first eye. I find that surgery on the second eye usually resolves most complaints following implantation of a multifocal lens in the first eye. For patients with monofocal pseudophakia in the fellow eye my experiences with multifocal IOLs has been mixed whereas that with Crystalens has been uniformly positive.

For residual ametropia I will most commonly perform LVC 6 to 8 weeks postoperatively (almost exclusively laser in situ keratomileusis [LASIK] in my practice). If the patient is otherwise happy with the quality of their vision I feel LVC represents both the safest and most cost-effective solution to correct refractive error. I counsel all of my patients preoperatively that in my practice there is about a 10% chance of requiring LASIK, and that if LASIK is necessary they will receive it at half price relative to other patients who present for LVC. In the event early PCO is present I often present the patient with the option of temporizing with glasses until YAG becomes necessary so that any refractive shift resulting from capsulotomy will occur prior to LVC.

A dilemma that occasionally arises with patients unhappy with their multifocal IOL vision is whether to perform YAG capsulotomy for PCO that does not seem overly impressive at the slit lamp or whether to perform an IOL exchange. My first step in such a scenario is to perform optical coherence tomography (OCT) testing to rule out subtle cystoid macular edema, and I also aggressively treat any dry eye conditions. If there is any ametropia I will prescribe single vision distance glasses that I tell the patient are for diagnostic purposes only and that these will be converted to sunglasses following a few weeks of wear to see if the patient's symptoms are diminished from treatment of the ametropia. If the aforementioned steps have been performed the decision of whether to perform a YAG capsulotomy or IOL exchange can be complex and many factors must be considered. Was the patient initially happier with their vision, or is the complaint increasing? In such case YAG is usually the answer. If I have significant doubt about which course of action to take I will usually employ tincture of time to help clarify the correct path to follow. A vital pearl is to involve the patient in the decision making; I tell patients that once YAG capsulotomy has been performed IOL exchange is no longer possible. Most importantly, in the small minority of patients having difficulty with neuroadaptation it is vital to continually reassure them that you are their partner and are committed to working through the problems until they are satisfied with the outcome. Significant neuroadaptation really does occur for as long as 2 years after surgery, and I stress to patients who are struggling that a positive mental attitude and viewing the glass as "half full" really does positively affect the speed and degree of neuroadaptation that occurs.

This area will continue to evolve rapidly with approval of the Tecnis multifocal IOL as well as improved designs for accommodating lenses that are in various phases of clinical testing and that will ultimately prove to be the wave of the future.

CHAPTER 124

WHY OFFER MULTIPLE PREMIUM IOLS?

Audrey Talley-Rostov, MD

Why Offer Multiple IOLs?

The introduction of presbyopia-correcting intraocular lenses (Pr-C IOLs) has shifted the emphasis of cataract surgery from just treating patients' functional symptoms to optimizing the refractive outcome of the procedure as well. Familiarity and facility with the variety of available Pr-C IOLs allows the surgeon to provide the patient with the best options for matching lifestyle needs and visual desires, thereby reducing dependence on glasses.

Current day Pr-C IOLs fall into 2 categories: multifocal IOLs and accommodating IOLs. Understanding a patient's occupation, recreational activities, hobbies, geographic location, frequency of night driving, and personality are crucial to providing the patient with the optimal IOL for his or her lifestyle. Educating the patient about IOL selection and the benefits and limitations of each IOL can help to temper patient expectations and hopefully increase patients' postoperative satisfaction. Just as there is no single refractive procedure that can provide all patients with perfect vision correction, there is no single Pr-C IOL that can provide all patients with their desired vision correction.

Multifocal IOLs

In 2005, the FDA approved 2 multifocal IOLs, a refractive IOL, the ReZoom (Advanced Medical Optics, Santa Ana, CA) lens and a diffractive IOL, the ReSTOR (Alcon, Fort Worth, TX) lens. The ReZoom IOL has 3.5 D of additional power for near, which translates to approximately 2.5 D in the spectacle plane. The ReSTOR IOL has 4.0 D of additional power for near, translating to approximately 3.2 D in the spectacle plane

Recent studies of the ReZoom lens, based on a European study that conformed to Food and Drug Administration (FDA) standards[1] indicated that 93.0% never or occasionally wore glasses. These patients reported needing glasses for reading fine print. In recent studies with the ReSTOR IOL,[2] patients achieved excellent visual acuity at distance and near and functional visual acuity in the intermediate range. A recent study[3] on "mix and match" technologies with the ReZoom IOL implanted in the dominant eye and the ReSTOR IOL implanted in the nondominant eye reported even greater spectacle independence and patient satisfaction.

Patients desiring good distance and intermediate vision, but who do not mind wearing glasses for close work such as prolonged reading or handiwork, may be better candidates for the ReZoom IOL. Patients desiring good distance and reading vision, but who are not as concerned about intermediate vision, and do not do a lot of computer work may be better candidates for the ReSTOR IOL. Consideration for the "mix and match" technique of ReZoom in the dominant eye and ReSTOR in the nondominant eye should also be discussed to maximize patient options and satisfaction.

A full discussion with the patient regarding multifocal IOLs should also include the potential for dysphotopsia, and specifically the perception of glare or halos around point sources of light at night. Although studies have shown that most patients will exhibit neuroadaptation to these phenomena with time (weeks to months)[4] patients who engage in frequent night driving (truckdrivers or patients living in remote, rural locations) may not be ideal candidates for multifocal IOLs. The use of brimonidine tartrate 0.2% has also been shown to be effective in decreasing night-vision disturbances in these patients.[5]

Pupil size can also be an issue in determining which IOL might be most appropriate for the patient. Patients with small pupils (less than 3 mm) may not achieve optimal results in the near to intermediate range with the ReZoom IOL because this lens is dominant for distance centrally. Small or eccentric pupils can also be an issue with the ReSTOR IOL, which has a near vision dominance, centrally. Patients with small or eccentric pupils may experience an increase in dysphotopsia with the ReSTOR lens and require laser pupilloplasty or mydriatics[6] to help remedy their symptoms.

Accommodating IOLs

The Crystalens AT-5 (Eyeonics, Inc, Aliso Viejo, CA) is the current design of the accommodating IOL that works by axial movement of a 5.0-mm optic on hinged haptics. The add power at the spectacle plane for this lens is approximately 1.0 to 2.5 D.

Studies of the Crystalens indicate that this IOL provides better uncorrected near and distance visual outcomes when compared with standard monofocal IOLs.[7] In a questionnaire distributed in an FDA study at 1 year after implantation with the Crystalens, 73% of patients never or rarely wore glasses, 15% wore them some of the time, and 11% wore them most to all of the time.[1] There are fewer complaints of the photic phenomena of night glare and halos with this lens.

Patients desiring good distance and intermediate vision, who may be concerned about the possibility of dysphotopsia, and who do not mind waiting a longer time to achieve the full benefit of the accommodative aspects of the lens, may be good candidates for the Crystalens.

Matching the Patient With the IOL

The first step in determining which IOL might be best for the patient is to determine the patient's preoperative visual needs and desires. The use of a questionnaire, such as the ones popularized by Maloney and Dell[8] can help the patient to evaluate the range of vision that best suits his or her lifestyle.

William Maloney, MD was the first to describe the concept of dividing vision into five lifestyle zones.[8] Zone 1 describes near vision tasks and would require near dominant vision, whereas Zone 5 describes distance vision and would require perfect emmetropia. Steven J. Dell, MD developed a now widely used patient questionnaire[8] that helps the physician to assess their visual needs and lifestyle demands. This questionnaire asks the patient to rank, in order of personal priority, the visual tasks most important to him or her. This further helps to establish the visual tasks and activities for which the patient would most like to be glasses independent.

The ReZoom or Crystalens would be the best IOL options for patients desiring good vision in the intermediate to distance range (Zones 2 to 4), who want to be able to do their activities of daily life such as walking around, driving, and using a computer, but who do not mind using glasses for prolonged reading, reading small print, or night driving. The Crystalens would also be the IOL of choice if the patient lives in a rural area, does a lot of night driving, or is particularly concerned about dysphotopsia. The patient should be made aware that with the Crystalens, their full range of vision for intermediate tasks may take as long as 6 months to achieve, that results are more variable, and that eye exercises (using their eyes for near tasks to promote accommodation) may be necessary. If dysphotopsia is not a particular concern, and if the patient desires more immediate benefit of the intermediate range of vision, the ReZoom lens should be considered as the lens of choice.

The ReSTOR lens would be the best option for patients desiring good near vision for activities such as reading and crafts (Zones 1 to 2), who do not do a lot of computer work and are not as concerned with intermediate range vision, and do not do a lot of night driving or have concerns about dysphotopsia.

A "mix and match" combination of a ReZoom IOL in the dominant eye and a ReSTOR IOL in the nondominant eye should be a primary consideration for patients who would like to have a full range of vision, with an intermediate to distance predominance, who do not do a lot of night driving or have concerns about dysphotopsias. The majority of my patients receive this "mix and match" combination.

Examples of Patient/IOL Customization and Management

INTERMEDIATE RANGE VISION

If the patient desires a full range of vision, with predominance of vision in the intermediate vision range, does not do a lot of night driving, and is not particularly concerned about dysphotopsia, then implantation of a ReZoom lens in the dominant eye is a good initial step (Figure 1). After the first eye is complete, there should be an assessment of the patient's satisfaction and functionality of vision. If the patient is satisfied with his or her vision, but desires an expanded near range of vision, then implantation of a ReSTOR lens should be planned for the nondominant eye. If the patient is satisfied with the vision and wants the exact same vision for his or her other eye, then consideration for a ReZoom lens should be made for the nondominant eye.

If the patient has a lot of complaints of dysphotopsia, surgery on the second eye should be delayed for at least 4 weeks to see if the symptoms are starting to resolve. Consideration for a Crystalens should be given for the patient's second eye. If after implantation of a Crystalens in the patient's nondominant eye the patient still has complaints of the dysphotopsia in the eye with the ReZoom lens, then consideration for an IOL exchange with a Crystalens or an aspheric lens should be considered. IOL exchange is technically easier if performed within 8 weeks of the initial surgery. If an IOL exchange is unable to be performed successfully without a significant risk of capsular bag rupture, then consideration can be given for implantation of a piggyback IOL in the sulcus, as this can also diminish symptoms of dysphotopsia.[9]

If the patient is desiring of intermediate range vision, does a lot of night driving, and/or is concerned about dysphotopsia and/or has small pupils, implantation with the Crystalens in the dominant eye should be considered. The patient needs to be made aware of the delay in obtaining the full range of vision expected, and the eye exercises that are necessary for the Crystalens to perform maximally. If the patient is happy after successful Crystalens implantation in the dominant eye, implantation of a Crystalens should be considered for the nondominant eye. A slight monovision approach with the Crystalens implantation in the nondominant eye having a

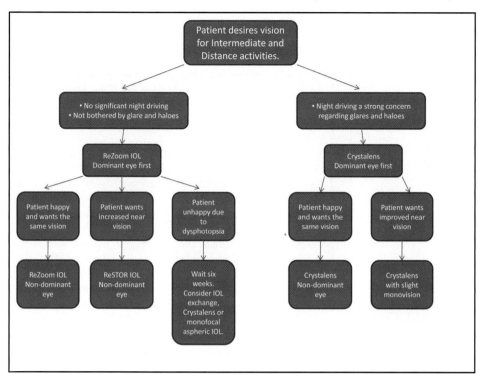

Figure 1. Evaluation of patient choosing intermediate and distance vision.

target of approximately −0.75 D can also be considered if the patient desires an improved range of near vision.

NEAR RANGE VISION

If the patient desires a full range of vision, with predominance of vision in the near vision range (reading or handiwork), does not do a lot of computer work, does not do a lot of night driving, and is not particularly concerned about dysphotopsia, then implantation of a ReSTOR lens in the nondominant eye is a good initial step (Figure 2). After the first eye is complete, there should be an assessment of the patient's satisfaction and functionality of vision. If the patient is satisfied with the vision and wants the exact same vision for his or her other eye, then consideration for a ReSTOR lens should be made for the dominant eye. If the patient is satisfied with his or her vision, but desires an expanded intermediate range of vision, then implantation of a ReZoom lens should be planned for the dominant eye.

If the patient has a lot of complaints of dysphotopsia, surgery on the second eye should be delayed for at least 4 weeks to see if the symptoms are starting to resolve. Consideration for a Crystalens should be given for the patient's second eye (in this case, the dominant eye). If after implantation of a Crystalens in the patient's dominant eye the patient still has complaints of the dysphotopsia in the eye with the ReSTOR lens, then consideration for an IOL exchange with a Crystalens or an aspheric lens to provide for monovision should be considered.

Conclusion

Pr-C IOLs have changed the landscape of cataract surgery, bringing it into the realm of refractive surgery. Surgeons should be knowledgeable about and have facility with the variety of available Pr-C IOLs in order to provide the patient with the best options for matching lifestyle needs and visual desires. Customizing IOL selection to the individual patient improves the surgeon's ability to manage preoperative expectations and postoperative results and can ultimately increase patient satisfaction with the procedure.

References

1. Packer M, Fine IH, Hoffman RS. Refractive lens exchange. *Focal Points*. 2007;xxv(6):1-8.
2. Blaylock J, Si Z, Vickers C. Visual and refractive status at different focal distances after implantation of the ReSTOR multifocal intraocular lens. *J Cataract Refract Surg*. 2006;32:1464-1473.
3. Akaishi L, Fabri PP. PC IOLs mix and match technologies: Brazilian experience. Presentation, World Ophthalmology Congress, Sao Paolo, Brazil, February 2006.
4. Artal P. Neural adaptation to aberrations. *Cataract and Refractive Surgery Today*. 2007;7:76-77.
5. McDonald JE 2nd, El-Moatassem Kotb AM, Decker BB. Effect of brimonidine tartrate ophthalmic solution 0.2% on pupil size in normal eyes under different luminance conditions. *J Cataract Refract Surg*. 2001;27:560-564.
6. Donnenfeld E. Cataract surgery in post refractive surgery patients. *Cataract and Refractive Surgery Today*. 2006;69-70.
7. Macsai M, Padnick-Silver L, Fontes B. Visual outcomes after accommodating intraocular lens implantation. *J Cataract Refract Surg*. 2006;32:628-633.
8. Dell S. Screening and evaluating presbyopic patients. *Cataract and Refract Surg Today*. 2007;81-82.
9. Ernst P. Severe photic phenomena. *J Cataract Refract Surg*. 2006;32: 685-686.

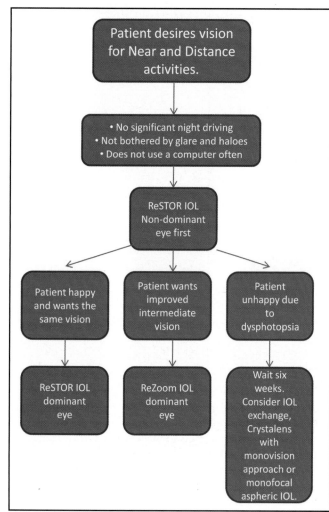

Figure 2. Evaluation of patient choosing near and distance vision.

CHARGES FOR PRESBYOPIA-CORRECTING IOLs AND ADDITIONAL REFRACTIVE PROCEDURES

In my practice, we charge a set amount for Pr-C IOLs and additional testing needed for the IOLs. Limbal relaxing incisions (LRI) are included in the price when performed at the time of cataract surgery. For astigmatism >0.75 D I routinely do LRIs.

If the patient desires additional refractive procedures (laser in situ keratomileusis [LASIK], photorefractive keratectomy [PRK], or conductive keratoplasty) after the initial cataract surgery with the Pr-C IOL, we charge half price for the additional refractive procedure. If there is a high likelihood of requiring an additional refractive procedure following the cataract surgery (eg, a patient with high astigmatism or one who had previous LASIK or PRK), the patient is informed of the likelihood of needing additional surgery to optimize his or her refractive outcome, and is provided with the information regarding the costs of the additional procedures (both the full cost as well as the 50% discount that they would receive if they require the additional procedure).

For the occasional case of a refractive surprise or a very unhappy patient requiring additional refractive procedures, I have charged a nominal fee, or no fee.

CHAPTER 125

WHY OFFER MULTIPLE PREMIUM IOLs?

Sheri L. Rowen, MD, FACS

Throughout my entire career, I could not wait to have access to presbyopia-correcting lenses. I had hoped presbyopia correction would be available to us before I retired, as I knew it would be one of our greatest challenges to master in the field of intraocular lens (IOL) surgery. It was and it is. It takes time, commitment, and patience to explain the options to our patients, and we can only hope they understand enough to work with us. There is no perfect lens system currently available so we have to be prepared to accommodate individual patient needs. Because there is no single procedure that will consistently reverse presbyopia, we should learn to use all of the refractive modalities and combinations of different options in order to maximize uncorrected vision while inducing a minimum of unwanted aberrations.

The most important principle, in my opinion, is to optimally correct the dominant eye, for distance, with excellent quality of vision. The source of most patient complaints relates to an inability to see clearly at distance, as opposed to being unable to see a J1+ font for print. For this reason, I overwhelmingly favor the use of the Crystalens (Eyeonics, Inc, Aliso Viejo, CA) for the dominant eye.

Scheduling

In a busy practice setting, it seemed impractical to plan to spend up to half an hour with a patient expressing interest in this new technology during their first visit, but doing so has been valuable and necessary. It does wreak havoc with the flow of the day's schedule, thereby creating an administrative nightmare, but it is truly time well spent. You must commit to mastering the available technology, and you must know and properly educate your patients before you operate on them. We must also allot adequate time at the 1-week visit to discuss lens selection for their second eye. Therefore, it is critical to arrange your schedule to allow for this added chair time. As our populace is becoming better educated about their health, increasing numbers of patients will call in advance to ask about these new IOLs. In these cases, our staff can assist us by explaining these options to patients, mailing out the

appropriate brochures, and arranging for a longer consultation to discuss the premium IOLs. More often, however, we learn through our screening measures that the patient did not know these lenses existed or did not understand the material that was sent, but are still curious about this new technology. Even if it requires scheduling a second appointment, it is important to adequately discuss the IOL options with these patients. I do think in the future, it will take less time to educate aging baby boomers, whose computer skills will enable them to review information online, or via a small informational CD that they receive in the mail. The IOL Counselor (Patient Education Concepts, Houston, TX) and other interactive computer programs can also help to explain these concepts to patients without requiring a significant amount of physician time.

Patient Selection

Whereas we have all been told how important it is, patient selection is an interesting and challenging process. It is almost impossible to predict who might want and would be willing to pay extra for this premium upgrade. I have been quite surprised by which patients select them. Never assume that they cannot afford it (based on the way they dress, for example), as you will find many patients who will put their hard-earned money toward something important that they desire. I first ask patients how they feel about needing glasses for near vision. Then, I explain that the advantages extend beyond reading alone, and will allow them to see many items within arms length, including their watch, cell phone, shopping labels, and so on. In fact, my standard question is, "How much would you spend for a car that will last 4 to 5 years? Answer: "At least ~$20,000." Then I reply, "it seems pretty reasonable to spend $5000 for vision that will last a lifetime." You will be shocked at how that analogy opens up their interest and the discussion.

We actually have an obligation to inform patients that these technologies are available, as they can become quite disturbed if they do not find out about these options until after the surgery. Patients who are already frustrated with bifocals, glasses, or contact lenses, will be much more receptive to the concept of presbyopia-correcting IOLs. Others really value the concept of visual freedom,. If, after introducing the topic, the patient says, "I have always worn glasses and don't mind wearing them" then you know that they like their eyeglasses, and that it is not necessary to spend much time educating them about premium IOLs. The more interested patients might volunteer, "I hate having to be dependent on glasses for everything I do," or "I hate having to constantly move my head up and down to see what I am doing through my glasses."

No matter what, beware of the self-described perfectionist, with a demanding personality. These individuals can be very critical and difficult to please, so we must really "under sell and try to over deliver." Also, we must emphasize that there are no guarantees that we can provide good vision at every distance.

Lens Selection

The choice of IOL boils down to the wants and needs of the patient. We have to consider the importance of the different focal distances and how each lens can match their personal lifestyle. No current lens provides absolute perfection, so we must pick the technology with the best balance of pros and cons for each individual. Many of us have found that most patients are happy if we can at least achieve excellent DISTANCE vision. Now, we have to maintain the level of satisfaction with distance vision experienced by our monofocal IOL patients, and try to provide that elusive NEAR vision as well.

One of my first questions is, "What do you do for a living?" Knowing this, I address the potential focal ranges needed and size of font that they would like to see clearly. I also ask about their avocation and hobbies. I try to get a feel for their personality, using the Dell questionnaire, and then ask additional questions. The patient learns that I care about him or her and will try to best satisfy his or her needs and desires for visual rehabilitation. This is a highly interactive process that spans the preoperative and postoperative periods.

How to Select the First Eye Lens

My preference is to address the dominant eye first, and target emmetropia with a Crystalens. With the new 5-0 Crystalens, hitting the refractive target is much easier than in the past.

We congratulate the patient when we achieve our goal. Patients typically get J3 near vision with the Crystalens, which equates to 20/40. Some patients are so satisfied with this result that they then request the same lens in the other eye. Others find that they are not able to read well up close, and we use a +.50 hand held trial lens, to see if this provides adequate near function. If this works, we can then implant a Crystalens with a −.50 or −.75 refractive target for their nondominant second eye. This strategy works quite well, and they may either eliminate or dramatically reduce their need for glasses (using them for fine details only). If, however, they do not achieve the clarity or the reading speed they desire (which does improve over time with all of the premium lenses), we can offer a multifocal IOL for the nondominant second eye.

Formerly myopic patients who loved holding reading material close to see would be good candidates for the new Aspheric ReSTOR (Alcon, Fort Worth, TX) in the second eye. So would someone who loves to read, and wants to see very clearly at near. The Crystalens can provide seamless clear distance, excellent intermediate, and fair to good near, without any light aberrations. The ReSTOR lens provides good distance and excellent near, but only fair intermediate vision. Cortical adaptation to mixed IOLs occurs fairly rapidly and patients assimilate the different images, which are usually not conflicting. In this way, they get the benefit of each lens as a summed result. These are some of the happiest patients, because they never need glasses for any range of distance. They do notice that the two eyes have a slightly different sharpness of vision, but acuity is fairly equal in the distance. The Crystalens takes the prize for outstanding distance clarity and clear intermediate vision. The ReSTOR, although having good, but not as sharp acuity in the distance and night vision, wins the prize for near. Remember, we see our best with binocularity. We must be aware that there are a few patients that truly discern the difference in color vision through the two lenses (especially seeing whites).

There are patient needs that are not met by this combination, as the Crystalens in the first eye may not perform that well for near, or even intermediate, in some patients. If this happens, especially for computer users, the ReSTOR is not the best combination lens for the second eye.

We could make them −.75 myopic with a Crystalens in the second eye, and can try this out on the dominant eye with trial lenses. However, if this strategy does not significantly improve their intermediate vision, I recommend the ReZoom lens (Advanced Medical Optics, Santa Ana, CA) for the second eye. The ReZoom IOL provides excellent distance and intermediate vision, and good near vision. It carries the potential downside of significant halos around lights, which can be quite bothersome. If good distance vision is achieved with the Crystalens, however, the halos from a ReZoom in the nondominant eye can be more easily ignored, and filtered out. Not every ReZoom patient complains about these aberrations, but they can be so bothersome, as to require removal. Most patients do eventually adapt, but it can take 6 to 8 months. With ReSTOR some patients do not see clearly, because their brain cannot tolerate this kind of multifocality. These patients may also require lens removal. In contrast, while the Crystalens can under perform with respect to accommodative range, optical aberrations are rare. It can therefore serve as the replacement lens following explantation of a multifocal IOL.

(Algorithm)

1. Crystalens for Dominant Eye. Aim for Plano to −.25 D.

2. Assess near vision, and determine if it is enough, or if it can be refined with an additional power of 0.5 to 0.75 D. Have patient use that power at distance to see if they will accept a slight myopia for the second eye. (Anecdotally, some patients see 20/20 with a Crystalens having a −.5 to −.1.0 D of myopia).

3. If the patient is satisfied, insert a Crystalens in the second eye. I have the least complaints of all with a bilateral Crystalens system, as long as they can function well enough at near.

4. If they have not achieved adequate near vision, consider a multifocal lens for the second eye (either ReSTOR or ReZoom based on the individual needs of the patient).

5. Use ReSTOR if better near vision is required. Use ReZoom if good intermediate vision is required.

6. Strive to implant matched IOL systems if possible, but prepare your patient in advance that adaptation will be necessary with mixed IOLs.

Special Considerations

THE MYOPIC EYE

The myopic eye, particularly the –1.5 to –2.5 D myope, presents a significant challenge as it is hard to duplicate the clarity and magnification that this patient already has at near. All ophthalmologists should try on a contact lens to see what having this refractive error is like, or in fact, what monovision is like. These patients are usually not satisfied with near vision that is less than perfect, so I often plan to use a Crystalens/ReSTOR combination, which should wow them for distance, and yet still maintain their near function. They are used to moving near objects close up to see, and generally adapt well to this strategy. They could also be candidates for ReSTOR/ReSTOR, but we must be careful of intermediate expectations in this situation. Never underestimate the need for intermediate vision, as we use this range for so many tasks that we perform on a daily basis. A ReZoom/ReSTOR combination can overcome this problem, but there will be halo/glare adaptation issues.

THE ASTIGMATIC EYE

We should also include toric lenses in our armamentarium. I have used the STAAR Toric lens (STAAR Surgical, Monrovia, CA) for years with great success. It has been an easy decision to provide great distance vision for patients with high cylinder that would have left them with a blurred image following traditional cataract surgery. No one sees well through spectacles with a >1 D Cylinder correction, because there is a sweet spot that we must align perfectly with the visual axis, and when they look to the side, the image immediately blurs. These patients are ecstatic, as they have never been able to see so effortlessly and clearly before. This attention to the corneal shape is critical for good outcomes. We now have the Alcon Acrylic Toric, which is also an excellent lens. It is easy to position and remains in the correct alignment, but any residual cortex can bind up the flexible haptics, which will shift the lens slightly out of position. For this reason, it is important to check for expansion of the haptics as you rotate the AcrySof Toric IOL in the capsular bag.

Measuring Devices

To achieve emmetropia, we need exquisitely accurate and reproducible technology. The IOL Master (Carl Zeiss Meditec, Jena, Germany) with its new upgrade is just that. The axial length will come out within .05 microns each time, and the suboptimal keratometry has also been improved with this software upgrade. We are in the process of analyzing results comparing Manual Ks to the upgraded IOL Master Ks, and so far they are very close. Topography is helpful to be able to adjust astigmatism on the correct axis, and look for any corneal irregularities. I use the Pentacam (Oculus Inc, Lynwood, WA) for this. Before we consider a multifocal lens, we must rule out any macular or corneal pathology, including epiretinal membranes, and macular edema or degeneration. Do a thorough clinical exam and use optical coherence tomography (OCT) to examine the macula. We can still consider a Crystalens in these situations, as it acts like a monofocal lens and does not reduce contrast sensitivity.

Planning

My personal preference is to start by implanting the Crystalens for the patient's dominant eye. I feel I can guarantee fantastic distance vision, great intermediate, and better near than any current monofocal lens. I then check the patient's near vision at the 1-week visit, when we carefully discuss the options. I pick the lens for the second eye based on their experience with the first IOL. It is important to have access to an excimer laser to tweak your outcomes when necessary. If you do not have one, develop a relationship with someone who does.

Management of patient expectations is critical for a happy patient, doctor, and staff. The preoperative and 1-week postoperative visits are crucial for building rapport, understanding, and acceptance on the part of our patients.

CHAPTER 126

MONOVISION WITH MONOFOCAL IOLs

William F. Maloney, MD

"Mind the Gaps": Managing the Missing Focus Zone

The popularity of mixing presbyopia-correcting intraocular lenses (IOLs) highlights our growing realization that we do not yet have an off-the-shelf comprehensive presbyopia-correcting IOL. Using my focus zone chart, no lens delivers all 5 zones. Typically, the ReSTOR (Alcon, Fort Worth, TX) misses zone 2 whereas the ReZoom (Advanced Medical Optics, Santa Ana, CA) and Crystalens (Eyeonics, Inc, Aliso Viejo, CA) fail to fully deliver zone 1 focus.

"Mixing" attempts to mitigate the effects of these fixed reading zone deficiencies by employing a complementary pair of refractive IOLs. It is my view that this approach works well and is readily accepted. These strategic IOL combinations also have solid support in current theories of the neurophysiology of binocular vision.

Physiologic Binocular Rivalry: Two Eyes Vying for the Mind's Eye

Strategic pairing of IOLs with different reading capabilities is effective because the "winner" with the better focus for the task at hand is instantly granted access to visual awareness whereas the ineffectual "loser" is readily suppressed and remains unnoticed. The moment that task changes—say from computer work to reading the stock charts—a rematch is instantly underway, this time with the opposite outcome. This continual interocular contest for visual awareness is binocular rivalry at work.

Along with fusion and stereopsis, rivalry is a regular aspect of physiologic binocular vision and our visual neural circuitry evolved to mediate precisely this sort of interocular contest.

That is right; we are hardwired to make effective use of these IOL pairings.

Pseudophakic Monovision: Focus Paired to Achieve Each Desired Result

Pseudophakic monovision is a category of IOL mixing of conventional IOLs with different focal lengths—each with just the right amount of myopic focus. The resulting anisometropic rivalry becomes the vehicle to ride these neural rails and deliver a made-to-order range of uncorrected focus selected to best meet each patient's particular goals.

A candidate's unique anisometropic "sweet spot" is unambiguously revealed by preoperative assessments including interocular defocus tolerance, suppression capacity, targeting, and oculomotor dominance. The most important test measures sensory dominance separately for near and far. With sensory dominance correctly identified, the vast majority of patients instantly and effortlessly accept 2 D or more of anisometropia. Usually, however, no more than 1.50 to 1.75 D of anisometropia is needed because of the additional 1 D of accommodative effect derived from pseudoaccommodation—a very useful property of every conventional IOL. Neuroadaptation is thus not experienced by authentic pseudophakic monovision patients who typically report that their results feel "completely natural" within 1 or 2 days. We are now learning that this is not the case with multifocal patients.

Neuroadaptation: The Foremost Concern With Multifocality

Mixing complementary multifocal IOLs can effectively address the particular focus zone deficiency inherent in each.

However, mixing does nothing to address the prolonged neuroadaptation period these lenses typically require.

Multifocality is fundamentally at odds with current theories of the neurophysiology of binocular vision. We have just seen that the structure and function of the visual cortex evolved to mediate interocular image disparity. Multifocality's intraocular disparity has no physiologic precedent. Without a neural template to separate out and convey the needed focus into awareness, a prolonged neuroadaptation period is required to put in place the necessary neural tracks. As that work goes on, the "smeared" vision emblematic of truncated focus distinction slowly moderates and often—but not always—gradually disappears. It is a testament to the astonishing plasticity of the visual cortex that this is ever accomplished at all, let alone within 6 to 12 months. When adaptation falls short and the patient loses faith explantation is sometimes the only answer, usually despite a technically perfect procedure. Clearly we must identify and exclude those patients who are less likely to neuroadapt, but how?

Monovision Misconceptions

A large part of the conventional wisdom concerning pseudophakic monovision is either incomplete or just plain off the mark. Here are some key misconceptions:

* *Pseudophakic monovision is like permanent contact lens monovision:* Despite the paucity of preoperative assessments and problems related to the contacts themselves, optometric monovision has an acceptance rate of over 65%. Authentic pseudophakic monovision following a comprehensive preoperative assessment has an acceptance rate of 99% in my experience. The difference results from the larger anisometropic "sweet spot" that results from pseudophakic pseudoaccommodation.

* *Surgeons cannot charge for pseudophakic monovision:* There is no noncovered device charge because this approach uses a conventional IOL. However, charges for surgeon's services in conjunction with presbyopia correction are for appropriate refractive assessments and procedures. These are noncovered and apply regardless of the IOL device employed.

* *Pseudophakic monovision creates troublesome visual compromise:* Part of a recent letter from a colleague is perhaps the best response here.

Dear Dr. Maloney

Your article about pseudophakic monovision in last week's issue of *Ocular Surgery News* reminded me to write to thank you for pointing out the advantages of monovision in pseudophakia.

One year ago when I faced cataract surgery, I was emboldened by your stance in favor of monovision in my decisions to choose monovision, even after carefully examining many ReSTOR lens, Crystalens and ReZoom lens patients in our practice. My partners could not imagine that I was going against the flow towards these multifocal pseudophakoi.

Now, one year later, I know that my decision was the correct one. I have strong monovision with −0.25 in my dominant right eye and −3.00 in my non-dominant left eye. I can read the finest print in dim light in an examination room, yet I can also drive an automobile without spectacles. In fact, the only time I even tried to use spectacles after my surgery was in the operating room, but now I find that it works just as well to simply dial my −3.00 into one ocular of the operating microscope.

Keep up the good work! I always enjoy reading your column…

(Name withheld for patient privacy)

I am particularly struck by this colleague's account of his pseudophakic monovision result for what it does not include:

* Any period of neuroadaptation
* Any compromise in stereopsis
* Any compromise in depth perception
* Any compromise in contrast sensitivity
* Any compromise in fine print reading
* Any compromise in intermediate focus
* Any need for "accommodating exercise"

The Right Question: "Which IOL Is Best for This Patient?"

Pseudophakic monovision is perhaps the most versatile approach to presbyopia correction because the accommodative effect is not fixed but rather entirely created. As our colleague's letter attests, it is worthy of your consideration.

Mixing introduces an important new degree of versatility to the premium IOL category as well. A comprehensive approach requires that we shift from emphasis on a single preferred approach where we ask the question, "Which patient is best for this IOL?"

Surgeons should be fully familiar with each alternative so as to be in a position to select the one best able to deliver each candidate's unique reading goals. That is, after all, what our patients assume we have already done when we inform them of this important new option.

Suggested Reading

Blake R, Logothetis, N. Visual competition. *Nature Rev/Neurosci.* 2002;31:1-11.

Blake R, Overton R. The site of binocular rivalry suppression. *Perception.* 1979;8:143-152.

Blake R. A neural theory of binocular rivalry. *Psychol Rev.* 1989;96:145-167.

Lehky S, Blake R. Organization of binocular pathways: modeling and data related to rivalry. *Neural Computation.* 1991;3:44-53.

Ooi TL, He ZJ. Binocular rivalry and visual awareness: the role of attention. *Perception* 1999;25:551-574.

Polonski A, Blake R, Braun J, Heeger J. Neuronal activity in human primary visual cortex correlates with perception during binocular rivalry. *Nature Rev/Neurosci.* 2000;3: 1153-1159.

Sengpiel F, Blakemore C, Harrad R. Interocular suppression in the primary visual cortex: a possible neural basis of binocular rivalry. *Vision Research.* 1995;35:179-195.

Tong F, Nakayama K, Vaughan JT, Kanwisher N. Binocular rivalry and visual awareness in human extra striate cortex. *Neuron.* 1999;21:753-759.

CHAPTER 127

MONOVISION WITH MONOFOCAL IOLS

Graham D. Barrett, MBBCh, FRANZCO, FRACS

Helmholtz was the first to describe the currently accepted mechanism that enables individuals to achieve a dynamic range of focus both for near and far objects. In the human eye this is accomplished by contraction of the ciliary muscle, which results in relaxation of the zonules allowing an increase in curvature of the elastic lens and capsule. The ability of the eye to change its focus for near gradually diminishes with age—a process known as presbyopia—and is no longer functional after cataract surgery.

Surgeons performing cataract surgery typically aim to achieve emmetropia so their patients have excellent unaided distance acuity. There are several options available to correct near vision after cataract surgery.

Spectacles

Monofocal intraocular lens (IOL) implants provide a single plane of focus. If emmetropia is achieved for distance in both eyes, reading glasses with an add power ranging from 2 to 3 D will be required for near vision after surgery. If we look critically at the quality of vision achieved with spectacles whether in the form of progressive, bifocal, or separate reading glasses, they do provide excellent acuity with high contrast sensitivity, perfect stereo-acuity and do not create significant dysphotopsia or unwanted optical images. These patients, however, are functionally dependent on optical aides. Published data on the expectations of patients prior to cataract surgery suggests a paradox.[1] The vast majority do expect to wear reading glasses but a similar proportion rate spectacle independence as being very important following cataract surgery.

Multifocal IOLs

One of the most widely practiced strategies to provide unaided distance and near vision following cataract surgery is the use of multifocal implants. These implants are based on diffractive or refractive optics that provide more than one focal plane. The optical principle is to provide simultaneous focus for near and distance vision. Central cortical processing allows most individuals to ignore the blurred image and concentrate on the image of regard. The superimposition of the defocused image, however, results in reduced contrast sensitivity compared to monofocal IOLs. A review of the literature comparing the results of multifocal IOLs[2] confirmed reduced contrast sensitivity as well as associated dysphotopsia, such as halos, particularly when driving at night. Multifocal IOLs perform well in visual tasks involving high-contrast targets in photopic conditions such as the measurement of Snellen visual acuity. They therefore provide good Snellen acuity and stereo-acuity but the reduced modulation transfer function and dysphotopsia are an important compromise compared to spectacles for near vision.

Accommodating IOLs

An alternative to multifocal implants are accommodating IOLs. These include lenses with hinged and anteriorly vaulted haptics as well as dual optic implants, which have a greater potential for accommodation. These lenses are an attractive alternative to multifocal implants as they do not have the same adverse effects on contrast sensitivity and incidence of dysphotopsia. The efficacy of this type of lens, however, is questionable. A comprehensive review[3] concluded that published objective data showed limited forward translation with single optic accommodating lenses and that convincing psycho visual data demonstrating efficacy was lacking. Furthermore, the fixation characteristics and posterior capsular opacification (PCO) prevention of many current accommodative lens designs are as yet unproven. Because of the limitations of multifocals and accommodating lenses it is worth considering an alternative concept to assist unaided near vision following cataract surgery—the monovision concept.

Monovision

In essence monovision in pseudophakia is aimed at achieving emmetropia in the dominant eye but creating a myopic defocus for near vision in the nondominant eye. Interocular suppression of the blurred image is dependent on higher cortical function. Monovision has been widely practiced with contact lenses since the 1960s with success in approximately 80% of cases.[4] Depending on the age, typically 1 to 2 D of induced myopia in the nondominant eye is employed by practitioners who practice monovision with contact lens correction. From the contact lens literature monovision presents several potential problems. Patients with high ocular dominance are often not able to fully suppress the blurred image. In particular high contrast, high frequency images proved to be troublesome, particularly in low illumination. Finally, there may be interference with binocular function and reduced stereo acuity.

Monovision is also widely practiced in patients undergoing refractive surgery. Generally all patients 40 years or older undergoing laser in situ keratomileusis (LASIK) are offered monovision as an alternative to having both eyes corrected for distance. My own experience concurs with the results published in the literature, which suggests that patients are highly satisfied with monovision correction after LASIK in the presbyopic age group.[5] Interestingly the data suggest that patients corrected for distance in both eyes were equally happy to those who selected monovision, emphasizing the importance of counseling patients and involving them in deciding what form of correction is preferred.

Monovision can be an effective solution for unaided near vision for pseudophakic patients. Surprisingly there is a paucity of published studies concerning pseudophakic monovision in the literature, but what is available demonstrates a very high success rate. In a study published by Greenbaum,[6] 92% of patients achieved 20/30 and J1 unaided acuity with a 90% acceptance rate. This raises the question whether modifying the degree of intended myopia in monovision for pseudophakia could increase patients' satisfaction and the overall acceptance rate. As indicated previously visual acuity testing with high contrast targets such as Snellen acuity is insufficient to explain patient satisfaction so more information is required to identify the limitations and to recommend which patients are best suited for monovision as a strategy in cataract surgery.

Required Myopic Defocus for Monovision in Pseudophakia

We have all been surprised to encounter patients in the waiting room who have had bilateral monofocal IOL implants who have excellent unaided distance acuity, and are happily reading the newspaper without glasses after cataract surgery. I decided to look at the refractive outcome in a series of my own patients in whom I performed cataract surgery with a monofocal lens to identify what degree of myopic defocus was required for adequate near vision. In my audit I recorded unaided near and distance acuity as well as the spherical equivalent refractive error. Previously I did not routinely encourage monovision so this group of patients was intended to be emmetropic with a small amount of residual myopia to assist with near vision. The mean spherical equivalent of myopia of this group of patients was −0.38 D with the majority of patients clustered between 0 and −0.50 D. This minor level of myopia provided excellent unaided distance acuity typically 20/20 or 20/25 with unaided near vision N10 (J6) or decimal 0.33 to 0.4, which is the print size of novels and magazines.

Examination of the patients who ended up more myopic at −1.00 D revealed that distance acuity was reduced to 20/40 but the unaided near vision improved to N5 (J1) or 0.67 equivalent to the smallest type in general use. The results suggested that pseudoaccommodation with monofocal implants does exist and −1.00 to −1.50 D of myopia should be sufficient for the majority of near vision tasks. I also noted that binocular summation is also a feature of monovision correction in that near acuity improved by approximately one line with binocular compared to monocular testing. These results proved helpful in planning a strategy to avoid the limitations of traditional monovision, which is usually aimed at a myopic defocus of −2.00 D in the nondominant eye.

Contrast Sensitivity, Stereo-Acuity, and Binocular Rivalry

Contact lens studies[7] have demonstrated that contrast sensitivity may be reduced with monovision. With binocular viewing, however, the reduction in contrast for near increases as the myopic defocus approaches −2.00 D and then improves at higher levels of difference between the dominant and nondominant eye. The reduction in contrast can therefore be minimized by limiting the myopic defocus to −1.50 D in the eye intended for near vision.

Stereo-acuity may also be compromised with monovision. The refractive surgical literature[8] demonstrated a significant reduction with the Titmus stereo-acuity test at levels of anisometropia of 2.00 D and greater. Once again the data suggest an upper limit of −1.50 D myopic defocus for monovision in pseudophakia.

Previous studies[9] evaluating ocular dominance and patient satisfaction in monovision noted that strong ocular dominance or rivalry may result in asthenopia, particularly when the anisometropia was greater than −2.00 D. This suggests that the level of myopic defocus should be limited to avoid this problem.

Recommendations

These insights have led to my current preferred practice for patients undergoing cataract surgery or clear lens replacement. I aim for emmetropia for distance in the first eye (preferably dominant eye) and if achieved I aim for −1.00 D of myopia in the second eye. I have found this level of myopia is sufficient to provide a high level of spectacle independence both for distance and near. The level of myopia, however, still provides reasonable distance acuity and preserves contrast sensitivity and stereo-acuity. Furthermore, limiting the difference in refraction to −1.00 D avoids symptoms of asthenopia due to binocular rivalry.

My experience suggests that is not as critical for the dominant eye to be targeted for distance as is the custom with higher levels of myopic defocus. I elect to perform surgery in the eye that has the greater degree of cataract and poorer vision and aim for emmetropia—even if this is not the dominant eye, which can be difficult to determine with significant cataract.

Bill Maloney has suggested an alternative approach where he classifies functional vision into different zones and discusses with patients their preference in relation to these zones to help determine lens power selection and the degree of intended monovision.[10] Zone 1 consists of activities requiring small print whereas zone 5 emphasizes distance acuity with low illumination. I think this is a useful alternative strategy and Bill recommends a myopic refraction of −2.00 D for Zone 1, −1 D for zone 2, and −0.50 for zone 3.

My preference, however, is based on the principle that a monofocal lens provides a good range of focus and −0.50 D adequately covers zone 2 to 4. In my experience −1.00 D of myopic defocus satisfied near vision requirements of most patients and is a well-tolerated form of monovision.

Prospective Study

In order to evaluate the strategy of modified monovision in more detail I have conducted a prospective study on monovision in pseudophakia with my current fellow, Dr Yaron Finkelman. In this study the first eye was targeted for emmetropia and if achieved the second eye had a target refraction of −1.00 D. The important outcomes measured included the unaided near and distance acuity, spherical equivalent refractive error, as well as a modified V14 questionnaire to evaluate the level of spectacle independence and patient satisfaction after surgery.

The unaided acuity achieved so far is encouraging in that 80% of patients have achieved N6 (J2) and 100% (J3) or better binocular near acuity. Similarly the unaided distance acuity is excellent with 80% 20/20 and 100% 20/30 or better unaided binocular distance acuity. The mean spherical equivalent refractive error in the distance eye was −0.19 D and for the near eye −1.36 D.

Patients were also asked to rate their need for contact lenses or glasses after surgery. The scale runs from 0 to 10 where 0 is "I am completely free from glasses or contact lenses" and 10 is "totally dependent on glasses or contact lenses." The average score was 1.3, demonstrating that the vast majority of patients considered themselves spectacle independent. On a similar scale patients were asked to estimate their satisfaction or dissatisfaction after surgery where 0 is "not satisfied at all" and 10 "very satisfied." An average score of 9.9 indicated that the vast majority of patients were highly satisfied with the refractive outcome.

Advantages of Monovision

Monovision is a viable alternative to improving unaided near vision in pseudophakia. In comparison to other strategies, modified monovision for near correction achieves excellent acuity. There is some reduction in contrast sensitivity although significantly less than occurs with multifocal implants. Although stereo-acuity may be diminished this does

not lead to subjective complaints if the intended degree of monovision is limited to −1.00 to −1.50 D. The most appealing aspect of monovision, however, is that it is reversible and full binocular vision can be simply restored with the aid of spectacles when required.

Patient Selection

I recommend aiming for −1.00 D of myopia in the non-dominant eye to avoid potential limitations that can occur at higher levels of anisometropia. One of the attractive features of monovision is the ability to easily demonstrate to patients the type of vision they can expect. After surgery in the first eye has been completed the amount of myopic defocus can be simply demonstrated with the addition of a +1.00 lens. The patient can immediately appreciate the effect on distance acuity as well as the amount of near vision they can expect if the target refraction is achieved. Patients need to be informed of their choices regarding options for unaided near vision when undergoing cataract surgery or lens replacement for refractive errors. Typically approximately 50% of patients will elect to have monovision rather than aim for emmetropia for distance in both eyes. The selection process for monovision is less demanding than multifocal implants and patients are better able to comprehend their choices.

Adaptation

Monovision occurs naturally in many individuals and is more physiological than the simultaneous near and distance focus images provided by multifocal implants. Patients who achieve modified monovision are able to appreciate the improved functionality in their near vision immediately without the period of neuroadaption, which is necessary in some patients who have had multifocal lenses implanted.

Patient Satisfaction

Most surgeons will have encountered unhappy patients who have had bilateral multifocal implants performed. Even with careful selection the compromise in quality of vision for some patients is unacceptable. In contrast modified monovision is widely accepted by patients and the degree of myopia can be altered with optical aids or LASIK if required.

Relatively minor levels of astigmatism, posterior capsular opacification, and macula dysfunction have a greater affect on visual acuity with multifocal implants compared to monofocal implants. Although multifocal IOLs may provide acceptable vision in the immediate postoperative period, complicating factors may become significant years after cataract surgery has been performed. Astigmatism can be corrected with limbal relaxing incisions but there is a tendency to against-the-rule change with time. Furthermore a decline in macula function can be expected with age. The quality of vision with modified monovision is less likely to be compromised by these factors.

All cataract and implant surgery regardless of the type of implant demands careful attention to the refractive outcome and the highest standard of surgery. Although "premium" is a description currently in vogue to refer to multifocal lenses it is a misconception that other solutions require any less care in planning and skill. Excellent outcomes for monovision require precision biometry and management of associated astigmatism, either with limbal incisions or toric monofocal IOLs. It is somewhat surprising that considering the limitations, multifocal IOLs are currently being embraced with enthusiasm, and monovision is not more widely practiced. The increased use of multifocal implants is to some extent driven by industry and has financial implications relating to reimbursement. It is important that these issues do not influence the consideration of alternative strategies for near vision in pseudophakia, such as monovision, in providing solutions to our patients.

References

1. Hawker MJ, Madge SN, Baddeley PA, Perry SR. Refractive expectations of patients having cataract surgery. *J Cataract Refract Surg.* 2005;31(10):1970-1975.
2. Leyland M, Zinicola E. Multifocal versus monofocal intraocular lenses in cataract surgery: a systematic review. *Ophthalmology.* 2003;110:1789-1798.
3. Burkhard Dick H. Accommodative intraocular lenses: current status. *Curr Opin Ophthalmol.* 2005;16:8-26.
4. Johannsdottir KR, Stelmach LB. Monovision: a review of the scientific literature. *Optometry Vision Sci.* 2001;78:646-651.
5. Goldberg DB. Laser in situ keratomileusis monovision. *J Cataract Refract Surgeons.* 2001;27:1449-1455.
6. Greenbaum S. Monovision pseudophakia. *J Cataract Refract Surgeons.* 2002;28:1439-1443.
7. Pardhan S, Gilchrist J. The effect of monocular defocus on binocular contrast sensitivity. *Ophthalmic Physiol Opt.* 1990;10(1):33-36.
8. Wright KW, Guemes A, Kapadia MS, Wilson SE. Binocular function and patient satisfaction after monovision induced by myopic photorefractive keratectomy. *J Cataract Refract Surgeons.* 1999;25:177-182.
9. Handa T, Mukuno K, Uozato H, Niida T, Shoji N, Minei R, Nitta M, Shimizu K. Ocular dominance and patient satisfaction after monovision induced by lens implantation. *J Cataract Refracti Surgeons.* 2004;30:769-774.
10. Maloney WF. Let the patient, not the technology, guide approach in presbyopia correction. *Ocular Surgery News,* Aug 15, 2004.

CHAPTER 128

MULTIFOCAL IOL IN ONE EYE?

Frank A. Bucci, Jr, MD

The question is frequently asked whether multifocal implants can be used successfully as a unilateral option. This chapter summarizes my experience using unilateral multifocal implants in 150 patients. All of these patients received either a ReSTOR (Alcon, Fort Worth, TX) (n = 46) or a ReZoom (Advanced Medical Optics, Santa Ana, CA) (n = 104) multifocal implant from June 2005 until June 2007. For a number of years prior to June 2005, I had selectively implanted the Array multifocal lenses (Advanced Medical Optics) on a unilateral basis. I specifically recall 3 internists who were able to perform their daily medical charting without spectacle correction with only one Array multifocal implant. Numerous cataract patients functioned well with one Array multifocal implant and one monofocal intraocular lens (IOL). The visual function of these patients strongly suggested that different types of optical systems are well tolerated if certain visual goals are achieved. Tolerating different optical systems has been the basis for the widespread success of mixing and matching multifocal implants. It is interesting to note that 3 of the unilateral Array patients referred to above were part of a group of 6 unilateral Array patients who eventually received a diffractive ReSTOR lens in their opposite eye years following their original implantation of the Array implant. The overall success of these Array/ReSTOR patients was the basis for subsequently pursuing ReZoom/ReSTOR in 126 patients with outstanding results. Just because the addition of the ReSTOR lens completed the patient's goal of full spectacle independence, we should not underestimate the contribution of one Array multifocal lens, which enhanced the independent visual performance of these presbyopic patients for years prior to receiving the ReSTOR lens.

The ReSTOR multifocal implant was my unilateral multifocal implant of choice from June 2005 until December 2005. The mean age of 21 cataract and 25 refractive lensectomy patients was 59 years. Twenty-two patients had a monofocal lens in their opposite eye and 24 patients were phakic in the opposite eye. Objectively, these eyes achieved excellent visual outcomes. Those patients with greater than 0.75 D of astig-matism received either astigmatic keratectomy (AK) or laser vision correction postoperatively to maximize their uncorrected visual acuity. Fourteen eyes underwent a postoperative microradial keratotomy (RK)/AK procedure whereas 4 eyes underwent laser vision correction (2 photorefractive keratectomy [PRK] and 2 laser in situ keratomileusis [LASIK]). The distance target refraction was plano to +0.25, with a goal of having less than 0.5 D of astigmatism. The mean postoperative spherical equivalent achieved was +0.17 D and the mean magnitude of postoperative astigmatism was +0.41 D. The preoperative refractive errors of these ReSTOR eyes were 41.0% hyperopia, 35.9% myopia, and 23.1% emmetropia.

Unfortunately, the subjective response of these patients was poor and did not contribute postoperatively to the overall multifocal lens experience of my practice. In general, the visual performance of the ReSTOR multifocal implant was disappointing to most patients. Patient satisfaction was very low, secondary to 1) poor intermediate vision and the inability to see their computers, desktops, and kitchen counters, etc.; 2) a focal point that they perceived as being too close to their face; 3) a generalized waxy vision, which was present both at distance and near; and 4) a subtle, but distinct, loss of uncorrected and/or best-corrected distance visual acuity.

Three patients had a very severe form of waxy vision, which I have reported on previously and call "Vaseline vision dysphotopsia".[1] Vaseline vision dysphotopsia in these 3 patients led to explantations and IOL exchanges for 3 ReZoom multifocal implants. All 3 unilateral ReSTOR explantations (for a ReZoom IOL) were emmetropic lensectomy patients with a mean age of 50 years. These disappointing results with unilateral ReSTOR multifocal implants (except as a mix-and-match combination with another multifocal) led to the abandonment of the ReSTOR at the end of 2005.

Subsequently, over the next 18 months, we successfully implanted 104 ReZoom multifocal implants. Fifty-three cataract and 51 refractive lensectomy patients received the ReZoom multifocal unilaterally. Fifteen patients had a monofocal lens in their opposite eye, whereas 89 patients were phakic in the opposite eye. The preoperative refractive errors for the ReZoom unilateral eyes were 31.5% hyperopes, 38.0% myopes, and 30.4% emmetropes. Distance target refraction was plano to –0.25 and the goal again was to have less than .5 D of astigmatism. Mean spherical equivalent postoperatively was –0.11 D of myopia and the mean amount of postoperative astigmatism was 0.38 D. Forty of 92 patients received a postoperative enhancement procedure for residual refractive error. Twenty-three patients had micro-RK/AK, 12 patients had LASIK, and 5 patients had PRK.

Although the actual objective visual outcomes between the ReZoom and ReSTOR are not extremely different (Table 1), the subjective response to the ReZoom lens was extremely different compared to that we experienced with the ReSTOR. Patients were happy to have clear distance vision, especially during the day, their intermediate vision was significantly enhanced, and they had a substantial amount of reading. Some patients continued to need spectacles for near vision or fine print, but because they were carefully counseled preoperatively, this was not a disappointment.

Neuroadaptation to halos during night driving progressed much more rapidly than was experienced with the Array multifocal lens. In addition, in the opposite eye these patients were either emmetropic or frequently corrected with a contact lens, which provided these patients a nonhaloed image while driving at night. In my experience, this dramatically reduces the overall patient complaints with regard to halos.

As with all potential multifocal implant patients, preoperative counseling, managing patient expectations, and careful overall patient selection are still critical in achieving success and high levels of patient satisfaction with unilateral multifocal implants. The unilateral ReZoom lens was an excellent prelude to a potential refractive/diffractive combination in the future presbyopic life of these patients. My practice currently contains over 50 patients functioning successfully with one

ReZoom lens and who are anticipating implantation of the Tecnis multifocal diffractive lens (Advanced Medical Optics) in their opposite eye upon Food and Drug Administration (FDA) approval. There are numerous European and South American surgeons who are reporting very high levels of success with the ReZoom/Tecnis multifocal IOL combination.

Conclusion

A unilateral ReZoom multifocal implant placed opposite a phakic or a pseudophakic eye is a viable first option in presbyopic cataract and refractive lensectomy patients. A unilateral multifocal is a viable option compared to 2 monofocals, 2 multifocals, monovision IOLs, or other means of correcting presbyopia without implants. Although my current experience with the new Crystalens 5.0 (Eyeonics, Inc, Aliso Viejo, CA) accommodating IOL is limited, I believe that it has the characteristics consistent with successful use as a unilateral presbyopia-correcting (Pr-C) IOL. It has excellent distance vision, both during the day and at night, it has excellent intermediate vision, and it provides the patient with substantial reading vision compared to the patient's preoperative implant status. The lack of fine detailed reading with the Crystalens 5.0 could easily be enhanced in the future presbyopic life of these patients with a Tecnis multifocal refractive implant as envisioned with the ReZoom IOL. Both the ReZoom and the Crystalens 5.0 have excellent intermediate vision, which complements the only minor weakness of the Tecnis multifocal lens, whereas the ability to read fine print independent of pupil size with the Tecnis multifocal complements the one weakness of the ReZoom and Crystalens 5.0. For the extremely halo-phobic patients, the Crystalens 5.0 might be the unilateral lens of choice before later being paired with the Tecnis multifocal lens, but still providing a nonhaloed image in one eye while driving at night throughout the life of the presbyopic patients.

It is my clinical impression that Pr-C IOLs with excellent intermediate vision (such as the ReZoom and Crystalens 5.0) should be the first lens implanted when a long delay is expected before the implantation of the second Pr-C IOL. The patients appear to prefer to have their refractive errors corrected in a descending order from distance, intermediate, to near. Patients with strongly corrected near vision, who are lacking intermediate vision, are frequently not comfortable with this experience. I believe this observation helps explain the divergent patient acceptance of the unilateral use of a ReSTOR multifocal versus a ReZoom multifocal lens.

As more multifocal implants become available with improved optical performances, use of a unilateral Pr-C IOL, either temporarily or permanently, continues to be a viable alternative for surgeons and their presbyopic patients.

IOLs Selection: Can I Implant a Multifocal IOL in Just One Eye?

Richard J. Mackool, MD

The key to implantation of a multifocal intraocular lens (IOL) in one eye of a patient whose other eye is either phakic, or pseudophakic with a monofocal lens, is informed consent. Such patients should be informed as to what they might expect, the problems that might arise, and what would be done if such a problem did occur.

Young patients who have a normal lens (not presbyopic) in their other eye are, in general, not excellent candidates for multifocal lens insertion. The latter will often be unfavorably compared to their "perfect" eye.

I have found that the overwhelming majority of patients who have a monofocal lens in one eye do extremely well with a multifocal ReSTOR (Alcon, Fort Worth, TX) lens in their other eye. These patients have already experienced the benefits and deficiencies of a monofocal IOL, and can readily understand the advantages of a multifocal lens. If the previously operated eye is essentially plano, I inform them that they might notice that they have slightly sharper distance vision in that eye but their unaided near vision will almost certainly be vastly superior in the eye receiving the multifocal lens. I also explain that, should they desire to read using both eyes, a near vision spectacle of approximately equal strength OU will be required (otherwise aniseikonia will occur).

If the previously operated eye has good uncorrected intermediate vision, eg, spherical equivalent refraction of –1.00 to –2.00, I inform them that distance and near acuity will be better in the multifocal eye, but intermediate acuity is likely to be best in the monofocal eye. I also explain that spectacles can be worn to make both eyes approximately equal at distance, intermediate, and near.

Lastly, and of greatest potential difficulty, if the previously operated eye has good uncorrected near vision, eg, spherical equivalent refraction of at least –2.25, I inform them that they will have absolute monovision for distance if a multifocal lens is implanted, and that wearing a distance vision correction for the monofocal eye would not be likely to produce satisfactory binocular distance vision (a contact lens could of course solve this problem). I also explain that intermediate vision is likely to remain "weaker" than both distance and near vision.

Regardless of the above, all patients who receive multifocal IOL technology should be informed that there is a small subset of patients who will not be satisfied with the results. In such cases, IOL exchange can be required and the patient should know this in advance.

CHAPTER 129

MIXING IOLs—
WHAT ARE THE OPTIONS?

Elizabeth A. Davis, MD, FACS and Richard L. Lindstrom, MD

If one described the perfect intraocular lens (IOL), it would include perfect quality vision without aberrations or contrast loss, seamless accommodation from distance to near, absence of dysphotopsias or posterior capsule opacification, and no loss of function with time. Unfortunately, no such IOL exists. Every currently available lens has benefits and disadvantages. Because of this, it may sometimes be useful to combine lenses of different types in a single patient to enhance his or her functional outcome, the overall goal being to maximize vision and to reduce unwanted side effects.

It is important for the ophthalmologist to understand the strengths and weaknesses of each IOL to best use complimentary ("mix and match") IOLs.

Available IOLs:
Strengths and Weaknesses

The standard monofocal IOL is the best economic value. It gives excellent distance, fair intermediate, and poor near vision. For example, uncorrected acuity might typically measure 20/20+, J4, and J7 at the 3 distances. The overall pseudoaccommodative amplitude is approximately 2 D, which means it has about 1 D of pseudoaccommodative amplitude toward the minus side. This means that if the patient is targeted for a −1.50 refractive outcome, he or she will be able to read as though he or she had a +2.00 to +2.50 reader. The lens has positive spherical aberration of approximately +0.10 μm, which is somewhat dependent on optic power and optic design. This type of pseudophakic spherical aberration is best used in patients who have negative spherical aberrations in the cornea. These would include posthyperopic laser in situ keratomileusis (LASIK) or keratoconus patients or those who have corneas with naturally occurring negative spherical aberration (10% to 20%).

Second, we have aspheric monofocal IOLs, including those with no spherical aberration (Bausch & Lomb Advanced Optic [Rochester, NY]) and those with negative spherical aberration (Advanced Medical Optics Tecnis [Santa Ana, CA], Alcon IQ [Fort Worth, TX]). The IOL with no spherical aberration is most forgiving of decentration and tilt and might be selected in patients whose decentration might occur such as in pseudoexfoliation, a capsular tear, or where an ideal capsulorrhexis is not available.

The implants with negative spherical aberration give better quality of vision, especially mesopic vision in the patient with a typical cornea with positive spherical aberration. They also provide superior performance in the patient that has undergone myopic keratorefractive surgery.

The accommodating IOL as designed by Eyeonics, Inc (Aliso Viejo, CA) (the Crystalens) gives excellent distance and intermediate vision. Typically, one can achieve 20/20+ and J1 at distance and intermediate, respectively. It provides good near acuity with a typical outcome being J3 or better. This lens has the least night vision symptoms, the least loss of contrast sensitivity, and the least color distortion of all presbyopia-correcting IOLs. It is also pupil size independent in its optical function. It is excellent for blended vision.

The zonal aspheric multifocal IOL manufactured by Advanced Medical Optics (the ReZoom) provides good distance acuity, good intermediate acuity, and good near acuity. Typical outcomes are 20/20 distance, J2 intermediate, and J2 at near. There are some night vision symptoms, some loss of contrast sensitivity, and some color distortion. This lens is pupil size dependent.

The aspheric diffractive multifocal IOL (Advanced Medical Optics Tecnis diffractive multifocal IOL) provides good distance acuity, fair intermediate, and excellent near acuity. Typical outcomes to be expected are 20/20- at distance, J4 at intermediate, and J1 at near. It also has the potential for night vision symptoms, decreased contrast sensitivity, and some color distortion. The decreased contrast sensitivity usually associated with a multifocal implant is reduced by the aspheric nature of the optic. This lens is not pupil-size dependent.

The apodized diffractive/refractive multifocal IOL (Alcon ReSTOR) provides good distance acuity, fair intermediate, and excellent near. Distance acuity might be expected to be 20/20-, intermediate J4, and near J1. This lens also potentially generates night vision symptoms, decreased contrast sensitivity, and color distortion. It is also pupil-size dependent as the lens becomes more distance dominant as the pupil dilates.

Mix and Match Options

There are presently 3 main categories of IOLs: monofocal (spheric, aspheric, and toric), accommodative, and multifocal. Amongst these lenses, there are 5 basic mixing combinations possible. The first combination is the use of 2 monofocal IOLs with differing focal points to achieve monovision. This can be a very successful option, particularly in patients who have worn such a correction in contact lenses. The exact focal point of the near eye can be chosen to suit the patient's needs. Targeting myopia of 1.0 to 1.75 D allows for functional intermediate vision, whereas a target of 2.0 to 2.5 D provides true near vision. The monovision approach requires neuroadaptation with suppression of the near eye when gazing at distant objects and suppression of the distance eye when focusing up close. The greater the disparity between eyes, the more difficult it is for the patient to adapt. Nevertheless, there is the benefit of maintaining high quality of vision with the monofocal optics. Pseudophakic monovision is a good option in patients who have the potential for development of eye diseases that impact contrast sensitivity (eg, glaucoma, macular degeneration, diabetic retinopathy). It is also a good option in an eye that has undergone keratorefractive surgery (eg, excimer laser ablation, incisional keratotomy) where corneal irregularities may already impact contrast acuity and visual quality.

The second mixing combination is a monofocal IOL with an accommodating IOL. This option provides excellent distance and intermediate vision and fairly good near vision (J3). If some myopia is targeted in the eye with the accommodating IOL, a stronger near point can be achieved, albeit with some sacrifice of distance acuity in that eye. This combination may be particularly useful when the patient has had prior lens surgery in one eye with a monofocal IOL and desires enhanced near vision in the second eye without sacrificing quality. This approach maintains high quality of vision with monofocal optics. It too is a good option in patients at risk for eye diseases or who have previously undergone corneal refractive surgery.

A third combination is a monofocal IOL with a multifocal IOL. Here, both eyes can achieve excellent distance vision with the added benefit of some pseudoaccommodation in the multifocal eye. The ReZoom multifocal IOL provides excellent intermediate vision and good near vision whereas the ReSTOR IOL provides excellent near vision but minimal intermediate vision. As with all multifocal IOLs, there is a chance for glare, halos and reduced contrast acuity. However, most patients find these symptoms to diminish with time. Additionally, should they occur, limiting their presence to only one eye may be mitigating.

The fourth option for mixing IOLs involves an accommodative IOL with a multifocal IOL. This is similar to the third option described in terms of quality of vision, but with enhanced intermediate vision.

Lastly, one can mix 2 multifocal IOLs of differing types. Many surgeons find this useful when the patient seems to be comfortable with and adaptable to multifocal optics but has a strong desire for improving both uncorrected intermediate and near vision. Mixing a ReZoom and ReSTOR IOL can achieve this result.

For all of these combinations it is imperative to treat any pre-existing conditions that may impair vision. This includes treatment or management of lid malposition, blepharitis, dry eye, and anterior basement dystrophy. Intraoperatively, attention to IOL centration/positioning is particularly important with the toric, accommodating, and multifocal IOLs. Improper positioning of these IOLs may not only reduce their effectiveness but may impair the visual outcome. Techniques that reduce the incidence of posterior capsular opacification (PCO) and capsular phimosis (adequate capsulorrhexis size, symmetric capsular shape, meticulous cortical cleanup, and capsular optic overlap) are also important. Use of nonsteroidal anti-inflammatory eye drops for several weeks postoperatively may prevent cystoid macular edema (CME), which even in subtle forms can impair contrast acuity. A plan to treat any corneal astigmatism of 0.75 D or greater is often required. If a toric IOL is not used, then incisional keratotomies, laser excimer ablation, or conductive keratoplasty should be considered.

As always, to achieve optimal outcomes for any of these choices, preoperative patient counseling is critical. The surgeon should understand the patient's needs and preferences. Additionally, the patient should be made aware of the limitations of all of these choices and the potential compromises and side effects. The patient should be informed of the potential need for additional enhancement surgeries and the associated costs and risks.

Outcomes With Mix and Match

Select recent clinical series of mix and match with some multifocal and accommodating IOLs provide insight into the outcomes that might be obtained. Leonardo Akaishi, MD and Pedro Paulo Fabri from Sao Paulo, Brazil have performed a comparative series of ReZoom/ReZoom, ReSTOR/ReSTOR, ReZoom/ReSTOR, and Tecnis Diffractive/ReZoom. Their outcomes are summarized in Table 1. The best outcomes were obtained with ReZoom/ReSTOR and ReZoom/Tecnis Diffractive Intraocular Lens combinations.

Rick Milne, MD from Columbia, SC has also performed a comparative series looking at patient satisfaction, spectacle independence, and daytime and nighttime halo. His outcomes are summarized in Table 2. Again, the ReZoom/ReSTOR outcomes generated higher patient satisfaction than the ReSTOR/ReSTOR outcomes in this series.

Frank A. Bucci, Jr MD from Wilkes-Barre, PA has also completed a series comparing ReSTOR/ReSTOR to ReZoom/ReZoom. His outcomes are summarized in Table 3. Of note is that his intermediate vision outcomes are significantly better with ReZoom/ReSTOR than with ReSTOR/ReSTOR and that his patient satisfaction is also higher.

Finally, Trevor Woodhams, MD from Atlanta, GA has a series of patients with Crystalens/ReSTOR use in alternate

Table 1

VISUAL OUTCOMES OF VARIOUS MIX AND MATCH COMBINATIONS

	ReZoom/ReZoom (N = 100)	ReSTOR/ReSTOR (N = 100)	ReZoom/ReSTOR (N = 88)	ReZoom/Tecnis Diffractive (N = 15)
Bilateral uncorrected distance	20/20	20/25	20/20	20/20
Bilateral uncorrected intermediate	J2.15	J3.85	J2.30	J2.10
Bilateral uncorrected near	J2.30	J1.40	J1.50	J1.10
Average reading speed (words per minute)	125	165	155	185
Spectacle independence	75%	89%	100%	100%
Halos/glare	2+	1+	1+	1-
MTF	0.20	0.12	0.18	0.38

Data from Leonardo Akaishi, MD and Pedro Paulo Fabri, MD.

Table 2

RESULTS OF PATIENT QUESTIONNAIRE FOR TWO MIX AND MATCH COMBINATIONS

	ReSTOR/ReSTOR (N = 30+)	ReZoom/ReSTOR (N = 30+)
Satisfied/very satisfied	83%	96%
Neutral dissatisfied	0	4%
Very dissatisfied	17%	0%
Would have procedure again, recommend to family and friends	70%	97%
Complete spectacle independence	65%	94%
Daytime halo	43%	18%
Nighttime halo	86%	71%
Requesting explants	6%	0%

Data from Rick Milne, MD.

eyes. Again, he found excellent distance, intermediate, and near vision with high patient satisfaction (Table 4).

Mixing IOLs is an established and successful strategy for many patients. All of the above combinations have been performed with excellent outcomes by the authors. The choice of which IOLs to use depends upon patient lifestyle, preference, and personality. Until the "perfect" IOL is developed, mixing IOLs will remain a useful strategy for correcting vision for our patients.

Table 3

VISUAL OUTCOMES AND DISTANCE, INTERMEDIATE, AND NEAR FOR TWO MIX AND MATCH COMBINATIONS

	ReSTOR/ReSTOR (N = 55+)	ReZoom/ReSTOR (N = 39+)	
Bilateral uncorrected distance	20/25	20/25	(P=NS)
Bilateral uncorrected intermediate	J3.81	J2.39	(P.001)
Bilateral uncorrected near	J1.00	J1.04	(P=NS)
Unhappy with intermediate	32%	0%	

Data from Frank A. Bucci, Jr, MD.

Table 4

VISUAL OUTCOMES FOR CRYSTALENS/RESTOR COMBINATION

	Crystalens/ReSTOR (N = 32)
Bilateral uncorrected distance	20/25
Bilateral uncorrected intermediate	J1.3
Bilateral uncorrected near	J1.3

Data from Trevor Woodhams, MD.

CHAPTER 130

BILATERAL MULTIFOCALS— MIXING VERSUS MATCHING

Con Moshegov, MD, FRANZCO, FRACS

Multifocal intraocular lenses (IOLs) are being increasingly used in both cataract and clear lens (refractive) surgery.

Surgeons should not underestimate the joy people derive from being able to do the following simple things:

* Read menus
* See price tags
* Put on eye make up
* Read messages on their cell phones
* Watch TV
* Drive a car

…without glasses!

Cataract surgery is increasingly being offered to much younger patients than in the past. These patients are well educated as to the possibility of spectacle independence with the procedure. Because they are very active, the prospect of being less dependent on glasses to perform daily activities is very attractive to them.

Furthermore, an increasing number of patients presenting for consideration of refractive surgery are in the older presbyopic age group. Refractive lens exchange (or clear lens extraction) is an increasingly popular alternative to laser refractive surgery in these patients.

One way to achieve relative spectacle independence is through bilateral multifocal IOL implantation. Some believe that the best results are achieved by implanting different presbyopia-correcting IOLs in each eye. The question is should we be mixing or matching multifocal IOL technologies?

Multifocal IOL Technology

My experience has been with 4 multifocal IOLs: Array (Advanced Medical Optics, Santa Ana, CA), ReZoom (Advanced Medical Optics), Tecnis multifocal (Advanced Medical Optics), and AcrySof ReSTOR (Alcon, Fort Worth, TX).

The first widely available multifocal IOL was the Array. This is a refractive multizonal multifocal lens with its center geared to distance vision. It has been associated with a higher degree of unwanted visual aberrations such as halos and glare. Additionally, with small pupils obscuring the reading portion of the lens, some patients implanted with the Array just cannot read at close range unless they wear glasses.

The more advanced ReZoom is characterized by a larger (distance weighted) central zone surrounded by a larger (but slightly more peripheral) near weighted zone. Because studies with this IOL have not been as exhaustive as with the Array (the Food and Drug Administration [FDA] did not demand as much investigation because the design of the lens closely resembled the previously approved Array), it is difficult to quantify the incidence but, though better, the problem of marked haloing and glare persists.

The AcrySof ReSTOR IOL (Figure 1) is now the most the most widely implanted multifocal IOL in the world. The benefits of this lens have been confirmed in numerous US and international studies.

The optic is designed with a central 3.6-mm diffractive component surrounded by a conventional refractive portion. The central part of the optic is designed to enable both distance and near vision, while the surrounding area is purely for distance vision correction. The idea was that the diffractive component would contribute less to the optical pathway of incoming light rays in the dark (when the pupil is large).

International data on the ReSTOR have indicated that the lens provides excellent near vision with little or no compromise to distance visual acuity. Reduction in contrast sensitivity is minimal and yet the reduction in spectacle dependence compared to monofocal controls is immense. Visual disturbances are easily tolerated.

In my experience, visual outcomes with the ReSTOR IOL are comparable to those of a monofocal single-piece AcrySof lens. Yet, 95% of patients see J4 almost immediately. The near point averages about 12 to 13 inches with this lens.

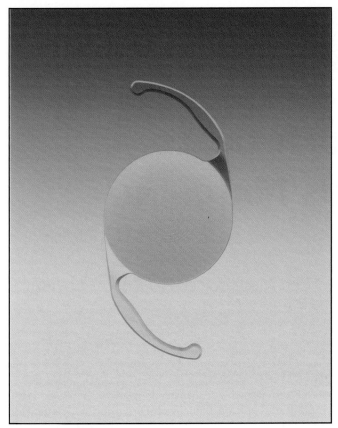

Figure 1. AcrySof ReSTOR IOL.

Intermediate vision can be less than optimal with the ReSTOR. If patients note difficulty seeing computer monitors (about 24 inches from the eyes), a pair of +1.00-D spectacle magnifiers can assist greatly. Often these can be discontinued after a few months by which time the patient adapts to the technology.

Fewer than 10% of patients with the ReSTOR complain of marked visual disturbances; the majority note only mild halos, glare, night vision problems, or no problems at all. However, it is always wise to counsel patients on potential side effects and visual limitations with any lens.

A significant feature of the ReSTOR that cannot be overlooked is protection against photo-toxic blue-light.[1] Cataract extraction may accelerate age-related macular degeneration (AMD).[1,2] The yellow chromophore in ReSTOR is designed to protect the macula against this by filtering the same amount of blue light as the natural adult human crystalline lens.

The AcrySof material and design in the ReSTOR have a record of very low incidence of posterior capsular opacification (PCO) and the subsequent need for laser capsulotomy.

New techniques of implantation of these lenses allow them to be implanted through wound sizes as small as 2.0 mm.

Careful selection of candidates maximizes the benefits of the ReSTOR lens. The ideal patient is a presbyopic hypermetrope who has lost not only his or her near vision but his or her unaided distance acuity as well. The patient's uncorrected distance vision should be 20/40 or less with a loss of near reading ability. Typically, these patients wear bifocal or progressive lens spectacles and are keen to be rid of them. Astigmatism interferes with the function of the lens and it is best to avoid

patients with significant cylindrical error. Pre-existing macular pathology or significant ocular surface disease may preclude a successful outcome.

Mixing Versus Matching: Improving Unaided Intermediate Vision

Patients with Array or ReZoom in both eyes usually have excellent distance and intermediate vision but can be dissatisfied with their near vision.

Patients with bilateral ReSTOR typically have superb distance and near vision but can be dissatisfied with their intermediate vision.

Toward the end of 2003 the thought came to me that the greatest range of unaided vision could be achieved by coupling a ReSTOR with either an Array or a ReZoom IOL in the fellow eye.

It was my previous experience that patients who had intolerable glare and halos with the Array usually had sufficient alleviation of their symptoms when the Array in their dominant eye was explanted. It was as though the halos in the nondominant eye were much less noticeable to the patient.

Early experience with the ReSTOR IOL confirmed it had fewer halos and glare than the Array so I felt it was the better choice for the dominant eye. On the other hand, as the Array was a little better for intermediate vision, I started implanting it in the fellow (nondominant) eye.

Personal Experience

I conducted a study in which I placed a ReSTOR in the dominant eye and an Array or ReZoom in the nondominant eye. My target was emmetropia for both eyes. The IOL Master (Carl Zeiss Meditec, Jena, Germany) was used for biometry, and the Haigis and SRK-T formulae were used for lens calculations. The surgery was performed with a clear corneal incision under topical anesthesia using either phacoemulsification or AquaLase (Alcon).

Fifty-six patients undergoing cataract or clear lens extraction took part in the study and were divided into 3 groups:

1. Group 1 (n = 17) had a ReSTOR IOL implanted in the dominant eye and an Array in the nondominant eye.

2. Group 2 (n = 9) had a ReSTOR implanted in the dominant eye and a ReZoom in the nondominant eye.

3. Group 3 (n = 30) had a ReSTOR implanted in each eye.

The refractive outcomes and uncorrected visual acuities were virtually the same among the groups at 6 months. I was more interested in patients' ability to perform their daily tasks under varying conditions. Just how much could they do without using spectacles and did certain conditions (such as driving at night or in the rain) cause any problems?

Severe difficulty in driving at night (or in the rain) was reported by 4 ReSTOR/Array patients (24%), 3 ReSTOR/ReZoom patients (33%), and 1 ReSTOR/ReSTOR patient (<1%).

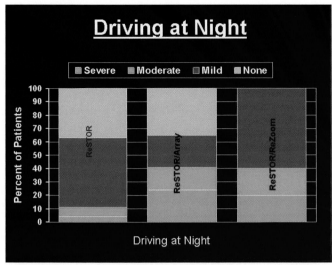

Figure 2. There was a tendency to more severe difficulty in driving at night in the mixed IOL groups.

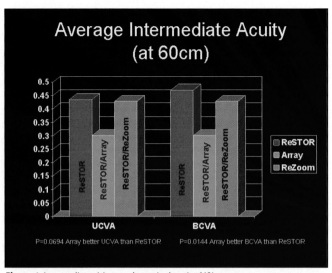

Figure 4. Intermediate vision was better in the mixed IOL groups.

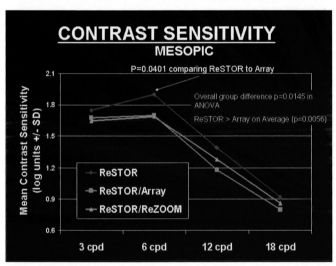

Figure 3.: Mesopic contrast sensitivity was slightly better in the group bilaterally implanted with ReSTOR.

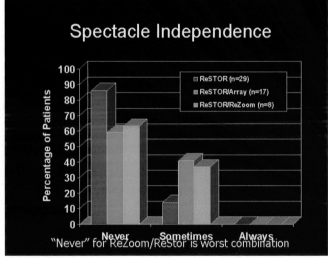

Figure 5. Spectacle independence was highest in the bilateral ReSTOR group.

ReSTOR/Array patients experienced the highest incidence of severe halos. None of these results reached statistical significance, but there was a tendency toward more halos and difficulty driving at night or in the rain in the groups with different IOLs (Figure 2).

Interestingly, there was a statistically significant difference in mesopic contrast sensitivity with the mixed group doing less well than the bilateral ReSTOR group (Figure 3).

The average intermediate acuity at 60 cm was better in the ReSTOR/Array group (Figure 4), but at the price of near vision at 30 cm. This was worse in the mixed groups compared to the ReSTOR/ReSTOR group.

Spectacle independence was achieved at 6 months in 87% of patients with AcrySof ReSTOR IOLs in both eyes.

In comparison, spectacle independence was achieved by only 61% of patients with the ReSTOR/Array combination and 56% of patients with the ReSTOR/ReZoom combination (Figure 5).

Although the ReSTOR/ReSTOR patients may have had to sit up a little closer to the computer screen to optimize their view of fonts, at least they were able to do so without glasses!

Others Find the Same

Richard Mackool, MD; Robert Lehman, MD; and Robert Kaufman, MD, have demonstrated 95%, 90%, and 100%, respectively, spectacle freedom with bilateral implantation of AcrySof ReSTOR in their independent postmarket studies.[3-5]

Richard Mackool, MD, said, "I have seen more dissatisfaction in my series of mixed technology patients versus those receiving bilateral ReSTOR implantation."[4]

Short-term and long-term FDA and postmarket studies in hundreds of patients implanted with the ReSTOR and ReZoom IOLs did not support mixing these lenses.[3] Kerry Solomon, MD said, "In clinical practice, the vast majority of patients do not require combined IOL technologies."[3]

The Role of Binocular Summation

Why are visual outcomes generally better with bilateral implantation? Two eyes performing the same visual task are always better than one. This is known as binocular summation. We know monovision patients still read better when the distance eye has a spectacle lens in front of it, allowing both eyes to read together.

There is a mismatch in the near points when you put a ReSTOR in one eye and an Array in the other eye. This interferes with binocular summation when reading.

Furthermore, patients who have a mixture of IOLs between the 2 eyes often perceive the asymmetry. If this is acceptable to them, then quite likely they could also have tolerated monovision. The intolerance to monovision is precisely the reason multifocal technology is chosen for many refractive and cataract patients.

When patients who have been bilaterally implanted with the ReSTOR IOL have difficulty with computer monitors or other intermediate vision tasks they can use a pair of simple +1.00 D magnifiers to help. However, they can also alter their posture a little so as to avoid the need for these. In other words, they can get by without glasses with some minor adjustments. On the other hand, patients who cannot see up close with a mixed combination of IOLs have no choice but to put on a pair of glasses.

Studies from around the world seem to show higher patient dissatisfaction with mixed IOL technologies, and so I believe that mixing and matching may not be the best option for our patients.

If you want to maximize the number of patients that can get by without needing glasses at all, the best combination is an AcrySof ReSTOR IOL in each eye.

References

1. Sparrow JR. Blue light-absorbing intraocular lens and retinal pigment epithelium protection in vitro. *J Cataract Refract Surg.* 2004;30: 873-878.

2. Wang JJ, Klein R, Smith W, Klein BE, Tomany S, Mitchell P. Cataract surgery and the 5-year incidence of late-stage age-related maculopathy: pooled findings from the Beaver Dam and Blue Mountains eye studies. *Ophthalmology.* 2003;110:1960-1967.

3. Solomon KD. Why not to mix and match IOLs. *Cataract & Refractive Surgery Today.* 2006;March:99-101.

4. Mackool RJ. The benefits of bilateral ReSTOR implantation. *Eyeworld Supplement.* 2006;2(3):8-11.

5. Lehmann RP. Combining liquefaction with ReSTOR technologies for safe and effective outcomes. Paper presented at: The Hawaiian Eye 2006 Meeting; January 16, 2006; Maui, HI.

CHAPTER 131

WHICH IOL COMBINATION? CLINICAL RESULTS

Jay S. Pepose, MD, PhD

The Options

The availability of 3 Food and Drug Administration (FDA)-approved intraocular lenses (IOLs) for the treatment of presbyopia gives the surgeon the capability of customizing binocular vision for a given patient. Recently, my colleagues and I[1] completed a prospective, nonrandomized 5-arm comparative trial of bilateral ReZoom zonal refractive multifocal IOL (Advanced Medical Optics, Santa Ana, CA), bilateral ReSTOR apodized diffractive multifocal IOL (Alcon, Fort Worth, TX), bilateral Crystalens accommodating IOL (Eyeonics, Inc, Aliso Viejo, CA), and Crystalens-ReZoom and Crystalens-ReSTOR combinations, with Crystalens implanted in the dominant eye.

The Outcomes

The monocular results paralleled the binocular findings and are summarized in Table 1. Briefly, there were no statistically significant differences in uncorrected distance vision in the 5 groups. Crystalens produced the best-corrected distance, distance-corrected and uncorrected intermediate, and best-corrected near vision. ReZoom gave statistically better uncorrected and distance-corrected intermediate vision than with ReSTOR. ReSTOR resulted in better uncorrected near vision, required the lowest reading add, but gave the lowest best-corrected distance vision and uncorrected and distance corrected intermediate vision.

Any patient with Crystalens in one or more eyes had the best intermediate vision. Any patient with ReSTOR in one or both eyes had better near vision. Contrast sensitivity testing was reduced at a number of spatial frequencies in patients with either multifocal IOL in one or both eyes and photic complaints were more prevalent. Patients with Crystalens in the dominant eye and ReSTOR in the nondominant eye had the best distance, intermediate, and near binocular vision, but somewhat more night glare complaints than patients with bilateral Crystalens on both quality of life and quality of vision surveys.

The Art

True customization of multifocal and/or accommodating IOLs for a given patient is an acquired art developed with some foundation in science. Despite technically flawless surgery, some patients may be highly dissatisfied with certain premium IOL channels, while other patients are ecstatic with the same IOL combination. This may reflect a composite of preoperative expectations, preoperative and postoperative refraction, degree of lens opacity, neural processing capabilities, foveal status combined with cone density and spacing, and overall personality traits. Directed, open-ended questions can identify patients' special needs, such as a woman with short arms who likes to sew or a man whose passion is to fly fish or perform other tasks at a very short focal length. Patients who work in low contrast situations, such as a radiology technician or a truck driver, may not be ideal or even suitable candidates for multifocality along with those with macular dysfunction or forms of optic neuropathy. Patients who spend extended periods of time on computers or cell phones or require intermediate vision with reasonably good image quality, which in our study was statistically better with Crystalens and ReZoom than with ReSTOR in eyes targeted for emmetropia.

Since multifocal lenses split light differently at different pupil diameters, pupil size, shape, and dynamics need to be evaluated in an effort to predict the performance of these lenses in an individual patient, or sometimes even an individual eye of a given patient. This can be assessed in a "low tech" qualitative manner using a penlight and pupil card. Alternatively, sophisticated devices such as the Procyon, Neuroptics, or Colvard pupillometers, or a wavefront aberrometer while varying the room lighting, can be used to make a more quantitative measurement. The assessment and impact of pupil size on the optical performance and choice of multifocal IOL is discussed in more detail in Chapter 152. Briefly, patients with small or irregularly shaped mesopic pupils with

Table 1

SUMMARY OF VISUAL OUTCOMES OF PATIENTS WITH VARIOUS ACCOMMODATING AND MULTIFOCAL INTRAOCULAR LENS COMBINATIONS

Monocular Testing Comparing Crystalens, ReZoom, and ReSTOR

- Crystalens eyes had statistically better BCD, UCI, DCI, BCN, but required the greatest reading add.
- ReZoom eyes had statistically better UCI and DCI than ReSTOR.
- ReSTOR eyes had statistically better UCN and required the lowest reading add but had statistically worse UCI and DCI.

Binocular Testing

- Any combination of Crystalens in one or both eyes was better for intermediate.
- Any combination of ReSTOR for one or both eyes was better for near.
- Crystalens-ReSTOR combination provided better mean intermediate and near visual acuities overall.

BCD = best-corrected distance; BCN = best-corrected near; DCI = distance-corrected intermediate; UCI = uncorrected intermediate; UCN = uncorrected near

little dynamic range may not obtain as much near vision with a multifocal that is dominant for distance centrally, such as ReZoom. A patient who has little dynamic range in pupil size, may obtain superior near vision with ReSTOR but may be more likely to have dysphotopsia and night-time complaints. These can sometimes be lessened with a mydriatic drop, along with excellent IOL centration with respect to the visual axis. A patient with large pupils who demonstrates a pupil center shift under mesopic or scotopic conditions may be better suited for a Crystalens or perhaps monovision with an aspheric, monofocal IOL. Patients with midsized pupils generally do well with Crystalens or ReZoom at most ranges of vision.

The Unknowns

There are a number of variables, which cannot be predetermined, that can affect the outcome of refractive cataract surgery besides an unanticipated intraoperative complication. These include postoperative changes in corneal wavefront, the final IOL position, tilt and decentration, residual defocus and astigmatism, pattern of higher-order aberrations and phase reversals, and neural adaptive capability. In comparison to the accommodating IOLs, more higher-order aberrations are generally introduced in eyes with multifocal IOLs, often making these patients less tolerant of residual second-order aberrations (ie, defocus and astigmatism). Such patients are more likely to require a postoperative enhancement, most often with a form of laser vision correction.

Part and parcel of the preoperative workup for all premium IOL candidates, therefore, is an initial laser in situ keratomileusis (LASIK) or laser surface treatment evaluation performed as a contingency plan. This should include an assessment of corneal topography, dry eye, and regional pachymetry. These studies may need to be expanded after phacoemulsification for the subset of patients who eventually require laser vision enhancement. This allows preoperative counseling regarding the manner by which an enhancement might be performed, be it through LASIK, surface treatment, or perhaps bioptics for those with high preoperative corneal astigmatism. As an illus-

trative case, a premium IOL patient anticipating good uncorrected distance and near vision was referred for a postoperative laser vision enhancement. Topographic analysis revealed that this patient had keratoconus and had not been diagnosed or counseled about this before cataract surgery. Preoperative topographic assessment after discontinuing contact lens use for an appropriate length of time can enhance the accuracy of keratometry, aid in planning astigmatism treatment during cataract surgery, and circumvent this unforeseen and unfortunate "postoperative surprise."

The Bottom Line

Surgeons offering premium channel IOLs must take ownership of the concept that achieving good uncorrected distance vision is a prerequisite to attaining a high level of patient satisfaction. Premium IOL patients who do not enjoy good uncorrected distance vision following primary cataract surgery will therefore require some form of postoperative enhancement, and this possibility should be planned for and discussed openly with all patients preoperatively. In general, under promising and then over delivering with regard to high-quality, uncorrected, binocular distance vision, along with functional intermediate and reasonable near vision represents a successful strategy. This can be accomplished with a bilateral accommodating IOL or mixed accommodating-multifocal IOL combinations, tailored to meet each patient's specific visual needs.

References

1. Pepose JS, Qazi MA, Davies J, Doane JF, Loden JC, Sivalingham V, Mahmoud AM. Visual performance of patients with bilateral versus combination Crystalens, ReZoom and ReSTOR intraocular lens implants. *Am J Ophthalmol.* 2007;144(3):347-357.
2. Hofeldt AJ, Weiss MJ. Illuminated near card assessment of potential acuity in eyes with cataract. *Ophthalmology.* 1998;105:1531-1536.

CHAPTER 132

MIXING IOLs—
HOW DO I GET STARTED?

John F. Doane, MD and Randolph T. Jackson, MD

"We never told anyone they could do that," an intraocular lens (IOL) sales representative stated regarding mixing presbyopia-correcting (Pr-C) IOLs. There are indeed no Food and Drug Administration (FDA) studies evaluating the combining of the ReSTOR (Alcon, Fort Worth, TX) with other PrC IOLs at present. Yet, time and again, necessity is the mother of invention. In medical care and surgery, necessity allows physicians to utilize the sacred privilege, the Practice of Medicine Act,[1] to achieve the best outcome for a given patient. One of ophthalmology's current arenas for the invocation of this act is the implantation of Pr-C IOLs. Although data from the FDA clinical trials for a given therapy establish a baseline level of safety and efficacy, the widespread postapproval usage by rank-and-file physicians is the ultimate barometer by which a therapy, medication, or device's real-world safety and efficacy are determined. I have had the honor of being involved in the FDA clinical trials for the Crystalens accommodating IOL (Eyeonics, Inc, Aliso Viejo, CA) since the year 2000. In that capacity, I have gained a tremendous amount of first-hand experience with and knowledge of the phenomenon of accommodation, its measurement, its loss due to presbyopia, and its treatment and potential return with man-made intraocular devices. I have been astounded by the postoperative results achieved with the Crystalens to such a level that I have recommended this IOL to family members, friends, and patients alike. This chapter describes my exploration into the mixing of the Crystalens with the AcrySof ReSTOR diffractive multifocal IOL (Alcon, Fort Worth, TX). I am certain many readers will relate to my initial feelings, concerns, reservations, and experiences.

My Introduction to Mixing IOLs

My first experiences mixing Pr-C IOLs occurred in the setting of a 5-site, controlled clinical study involving 4 other surgeons (James Davies, MD, of Carlsbad, California; James C. Loden, MD, of Nashville, Tennessee; Jay Pepose, MD, PhD, of St. Louis, Missouri; and Varunan Sivalingam, MD, of Medford, New Jersey). In this study sponsored by Eyeonics, Inc, we evaluated 5 different bilateral IOL scenarios: group 1, bilateral AcrySof ReSTOR IOLs; group 2, bilateral ReZoom IOLs (Advanced Medical Optics, Santa Ana, CA); group 3, bilateral Crystalens IOLs; group 4, a Crystalens in one eye and an AcrySof ReSTOR lens in the other; and group 5, a Crystalens in one eye and a ReZoom lens in the other.[2] I felt I could translate the findings from this investigation into my clinical practice.

Real-World Experience

Although my experience with bilateral Crystalens implantation has generally been excellent, a subset of my patients were less than pleased with one aspect of their overall visual function, despite my careful counseling. They were very happy with their distance and intermediate vision but were hoping for better near vision. Despite waiting 1 to 2 years in most cases to see if they would adapt, these patients eventually concluded that they did not achieve the outcome for which they had hoped: nearly complete independence from spectacles for distant, intermediate and near focal points.

Getting Started
Mixing Pr-C IOLs

After my experience in the Eyeonics study, I believed that the best solution would be to implant an AcrySof ReSTOR IOL in the nondominant eye and the Crystalens in the dominant eye of these patients. My experience in the trial gave me confidence in this approach that I otherwise would not have had. Earlier on in my PrC IOL clinical experience and mental preparation, I was concerned about splitting light with a multifocal IOL, with the resulting induction of halos and loss of contrast sensitivity. Loss of contrast sensitivity in scotopic environments is of particular concern with younger patients who have decades of night driving ahead of them.

My experience with the mixing study led to my decision to leave the Crystalens in patients' dominant eyes and to implant the AcrySof ReSTOR in their nondominant eyes. My rationale was that any perception of halos would probably be less bothersome in a person's nondominant eye. Furthermore, I felt these patients would be happiest if their dominant eyes had the best quality and quantity of distance vision.

So what happens in the clinic? If a patient has interest in computer work, night driving, and high-quality vision in low light, and wants to have a PrC IOL, the Crystalens is an excellent binocular solution without mixing. A certain percentage of bilateral ReSTOR patients would be disappointed with their unaided computer vision and may have some unwanted scotopic optical issues as well. This type of patient could do extremely well with a Crystalens in their alternate eye in order to provide functional intermediate vision for the dashboard and computer screen for example. Two approaches can be taken when mixing the Crystalens and ReSTOR. One can plan from the outset to implant the ReSTOR in the nondominant eye and the Crystalens in the dominant eye. This by and large works very nicely. As with all PrC IOLs, the end refraction needs to be very close to emmetropia with no residual astigmatism. If the patient does not occlude one eye or the other, they should note excellent distance, intermediate, or near vision. A second approach is to perform the first eye surgery and assess the visual result before deciding on the IOL for the second eye. Let us say the first eye receives the Crystalens and this eye does very well at distance, intermediate, and near. In this case, a Crystalens can be implanted in the second eye. If the first eye does not have enough uncorrected reading vision, then a ReSTOR can be implanted in the second eye. On the other hand, if a ReSTOR is implanted in the first eye and the patient is satisfied at all focal points, then a ReSTOR can be implanted in the second eye. On the contrary, if the first eye does not have sufficient intermediate vision, the Crystalens can be implanted in the second eye in an effort to improve intermediate function for this patient.

As for all Pr-C IOLs, I believe that it is necessary to reduce patients' corneal astigmatism to less than 0.50 D postoperatively. If they have less than 2.50 D of corneal astigmatism preoperatively, I will perform concurrent limbal relaxing incisions at the time of the lens extraction and IOL placement. For more than 2.50 D of preexisting corneal astigmatism, I plan a 2-stage procedure; I place the IOL first and perform laser vision correction at a later date. After the appropriate IOL placement, my patients have mixed astigmatism with a spherical equivalent near plano. My desire is for the spherical equivalent after the IOL implantation but before laser vision correction is for it to be slightly myopic (−0.50 to −1.00 D). I believe it is easier to treat low myopia with an excimer laser than a hyperopic spherical equivalent. Approximately 20% of the eyes I treat require some form of laser vision correction to achieve the optimal result from Pr-C IOLs. The vast majority of these ablations are for minor refractive errors, but they make a significant difference in patients' degree of satisfaction.

Patient Selection

At present, my colleagues and I at Discover Vision Centers in Kansas City, Missouri decide on a per-case basis whether to implant the Crystalens IOL bilaterally or to combine this IOL with an AcrySof ReSTOR lens. I do not implant the AcrySof ReSTOR IOL bilaterally because I personally do not find that this approach provides recipients with adequate intermediate function in general. Our stance is that a patient who wants the highest quality of vision and does not mind occasionally wearing low-power reading spectacles should receive bilateral Crystalenses. If a patient never wishes to wear spectacles and would be significantly disappointed if they were necessary, we consider mixing the 2 lenses. For the ReSTOR/Crystalens patients, we have found that it is necessary to discuss 2 issues specific to the ReSTOR lens preoperatively. We had originally thought halos would be a significant issue for eyes that received this IOL. Although some patients notice the phenomenon, the incidence is far less than I anticipated. Another unanticipated but significant complaint is that of waxy vision, which we have attributed to an alteration in contrast sensitivity by the diffractive optic. I explain the benefits and drawbacks of the ReSTOR lens to patients. They will have a high likelihood of being able to read even the smallest print, but they must be willing to risk the possibilities of seeing halos or having waxy vision in that eye. This dysphotopsia is symptomatic in approximately 10% of patients in our experience, and it tends to lessen with time. Thanks to a thorough informed-consent process, I have not yet had to explant an AcrySof ReSTOR IOL for dysphotopsia. Of course, I also explain the advantages and disadvantages of the Crystalens-accommodating IOL to patients in depth. I tell them that their quality of vision with this lens will be excellent but that total independence from spectacles, although common among my patients, is not guaranteed.

Outcomes and Patient Opinions

Now that we have established the theoretic and clinical basis for mixing PrC IOLs, let's look at visual outcomes and review patient opinions. We performed 52 consecutive bilateral Crystalens/ReSTOR surgeries for either cataract or refractive lens exchange. Thirty-one patients (60%) returned a survey. The follow-up time ranged from 33 to 546 days. In our patients, the preoperative refraction spherical equivalent ranged from −9.00 to +3.00, whereas astigmatism averaged 0.86 D (ranging up to 4.25 D, with the standard deviation being 0.74 D).

Secondary procedures are sometimes needed to help achieve optimum results. Twenty-eight percent of eyes received limbal relaxing incisions. Twenty-six percent of eyes had laser vision correction either with a planned bioptic flap (4%) cut at the time of IOL surgery, or as a later secondary procedure (22%). Due to heightened expectations, yttrium-aluminum-garnet (YAG) capsulotomies are often performed at an earlier stage in PrC IOL patients, in our experience. In 29% of eyes a YAG capsulotomy had been performed.

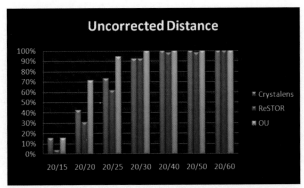

Figure 1. Uncorrected distance visual acuity for each eye and using both together.

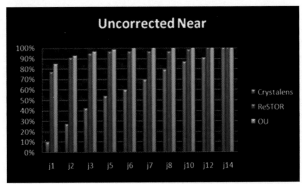

Figure 2. Uncorrected near visual acuity for each eye and using both together.

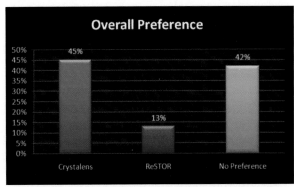

Figure 3. Percentage of patients with an overall preference for each eye.

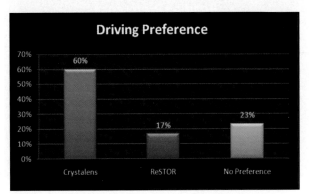

Figure 4. Percentage of patients preferring each eye for driving.

As seen in Figure 1, distance visual acuity is excellent with both lenses, but the Crystalens more often produced 20/15 vision. Using both eyes together, over 90% saw at least 20/25 unaided for distance. Near visual acuity was measured at the patient's self-selected distance, which in many cases was a bit closer than they preferred when using the eye with the ReSTOR lens. Figure 2 reveals that small optotype print was read better in the ReSTOR eye and binocular near vision was excellent with over 90% reading J2 or better.

An interesting question is, what was the patients' overall preference of lens style? The Crystalens had a clear lead with 45% of patients, whereas only 13% preferred the ReSTOR and 42% had no preference (Figure 3). It is interesting to look at results broken down by activity, such as driving, using the computer, and reading. Good unaided binocular driving vision is a key objective with PrC IOLs, which makes them superior to simple monovision. Reading street signs and driving at night are common patient concerns. In our survey, a majority of patients, (60%) preferred the Crystalens for driving vision, versus 17% preferring the ReSTOR and 23% reporting no preference (Figure 4). With the importance of computers and cell phones today, intermediate visual function is another critical element to provide with any refractive surgical procedure in presbyopic patients. Based on design alone, it would be expected that the Crystalens would provide better intermediate function than the ReSTOR. This was supported by the patient questionnaire data in which 47% of the patients preferred the Crystalens, versus 17% for the ReSTOR and 37% who had no preference (Figure 5). Reading ability is where the trend reversed and this is where the utility of the ReSTOR as a second lens becomes apparent. An overwhelming 72% of

patients prefer the ReSTOR for reading vision, versus 17% for the Crystalens and 10% who had no preference (Figure 6).

Many surgeons have avoided recommending and implanting multifocal intraocular lenses due to an increased risk of glare, halos, and problems with night driving. To evaluate and compare any potential differences, we asked patients to rate the severity of visual side effects on a scale from 0 (none) to 10 (severe). The results can be seen in Figure 7. Frequency and severity of visual symptoms was low for both lenses. One symptom that some patients did report with the ReSTOR is "waxy" vision, but the severity was mild. None of the patients requested that either of the lenses be exchanged for the alternate, or any other, lens.

The Quick "To-Do" List Before You Mix

We do have a few suggestions for those interested in mixing PrC IOLs. We doubt anyone would do this with their first PrC IOL patients. An interest in mixing would likely come from experiences with some dissatisfied patients who have the same PrC lens in each eye. Once you have decided to try PrC IOL mixing, you must first determine the "dominant" eye for distance. It is not written in stone that the Crystalens has to be placed in the dominant eye or the ReSTOR in the nondominant eye; yet, this has been our preference to date. Our technique for determining the dominant eye for distance is to use a "hole" card that the patient can hold at arm's length in front of their face. This is simply a small piece of paper with a round hole cut out of the center. The patient centers a distance target

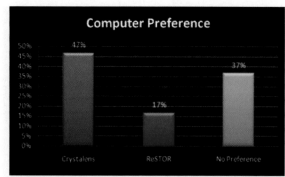

Figure 5. Percentage of patients preferring each eye for computer use.

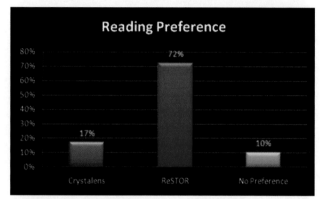

Figure 6. Percentage of patients preferring each eye for reading.

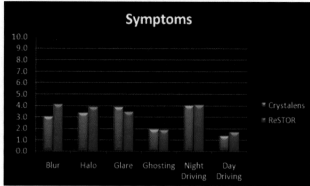

Figure 7. Average severity of visual symptoms with each eye. Results tablulated from visual analog scale ranging from 0 (none) to 10 (severe).

through the hole with both eyes open and then brings the card back to their face. The eye that ends up with the hole in front of it is the dominant eye. There are, of course, other methods to assess dominance as well.[3]

Which patients should you start with? In our experience this question is typically answered by the patient's history. A patient who wants to see at all focal points without glasses, and would be dissatisfied if this did not occur, is a prime candidate for mixing. Thus, the selection of in whom to mix IOLs will essentially be prompted by patient's preoperative expectations. How do you convey the rational of mixing IOLs to patients and is it too time consuming to communicate this in a busy clinical setting? It usually only takes me 2 to 3 minutes to describe why I want to mix PrC IOLs. I typically make simple drawings with a pen and paper illustrating that we need 3 focal points to function: far distance (8 feet to the horizon), intermediate (2 to 8 feet for computer, cell phone, cooking), and near (within 2 feet for reading). I tell them that bilateral Crystalens will perform exceptionally well for the distance and intermediate foci, but approximately 25% of patients will require low-power readers. On the other hand, bilateral ReSTOR patients may do well at distance and within 12 inches, but not do so well at intermediate distances. I next show them on paper that both the Crystalens and ReSTOR will provide good distance vision for each eye, the dominant (Crystalens) eye will provide intermediate vision, and the ReSTOR and to a lesser extent the Crystalens eye will both assist with near. The patients universally comprehend this rationale. I tell them that with both eyes open they will not be able to tell which eye is doing

which. A frequent question is "this sounds like monovision." I nip this topic in the bud early. With monovision one eye sees near and the other sees distance. With mixing, both eyes see distance and both see up close, so PrC IOLs are a binocular system. Is it truly important which eye, dominant or nondominant, gets which lens? We do not know for sure, and although the conventional wisdom is currently that the multifocal lens should be placed in the nondominant eye, there is at least one small study that indicates multifocal lenses may be more effective in the dominant eye.[4] The same principle may hold for Crystalens/ReSTOR IOL mixing. Another question is, do you target the Crystalens for –0.25 to –0.50 D of residual sphere? Although we might do this for the nondominant eye with bilateral Crystalens implantation, we do not do this with the mixing scenario. With mixing, we feel the Crystalens eye generally needs to be plano in order to provide exceptional distance vision. It is important with the ReSTOR that less than 0.5 D of residual astigmatism be present. We have seen patients with a refractions such as plano +0.75 × 090 that have 20/50 uncorrected distance visual acuity and 20/20 best spectacle-corrected distance vision. It is felt that with the diffractive optic any residual astigmatism will decrease the best unaided vision much more than would be anticipated when compared to the same residual astigmatism with a monofocal intraocular lens. If the ReSTOR eye has no cylinder but some residual sphere, we would prefer this be between plano to +0.50. Any more residual hyperopia will diminish the uncorrected distance visual acuity. Slight hyperopia also tends to move the near point further away, and is beneficial for those patients for whom reading at 12 inches is too close.

Conclusion

In summary, mixing different PrC IOLs can improve the range of visual function that many patients want in their everyday lives. We believe most would agree that no single PrC IOL is perfect for all patients in all instances. Likewise we think that practitioners who are involved with PrC IOLs would agree that there is somewhat of an "art" to selecting the best plan for each individual patient with respect to their daily visual requirements and preferences. To this end a mixing technique may be the best solution.

References

1. Section 906. [21 U.S.C. 396] Practice of Medicine. Available at http://www.fda.gov/opacom/laws/fdcact/fdcact9.htm. Accessed July 10, 2007.

2. Pepose, JS. Mixing versus matching IOLs. *Cataract Refract Sur Today.* 2007;August:65.

3. Probst LE, Doane JF (eds). *Ocular Evaluation. Refractive Surgery: A Color Synopsis.* Thieme; 2001.

4. Shoji N, Shimizu K. Binocular function of the patient with refractive multifocal intraocular lens. *J Cataract Refract Surg.* 2002;28:1012-1017.

CHAPTER 133

MIXING MULTIFOCAL IOLs— CLINICAL RESULTS

Frank A. Bucci, Jr., MD

Spectacle independence and high levels of patient satisfaction are the goals when using implants to surgically correct presbyopia. The surgeon must create what I call "the 4 essential visual elements of success" if he/she hopes to produce highly satisfied cataract or refractive lensectomy patients. The 4 elements include 1) high-quality distance vision; 2) functional intermediate vision—the patient must be able to see his computer; 3) functional near vision in both bright and moderate light—the patients must be able to read the newspaper; and 4) functional driving at night after neuroadaptation—the light phenomena should be acceptable to the patient.

The Array multifocal implant (Advanced Medical Optics, Santa Ana, CA) had excellent distance and intermediate vision, but was lacking with regard to near vision and night halos. The ReSTOR implant (Alcon, Fort Worth, TX) was a valiant attempt to create a multifocal intraocular lens (IOL) with strong reading and fewer halos at night. Unfortunately, these characteristics were achieved at a substantial cost.

While attending the 2004 European Society of Cataract and Refractive Surgery (ESCRS) meeting in Paris, I heard numerous papers about the "success" of the ReSTOR IOL. Reports of less halos and better reading than the Array with adequate intermediate vision were delivered repeatedly. I began wait listing my multifocal IOL patients until the ReSTOR was available on June 1, 2005. I quickly established a cohort of 55 bilateral ReSTOR patients in only a 3-month period. Sixty-three percent of these patients were elective refractive lensectomy surgeries. Because the refractive lensectomy patient is the true test for presbyopia-correcting (Pr-C) IOLs, I quickly learned the strengths and weaknesses of the ReSTOR IOL in the summer of 2005.

The driving force behind originally "mixing" the ReZoom (Advanced Medical Optics, Santa Ana, CA) and the ReSTOR was that the visual performance with bilateral ReSTOR IOLs grossly failed to meet my patient's needs.

The inadequate results were more immediate and magnified in the younger, more demanding refractive lensectomy patients compared to the cataract patients. However, the relative deficiencies of bilateral ReSTOR (poor intermediate, less than excellent distance, poor reading in moderate light, hyperclose near point, and diffuse "waxy" vision) were soon experienced by all types of patients.

Seventeen of the original 53 bilateral ReSTOR patients offered early and strong spontaneous complaints regarding their intermediate vision. More than 1 out of 3 of all lensectomy patients had major complaints with intermediate vision. It became apparent very quickly that baby boomers and younger cataract patients would not tolerate the obvious absence of functional intermediate vision after paying in excess of $8000. During this same time period, I evaluated several unilateral Array patients who were waiting for another IOL that would give them better detailed reading without additional halos. Five patients received a ReSTOR in their opposite eye. These patients were extremely happy and completely free of glasses. It made sense to try ReZoom/ReSTOR (RZ/RS) to solve my patient's intermediate visual problems because the ReZoom is a significant upgrade of the Array.

This resulted in a second cohort of RZ/RS patients (*n* = 110) who achieved statistically and clinically better bilateral intermediate vision (RZ/RS J2.44 versus ReSTOR/ReSTOR [RS/RS] J3.60), resulting in no spontaneous complaints related to intermediate vision (Figures 1 and 2). The subjective response to the surgery for the RZ/RS patients appeared to be more positive above and beyond just having superior intermediate vision. The RZ/RS patients seem to have the "Wow" factor that we frequently observe in laser in situ keratomileusis (LASIK) patients. Even the so-called successful or satisfied RS/RS patients seemed to be relatively "underwhelmed." I have observed other relative deficiencies in the ReSTOR lens compared to the ReZoom lens after implanting 300 ReSTOR and 400 ReZoom lenses.

There were no statistically significant differences with bilateral near vision between the 2 cohorts. However, the RZ/RS patients frequently reported a more comfortable reading distance compared to RS/RS patients, who often thought

Figure 1. ReZoom/ReSTOR versus ReSTOR/ReSTOR bilateral intermediate.

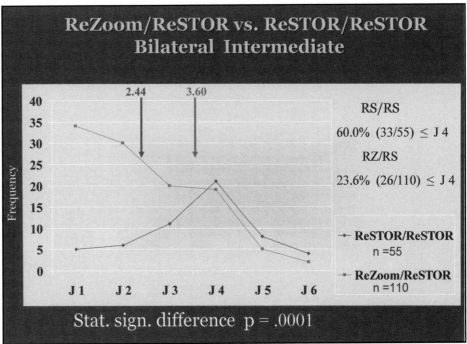

their near point of focus was too close. I, and others, including Akaishi and Fabri,[1] at the World Cornea Congress (2006) have observed subtle but significant losses in best-corrected and uncorrected distance visual acuities with the ReSTOR lens. Reports of "waxy vision" have been prevalent since the release of the ReSTOR lens.

I have recently reported[2] a group of patients with a severe form of waxy vision, which I call "Vaseline vision dysphotopsia" (VVD). Although this severe form of waxy vision occurred in only 4.33% of 300 ReSTOR eyes, it appears that explantation is required to achieve an adequate relief in symptoms.

Why were the deficiencies in the ReSTOR IOL slow to be reported compared to my early observations? Why might the levels of patient's satisfaction for the Food and Drug Administration (FDA) ReSTOR patients have been misinterpreted? The typical American surgeon using the ReSTOR lens has a ratio of over 20/1 cataract to lensectomy patients. Visual expectations related to culture and other factors with cataract patients versus lensectomy patients are extremely different. The criteria for success with a 75-year-old dense nuclear sclerotic cataract patient versus a 50-year-old baby boomer refractive lensectomy patient are very different. The perception of visual improvement by cataract patients averaging 70+ years in age is dominated by the results directly tied to the extraction of the cataract, irrespective for the type of IOL implanted. The FDA ReSTOR patients were cataract patients. In addition, these ReSTOR cataract patients now have some uncorrected near vision that they never had before, improved uncorrected distance vision, and paid nothing for their surgery. Their modest expectations were frequently exceeded and this scenario of free surgery with a typical postcataract result will rarely elicit major complaints.

Patient expectations are always tied to the levels of payment required. As stated above, the FDA ReSTOR cataract patient paid nothing for their surgery. Even post-FDA ReSTOR cataract patients pay almost 60% less than elective

lensectomy patients. So to say that there was an 80% "success rate" for these bilateral ReSTOR patients in the FDA study tells us very little about how this IOL might perform in the 40- to 60-year-old lensectomy or young cataract patient.

The original targeted market for these Pr-C IOLs was not the cataract patient. It was the precataract presbyopes. Because all these patients, including the cataract patients, are paying "out of pocket," all these procedures are now officially "refractive surgeries." An 80% success rate for any refractive surgery is unacceptable. Can you imagine if you told your LASIK patients that they had an 80% chance of functioning without glasses after paying $3000 to $5000 for surgery?

The results of my RS/RS versus RZ/RS study and the result of my VVD investigation have led me to 2 core conclusions about multifocal IOLs. The first conclusion is that mixing a refractive multifocal IOL with a diffractive multifocal IOL will produce the highest levels of patient satisfaction and spectacle independence. The second conclusion is that the ReSTOR IOL is not the optimum diffractive lens of choice for the refractive IOL/diffractive IOL combination. The Brazilian group, Akaishi and Fabri, have already reported ($n = 45$) superior reading speeds, greater pupillary independence, better quality distance vision, and less halos and glare with the ReZoom/Tecnis multifocal (TMF; Advanced Medical Optics, Santa Ana, CA) combination versus the RZ/RS combination. Numerous European surgeons have reported identical findings as well.

The diffractive rings of the TMF are spread throughout the entire optic, unlike the ReSTOR, which has all the rings located within the central 3.6 mm. Some investigators have hypothesized that the central "crowding" of the rings may be responsible for the waxy vision (VVD) associated with the ReSTOR. Also, eyes with the ReSTOR IOL only read well in bright light (small pupils) because of the centrally located rings. The TMF lens has excellent reading in both bright and moderate illumination because the diffractive rings are spread

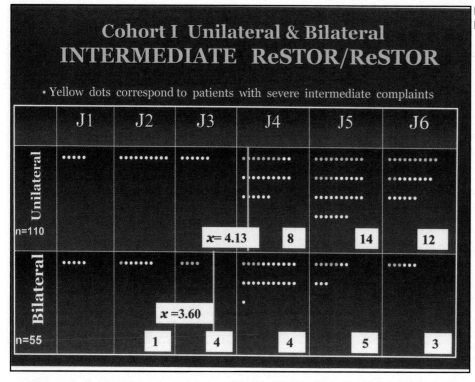

Figure 2. Cohort unilateral and bilateral intermediate ReSTOR/ReSTOR.

throughout the entire optic, making it pupillary independent. Although the TMF is a diffractive IOL with numerous rings, there have been no reports of waxy vision of any kind associated with its visual performance.

The aspheric surface of the TMF compared to the ReSTOR lens also contributes to its superior distance vision. Many patients have reported a wider near focal range when reading with bilateral TMF implants compared to bilateral ReSTOR. Mixing the positive qualities of the diffractive TMF IOL with the superior intermediate vision of the refractive ReZoom IOL provides a surgeon with an extremely effective tool for meeting even the highest expectations of both lensectomy and cataract patients.

High levels of success with Pr-C IOLs takes more than just correct IOL selection to achieve good distance, intermediate, and near vision. Proper patient selection and managing patient expectations are dependent on establishing meaningful communication during the preoperative consultation. The preoperative examination should confirm full visual potential, with special attention to the cornea and the retina. The surgeon should also strive to continually upgrade his phaco skills and surgical skills for correcting residual refractive errors, such as corneal astigmatism.

When all these issues have been addressed, the surgeon has created an environment consistent with very high levels of spectacle independence. Although optimum IOL selection is a critical element, it is still only one of many essential building blocks (see Figure 2) necessary for producing a satisfied presbyopic IOL patient. In Europe and South America, many elderly cataract patients are doing well with bilateral TMF (+0.25 OU), and younger lensectomy patients with high intermediate requirements are doing well with bilateral ReZoom (plano/–0.50). However, I believe that the ReZoom/TMF refractive/diffractive combination will be the optimum choice for both cataract and lensectomy patients once TMF is approved by the FDA.

References

1. Akaishi and Fabri
2. ARVO 2007.

CHAPTER 134

MIXING TECNIS AND REZOOM MULTIFOCAL IOLS

Michael C. Knorz, MD

In this chapter, I will review some of the currently available multifocal intraocular lenses (IOLs) and then discuss some of my experience and thoughts on mixing and matching them. In addition to the 2 multifocal IOLs currently available in the United States, the ReZoom (Advanced Medical Optics, Santa Ana, CA) and the ReSTOR (Alcon, Fort Worth, TX), here in Europe we have 5 additional multifocals available for use in cataract surgery and refractive lens exchange (RLE).

Diffractive Multifocal IOLs

ACRYSOF RESTOR

This 1-piece diffractive acrylic IOL has a 6-mm optic and can be injected through a 2.8-mm incision. The apodized diffractive design has 12 "zones," with a total add of 4 D at the IOL plane. It comes in either a blue blocker/ultraviolet (UV) model or UV blocking only. It is available in a power range of 10 to 30 D.

**ACRI.LISA 366D

This is a 1-piece, aberration-correcting, aspheric hydrophobic acrylic, microincision IOL. The *Acri.LISA (*Acri.Tec, Hennigsdorf, Germany) is actually more of a hybrid multifocal in that LISA stands for (L) light intensity distribution of 65% (refractive) far and 35% (diffractive) near; (I) independent from pupil size; (S) smooth refractive/diffractive surface profile; and (A) optimized aspheric surface. The IOL has a total add power of +3.75 D. It is designed to be injected through a sub-2-mm cataract incision using the *Acri.Tec A2-2000 injector. It is available in a power range of 10 to 32 D in 0.50-D increments. IOLs in 1-D increments can be specially made with an 8-week lead time.

*ACRI.LISA 356D

This is essentially the same diffractive/refractive multifocal design as the 366D, with the exception that the 356D is designed to go through a larger incision. It is available in 0.5-D increments of 10 to 30 D, with IOLs of 0.0 to 9 D and 31 to 44 D available with 8 weeks lead time.

TECNIS ZM900

This is a 3-piece, diffractive multifocal, silicone IOL with a 6-mm optic. The diffractive design on the posterior surface creates two focal points that are 4 D apart. As a result, light entering into the eye is evenly distributed between near and distance vision that is independent of pupil size. Additionally, the Tecnis ZM900 (Advanced Medical Optics) has a modified, prolate anterior surface that is designed to compensate the spherical aberration of the cornea, creating an optical system that is ideally free of spherical aberration. This should lead to better focusing and sharper vision. The Tecnis ZM900 is available in 0.50-D increments from 5 to 34 D.

Refractive Multifocal IOLs

REZOOM MULTIFOCAL IOL

This refractive multifocal is a 3-piece acrylic with 5 refractive zones: (moving from the outer zone, inwards) a low-light/distance-dominant zone, a near-dominant zone, a distance zone, another near-dominant zone, and a bright-light/distance-dominant zone. Transitions provide intermediate vision. With a design the company calls "Balance View Optics," the ReZoom multifocal is intended to have 100% light transmission over all 5 optical zones. The ReZoom has a total near add of +3.5 D and is available from 5 to 30 D in 0.50-D increments.

MF4 IOL

This refractive multifocal is a 1-piece, hydrophilic acrylic with a 4-zone optic with a tripod design. It has a 6-mm optic and has a total near add of +4 D. Carl Zeiss Meditec (Jena, Germany) describes the lens as an "autofocus" multifocal IOL. Although this lens was first introduced about 4 years ago by IOLTech, there has not been a great deal published on the results. The MF4 multifocal IOL is available from 15 to 26 D in 0.5-D increments.

M-FLEX MULTIFOCAL IOL

This is the newest multifocal in the European market. The M-Flex (Rayner, Hove, East Sussex, UK) is a hydrophilic acrylic IOL with a 6.25-mm, multizone aspheric optic. The IOL comes with either 4 or 5 zones, depending on the IOL base power that is needed. It is distant dominant with a +3-D near add. The first of these lenses were implanted in 2005, although no results have been published to date. The MFlex is available in powers from 14 to 25 D in 1-D increments and in 18.5 to 23.5 D in 0.50-D increments.

With such a wide range of multifocal IOLs available in Europe, it is interesting to note that the concept of combining different types of multifocals in the same patient remains a fairly new one.

The fact that the idea of mixing and matching has not been widely discussed is likely due to lingering doubts over multifocal IOL technology in general. Many surgeons still remember the visual disturbances and unhappy patients encountered with first generation multifocals. However, what I have experienced in the use of second-generation multifocals, including the Tecnis ZM900, the ReZoom, the AcrySof ReSTOR, and the *Acri.LISA, is that these IOLs provide very good visual results without the level of complaints about glare and halos that we saw with the "old" designs. I have no personal experience with the other designs mentioned in this article.

Mixing and Matching

I routinely use the ReZoom and the Tecnis multifocal IOL as my IOLs of choice. Both have unique properties, and both are needed in my clinical practice. The ReZoom, being a distant-dominant design, provides very good distance vision, which is slightly better than the Tecnis multifocal or the ReSTOR. Intermediate vision with the ReZoom is good, and also better than that achieved with the Tecnis multifocal or the ReSTOR. Near vision is somewhat lower, not as good as with the Tecnis multifocal or the ReSTOR.

The Tecnis multifocal, on the other hand, provides excellent near vision in all patients, but some can be frustrated by the lack of intermediate vision, or so-called "computer vision."

Being, for years, an advocate of bilateral implantation of the same IOL design, I recently changed because of the complaints of some of my patients regarding a reduction of intermediate vision whenever I used a diffractive IOL design such as the Tecnis multifocal IOL. The benefit of the mix and match approach is that it enables surgeons to play the strengths and weaknesses of these multifocals off one another in order to provide cataract and refractive lens exchange patients with the best possible range of vision.

Patient Selection

In my own practice, mixing and matching of multifocal IOLs is more frequently becoming my standard of care. The key, as always in multifocal IOLs, is patient selection. As a general rule, patients must be willing to accept some side effects—mainly halos and glare—in exchange for the benefits of reduced dependence from spectacles. Once this is established, patients are questioned about their visual tasks. Patients who mainly want to read are ideal candidates for a Tecnis multifocal IOL in both eyes. Patients who read little and just require excellent distance and some intermediate vision are ideal candidates for a ReZoom in both eyes. The majority of patients, however, is best served by a mix and match approach, using the ReZoom IOL in the dominant eye and the Tecnis multifocal IOL in the nondominant eye.

My Approach to Mix and Match

In a refractive lens exchange or a cataract patient in whom I am primarily considering a mix and match approach, I will always operate on the dominant eye first. I will implant a ReZoom multifocal IOL in the dominant eye because of its excellent distance vision and good intermediate. During the postoperative follow up, I will then ask the patient how happy he is with his near vision. Usually, about 50% of patients can read well with a ReZoom IOL in addition to a good intermediate vision. If the patient is happy with his reading ability, I will also implant a ReZoom IOL in the second eye. Because reading will always be better when both eyes are implanted, it is therefore safe to do so if the patient is already happy with the reading ability in his first eye. Should the patient tell me that his near vision is not good enough, I will implant a Tecnis multifocal IOL in the second, nondominant eye. If the patient is unsure, I will also use a Tecnis multifocal IOL in the second eye. This approach has proved to be very helpful. There have been no more complaints of patients who cannot see their laptop or computer screens at intermediate distance. Statistically, about 50% of the patients will end up with a ReZoom in both eyes and 50% with mix and match.

Refractive Enhancements

A basic requirement with multifocal IOLs is achieving spectacle independence: it is the "selling point," as we recommend these IOLs to our patients who do not want to wear spectacles. They have to pay a price for this, which is to accept visual side effects such as halos and glare. All multifocal IOLs will only perform as designed if emmetropia is achieved. As emmetropia cannot be achieved in all eyes after the implantation of a multifocal IOL, there will always be a certain number of eyes requiring refractive enhancement (about 10% to 20%). I will typically perform laser in situ keratomileusis (LASIK) in these eyes about 3 months after the IOL implantation. In eyes with a Tecnis multifocal IOL, I will perform a wavefront-guided LASIK using the Visx STAR S4 (Santa Clara, CA) with iris registration. In eyes with a refractive multifocal IOL such as the ReZoom, aberrometry is not reliable with current aberrometers, and I will therefore perform a standard LASIK in these eyes.

Another approach is used in eyes with relatively high corneal astigmatism prior to IOL surgery. In my hands, this means eyes with 2 D or more of astigmatism. In these eyes, I will use the IntraLase FS 60 laser to cut a flap (100 μm, 9 mm) immediately prior to the refractive lens exchange or cataract surgery.

I will not lift this flap, but perform lens surgery. As the flap is not lifted, the lens surgery proceeds without any additional difficulty. About 4 weeks later, I will lift the flap and perform the laser enhancement. This technique shortens the time interval between lens and laser surgery, which means faster visual recovery for the patient.

CHAPTER 135

MIXING MULTIFOCAL IOLs— STAGED IMPLANTATION

Kerry K. Assil, MD and William K. Christian, MD

To obtain a full-range of optimal, functional vision some patients may need a different type of multifocal lens in each eye. Custom matching, or custom lens selection with staged implantation is a process of customizing and selecting the best type of intraocular lenses (IOLs) according to a patient's lifestyle and individual visual needs.

Mixing IOLs

Although mixing refractive and diffractive lens technologies can be a successful approach and a viable option for the right patient, it is not necessarily the best strategy for everyone (Table 1).

Combining diffractive and refractive IOLs in the same patient can provide a full range of vision by combining the benefits of both technologies. Refractive multifocal IOLs, while providing multiple focal points, are typically distance dominant. There is little or no loss of available light rays to diffraction. Therefore, the refractive range is balanced for optimal vision at multiple distances and lighting conditions. Diffractive multifocal IOLS also provide multiple focal points and are typically near dominant. These patients achieve excellent near vision, but the diffractive multifocal IOL has no refractive element for intermediate vision. Furthermore, the diffractive design may decrease contrast acuity in certain lighting conditions. This may be problematic for refractive lens exchange patients who do not have a cataract and are therefore used to excellent quality of vision.

Ideal candidates for mixing IOLs include: patients desiring spectacle independence at all times; patients with either very small or very large pupils; patients who are less tolerant of halo and glare (especially for night driving); and patients unsatisfied with vision in the first implanted eye, yet with realistic expectations.

In our clinic, patients who receive custom matching usually have a refractive multifocal IOL placed in the distance dominant eye (aiming for plano to −0.25 D), and a diffractive multifocal IOL implanted in the nondominant eye (aiming for plano to +0.25 D).

Physician/Patient Discussions

Patients who select premium multifocal IOLs are not paying for the privilege of receiving a special type of lens. Instead, they are paying the premium to be able to see without glasses. Thus, the preoperative discussion about their visual needs and potential lifestyle liberation is critical.

The surgeon and staff should not use highly technical terms initially. Instead, after it has been established that a patient will have cataract surgery they should be asked the simple question: "Would you like to see everything without glasses?" Then, wait and listen to the patient talk about their visual needs and desires. This way, the patient drives this portion of the discussion, and the surgeon receives the input that helps to determine the best multifocal option. If they are a candidate for custom lens selection, the approach can then be explained and the surgeon and patient can talk about reasonable expectations and expected outcomes.

Staged Implantation

With staged implantation a surgeon implants the primary lens in the first eye and assesses patient satisfaction with this eye at 1 to 2 weeks postoperatively. If the patient is dissatisfied, find out why. The IOL for the fellow eye is then chosen based on the patient's feedback. This approach customizes lens selection to patient lifestyle; provides a safety net; allows the patient to participate actively in the process; and allows us to better maximize patient satisfaction (Table 2 and Figure 1).

A key consideration in choosing your primary presbyopia-correcting IOL is to make clear distance vision the first priority. Patients pay for near vision, but they expect good distance vision. Patients also need and want a functional range of vision because older generations are staying active longer and are using computers on a regular basis.

Table 1

EVALUATING IOL ALTERNATIVES: RESULTS WITH MIXING IOLS

	ReSTOR/ ReSTOR n = 55 pts	ReZoom/ ReSTOR n = 128 pts	ReZoom/ ReZoom n = 30 pts
Mean age	59	61	54
J near	1.17		1.39
J near OU	1.00	1.09	1.27
J Intermediate	4.21		3.07
J Intermediate OU	3.81	2.39	2.04
Mean follow-up	19 months	13 months	3 months
Cat/RL %	38/62	48/52	53/47

Mixing refractive and diffractive lens technologies can be a successful approach for the right patient.

Data courtesy of Frank A. Bucci, Jr, MD.

Table 2

STAGED IMPLANTATION: HOW IT WORKS

	ReZoom	ReSTOR	Crystalens
Distance	Excellent	Good	Excellent
Intermediate	Good	Poor	Good
Near	Good	Excellent	Variable
Effective add power	+2.6	+3.2	Variable

For cataract patients, the dominant eye should be implanted first, except in cases in which the best-corrected visual acuity (BCVA) is much worse in one eye, in which case, this eye is operated on first.

For precataract patients, determine ocular dominance and then implant the primary multifocal lens in the dominant eye. Implant the nondominant eye 1 to 2 weeks after the dominant eye.

Surgeons, of course, want to maximize patient satisfaction. Although the majority of patients with mid-sized pupils will be satisfied receiving bilateral refractive multifocal IOLs, patients with miotic or large pupils may do better with a mixed multifocal IOL implantation strategy.

Being up front with patients helps them to have realistic expectations. Be sure to communicate that the visual benefits of premium lenses are maximized with binocular presbyopia-correcting IOL implantation. Discuss the expected halo effect. For example, I tell every patient that they may have some halos at night forever and they will get less obvious with time, but may persist. My staff and I try to turn a negative into a positive: I tell patients that the halos are a natural result of the lens design that enables vision freedom.

In addition, devices like the IOL Counselor's Halo Simulator (Patient Education Concepts, Houston, TX) can help illustrate what a patient may experience. Alphagan also can give a bit of help if they have difficulty dealing with halos and glare postoperatively.

Finally, it is also important to mentally prepare patients for the possibility of a refractive enhancement. The surgeon's capability to do subsequent procedures, such as limbal relaxing incisions, laser enhancement, and/or yttrium-aluminum-garnet (YAG) capsulotomies is a key component of successful multifocal IOL implantation.

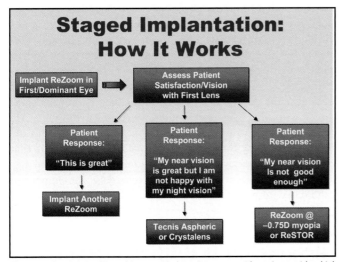

Figure 1. Custom matching with stage implantation can provide patients with a high quality full range of vision.

CHAPTER 136

PEARLS FOR MIXING MULTIFOCAL IOLs

Angel López Castro, MD

Why Mixed IOLs?
Why Mix and Match?

With the recent availability of multifocal and accommodating intraocular lenses (IOLs), surgeons now have the ability to potentially provide glasses-free vision at all distances for our cataract and refractive lens exchange patients. It is a very exciting time, but also a confusing time, given the various properties of the available IOLs and the varied needs and expectations of patients. So far, all of the new presbyopia-correcting IOLs come with trade-offs.[1] Some provide better distance vision,[2] whereas others are better for up-close vision.[3] None of them are perfect.[4] I have been drawn to the concept of combining 2 IOLs with different optical properties to maximize the patient's range of vision. One might consider a variety of lens combinations, including monofocal-multifocal combinations. To me, mixing one diffractive and one refractive multifocal IOL makes the most sense intuitively, given the synergistic strengths of these technologies. In this chapter, I will review what I have learned about custom matching IOLs.

Improving Intermediate Vision

To date, my experience with custom matching has been primarily with the combination of a ReZoom (Advanced Medical Optics, Santa Ana, CA) refractive multifocal IOL in the dominant eye and a Tecnis (Advanced Medical Optics) aspheric diffractive multifocal IOL in the other eye. My original goal in combining these lenses was to improve intermediate vision,[3,4] which was weak in patients with bilateral diffractive IOLs. However, I also found that this combination provides other advantages, primarily by extending the range of vision under different lighting conditions. The refractive ReZoom lens provides the intermediate vision that is missing with bilateral implantation of diffractive IOLs. In bright light, it provides superior distance visual acuity (VA) with no loss of light trans-

mission, whereas the diffractive multifocal Tecnis provides excellent near VA with the aspheric Tecnis platform. In dim light, ReZoom provides better reading capability in the middle range of the pupil. Meanwhile, the outer portion of the Tecnis multifocal lens becomes dominant, providing better distance vision and decreasing nighttime photic phenomena. Thus, combining the optical properties of these two lenses provides patients with a full range of vision under most lighting conditions. Previously, I would have recommended refractive lenses for light-to-moderate readers, computer users, people who primarily drive during the day, and those who enjoy sports, playing cards or other indoor activities. I would have chosen diffractive lenses for patients who are heavy readers, drive or work at night, or who enjoy going to the movies. But the night driver who also uses a computer presented a difficult case because neither option would fully meet his or her lifestyle needs. The great thing about custom IOL matching is that a diffractive-refractive IOL combination suits most activities for any given patient, allowing you to increase the number of candidates for multifocal IOLs in your practice.

Chair Time:
Discussing It With the Patient

Suggesting a clear lens surgery with multifocal lenses in general, and with the mix and match method in particular requires spending much more time with patients when they come to our office for an evaluation. The reason for this is that in addition to performing the exam, we need to become familiar with our patient's personality, occupation, and lifestyle (daily activities). For example, we must determine whether they are security guards or hunters, what their priorities are regarding vision, whether they are heavy readers or PC users, play cards or drive at night, and whether they have any other specific visual requirements—in other words, we must become intimately familiar with our patient's visual needs and requirements. We have to explain to them what the available options

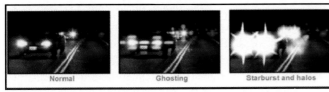

Figure 1. Dysphotopsia simulations.

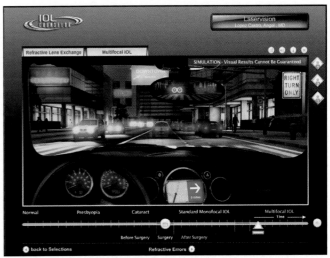

Figure 2. IOLCounselor halo simulation with a multifocal lens.

are and what they will be getting: two monofocal lenses, monovision, 2 equal multifocal lenses, either diffractive or refractive (custom match), or diffractive-monofocal and diffractive–refractive asymmetrical implants. It is very important to explain what outcome can reasonably be expected, and what the postoperative period will be like. This will help to rule out poor candidates, to allay excessive patient concerns during the postoperative period, and to prevent patient dissatisfaction.

Before making a decision, patients should become familiar with the available options.[3,4] We make use of videos and/or photographs (Figure 1 [IOL Counselor, Patient Education Concepts, Houston, TX, www.iolcounselor.com] and Figure 2), that simulate vision with these lenses, and administer personality questionnaires (Dr. Dell questionnaire [Appendix A]), including questions about each patient's visual preferences, functional expectations, and their tolerance of visual side effects.

Before surgery we tell our patients in writing what the advantages are that they will receive (less dependence on glasses, improved quality of life) along with the potential disadvantages and side effects, including halos, glare, and loss of contrast sensitivity.[5]

We must make sure we have understood our patient's wishes, and that they, too, have understood what they will get and how that will be achieved.

What Should Patients Know Before Surgery Regarding the Postoperative Period?

* Postoperative far vision is acceptably good within a few days after surgery with both types of multifocal lenses, especially with ReZoom, and it continues to improve over time.
* It usually takes several weeks for near vision to improve, especially in the ReZoom lens eye.
* Binocular near vision continues improving beyond a 2-month-long period.
* The younger the patient, the sooner optimum near vision is achieved.
* The patient will notice halos, glare, or double vision, especially in dim light (mesopic light levels). This is related to multifocality, and the second image is responsible for this problem. Patients should be warned of the fact that dysphotopsia[6] is more pronounced during the first several months and may cause problems with night driving. It then gradually subsides because of the neuroadaptation process, and eventually very few patients continue to have ghosting or clinically significant dysphotopsia[6] by 6 months after surgery.
* Multifocality causes a mild loss of contrast sensitivity (poorer vision) under mesopic conditions. However, there are published studies that compared contrast sensitivity six months after surgery between eyes with monofocal and multifocal lenses, and no significant differences were found.[5]
* Patients may have multifocality problems at first (difficulties in choosing the image of interest out of two available images), because they will require visual retraining. Fortunately, this will gradually improve with neuroadaptation, which can take up to six months to a year to occur.
* Reading speed[7] may initially be reduced, but this also improves over time, and significant reductions are rare.
* There will be visual differences between both eyes if the mix and match technique is used, but this is what should be expected as the goal is to have complementary differences between both eyes.
* For reading, good lighting is important.
* The patient will probably require a new excimer laser intervention in the event of clinically significant residual refractive error.
* If there is significant preoperative corneal astigmatism, corrective eyeglasses will be necessary until the laser intervention is performed (usually two months after clear lens surgery).

Rarely, it may be necessary to explant one or both lenses in order to solve intolerable side effects.

What Should the Physician Know Before Recommending Implantation of a Multifocal Lens?

* Multifocal lenses should not be offered to a patient who is not interested in discontinuing the use of eyeglasses.

* They should not be offered to a patient who is not willing to accept halos.

* This procedure should not be offered to a patient with a type A personality.

* Implantation of these lenses requires more postoperative trips to the office, and visits usually require increased chair time and discussions with patients.

* The physician should anticipate potential explanations for common complaints. (Be prepared!)

* Emmetropia must be achieved: the physician should have an Excimer laser available, either for photorefractive keratectomy (PRK) or laser in situ keratomileusis (LASIK), and the patient must meet corneal requirements for the procedure to be performed. Any residual refractive error can be corrected with laser after 2 months. Postoperative ametropia greater than 0.5-D sphere or a 0.75-D cylinder is poorly tolerated, especially in the eye with the diffractive lens. The refractive accuracy is far more important than when using a monofocal lens.[8]

* Like all refractive lenses, ReZoom is more forgiving of residual ametropia than diffractive multifocal lenses; it works better with slightly myopic outcomes than slightly hypermetropic ones.

* The physician should speak clearly and honestly with the patient.

* The physician should not mislead patients into expecting that the results will be perfect.

* The physician should not lie to a dissatisfied patient.

* A yttrium-aluminum-garnet (YAG) laser should be available, because a capsulotomy should be performed (a reasonable time after the intervention) in case of even mild clinically significant capsule opacity, especially in eyes with diffractive multifocal IOLs.

* The patient should not expect to eliminate wearing glasses altogether, but instead expect to achieve less spectacle dependence. This must be emphasized, because patients may interpret the use of glasses for very specific activities as a failure of the surgery.

* We should have a predefined mix and match plan that is not dependent upon the patient's initial satisfaction or dissatisfaction with the first eye's result. This is because both near and far vision will improve over time and the 2 IOLs will have an additive effect).

* The refractive lens should be implanted in the dominant eye and the diffractive lens in the non-dominant eye.

* Optical coherence tomography should be available in case a patient has poor vision due to subclinical cystoid macular edema or macular thickening that cannot be detected with sterior biomicroscopy.

* Many medical and surgical accommodations may be necessary: same-day surgery for each eye, temporary glasses for astigmatism, excimer laser treatment, and perhaps an early YAG capsulotomy.[8] All costs should be clearly spelled out in the written estimates provided to the patient.

* We charge a fixed global sum for the entire process, whether complementary enhancement procedures are required or not, because an extra charge accompanying the extra enhancement procedures may make the patient even more unhappy.

* A patient's visual quality cannot be assessed with standard high contrast optotypes, with good ambient lighting and a miotic pupil. We should bear in mind that even if patients have a 1.0 visual acuity result in these conditions, they may be bothered by halos, glare, or double vision at night, which, if coupled with low contrast sensitivity, may lead to functionally poor vision and difficulties in night driving.[5]

  Contrast sensitivity tests (Sinewave contrast sensitivity test, ETDRS (Early Treatment Diabetic Retinopathy Study), Pelli-Robson or Regan) performed at different ambient light levels, with and without glare, are more representative of real-life situations. They are very useful to simulate visual function in the real world.[5]

* As with all refractive procedures, dissatisfied patients should be seen frequently, and they should be reassured; explain to them that outcomes typically improve over the course of several weeks to months.

* This is still not a universally perfect solution for presbyopia.

How To Get Started and Who Are the Best Candidates?

The initial question when I first considered mixing dissimilar optics was whether the patient would tolerate and integrate these disparate images. Initially, we implanted a diffractive lens in the second eye of patients who already had a monofocal lens in their first eye. After reading the initial positive experiences that others had achieved with IOL mixing, we decided to start using the mix and match strategy, and we have not received a single complaint so far in terms of visual integration of both types of images. Patients tolerate the combination of both lenses perfectly well.

The following is a list of the best candidates for this procedure:

* Patients who have cataracts[2]

* Hyperopic presbyopia patients

* Moderately myopic presbyopes (second only to hyperopes in terms of satisfaction rates)

* Patients who are not wearing full spectacle correction

* Refractive patients who are contact lens intolerant

Figure 3. Key points for patient selection.

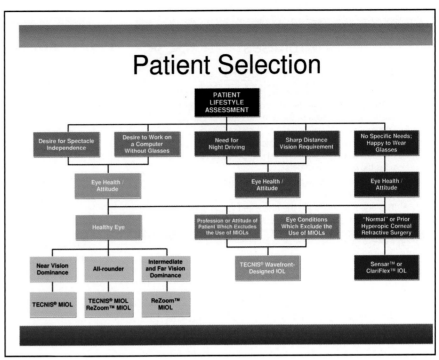

* Relatively young refractive patients requesting spectacle independence
* Patients who are generally tolerant and conformist
* Patients with a good tear film
* Patients who are not professional drivers
* Patients with low preoperative astigmatism
* Poor starting candidates are refractive patients with no cataract and with low myopia

Patient Selection

WHEN TO USE MULTIFOCAL LENSES

Patient selection is critically important for multifocal implants, and is a critical determinant of whether the procedure will be a success or failure. Special attention should be paid to the preliminary office consultation, in which the physician gets to know the patient's personality and habits (Figure 3).

A basic premise is that patients should desire freedom from eyeglasses, for both near and far vision. We should always ask, "Do you really want to avoid wearing eyeglasses?" If patients say they do not mind wearing glasses, we should implant monofocal lenses instead (Figure 4).

EXCLUSION CRITERIA

* Eye disease: multifocal lenses should not be implanted in patients with any eye disorder.
  * Macular disease of any type.
  * Impaired ocular motility: tropias, phorias, convergence problems, eccentric fixation, or impaired fusion due to any cause.
  * Moderate to deep amblyopia: because of the problems they would have in near vision, because the diffractive lens is implanted in the non-dominant eye and this eye is used for reading. In case of an amblyopic eye, and if patients require uncorrected near vision (very common in myopic people), a bilateral implant with two diffractive lenses will be performed.
  * Moderate or severe dry eye. A patient with poor tear quality may have poor vision, especially in the eye with the diffractive lens.
  * Any abnormality in corneal transparency or regularity: leukomas or ecstatic diseases (keratoconus, pellucid marginal degeneration).
  * If pupil size is abnormally small at low light levels (<4 to 4.5 mm) or extremely large with light (>6 mm).
  * Avoid multifocal implants in eyes with eccentric pupils (because the IOL centered within the capsular bag will not be aligned with the center of the pupil).
  * Glaucoma. Glaucomatous neuropathy impairs the visual perception and neuroadaptation process. These patients in particular are poor candidates for diffractive multifocal lenses.
  * Pseudoexfoliation. The lens may become subluxated or dislocated during the early or late postoperative period.
* Related to lifestyle and occupation:
  * Unrealistic visual expectations.
  * Patients demanding high visual precision:
    * Those who require high levels of contrast sensitivity (pilots, photographers), especially in dim lighting conditions (professional drivers).

Premises

- **THE PATIENT MUST DESIRE INDEPENDENCE FROM EYEGLASSES**
- Must agree to or tolerate the side effects that might occur, such as halos or glare in the night, or dim light conditions.
- It requires extra time in the office, to speak with and to make clear to the patient what can be achieved and the possible unwanted effects
- They are lenses designed to allow for good vision at different distances.
- The major problem are the unwanted visual symptoms, not the ability for near and distant vision

Figure 4. Patient selection matrix.

Key Success Factors

- Careful patient selection
- Comprehensive patient information
- Careful selection of appropriate MIOLs
- Accurate biometry with optimized A-constants
- Measures to reduce postoperative astigmatism (LRI, LASIK touch-up)
- Clean capsule
- **Tear film**

Figure 5. Key points for success.

⊙ Need for highly precise near vision (neither a watchmaker nor a jeweler are good candidates) or far vision (sharpshooters).

⊙ Patients who work under poor lighting conditions (neither professional drivers nor air traffic controllers are good candidates).

❖ Patients who are satisfied with their reading glasses.

❖ Caution is advised with people over 70 years of age, because their neuroadaptation may be unpredictable.

✱ Related to personality:
- ❖ Altered mental or psychiatric status of any type.
- ❖ Patients who are never satisfied with their progressive glasses.
- ❖ Stroke.
- ❖ Dyslexia.
- ❖ Patients with type A personality (perfectionist, intolerant, obsessive, demanding, self-critical).

✱ Preoperative refraction:
- ❖ Patients with low myopia or with emmetropia and presbyopia, especially in the case of clear lens surgery, are very poor candidates (they will notice loss of far vision contrast sensitivity compared with prior to correction).
- ❖ Requirement for an IOL power beyond that which is available: Tecnis +5 to +34, ReSTOR (Alcon, Fort Worth, TX) +10 to +30, and ReZoom +6 to +30.

✱ Surgical complications:
- ❖ Relative exclusion:
  - ⊙ Capsular tear (the lens can still be implanted in sulcus if it is a Tecnis or a ReZoom lens but not a ReSTOR one). Special care should be taken with myopic patients because the sulcus may be larger than normal and may increase the incidence of lens decentration.
  - ⊙ Inability to remove a fibrous plaque from the posterior capsule during surgery.
- ❖ Absolute exclusion:

⊙ A lens that is off center (dislocated) due to any cause should not be left in.

⊙ A splintered or cracked lens should not be left in (Figures 5 and 6).

When to Use Custom Match?

✱ Bilateral ReZoom
- ❖ Lifestyle: mostly outdoors
- ❖ Preoperative refraction: High hyperopia
- ❖ Pupil size: small
- ❖ Moderate or occasional readers
- ❖ Computer users
- ❖ Day drivers
- ❖ Sportspeople
- ❖ Card players, cooks, shoppers

✱ Bilateral Tecnis
- ❖ Lifestyle: heavy readers, craftspeople
- ❖ Preoperative refraction: Low myopia
- ❖ Pupil size: large
- ❖ Night and day drivers
- ❖ Film lovers
- ❖ People who work at night (guards)

Clear Lens Extraction: Special Considerations

I do not currently recommend multifocal lenses for emmetropic refractive patients (without cataract[s]) who are only interested in avoiding reading eyeglasses.

Patients with previous ametropia who are interested in refractive surgery should be warned of the risks of intraocular surgery, as compared to LASIK. They should also be told that enhancement with excimer laser correction may eventually be required.

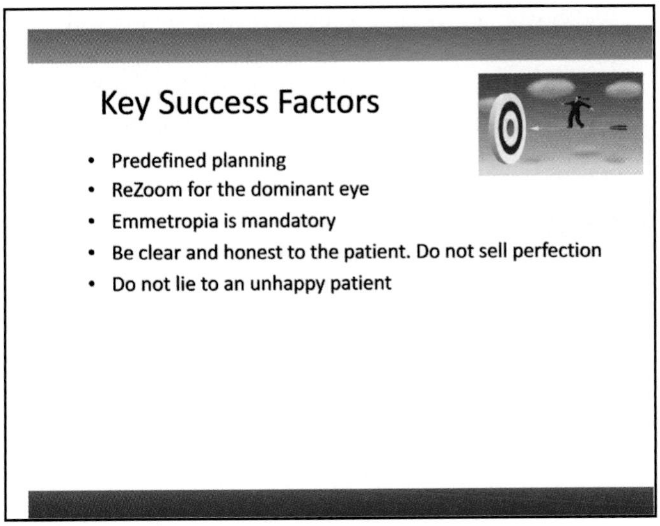

Key Success Factors

- Predefined planning
- ReZoom for the dominant eye
- Emmetropia is mandatory
- Be clear and honest to the patient. Do not sell perfection
- Do not lie to an unhappy patient

Figure 6. Key points for success.

* Our indications for clear lens surgery in terms of preoperative refraction and age are the following:
* Hypermetropia with a spherical equivalent greater than 4 D in people older than 45 years of age.
* Myopia with a spherical equivalent greater than 8 D in people older than 45 years of age.
* Myopia with a spherical equivalent greater than 6 D in people older than 50 years of age.

Special Cases

* Pediatric cataract: We have had very positive (although limited) experience using multifocal IOLs in patients with congenital or cortisone-induced cataracts, provided that the aforementioned general premises are met. We currently recommend multifocal IOLs for these younger patients because they benefit greatly from not wearing reading glasses, and they have excellent neuroadaptation.
* Traumatic cataract: We also consider multifocal IOLs in these eyes provided that the cornea is transparent, there is no irregular astigmatism, and the zonules and capsular bag are strong and secure enough to provide proper IOL centration and stability.[2]
* Previous refractive surgery: We do not think that prior keratorefractive surgery is an absolute contraindication to using multifocal IOLs,[2] especially if the cornea can still undergo Excimer laser ablation surgery to enhance residual refractive error. This principle also holds true for eyes that have undergone prior radial keratotomy. Nowadays intraocular lens calculation following previous Excimer laser corneal surgery can be done using methods such as the Haigis–L formula, the double-K method, the Best formula, and others.

The Physician's Game Plan for a Dissatisfied Patient

* Try to define the problem and act if it can be resolved.
* Make sure that a problem truly exists.
* If the cause of the patient's complaint is not clear, perform a contrast sensitivity test, with and without glare.
* Frequent exams should be performed and patients should be reassured (patient visits and discussions should not be put off), and they should not be referred to another ophthalmologist. The surgeon who operated on the patient should perform the examination.
* Patients should feel they are not alone with this problem and that the physician cares for them and is committed to helping them.
* Patients should be reassured that in our experience, adverse effects usually disappear or improve over time.
* Tell patients that dysphotopsia6 is inherent to multifocality—that is the price they have to pay for good uncorrected far and near vision. Show patients a photograph of a multifocal lens where the rings or the various optical zones are displayed, and use this to explain that although these lenses allow for far and near vision, they cause these halos in low ambient light.
* Speak clearly and honestly with your patient.
* Do not lie to a dissatisfied patient.
* Complaints about the first eye usually improve when the second eye is operated on.
* Avoid desperate and drastic solutions; problems usually resolve in the first 6 months.
* If faced with a very upset patient who has an untreatable problem inherent to the multifocal lens, pose the following challenge: simulate for the patient what vision with near vision with a monofocal lens would be like, if an IOL exchange were to be performed: most of them will back out because they will not want to lose their near vision.

What Points Should We Check?

* Is there residual correction?
* Is the posterior capsule transparent?
* Is the lens properly centered with respect to the pupil?
* Is there a quality ocular surface?
* Check tear quality and quantity.
* Rule out macular edema through OCT.

When to Explant

When you are convinced that the multifocal lens is responsible for persistent patient complaints about halos, doubled images, glare, acuity or definition loss, an IOL explantation and exchange may be suggested. One must rule out other causes of visual impairment, and one should make sure that a reasonable amount of adjustment has been attempted, which may take up to one year. It is best to simulate the likely new situation for far and near vision with the replacement IOL.

Slight lens decentration is usually not a reason to explant the IOL, Kazuno et al[9] study concluded that up to 1-mm decentrations of multifocal lenses do not affect the quality of the retinal image significantly.

If the patient is unhappy with their mixed vision, try to determine which IOL produces the most bothersome vision, and which IOL is the better tolerated. The lens causing the greatest discomfort should be detected. Typically, it is the diffractive lens that is most bothersome, and there is good tolerance of the refractive multifocal lens. In this case, discuss exchanging the diffractive IOL for a refractive multifocal to avoid losing intermediate and near vision. If the refractive lens causes more difficulties, it should be changed for a monofocal lens in one eye first, to assess the situation, and then in the other eye, if necessary.

Conclusion

Newer multifocal lenses are growing in popularity for the treatment of presbyopia. We have gone from using them in 2% of all lenses implanted 3 years ago to 15% to 20% nowadays.

The decision to implant these lenses requires careful patient selection following a thorough ophthalmologic examination, in which poor candidates are dismissed. Despite this, some patients do not tolerate multifocality well, and we cannot always predict in advance who these patients will be.

We should not confuse natural accommodation with "near vision" provided by multifocality. Multifocality is not without optical drawbacks. There is an unavoidable reduction of contrast sensitivity due to light scattering with any multifocal IOL.[5]

References

1. Olson RJ, Werner L, Mamalis N, Cionni R. PERSPECTIVES: New intraocular lens technology. *Am J Ophthalmol.* 2005;140:709-716.

2. Bellucci R. Multifocal intraocular lenses. *Curr Opin Ophthalmol.* 2005;16:33-37.

3. Kohnen T, Allen D, Boureau C, Dublineau P, Hartmann C, Mehdorn E, Rozot P, Tassinari G. European multicenter study of the AcrySof ReSTOR apodized diffractive. *Ophthalmology.* 2006;113(4):578-584.

4. Blaylock JF, Si Z, Vickers C. Visual and refractive status at different focal distances after implantation of the ReSTOR multifocal intraocular lens. *J Cataract Refract Surg.* 2006;32:1464-1473.

5. Montés-Micó R, Alió JL. Distance and near contrast sensitivity function after multifocal intraocular lens implantation. *J Cataract Refract Surg.* 2003;29:703-711. 2003

6. Schwiegerling J. Recent developments in pseudophakic dysphotopsia. *Curr Opin Ophthalmol.* 2006;17:27-30.

7. Hütz WW, Berthold Eckhardt H, Röhrig B, Grolmus R. Reading ability with 3 multifocal intraocular lens models. *J Cataract Refract Surg.* 2006;32:2015-2021.

8. Leccisotti A. Secondary procedures after presbyopic lens exchange. *J Cataract Refract Surg.* 2004;30:1461-1465.

9. Negishi K, Ohnuma K, Ikeda T, Noda T. Visual simulation of retinal images through a decentered monofocal and a refractive multifocal intraocular lens. *Jpn J Ophthalmol.* 2005;49:281-286.

CHAPTER 137

PEARLS FOR MIXING MULTIFOCAL IOLs

Matteo Piovella, MD

The challenge with multifocal intraocular lenses (IOLs) is to select good candidates preoperatively and exclude those who are likely to be dissatisfied with the surgery. Optimal patient selection is the main goal for surgeons who are already able to achieve good refractive outcomes with their standard cataract surgery practices. I believe the main reason only 3% to 4% of IOLs implanted today are presbyopia-correcting (Pr-C) IOLs is that surgeons are afraid to embark on new and difficult procedures that entail a higher risk of patient dissatisfaction in exchange for minimal benefits to the surgeon. By following the steps for custom matching that I outline in this chapter, 94% of my multifocal IOL patients are happy with their results for far and near vision. However, the most important advantage has been the benefit my practice has derived from the multifocal IOL experience.

It is necessary to fully understand the patient's needs when using multifocal IOLs. For patient satisfaction and for the benefit of the practice, the time and resources that this step-by-step process entails must be taken into account. After years of not seeing my practice develop because I was not pushing myself to look beyond the "safe haven" of standard cataract surgery, multifocal IOL technology came as a revolution that led to the introduction of new minimum quality requirements that increased benefits for the entire practice. This new technology has helped me and my practice improve our results in every area, so that we have reduced the number of surgical complications and surgeon-patient misunderstandings in more routine cataract surgery as well as with specialized lenses.

New technology, new concepts, new examination methods, more consultation time, and better patient education are crucial. The patient and his or her unique visual needs become the center of attention for me and my staff. This includes utilizing the best available technology for the examination and the surgery. It includes I and my staff being reassuring, understanding, and supportive to the patient and the patient's family at every opportunity.

I would like to share some simple examples of this new approach of custom-matching multifocal IOLs. It is very important to provide the patient with clear and simple information. Do not promise 100% spectacle independence. Explain to patients that there will be an adjustment period for all IOLs, but especially with premium IOLs. The patients must understand that the visual system works best when both eyes have had surgery and are working together.

Identification of the dominant eye is very helpful in deciding the best options for the patient. I prefer to apply the simple rules that conductive keratoplasty (CK) treatments have demonstrated to be very effective. I always start with a diffractive Tecnis multifocal IOL (Advanced Medical Optics, Santa Ana, CA) in the nondominant eye and, in most situations, implant a refractive ReZoom multifocal IOL (Advanced Medical Optics) in the dominant eye. These lenses are complementary. The refractive ReZoom provides excellent distance vision, especially in the dominant eye, and good intermediate vision. The diffractive Tecnis IOL (Figures 1 and 2) provides very good near acuity and it is less pupil dependent than the ReZoom lens (Figure 3). This last point is important if you are routinely using mydriatics in the postoperative period. Implanting a Tecnis multifocal IOL, which is relatively pupil size independent, decreases the patient's stress about the perception of halos and glare immediately after the surgery. I prefer to implant the second fellow eye 1 week after the first eye surgery is done. The sooner the second eye is done, the quicker the patient will have the benefit of both lenses. In between the first and second eyes, I evaluate the patient's satisfaction and make the final choice of the second IOL.

When I began implanting multifocal IOLs, I became very interested in achieving outstanding unaided near visual acuities and avoiding any significant decrease in the quality of vision. I minimize patient complaints of poor visual quality by matching the multifocal IOL to the patient's pupil size (Tables 1 and 2). For example, if the pupil size under mesopic conditions is over 5.2 mm, I prefer bilateral Tecnis implantation. In my experience, even cataract patients with 6.0-mm pupils who are implanted with monofocal IOLs may experience visually significant glare and halos. I also choose bilateral Tecnis

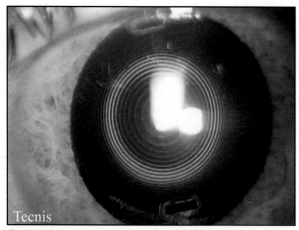

Figure 1. Slit-lamp view of a Tecnis-implanted eye.

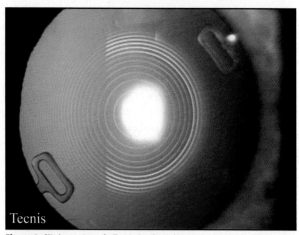

Figure 2. Slit-lamp view of a Tecnis-implanted eye.

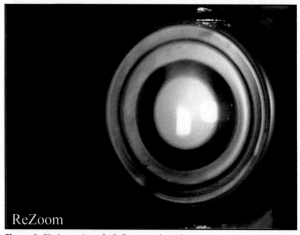

Figure 3. Slit-lamp view of a ReZoom-implanted eye.

Table 1

CLINICAL PREOPERATIVE DATA OF THE STUDY EYES

	Tecnis 40 eyes (mean ± S.D.)	ReZoom 40 eyes (mean ± S.D.)
UCVA	0.41 ± 0.22	0.33 ± 0.18
IOP (mmHg)	15.73 ± 3.52	15.89 ± 3.85
Endothelial Cell Counts/mm2	2424 ± 298	2402 ± 281
Pupil diameter (mm)	4.60 ± 0.65	4.74 ± 0.66
IOL power (diopters)	22.03 ± 3.70	21.01 ± 3.40

Table 2

ONE-MONTH CLINICAL DATA OF THE STUDY EYES

	Tecnis 40 eyes (mean ± S.D.)	ReZoom 40 eyes (mean ± S.D.)
IOP (mmHg)	15.73 ± 3.52	13.08 ± 2.97
Endothelial Cell Counts (ECC)	2170 ± 425	2313 ± 320
% ECC decrease	-7.09	-2.2
Pupil Diameter (mm)	4.53 ± 0.66	4.48 ± 0.68

Integrating Multifocal IOls Into the Practice

There is no question that certain changes are required from a standard cataract practice to properly integrate multifocal IOLs. It is important to have the best possible equipment to obtain the most accurate measurements in order for the surgeon to obtain the best possible results. Biometry needs to be improved. It is ideal to obtain 2 different sets of measurements with 2 different technologies in order to compare the results and avoid errors. I prefer the IOL Master (Carl Zeiss, Jena, Germany) and contact A-scan. In addition to advanced biometry, mesopic pupillometry is very helpful. I prefer to use an aspheric IOL with larger pupil sizes. I spend much more time counseling patients, both pre- and postoperatively. I anticipate this need and adjust my schedule accordingly. We have obtained a new computer instrument (Figures 4, 5, and 6) (Eyevispod Analysis System, PGB srl, Milano, Italy) to test near vision and to determine reading speed at 1 week, 1 month (Table 3), and 6 months after surgery. We typically see 14% improvement in reading speed during the first month alone. Essentially, all of this extra attention means that our multifocal IOL patients receive much more information and support from me and my staff.

multifocal IOLs for patients with equal dominance in both eyes and for those who seem to be especially sensitive to glare and halo. However, bilateral Tecnis IOLs may not be the best choice for heavy computer users. A refractive lens that provides more intermediate vision is desirable for these patients.

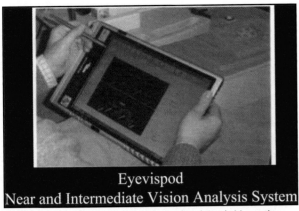

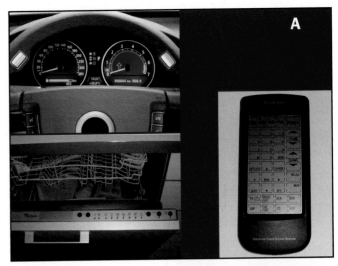

Figure 4. Eyevispod device for near and intermediate (60 cm) vision testing.

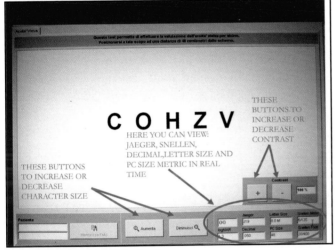

Figure 5. Near vision test with Eyevispod.

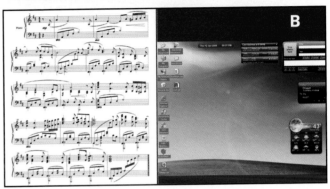

Figure 6. Intermediate vision test with Eyevispod.

I have a lower threshold for intervention in the event of unsatisfactory results. For example, neodymium:yttrium-aluminum-garnet (Nd:YAG) capsulotomy should be performed sooner rather than later if there is any posterior capsular opacification (PCO). Specific attention is needed if silicone IOLs are implanted. I have a low threshold to do a laser vision correction enhancement over a multifocal IOL. I have also found that even minor corrections of residual sphere or cylinder can dramatically improve the patient's vision if he or she is especially bothered by glare and halos. If the residual refractive error is mild (within 0.75 D), I will usually prescribe low-power "emergency spectacles" 1 month postoperatively. For larger errors, I will perform a laser enhancement after 6 months. Surgeons who cannot or will not incorporate these new strategies should consider not implanting multifocal IOLs. However, for those who are willing to invest their time and attention, it is certainly possible to achieve a successful multifocal IOL practice with high rates of patient satisfaction.

One of the most important concepts to keep in mind when treating patients with multifocal IOLs is the following: "Many things that patients report in the postoperative period are really observations they are making about their vision. They are not necessarily complaining, but want to be reassured that this is normal" (Rich Tipperman, MD; oral communication; 2007). As I see it, we are undergoing a positive revolution com-

Table 3

ONE-MONTH VISUAL ACUITY DATA OF THE STUDY EYES

	Tecnis 40 eyes (mean ± S.D.)	ReZoom 40 eyes (mean ± S.D.)
UCVA	0.81 ± 0.17	0.88 ± 0.15
BSCVA	0.95 ± 0.10	0.98 ± 0.06
SE	-0.12 ± 0.54	-0.30 ± 0.39
Near Binocular Visual Acuity (Jaeger) (Eyevispod)	1.69 ± 0.86	
Monocular Visual Acuity (Jaeger) (Eyevispod)	4.19 ± 1.75	5.13 ± 2.29
Intermediate (60 cm) Binocular Visual Acuity (Eyevispod)	6.27 ± 1.35 (number of slides out of 8 presented slides)	
Words per minute, binocular vision (Eyevispod)	93.88 ± 27.16	

parable with that in the early 1980s when eye surgeons around the world had the excellent results of extracapsular cataract extraction and at the same time had to switch to phacoemulsification. Passing on this chance means missing out on a very important opportunity.

Frequently Asked Questions by Patients With Selected Answers

Question: Why do my 2 eyes see differently?

Answer: This is a real observation and it is normal with mixing different IOLs. Multifocal vision is not a simple technology. Each eye has to perform a different task in order to allow perfectly integrated results for reading far, intermediate, and near without glasses. Also, people who have never experienced eye surgery are now looking with both eyes open! Interestingly, in my experience, the only patient who complained of differences between both eyes after 3 months had the same IOL type implanted bilaterally.

Question: An eye doctor I met on the beach this summer told me that all my problems are due to the fact that I have multifocal IOLs. Is this true?

Answer: Many surgeons are uncomfortable or lack experience with multifocal IOL implantation. Therefore, they naturally do not understand its potential.

Question: I am unhappy with the results. Why can't I see any improvement?

Answer: Some people are negative by nature, and find faults even if something is perfectly fine. Be supportive and confident, and reassure the patient that everything will be OK.

Question: I am scheduled to undergo surgery in my second eye within a week. Can I avoid this?

Answer: Do not be afraid. Some patients are perfectly happy after just one eye surgery. After a few months they will come back for the fellow eye surgery with further improvement. Normally, patients with specific sensitivities that are difficult to manage ask for immediate fellow eye surgery.

Question: I do not want to have multifocal IOLs. Can I avoid them?

Answer: Many patients who have had difficulties with multifocal glasses are afraid that they will experience the same problems with multifocal IOLs. You need to explain the differences, but remember that these patients will be hesitant towards multifocal implants. If the patient has significant reservations, do not persist in recommending multifocal IOLs.

Bibliography

Piovella M, Kusa B, Camesasca FI. Mix and Match Cataract Surgery with Refractive (ReZoom) and Diffractive (Tecnis) Multifocal IOL Implantation. Scientific poster (271) presented at AAO Annual meeting; 2007.

CHAPTER 138

MIXING ACCOMMODATING AND MULTIFOCAL IOLS

J. Trevor Woodhams, MD

The advent of presbyopia-correcting intraocular lenses (Pr-C IOLs) opened a door for precataract baby boomers. Reportedly, these individuals have independent lifestyles and a willingness to undergo elective surgical procedures that promise to enhance their standard of living. Serendipitously, refractive lens exchange is often easier and safer to perform than traditional cataract surgery, which may pose the increased challenges of denser nuclei. A patient whose visual acuity can be readily refracted to nearly 20/20 (or better) prior to surgery, however, is deservedly more demanding of his or her postoperative visual outcome than one whose cataract has severely compromised visual acuity, night vision, and contrast sensitivity. This chapter discusses my experience with Pr-C IOLs in the context of presbyopic lens exchange surgery as a primarily refractive procedure. The emphasis will be on mixing the Crystalens (Eyeonics, Inc, Aliso Viejo, CA) and the AcrySof ReSTOR lens (Alcon, Fort Worth, TX).

Two Presbyopia-Correcting IOLs

Currently, there are 2 distinct categories of Pr-C IOLs: accommodating and multifocal (both refractive and diffractive). These lenses work in significantly different fashions and both have their weaknesses and strengths. For the traditional cataract surgeon, applying the skills necessary for refractive surgery with such things as patient selection and IOL choice is highly important in order to establish an early track record of success.

The Crystalens

The Crystalens was the first accommodating IOL on the US market and presented surgeons with a steep learning curve but allowed them to provide patients with high-quality distance and intermediate vision, albeit with mixed results in terms of consistent reading ability. Although most patients were quite pleased with the Crystalens, many still needed supplemental readers postoperatively for sustained near work. A formerly +3.00-D hyperopic presbyope may not mind wearing reading glasses, but a former –3.00-D myope most assuredly will and will take up much of your time describing what he or she could see up close prior to your surgery! While a preoperative explanation of the serendipity of near vision in the presbyopic myope is mandatory, even this is often inadequate to offset patient expectations in the real world.

The Crystalens works through a combination of actual anterior movement of the optic along with lens arching. Its accommodative effect increases with time, presumably due to increased strength and tone in the ciliary muscle from being repeatedly used.

The AcrySof ReSTOR Lens

The AcrySof ReSTOR lens, introduced 1 year after the Crystalens, employs an entirely different approach to presbyopia correction. Multifocality at near and distance is achieved by concentric rings of varying dioptric power, which are apodized to suppress image confusion and internal reflectivity. This lens provides slightly greater than a +3.00-D add at a typical (though somewhat close) reading distance of approximately 12 inches. Undesirable optical side effects include an unsatisfactory intermediate focal point (18 to 35 inches) and what many early recipients of the lens described as *"waxy" vision*.

The source of this "wax paper" effect can be identified by comparing the modulation transfer function (MTF) of 2 Pr-C IOLs—one accommodating, the other multifocal—under optical bench conditions (Figure 1). The steep drop-off the MTF curve is indicative of a significant loss of contrast across a wide range of frequencies that is perceived as (among other things) a loss of crisp edges and a general difficulty in perceiving objects with less than brightly lit backgrounds. This reduction in the area under the curve is roughly equivalent to the Strehl ratio, a measure of the overall quality of any optical device, and is also perceptible *in vivo* as decreased edge recognition and contrast sensitivity (ie, "waxy" vision). While

Figure 1. The source of this "wax paper" effect can be identified by comparing the modulation transfer function (MTF) of 2 Pr-C IOLs—one accommodating, the other multifocal— under optical bench conditions.

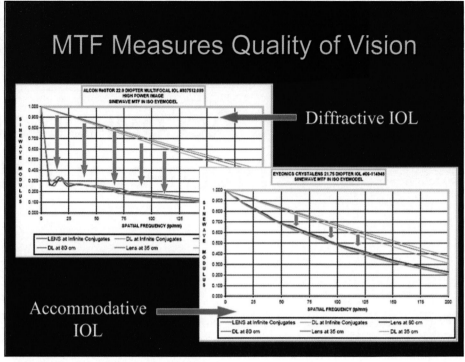

the "area under the curve" is by itself highly significant clinically, we can also recognize another serious compromise in visual acuity itself (ie, resolution). This refers to how far a patient can read down a typical 100% contrast eye chart. This is the "cutoff" where the MTF curve drops to the x-axis (abscissa). It corresponds to fine optical acuity found at the bottom of the typical eye chart. The cutoff can also be objectively determined in vivo using the double-pass technique employed by the Optical Quality Assessment System (Visiometrics, SA, Terrassa, Spain)

Mixing IOLs

The rationale for combining the Crystalens and the AcrySof ReSTOR IOL in a single patient is 2-fold. First, the pairing provides *maximum visual acuity* and performance *at distance* because of the higher resolving ability and better optical performance of a nonmultifocal accommodative IOL. While the quality of distance vision with an apodized, diffractive multifocal IOL can be excellent, it does not perform as well as a monofocal IOL under low light (mesopic) and nighttime (photopic) conditions. Surgical planning, then, typically dictates putting the Crystalens in the patient's dominant eye and the AcrySof ReSTOR in his or her fellow eye. Secondly, this strategy achieves a better range of visual performance at intermediate and close reading distances than would typically be the case using maximally distance-targeted accommodative or multifocal IOLs bilaterally.

Assuming that the patient tolerates the different optics of the 2 IOLs, both of his or her eyes will perceive equal levels of acuity at distance under bright lighting conditions based on my experience. The dominant eye's perceived image, however, may have significantly higher levels of contrast sensitivity, thereby providing finer levels of visual discrimination that

would otherwise be adversely affected under dim lighting conditions (the depressed MTF from the multifocal IOL). At close reading distances (11 to 13 inches), however, the AcrySof ReSTOR can relieve the accommodative strain on the ciliary muscle through the higher magnification inherent in its design. At intermediate distances, there is typically enough accommodation associated with the Crystalens to comfortably meet my patients' moderate accommodative demand over a wide range of intermediate distances, especially when they perform tasks such as using the computer. In my experience, bilateral AcrySof ReSTOR patients are quite pleased with their distance and near acuity, but usually complain about inadequate intermediate distance visual performance. Once again, the mixed IOL strategy can effectively address this problem.

Does mixing the Crystalens with the AcrySof ReSTOR lens work in the real world? Although it is probably not the best possible solution to meet every patient's needs, we find the combination to be effective and often better than bilaterally matched Pr-C IOLs in many, if not most, patients (Figure 2).

Prospective Evaluation of Mixed IOL Strategy

We performed a prospective, nonrandomized study of 60 consecutive patients undergoing refractive lens exchange with the mixed IOL strategy described above (currently in preparation in submission for publication). One hundred percent (100%) saw at least 20/32 binocularly. Limbal relaxing incisions but not laser refractive surgery was employed for astigmatism control. J8 (roughly the equivalent of 20/40 at near) was achieved at near in almost 100% of patients with over 70% able to read J3 (about 2/25 equivalent). Intermediate vision is a traditionally underrated aspect of visual functioning whose importance is coming to be more appreciated. Here,

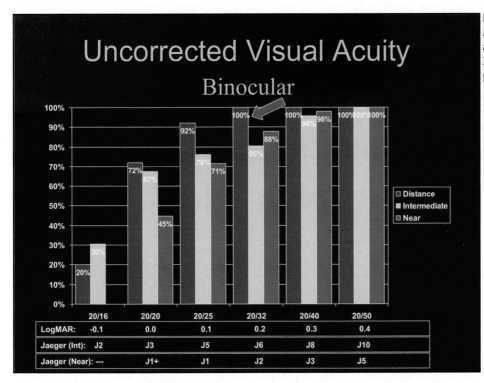

Figure 2. The mixing of the Crystalens with the AcrySof ReSTOR lens demonstrates the degree of acuity at 1) distance, 2) intermediate distance, and 3) near when the patient is allowed to choose his or her preferred range.

over three-fourths of patients could read J5 (the equivalent of 20/25) and over two-thirds were able to read the equivalent of 20/20 at a typical computer screen distance! At both near distance these results compare with 2 series (see Figure 2).

As expected, near vision was better in patients with bilateral AcrySof ReSTOR lenses and intermediate vision over an impressive range of distances was best in patients with bilateral Crystalens IOLs.

Postoperative Vision

What may dissatisfy patients about a mixed IOL approach? I find it is rarely a perceptual disparity in distance viewing. An occasional person will spontaneously mention a waxy image through the multifocal IOL. Even when questioned about waxy vision specifically, those who notice a difference will relate it more often to the close reading distance and describe letters as having "ghost image" edges. The high degree of magnification with the AcrySof ReSTOR lens at about 12 inches will often be compared advantageously to that of the Crystalens at that same distance.

Intermediate distance vision is almost never a source of complaints in my patients with mixed IOLs. Most are not even aware that their 2 eyes see differently at the 14- to 46-inch range. This finding, coupled with my patients' extremely high satisfaction with distance vision under even low-light conditions, has convinced me that the AcrySof ReSTOR/Crystalens combination works well for refractive lens exchange in most patients over age 50 (my rough cutoff age when selecting patients for this surgery). When might this combination not be advisable? First, this disclaimer: no IOL available today performs as well as the native, emmetropic crystalline lens. Patients with night driving demands (truck drivers) and rapid, repetitive near tasks (scanning driver's ID in security lines)

should be approached with caution. Furthermore, I find that refractive lensectomy patients in approximately the +1- to −3-D preoperative range (as mentioned previously) are the most challenging and will often have expectations that cannot always be met with current generation accommodative IOLs (Crystalens 5.0), even when paired with the ReSTOR. Conversely, high myopes (>−6 D) and hyperopes (>+3 D) are often more satisfied with their overall vision with bilateral accommodative IOLs, especially when a small amount of myopic offset (−0.50 to −0.75 D) is achieved (eg, modified monovision).

Conclusion

I anticipate combining the Crystalens and AcrySof ReSTOR lens at least until Alcon releases a "mid-range" (±1.50 D) add model of its multifocal IOL. It will be interesting to see whether the company's recently available aspheric ReSTOR will significantly improve its MTF. If so, the current drawbacks of bilaterally implanting the AcrySof ReSTOR lens will decrease dramatically.

As manufacturers improve the degree of dioptric or linear magnification at near with accommodating IOLs like the Crystalens, the relative advantage of multifocal Pr-C IOLs such as the AcrySof ReSTOR lens will likely disappear. Once accommodating IOLs provide a dependable range of magnification at near without excessive demand on accommodative reserve, I believe that they will completely replace multifocal IOLs because of their superior optical performance, as documented objectively by modulation transfer function and subjectively by patient satisfaction. In the meantime, judicious use of a "mixed" format in presbyopic, refractive IOL surgery offers a rewarding trade-off in benefits.

CHAPTER 139

MIXING OR MATCHING IOLs— WHY I DO NOT MIX

Richard Tipperman, MD

Multifocal intraocular lens (IOL) surgery has many similarities to traditional refractive surgery. One of the fundamental principles common to both of these fields is the concept of "20/happy." In reality, our goal as cataract surgeons utilizing presbyopia-correcting (Pr-C) IOLs is not to have a patient who "never wears glasses" nor a patient who is "20/20" for a specific distance but rather it is to have a patient who is "20/happy." Proponents of multifocal IOL mixing proclaim that it creates a greater percentage of happy patients while other clinicians seem to obtain excellent results by almost exclusively matching Pr-C IOLs.

In examining the subject of mixing and matching IOLs, one must first review the proposed benefits and downsides of each approach. I will discuss in this chapter why "mixing" of multifocal IOLs does not produce a greater percentage of happy patients and in the long run is more likely to produce a greater percentage of unhappy patients. Patients are happiest following multifocal IOL surgery if they can function normally on a day-to-day basis with minimal dependence on spectacles.

Multifocal IOls and Night Time Visual Disturbances

One of the reasons I prefer the ReSTOR multifocal lens (Alcon, Fort Worth, TX) platform is that it produces fewer difficulties with night time glare and halos than those seen with the ReZoom zonal refractive IOL (Advanced Medical Optics, Santa Ana, CA). I presented a paper at the American Society of Cataract and Refractive Surgery (ASCRS) meeting in 2007 describing the results of an optical bench evaluation of the night time visual symptoms with various multifocal IOLs. As the reader can see from Figure 1, the least distortion is seen with the ReSTOR platform. These results are similar to a poster that was presented at the 2007 European Society of Cataract and Refractive Surgeons (ESCRS) meeting and analyzed visual disturbances in a simulated night-driving environment. Again in Figure 2 it is clear that the least amount of visual disturbanc-

es are seen with the ReSTOR platform. Obviously, in order to justify placing a ReZoom IOL in a fellow eye, the surgeon must feel the known disadvantage of night time dysphotopsia will be offset by a significant improvement in another parameter of visual function.

Multifocal IOls and Intermediate Vision

Proponents of mixing IOLs with the ReSTOR platform propose that it improves intermediate vision without any disadvantages because the brain shifts into the clearer image.

In my own practice I have rarely noted any patients with *significant* midrange vision problems with bilateral ReSTOR implantation. This may be for several reasons, including the following:

* My approach to preoperative counseling, which is critical to the success with multifocal IOLs. Preoperatively, each patient should understand that this technology needs to be viewed as a bilateral procedure and he or she will function best once he or she has the second eye surgery completed.

* I educate patients about the improved vision that occurs both with bilateral summation and neuroadaptation and counsel them that their intermediate vision will improve with time.

* I physically show the patient where his or her near point will be immediately after surgery. (I actually hold their hands and move them approximately 12 to 14 inches from their face and say, "Early on this is where you will see best up close. Over time the focal point will move further out."). It is important for patients to understand this phenomenon preoperatively so that he or she will be comfortable in the postoperative period.

* Finally, I do address midrange vision by telling the patient that the lens design has a peak for vision reading

Figure 1. The least distortion is seen with the ReSTOR platform.

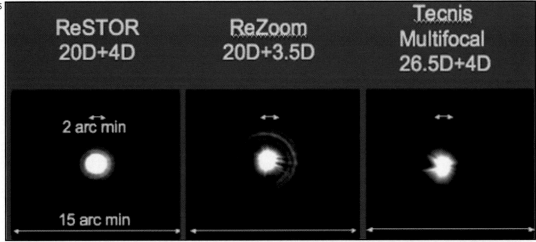

Figure 2. It is clear that the least amount of visual disturbances are seen with the ReSTOR platform.

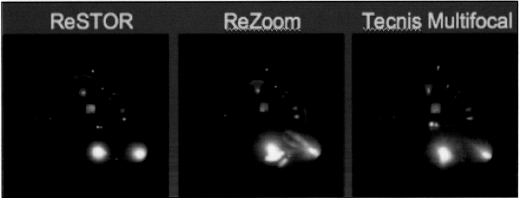

up close and in the distance, and it is not quite as strong (but still very functional) for midrange vision.

Data from other clinicians also demonstrate that the midrange "difficulties" of the ReSTOR lens have been over estimated. A prospective study by Dr. David Chang of his cohort of bilateral ReSTOR, bilateral ReZoom, and retrospective study of his bilateral Crystalens (Eyeonics, Inc, Aliso Viejo, CA) patients revealed that the bilateral ReSTOR patients actually had the strongest midrange vision (at 50 cm) of the 3 lens platforms when the patients were fully corrected for distance vision.

Another study reviewed the data from a group of ophthalmologists including Drs. Robert Cionni, Stephen Lane, Eric Donnenfeld, Kerry Solomon, Jim McCulley, and David Chang. One of the strengths of this study is that it includes multiple surgeons who have experience using a variety of Pr-C IOL platforms. This included over 150 patients at 6 months with bilateral ReSTOR IOL implantation and found the patients had an extremely high degree of satisfaction with their overall visual function for distance, intermediate, and near. The patients reported a high degree of satisfaction when specifically queried regarding computer use.

Intermediate Vision: Observations Versus Complaints

How then do we reconcile the disparate experience of some clinicians? This brings up the concept of patient "observations" versus "complaints." Ophthalmologists live with cataract surgery day in and day out and everything that occurs is usually expected and ordinary. However, it is a unique experience for the patient, and he or she has no frame of reference to determine if a symptom is "normal or not." As a result, the patient may have a multitude of questions or observations because he or she is not sure if what he or she is experiencing is expected or unusual. In almost all cases these are not "complaints" but instead "observations" the patient is making for which he or she would like reassurance.

For example, it is not uncommon for a cataract patient to remark following surgery "My eye feels scratchy." In this instance, the patient is not complaining but instead is bringing an observation up to the treating surgeon because he or she wants to know if it is normal or not. Typically, once patients hear, "The scratchiness is a normal part of healing," they are relieved.

An identical process can happen with intermediate vision following ReSTOR cataract surgery. Usually, the patients who make an observation regarding their midrange vision are those with the sharpest overall vision (eg, 20/20, J1). In these instances, their vision is so strong at distance and near that they can often notice the drop off in mid-range. They will often state something such as, "How come it is not as clear out there?" while pointing at midrange. Understanding that this is an observation rather than a complaint, I will answer, "That is normal. Remember we discussed prior to surgery that early on your best sweet spots for vision would be at near and distance but that the midrange would improve overtime?" Typically, the patient will nod his or her head and answer, "Oh yes. That is right. We did discuss that."

Studies Evaluating "Mixing"

Dr. Richard Mackool performed a prospective study of mixing multifocal IOLs. His series consisted of 15 consecutive patients (13 with cataract and 2 undergoing refractive lens exchange [RLE] for hyperopia). The patients were queried as to which eye they preferred for distance, intermediate, or near and the overall quality of their vision. There was no difference in postoperative measured or subjective distance acuity with either lens platform. Nearly all patients preferred their ReSTOR eye for near and many favored their ReZoom eye for intermediate. One patient requested removal of his or her ReZoom lens because of poor distance, near, and intermediate vision, and 4 patients (including the 2 RLE patients) insisted on removal of the ReZoom lens because of poor near vision. Two of these patients also listed symptoms of nocturnal glare and halo as an additional reason for explantation. No patients requested removal of their ReSTOR lens and all patients that had their ReZoom lens explanted were happy as bilateral ReSTOR patients.

Dr. Kerry Solomon also performed a prospectively randomized study on mixing and matching multifocal IOL platforms. He noted that bilateral ReSTOR had the best overall reading and near vision, the best visual summation, and the least night vision symptoms at 3 and 6 months. Mixing and a "Blaylock" approach (bilateral ReSTOR with a planned myopia of approximately 1 D aim in nondominant eye) provided better range of vision *at the expense of near vision and night vision symptoms.*

An additional study by Dr. Paul Mann evaluated his personal experience with 205 patients with Pr-C IOLs (32 received bilateral Crystalens implantation, 82 received bilateral ReSTOR lenses, 49 received bilateral ReZoom implantation, and 42 patients received a ReSTOR lens in one eye and a ReZoom lens in the fellow eye). He had patients evaluate numerous parameters, including visual function at all distances (including intermediate, night time glare and halos, spectacle independence, and general satisfaction). The majority of the patients in all groups were pleased with the outcome of their procedure and would recommend it to a family member or friend. There was clear data that mixing ReSTOR/ReZoom did not yield higher levels of spectacle independence than bilateral implantation of either lens. Prior to evaluating the data, Dr. Mann felt that mixing ReSTOR/ReZoom was beneficial. He reports that as a result of the study, however, he is now less likely to mix and match the ReZoom/ReSTOR lenses and more likely to implant 1 of the 3 lens options bilaterally. Overall, he is inclined to implant the ReSTOR lens bilaterally in most of his patients who desire spectacle independence.

In contrast to the excellent results reported above with bilateral ReSTOR and the poorer results demonstrated with mixing, a few physicians have reported superior results with mixing ReSTOR/ReZoom IOLs. I cannot reconcile these clinical findings with either my own clinical experience or that of the physicians noted above. Lowered patient and/or physician expectations may play a role in the reported "success" of these patients. I have, in fact, had an opportunity to see a number of these "mixed" patients and to document their unhappiness with this approach.

Conclusion

It is possible to have happy patients with any of the Pr-C platforms or even combination of Pr-C platforms. There is no question that each IOL has its own particular strengths and weaknesses, and some of the variances seen from different investigators may represent variances in the ways these particular physicians counsel and manage their patients. Each physician needs to objectively evaluate the benefits of these technologies and decide on the most reasonable approach.

I believe that when one carefully reviews the hard objective data it is clear that bilateral ReSTOR implantation will lead to the greatest percentage of happy patients *and more importantly the least likelihood of significant clinical problems.* Theoretical or occasional clinical issues with mid-range vision with any Pr-C IOL can be resolved with optical correction. However, glare, halo, and dysphotopsia, which are more common with the ReZoom IOL than any other Pr-C IOL, might only be ameliorated with an IOL exchange. As such there seems to be little support for mixing the ReSTOR apodized diffractive IOL with a zonal refractive IOL such as the ReZoom.

It is likely that the improved clinical results seen with the aspheric ReSTOR (which are described elsewhere in this book) will only strengthen the rationale for bilateral ReSTOR implantation.

Addendum: When I Do Consider Mixing

With this strong a rationale for bilaterally matched multifocal IOLs presented above, the reader might wonder for which patients do I mix multifocal IOLs? First off, I am very comfortable placing a ReSTOR IOL in the second eye of a patient that has been previously implanted with a monofocal IOL. Again, one of the critical aspects of multifocal IOL success is appropriate patient education. Patients previously implanted with a monofocal IOL have the best personal understanding of the absolute presbyopia that accompanies pseudophakic emmetropia. Many patients implanted when monofocal IOLs were the only available option are very interested in and are excellent candidates for ReSTOR IOL implantation when having surgery on their second eye.

The other group of patients for whom I will mix different IOLs are those with excellent vision following ReSTOR implantation in their first eye but who are bothered by dysphotopsias. Most of these patients will "neuroadapt" and eventually cease to visualize or be bothered by the halos. There is a subgroup of patients, however, where the dysphotopsias do not lessen (fortunately this is uncommon).

If the patient otherwise has excellent vision for distance and near in his or her multifocal eye, he or she may desire to keep the lens and try and manage with the dysphotopsias. In these cases, placing a monofocal IOL in the fellow eye and targeting distance vision can often significantly improve the overall clinical function because the pure distance image from the monofocal IOL will allow the patient to suppress the distance vision dysphotopsias in the multifocal IOL eye. Others would consider the placement of a Crystalens in the fellow eye. Up to now, I have avoided this lens platform for the same reasons I have chosen not to implant plate-haptic design lenses in general.

Another group that may require "mixing" of different IOLs is patients with extreme midrange concerns (professional musicians, auto mechanics who work under a car hood doing repairs at midrange). If they are pleased with the overall vision following the first ReSTOR IOL implantation, I will go ahead and match the second eye to the first. If they have concerns regarding midrange vision, then I would adjust the second eye in the manner described by Blaylock where a mild myopic error (−1.00 D) is targeted in the nondominant eye to improve the midrange vision. Others would take the approach of placing a ReZoom in the second eye, but in this situation I would warn the patient that he or she will most likely have more night time visual disturbances.

CHAPTER 140

MIXING VERSUS MATCHING— WHO IS MORE SATISFIED?

Paul Mann, MD

Presbyopia-correcting intraocular lenses (Pr-C IOLs) are gaining in popularity for several reasons. Today's cataract patients are young and active, and they want freedom from spectacles. Additionally, these lenses offer a better range of vision than monovision or blended-vision laser in situ keratomileusis (LASIK).

Three Pr-C IOLs are currently available in the United States, and each has its advantages. Although it may be tempting to mix and match IOLs to gain the benefits of 2 models, I have found that patients achieve optimal vision when they receive the same multifocal lens in both eyes.

The Available Presbyopia-Correcting Lenses

The ReZoom (Advanced Medical Optics, Santa Ana, CA) is a zonal refractive multifocal lens. Its power alternates from the center to the periphery of the optic, and an altered curvature on the front of the IOL allows for multiple points of focus. The AcrySof ReSTOR (Alcon, Fort Worth, TX) is an apodized diffractive multifocal lens that is based on the AcrySof single-piece lens platform. The diffractive grading is limited to the central 3.6 mm of the lens, while the periphery of the IOL is purely refractive, just like that of a monofocal lens. Additionally, the diffractive step heights are larger (approximately 1.3 µm) in the center of the AcrySof ReSTOR lens and gradually become smaller toward the periphery. The Crystalens (Eyeonics, Inc, Aliso Viejo, CA) is a modified plate-haptic lens with a biconvex optic. This implant has hinges that allow it to move forward and backward along the axis of the eye.

Postoperative Phone Survey

METHODOLOGY

Our practice began implanting the Crystalens in February 2004, the AcrySof ReSTOR lens in July 2005, and the ReZoom lens a few months later. We began mixing and matching the AcrySof ReSTOR and ReZoom in the fall of 2005 to try and achieve greater independence from glasses for our patients. In 2006, my practice conducted a study to determine patients' satisfaction with these 3 IOLs. All respondents underwent IOL implantation between January 1 and December 31, 2006. My staff contacted these individuals 3 months after their last procedure (see Survey Questions on p. 499).

Our study included 205 patients. Thirty-two had received bilateral Crystalenses, 82 had received bilateral AcrySof ReSTOR IOLs, 49 had received bilateral ReZoom lenses, and 42 had received an AcrySof ReSTOR lens in one eye and a ReZoom IOL in their fellow eye.

RESULTS

My staff and I asked patients to rate their vision on a scale of 1 to 5, with 5 being the best. Those who had received the AcrySof ReSTOR or ReZoom lens bilaterally or the 2 IOLs in combination rated their distance vision similarly (Figure 1). The Crystalens patients had the best intermediate vision, and the AcrySof ReSTOR patients had the best reading vision.

Patients who received the AcrySof ReSTOR in one eye and the ReZoom lens in their fellow eye had slightly better nighttime (3.73), daytime (4.14), and overall vision (3.82) than the patients in the other groups. The scores for overall vision were 3.73 in the Crystalens group, 3.76 in the AcrySof ReSTOR group, and 3.69 in the ReZoom group.

When asked, 36% of the Crystalens, 47% of the AcrySof ReSTOR, 84% of the ReZoom, and 60% of the AcrySof ReSTOR/ReZoom patients reported difficulty with halos. Problems with glare were reported by 31% of the Crystalens, 35% of the AcrySof ReSTOR, 16% of the ReZoom, and 19% of the AcrySof ReSTOR/ReZoom patients.

Interestingly, 100% postoperative independence from spectacles was reported by 78% of the AcrySof ReSTOR, 55% of the ReZoom, 51% of the AcrySof ReSTOR/ReZoom, and 45% of the Crystalens patients (Figure 2).

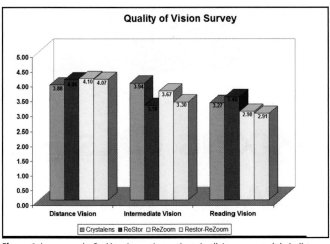

Figure 1. In a survey by Dr. Mann's practice, patients in all 4 groups rated their distance, intermediate, and reading vision after receiving IOLs in both eyes.

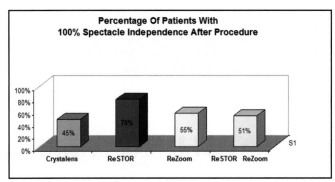

Figure 2. The survey determined how many patients achieved 100% independence from their spectacles after bilateral IOL surgery.

Patients' Satisfaction

Surprisingly, quality of vision and spectacle independence did not always correlate with patients' satisfaction. When asked, 82% of the Crystalens, 78% of the AcrySof ReSTOR, 78% of the ReZoom, and 74% of the AcrySof ReSTOR/ReZoom patients said that they would recommend the procedure. Additionally, 76% of the AcrySof ReSTOR, 76% of the ReZoom, 70% of the Crystalens, and 63% of the AcrySof ReSTOR/ReZoom patients answered that the benefit of lens implantation was worth the monetary cost.

Eighty-five percent of Crystalens, 77% of AcrySof ReSTOR/ReZoom, 69% of AcrySof ReSTOR, and 69% of ReZoom patients stated that they were properly educated about the procedure. Because we started implanting the Crystalens 1.5 to 2 years before the other 2 lenses, I feel that our organization has more experience with this lens. This experience may have helped us to better create realistic expectations for our patients with the Crystalens as opposed to the other groups. Perhaps this is why 82% of the patients would recommend the procedure to friends and family while only 45% were completely independent of spectacles.

Conclusion

None of the 3 Pr-C IOLs offers perfect vision for each patient. Each appears to have weaknesses. For instance, many AcrySof ReSTOR patients have difficulty with their intermediate vision, while the majority of ReZoom patients have halos at night. Crystalens patients often complain of poor near vision. Because of these inadequacies, it is very important for the surgeon to understand the visual needs of his or her patients when selecting implants for patients. Educating patients to create realistic expectations is crucial to the success of these implants. We are constantly working within our own practice to improve our abilities to educate patients about these implants and we certainly have more work to do.

In our study, the majority of patients in all 4 groups were pleased with their outcomes and would recommend the proce-

dure to others. It is important to note the mix and match group had similar satisfaction rates as the other groups. Interestingly, mixing and matching the AcrySof ReSTOR and ReZoom lenses did not yield a higher level of spectacle independence than the bilateral implantation of either lens. Because of my desire to create spectacle independence for patients who choose to pay a premium price for Pr-C IOLs, I am less likely to mix and match these IOLs and prefer to implant the 3 lens models bilaterally.

Currently, when patients strongly desire independence from spectacles, I am more inclined to implant the AcrySof ReSTOR lens bilaterally. We have not implanted many patients with the AcrySof ReSTOR and Crystalens combination in our practice. Anecdotally, reports have surfaced that these patients may have a high rate of spectacle independence. I am looking forward to seeing data from surgeons' experiences mixing the AcrySof ReSTOR with the Crystalens.

Survey Questions

We asked patients to rate their answers to the following questions on a scale of 1 to 5 (1 = poor, 2 = below average, 3 = satisfactory, 4 = good, 5 = excellent).

* How would you rate the quality of your vision?
  ❖ Distance vision
  ❖ Computer/intermediate
  ❖ Reading
  ❖ Nighttime
  ❖ Daytime
  ❖ Overall
* Do you have difficulty with halos/glare?
* Do you ever wear glasses?
* Would you recommend cataract surgery to your family and friends?
* Do you feel that the benefit of this surgery was worth the investment?
* Do you feel that you were adequately informed before surgery about possible visual outcomes?

CHAPTER 141

MATCHING VERSUS MIXING IOLs— CLINICAL COMPARISON

Richard J. Mackool, MD and Richard J. Mackool, Jr, MD

In attempting to determine whether or not an individual patient is best served by bilateral implantation of the same intraocular lens (IOL) or implantation of a different IOL in each eye, the benefit of each method must be weighed against any potential disadvantages.

In a previous study[1] we found that uncorrected near visual acuity was significantly better after binocular ReSTOR lens (Alcon, Fort Worth, TX) implantation than after monocular implantation of this IOL (Figure 1). In 45 patients (90 eyes) receiving bilateral ReSTOR implantation, uncorrected near visual acuity in the first eye at 6 months postoperatively was 20/20 or better in 44% of eyes. However, uncorrected binocular near visual acuity was 20/20 or better in 82% of eyes (with best distance correction in place, 90% of patients achieved near visual acuity of 20/20 or better). This data clearly demonstrates that binocular near visual acuity (VA) is better than monocular near VA; that is, 2 eyes really are better than one. Consistent with this finding, Solomon[2] found that reading speed was superior in patients with bilateral ReSTOR implantation as compared to those with a ReSTOR and ReZoom implant in each eye.

We therefore undertook the following prospective randomized study of mixing different multifocal IOLs. Note that as of October 2007, all other reports concerning results of implantation of a different multifocal IOL in the same patient have been anecdotal; that is, there have been no prior prospective, randomized studies with regard to the "mix and match" technique.

Fifteen patients (30 eyes) between the ages of 37 and 82 years of age were enrolled in this study. As a requirement of entry, patients could not have any ocular pathology or condition that might affect the outcome of surgery. Thirteen patients (26 eyes) underwent cataract extraction with IOL implantation in both eyes at an interval of 2 to 4 weeks, and 2 patients (4 eyes) underwent refractive lens exchange procedures on both eyes at an interval of 2 weeks.

The first eye undergoing surgery was randomly selected to receive either a ReSTOR or ReZoom (Advanced Medical Optics, Santa Ana, CA) IOL. The other eye received the lens style that was not implanted in the first eye. All patients were advised preoperatively that, should they be dissatisfied with the performance of either or both lenses at 2 months or later after the second eye was operated, IOL exchange could be performed and either a) their preferred lens of choice or b) a monofocal lens would be implanted.

The following "objective" data were collected at 1 and 3 months after the second eye was operated. Best uncorrected and corrected distance visual acuity, best intermediate visual acuity at 50, 60, and 70 cm with best distance correction, and best near vision at the distance preferred by the patient with best distance correction.

Subjectively, the patients also completed a questionnaire indicating which eye, if any, they preferred for distance, intermediate, and near vision when wearing their best distance correction.

Fourteen patients (28 eyes) completed the study by returning for the follow-up examinations at 1 and 3 months. One patient was lost to follow-up. The 3-month postoperative data are presented in this report. Five patients underwent IOL implant exchange at 3 to 4 months after surgery because of dissatisfaction with one of the IOLs, and their results are also reported.

Table 1 indicates the best corrected distance vision results in these patients. Six patients achieved better objective visual acuity with the eye receiving the ReSTOR lens (the "ReSTOR eye"), 4 patients achieved better acuity with the ReZoom eye, and 4 patients had no difference in acuity between eyes. Subjectively, 3 patients preferred the ReSTOR eye for distance vision, 3 patients preferred the ReZoom eye, and 8 patients could discern no difference between eyes. Therefore, there was no objective or subjective difference with regard to the number of patients who preferred the ReSTOR or ReZoom IOL for distance vision.

Table 2 demonstrates the results with regard to intermediate vision. Two patients achieved better visual acuity at intermediate distances with the ReSTOR lens, 7 patients achieved

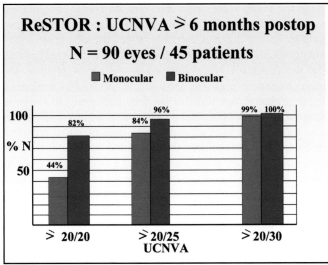

Figure 1. A previous study found that uncorrected near visual acuity was significantly better after binocular ReSTOR lens implantation than after monocular implantation of this IOL.

Table 1

BEST-CORRECTED DISTANCE VISUAL ACUITY AT 3 MONTHS

Preference	Obj/Subj @ 3 mos
RS	6/3
RZ	4/3
None	6/8

Summary: No objective or subjective difference in DV with RS or RZ eye.

Table 2

INTERMEDIATE VISUAL ACUITY AT 3 MONTHS

Preference	Obj/Subj @ 3 mos
RS	2/2
RZ	7/6
None	5/6

Summary: RZ performed better than RS, objectively and subjectively, for Int VA.

Table 3

NEAR VISUAL ACUITY AT 3 MONTHS

Preference	Obj/Subj @ 3 mos
RS	12/13
RZ	1/1
None	1/0

Summary: RS performed better than RZ, objectively and subjectively, for near VA.

better acuity with the ReZoom lens, and 5 patients had no difference in acuity between eyes. Subjectively, 2 patients preferred the ReSTOR eye, 6 preferred the ReZoom eye, and 6 had no preference. In these eyes, the data therefore indicated that the ReZoom performed better than the ReSTOR lens, both objectively and subjectively, for intermediate vision.

Table 3 indicates the results at near (reading). Twelve patients achieved better near vision with the ReSTOR eye, 1 patient achieved better near vision with the ReZoom eye, and 1 patient had equal vision at near with each eye. Subjectively, 13 patients preferred the ReSTOR eye, and 1 patient preferred the ReZoom eye for reading. No patients stated that both eyes read equally well. This data indicates that the ReSTOR lens performed better than the ReZoom lens for reading, both objectively and subjectively.

IOL exchange. Five eyes (5 patients) underwent an IOL exchange at 3 to 4 months after surgery because of dissatisfaction with one of their lens implants. Three patients (3 eyes) had undergone cataract-implant surgery, and 2 patients (2 eyes) had undergone refractive lens exchange. All of the patients had exchange procedures in which the ReZoom IOL was removed and the ReSTOR lens was implanted.

The indication(s) for and results of IOL exchange are shown in Table 4. All 5 patients reported that poor near vision was the primary reason that they requested IOL exchange. However, 1 of the 5 patients also stated that intermediate vision was poor with the ReZoom lens, 2 patients complained of poor distance vision with the ReZoom lens, and 2 patients complained of severe glare and halo with the ReZoom lens. These 5 patients were followed for 6 months after undergoing IOL exchange, and all of their complaints were resolved both objectively (by measured acuity) and subjectively after exchange of the ReZoom IOL to the ReSTOR lens.

Case Reports

The following case reports are illustrative of the complaints of the patients undergoing IOL exchange.

CASE 1

A 50-year-old surgical operating room (OR) technician underwent refractive lens exchange OU. Preoperatively, refraction was +1.25 in each eye (OU) and he wore progressive spectacles. Best corrected visual acuity (BCVA) was 20/20 OU. After ReZoom implantation in the right eye (OD) and ReSTOR implantation left eye (OS), best corrected distance vision (BCDV) was 20/20–1 OU, near vision with best distance correction was 20/50 OD and 20/16 OS, and mean intermediate vision at 50, 60, and 70 cm was 20/25 OD and

Table 4	
INTRAOCULAR LENS EXCHANGE (N = 5)	
Indication: N	*Results at 1 and 12 mos*
Poor NV: 5	0/5
Poor Int V: 1	1/5
Poor DV: 2	0/5
Glare/Halo: 2	0/5

20/30 OS. The patient complained of poor near vision in the right eye, and stated that distance vision was good in both eyes. He preferred the ReSTOR eye for distance vision and the ReZoom eye for intermediate vision. He was particularly disturbed by the absence of stereopsis at near and intermediate distances. After IOL exchange OD (ReZoom explantation and ReSTOR implantation), near vision OD improved to 20/20, intermediate vision improved to 20/20 when viewing with both eyes simultaneously (it had been 20/25 prior to IOL exchange), and he noted the return of normal stereopsis at near. He was able to function as a surgical OR technician without correction (prior to exchange he required near vision spectacles in order to do this).

CASE 2

A 49-year-old mailman underwent refractive lens exchange OU. Preoperatively he had hyperopia/presbyopia with BCVA of 20/20 OD and 20/15 OS. Three months after uneventful ReZoom implantation OD and ReSTOR implantation OS, BCDV was 20/25 OD and 20/16 OS. With best distance correction, intermediate vision was 20/50 OD and 20/40 OS, and near vision was 20/50 OD and 20/16 OS. The patient complained of poor distance, near and intermediate vision OD, and also severe halos OD. After IOL exchange OD (ReZoom explantation and ReSTOR implantation), BCDV improved from 20/25 to 20/20 OD, intermediate vision with best distance correction improved from 20/50 to 20/40, and near vision improved from 20/50 to 20/20. He also reported that the halo problem had resolved.

Conclusion

Our findings clearly indicate that randomized implantation of the ReSTOR and ReZoom IOLs produced results that were unsatisfactory in a significant minority (5 of 15) patients.

This study was not designed to determine the results of methods such as intentional implantation of either IOL in the dominant or non-dominant eye. In fact, although successful reports of mixing and matching various IOLs have been reported,[3] these communications typically describe insertion of the ReSTOR IOL in the non-dominant eye. Such techniques may yield dramatically different results from those obtained by us because, among other possible factors, the implant inserted into the non-dominant eye would be at a comparative disadvantage to that inserted in the dominant eye. This could

cause the study subjects to feel very differently about their outcome (for example, they might prefer their dominant eye for distance) and could certainly affect the objective acuity measurements as well. In other words, the patient might find that the dominant eye performed as well or better than the non-dominant eye simply because the former has a superior inherent acuity regardless of the lens implanted. In order to obtain data that would offer a valid comparison of such strategies, a study in which patients were randomized to receive a predetermined lens in their dominant and non-dominant eyes would be required. In addition, these 2 groups would need to be compared to patients randomly selected to receive the same implant style in both eyes. Such a study has yet to appear in the literature.

In our opinion, the results of this study provide compelling evidence that randomized implantation of a ReSTOR and ReZoom lens in each eye of a patient can create severe problems including reduced near visual acuity, absence of stereopsis at near and intermediate distances, and increased glare. These issues caused 5 of our patients to insist on undergoing an IOL exchange procedure.

A potential advantage of "mixing and matching" these multifocal lenses is the possible creation of better intermediate visual acuity as a result of the lower power add designed in the ReZoom IOL. It has been postulated that this arrangement would result in reduced need for spectacle wear. However, this has not been demonstrated in randomized prospective studies, and one of our patients (case 1) actually obtained improved binocular intermediate visual acuity after IOL exchange from a ReZoom to a ReSTOR IOL. This patient was one of the 2 hyperopic patients who had undergone refractive lens exchange, both of whom subsequently underwent the IOL exchange procedure because of poor near vision and absent near stereopsis. The above patient's occupation (ophthalmic surgical operating room technician) was compromised by the lack of stereopsis at near, and his ability to perform near vision tasks that required stereopsis returned after IOL exchange. Such findings should at the very least cause one to approach mixing and matching with caution and to obtain well-documented informed consent.

The results of this study do not shed any light on the question as to when or if the use of IOLs with different power near adds is appropriate. More randomized studies are needed to determine, for example, whether or not a patient who complains of poor intermediate vision after ReSTOR implantation in the first eye is better served with implantation of the same or another type of IOL (ReZoom, Crystalens [Eyeonics, Inc, Aliso Viejo, CA], monofocal, etc) in the second eye. Similarly, what is the best course of action for a patient who receives a ReZoom lens in the first eye and complains of poor near vision? Will that patient be more likely to fare better if a ReZoom, ReSTOR, or monofocal lens is implanted in the second eye? There may be a subset of patients who are better served with implantation of multifocal IOLs of different power, and this may be particularly true if both IOLs utilize similar optics. At the present time, we do not believe that a satisfactory method for identifying such patients exists because such a method can only be derived from additional randomized studies. As discussed in this report, these studies do not exist.

References

1. Mackool, RJ. Pros and cons of symmetric vs "mixing and matching" multifocal IOLs. Presented at The Storm Eye/ASCRS Annual Meeting; June 2006; Kiawah, SC.

2. Solomon KD, Fernandez de Castro LE, Vroman DT, Sandoval HP. Mix and match versus bilateral implantation of a diffractive multifocal IOL. Presented at the Annual Meeting of the ASCRS; April 2007; San Diego, Calif.

3. Pepose JS, Qazi MA, Davies J, Daone JF, Loden JC, Sivalingham V, Mahmoud AM. Visual performance of patients with bilateral vs combination Crystalens, ReZoom, and ReSTOR intraocular lens implants. *Am J Ophthalmol.* 2007;144(3):347-357.

CHAPTER 142

REFRACTIVE IOL SELECTION— EUROPEAN PERSPECTIVE

H. Burkhard Dick, MD

Refractive intraocular lenses (IOLs) have been a surgical option for European cataract and refractive surgeons for more than 20 years. However, trade-offs in visual outcomes and skepticism about patient acceptance has limited their use until more recently.[1-8] With the availability of newer technology, as well as better understanding about proper patient selection, use of refractive IOLs has grown dramatically in the past couple of years.

The increased usage of these refractive IOLs, including accommodative, multifocal and toric IOLs, however, presents new challenges. Surgeons must achieve emmetropia, or come as close to emmetropia as possible. There are also reimbursement issues in countries where healthcare is publicly funded and where these IOLs are deemed to be too expensive to cover.

In this chapter, I will briefly look at refractive IOLs from a historical perspective, followed by an overview of IOLs currently available to European surgeons. Next, I will explore how the use of refractive IOLs has evolved as the technology, and our understanding of how to use it, has changed. Finally, I will look at the challenges of reimbursement in Europe in light of growing patient demand, but government restraints.

The Historical View

Although the recent introduction of certain multifocal IOLs (ReZoom [Advanced Medical Optics, Santa Ana, CA] and ReSTOR [Alcon, Fort Worth, TX]) have reignited the interest in refractive lens surgery, refractive IOLs, and specifically multifocal IOLs, have been implanted for more than 20 years now in Europe.

Beginning with a diffractive multifocal (3M) and 2– to 3–refractive zone designs (IOLab and Domilens, among others), these IOLs received a great deal of attention in the late 1980s and early 1990s. As clinical results were presented, it became clear that there were a number of challenges facing this technology. These included high levels of induced astigmatism due to the nonfoldable polymethylmethacrylate (PMMA) material

and cataract surgical techniques used at that time, as well as a tendency for IOL decentration. From a vision standpoint, there was also reduced contrast sensitivity and increased glare in many of the early multifocal IOL patients. Writing in a 1997 edition of Current Opinions of Ophthalmology, Pearce noted that 10 years after he implanted the first multifocal IOL, there was a "gradual lessening of the commitment to this modality by the ophthalmic community." Pearce maintained that this lack of interest was due, in part, to the US Food and Drug Administration (FDA)'s continual delay of approving multifocal IOLs, despite his belief that there was "more than adequate clinical data."[2]

However, there were also reports such as one that appeared in 1993 in the German journal *Klinische Monatsblätter für Augenheilkunde* in which investigators at the University Eye Clinic of Giessen concluded that implantation of multifocal IOLs should be limited to special indications such as a "distinct patient request to dispense with wearing near or bifocal glasses." They added that because of reductions in contrast sensitivity and mesopic vision, as well as an increase in glare, multifocal IOLs should not be implanted in patients with demanding needs, such as professional car drivers.[3] The widespread release of the Array Multifocal (Advanced Medical Optics, Santa Ana, CA) in the mid 1990s, also contributed to the decline in interest in the first generation of multifocal IOLs.

Despite these early setbacks, many refractive and cataract surgeons maintained the belief that improving technology should result in better refractive IOL technologies. In 2001, we published a review article in the German journal *Der Ophthalmologe* that concluded that newer generations of multifocal IOLs, using multizonal, progressive technology, along with foldable materials and small-incision cataract surgery, were helping to overcome the drawbacks first encountered with these lenses.[5]

As Mark Packer and colleagues noted in the introduction to a review of multifocal IOLs that appeared in 2006 in *Ophthalmology Clinics of North America*, "The fundamental challenge of multifocality remains the preservation of optical quality. Another significant challenge for multifocal technology continues to be the reduction or elimination of unwanted photopic phenomena, such as halos."[9]

Refractive IOL Technology in Europe Today

There is little doubt that in the intervening 20 years, a proliferation of refractive IOLs has become available. This is particularly so in Europe where medical devices are able to reach the market without the lengthy clinical study and approval process required by the US FDA. In Europe, medical device manufacturers must demonstrate conformity to the appropriate established regulations set up by the European Union for CE marking (Officially, CE has no meaning as an abbreviation, but may have originally stood for Communauté Européenne or Conformité Européenne, French for European Conformity). Although quite rigorous, the path to regulatory approval in Europe is shorter, which means we have much earlier access to new products.

As of this writing, there are more than 30 different types of refractive IOLs on the market in Europe in the categories of multifocal, toric, refractive and accommodative (Table 1).

Multifocal IOLs

Available multifocal IOLs can primarily be categorized into 2 types: refractive and diffractive. However, there also one multifocal now available that is described as a refractive-diffractive IOL and another that is a combination of a multifocal and accommodative IOL.[10,11]

REFRACTIVE MULTIFOCAL IOLS

ReZoom Multifocal Intraocular

This IOL is a 3-piece hydrophobic acrylic IOL with 5 refractive zones (Figure 1): (moving from the outside zone to the center) a low-light/distance-dominant zone, a near zone, a distance zone, a second near zone, and a bright-light/distance-dominant zone in the center. Transitional optics between the zones provides intermediate distance vision. The manufacturer states that ReZoom's "Balance View Optics" allows for 100% light transmission over all five optical zones (Figure 2). The ReZoom has a rounded anterior and a sharp posterior edge design (OptiEdge). I conducted a prospective, randomized, masked clinical trial to compare the ReZoom (n = 24) and the first-generation Array (n = 18) IOLs. Outcomes with the former proved superior in several regards.

The mean defocus acuity curves for both IOLs were similar; they demonstrated acceptable near vision and excellent intermediate vision, which is not achieved with current diffractive multifocal IOL designs. Patients who received the ReZoom lens reported that they saw comfortably without glasses at distance (100%), intermediate distance (95%), and near (71%). Sixty-seven percent of my ReZoom patients never wore glasses at 6 months postoperatively. All ReZoom patients reported driving easily, and they expressed great satisfaction with their

depth and color perception, neither of which deteriorated during 6 months of follow-up.

Regarding distance-corrected near visual acuity, 83.3% of ReZoom patients saw 20/40 or better. The group's mean binocular distance UCVA was 20/20, and the mean binocular distance BCVA was 20/17. These patients' mean near UCVA at 40 cm was 20/42, and their distance-corrected visual acuity at 40 cm was 20/35. All ReZoom eyes had a binocular distance BCVA of 20/25 or better.

Compared to the Array IOL (Advanced Medical Optics), the ReZoom IOL produced fewer photic phenomena. Specifically, the incidence of halos with the ReZoom was one-third that with the Array lens. The former was also associated with distinctly fewer incidences of starbursts. Photic phenomena were less of a problem with the ReZoom IOL versus the multifocal Array lens.

M-Flex Multifocal IOL

This refractive multifocal (Rayner, Hove, East Sussex, UK) is relatively new to the European market. The M-Flex is a hydrophilic acrylic with a multi-zone aspheric optic (Figure 3). Depending on the IOL base power, there are 4 or 5 zones. This IOL has a distant dominant design with a +3-D near add. Our first 25 patients demonstrated very satisfactory outcomes with this new IOL.

MF4 IOL

This lens (Carl Zeiss Meditec, Jena, Germany) is a one-piece, hydrophilic acrylic IOL with a 4-zone optic, which the manufacturer describes as an "autofocus" multifocal. First developed and introduced by IOLTech (La Rochelle, France), little has been published in the way of clinical results.

DIFFRACTIVE MULTIFOCAL IOLS

AcrySof ReSTOR

Based on one of the original multifocal IOL designs (the 3M diffractive), this lens (Alcon) is a one-piece hydrophobic acrylic that is capable of being injected through a 2.8-mm incision. The manufacturer calls the ReSTOR an apodized diffractive and it has 12 zones with a total near add of 4 D (Figure 4).

Tecnis ZM900

This lens (Advanced Medical Optics) is the only 3-piece silicone multifocal IOL on the market in Europe. It is also available in a hydrophobic acrylic material. The diffractive design on the posterior surface creates two focal points that are 4 D apart (Figure 5). The anterior surface has a modified prolate design that is intended to compensate for spherical aberration (Figure 6). The manufacturer claims that this design leads to better focusing and sharper vision. The haptics consist of clear PVDF (poly-vinylidenfluoride) with a C-design, staked into the middle of the sharp optic edge.

*Acri.Twin Multifocal

These diffractive multifocals (*Acri.Tec, Henningsdorf, Germany) are actually a set of 2 IOLs. One IOL is a distant-dominant multifocal (70% distance and 30% near) and the other is a near dominant multifocal (30% distance and

Table 1

IOLs Currently Available in the European Market

Company	Model	Material	Design	Indication	Features/Benefits	Available Powers
*Acri.Tec	Acri.Comfort 643TLC	Hydrophobic acrylic	Tripod, 6 mm optic w/overall diameter of 10 mm	Toric IOL	Good rotational stability and centration. Aspheric optic increases image quality of depth of sharpness	0 to +40 D and +1 to +12 D, cylinder
	Acri.Comfort 646TLC	Hydrophobic acrylic	Plate, 6 mm optic w/overall diameter of 11 mm	Toric IOL	As described above	0 to +32 D and +1 to +12 D, cylinder
	*Acri.lisa 356D	Hydrophobic acrylic	One piece, c-loop, 6 mm optic w/overall diameter of 11.5 mm	Multifocal IOL	Refractive-Diffractive surface w/optimized aspheric optic. Asymmetrical light distribution. Pupil independent. Good visual acuity at near, intermediate and distance. Patient satisfaction of more than 96%	0 to +44 D
	*Acri.lisa 366D	Hydrophobic acrylic	Plate, 6 mm optic w/overall diameter of 11 mm	Multifocal IOL	As described above	0 to +32 D
	*Acri.lisa 536D	Hydrophobic acrylic	3-piece c-loop, 6 mm optic w/overall diameter of 12.5 mm	Multifocal IOL	As described above	0 to +44 D
	*Acri.Twin 447D/443D	Hydrophobic acrylic	Plate, 6 mm optic w/overall diameter of 11 mm	Multifocal IOL	Twin system contains distance dominant and near dominant IOLs to improve binocular visual acuity. Asymmetrical distribution of light. Pupil independent. Diffractive surface profile	0 to +44 D

Table 1 (continued)

IOLs Currently Available in the European Market

Company	Model	Material	Design	Indication	Features/Benefits	Available Powers
	*Acri.Twin 527D/523D	Hydrophobic acrylic	3-piece c-loop, 6 mm optic w/overall diameter of 13 mm	Multifocal IOL	As described above	0 to +44 D
	*Acri.Twin 737D/733D	Hydrophobic acrylic	3-piece c-loop, 6 mm optic w/overall diameter of 12.5 mm	Multifocal IOL	As described above	0 to +44 D
						+10 to +30 D
Alcon Labs	ReStor SN60D3	Hydrophilic acrylic	1-piece modified L w/ blue and UV blocking	Multifocal IOL	Diffractive optic w/12 zones for a total add of 4 D.	+10 to +30 D
	ReStor SA60Ds	Hydrophilic acrylic	1-piece modified L w/UV blocking	Multifocal IOL	As described above	
	AcrySof SA60TT	Hydrophilic acrylic	1-piece modified L w/ blue and UV blocking	Toric IOL	Available in three cylinder options: 1, 1.5 and 2.25 D. Customized software program helps surgeon to determine appropriate lens for each eye	??
Advanced Medical Optics (AMO)	Tecnis ZM900	Silicone	3-piece c-loop, 6 mm optic w/overall diameter of 12 mm	Multifocal IOL	Diffractive posterior surface and prolate anterior surface. Light is split evenly between near and distance vision that is pupil independent. Prolate design compensates for spherical aberrations	+5 to +34 D

Table 1 (continued)

IOLs Currently Available in the European Market

Company	Model	Material	Design	Indication	Features/Benefits	Available Powers
	ReZoom	Hydrophobic acrylic	3-piece c-loop, 6 mm optic w/overall diameter of 12 mm	Multifocal IOL	Refractive with a combination of 5 near and distance zones and transitions to provide intermediate vision. Designed to provide full range of vision with 100% light transmission	+5 to +30 D
	Verisyse VRSM50	PMMA	Iris fixated, anterior chamber lens, 5 mm optic w/overall diameter of 8.5 mm	Myopic IOL	Iris-fixated IOL for correction of higher levels of myopia	-3 to -23.5 D
	Verisyse VRSM60	PMMA	Iris fixated, anterior chamber lens, 6 mm optic w/overall diameter of 8.5 mm	Myopic IOL	As described above	-3 to -15.5 D
	Verisyse VRSH50	PMMA	Iris fixated, anterior chamber lens, 5 mm optic w/overall diameter of 8.5 mm	Hyperopic IOL	Iris-fixated IOL for correction of hyperopia	+1 to +12 D
	Verisyse Toric	PMMA	Iris fixated, anterior chamber lens, 5 mm optic w/overall diameter of 8.5 mm	Toric IOL	Iris-fixated, negative and positive cylinder IOL for correction of astigmatism	-2 to -7 D and '+2 to +7.5 D
	Veriflex	Silicone	Claw design PMMA haptics, 6 mm optic w/overall diameter of 8.5 mm	Myopic IOL	Iris-fixated IOL for correction of myopia	-2 to -14.5 D
Carl Zeiss Meditec	MF4	Hydrophilic acrylic	1-piece, tripod design, 6 mm optic	Multifocal IOL	4-zone optic with total near add of +4 D with "autofocus"	+15 to +26 D

Table 1 (continued)

IOLs Currently Available in the European Market

Company	Model	Material	Design	Indication	Features/Benefits	Available Powers
Human Optics	MicroSil MS6116 TU	Silicone	3-piece w/Z-design PMMA haptics	Toric IOL	Spherical anterior surface and toric posterior surface. For use to correct astigmatism with high levels of hyperopia and myopia	+15 to +25 D, '3 to +14 D, +26 to +31 D and +2 to +12 D, cylinder
	MicroSil MS6116T-Y	Silicone	3-piece w/Z-design PMMA haptics	Toric IOL	Spherical anterior surface and toric posterior surface with blue light filtration. For use to correct astigmatism with high levels of hyperopia and myopia	+15 to +25 D, '3 to +14 D, +26 to +31 D and +2 to +12 D, cylinder
	MicroSil MS 614T	Silicone	3-piece w/C-loop PMMA haptics	Toric IOL	Spherical anterior surface and toric posterior surface. Intended for sulcus fixation. For use to correct astigmatism with high levels of hyperopia and myopia	+15 to +25 D, '3 to +14 D, +26 to +31 D and +2 to +12 D, cylinder
	Akkommodative 1CU	Hydrophilic acrylic	1-piece with 4 haptics	Accommodative IOL	Designed to provide accommodation and reduce need for reading glasses	+16 to +35 D
Morcher	BioComFold 43E	Hydrophilic acrylic	1-piece, ring-haptic IOL, 5.8 mm optic w/overall diameter of 10.20 mm	Accommodative IOL	Accommodative IOL with a 5-degree, forward angled ring haptic	10 to 30 D
	BioComFold 43S	Hydrophilic acrylic	1-piece, ring-haptic IOL, 5.8 mm optic w/overall diameter of 10.20 mm	Accommodative, Multifocal IOL	Hybrid accommodative IOL with a refractive multifocal optic	10 to 30 D

Table 1 (continued)

IOLs Currently Available in the European Market

Company	Model	Material	Design	Indication	Features/Benefits	Available Powers
Ophtec	Artiflex AC 401	Silicone	Claw design PMMA haptics, 6 mm optic w/overall diameter of 8.5 mm	Myopic IOL	Iris-fixated IOL for correction of myopia	-2 to -14.5 D
	Artisan 202	PMMA	Claw design PMMA haptics, 5 mm optic w/overall diameter of 7.5 mm	Myopic IOL	Iris-fixated IOL for correction of myopia	-3 to -23.5 D
	Artisan 204	PMMA	Claw design PMMA haptics, 6 mm optic w/overall diameter of 8.5 mm	Myopic IOL	Iris-fixated IOL for correction of myopia	-1 to -15.5 D
	Artisan 206	PMMA	Claw design PMMA haptics, 5 mm optic w/overall diameter of 8.5 mm	Myopic IOL	Iris-fixated IOL for correction of myopia	-1 to -23.5 D
	Artisan 203	PMMA	Claw design PMMA haptics, 5 mm optic w/overall diameter of 8.5 mm	Hyperopic IOL	Iris-fixated IOL for correction of hyperopia	+1 to +12 D
	Artisan Toric	PMMA	Claw design PMMA haptics, 5 mm optic w/overall diameter of 8.5 mm	Toric IOL	Iris-fixated IOL for correction of astigmatism	2 to 7 D
Rayner	M-Flex 630F	Hydrophilic acrylic	1-piece, 6.25 mm optic w/overall diameter of 12.5 mm	Multifocal IOL	4 or 5 zone aspheric lens (depending on dioptric power) with distance dominant focus and a total add of +3 D. Anatomically correct for highly myopic eyes	+14 to +25 D and +18.5 to +23.5 D

Table 1 (continued)

IOLs Currently Available in the European Market

Company	Model	Material	Design	Indication	Features/Benefits	Available Powers
STAAR Surgical	Myopia ICL	Collamer	Optics and overall diameter vary with refractive power	Myopic PCIOL	4th generation of ICL designed to provide adequate vaulting over crystalline lens	-3 to -23 D
	Hyperopia ICL	Collamer	Optics and overall diameter vary with refractive power	Hyperopic PCIOL	As described above	+3 to +21 D
	Toric ICL	Collamer	Optics and overall diameter vary with refractive power	Toric PCIOL	As described above	-6 to -23 D and +1 to +6 D, cylinder
	Toric IOL AA4203TF	Silicone	One-piece plate haptic, 6 mm optic w/overall diameter of 10.8 mm	Toric IOL	Designed to correct between 1.4 and 2.3 D of astigmatism during cataract surgery	24 to 28.5 D, 2 and 3.5 D, cylinder
	Toric IOL AA4203TL	Silicone	One-piece plate haptic, 6 mm optic w/overall diameter of 11.2 mm	Toric IOL	As described above	9.5 to 23.5 D, 2 and 3.5 D, cylinder
Visiogen	Synchrony IOL	Silicone	Dual optic IOL connecting a 5.5 mm high power anterior optic with a 6 mm negative power posterior optic	Accommodative IOL	Designed to provide accommodation and reduce need for reading glasses following cataract surgery or in cases of presbyopia	

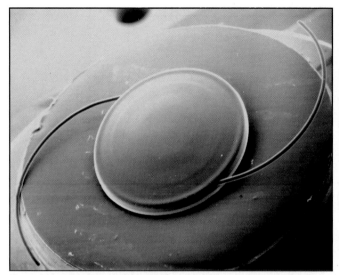

Figure 1. Overview of the ReZoom multifocal IOL photographed at high magnification using scanning electron microscopy (SEM).

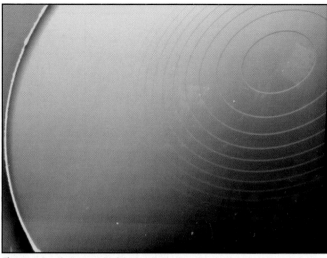

Figure 4. Detail photograph of the apodized anterior optic of the ReSTOR multifocal IOL using SEM.

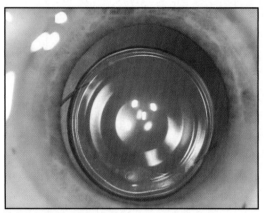

Figure 2. Intraoperative photograph of the zonal distribution in the ReZoom optic.

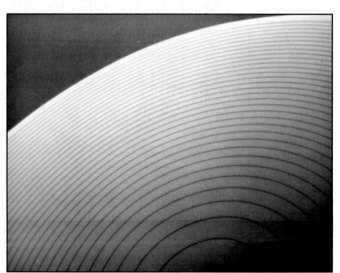

Figure 5. Posterior surface of the Tecnis multifocal optic showing diffractive rings over the entire 6 mm surface using SEM.

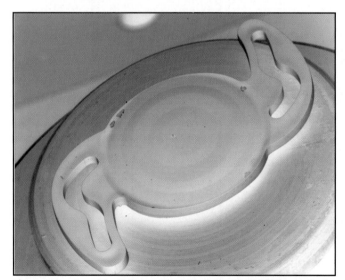

Figure 3. Overview of the M-Flex multifocal IOL photographed at high magnification using SEM.

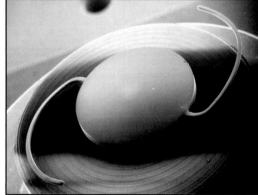

Figure 6. Prolate anterior surface of the Tecnis multifocal IOL (SEM).

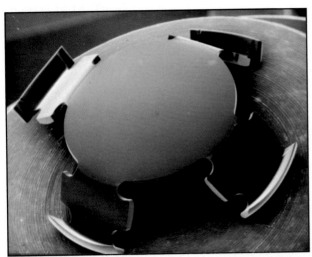

Figure 7. 1CU IOL with 4 opposing haptics (SEM).

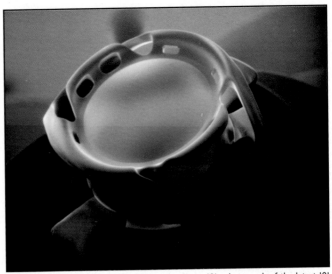

Figure 9. Dual-optic single-piece silicone Synchrony IOL: photograph of the latest IOL version (SEM).

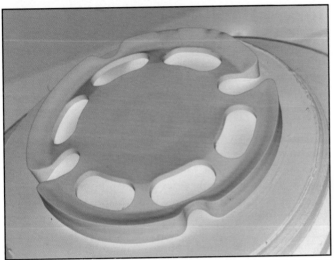

Figure 8. BioComFold 43S: a hybrid of accommodative and multifocal IOL technology (SEM).

70% near). The idea is to provide more effective pseudoaccommodation, according to the manufacturer. The IOLs have a total near add of +4 D.

COMBINATION REFRACTIVE-DIFFRACTIVE MULTIFOCAL IOLS

*Acri.LISA 366D, 356D, & 536D

These hydrophobic acrylic multifocal IOLs (*Acri.Tec, Henningsdorf, Germany) are a hybrid design with both refractive and diffractive components. LISA actually stands for: (L) light intensity distribution of 65% far (refractive) and 35% near (diffractive); (I) independent from pupil size; (S) smooth refractive/diffractive surface profile; and (A) optimized aspheric surface. There are 3 available designs: a 1-piece c-loop (356 D), a plate-style (366 D), and a 3-piece c-loop (536 D). All the lenses have a total near add of +3.75 D.

Accommodative IOLs

Much attention is now being paid to this category of refractive IOLs given the increased interest and awareness of presbyopia.[12] As of this writing, there are 4 accommodative IOLs offered in Europe: The Human Optics Akkommodative 1CU, the Morcher BioComFold 43E, the Visiogen Synchrony, and the Crystalens. A fifth IOL, the Morcher BioComFold 43S, is a hybrid of accommodative and multifocal technology.

AKKOMMODATIVE 1CU

This (Human Optics, Erlangen, Germany) is a hydrophilic acrylic, single-piece IOL with 4 opposing haptics that taper at the transition from optics to haptics (Figure 7). The design mechanism that creates accommodation relies on the relaxation of the zonular fibers as the ciliary body contracts, leading to relaxation of the capsular bag and the forward movement of the IOL.[13] IOLs that are lower in lens power will generate less accommodation than those in the higher power ranges.

BIOCOMFOLD 43E AND 43S

This lens (Morcher, Stuttgart, Germany) is a single-piece, hydrophilic acrylic with a disc-like shape and a peripheral bulging, discontinuous ring. This ring is connected to the optic with an intermediate, forward-angled perforated ring section. The optic is positioned in front of the ring that results in a forward shift when the ciliary muscle contracts on the haptic. The 43S operates on the same principle but has a refractive multifocal optic (Figure 8).[5]

SYNCHRONY

A dual-optic, single-piece, silicone IOL, the Synchrony (Visiogen, Irvine, CA) has a 5.5-mm high-power, anterior optic that is connected to a 6-mm, negative-power optic by haptics

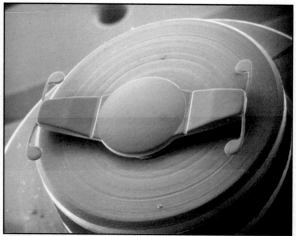

Figure 10. Overview photograph of the Crystalens accommodative IOL (SEM).

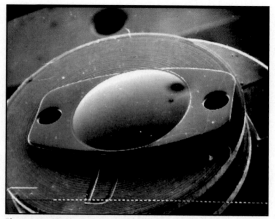

Figure 11. STAAR plate-haptic silicone IOL with broader fenestration holes (SEM).

that have a spring-like action (Figure 9). Once implanted inside the capsular bag, the tension of the bag compresses the optics, reducing the distance between them. When the zonules relax during accommodation, anterior displacement of the anterior optic occurs, helping to improve accommodation.

CRYSTALENS (AT-45)

The IOL (Eyeonics, Inc, Aliso Viejo, CA) is made of silicone with a 1.43 index of refraction. It has a 4.5-mm optic and features grooved plate haptics with ends made of poly-amide (Figure 10). In the investigational FDA clinical trials, the Crystalens allowed approximately 73% of the subjects to remain essentially free of spectacles. The overall diameter of this IOL is 11.5 mm, which is normally larger than the diameter of the capsular bag, and the IOL is flexed at the 2 hinges. This configuration results in the 4.5-mm optic vaulting posterior as soon as the IOL is implanted in the capsular bag. To prevent anterior luxation of the optic through the pupil, immediately postoperatively and on the first postoperative day, one drop of atropine is applied topically.

The new Crystalens Five-0 has been redesigned to include several new features. The optic size has been increased from 4.5 to 5.0 mm and the plates are parallel rather than trapezoi-dal. There is 17% greater surface area for contact between the optic, plates and capsular bag, and the plate arc length has been increased by 90%.

Surgeons' preference for a larger optic led to the develop-ment of the redesign. The parallel pockets, formed by capsular fusion when the capsulorrhexis is made larger than the optic, might lead to greater plate motion by creation of a uniform width pocket in the capsular bag. The increase in surface area and arc length might further enhance predictability and capsular bag support. Crystalens Five-0 can be inserted with an injector through a 2.8 mm incision. This feature intends to increase the ease with which surgeons can implant the lens. This IOL is expected to be available in Europe in the begin-ning of 2009.

Toric IOLs

Lens rotation remains one of the most critical factors when implanting a toric IOL—and there are a wide variety of designs available in Europe with the intent to ensure that these IOLs remain aligned to the proper axis.

STAAR TORIC IOL

This IOL (STAAR Surgical, Monrovia, CA) was the first toric IOL to enter the marketplace in the late 1990s. Designed to correct astigmatism following cataract surgery, the first design of this lens, with an overall length of 10.8 mm, was found to have some problems with rotational stability. The company subsequently released a longer version of this toric IOL and increased the size of the fenestration holes in order to encourage quicker capsular fibrosis (Figure 11).[14]

STAAR TORIC IMPLANTABLE COLLAMER/ CONTACT LENS

This collamer phakic IOL (STAAR Surgical, Monrovia, CA) is implanted between iris and the crystalline lens. Earlier versions of the lens had a tendency to come into contact with the natural lens, potentially causing cataract to develop. The fourth generation of the product, according to the manufac-turer, now has a vaulted design to ensure clearance over the natural lens (Figure 12).

ACRI.COMFORT 643TLC AND ACRI.COMFORT 646TLC

*Acri.Tec's (*Acri.Tec, Hennigsdorf, Germany) solution for astigmatic correction is a hydrophobic acrylic available in 2 styles: A tripod design with a 6-mm optic and overall diam-eter of 10 mm and a 1-piece plate design with a 6-mm optic and overall diameter of 11 mm. The manufacturer claims that both designs offer good rotational stability. Further, it says that the aspheric optic increases image quality and depth of sharpness.

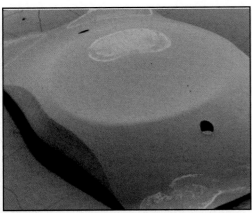

Figure 12. ICL (fourth generation): overview (SEM).

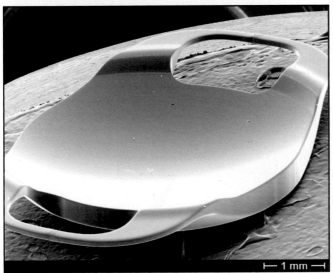

Figure 13. Backside of the Verisyse Toric PMMA phakic IOL with a view on the torus (SEM).

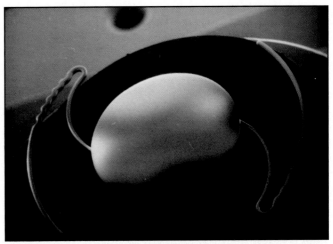

Figure 14. Silicone toric MS6116TU with Z-shaped haptic for improved rotational stability (SEM).

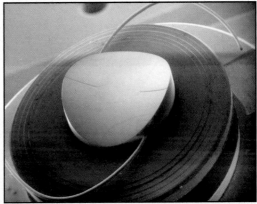

Figure 15. Silicone toric MS614T (a high torus can be observed) with long C-shaped haptics for sulcus implantation (SEM).

ACRYSOF SA60TT

This hydrophobic acrylic is a one-piece IOL with modified "L" haptics and comes with both blue and ultraviolet (UV) blocking filters. It is available in 3 cylinder powers: 1, 1.5, and 2.25 D.

VERISYSE TORIC

This PMMA, iris-fixated, claw phakic lens (Advanced Medical Optics, Santa Ana, CA) is available in both negative and positive cylindrical powers for the correction of astigmatism (Figure 13). It is also offered by Ophtec as the Artisan Toric.[15,16]

MICROSIL MS6116TU, MICROSIL MS6116T-Y, AND MICROSIL MS614T

These silicone toric IOLs (Human Optics, Erlangen, Germany) have spherical anterior surfaces and toric posterior surfaces and are intended to correct higher levels of astigmatism.[17,18] Two models (MS6116TU and MS6116T-Y) have undulated "Z"-loop shaped PMMA (MicroPlex) haptics (Figure 14), whereas the third model (MS614T) has long "C"-shaped PMMA haptics and is intended for sulcus fixation. The total diameter is 14.0 mm and the optic diameter is 6.0 or 7.0 mm with or without blue light protection in the optic (Figure 15).[19,20]

Posterior Chamber Implantable Collamer/Contact Lenses

STAAR Surgical also offers the phakic implantable collamer/contact lenses (ICLs) for myopic and hyperopic correction. Like the Toric ICL model, these lenses are also implanted between the iris and the crystalline lens/IOL. The manufacturer states that one of the benefits of the ICL is that it can correct higher levels of refractive error than laser vision correction procedures.

Anterior Chamber Phakic IOLs

The most commonly used types of anterior chamber IOLs currently used in Europe are the iris-fixated, claw design lenses first developed by a Dutch surgeon, Jan Worst, MD. These lenses are available through Worst's company, Ophtec, as the Artisan lenses (PMMA) and the Artiflex (silicone). They are also available from Advanced Medical Optics under the brand

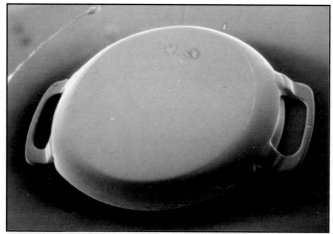

Figure 16. Overview of the Artiflex/Veriflex phakic IOL (SEM).

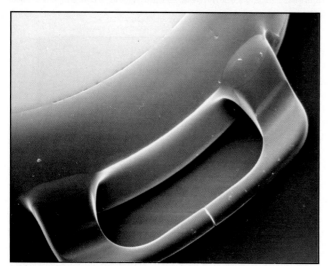

Figure 17. Optic haptic junction area with the angulated PMMA claw of the foldable Artiflex/Veriflex phakic IOL (SEM).

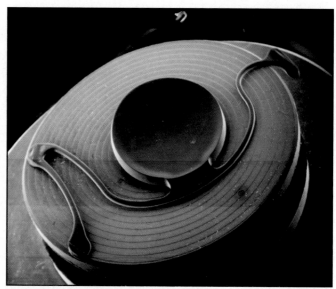

Figure 18. Foldable hydrophilic acrylate Vivarte phakic IOL with soft haptic ends for sizing error compensation (SEM).

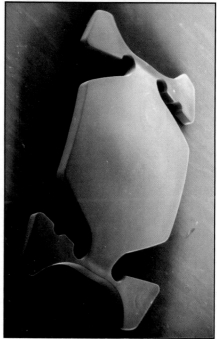

Figure 19. Overview of the hydrophilic acrylic Icare phakic IOL for angle fixation in myopic eyes (SEM).

names of Verisyse (PMMA) and Veriflex (silicone) (Figures 16 and 17).

It is interesting to note that in the summer of 2007, based on clinical data, the French government took the step of banning the sale of angle-supported phakic IOLs. The ban was instituted because of high levels of endothelial cell loss in eyes with the Vivarte phakic IOL (Figure 18), typically occurring at approximately 3 years after implantation.[21]

The Vivarte IOL (also under the name GBR) was a 1-piece phakic IOL manufactured from a mixture of acrylate with a refractive index of 1.47. The foldable optic had a 5.5 mm diameter and the IOL was available in diameters of 12.0, 12.5, and 13.0 mm for myopia only.

The Icare phakic anterior chamber angle-fixated IOL was a 1-piece hydrophilic foldable IOL with a convexoncave optic of 5.75 mm diameter and a range of total diameters measuring 12.0 to 13.5 mm in 0.5-mm steps (Figure 19). It had 4 flexible haptics and was available only for myopia.

The PRL was a 1-piece posterior chamber phakic IOL made from silicone (refractive index: 1.46) with a total length of 10.6 mm for hyperopia (Figure 20) and 10.8 and 11.3 mm for myopic eyes (Figure 21). The optic diameter valued 4.5 to 5 mm with an IOL width of 6 mm.

Evolution of Use of Refractive IOLs

The interest in refractive IOLs in Europe has followed a pattern similar to what has been seen in other countries. At first, primarily refractive surgeons used these IOLs, most frequently in patients who were not appropriate candidates for laser vision correction. However, as the technology has improved and the choice of refractive IOLs has expanded, so has the interest in implanting these IOLs grown. The vast majority of European countries are now seeing an increase in implantation rates in refractive IOLs. In Belgium, for example, the percentage of multifocal IOLs implanted has increased by almost 3% in just 1 year.[22] Similar increases have been reported in Norway and

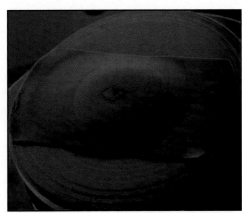

Figure 20. Overview of the 1-piece silicone PRL for hyperopia (SEM).

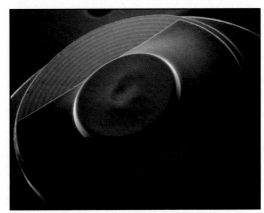

Figure 21. Overview of the 1-piece silicone PRL for myopia (SEM).

France.[23,24] In fact, this 2006 French survey showed that for the first time refractive lens exchange was the most popular treatment for presbyopia, accounting for 15% of presbyopic surgeries, compared to 12% for presbyLASIK. The survey found that multifocal IOLs were used in 21% of cases in 2006, compared to 13% in 2004.

Helping to drive this growth is increased patient awareness about refractive IOLs and treatment options. As is the case in the rest of the world, European consumers now rely heavily on the Internet to research and learn about new technologies.

However, this increased interest and awareness on the part of consumers presents a unique challenge in Europe where the vast majority of healthcare treatments are provided under public health systems. As most are aware, these refractive IOLs carry a much higher cost than traditional, monofocal IOLs. At the same time, many governments, including those in Germany, the United Kingdom, and Italy are looking to cut the rising cost of healthcare and pressuring physicians and hospitals to reduce costs and become more efficient. In Germany, for example, the recently instituted diagnosis-related groups (DRGs) now designate a universal, single payment for procedures based on whether the procedure is extraocular, intraocular, or laser surgery.[25] Because of these increased cost pressures, and the government's decision not to include premium priced IOLs, when a patient opts for one of these lenses, it becomes a private pay procedure.

What is interesting about this position taken by many of the European governments is that a number of studies, including one the author was involved in, have demonstrated that multifocal IOLs are cost effective. One study used 3 different meta-analyzes to review previously published studies, evaluating visual outcomes and cost effectiveness. The conclusion reached was that multifocal IOLs added an incremental cost of 63 Euros per additional line of near visual acuity gained and were a cost effective alternative to the standard monofocal IOL.[26] A prospective Dutch study compared direct and associated costs between a monofocal group and a multifocal IOL group. This study found no significant differences in total patient costs between the 2 groups. Further, they found that the monofocal patient group spent more money on spectacles because of the need for bifocal or multifocal lenses.[27]

Conclusion

Based on the survey results discussed, as well as anecdotal findings, it is quite clear that the popularity of refractive IOLs is on the rise for both refractive lens exchange and cataract surgery. Particularly, with the increasing availability of small-incision refractive lenses that provide predictable outcomes, more surgeons will come to rely on these IOLs as important tools in their refractive-cataract surgery armamentarium. The challenge in Europe will be to convince regional governments of the added value these IOLs bring to patients in order to increase their availability to greater numbers of consumers.

References

1. Eisenmann D, Jacobi FK, Dick B, Jacobi KW. The Array silicone multifocal lens: experiences after 150 implantations. *Klin Monatsbl Augenheilkd.* 1996;208:270-272.

2. Pearce JL. Multifocal intraocular lenses. *Curr Opin Ophthalmol.* 1997;8:2-5.

3. Hessemer V, Eisenmann D, Jacobi K. Multifocal intraocular lenses: an assessment of current status (in German). *Klin Monatsbl Augenheilkd.* 1993;203:19-33.

4. Häring G, Dick HB, Krummenauer F, Weissmantel U, Kröncke W. Subjective photic phenomena with refractive multifocal and monofocal intraocular lenses: results of a multicenter questionnaire. *J Cataract Refract Surg.* 2001;27:245-249.

5. Auffarth G, Dick B. Multifocal intraocular lenses: a review (in German). *Ophthalmologe.* 2001;98:127-137.

6. Dick HB, Gross S, Tehrani M, Eisenmann D, Pfeiffer N. Refractive lens exchange with an Array multifocal intraocular lens. *J Refract Surg.* 2002;18:509-518.

7. Dick HB, Krummenauer F, Schwenn O, Krist R, Pfeiffer N. Objective and subjective evaluation of photic phenomena after monofocal and multifocal intraocular lens implantation. *Ophthalmology.* 1999;106:1878-1886.

8. Schmitz S, Dick HB, Krummenauer F, Schwenn O, Krist R. Contrast sensitivity and glare disability by halogen light after monofocal and multifocal lens implantation. *Br J Ophthalmol.* 2000;84:1109-1112.

9. Packer M, Hoffman RS, Fine IH, Dick HB. Refractive lens exchange. *Int Ophthalmol Clin.* 2006;46:63-82.

10. Lane S, Morris M, Nordan L, Packer M, et al. Multifocal intraocular lenses. *Ophthalmol Clin N Am.* 2006;19:89-105.

11. Bellucci R. Multifocal intraocular lenses. *Curr Opin Ophthalmol.* 2005;16:33-37.

12. Dick H. Accommodative intraocular lenses: current status. *Curr Opin Ophthalmol.* 2005;16:8-26.

13. Dell S, Dick HB. Single-optic accommodative intraocular lenses. *Ophthalmol Clin North Am.* 2006;19:107-124.

14. Schwenn O, Kottler U, Krummenauer F, Dick HB, Pfeiffer N. Effect of large positioning holes on capsule fixation of plate-haptic intraocular lenses. *J Cataract Refract Surg.* 2000;26:1778-1785.

15. Tehrani M, Dick HB. Iris-fixated toric phakic lens: three-year follow-up. *J Cataract Refract Surg.* 2006;32:1301-1306.

16. Dick HB, Alio J, Bianchetti M, et al. Toric phakic intraocular lens: European multi-center study. *Ophthalmology.* 2003;110:150-162.

17. Dick HB, Augustin AJ. Lens implant selection with absence of capsular support. *Curr Opin Ophthalmol.* 2001;12:47-57.

18. Warlo I, Krummenauer F, Dick HB. Rotational stability in intraocular lenses with C-loop haptics versus Z-haptics in cataract surgery. A prospective randomized comparison. *Ophthalmologe.* 2005;102:987-992.

19. Tehrani M, Stoffelns B, Dick HB. Implantation of a custom intraocular lens with a 30-diopter torus for the correction of high astigmatism after penetrating keratoplasty. *J Cataract Refract Surg.* 2003;29:2444-2447.

20. Tehrani M, Dick HB. Incisional keratotomy to toric intraocular lenses: an overview of the correction of astigmatism in cataract and refractive surgery. *Int Ophthalmol Clin.* 2003;43:43-52.

21. Ocular Surgery News Europe/Asia Edition, July 2007.

22. Goes F. Belgium: Bladeless LASIK, New IOLs becoming popular. Cataract & Refractive Surgery Today Europe, Summer 2007).

23. Thilesen T. No Regulations on private surgery, refractive surgery in Norway. Cataract & Refractive Surgery Today Europe, Summer 2007.

24. McGrath D. Survey charts evolution in French practice habits. Eurotimes, July 2007).

25. German eye surgeons losing patients because of new laws. Eurotimes, May 2005.

26. Pagel N, Dick HB, Krummenauer F. Incremental cost effectiveness of multifocal cataract surgery (in German). *Klin Monatsbl Augenheilkd.* 2007;224:101-109.

27. Dolders M, Nijkamp M, Nuijts R, van den Borne B, Hendrikse F, Ament A, Groot W. Cost effectiveness of foldable multifocal intraocular lenses compared to foldable monofocal intraocular lenses for cataract surgery. *Br J Ophthalmol.* 2004;88:1163-1168.

CHAPTER 143

REFRACTIVE IOL SELECTION— SOUTH AMERICAN PERSPECTIVE

Leonardo Akaishi, MD

Ophthalmology in South America is now at a special place in time. The introduction of new intraocular lenses (IOLs) for presbyopia and cataracts provides a wide range of alternatives, both for patients and for doctors. The possibility of a patient choosing and paying for a premium IOL enables doctors to be appreciated and compensated for the true value of their work. Refractive IOLs therefore provide an opportunity for some ophthalmologists to differentiate themselves from others.

Until recently, we basically had only one IOL alternative. There was no need to understand very much about each individual patient's lifestyle. Cataract surgeons, therefore, were able to perform a large number of surgeries with maximal speed and efficiency. As a result, the value of cataract surgery became diminished in the minds of the payers. It was common practice for patients and health insurance providers to look for ways to lower costs, particularly in Latin America. Most of the time, there was no major perceived difference between providers. Today, because there are many IOL alternatives, the emphasis is shifting to selecting the best IOL and offering state-of-the-art surgery.

At this point, there is no single IOL that can meet all of our patients' needs. A patient must select the right lens and build a good relationship with his or her doctor before surgery in order to achieve success and have his or her refractive expectations met. We have the opportunity to enrich the patient's life through refractive IOLs and this is our goal.

Unfortunately—or maybe fortunately—cataract surgery has essentially become refractive surgery, imposing a higher standard with regard to outcomes. If the patient has unrealistic expectations, dissatisfaction and subsequent lawsuits may follow. It is my opinion that presbyopia-correcting surgery will become, in the short-term, the most common cause of ophthalmology-related lawsuits worldwide.

The indiscriminate dissemination of clear lens extraction for correcting presbyopia is of concern because we do not know enough about the visual quality of multifocal lenses in purely presbyopic refractive patients.

There is a common opinion that patients with >1.5 D of hyperopia will be happy with a refractive lens exchange and implantation of a multifocal IOL. In my clinical experience, this is not always true. Even though they read 20/20 on the acuity chart following multifocal IOL implantation, some patients experience quality of vision that is worse than their corrected vision was preoperatively. It is necessary to use other measures of quality of vision, such as contrast sensitivity and higher-order aberrations (HOA) to understand how our multifocal IOL patients see. It is also important to understand the patient's true expectations of their surgery.

The preoperative modulation transfer function (MTF) measurement helps to determine if surgery is necessary because it is another indicator of ocular optical quality. The optical quality of a normal crystalline lens is better than the optical quality of monofocal IOLs, and these in turn are better than multifocal IOLs. Consider the internal aberrations of an eye with good quality high-order MTF, even with ametropia that is corrected with spectacles. The optical quality of this eye can be worse after a multifocal IOL is implanted, which would be manifest as visual complaints.

When we perform presbyopia-correcting IOL surgery, an emmetropic patient must be informed preoperatively whether his or her distance vision will become worse in terms of visual quality with halos and glare. We must spend more time with a patient during the preoperative consultation, selecting the most appropriate lens and emphasizing realistic expectations. The time we spend with a patient preoperatively is critical for achieving patient satisfaction postoperatively. It is imperative that doctors talk more with their patients preoperatively, conducting a thorough evaluation, that lets them become familiar with their patients' desires, habits, and lifestyles. Anatomical factors, such as anterior chamber depth and pupil size should also be taken into account.

The key to surgical success is stressing preoperatively what the patient should realistically expect postoperatively.

We have implanted more than 1000 ReSTOR (Alcon, Fort Worth, TX), 1400 Tecnis MF (Advanced Medical Optics, Santa Ana, CA), and 250 ReZoom (Advanced Medical Optics)

Table 1

MULTIFOCAL IOL CHARACTERISTICS

	Far Vision	Intermediate Vision	Near Vision	Halos	Pupil Size	Light Level
ReSTOR	++++ +	+	++++	+	++	+++
ReZoom *	++++ +	+++	++	++	+++	-
Tecnis	++++	++	+++++	++	−	−

Personal Experience

I have implanted more than 2500 multifocal IOLs. I started with the Array (Advanced Medical Optics) and now I have been working with the ReSTOR, ReZoom, and Tecnis multifocal.

My experience and perception say:

- The best visual acuity for far is the ReSTOR IOL due to apodization and the fact that part of the IOL is refractive.
- The best visual acuity for intermediate is the ReZoom; the worst is the ReSTOR.
- The best visual acuity for near is the Tecnis. The near vision of the Tecnis is unbelievable
- The ReSTOR near vision is too close and the patient must have alot of light to read. It is almost impossible to read a menu in a restaurant.
- In relation to halos, all multifocals have them. The ReSTOR has a little bit less because of the apodization and refractive zone.
- Concerning pupil size, the ReZoom IOL does not work with pupil sizes less than 3.0 mm. We should remember that the pupil size reduces with aging. I am not sure how these patients with ReZoom will be in the future.
- The ReSTOR IOL is pupil size dependent. I have a patient that had a paralytic pupil after glaucoma block. I implanted a ReSTOR IOL 3 years ago in a patient and she complained about double vision for near. I reduced the pupil size to 3 mm with stitches, the double vision disappeared.
- The Tecnis multifocal is totally pupil independent.

IOLs in the last 4 years, and we observed the following (Table 1):

* Distance vision: The ReSTOR IOL provides the best quality vision of the 3 multifocals presumably due to its refractive (monofocal) periphery.

  The Tecnis MF IOL is very sensitive to small amounts of residual myopia; for example, −0.50 D of myopia worsens distance vision much more when compared to ReSTOR and ReZoom IOLs.

* Intermediate vision: The ReZoom IOL performs the best at this range. In most patients with pupils larger than 3.5 mm, we find J3 intermediate vision, which approximates to an Arial 10-point font on a computer. When their refraction is +0.50 D of hyperopia, patients with the Tecnis MF IOL achieve intermediate vision comparable to that with ReZoom lenses, while still maintaining good distance vision. This is my current target: +0.50 with the Tecnis MF IOL.

* Near vision: The Tecnis MF IOL performs the best at near because it provides the most comfortable reading distance and does not require very bright reading illumination. A patient is able to read a menu in a restaurant under mesopic conditions, as opposed to the ReSTOR lens, which requires much brighter illumination for reading activities.

Although some patients with the ReZoom IOL are able to read J1 to J2, most still need reading glasses. Reading speed and reading clarity with the ReZoom IOL are significantly lower when compared to the diffractive multifocals.

* Halos: All of these IOLs cause halos. The ReSTOR IOL is associated with the lowest number of halo complaints due to its design. Patients with the ReZoom IOL complain most frequently about this phenomenon.

* Pupil size: ReZoom and ReSTOR IOLs are pupil size-dependent. Patients with pupil sizes smaller than 3.5 mm implanted with ReZoom lens were unsatisfied with their near and intermediate vision because the central optical zone is targeted for distance vision.

We also notice that patients with pupils larger than 4.5 mm have better intermediate vision than the ones with small pupils.

We know that pupil size is reduced with age. What will happen to patients implanted with pupil size-dependent multifocal lenses in the long term? Could neurosensory adaptation really offset this loss?

We know little about the relationship between pupil size, accommodative miosis, neurosensory adaptation, quality of vision, and multifocal IOLs. Why do American and Canadian patients show higher levels of satisfaction with the ReZoom lens than Latin and South American patients? Is it because most North Americans are taller and so their reading distance is further away? Would it be because Caucasians have larger pupils by nature?

Multifocal lens implantation in patients who had previously undergone refractive surgery (photorefractive keratectomy [PRK], laser in situ keratomileusis [LASIK], radial keratotomy [RK]) yielded very good results: We prefer to implant the Tecnis MF IOL (negative spherical aberration) in patients who have had previous myopic PRK, LASIK, or RK, in order to offset the oblate corneal shape. We recommend the spherical ReSTOR lens in patients who have had previous hyperopic LASIK or PRK in order to not to increase negative spherical aberration.

We found a mean uncorrected visual acuity of 20/35 in 55 postrefractive surgery eyes, with 8 eyes (14.5%) requiring an excimer laser enhancement to correct residual ametropia. The satisfaction rate in this group was 84% and, so far, there have been no multifocal IOL explantation cases.

* Multifocal lens implantation in patients with monofocal IOLs in the fellow eye: Due to the quality of vision afforded by multifocal IOLs, patients can adjust to either a monofocal or multifocal IOL.

If the patient is left with mild myopia in the eye implanted with the monofocal IOL, his or her intermediate vision is improved. Those patients must be informed that they will need glasses in some situations. We have implanted a multifocal lens in one eye and a monofocal IOL in the contralateral eye of 56 patients, and the results were amazing.

The halo symptoms in these patients were significantly less than in those patients with bilateral multifocal IOLs, and most patients wear glasses only for prolonged reading.

* Astigmatism is not an absolute contraindication for multifocal IOLs provided that the cornea is amenable to laser bioptic astigmatism correction, and the patient is willing to undergo a second procedure.

At this point in time, in over 50% of my surgeries with MF IOLs, I do limbal relaxing incisions (LRI) at the same surgical setting, even for those patients whose have more than 2.0 D of corneal astigmatism. I prefer to diminish the astigmatism with an LRI and then if necessary, achieve further correction with excimer laser.

I have noticed that when you at least partially reduce the patient's astigmatism with LRIs at the time of IOL surgery, he or she is happier and more patient and can wait for excimer laser treatment to correct the final residual cylinder. Prescribing temporary glasses is very important so that the patient can still have good vision for near and far as they await the optimal time for laser vision enhancement.

* Implanting 2 lenses with different designs surely improves the final refractive outcome.

After an extensive preoperative assessment, we select the first lens. Then, we assess the patient's satisfaction 7 to 15 days following the first surgery.

Example 1. If we select, for example, a Tecnis MF for the first eye, and, 15 days later, the patient thinks his or her distance vision is not satisfactory, we implant a ReSTOR lens in the fellow eye. We know that the ReSTOR IOL provides better distance vision due to its refractive periphery and because it is less sensitive to subtle amounts of residual refractive error when compared to the Tecnis MF. A patient implanted with

a Tecnis IOL with 0.5 degree of residual myopia has worse functional vision than a ReSTOR patient with the same degree of myopia. With the ReSTOR halos are also less frequent than with the Tecnis MF.

On the other hand, if the intermediate vision is not adequate following Tecnis MF implantation in the first eye, we can implant a ReZoom lens in the fellow eye. The ReZoom IOL provides better intermediate vision compared to other multifocal IOLs, but the pupil should be larger than 3.5 mm.

Another alternative for improving intermediate vision is to implant a second Tecnis MF IOL and leave the patient with a final hyperopic refraction of +0.50 D.

Example 2. If we implant a ReSTOR IOL for the first eye and the near vision is too close, particularly in tall patients (long arms), the second lens should be a Tecnis MF or ReZoom IOL. Some patients with the ReSTOR IOL complain about the need for brighter lighting order to read, as illustrated by the fact that they cannot read a menu in a dimly lit restaurant. In these cases, we would implant a Tecnis MF in the fellow eye because its reading function is fully pupil-independent.

Patients with multifocal IOLs should be advised preoperatively that they will likely need glasses for intermediate tasks, such as computer use. This is especially true if they have longer arms, or smaller pupils (<3.0 mm).

We prefer to implant a ReSTOR IOL in the dominant eye and a Tecnis MF IOL in the other eye in patients who drive at night, use computers, and read intensely.

In 40 patients in whom we mixed the Tecnis MF IOL and a ReZoom IOL, we were able to achieve near vision of J3 at 60 cm, which corresponds to 10-point computer font. So far, multifocal lenses seem to be the best way to help patients achieve independence from glasses (Figure 1).

Absolute Contraindications to Multifocal IOLs

* Patients with potential <20/40 in both eyes
* Maculopathy
* Uncorrectable astigmatism (keratoconus, pellucid marginal degeneration, corneal ecstasia)
* Corneal opacity
* Hypercritical patients
* Vitreous opacities (these are more likely to bother patients with multifocal rather than monofocal IOLs. Whenever necessary, the possibility of vitrectomy surgery needs to be discussed).
* Retinal drusen and diabetic retinopathy (we should evaluate the patient's age and prognosis)
* Only eye (in patients with mental and physical problems)

Pearls for Managing Complications

Many times, a secondary procedure will be required for optimizing a multifocal IOL's full performance. Examples

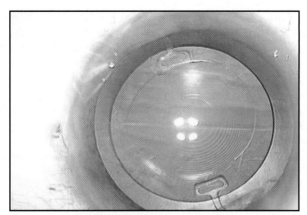

Figure 1. Tecnis MF in nondominant eye.

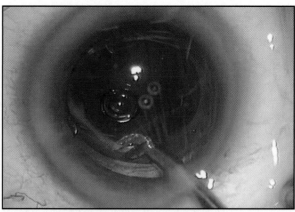

Figure 3. Cutting anterior capsule.

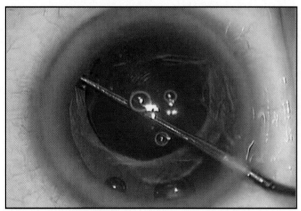

Figure 2. Centralization OD IOL.

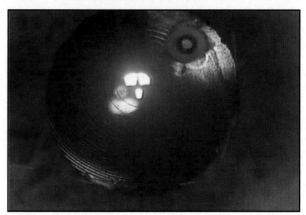

Figure 4. IOL centralized.

might include the correction of residual ametropia, or improving IOL centration.

* Decentered IOL
  * Correct surgically as soon as possible (Figures 2, 3, and 4).
* Complaints of poor intermediate visual acuity (mainly for computer users):
  * Treat posterior capsule opacification (yttrium-aluminum-garnet [YAG])
  * Verify refraction even though visual acuity is 20/20 uncorrected
* Complaint of good vision in the morning but worsening vision in the afternoon:
  * Screen for dry eye.
* Complaint of intense halos:
  * Check refraction (remember ametropia increases halos)

  * Treat posterior capsule opacification
  * Treat dry eye or keratitis
* Complaint of visual fatigue despite 20/20 uncorrected acuity
  * Treat residual refractive error with laser vision enhancement (eg, 0.75 D of astigmatism, or −0.50 D myopia in a ReSTOR patient)
* Complaint of poor near vision in patients who have residual hyperopia (eg, +1.0 D with the Tecnis or ReZoom IOL)
  * We can correct this by surgically repositioning the IOL optic in front of the capsulorrhexis. The haptics should remain inside the bag. Doing this will induce myopia with the need to exchange the IOL, but the procedure must be done before significant contracture of the capsulorrhexis.

CHAPTER 144

REFRACTIVE IOL SELECTION— ASIAN PERSPECTIVE

Jerry Tan Tiang Hin, MBBS, FRCS, FRCOphth

"The number of Japanese aged 100 years or older will reach a record of more than 32,000 by next month, according to a Japanese government survey.

One in 5 Japanese is now aged 65 years or above, and by mid century, that figure will nearly double" (Reuters, 15 September 2007).

Asia is a paradox. On one hand it has countries like Japan and Singapore, with modern economies and life expectancies of 80 years. Asia also has countries such as Cambodia and Bhutan with third-world economies and a life expectancy of approximately 60 years (Table 1).

Even within a single country such as China, there are thousands of millionaires as well as thousands of people living below the poverty line.

The rich and powerful in Asia are global citizens, and with the Internet, they are well informed. They demand the best and can get it, whereas the poor are so deprived that even receiving cataract surgery is a matter of luck and hope. Cataract camps operate on thousands of under-privileged Asians and there is no choice of an implant except a single piece monofocal intraocular lens (IOL), if at all.

In this age of globalization, multifocal IOL implants from companies like Alcon and Advanced Medical Optics are readily available in almost all Asian countries.[1-4] However, many intraocular implants from India are also available to the poorer Asian citizens.[5]

The Asian patient is no different from any other patient from Europe and America. The rich and intelligent are demanding, especially when the cost of such a surgery is high.

The Asian Patient

The ideal patient for multifocal lens implantation is a highly motivated individual that is willing to sacrifice some contrast sensitivity and would not mind wearing reading glasses occasionally.[6-18]

The least suitable patient for this surgery has a Type A personality, and is not willing to take time to understand the technology and its limitations.[19,20] Certain professionals such as architects and accountants and, in general, fussy patients are the least likely to be happy with a multifocal IOL.

Unfortunately, many Asian patients completely trust their doctor and do not want to learn about any details of the surgery until after complications occur or when their expectations and goals have not been met.

The "new" wealthy Asian patient has a mixture of Asian values but with a Western mentality (Table 2). Malpractice litigation, which was previously unheard of, is now more commonplace. Baby boomers have extremely high expectations: they want the best for themselves and their parents, and can be unforgiving when expectations are not met. Herein lies the problem—whenever costs are high, expectations are higher.

Conditions for the Perfect Multifocal IOL Surgery

Implantation of multifocal IOLs requires not only a suitable patient, but suitable "hardware" and "software" for a successful outcome. Unfortunately, some of this technology is not readily available in many Asian countries, nor do the cataract surgeons possess all of these requisite skills (Table 3).

PERFECT BIOMETRY

Partial coherence interferometry with the IOL Master (Carl Zeiss Meditec, Jena, Germany) has been proven to produce the most accurate biometry. Unfortunately, many Asian countries do not have this technology available.

In addition, IOL Master measurements may not be possible through very dense cataracts, which are more common in Asia.

Immersion biometry is an alternative but is less accurate than partial coherence interferometry. Well trained ophthalmic technicians are essential for the use of immersion and contact biometry.

Table 1

ASIAN LIFE EXPECTANCY – 2007

Country	Life Expectancy (in years)	Population	GDP (Millions)
Bangladesh	64	142 million	60,000
Bhutan	64	637,000	844
Cambodia	57	14 million	6,187
China	72	1.3 billion	2,234,000
India	64	1.095 billion	860,000
Indonesia	68	221 million	287,000
Japan	82	128 million	4,534,000

Source: Adapted from The World Bank: World Development Indicators 2007.

Table 3

REQUIREMENTS FOR DELIVERING THE "PERFECT" MULTIFOCAL IOL RESULT

- Laser interferometry for biometry
- Phacoemulsification with continuous capsulorrhexis
- Correction of astigmatism
    - LRI (limbal relaxing incisions)
    - SIA (Surgically induced astigmatism)
    - LVC (Laser vision correction)
- Personalized A-constant
- No macular disease—Increasing incidence as population increases
- Posterior capsulotomy—Availability of the yttrium-aluminum-garnet (YAG) laser
- Optimum pupil size—Pupillometer needed to detect very small or large pupils
- Educated and motivated patient

Table 2

"NEW" VERSUS "OLD" ASIAN PATIENTS

"New" Asian Patient	"Old" Asian Patient
1. Trusting until a complication occurs	1. Trusting
2. Willing to pay top dollar but wants the best	2. Frugal—does not want to spend on health
3. Pro-active	3. Fatalist—what will be will be
4. Willing to learn about illness and surgery but would rather not hear about risks and complications	4. Does not want to understand the details and is willing to accept complications
5. Litigious—"Western" in outlook	5. Litigation against doctors unheard of
6. Complains more often	6. Seldom complains

PHACOEMULSIFICATION WITH CONTINUOUS CAPSULORRHEXIS

Phacoemulsification and a continuous capsulorrhexis (CCC) are essential prerequisites for implanting multifocal IOLs. The majority of cataract patients in Asia still undergo extra-capsular cataract extraction. IOL decentration is more likely without a continuous capsulorrhexis. The cost of phacoemulsification and the multifocal IOL is another major stumbling block. Manual small incision cataract surgery (SICS) is a possible solution. Most SICS techniques, however, do not preserve a continuous anterior capsule edge and are not astigmatically neutral.[21-23]

CORRECTION OF ASTIGMATISM

Toric multifocal IOLs are not available worldwide. As a result, patients with significant astigmatism are not ideal candidates for multifocal IOLs.

The use of limbal relaxing incisions (LRI) or astigmatic keratotomy has not gained popularity in Asia. This is probably due to lack of training, lack of experience, the unavailability of corneal topography, inconsistent results, and the lack of patient assessment time due to the high volume of cataract examinations.

Laser in situ keratomileusis (LASIK) after multifocal IOL surgery is gaining limited popularity in Asia because of its relative simplicity and accuracy. However, cost is still a major hurdle and many Asian patients are innately reluctant to have multiple surgeries to achieve a singular goal.

PERSONALIZED NORMOGRAM

Accurate postoperative quantitative analysis of surgical outcomes is an important factor in consistently achieving emmetropia. An under- and over-correction of −0.50 D will negate many of the benefits of multifocal IOL surgery.

Determination of a personalized A-constant or of surgically induced astigmatism are important elements for refractive IOL success. Such outcome analysis requires a conscientious and well-trained staff for accurate data input, along with computers and specialized software programs. These are luxuries that are too costly and time consuming for many Asian eye centers.

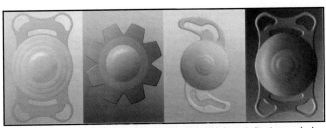

Figure 1. Various multifocal and accommodative IOLs made by an Indian intraocular lens manufacturer.

MACULAR DISEASE

The aging of the population and the changing dietary habits in Asia will increase the incidence of macular degeneration and diabetes mellitus. Unfortunately, smoking is still popular in many parts of Asia. Macular abnormalities will certainly disqualify many from being multifocal IOL candidates.

POSTERIOR CAPSULOTOMY

YAG laser capsulotomy may need to be performed much earlier in patients with multifocal IOLs because of the specialized optics. YAG lasers are now available in most Asian ophthalmological clinics, but there are still poor communities and countries where access to a YAG laser is limited.[24,25]

PUPILLOMETRY

Laser vision correction has certainly improved our understanding of clinical optics.

The size of the pupil is an important factor for the function of a multifocal IOL and the incidence of optical aberrations. A very small pupil negates the multifocality,[26,27] whereas a very large pupil may increase the incidence of halos and glare.[28]

In Asia, pupillometry is not usually performed for the preoperative cataract patient.

EDUCATED AND MOTIVATED PATIENT

Generally, little attention is paid to patient education in Asia. Historically, patients simply put their trust in the "doctors' hands." However, with increasing Westernization, patients are now more willing to participate in medical decision making. It is certainly mandatory for patients to understand and accept the limitations of current multifocal IOL technology.

The disinterested or overly trusting patient can quickly turn into a very angry patient if the results are disappointing. It is therefore important that the surgeon not over-sell the technology as this may raise expectations to an unreasonable level—especially in the case of refractive lens exchange.

Asian Experience With Accommodative IOLs

Accommodative IOLs, like the AT-45 Crystalens (Eyeonics, Inc, Aliso Viejo, CA) and the Humanoptics 1CU (Erlangen, Germany), have not achieved much popularity in Asia.[29] As with multifocal IOLs, early experience with these implants again underscored the importance of performing flawless cataract surgery.[30,31] In addition to all the requirements needed for successful multifocal IOL implantation, accommodating IOLs

necessitate achieving a "perfect" capsulorrhexis. Too small an opening can result in capsulophimosis with infolding of the flexible haptics of the Humanoptics 1CU lens. Too large an opening may impair anterior or posterior movement of the accommodative IOL.[32] Experience has shown that these accommodating lenses are most successful in hyperopic individuals with short axial lengths, because the higher the IOL dioptric power, the greater the accommodative effect from a small amount of axial movement.

The inability to predict the final intraocular axial position of these flexible implants results in variable postoperative refractions. Finally, the anterior flexing and vaulting of implants such as the Humanoptics 1CU often results in rapid and severe Elschnig pearl formation. Without apposition of the optic to the posterior capsule, lens epithelial cells can readily migrate across the central posterior capsule.

Asian Multifocal IOLs

There are a few Asian countries that are currently producing multifocal IOLs. Some of these have unique designs (Figure 1), but there have been no prospective published studies to date, on the efficacy of these IOLs.

An example of one such lens is the Ultrasmart Acryfold lens made by Appasamy Associates, India. This is an ultra thin lens with elements that reportedly reduce spherical aberration and provide a pseudo-accommodative effect.

As Asia progresses economically, we will definitely see more multifocal IOLs designed and manufactured in Asia, and we anxiously await studies detailing clinical results with these refractive IOLs.

Multifocal IOL Implantation in Children in Asia

Many Asian countries do not regulate the use of multifocal IOLs in children.

Monofocal IOL implantation in children is now well accepted worldwide.[33-38] However, the use of multifocal IOLs for pediatric cataract is less well established.[39,40]

Studies in India, and other Asian countries, are showing promising results for the use of Array (Advanced Medical Optics), ReZoom (Advanced Medical Optics), ReSTOR (Alcon), and Presiol (an Indian-made multifocal IOL) in pediatric eyes. A study done by Mehta et al[41] showed 88% of children with bilateral multifocal IOLs achieving 6/12 or better vision as well as a near vision of at least N8 with correction. One-hundred percent of patients with unilateral multifocal IOL implantation achieved 6/18 or better. The complications that they reported from this study are listed in Table 4.

Asian Surgeon's Perspective on Multifocal IOLs

A survey was sent out via eblast to Asian ophthalmologists. A total of 50 responses were received from doctors in countries like India, Singapore, and China.

Table 4		
COMPLICATIONS OF MULTIFOCAL IOL IMPLANTATION IN CHILDREN IN ASIA		
Complications n = 157		
Complication	No.	%
Corneal abrasion	03	1.9
Shallow A/C	11	7.0
Iritis mild	12	7.6
Iritis severe	03	1.9
Raised IOP—temporary	15	9.6
Raised IOP—needed surgery	02	1.3
Hyphema	07	4.4
IOL decentered requiring surgery	09	5.7

The results are summarized as follows:

* 39% of responding doctors did not implant multifocal IOLs. These doctors were waiting for longer term results and were also not confident in the optical quality of current multifocal IOLs.

* 61% of responding doctors implanted multifocal IOLs; 64% implanted these lenses in 5% to 20% of their cataract cases. There were no doctors implanting these lenses in 100% of their patients. The main reason for not implanting more multifocal IOLs was the inability of the lenses to satisfy higher patient expectations. Surprisingly, the added cost of the multifocal lens was a less important factor in its usage.

Conclusion

Although multifocal IOLs are a step in the right direction, a toric, truly accommodating intraocular lens will be the ultimate cure for cataracts <u>and</u> presbyopia. In a final bit of irony, this "perfect" IOL is particularly suited for the world's poorest population who, because of cost, do not have access to spectacles. A toric accommodating IOL would be a perfect solution—able to eliminate the patient's myopia or hyperopia, astigmatism, and presbyopia.

References

1. Bellucci R. Multifocal intraocular lenses. *Curr Opin Ophthalmol.* 2005;16(1):33-37.

2. Blaylock JF, Si Z, Vickers C. Visual and refractive status at different focal distances after implantation of the ReSTOR multifocal intraocular lens. *J Cataract Refract Surg.* 2006;32(9):1464-1473.

3. Chiam PJ, Chan JH, Aggarwal RK, Kasaby S. Restor intraocular lens implantation in cataract surgery: quality of vision. *J Cataract Refract Surg.* 2006;32(9):1459-1463.

4. Kohnen T, Allen D, Boureau C, et al. European multicenter study of the AcrySof ReSTOR apodized diffractive intraocular lens. *Ophthalmology.* 2006;113:575-584.

5. Mehta KR, Mehta CK. Mastering the presbyopic surgery lenses & phakic IOLs. *Multifocal IOLs in Children: A Long-Term Analysis.* 2007;40:547-563

6. Arens B, Freudenthaler N, Quentin CD. Binocular function after bilateral implantation of monofocal and refractive multifocal intraocular lenses. *J Cataract Refract Surg.* 1999;25:399-404.

7. Dick HB, Krummenauer F, Schwenn O, et al. Objective and subjective evaluation of photic phenomenon after monofocal and multifocal intraocular lens implantation. *Ophthalmology.* 1999;106:1878-1886.

8. Gimbel HV, Sanders DR Raanan MG. Visual and refractive results after multifocal intraocular lenses. *Ophthalmology.* 1991;98:881-888.

9. Holladay JT, Van Dijk H, Land A, et al. Optical performance of multifocal intraocular lenses. *J Cataract Refract Surg.* 1990;16:413-422.

10. Holladay JT, Piers PA, Koranyi G, et al. A new intraocular lens design to reduce spherical aberration of pseudophacic eyes. *J Cataract Refract Surg.* 2002;18:683-691.

11. Javitt JC, Steinert RF. Cataract extraction with multifocal intraocular lens implantation: a multinational clinical trial evaluating clinical, function and quality-of-life outcomes. *Ophthalmology.* 2000;107:2040-2048.

12. Liekfeld A, Pham DT, Wollensack J. Functional results in bilateral implantation of a foldable multifocal posterior chamber lens. *Klin Mbl Augenheilkd.* 1995; 207:283-286.

13. Mester U, Dillinger P, Anterist N. Impact of a modified optic design on visual function: clinical comparative study. *J Cataract Refract Surg.* 2003;29:652-660.

14. Pieh S, Lackner B, Hanselmayer G, et al. Halo size under distance and near conditions in refractive multifocal intraocular lenses. *Br J Ophthalmol.* 2001;85:816-821.

15. Pieh S, Marvan P, Lackner B, et al. Quantitative performance of bifocal and multifocal intraocular lenses in a model eye: point spread function of multifocal intraocular lenses. *Arch Ophthalmol.* 2002;120:23-28.

16. Post CT Jr. Comparison of depth of focus and low-contrast acuities for monofocal versus multifocal intraocular lens patients at 1 year. *Ophthalmology.* 1992;99:1658-1663.

17. Ruther K, Eisenmann D, Zrenner E, et al. Effect of diffractive multifocal lenses on contrast vision, glare sensitivity and colour vision. *Klin Monatsbl Augenheilkd.* 1994;204:14-19.

18. Walkow T, Klemen U. Patients satisfaction after implantation of diffractive designed multifocal intraocular lenses in dependence on objective parameters. *Greafes Arch Clin Exp Ophthalmol.* 2001;239:683-687.

19. Klemen UM, Hahsel B, Lackinger B. Refractive versus Diffractive: A Comparison of 4 Multifocal Intraocular Lenses. *Kongreß der DGII,* Biermann Verlag; 2006:345-349.

20. McBridge DK, Matson W. Assessing the significance of optically produced reduction in braking response time: possible impacts on automotive safety among the elderly. *Potomac Institute for Police Studies.* April 1, 2003.

21. Guirao A, Tejedor J, Artal P. Corneal aberrations before and after small-incision cataract surgery. *Invest Ophthalmol Vis Sci.* 2004;45(12):4312-4319.

22. Kohnen T, Kasper T. Incision sizes before and after implantation of foldable intraocular lenses with 6 mm optic using Monarchand Unfolder injector systems. *Ophthalmology.* 2005;112:58-66.

23. Wan I, Dai E, Koch DD, et al. Optical aberrations of the human cornea. *J Cataract Refract Surg.* 2003;29(8):1514-1521.

24. Buehl W, Menapace R, Sacu S, et al. Effect of a silicone intraocular lens with sharp posterior edge on posterior capsule opacification. *J Cataract Refract Surg.* 2004;30:1661-1667.

25. Mester U, Fabian E, Gerl R, et al. Posterior capsule opacification after implantation of CeeOn Edge 911A, Phacoflex SI-40NB, and AcrySof MA60BM lenses. *J Cataract Refract Surg.* 2004;30:979-985.

26. Koch DD, Samuelson SW, Villareal R, et al. Changes in pupil size induced by phacoemulsification and posterior chamber lens implantation: consequences for multifocal lenses. *J Cataract Refract Surg.* 1996;22:579-584.

27. Koch DD, Samuelson SW, Haft EA, et al. Pupillary size and responsiveness: implications for selection of abifocal intraocular lens. *Ophthalmology.* 1991;98:1030-1035.

28. Hayashi K, Hayashi H, Nakao F. Correlation between papillary size and intraocular lens decentration and visual acuity of a zonal-progressive multifocal lens and a monofocal lens. *Ophthalmology.* 2001;18:2011-2017.

29. Humming JS, Slade SG, Chayet A, AT-45 Study Group. Clinical evaluation of the model AT-45 silicone accommodating intraocular lens: results of feasibility and the initial phase of the FDA Clinical Trial. *Ophthalmology.* 2001;108:2005-2010.

30. Kuchle M, Seitz B, Langenbucher A, Gusek-Schneider GC, Martus P, et al. The Erlangen Accommodative Intraocular Lens Study Group. Comparison of 6 months results of implantation of the 1CU accommodative intraocular lenses with conventional intraocular lenses. *Ophthalmology.* 2004;111:825-834.

31. Weghaupt H, Pieh S, Skorpik C. Comparison of pseudoaccommodation and visual quality between a diffractive and refractive multifocal intraocular lens. *J Cataract Refract Surg.* 1998;24:663-665.

32. Findl O, Kiss B, Petternel V, Menapace R, Georgopoulos M, et al. Intraocular lens movement caused by ciliary body contraction. *J Cataract Refract Surg.* 2003;29:669-676.

33. Ahmadieh H, Javadi MA. Intraocular lens implantation in children. *Curr Opin Ophthalmol.* 2001;12(1):30-34.

34. Crouch ER, Crouch ER, Pressman SH. Prospective analysis of pediatric pseudophakia: myopic shift and postoperative outcomes. *J AAPOS.* 2002;6(5):277-282.

35. McClatchey SK, Dahan E, et al. A comparison of the rate of refractive growth in pediatric aphakic and pseudophakic eyes. *Ophthalmology.* 2000;107(1):118-122.

36. Menezo JL, Taboada J. Assessment of intraocular lens implantation in children. *J Am Intraocul Implant Soc.* 1982;8(2):131-135.

37. Peterseim MW, Wilson ME. Bilateral intraocular lens implantation in the pediatric population. *Ophthalmology.* 2000;107(7):1261-1266.

38. Speeg-Schatz C, Flament J, Weissrock M. Congenital cataract extraction with primary aphakia and secondary intraocular lens implantation in the ciliary sulcus. *J Cataract Refract Surg.* 2005;31(4):750-756.

39. Jacobi PC, Dietlein TS, Jacobi FK. Scleral fixation of secondary foldable multifocal intraocular lens implants in children and young adults. *Ophthalmology.* 2002;109(12):2315-2324.

40. Jacobi PC, Dietlein TS, Konen W. Multifocal intraocular lens implantation in pediatric cataract surgery. *Ophthalmology.* 2001;108(8):1375-1380.

41. Mehta KR, Mehta CK. Multifocal IOLs in Children: A long term analysis. *Mastering The Presbyopic Surgery Lenses & Phakic Iols.* 2007;40:546-563.

CHAPTER 145

CASE STUDIES—WHAT WOULD YOU DO?
HOW WOULD YOU COUNSEL THESE PATIENTS SEEKING MAXIMUM SPECTACLE INDEPENDENCE?

David F. Chang, MD; Steven J. Dell, MD; Warren E. Hill, MD, FACS; Richard L. Lindstrom, MD; and Kevin L. Waltz, OD, MD

1. **A 68-year-old hyperope (+1.50) with visually significant bilateral cataracts, who uses a computer at work most of the day.**

   David F. Chang: For this patient I would suggest bilateral ReZoom (Advanced Medical Optics, Santa Ana, CA) intraocular lenses (IOLs), which provide good odds of being able to work at a desktop computer without glasses. Although the reading add is lower than that of the ReSTOR (Alcon, Fort Worth, TX), this person will probably be happy with their reading performance, because they have no such ability preoperatively. I would warn that prioritizing spectacle independence means accepting the compromise of halos at night. If this was a concern, I would implant the ReZoom in the nondominant eye first, leaving the option of a Crystalens 5.0 (Eyeonics, Inc, Aliso Viejo, CA) in the dominant eye should the patient be unhappy with halos during night driving.

   Steven J. Dell: Intermediate vision is superb with the Crystalens 5.0, and I would suggest this lens bilaterally. Targeting the dominant eye for –0.25 D, and the nondominant eye for –0.75 D will provide high grade distance, intermediate, and near vision without the photic phenomena associated with multifocals.

   Warren E. Hill: I would implant bilateral ReZoom IOLs for the obvious optimization of intermediate vision. An alternative would be modified monovision using a high quality aspheric with negative spherical aberration correction. The dominant eye would be targeted for –0.25 D and the nondominant eye would be targeted for –1.25 D. Jay McDonald in Fayetteville, Arkansas has taught us that for these patients binocular vision is typically preserved at 60 seconds of arc or better and intermediate vision is excellent.

   Richard L. Lindstrom: My preference would be the Crystalens 5.0 in a 68-year-old hyperope (+1.50) who wants good computer working distance. I would seek an outcome of –0.25 in one eye and –0.75 in the other eye. An alternative would be monofocal monovision with a target of –0.25 and –1.75.

   Kevin L. Waltz: This is an ideal patient for a bilateral Crystalens, leaving one eye slightly myopic. The slightly myopic eye will enhance the near vision, but just as importantly will allow the patient to see the computer screen with little or no accommodative effort. It is important to remember that when an accommodating IOL works it requires muscular input, which gives the potential of accommodative fatigue. A slight amount of myopia reduces this potential for accommodative fatigue.

2. **A 42-year-old emmetrope with monocular cataract.**

   David F. Chang: This patient will be harder to please because he or she has never experienced presbyopia, and we cannot truly match the visual quality and accommodative range of the phakic eye. I would stress this point preoperatively, and implant a ReSTOR if the patient seemed accepting of the inherent compromises (weaker intermediate function, some ghost images, and reduced quality of vision at night). I would stress that the ReSTOR would provide greater spectacle freedom than a monofocal IOL, and much better clarity than their cataract, but that we have nothing that can duplicate their noncataractous eye. Furthermore, they will appreciate the multifocal IOL much more when their phakic eye becomes more presbyopic. If the patient had a demanding or compulsive personality, however, a Crystalens with slight myopia to produce monovision might be the safest choice.

Steven J. Dell: This is a tough situation because the patient really has not experienced the full ravages of presbyopia yet. The patient is also young enough to easily notice unwanted images from a multifocal. The first step is to determine the reason for the unilateral cataract. Trauma, inflammatory conditions, and other unusual circumstances should be investigated. A unilateral Crystalens 5.0 is certainly an option. Distance and intermediate vision would be good, but near acuity would be inferior to a bilateral implantation.

Warren E. Hill: Here, an aspheric IOL with negative spherical aberration correction would be a good choice. This strategy would give the highest quality vision and would not be a departure from what is required for the fellow, noncataractous eye.

Richard L. Lindstrom: My first choice for this patient would be the Crystalens 5.0 with a target of −0.25. To me distance vision is the first priority, intermediate vision second, and near vision is third. Quality of vision is important as well. As an alternative I would consider an aspheric monofocal IOL with a target of −0.25.

Kevin L. Waltz: This is a difficult patient. There is likely no significant presbyopia. It is unlikely any of the presbyopia-correcting IOL options available in 2007 will be completely satisfactory. I would choose the lens with the least objectionable side-effect profile rather than try to emphasize the most effective aspects of a given lens.

3. A 66-year-old myopic (−3.00) homemaker with bilateral cataracts who does some night driving and currently reads without any glasses.

David F. Chang: Bilateral ReSTOR lenses will provide the best near vision at the reading distance that this myopic patient is accustomed to using. I would be confident that she would be able to drive well at night after a fairly minimal period of adaptation.

Steven J. Dell: In this situation, bilateral Crystalens implantation may result in an unhappy patient. The patient's habitual myopia has provided extremely high grade near vision for many years, and the Crystalens is unlikely to match that level of near acuity. Upon further counseling, the patient might elect to preserve her bilateral myopia, or might opt for monovision. If maximum spectacle independence remains her goal, a strategy of using the Crystalens in the dominant eye and a diffractive multifocal such as the ReSTOR in the nondominant eye has worked surprisingly well in my patients.

Warren E. Hill: The moderate myope who loves to read without glasses often does best with bilateral monofocal IOLs. These patients have been used to clear vision at near without glasses for most of their life and may feel that the small visual compromise with a multifocal IOL is unacceptable. And even though the new aspheric ReSTOR seems to have fewer problems with halos at night, I think that for this patient, monofocal IOLs may be the best solution.

Richard L. Lindstrom: A 66-year-old myopic homemaker who is happy with her vision prior to cataract development would likely do well with aspheric IOLs and a target of −2.75 D. Using a near dominant multifocal such as the ReSTOR or Tecnis multifocal is also a reasonable option. Finally, monovision can work well in many of these patients.

Kevin L. Waltz: A myopic presbyope who likes to read without glasses is a special situation. The story tells you the patient prefers a flat wavefront with little to no higher-order aberrations (HOAs) at distance and near. There is only one technology in 2007 that can satisfy these requirements—glasses, preferably wavefront-corrected glasses. I would be very reluctant to operate on this patient.

4. A 70-year-old −12.00 D myope with bilateral cataracts, who has worn monovision rigid gas permeable contact lenses (RGPs) for 30 years (1.5 cylinder by keratometry)

David F. Chang: Multifocal IOLs would only be an option if the patient were willing to undergo a secondary laser enhancement, which could not be done for 4+ months to allow for refractive stability. Because the patient is well adapted to monovision already, I would then favor bilateral Crystalens implants as a means to achieve monovision with greater depth of focus than would be expected with monofocal IOLs. Assessing the patient's accommodative or pseudoaccommodative ability in the first eye (targeting emmetropia in the same that wore the distance RGP), would help me to decide how much myopia to target in the nondominant second eye. I would repeat the keratometry after a 2-week hiatus from contact lenses. I would explain that residual latent astigmatism is a virtual certainty, but could be corrected with spectacles or rigid contact lenses, or with a laser procedure that could be done at any future time. I would perform limbal relaxing incisions (LRI) at the time of surgery explaining that at worst, it would reduce the severity of astigmatism, and at best, it might preclude the need to correct residual astigmatism with laser vision enhancement or a contact lens. Even if the patient were content to wear monovision contact lenses for the rest of his or her life, the Crystalens would add the upside potential for improving binocularity by providing greater range of focus for each individual eye.

Steven J. Dell: The true nature of this patient's corneal cylinder will take months of contact lens abstinence to sort out, but I expect the astigmatism will increase significantly as the corneal warpage subsides. This case points out the importance of preoperative topography. Some of these patients have unrecognized forme fruste keratoconus, which would alter my plans considerably. Let us assume the topography is normal. This patient is accustomed to extremely high quality visual acuity, and I believe it is a mistake to steer the patient away from monovision. Pseudophakic monovision with a toric IOL might be the best option in this case. Residual astigmatism would require laser vision correction. Note that a toric IOL implantation eliminates the option of a future rigid gas permeable contact lens (RGP). This is because the intraocular neutralization of the corneal cylinder would be incompatible with future RGP neutralization of the corneal cylinder by means of the toric tear film under the RGP.

Warren E. Hill: I would approach this in the form of monofocal IOLs with a monovision strategy in the form of a toric, or an aspheric with LRI. It has been my experience that those who have used monovision for many years tend to like staying with that approach.

Richard L. Lindstrom: In a 70-year-old who has been happy long term with monovision I would favor monovision with an aspheric IOL, targeting -0.25 and -1.75. As an alternative I would offer the Crystalens with -0.25 and -0.75 as the targets. I would treat the astigmatism with a combination of on axis incision and Arc-T astigmatic keratotomy at an 8-mm optical zone. If required, I would do a laser in situ keratomileusis (LASIK) or photorefractive keratectomy (PRK) enhancement postoperatively.

Kevin L. Waltz: I would offer bilateral crystalens with a slight residual myopia in one eye. I would treat the keratometric cylinder with corneal relaxing incisions (CRIs) and attempt to leave about 0.5 D of residual cylinder to improve depth of focus. Patients who require low power Crystalenses tend to develop an impressive amount of accommodation.

5. A 56-year-old high myope wearing glasses (OD −8.00+3.00 x 90; OS −5.00 + 3.25 x 95). He has 3+ nuclear cataract in 20/70 right eye, and 1 to 2+ nuclear sclerosis (NS) in 20/25 left eye.

David F. Chang: Compared to patients older than 70, incisional keratotomy is much less effective and more unpredictable in patients in their 50s. Although the patient could have a presbyopia-correcting IOL with planned bioptics laser enhancement, I would emphasize the difficulty that their astigmatism poses. I would then present the option of a toric IOL with a target of emmetropia. The patient would then wear a toric soft contact lens in the left eye with the option of reversibly trying monovision. My guess is that most patients would elect this option rather than undergoing a second non-covered laser surgical procedure. Explaining that keeping their natural lens in the left eye has some advantages (lower risk of retinal detachment than the pseudophakic eye) usually gives the reluctant patient sufficient motivation to try a monocular contact lens. In the unlikely event that a monocular contact lens proved to be intolerable, the presence of an early cataract would dictate lens exchange instead of LASIK or a phakic IOL to resolve the anisometropia. We all know that the left eye will likely develop a progressive NS cataract before very long.

Steven J. Dell: Given the circumstances, I would approach this case as though it were headed for bilateral surgery in the near future. Glare testing and the patient's visual complaints would dictate the timing of surgery on the left eye. After a retinal consultation, I would offer bilateral Crystalens 5.0 implantation with a slightly myopic outcome of -0.75 D in the nondominant eye. If the astigmatism were mostly corneal, I would anticipate LASIK with a femtosecond flap as a planned second procedure. This can be safely performed at about 60 days postoperatively in the context of small incision clear corneal surgery. Preoperative artificial tears, punctual occlusion, oral omega-3 fatty acid supplementation, and topical cyclosporine are extremely helpful in these patients undergoing LASIK.

Warren E. Hill: This would be a good place for a toric IOL combined with LRI to pick up the extra 1.00 D of corneal astigmatism. This would be too much corneal astigmatism to go after with LRI alone.

Richard L. Lindstrom: I prefer Crystalens 5.0 with a target of -0.25 and -0.75 for this patient. I would treat the astigmatism with on axis incision and Arc-T astigmatic keratotomy at an 8-mm optical zone. He would require a 3-mm or 45-degree cut opposite the incision and a 2-mm or 30-degree cut on the same side as the incision. A LASIK or PRK enhancement might be needed.

Kevin L. Waltz: This is my favorite patient of the group. This patient is handicapped with or without their glasses. You will do them a huge favor with any of the presbyopia-correcting IOLs and a laser vision correction (LVC) procedure to correct the astigmatism. I prefer to treat all of the cylinder and a small amount of the sphere first with bilateral same day LASIK. I begin the lens surgery about one month later and do each eye about 1 week apart. There is a chance of needing an enhancement, but the overall result is so spectacular that the patients are uniformly thrilled with the process.

6. 52-year-old nearly emmetropic stockbroker who loves to play golf. He has clear lenses and wants not to be spectacle-dependent at all costs.

David F. Chang: This is a patient with demanding visual needs (golf ball at distance and newspaper stock prices at near). I also worry when patients exhibit traits of an excessive feeling of entitlement. An uncompromising personality who wants a normal aging process to be fixed "at all costs" may be quite dissatisfied with the optics of our current presbyopia-correcting IOLs. I would stress that if it were me, I would be determined to adapt to contact lens monovision "at all costs" and wait for a future generation accommodating IOL to be approved.

Steven J. Dell: This is an extremely challenging patient. Golf requires good binocular acuity, and his profession requires excellent intermediate vision. As a further challenge, the patient has excellent uncorrected distance acuity preoperatively. In my experience, there are many ways I could imagine making this patient unhappy postoperatively. While I might be able to offer the patient a larger quantity of vision, it would be at the expense of some quality of vision. I think the surgical solution to this patient does not currently exist, so I would counsel the patient not to have surgery at this time.

Warren E. Hill: I would discuss with this patient placing a Crystalens in the dominant eye and aspheric ReSTOR in the nondominant eye. Highly motivated individuals are often willing to accept/adapt to a non-standard strategy in order to meet their visual objectives. Here, mix and match would be a first consideration.

Richard L. Lindstrom: Today the 52-year-old emmetropic golfing stock broker with clear lenses in my practice is told to keep golfing, wear readers, or try monovision or multifocal contact lenses. In regards to surgery, he is told to wait for better technology or the development of a cataract.

Kevin L. Waltz: I would consider treating one eye with conductive keratoplasty or monovision LVC after a successful trial of contact lenses. I would also consider a mix and match strategy with the dominant eye set for distance with a Crystalens. I would consider a diffractive multifocal IOL for the fellow eye, preferably a Tecnis multifocal to allow excellent near vision in all lighting conditions.

SECTION IX

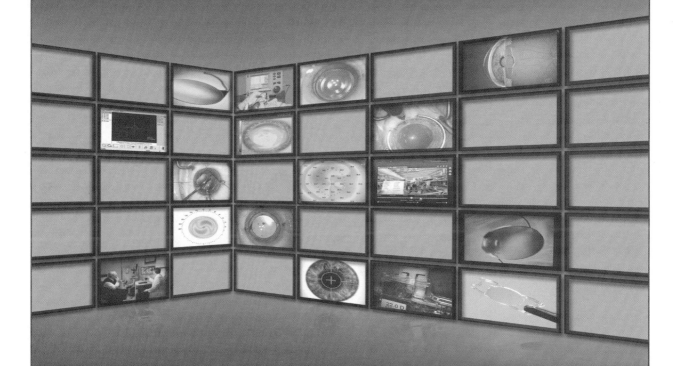

Preoperative
Ocular Assessment

CHAPTER 146

HITTING EMMETROPIA

Warren E. Hill, MD, FACS

Well, here it is. One of the most important parts of mastering presbyopia-correcting intraocular lenses (Pr-C IOLs): hitting emmetropia. These days there is no middle ground, no "close is good enough," and nowhere to hide if you miss the refractive target. If you have not done so already, it is time to get your game face on. Let us get started.

There are a number of common misconceptions regarding how best to achieve highly accurate postoperative refractive outcomes. The first and most common misconception is that optimizing one part of the measurement and calculation process will take you all the way to the end. I wish it was this easy.

How many times have you heard someone say: "I just bought this expensive piece of equipment (new biometer, fancy keratometer, or sophisticated formula software) and my refractive outcomes are not really that much better." You may have even experienced this yourself.

The hard reality of consistently achieving highly accurate IOL power calculations is that this is a multi-part process, with the final outcome dependent on each and every part. Here is how it works.

The Big Picture

Let's look at the big picture, which is more than just doing some measurements and running them through a formula, but rather all that's required in order to consistently arrive at our target for the final refractive result. The ability to hit your refractive target is dependent on the following:

1. Axial length, increasing in accuracy from applanation to immersion to optical coherence biometry. For Pr-C IOLs, immersion biometry, or optical coherence biometry are generally required for satisfactory results. The use of applanation biometry is to be avoided.

2. Central corneal power in keratometric diopters, ideally measured with the same calibrated instrument for all cases. For autokeratometry, the validation criteria requires that we produce 3 measurements for eyes within 0.25 D in each of the principal meridians. Simulated keratometry by topography generally lacks the required accuracy.

3. The accuracy of the formula being used at the parameters of the eye being measured. All 2-variable formulas have well-known shortcomings in their ability to estimate the effective lens position, which typically limits their calculation range. For example, in the setting of axial hyperopia, or very flat Ks, using the SRK/T formula may result in unanticipated postoperative hyperopia. More modern formulas, such as Haigis and Holladay 2, require additional measurements, such as anterior chamber depth for improved accuracy.

4. Configuration of the capsulorrhexis, which maintains a consistent postoperative distance of the IOL optic from the cornea, which is also known as the effective lens position. The capsulorrhexis should be as round as possible, centered, and slightly smaller than the optic of the IOL so that it remains contained within the capsular bag and at the plane of the zonules. Although we do not generally think of the capsulorrhexis as being part of the determination of IOL power, its proper, or improper, configuration has the potential to exert a greater impact on the final refractive outcome than the measurement of axial length. With a capsulorrhexis larger than the optic of the IOL, as the forces of capsular bag contraction are brought to bear, the optic of the IOL may be displaced anteriorly. To keep things in perspective, only 0.5 mm of anterior displacement at physiologic IOL powers is required for −1.00 D of unanticipated myopia.

5. Variations in retinal thickness around the foveal center. Ultrasound-based methods for the measurement of axial length (applanation, immersion, and A/B-biometry) measure from the corneal vertex to the vitreoretinal interface. Unfortunately, the retinal thickness around

the foveal center is not constant. This is a small but additional potential error in the measurement of axial length. When measuring the axial length by optical coherence biometry, variations in retinal thickness around the foveal center are not a factor.

6. Tolerance of IOL manufacturing at the power to be implanted. In general, the tolerances involved in IOL manufacturing become less accurate with increasing IOL power. Fortunately, at physiologic IOL powers, manufacturing tolerances for IOLs produced by most of the major manufacturers are quite good, and generally range somewhere between 0.15 D and 0.20 D.

The paradox of IOL power calculations is that you can have one of the aforementioned six components perfect (such as axial length after purchasing an IOL Master [Carl Zeiss Meditec, Jena, Germany]), and still have a large deviation from what was expected. In other words, improving one single item may not produce a noticeable improvement. The item with the highest mean absolute error (MAE) drives the final result. Here is how this works.

Understanding Mean Absolute Error

The most effective way to begin to look at the process of IOL power calculations is to think in terms of the *MAE* of each component part, which is something akin to accuracy. In order to arrive at a MAE, we need to look at the difference between a measured value and what we know to be the actual value. The actual value can be obtained from a highly accurate reference instrument, or can be back calculated after the surgery has been completed.

For example, let us say that we measure the central corneal power of 20 eyes using an older, manual keratometer. We then remeasure these same 20 eyes with a reference instrument, which we know to be much more accurate. We then look at the difference between the two, and perhaps also compare the original measurements obtained with the standard keratometer to a back-calculated value.

Let us call this difference between what we measure and what we determine to be the correct value our measurement error. A mean error would simply be the sum of all errors divided by the number of observations. But because some errors may be greater than the reference value, whereas others may be less, looking at a mean (average) value can be very misleading. The mean, or average of −0.38 D, +0.75 D, +0.13 D, and −0.50 D would be 0.00 D, falsely suggesting that the measurement process for this series has no error.

However, by removing the + and − signs from our measurement error values, we now have what is referred to as the *absolute error*, which is similar to variance. The *MAE* for −0.38 D, +0.75 D, +0.13 D, and −0.50 D would be 0.44 D, rather than 0.00 D. By looking at the MAE, we are provided with a better picture of how far from the correct answer we may be.

How Does This Work?

For a series of patients, if the largest MAE is 0.50 D, the absolute error of the entire multi-part process would not 0.50 D, but rather the square root of the sum of the individual squares of the mean absolute errors. This basic form of error analysis can be used to help us better understand how we can improve our refractive outcomes.

So, let us say that we measure the axial length for a series of 100 patients using an applanation technique with a MAE of 0.34 D, our Ks with an older manual keratometer are within 0.32 D, the 2-variable formula we like to use has a MAE of 0.25 D near schematic eye parameters, the capsulorrhexis is perfect for every case, variations in retinal thickness around the fovea add a MAE of 0.10 D, and the tolerance of manufacturing for the IOL is within 0.17 D. The absolute error for this series would be: 0.57 D, which is probably not good enough for consistent results using a Pr-C IOL.

If you are unconvinced, ask any practice to honestly track the absolute errors of their outcomes for 100 consecutive patients measured in the aforementioned manner and then calculate the mean absolute deviation from predicted. You will be surprised how close their numbers will be to this estimate. And do not be surprised if it is slightly larger, as the mean absolute errors listed herein represent an ideal value.

OK, we are now convinced of the need for improved outcomes and make the decision to buy the newest version of the IOL Master employing digital signal processing technology to measure axial length. Everything else remains the same, except that variations in retinal thickness are no longer a factor because we are measuring to the retinal pigment epithelium. With an axial length MAE of 0.02 D, the absolute error for this series improves by only 0.13 D, which is below our level of detection when refracting patients in 0.25 D steps. In other words, spending a lot of money to optimize one part did not dramatically increase the accuracy of the refractive outcomes.

To tighten our accuracy even more, in addition to measuring the axial length with the IOL Master, we now measure the central corneal power with a more accurate autokeratometer (such as with IOL Master software version 5.02) with a MAE of 0.13 D and use the Holladay 2 formula with a MAE of about 0.13 D near schematic eye parameters. Our MAE for this series now falls 0.24 D, which is well within in the range necessary for the use of Pr-C IOLs. This increased accuracy means that fewer patients will need to undergo laser in situ keratomileusis (LASIK) touch-ups, IOL exchanges, or placement of a piggyback IOL.

Conclusion

The paradox of IOL power calculations is that perfecting just one component of the IOL power calculation process will not result in a dramatic improvement in refractive outcomes. But if one part is very bad, a refractive surprise will almost certainly be assured. In order to consistently achieve the level of refractive accuracy required for Pr-C IOLs, each part of the calculation process must be optimized to the greatest extent possible.

CHAPTER 147

BIOMETRY PEARLS

Steven J. Dell, MD

Optimizing biometry is a complex process. There are so many possible sources for error. A great deal of time and money is spent obtaining the best information possible simply because the stakes are so high. A biometry miss in a presbyopia-correcting intraocular lens (IOL) patient will likely require an enhancement with multiple additional postoperative visits and possibly reduced patient satisfaction. In the worst case, litigation could result. The science of axial length determination has advanced considerably with technologies such as laser interferometry and immersion A-scan ultrasound, which avoid the globe compression errors seen in contact A-scan ultrasound.

With modern IOL formulae and highly accurate axial length determinations, the largest sources of error now have become poor keratometry information and incorrect data entry. Other sources of error include the capsulorrhexis size and the small variance of the actual versus the labeled IOL power, of which many surgeons are unaware. Surgeons have little control over this last variable.

The single easiest thing any surgeon can do to improve the odds of hitting the refractive target is to simply perform all measurements twice and average the values obtained. This alone will boost accuracy. This practice highlights errors and forces the technician and surgeon to explain why the 2 values differ. If they differ significantly, at least one of the values is incorrect, suggesting the need for more testing.

Optimizing the ocular surface prior to any measurements is perhaps the most neglected component of good data acquisition. Ideally, IOL measurements cannot be taken following a full ophthalmological exam with applanation tonometry and dilation. At the initial consultation, I place virtually all patients on artificial tears. The majority of patients also receive oral omega-3 fatty acid supplementation. Higher risk patients receive topical cyclosporine with or without punctual occlusion and a short course of topical steroids. Patients are brought back in 1 to 3 weeks for definitive measurements depending on the severity of their condition. The accuracy of topography or keratometry data is greatly enhanced with these measures. Since this is the source data for both the IOL calculation and for any astigmatic management such as limbal relaxing incisions or toric IOLs, this is a very, very critical issue.

The 2 axial length measurements obtained with the IOL Master (Carl Zeiss Meditec, Jena, Germany) often agree to the 0.01-mm level. This begs the question of why we repeat the measurements and average them in the first place. It is done simply to confirm that the values are accurate. Regarding keratometry, the data from the IOL Master are also very good, especially with the most recent software version. Repeating this measurement and averaging the 2 values regresses the measured value toward the true value. Alternatively, a second source of keratometry data can be used for comparison. One good way of doing this is to examine the mean corneal power from the numeric maps of the Carl Zeiss Meditec Inc Atlas topographer (Dublin, CA) at the 0- and 2-mm zones. Other topographers have similar capabilities. Once again, comparing the averages of multiple values improves accuracy. The key to any system is to perform measurements in a consistent way, so appropriate adjustments can be made based upon your individual outcomes.

Data entry errors can be reduced by directly importing measured values into data fields electronically or through the use of preprinted forms with flags for error detection. No matter how automated the process, the possibility of human error remains. Inputting data from 2 measurements into preprinted forms coerces stereotypical data entry and highlights differences between the 2 measurements of each eye. The results of the right and left eye can also be compared.

A surgeon factor can account for some variability as well. Assuming 2 surgeons practice together and use the same IOL measurement methods, any differences between their outcomes is likely related to capsulorrhexis size. This variable is more important with some IOL styles than others. Placing a 6.0-mm optical zone marker on the cornea and using this as a sizing guide will result in an approximately 5.5-mm capsulorrhexis size. This will vary slightly based upon anterior chamber depth and keratometry, but the consistency of the capsulorrhexis size will be considerably improved with this technique.

Implementing these measures has significantly improved my IOL calculation accuracy.

CHAPTER 148

MEASURING AXIAL LENGTH

Warren E. Hill, MD, FACS and Thomas C. Prager, PhD, MPH

In the early days of intraocular lens (IOL) implantation, and prior to commercially available biometers, the strategy for achieving emmetropia with a posterior chamber IOL was simply to add +18.0 D to the precataractous refraction. Equally primitive were early IOL power calculation formulas, which would often produce large refractive errors for long and short eyes. Thirty years later, both technology and patient expectations have dramatically changed and gone forever are the days when just being close to the refractive target was good enough. For the cataract surgeon implanting presbyopia-correcting (Pr-C) IOLs, one important part of the overall success of this procedure is the accurate preoperative measurement of axial length.

Applanation Biometry

Contact, or applanation, biometry, begins with the ultrasound probe being placed directly on the surface of the cornea. Even the most experienced technician may encounter problems with alignment, resulting in a measurement that is off axis by small or large amounts. When attempting to center the probe on the cornea, there will always be some degree of corneal compression, especially for patients with reduced intraocular pressure. It is this unavoidable artifact of variable corneal compression that generally makes the accuracy of the applanation technique less than adequate for Pr-C IOLs.

Immersion Biometry

In contrast to applanation biometry, with the immersion technique the ultrasound probe does not touch the cornea and instead is coupled to the surface of the cornea through a fluid interface between the eye and the ultrasound probe. This fluid coupling eliminates the artifact of variable corneal compression, making the measurement more consistent.

Immersion biometry may be performed with an open cylinder using a Hansen Shell (Hansen Ophthalmic Development Laboratory, Coralville, IA) filled with Goniosol, or with a fixed

immersion shell, the most commonly used being the Prager Shell (ESI, Plymouth, MN). The Prager Shell is modified from a design of an immersion shell first created by Jackson Coleman, MD more than 25 years ago.

Using a fixed immersion shell is a one-handed procedure. This is much easier to master than the open shell technique, which requires a certain level of dexterity in order to position the probe at the appropriate distance from the cornea while simultaneously being perpendicular to the retina and directing sound waves through the center of the cornea and lens. The fixed immersion technique minimizes significant variables such as corneal compression, alignment of the ultrasound beam and probe insertion, leading to more consistent results.

Appropriate fixation while performing an immersion scan may be a problem due to light scatter as a consequence of a dense cataract. This can be overcome by using patient proprioceptive feedback or simply having the patient fixate on their thumb extended to arms length. When judging the quality of the measurement of axial length by immersion biometry, the cornea, lens, and retinal spikes should be high and steeply rising, indicating perpendicularity of the incident sound wave to the acoustic interface (Figure 1). Spikes that are poorly formed, or of low amplitude, suggest poor alignment with the visual axis and may lead to errors in axial length.

When using the immersion technique, if the tops of the spikes appear flattened, this suggests that the amplifier gain is set too high, which may also result in inaccurate measurements. With very long eyes such as in those with a peripapillary staphyloma, the macula may be located on the sloping wall of the staphyloma and the retinal spike may be much lower than the corneal spikes. In normal eyes, however, the retinal/scleral spikes are often equal the height of the corneal spikes. Detection of orbital fat spikes behind the retina is required to ensure that the measurement was through the macula and not through the optic nerve head.

Although immersion biometry has cost advantages over optical coherence biometry, a study from 34 centers showed the potential for the equipment to transfer microorganisms

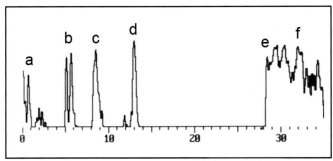

Figure 1. Typical immersion A-scan. a = probe tip; b = double peak of the cornea; c and d = the anterior and posterior lens capsule; e = retina spike; f = orbital fat.

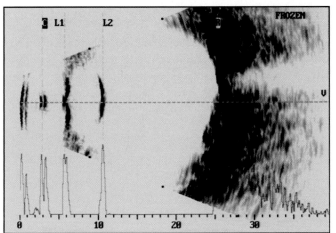

Figure 2. High quality immersion vector A/B-scan. A horizontal B-scan is aligned with the visual axis. With the vector A-scan passing through the middle of the cornea and the middle of the lens, it will then pass through the middle of the macula. With the void of the optic nerve appearing in the proper location, the A/B scan measures the refractive axial length rather than the anatomic axial length.

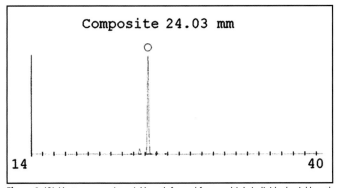

Figure 3. IOL Master composite axial length formed from multiple individual axial length measurements by digital signal processing technology.

from patient-to-patient. In this study 53% of swabs from the shell or tubing grew organisms associated with endophthalmitis or keratitis. These concerns can be readily eliminated by soaking the shell in alcohol for 5 minutes and using new tubing for each patient. This potential problem is avoided by using optical coherence biometry.

The immersion technique has been compared to optical coherence biometry with the IOL Master (Carl Zeiss Meditec, Jena, Germany) and for normal eyes there is little clinical difference in outcomes. However, for very long eyes with a peripapillary posterior staphyloma, or very short eyes where even small errors in axial length can produce disproportionately large postoperative refractive errors, optical coherence biometry is more precise.

Immersion biometry has the advantage of affordable instrumentation, clinical accuracy approaching that of optical coherence biometry, and the ability to measure the axial length through almost any axial opacity.

A/B Biometry

For those wishing to remain with an ultrasound-based method of axial length measurement, combining a horizontal B-scan with a vector-directed A-scan offers some important advantages. The main difficulty with an immersion A-scan is maintaining alignment with the visual axis so that the refractive axial length is being measured. This is especially important when the posterior segment has more than one radius of curvature, as with a peripapillary posterior staphyloma. With A/B-biometry, the anterior and posterior segments are imaged with a 10-MHz horizontal B-scan such that a simultaneous A-scan passes through the center of the cornea and the center of the lens. With the void of the optic nerve properly positioned, the vector of the A-scan is then directed to the location of the center of the macula. In this way, there is no doubt as to the alignment of the A-scan, and the biometrist can inspect for the presence of pathology at the same time. Although originally expensive, this technology is now becoming more commonplace and affordable (Figure 2).

Optical Coherence Biometry

Optical coherence biometry (OCB) using the IOL Master has become increasingly popular since its introduction in 2000. For surgeons implanting Pr-C IOLs, it is rapidly becoming the standard for axial length accuracy (Figure 3).

OCB is a noncontact method of axial length measurement with a resolution several orders of magnitude greater than 10-MHz ultrasound biometry. OCB measures from the corneal vertex to the retinal pigment epithelium and variables such as corneal compression and variations in retinal thickness around the fovea are non-issues. Alignment with the visual axis is far less of a problem than with immersion biometry. As long as the patient is looking directly at the small red fixation light, the measurement is directed to the center of the macula, registering the refractive axial length, rather than the anatomic axial length.

Because the axial length produced by OCB can be somewhat longer than that with immersion biometry, different lens constants are usually required. It is still a common practice for IOL manufacturers to list only applanation ultrasound lens constants for their IOLs. When measuring the axial length with OCB and using an IOL for the first time, one of the very first steps the surgeon should take is to individually optimize the lens constants for the formulas used.

The latest version of the IOL Master software now generates a highly accurate composite axial length from as many as 20 individual axial length measurements.

The validation criteria for optical coherence biometry are beyond the scope of this chapter. The IOL Master user's manual, or the online reference at www.doctor-hill.com should be consulted and followed closely.

Getting it Right

Regardless of whether the axial length is being measured by the immersion technique, or optical coherence biometry, several simple steps for reviewing the data will result in more precise outcomes.

For the great majority of patients, both eyes should show an axial length within 0.3 mm of each other. If the difference between eyes is greater than this amount, it is best to have a different person repeat the measurements for the sake of confirmation. It is also a good practice that when a significant difference in axial length is seen between eyes, following confirmation of this difference, a note should be placed in the chart stating that the "measurements are outside normal physiological findings."

If repeat measurements confirm that there is a significant difference in axial length between eyes, it is sometimes helpful to confirm this difference by other means. One method is to use the current glasses prescription to estimate the anticipated axial length difference. The average eye axial length is approximately 23.49 mm. Assuming that the central corneal power is the same for each eye, at normal axial lengths, for every 1 mm of axial length difference, there would be anticipated a 3 diopter difference in the refractive error.

Also, assuming that lens-induced myopia is not present, the axial length should correspond with the preoperative refractive error. For example, it would be highly unlikely for a +4.00 D refractive hyperope to have an axial length of 26.0 mm.

The precise measurement of axial length requires either a fixed immersion technique or optical coherence biometry using the IOL Master. Although both techniques have their advantages and disadvantages, to enhance patient satisfaction and to prevent a possible lens exchange clinicians should avoid applanation biometry when implanting Pr-C IOLs.

CHAPTER 149

IOL Power Calculations for Multifocal Lenses

Jack T. Holladay, MD, MSEE, FACS

The expectations of patients receiving multifocal intraocular lenses (IOLs) are high because they have been promised very little or no dependence of spectacles or contact lenses. Fulfilling this promise requires eliminating ocular astigmatism and achieving a precise postoperative refraction within ±0.25 D of plano. Techniques for determining the proper IOL power for multifocal IOLs are presented.

Several measurements of the eye are important for determining the appropriate IOL power to achieve a desired refraction. These measurements include central corneal refractive power (k-readings), axial length (biometry), horizontal corneal diameter (horizontal white-to-white), anterior chamber depth, lens thickness, preoperative refraction, and the patient's age. The accuracy of predicting the necessary power of an IOL is directly related to the accuracy of these measurements.[1,2]

Theoretical Formulas

Fyodrov and colleagues first estimated the optical power of an IOL using vergence formulas in 1967.[3] Between 1972 and 1975, when accurate ultrasonic A-scan units became commercially available, several investigators derived and published the theoretical vergence formula.[4-9] All of these formulas were identical,[4] except for the form in which they were written and the choice of various constants such as retinal thickness, the optical plane of the cornea, and the optical plane of the IOL. These slightly different constants accounted for less than 0.50 D in the predicted refraction. The variation in these constants was a result of differences in lens styles, A-scan units, keratometers, and surgical techniques among the investigators.

Although several investigators have presented the theoretical formula in different forms, there are no significant differences except for slight variations in the choice of retinal thickness and corneal index of refraction. There are 6 variables in the formula: 1) corneal power (K), 2) axial length (AL), 3) IOL power, 4) effective lens position (ELP), 5) desired refraction (DPostRx), and 6) vertex distance (V). Normally,

the IOL power is chosen as the dependent variable and solved for using the other five variables, where distances are given in millimeters and refractive powers given in diopters:

$$IOL = \frac{1336}{AL - ELP} - \frac{1336}{\dfrac{1336}{\dfrac{1000}{\dfrac{1000}{DPostRx} - V} + K} - ELP}$$

The only variable that cannot be chosen, or measured preoperatively, is the effective lens position (ELP). The improvements in IOL power calculations over the past 30 years are a result of improving the predictability of the variable ELP. Figure 1 illustrates the physical locations of the variables. The optical values for corneal power (Kopt) and axial length (ALopt) must be used in the calculations to be consistent with current ELP values and manufacturer's lens constants.

The term "effective lens position" was recommended by the Food and Drug Administration (FDA) in 1995 to describe the position of the lens in the eye, because the term anterior chamber depth is not anatomically accurate for lenses in the posterior chamber and can lead to confusion for the clinician.[5] The ELP for IOLs before 1980 was a constant of 4 mm for every lens in every patient (first-generation theoretical formula). This value actually worked well in most patients because the majority of lenses implanted were by iris clip fixation, in which the principal plane of the IOL averages approximately 4 mm posterior to the corneal vertex. In 1981, Binkhorst improved the prediction of the ELP by using a single-variable predictor, the axial length, as a scaling factor for the ELP (second-generation theoretical formula).[6] If the patient's axial length was 10% greater than normal (23.45 mm), he would increase the ELP by 10%. The average value of the ELP was increased to 4.5 mm because the preferred location of an implant was in the ciliary sulcus, approximately 0.5 mm deeper than the iris plane. In addition, most lenses were convex-plano, which was similar to

Figure 1. ELP is measured from the corneal vertex plane to the plane of the thin lens IOL.

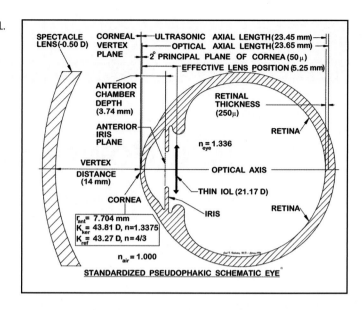

Table 1

CLINICAL CONDITIONS DEMONSTRATING THE INDEPENDENCE OF THE ANTERIOR SEGMENT AND AXIAL LENGTH

Anterior Segment Size	Axial Length		
	Short	**Normal**	**Long**
Small	Small eye Nanophthalmos	Microcornea	Microcornea + axial myopia
Normal	Axial hyperopia	Normal	Axial myopia
Large	Megalocornea Axial hyperopia	Megalocornea	Large eye Buphthalmos + axial myopia

---

the shape of the iris-supported lenses. The average ELP in 2007 has increased to 5.25 mm. This increased distance has occurred primarily for 2 reasons: the majority of implanted IOLs are biconvex, moving the principal plane of the lens even deeper into the eye, and the desired location for the lens is in the capsular bag, which is 0.50 mm deeper than the ciliary sulcus.

In 1988 my colleagues and I[7] proved that using a 2-variable predictor—axial length and keratometry—could significantly improve the prediction of ELP, particularly in unusual eyes (third-generation theoretical formula). The original Holladay 1 formula was based on the geometrical relationships of the anterior segment. Although several investigators have modified the original 2-variable Holladay 1 prediction formula, no comprehensive studies have shown any significant improvement using only these 2 variables.

In 1995, Olsen and colleagues published a 4-variable predictor that used axial length, keratometry, preoperative anterior chamber depth, and lens thickness.[8] His results did show improvement over the current 2-variable prediction formulas. The explanation is very simple. The more information we have about the anterior segment, the better we can predict the ELP. This explanation is a well-known theorem in prediction theory where the more variables that can be measured describing an event, the more precisely one can predict the outcome.

In a recent study,[9] my colleagues and I discovered that the anterior segment and posterior segment of the human eye are often not proportional in size, causing a significant error in the prediction of the ELP in extremely short eyes (<20 mm). We found that even in eyes shorter than 20 mm, the anterior segment was completely normal in the majority of cases. Because the axial lengths were so short, the 2-variable prediction formulas severely underestimated the ELP, explaining part of the large hyperopic prediction errors with current 2-variable prediction formulas. After recognizing this problem, we began to take additional measurements on extremely short and extremely long eyes to determine if the prediction of ELP could be improved by knowing more about the anterior segment. Table 1 shows the clinical conditions that illustrate the independence of the anterior segment and the axial length.

For 3 years, we gathered data from 35 investigators around the world. Several additional measurements of the eye were taken, but only 7 preoperative variables (axial length, corneal power, horizontal corneal diameter, anterior chamber depth, lens thickness, preoperative refraction, and age) were found to be useful for significantly improving the prediction of the ELP in eyes ranging from 15 to 35 mm (Figure 2).

The improved prediction of the ELP is not totally due to the formula, but is also a function of the technical skills of

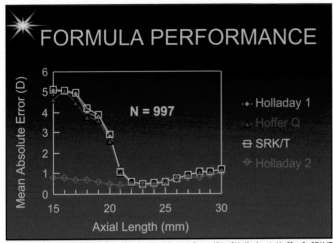

Figure 2. Comparison of Mean Absolute Prediction Error (D) of Holladay 1, Hoffer Q, SRK/T (2 variable ELP predictors using Ks & AL) versus Holladay 2 (7 variable ELP predictor using Ks, AL, WTW, ACD, LT, Age & Refraction).

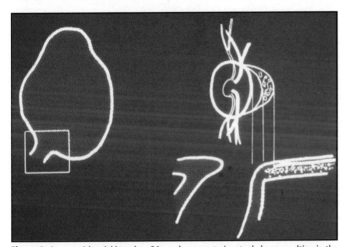

Figure 3. An eye with axial length > 26 mm has a posterior staphyloma resulting in the anatomic axial length measured from the anterior to posterior pole much different than the optical axial length from the corneal vertex to the fovea.

the surgeons who are consistently implanting the lenses in the capsular bag. A 20-D IOL that is 0.5 mm axially displaced from the predicted ELP will result in approximately a 1.0-D error in the stabilized postoperative refraction. However, when using piggy-back lenses totaling 60 D, the same axial displacement of 0.5 mm will cause a 3-D refractive surprise; the error is directly proportional to the implanted lens power. This direct relationship to the lens power is why the problem is much less evident in extremely long eyes, because the implanted IOL is either low plus or minus to achieve emmetropia following cataract extraction.

The Holladay 2 Formula provides more predictable results in unusual eyes. Once these additional measurements become routine among clinicians, a new flurry of prediction formulas using 7 or more variables will emerge, similar to the activity following our two variable prediction formula in 1988.[2] The standard of care will reach a new level of prediction accuracy for extremely unusual eyes, just as it has for normal eyes. Calculations on patients with axial lengths between 22 and 25 mm with corneal powers between 42 and 46 D will do well with current third generation formulas (Holladay 1[2], SRK/T,[10]

and Hoffer Q[11]). In cases outside this range, the Holladay 2 should be used to assure accuracy.

PRIMARY CATARACT SURGERY OR REFRACTIVE LENSECTOMY

The intraocular power calculations for refractive lensectomy are no different than the calculations when a cataract is present. The refractive lensectomy is usually reserved for patients who are outside the range for other forms of refractive surgery and, consequently, the measurements of axial length, keratometry, etc., are usually quite different from those of the typical cataract patient because of the exceptionally large refractive error and younger age of the patient. In most of the cases with high myopia, the axial lengths are extremely long (>26 mm). In cases of high hyperopia, the axial lengths are very short (<21 mm).

In patients with myopia exceeding 20 D, removing the clear lens often results in postoperative refractions near emmetropia with no implant. The exact result depends on the power of the cornea and the axial length. The recommended lens powers usually range from –10 to + 10 D in the majority of these cases. The correct axial length measurement is very difficult to obtain in these cases because of the abnormal anatomy of the posterior pole. Staphylomas are often present in these eyes, and the macula is often not at the location in the posterior pole where the A-scan measures the axial length (Figure 3).[12] In these cases, it is especially important to measure the axial length by optical coherence biometry using the IOL Master (Carl Zeiss Meditec, Jena, Germany) to assure that the measurement is from the corneal vertex to the center of the macula, which is the refractive axial length rather than the anatomic axial length. I have personally seen 3- to 4-D surprises because the macula was on the edge of the staphyloma, and the A-scan measured to the deepest part of the staphyloma. Such an error results in a hyperopic surprise because the distance to the macula is much shorter than the distance to the center of the staphyloma. The third-generation theoretical formulas yield excellent results if the axial length measurement is accurate and stable. In eyes shorter than 21 mm, it is equally important to use optical coherence biometry because the measurements must be more precise than with normal eyes to achieve the same accuracy in the postoperative refraction.

PIGGY-BACK IOLS TO ACHIEVE POWERS ABOVE 34 D

Patients with axial lengths shorter than 21 mm should be calculated using the Holladay 2 formula. In these cases, the size of the anterior segment has been shown to be unrelated to the axial length. In many of these cases, the anterior segment size is normal and only the posterior segment is abnormally short. In a few cases, however, the anterior segment is proportionately small to the axial length (nanophthalmos). The differences in the size of the anterior segment in these cases can cause an average of 5 D hyperopic error with third-generation formulas because they predict the depth of the anterior chamber to be very shallow. Using the newer formula can reduce the prediction error in these eyes to less than 1 D.

Accurate measurements of axial length and corneal power are especially important in these cases because any error is magnified by the extreme dioptric powers of the IOLs. With foldable IOLs, one IOL is placed in the capsular bag and the other in the ciliary sulcus to avoid interlenticular membranes and posterior capsule opacification. When piggy-backing a multifocal IOL, the multifocal IOLs may be placed in front or behind the monofocal IOL to achieve the best results, although the stronger power IOL is usually placed in-the-bag and the weaker IOL in the sulcus. Never piggy-back 2 multifocal IOLs or the near power will be double the intended power. Choosing a monofocal IOL with a lens constant equal to the multifocal IOL reduces the variability in the piggy-back calculation.

Choosing the Desired Postoperative Refraction Target

Determining the desired postoperative refractive target for multifocal IOLs is slightly different than monofocal IOLs, where a slight amount of myopia may be beneficial. With the ReZoom (refractive multifocal) (Advanced Medical Optics, Santa Ana, CA) and ReSTOR (diffractive multifocal) (Alcon, Fort Worth, TX) IOLs, the refractive target should be exactly zero (plano) or the nearest hyperopic choice that is closest to zero. The near vision with each of these lenses is excellent and slight myopia moves the near point too close for comfortable reading.

For the Crystalens (Eyeonics, Inc, Aliso Viejo, CA), the refractive target may be set slightly myopic (–0.50 D) for the "reading eye" in order to achieve slightly better near vision. This choice must be discussed with the patient, especially if they may compare the two eyes for distance, and to help the patient understand that there may be a small sacrifice in depth perception.

Personalized Lens Constant

Every surgeon offering premium IOLs (aspheric and multifocal) must personalize their IOL constants for these highly sophisticated lenses. Although the design of the IOL is the primary factor in the constant, variations in surgery such as placement of the IOL, location and design of the incision, as well as variations in calibration and design of axiometers and keratometers also effect the personalized lens constant (PLC). It usually takes from 20 to 40 cases for the surgeon to personalize the lens constant, but it is the only way to achieve superior results with these IOLs and accuracy within ±0.25 D for 95% of the patients.

Conclusion

Optimal refractive outcomes with multifocal IOLs can only be achieved when the appropriate patients are selected, the measurements are precise with keratometry/topography and axiometry (preferably by optical coherence biometry using the IOL Master), and the other 5 variables (white-to-white, anatomic anterior chamber depth, crystalline lens thickness, age, and preoperative refraction) used to assure accurate sizing of the anterior segment and ELP have been taken. Personalizing the lens constant is critical for eliminating systematic variations that are present in all of our instruments and surgical techniques. By using these techniques, excellent results and happy patients should be the rule with these new refractive IOLs.

References

1. Holladay JT, Prager TC, Ruiz RS, Lewis JW. Improving the predictability of intraocular lens calculations. *Arch Ophthalmol.* 1986;104: 539-541.

2. Holladay JT, Prager TC, Chandler TY, Musgrove KH, Lewis JW, Ruiz RS. A three-part system for refining intraocular lens power calculations. *J Cataract Refract Surg.* 1988;13:17-24.

3. Fedorov SN, Kolinko AI, Kolinko AI. Estimation of optical power of the intraocular lens. *Vestnk Oftalmol.* 1967;80:27-31.

4. Fritz KJ. Intraocular lens power formulas. *Am J Ophthalmol.* 1981; 91:414-415.

5. Holladay JT. Standardizing constants for ultrasonic biometry, keratometry and intraocular lens power calculations. *J Cataract Refract Surg.* 1997;23:1356-1370.

6. Binkhorst RD. *Intraocular Lens Power Calculation Manual. A guide to the Author's TI 58/59 IOL Power Module,* 2nd ed. New York: Richard D Binkhorst; 1981.

7. Holladay JT, Prager TC, Chandler TY, Musgrove KH, Lewis JW, Ruiz RS. A three-part system for refining intraocular lens power calculations. *J Cataract Refract Surg.* 1988;14:17-24.

8. Olsen T, Corydon L, Gimbel H. Intraocular lens power calculation with an improved anterior chamber depth prediction algorithm. *J Cataract Refract Surg.* 1995;21:313-319.

9. Holladay JT, Gills JP, Leidlein J, Cherchio M. Achieving emmetropia in extremely short eyes with two piggy-back posterior chamber intraocular lenses. *Ophthalmology.* 1996;103:1118-1123.

10. Retzlaff JA, Sanders DR, Kraff MC. Development of the SRK/T intraocular lens implant power calculation formula. *J Cataract Refract Surg.* 1990;16:333-340.

11. Hoffer KJ. The Hoffer Q formula: a comparison of theoretic and regression formulas. *J Cataract Refract Surg.* 1993;19:700-712.

12. Zaldiver R, Shultz MC, Davidorf JM, Holladay JT. Intraocular lens power calculations in patients with extreme myopia. *J Cataract Refract Surg.* 2000;26;668-674

CHAPTER 150

REFINING YOUR A-CONSTANT

Guy M. Kezirian, MD, FACS

Refractive predictability is a sine qua non for a successful premium intraocular lens (IOL) practice. Many factors contribute to your ability to achieve excellent refractive predictability and it is important to optimize all of them in your practice to achieve optimal results. Biometry must be meticulously performed, your equipment must be up to date and well calibrated, your refractions must be accurate, and your surgical technique consistent. Assuming these elements are in place, you are ready to refine your lens constants and improve the accuracy of your IOL calculations. Conversely, if you have not standardized your clinical and surgical procedures, then don't bother trying to refine A-constant; the effort will be futile.

The approach to refining your lens constants is the same regardless of the instruments or IOL equation you use. The SRK II and SRK/T[1] formulae use an "A-constant," the Holladay 1 formula uses a "Surgeon Factor," the Holladay II and Hoffer-Q[2] formulas use "anterior chamber depth," and the Haigis[3] approach uses 3 constants that attempt to improve the prediction of the effective lens position rather than a single number. In all cases, the lens constants are used to predict the position of the lens in the eye after surgery and are used with the various IOL formulas to calculate the IOL power.

Few surgeons attempt to calculate their own lens constants.[4] Instead, they rely on commercially available software such as the Holladay IOL Consultant,[5] which does it for them. All the surgeon has to do is enter valid information—and therein lies the challenge.

The ability to obtain reliable information is critical to developing a useful lens constant.

IOL software applications that develop personalized lens constants rely on accurate preoperative, intraoperative, and postoperative information. Any inaccuracies in these data points will prevent reliable lens constant refinements. All IOL calculators assume that the data provided have been collected using standardized methods. If not, the results are unreliable,

no matter how accurate the mathematical processing in the software is.

Most IOL software programs require measurements of axial length, anterior chamber depth, keratometry, and (for the Holladay 2) white-to-white diameters. To obtain reliable measurements, your staff must be well trained and your equipment properly calibrated. Obtaining consistent biometry is common source of frustration in many centers.

For the measurement of axial length, the surgeon should adjust the ultrasound velocity settings according to personal preferences. A recommended technique is to use 1532 m/s and add 0.32 mm to the measured result to obtain the axial length. This method adjusts for the variability in transmission velocity in the cornea and lens, rather than assuming an average velocity such as 1548 m/s.

Intraoperative data include the IOL model and power, but the assumption of all IOL calculation software programs is that your surgical technique is consistent. For example, capsulorrhexis size and shape can affect the final lens position, so if you change your rhexis, you can expect your A-constant to change and you should start with a new set of eyes for lens constant development. Alternatively, eyes with intraoperative complications (torn capsules, vitrectomies, etc) will not yield useful information about your usual outcomes. Such eyes should not be used in the IOL software for lens constant refinements.

The key postoperative data point is the manifest refraction. Unfortunately, this is one of the least reliable data points in many practices. Many surgeons simply ignore the postoperative refraction in happy patients, or just perform a cursory, approximate refraction if there is no indication that refractive enhancement will be needed. Another challenge is obtaining a reliable refraction at the appropriate time point (1 month or later from surgery) or at the right time during an examination (before cycloplegia). Finally, the refractive technique is more difficult in multifocal lenses. Only experienced refractionists should be trusted to obtain this critical information and they should be directed to use plus-to-blur as the refraction end point. An accurate refraction is needed in order to correctly refine your lens constants. You don't need serial refractions; you just need one accurate refraction performed after the eye has stabilized.

Some surgeons use different IOL formulas based on axial length. In these cases, the eyes should be kept in separate cohorts to prevent mixing of data from each group. Doing so allows the IOL software to refine your lens constants based on similar data and avoids introducing confounding variables into each subset. It is also helpful to remember that the accuracy of IOL power calculation formulas is not only affected by axial length. For example, very steep or flat corneal powers may also lead to inaccuracies, more for some formulas than for others.

A reasonable approach to refining your lens constants is to start by reviewing your current outcomes to see if your current outcomes are reaching a threshold of clinical accuracy that will support the effort. For example, with most monofocal IOLs, the standard deviation (SD) of the prediction error of the postoperative spheroequivalent refractions should be 0.75 diopter (D) or less. Assuming your current results are meeting this threshold, you may be ready to start refining your lens constants. If not, then you need to evaluate your clinical and surgical consistency and eliminate the sources of error that are responsible for your current results (see Assessing Your

Refractive Predictability below).

Premium IOLs rely on excellent refractive outcomes, and refining your lens constants is an essential component to improving your refractive predictability. The key to developing your own lens constants is consistency—both in the clinic and in the operating room.

References

1. Sanders DR, Retzlaff JA, Kraff MC, Gimbel HV, Raanan MG. Comparison of the SRK/T formula and other theoretical and regression formulas. *J Cataract Refract Surg.* 1990;16:341-346.
2. Hoffer KJ. The Hoffer Q formula: a comparison of theoretic and regression formulas. *J Cataract Refract Surg.* 1993;19:700-712.
3. Haigis W. [Critical corneal radii may skew correct IOL calculation by using the SRK/T formula.] [In German.] *Ophthalmologe.* 1993;90:703-707.
4. Holladay JT. Standardizing constants for ultrasonic biometry, keratometry, and intraocular lens power calculations. *J Cataract Refract Surg.* 1997;23:1356-1370.
5. Holladay JT. Holladay IOL consultant & surgical outcomes assessment. http://www.docholladay.com. Accessed December 07, 2007.
6. Holladay JT, Moran JR, Kezirian GM. Analysis of aggregate surgically induced refractive change, prediction error, and intraocular astigmatism. *J Cataract Refract Surg.* 2001;27:61-79.

ASSESSING YOUR REFRACTIVE PREDICTABILITY

You can use descriptive statistics to evaluate current refractive outcomes after cataract surgery, and each statistic has its own application. Holladay coined the term *prediction error*[6] to describe the difference between the refractive outcome predicted by the IOL formula, and the actual refractive outcome experienced by the patient. The mean prediction error describes the average difference between the expected and achieved spheroequivalent refraction. The standard deviation (SD) of the prediction error describes the amount of scatter that exists around the mean result, and the standard error of the prediction error is a measure of the reliability of your statistics based on sample size. With larger samples (more eyes), the standard error goes down, indicating that the results are more reliable and probably predict the real situation. However, the SD is not affected by sample size, so the SD can be estimated from a relatively small data set, such as 20 eyes.

The SD statistic assumes a normal (Gaussian) distribution of the data, which is a reasonable assumption in most cases. One SD is the measure of the spread around the mean that encompasses two-thirds of the data. So with a data set that has a mean of −0.25 D and a SD of −0.75 D, two-thirds of the eyes had refractions that fell between −1.00 and +0.50 D. With most monofocal IOLs, the SD of the prediction error of the postoperative spheroequivalent refractions should be 0.75 D or less.

In order to obtain a reliable assessment of the SD of your outcomes, it is necessary to qualify the data that you will use in your analysis to be sure it is representative of your outcomes. For example, don't use eyes with extreme axial lengths or extreme preoperative refractions, or eyes that experienced an intraoperative complication.

Use a spreadsheet program such as Microsoft Excel to calculate your results (Table 1). To determine your SD, enter the 1-month refraction from 20 eyes that had average axial lengths, done with the same IOL model using the same surgical techniques and calculated using the same IOL equation. In the SurgiVision–Eyeonics IOL DataLink Registry, the mean axial length in over 18,000 eyes is 23.93 ± 1.47 mm, and the average mean K values were 43.4 ± 3.2 D, so a reasonable approach would be to use eyes with axial lengths between 22.5 and 25.4 mm and mean keratometry values between 40.2 and 46.6 D.

Next, enter the predicted postoperative refraction for the IOL that was used for each eye, and the spheroequivalent postoperative refraction obtained at least 1 month after surgery. Subtract the difference between those 2 numbers to obtain the spheroequivalent prediction error, and Analysis Tool Pack's Descriptive Statistics or the STDEV function to calculate the SD of your results.

Refining your A-constant will improve your mean prediction error but it will not affect the SD of your results. If the SD of your spheroequivalent prediction error is 0.75 D or less, you are ready to start refining your lens constants. If not, it is time to review your clinical and operative procedures to improve your refractive predictability.

Table 1

CALCULATION OF THE STANDARD DEVIATION OF THE SPHEROEQUIVALENT PREDICTION ERROR FOR 20 EYES WITH THE CRYSTALENS AT FIVE-0 LENS

Preoperative Characteristics			*Prediction Error Calculation*		
Axial Length	Preop SE	Mean K	Predicted Postop SE	Actual Postop SE	Prediction Error
22.50	1.88	45.13	−0.25	−0.88	−0.63
22.71	2.63	43.88	−0.25	−0.13	0.13
23.00	1.50	44.38	0.00	0.00	0.00
23.00	1.75	43.88	−0.25	−0.63	−0.38
23.03	0.00	45.19	0.00	−1.75	−1.75
23.21	1.13	42.75	−0.50	−0.13	0.38
23.36	0.25	46.00	0.00	−0.50	−0.50
23.41	0.25	45.88	0.00	0.25	0.25
23.43	0.00	44.81	0.00	−1.75	−1.75
23.57	0.00	43.88	0.00	−0.88	−0.88
23.66	1.25	44.31	−0.25	0.50	0.75
23.76	2.38	43.56	−0.25	−0.13	0.13
23.77	2.75	42.25	−0.25	−0.38	−0.13
24.00	1.63	43.86	−0.25	−0.25	0.00
24.07	0.00	42.87	−0.25	0.75	1.00
24.13	1.00	43.31	0.00	−0.38	−0.38
24.16	1.63	42.88	−0.63	−0.63	0.01
24.23	0.75	42.80	0.00	−0.75	−0.75
24.66	0.25	41.34	0.00	−0.63	−0.63
25.40	2.88	40.50	−0.25	−0.38	−0.13

The preoperative data have been filtered to select for "average" eyes—those with axial lengths and mean keratometry values within 1 SD of average and refractions between −5 and +3 D. The postoperative spheroequivalent predicted by the IOL formula is subtracted from the actual postoperative spheroequivalent obtained for each eye. The last column shows the result, which is the spheroequivalent prediction error for each eye. Using the STDEV function in Microsoft Excel (Microsoft Corp, Redmond, WA), the SD of the prediction error is found to be 0.70 D. Because this falls within the threshold of ±0.75 D, this data set could be reasonably used to start modifying the lens constant for this surgeon.

CHAPTER 151

IOL CALCULATION AFTER PRIOR REFRACTIVE SURGERY

Kenneth J. Hoffer, MD, FACS

What could possibly be more important for patients choosing a refractive or multifocal intraocular lens (IOL) than the accurate calculation of the IOL power? This subject is considered a routine affair in most practices and the results are usually acceptable in the standard cataract patient. That may not be true in patients who are expecting (perhaps demanding) perfection and possibly paying extra for the IOL. It behooves every surgeon entering this area of surgical treatment to become completely familiar with every method to improve the accuracy of IOL power calculation in their practice.

A special dilemma arises in eyes that have previously had refractive surgery; either by corneal surgery or by a phakic IOL. Let us solve the biphakic eye problem first.

Biphakic Eyes (Phakic Eye With a Phakic IOL)

The problem here is eliminating the effect of the sound velocity through the phakic lens when measuring the axial length (AL) using ultrasound. I published a method[1] to correct for this potential error by using the following formula:

$$AL_{CORRECTED} = AL_{1555} + C \times T$$

where AL_{1555} = the measured AL of the eye at sound velocity of 1555 m/sec, T = the central axial thickness of the phakic IOL and C = the material-specific correction factor of +0.42 for PMMA, −0.59 for silicone, +0.11 for collamer, and +0.23 for acrylic.

My publications[1,2] on this subject contain tables showing the central thickness based on the dioptric power for each phakic IOL on the market today. The least error is caused by a very thin myopic collamer lens (eg, ICL) and the greatest error is seen with a thick hyperopic silicone lens (eg, PRL).

Corneal Refractive Eyes

INSTRUMENT ERROR

The problem of IOL power calculation errors in corneal refractive surgery eyes was first described by Koch et al[3] in 1989. The first problem that arises is that the instruments we use cannot accurately measure the corneal power needed in the IOL power formula in eyes that have had radial keratotomy (RK), photorefractive keratectomy (PRK), laser-assisted intrastromal keratomileusis (LASIK) and laser-assisted epithelial keratomileusis (LASEK). This major cause of error is due to the fact that most manual keratometers measure at the 3.2 mm zone of the central cornea, which often misses the central flatter zone of effective corneal power; the flatter the cornea, the larger the zone of measurement and the greater the error. The instruments usually overestimate the corneal power, leading to a hyperopic refractive error postoperatively.

INDEX OF REFRACTION ERROR

The second problem is that the assumed index of refraction of the normal cornea is based on the relationship between the anterior and posterior corneal curvatures. This relationship is changed in PRK, LASIK, and LASEK but not in RK eyes. RK causes a relatively proportional equal flattening of both the front and back surface of the cornea, leaving the index of refraction relationship relatively the same. The other refractive procedures flatten the anterior surface but not the posterior surface thus changing the refractive index calculation, which creates an overestimation of the corneal power by approximately 1 D for every 7 D of refractive surgery correction obtained. A manual keratometer measures only the front surface curvature of the cornea and converts the radius (r) of curvature obtained to diopters (D) using an index of refraction (IR) of usually 1.3375. The formula to change from D to radius is [r = 337.5/D] and from radius to D is [D = 337.5/r].

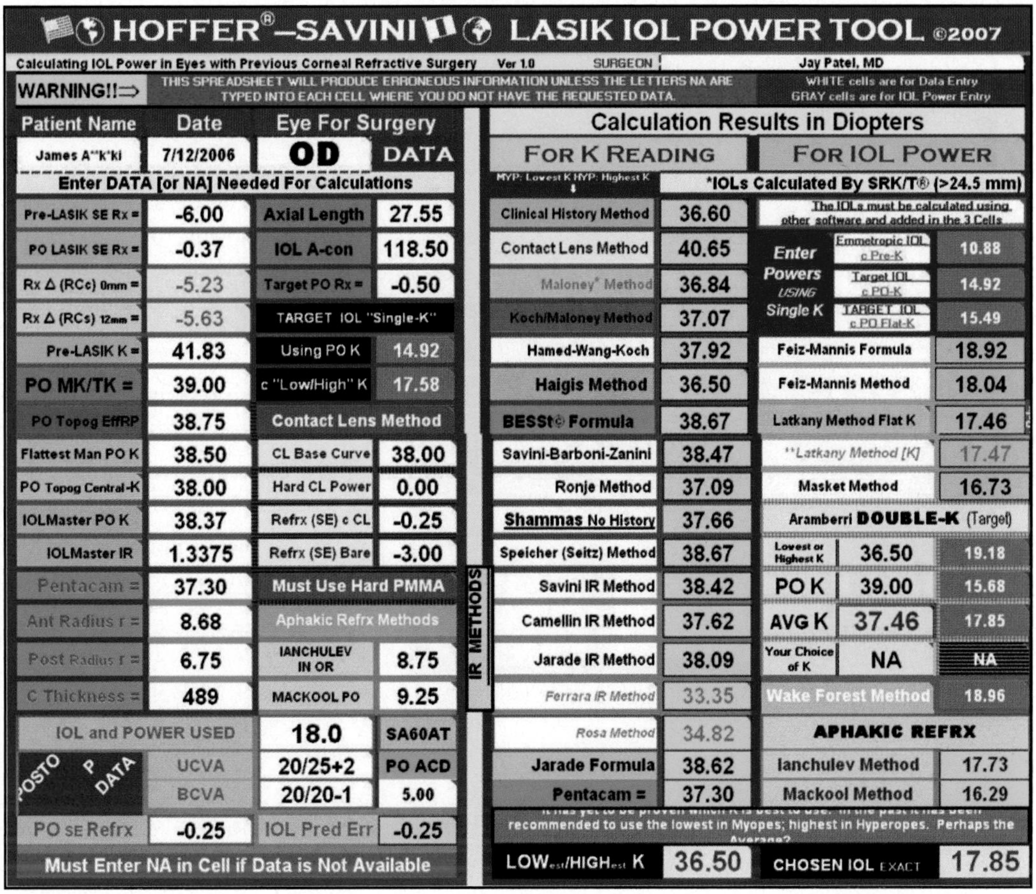

Figure 1. Hoffer/Savini LASIK Tool for IOL power calculation in refractive surgery eyes.

FORMULA ERROR

The third problem is that most of the modern IOL power formulas (Hoffer Q,[4] Holladay 1,[5] and SRK/T[6] but not the Haigis[7]) use the AL and corneal power (K) reading to predict the position of the IOL postoperatively. The flatter than normal K in RK, PRK, LASIK, and LASEK eyes causes an error in this prediction because the anterior chamber dimensions do not really change in these eyes.

History of Solutions

In 1989, Holladay[8] was the first to publish and popularize two methods to attempt to predict the true corneal power in refractive surgery eyes. I referred to them as the clinical history method and the contact lens method.[9,10] The latter was first described by Frederick Ridley[11] in the United Kingdom in 1948 and introduced in the United States by Soper and Goffman[12] in 1974. Over the years many researchers and authors have proposed multiple methods to solve this problem. No one procedure has yet to be proven to be the most accurate in all cases.

In this regard Giacomo Savini of Bologna, Italy and I collaborated , over a 2-year period to create an Excel (Microsoft Corp, Redmond, WA) spreadsheet tool that would automatically calculate most all the proposed methods and also provide a place to store all the data collected and entered. All the information could be stored in one place and it could be printed out on one sheet and stored in the patient's chart. The

Hoffer/Savini LASIK IOL Power Tool (Figure 1) was finished on July 4, 2007 and can be downloaded at no cost from www. EyeLab.com by clicking on the IOL Power button and then the Hoffer/Savini button.

In the creation of the tool, we divided all the published methods into those that attempt to predict the true power of the cornea and those that fudge the target IOL power calculated with the standard data. We then divided each group into those methods that need historical data regarding the status of the patient's eye prior to refractive surgery and those that do not need any historical data.

Before finishing the Tool, we asked each formula author to beta test it to make sure they agreed with our calculations and assumptions. We have converted formula abbreviations to maintain consistency. The legend for these abbreviations is listed on Sheet #3 in the Tool and at the end of this discussion.

METHODS TO ESTIMATE TRUE POSTOPERATIVE CORNEAL POWER

Those Needing Clinical History

Clinical History Method

$$K = K_{PRE} + R_{PRE} - R_{PO} \text{ or } [K = K_{PRE} + RC_C]$$

This method[1-9] is based on the fact that the final change in refractive error the eye obtains from surgery was due only to a change in the effective corneal power. If this refractive change

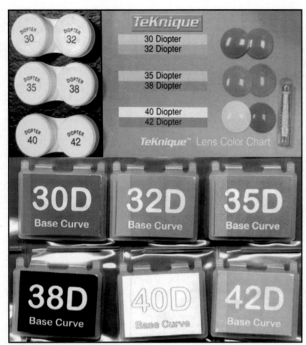

Figure 2. Plano contact lens kits commercially available for performing the contact lens method.

the patient experienced is algebraically added to the presurgical corneal power, we will obtain the effective corneal power the eye has now. Obviously this requires knowledge of the K reading and refractive error prior to refractive surgery.

Originally it was recommended to vertex-correct the refractive errors to the corneal plane. Odenthal et al[13] showed that clinical results were better if they were not corrected. We have decided to use vertex correction in the Hoffer/Savini Tool because this is more scientifically accurate. Several IOL power calculation computer programs calculate the Clinical History method automatically when needed [Hoffer® Programs and Holladay® IOL Consultant].

Hamed-Wang-Koch Method

$$K = TK_{PO} - (0.15*RC) - 0.05$$

This method[14] requires knowledge of the refractive change from the surgery and the postoperative Sim-K from the topography unit.

Speicher (Seitz) Method

$$K = 1.114*TK_{PO} - 0.114*TK_{PRE}$$

This method[15-17] requires obtaining the pre- and postoperative topographic Sim-Ks.

Jarade Formula

$$K = TK_{PRE} - (0.376*(TK_{POr} - TK_{PREr})/(TK_{POr}*TK_{PREr})$$

This method[18] requires obtaining the pre- and postoperative topographic Sim-Ks in radius of curvature, not D.

Ronje Method

$$K = K_{POFLAT} + 0.25*RC$$

This method[19] requires knowledge of the refractive change from the surgery and the postoperative flattest K reading measured now.

Adjusted Refractive Index Methods

These methods attempt to "correct" the index of refraction to better predict the corneal power. The first 2 methods require knowing the surgically induced refractive change at the spectacle plane and the average radius of curvature of the cornea now. The third method requires knowing the surgically induced refractive change at the corneal plane and the average radius of curvature of the cornea now.

* Savini[20] Method:
  $$K = ((1.338 + 0.0009856*RC_S) - 1)/(K_{POr}/1000)$$
* Camellin[21] Method:
  $$K = ((1.3319 + 0.00113*RC_S) - 1)/(K_{POr}/1000)$$
* Jarade[22] Method:
  $$K = ((1.3375 + 0.0014*RC_C) - 1)/(K_{POr}/1000)$$

Those Not Needing Clinical History

Contact Lens Method

$$K = B_{CL} + P_{CL} + R_{CL} - R_{NoCL}$$

The Contact Lens Method[11,12] was first described by Frederick Ridley[11] of England (the inventor of NaOH IOL sterilization) in 1948 and taught by Jospeh Soper[12] in 1974. This method is based on the principle that if a hard PMMA (not rigid gas permeable) contact lens (CL) of plano power (P_{CL}) and a base curve (B_{CL}) equal to the effective power of the cornea is placed on the eye it will not change the refractive error of the eye. Therefore, the difference between the manifest refraction with the contact lens (R_{CL}) and without it (R_{NoCL}) is zero. The formula above computes the effective corneal power if there is a difference in any of these parameters.

Originally it was recommended to vertex-correct the refractive errors to the corneal plane. Odenthal et al[13] showed that clinical results were better if they were not corrected. We have decided to use vertex correction in the Hoffer/Savini Tool because this is more scientifically accurate. Several IOL power calculation computer programs calculate this method and the clinical history method automatically when needed [Hoffer® Programs and Holladay® IOL Consultant]. Plano contact lens sets for performing this procedure are commercially available (Figure 2).

Obviously, this method is impossible if the cataract precludes performing an accurate refraction whereby the visual acuity is worse than 20/80.

Maloney Central Topography Method

$$K = 1.1141*TK_{PO-CTRI}* - 5.5$$

Based on his analysis of post-LASIK corneal topography central Ks (TK) on LASIK eyes, Maloney[23] developed a formulation to predict true corneal power using only the single central postoperative reading $TK_{PO-CTRI}$

Table 1

ROSA CORRECTION FACTOR CONVERSION TABLE BASED ON AXIAL LENGTH

22 to <23	1.01
23 to <24	1.05
24 to <25	1.04
25 to <26	1.06
26 to <27	1.09
27 to <28	1.12
28 to <29	1.15
>29	1.22

Koch/Wang Method

$$K = 1.1141*TK_{PO} - 6.1$$

Koch and Wang[24] analyzed several of these methods and obtained the best results using the Maloney method (discussed earlier) but only after increasing the constant from 5.5 to 6.1. They also offered a second method to calculate true corneal power if the change in the patient's refractive error (RC) is known. The formula is:

$$K = Kt_{PO} - (0.19 \times RC)$$

Savini-Barboni-Zanini Method

$$K = 1.114* Kt_{PO} - 4.98$$

This method[25] only requires the postoperative Sim-K from topography.

Shammas No History Method

$$K = 1.14*K_{PO} - 6.8$$

Shammas[26] studied a series of eyes that had had LASIK. His analysis led him to propose a formula to predict the effective power of the cornea without needing any of the patient's clinical history, only the postoperative K reading obtained with manual keratometry.

Adjusted Refractive Index Methods

Ferrara Method

$$K = ((-0.0006*AL^2 + 0.0213*AL + 1.1572) - 1)/(K_{POr}/1000)$$

This method[27] requires the AL measurement and the postoperative K reading in radius of curvature.

Rosa Method

$$K = (1.3375-1)/((K_{POr}*RCF)/1000)$$

This method[28] requires the postoperative K reading in radius of curvature and the use of a table (Table 1) to obtain a factor (RCF) based on AL. Unfortunately, they used the SRK II regression formula in their computation, which I disagree with.

Haigis Method

$$K = -5.1625*K_r +82.2603 -0.35$$

This method[29] requires only the postoperative K reading from the IOL Master (Carl Zeiss Meditec, Jena, Germany) in radius of curvature (or converted to D using the index of refraction setting in the IOL Master.)

Pentacam

A new comprehensive Eye Scanner, the Oculus Pentacam (Oculus, Inc, Lynwood, WA) (www.oculususa.com) images the anterior segment of the eye by a rotating Scheimpflug camera measurement. This rotating process supplies pictures in three dimensions, provides a topographic analysis of the corneal front and back surfaces as well as central corneal thickness and generates a TrueNetPower map of the cornea.

The TrueNetPower map of the postoperative cornea produced has been proposed as an accurate measure of the true corneal power. Initial results were disappointing and the software was reconfigured in early 2007. Several studies on the new software have also not lived up to expectations as of September 2007 and newer changes are being proposed.

The BESSt© Formula

Published by Borasio,[30] it uses the anterior and posterior corneal curvatures as well as the central pachymetry from the Pentacam unit to produce a predicted central corneal power. The formula is quite complicated but it is incorporated into the Hoffer/Savini LASIK Tool.

METHODS TO ADJUST/CALCULATE THE TARGET IOL POWER

Those Needing Clinical History

Aramberri Double-K Method

Use K_{PRE} to calculate ELP and K_{PO} to calculate IOL power

One of the most important developments to improve the prediction of corneal power in eyes that have had refractive surgery was proposed in 2001 and is termed the "Double-K" method by Aramberri[31] of San Sebastian, Spain. His proposal makes eminent sense. The modern theoretic formulas (except the Haigis) use the input of corneal power for two purposes; the first is to predict the ultimate position of the IOL (ACD or ELP) and the second (along with AL, target refraction, and ELP) is to calculate the power of the IOL. The formulations and algorithms used to predict the ELP are based on the anatomy of the anterior segment, which is not changed by corneal refractive surgery (only the center is flattened and thinned). Therefore, if the postoperative refractive surgery K reading (which is flatter) is used to calculate the ELP it will produce an erroneous ELP value. Because the anatomy has not changed, Aramberri recommends the use of the preoperative K reading to calculate the ELP. The IOL power is then calculated using the postoperative K reading, thus the use of 2 K readings ("Double-K"). His analysis of a small series of eyes proved the benefit of this idea.

Table 2

EXAMPLES OF CALCULATIONS OF THE MASKET METHOD IN A MYOPIC AND HYPEROPIC LASIK EYE

Myopic Eye	Hyperopic Eye
SRK/T calculates 16.0 D IOL	Hoffer Q calculates 22.0 D IOL
Change in Rx = −6.0 D	Change in Rx = +3.0 D
−0.323*(−6) + 0.138 = +2.076	−0.323*(+3) + 0.138 = −0.82
P = 16.0 + 2.0 = 18.0 D	P = 22.0 − 1.0 = 21.0 D

Feiz-Mannis Formula

$P = P_E - RC_S/0.7$

In this method[32] you calculate the emmetropic IOL power using the preoperative K reading and adjust that value (P_E) using the surgically induced refractive change.

Feiz-Mannis Method

This method[33] utilizes the change in refractive error to offset the calculated target IOL power. There is one formula for myopic eyes and another for hyperopic:

Myopic Eye $\quad P = P_{TARG} - 0.595*RC_C + 0.231$
Hyperopic Eye $\quad P = P_{TARG} - 0.862*RC_C + 0.751$

Latkany Methods [Myopic Eyes Only]

$P = P_{TARG\ FlatK} - 0.47*R_{PRE} + 0.85$

This method[34] requires knowledge of the pre-LASIK refractive error and the calculation of the target IOL power using the flattest postoperative K rather than the usual average K.

Masket Method

$P = P_{TARG} - 0.326*RC_C + 0.101$
[SRK/T: myopes; Hoffer Q: hyperopes]

This method[35] is a play on the Latkany method, which adjusts the power of the IOL calculated using the postoperative measured data using the knowledge of the surgically induced refractive change. He recommends using the SRK/T formula for myopic ALs and the Hoffer Q for hyperopic ALs. Example calculations are shown in Table 2.

In a series of 28 post-LASIK eyes, he reported 43% of the eyes obtaining a postoperative refractive error of plano, 95% within ±0.50 D of prediction and a total error range from −0.75 D to +0.50 D.

Wake Forest Method

Use R_{PRE} as the RX_{TARG} using measured AL and K_{PRE}

In 2005, Gagnon et al,[36] from Wake Forest University, published an alternative calculation method that has been discussed by others over the past 20 years. This method simply uses the patient's preoperative refraction before LASIK as the target or "desired" PO refraction in the calculation and the measured AL and K readings without modification.

Those Not Needing Clinical History

Aramberri Double-K Method

Use 43.5 or 44.00 to calc ELP and K_{PO} to calc IOL power.

The use of a standard normal K reading in the Double-K method is a great improvement over using the calculated very flat K reading.[31]

Ianchulev Intraoperative Aphakic Refraction Method

$P = 2.02*AR + (A - 118.4)$

In 2003, Ianchulev et al[37] proposed calculating IOL power by performing an aphakic refraction on the operating room table using a hand-held automated refractor immediately after the cataract has been removed and the AC is inflated to normal status. The resultant refraction is modified by the formula.

His early results are quite promising. This method would completely eliminate the need for AL, corneal power measurements, and the problems with LASIK and silicone oil-filled eyes. However, it would require a large IOL inventory in the operating room.

Mackool Secondary Implant Method

$P = 1.75*AR + (A - 118.84)$

This method[38] is similar to the above except the patient is removed from the operating room without an IOL implanted, then refracted in a refraction lane and then taken back to the operating room for secondary lens implantation. It is my impression that this method would not be popular with most surgeons.

Formula Legend

A = The IOL A constant for planned IOL style.

AL = Axial Length

AR = aphakic refractive error (SE).

B = base curve, P_{CL} = power of CL, NoCL = bare refraction.

CL = contact lens

K = predicted PO corneal power

K_{PO} = the average PO corneal power by manual keratometry (in diopters D)

K_{POFLAT} = flattest measured PO manual keratometry

K_{POr} = the average PO corneal power by IOL Master (in radius r [mm])

K_{PRE} = refractive surgery preoperative corneal power (K readings)

TK_{CTR} = exact singular PO topography central K

P = IOL Power

P_{EMM} = the IOL power calculated for emmetropia

P_{FlatK} = IOL power calculated for RxTARG using the PO flat-test K

P_{TARG} = the target IOL power to produce the PO desired refractive error

R = refractive error, PRE = preoperative, PO = postoperative

RC_C = surgical change in refractive error (SE) vertexed to Corneal Plane

RCF = Rosa Correction Factor based on Axial Length

RC_S = surgical change in refractive error (SE) at Spectacle Plane

R_{PO} = refractive surgery PO refractive error (spherical equivalent)

R_{PRE} = refractive surgery preoperative refractive error (spherical equivalent)

Rx_{TARG} = planned postoperative Target refractive error

TK = average PO topography central Sim-K or EffRP

Important Things to Keep in Mind

* Be sure the Index of Refraction is set to 1.3375 in the Setup screen of the IOL Master computer for the Hoffer Q formula to operate properly for hyperopic refractive eyes.
* If the AL is very difficult to obtain and the eye appears to have a length greater than 25 mm, suspect a staphyloma.
* Hard contact lenses (including gas permeable) should be removed permanently for at least 2 weeks prior to measuring corneal power for IOL power calculation on at least one eye.

* All patients having corneal refractive surgery should be given the following data to maintain in their personal health records: 1) Preoperative corneal power, 2) preoperative refractive error, 3) postoperative healed refractive error (before lens changes effected it). They should be told to give it to anyone planning to perform cataract/IOL surgery on them.

What Formula to Use

My study[4] of 450 eyes (by one surgeon using one IOL style) showed that in the normal range (72%) of AL (22.0 to 24.5 mm) almost all formulas function adequately, but that the SRK I formula is the leading cause of poor refractive results in eyes outside this range. Koch warned against the use of regression formulas in refractive surgery eyes way back in 1989.

It also showed that the Holladay 1 formula was the most accurate in medium long eyes (24.5 to 26.0 mm) (15%) and the SRK/T was more accurate in very long eyes (>26.0 mm) (5%). In short eyes (<22.0 mm) (8%) the Hoffer Q formula was most accurate and this was confirmed (p > .0001) in an additional large study of 830 short eyes as well as in a multiple-surgeon study by Holladay. Holladay has postulated that the other formulas overestimate the shallowing of the effective lens position (ELP) in these very short eyes.

We performed a later study[39] on 317 eyes, which showed that the Holladay 2 formula (unpublished) equaled the Hoffer Q in short eyes but was not as accurate as the Holladay 1 or Hoffer Q in average and medium long eyes (Table 3). It appears that in attempting to improve the accuracy of the Holladay 1 formula, the addition of more biometric data input has improved the Holladay 2 formula in the extremes of AL but deteriorated its excellent performance in the normal and medium long range of eyes (22.0 to 26.0 mm), which accounts for 82% of the population.

Therefore, because the majority of refractive surgery eyes are high myopes (>26 mm), I would recommend the use of the SRK/T formula. In those eyes between 24.5 to 26.0 mm, I recommend the Holladay 1 (not the Holladay 2). Use the Hoffer Q in hyperopic eyes less than 22 mm in length.

How to Handle Problems and Errors

The major problem is an unacceptable postoperative refractive error. The sooner it is discovered, the sooner it can be corrected and the patient made happy. Therefore, it is wise to perform K readings and a manifest refraction on the first postoperative day in these demanding patients. Immediate surgical correction (24 to 48 hours) will allow easy access to the incision and the capsular bag, a single postoperative period, and excellent uncorrected vision.[40] The majority of medico-legal cases today are due to a delay in diagnosis and treatment of this iatrogenic problem.

Up to now, we could only correct this problem by lens exchange, which creates the dilemma of determining which factor created the IOL power error; AL, corneal power, or mislabeled IOL or a combination of the above. Today, with the advent of low-powered IOLs, the best remedy may be a

Table 3

RESULTS OF ACCURACY OF 4 THEORETICAL FORMULAS ON 317 EYES USING THE HOLLADAY IOL CONSULTANT FOR ANALYSIS

Formula	Mean Absolute Error						All 317 Eyes	
	Short <22.0	Normal 22.0 to 24.5	M-long 24.5 to 26.0	V-long >26.0	Long <24.5	All Eyes	Max Error	>± 2D Error
Holladay 2	0.72	0.56	0.51	0.49	0.50	0.55	−1.60	0%
Holladay 1	0.85	0.42	0.37	0.56	0.43	0.43	−1.44	0%
Hoffer Q	0.72	0.43	0.47	0.58	0.50	0.45	−1.61	0%
SRK/T	0.83	0.46	0.35	0.44	0.36	0.44	−1.45	0%
Average	0.78	0.47	0.42	0.52	0.45	0.47		
Best	H-Q H-2	H-Q H-1	S/T H-1	S/T	S/T			

M-Long = medium long, V-Long = very long, Long = all long eyes, Max = maximum.

Shaded = recommended formulas.

piggyback IOL. Using a piggyback IOL, it is not necessary to determine what caused the error or to remeasure the AL of the freshly operated pseudophakic eye.

Conclusion

IOL power calculation is a real problem in eyes that have had refractive surgery. Because it has yet to be proven which proposed method works best in all eyes, it behooves the surgeon to use as many methods as data is available and carefully evaluate the results. The Hoffer/Savini Tool is an attempt to make this process easier. If surgeons using the Tool forward their results to us, we may be able give an accuracy weight to each of the methods.

References

1. Hoffer KJ. Ultrasound axial length measurement in biphakic eyes. *J Cataract Refract Surg.* 2003;29:961-965.

2. Hoffer KJ. Addendum to ultrasound axial length measurement in biphakic eyes: factors for Alcon L12500–L14000 anterior chamber phakic IOLs. *J Cataract Refract Surg.* 2007;33: 751-752.

3. Koch DD, Liu JF, Hyde LL, et al. Refractive complications of cataract surgery after radial keratotomy. *Am J Ophthalmol.* 1989;108:676-682.

4. Hoffer KJ. The Hoffer Q formula: a comparison of theoretic and regression formulas. *J Cataract Refract Surg.* 1993;19:700-712. ERRATA: 1994; 20:677, ERRATA: 2007;33:2-3.

5. Holladay JT, Prager TC, Chandler TY, Musgrove KH. A three-part system for refining intraocular lens power calculations. *J Cataract Refract Surg.* 1988;14:17-24.

6. Retzlaff J, Sanders DR, Kraff MC. Development of the SRK/T intraocular lens implant power calculation formula. *J Cataract Refract Surg.* 1990;16:333-340. ERRATA: 1990;16:528.

7. Haigis W. The Haigis Formula. In: Shammas, HJ, ed. *Intraocular Lens Power Calculations.* Thorofare, NJ: Slack Inc. Publishers; 2003:41-57.

8. Holladay JT. IOL calculations following radial keratotomy surgery. Questions and answers. *Refractive & Corneal Surg.* 1989;5:36A.

9. Hoffer KJ. Intraocular lens power calculation for eyes after refractive keratotomy. *J Refract Surg.* 1995;11:490-493.

10. Hoffer KJ. Calculating intraocular lens power after refractive surgery. (Guest Editorial) *Arch Ophthalmol.* 2002;120:500-501.

11. Ridley F. Development in contact lens theory. *Trans Ophthalmol Soc UK.* 1948;68:385-401.

12. Soper JW, Goffman J. Contact lens fitting by retinoscopy. *Contact Lenses,* Stratton Intercontinental Medical Book Corp., Ed: Soper JW, New York, NY, 1974, pp 99.

13. Odenthal MTP, Eggink CA, Melles G, Pameyer JH, Geerards AJM, Beekhuis WH. Clinical and theoretical results of intraocular lens power calculation for cataract after photorefractive keratectomy for myopia. *Arch Ophthalmol.* 2002;120:431-438.

14. Hamed AM, Wang L, Misra M, Koch D. A comparative analysis of five methods of determining corneal refractive power in eyes that have undergone myopic laser in situ keratomileusis. *Ophthalmology.* 2002;109:651-658.

15. Speicher L. Intra-ocular lens calculation status after corneal refractive surgery. *Curr Opin Ophthalmol.* 2001;12:17-29.

16. Seitz B, Langenbucher A, Nguyen NX, Kus MM, Kuchle M. Underestimation of intraocular lens power for cataract surgery after myopic photorefractive keratectomy. *Ophthalmology.* 1999;106:693-702.

17. Seitz B, Langenbucher A. Intraocular lens power calculation in eyes after corneal refractive surgery. *J Refract Surg.* 2000;16:349-361.

18. Jarade EF, Abi Nader FC, Tabbara KF. Intraocular lens power calculation following LASIK: determination of the new effective index of refraction. *J Refract Surg.* 2006;22:75-80.

19. Ronje. LASIK IOL Calculation, *Eyenet Magazine.* 2004;20:23-24.

20. Savini G, Barboni P, Zanini M. Intraocular lens power calculation after myopic refractive surgery: theoretical comparison of different methods. *Ophthalmology.* 2006;113:1271-1282.

21. Camellin M, Calossi A. A new formula for intraocular lens power calculation after refractive corneal surgery. *J Refract Surg.* 2006;22:187-199.

22. Jarade EF, Tabbara KF. New formula for calculating intraocular lens power after laser in situ keratomileusis. *J Cataract Refract Surg.* 2004;30:1711-1715.

23. Smith RJ, Chan WK, Maloney RK. The prediction of surgically induced refractive change from corneal topography. *Am J Ophthalmol.* 1998;125:44-53.

24. Koch D, Wang I. Calculating IOL power in eyes that have had refractive surgery. *J Cataract Refract Surg.* 2003;29:2039-2042.

25. Savini G, Barboni P, Zanini M. Correlation between attempted correction and keratometric refractive index of the cornea after myopic excimer laser surgery. *J Refract Surg.* 2007;23:461-466.

26. Shammas HJ, Shammas MC, Garabet A, Kim JH, Shammas A, LaBree L. Correcting the corneal power measurements for intraocular lens power calculations after myopic laser in situ keratomileusis. *Am J Ophthalmol.* 2003;136:426-432.

27. Ferrara G, Cennamo G, Marotta G, Loffredo E. New formula to calculate corneal power after refractive surgery. *J Refract Surg.* 2004;20:465-471.

28. Rosa N, Capasso L, Lanza M, Iaccarino G, Romano A. Reliability of a new correcting factor in calculating intraocular lens power after refractive corneal surgery. *J Cataract Refract Surg.* 2005;31:1020-1024.

29. Haigis W, Lege BAM. IOL-Berechnung nach refraktiver Laserchirurgie aus aktuellen Messwerten. In: 20.Kongress der Deutschsprachigen Gesellschaft für Intraokularlinsen-Implantation und Refraktive Chirurgie, Heidelberg, 03.-04.03.2006, hrsg. v. Kohnen T, Auffarth GU, Pham DT, Biermann Verlag Köln, 383-387, 2006. (Haigis W: IOL calculation after refractive surgery for myopia: the Haigis-L formula, *J Cataract Refract Surg,* in press.)

30. Borasio E, Stevens J, Smith GT. Estimation of true corneal power after keratorefractive surgery in eyes requiring cataract surgery: BESSt formula. *J Cataract Refract Surg.* 2006;32:2004-2014.

31. Aramberri J. Intraocular lens power calculation after corneal refractive surgery: double-K method. *J Cataract Refract Surg.* 2003;29:2063-2068.

32. Feiz V, Mannis MJ, Garcia-Ferrer F. Intraocular lens power calculation after laser in situ keratomileusis for myopia and hyperopia. A standardized approach. *Cornea.* 2001;20:792-797.

33. Feiz V, Moshirfar M, Mannis MJ, Reilly CD, Garcia-Ferrer F, Caspar JJ, Lim MC. Nomogram-based intraocular lens power adjustment after myopic photorefractive keratectomy and LASIK: a new approach.. *Ophthalmology.* 2005;112:1381-1387.

34. Latkany RA, Chokshi AR, Speaker MG, et al. Intraocular lens calculations after refractive surgery. *J Cataract Refract Surg.* 2005;31:562-570.

35. Masket S, Masket SE. Simple regression formula for intraocular lens power adjustment in eyes requiring cataract surgery after excimer laser photoablation. *J Cataract Refract Surg.* 2006;32:430-434.

36. Walter KA, Gagnon MR, Hoopes PC Jr., Dickenson PJ. Accurate intraocular lens power calculation after myopic laser in situ keratomileusis, bypassing corneal power. *J Cataract Refract Surg.* 2006;32:425-429.

37. Ianchulev T, Salz J, Hoffer KJ, et al. Intraoperative optical intraocular lens power estimation without axial length measurements. *J Cataract Refract Surg.* 2005;31:1530-1536.

38. Mackool RJ, Ko W, Mackool R. Intraocular lens power calculation after laser in situ keratomileusis: the aphakic refraction technique. *J Cataract Refract Surg.* 2006;32:435-437.

39. Hoffer KJ. Clinical results using the Holladay 2 intraocular lens power formula. *J Cataract Refract Surg.* 2000;26:1233-1237.

40. Hoffer KJ. Early lens exchange for power calculation error. *J Cataract Refract Surg.* 1995; 21:486-487.

CHAPTER 152

PUPIL ASSESSMENT FOR REFRACTIVE IOLs

Mujtaba A. Qazi, MD and Jay S. Pepose, MD, PhD

Pupil Size and Presbyopia-Correcting IOLs

With the availability of zonal refractive (ReZoom; Advanced Medical Optics, Santa Clara, CA) and apodized diffractive (ReSTOR; Alcon, Fort Worth, TX) multifocal intraocular lenses (IOLs), as well as accommodative IOLs (Crystalens AT-45, AT-50; Eyeonics, Inc., Aliso Viejo, CA), a multitude of ocular and patient-specific factors contribute to the decision-making process for matching the "optimal" premium IOL to a patient's visual functional needs. This IOL to patient customization is based upon an assessment of vocational and avocational pursuits, preferred near point, and, quite importantly, pupil dynamics.[1-3]

The distribution of light, by definition, varies significantly with pupil size for multifocal IOLs.[2,4,5] The ReZoom, a distance-dominant IOL adapted from the zonal-progressive design of the Array (Advanced Medical Optics, Santa Ana, CA), has 5 concentric refractive zones alternating for distance (zones 1, 3, and 5) and near (zones 2 and 4), with aspheric transitions that allow for intermediate vision (Figure 1). Approximately 83% of light with the ReZoom is directed to the distant focus and 17% to intermediate with a 2-mm pupil. At a 5-mm pupil, about 60% of light is directed to the distance, 30% to near, and 10% to intermediate focus.[6] The ReSTOR IOL has a central 3.6-mm apodized anterior surface, with 12 diffractive step heights from center to periphery, resulting in an energy continuum for light to be directed primarily at near to distance and at a lower intensity for intermediate vision.[7] For a 2-mm pupil, this IOL distributes approximately 40% of light at near, 40% at distance, and 20% lost to higher diffraction orders. With a 5-mm pupil, 84% of light is focused at distance, 10% at near, and only 6% lost.

Multifocal IOL designs, despite recent advances, still have higher associated halos and glare (20% to 25%) than reported with monofocal or accommodative lenses (3% to 9%), along with induction of higher-order aberrations and reduced contrast sensitivity.[8,9] Many, but not all, patients may neurally adapt to these photic phenomena. Thus, despite high overall patient satisfaction and reduced dependence on spectacles, the surgeon must weigh the specific advantages and disadvantages of each lens in selecting either bilateral implantation or mixing of these different IOL technologies in an effort to customize the treatment plan for each patient. To provide more data for the implanting surgeon upon which to base such complex decisions, pupil evaluation in different lighting conditions should therefore be an integral part of the preoperative assessment of a candidate for a premium IOL, particularly if a multifocal modality is being considered. Postoperatively, pupil assessment, including at the slit lamp, is needed to confirm the centration and position of the premium channel IOL. IOL repositioning or argon laser iridoplasty[10] may be a consideration in cases of multifocal IOL decentration relative to the pupil center.

Infrared Pupillometry

There are a number of pupillometers that utilize infrared tubes or cameras available commercially to assist the surgeon with this assessment, including the Colvard (Oasis Medical, Glendora, CA), Procyon (P2000SA, P3000SA; Procyon Instruments, United Kingdom), and NeurOptics (PLR-100; Neuroptics, San Clemente, CA) pupillometers.[11,12] Hand-held pupillometers such as the Colvard can be used to record the full range of scotopic, mesopic, and accommodative pupil sizes. Pupil sizes should be monocularly recorded with the lights on and off and the contralateral eye fixating first on a distance, and then on a near target. The Procyon pupillometer binocularly measures pupil size at 3 fixed illumination levels: scotopic at 0.04 lux, mesopic low at 0.4 lux, and mesopic high at 4.0 lux.[11] It therefore produces a full range of pupil sizes in multiple lighting conditions in a binocular and reproducible fashion that has been demonstrated to correlate more closely to physiologic variations in pupil size than hand-held, monocular testing tools such as the Colvard.[11,13,14] The hand-held

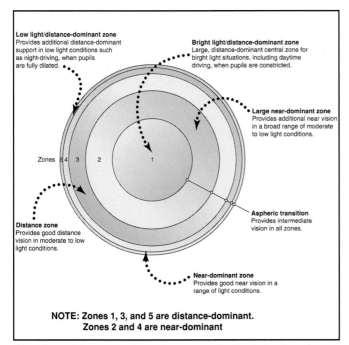

Figure 1. The ReZoom intraocular lens has a zonal diffractive design that is distance-dominant centrally.

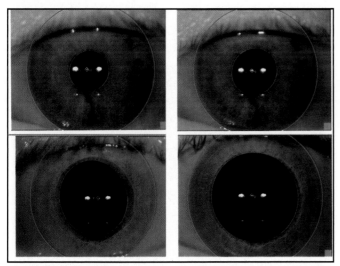

Figure 2. Pupil capture during aberrometry with (left) and without (right) ambient lighting. The top row illustrates a patient with small photopic and scotopic pupil sizes and a small dynamic range. The bottom row shows an eye with large photopic and scotopic pupil sizes, with a large dynamic range.

NeurOptics pupillometer monocularly records pupil dynamics in different lighting situations, controlling for corneal magnification of the pupil image by adjusting for vertex distance.[12] It records 3 seconds of data to ensure the effects of hippus are minimized and then reports average pupil size and standard deviation, maximum pupil size, minimum pupil size, percent constriction, average constriction velocity, maximum constriction velocity, and dilation velocity. Numerical results are displayed on a color liquid crystal display (LCD) and can be transferred to a portable printer wirelessly.

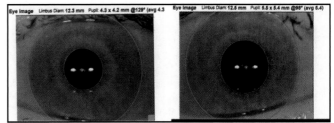

Figure 3. Different pupil shape and size of the right and left eye of a single patient are noted, highlighting the importance of assessing each eye independent of the other when selecting a presbyopia-correcting IOL.

Another resource readily available to the refractive surgeon is the infrared pupillometer built into the wavefront aberrometer. Several series report good correlation between the pupillometers listed earlier and pupil readings reported by aberrometers.[15-17] In addition to the usual scotopic readings routinely recorded during standard wavefront capture procedures, a second reading with the room light turned on can help define the pupil size with ambient lighting conditions. Although aberrometers generally have internal nonaccommodative targets, the patient can be instructed to focus on the target stimulus to provide information on accommodative pupil size. Another advantage of pupil testing via wavefront aberrometers, and with the Procyon as well, is that an image of the pupil is provided (Figure 2) so that the surgeon can evaluate for pupil size, shape, and position, as these parameters may impact the decision to place a multifocal IOL.

Conclusion

Given that an integral part of the preoperative assessment of a candidate for a presbyopic IOL is an evaluation for excimer refractive surgery, in anticipation for potential treatment of residual spherical error and/or astigmatism post cataract surgery, we routinely incorporate pupillometry testing in our assessment of premium channel IOL patients. In the interest of optimizing patient flow, we presently utilize wavefront aberrometry, with the technique described above, to record scotopic, photopic, and "accommodative" pupil sizes. With this information, important clinical decisions can be made during the informed consent and IOL selection process. Patients with small mesopic pupils with little dynamic range (Figure 2, top row) or small, irregularly shaped pupils may not obtain as significant near vision improvement with a multifocal IOL that is distant dominant centrally, such as the ReZoom, but may achieve more superior near vision with the ReSTOR. A patient with large pupils (Figure 2, bottom row), or those with a pupil center shift under mesopic or scotopic conditions, may be better suited for an accommodative IOL, such as the Crystalens, or perhaps an aspheric, monofocal IOL, in order to avoid nighttime dysphotopsia. Some patients may have distinctly different pupil sizes, shapes, or dynamics between their 2 eyes (Figure 3), requiring independent assessment of each eye when deciding on the most appropriate IOL. These and other examples highlight the importance of accurate pupillometry at different and standardized lux settings in the preoperative evaluation of the premium IOL candidate.

References

1. Pepose JS, Qazi MA, Davies J, et al. Visual performance of patients with bilateral vs combination Crystalens, ReZoom, and ReSTOR intraocular lens implants. *Am J Ophthalmol.* 2007;144(3):347-357.

2. Alfonso JF, Fernandez-Vega L, Baamonde MB, Montes-Mico R. Correlation of pupil size with visual acuity and contrast sensitivity after implantation of an apodized diffractive intraocular lens. *J Cataract Refract Surg.* 2007;33:430-438.

3. Mester U, Honold W, Wesendahl T, Kaymak H. Functional outcomes after implantation of Tecnis ZM900 and Array SA40 multifocal intraocular lenses. *J Cataract Refract Surg.* 2007;33:1033-1040.

4. Kawamorita T, Uozato H. Modulation transfer function and pupil size in multifocal and monofocal intraocular lenses in vitro. *J Cataract Refract Surg.* 2005;31:2379-2385.

5. Hayashi K, Hayashi H, Nakao F, Hayashi F. Correlation between pupillary size and intraocular lens decentration and visual acuity of a zonal-progressive multifocal lens and a monofocal lens. *Ophthalmology.* 2001;108:2011-2017

6. Lane SS, Morris M, Nordan L, Packer M, Tarantino N, Wallace RB. Multifocal intraocular lenses. *Ophthalmol Clin N Am.* 2006;19:89-105.

7. Davison JA, Simpson MJ. History and development of the apodized diffractive intraocular lens. *J Cataract Refract Surg.* 2006;32:849-858.

8. Pieh S, Lackner B, Hanselmayer G, et al. Halo size under distance and near conditions in refractive multifocal intraocular lenses. *Br J Ophthalmol.* 2001;85:816-821.

9. Zeng M, Liu Y, Liu X, et al. Aberration and contrast sensitivity comparison of aspherical and monofocal and multifocal intraocular lens eyes. *Clin Exp Ophthalmol.* 2007;35:355-360.

10. Donnenfeld ED. Patients unhappy with presbyopia-correcting IOLs. *Cataract Refract Surg Today.* 2007;7:54-56.

11. Bootsma S, Tahzib N, Eggink F, de Branbrander J, Nuijts R. Comparison of two pupillometers in determining pupil size for refractive surgery. *Acta Ophthalmol Scand.* 2007;85:324-328.

12. Michel AW, Kronberg BP, Narvaez J, Zimmerman G. Comparison of 2 multiple-measurement infrared pupillometers to determine scotopic pupil diameter. *J Cataract Refract Surg.* 2006;32:1926-1931.

13. Kohnen T, Terzi E, Buhren J, Kohnen EM. Comparison of a digital and a handheld infrared pupillometer for determining scotopic pupil diameter. *J Cataract Refract Surg.* 2003;29:112-117.

14. Kurz S, Krummanauer F, Pfeiffer N, Dick HB. Monocular versus binocular pupillometry. *J Cataract Refract Surg.* 2006;32:374-375

15. McDonnell C, Rolincova M, Venter J, McDonnell C, Rolincov M, Venter J. Comparison of measurement of pupil sizes among the Colvard pupillometer, Procyon pupillometer, and NIDEK OPD-scan. *J Refract Surg.* 2006;22:S1027-S1030.

16. Kohnen T, Terzi E, Kasper T, Kohnen E, Buhren J. Correlation of infrared pupillometers and CCD-camera imaging from aberrometry and videokeratography for determining scotopic pupil size. *J Cataract Refract Surg.* 2004;30:2116-2123.

17. Wickremasinghe SS, Smith GT, Stevens JD. Comparison of dynamic digital pupillometry and static measurements of pupil size in determining scotopic pupil size before refractive surgery. *J Cataract Refract Surg.* 2005;31:1171-1176.

CHAPTER 153

CORNEAL TOPOGRAPHY— IS IT NECESSARY?

Matthew C. Caldwell, MD and Natalie A. Afshari, MD

For years, the goal of cataract surgery has been to return patients to their best-corrected visual acuity. Significant advances made in surgical techniques and instrumentation have paved the way for a greater level of visual improvement. Phacoemulsification, foldable intraocular lenses (IOLs), and small incision surgery have shortened the recovery time to only several days on average. As patient expectations have increased, the goal has shifted from improvement of best-corrected visual acuity to refinement of uncorrected acuity as well.[1] The primary refractive effect of cataract surgery is on the lens. The lens, however, is responsible for only one third of the eye's total refractive power, with the remaining two thirds derived from the cornea.[2] Accurately measuring corneal shape and power is of the utmost importance if one is to achieve the optimal refractive outcome in cataract surgery.

Advances in corneal topographers have greatly increased the speed, ease, and accuracy of obtaining topographic data. Simplified estimates and qualitative descriptions of corneal shape have been available for many years with manual keratometry and photokeratoscopy.[2] The development of computerized analysis with videokeratoscopy, however, provides quantitative analysis of a much larger area of the cornea.[3] The rapid development of newer projection-based instruments, driven by the refractive industry, has led to increased accuracy by direct measurement of corneal shape, corneal thickness, and posterior corneal curvature.[2] The benefit of these instruments is evident in clinical research where they have illuminated the effects of surgery and incisions on corneal shape.[4,5] Current generation corneal topographers are noninvasive, quick, and easy to use; however, they can be a significant added expense for a practice that does not already own one. The importance of topography in routine cataract surgery, where many surgeons are already achieving excellent refractive results with keratometry readings and axial length measurements alone, may be a question for debate.

The roles for topography in cataract surgery can be divided into pre- and postoperative applications. Before surgery, topography can be helpful in the calculation of IOL power.

An accurate understanding of corneal shape is also valuable for planning the most appropriate incision location, as well as any adjunctive astigmatism reducing procedures. After surgery, corneal topography can be used to evaluate the refractive outcome, and aids in the evaluation of patients who fail to obtain expected levels of visual acuity. When needed, it can be helpful in postoperative suture adjustment. In the blossoming era of multifocal IOLs, topography is important whenever post cataract laser refractive procedures are used in a bioptics approach to fine tune refractive results.[6-8]

The value of topography in the calculation of IOL power is becoming more evident. A number of different theoretical and empirical formulas can be used to determine the required lens power. These will take axial length, corneal curvature, and sometimes additional data such as anterior chamber depth into account. From the simple SRK formula, $P = A - 2.5L - 0.9K$, it can be seen that the relationship between lens power (P) and cornea power (K) is approximately 1 to 1. For each diopter of error in keratometry, one would expect approximately 1 D of resultant error in lens power. Traditionally, these corneal measurements are obtained by keratometry, which measures only 4 data points in 2 perpendicular meridians near the 3-mm zone.[2] For the normal healthy prolate cornea, this approach works quite well, but the same cannot be said for abnormal corneas.[1,9] The postrefractive cornea, for example, tends to be oblate (following myopic laser in situ keratomileusis [LASIK]). Standard keratometry measurements taken at the 3-mm optical zone are not representative of true central corneal power in this case, and will result in a hyperopic refractive error after cataract surgery.[10-13] As an alternative, the clinical history method of calculating IOL power in the postrefractive patient bypasses the need for direct corneal measurements.[14] However, its results may not be valid in the patient who has had progressive lenticular or corneal changes because surgery, such as a radial keratotomy patient with hyperopic drift.[15] Additionally, prerefractive surgery data are frequently unavailable.

Current generation topographers are able to sample thousands of data points over nearly the entire cornea, including the central and far peripheral areas.[2] Many topographers are also able to calculate the actual posterior corneal curvature, which traditionally was only estimated by taking a percentage of the anterior curvature. This latter estimate has been another source of IOL calculation error in patients with an abnormal ratio of anterior to posterior curvature, such as LASIK patients who have had selective ablation of the anterior corneal surface. In the atypical cornea, topography is able to more accurately determine the true corneal power to be used for calculating the required IOL power. To date, these abnormal corneas have represented the exception to the rule. With the prolific increase in refractive surgery, however, these patients soon will make up a substantial portion of the cataract population.

An accurate preoperative assessment of corneal shape provides an understanding of preexisting corneal aberrations that might affect visual outcome. This allows the surgeon to plan the incision in such a way as to minimize its effect or even counteract normal physiologic aberrations. It has long been recognized that small changes in corneal curvature can greatly impact the focus of light on the retina. Topography has been used in clinical research to evaluate incision architecture and refractive impact.[5] Smaller incisions placed further from the visual axis have less impact on corneal shape. Multiplanar incisions may produce a water-tight closure without the need for sutures and the associated corneal distortion. Small incision cataract surgery with a 3.2-mm wound has been shown to induce less than half a diopter of astigmatism.[2] However, if this is added to preexisting astigmatism, the net increase in astigmatism may disappoint a patient desiring spectacle-free vision. Conversely, the wound can be placed over the steep axis in order to reduce preexisting astigmatism.[16] For greater amounts of astigmatism, the effect of the incision can be augmented by employing a Langerman's hinge or incorporating it into a relaxing incision. Topography can also help determine how much of the astigmatism evident by refraction is actually lenticular. Because this component will disappear with cataract extraction, it need not be treated.[17]

There are several applications of topography in the postoperative management of cataract patients. Many topographers have a "change" map that can be used to compare preoperative to postoperative topographies. Topography is important in the assessment of residual astigmatism, whether preexisting or surgically induced, which may be addressed postoperatively with relaxing incisions or a laser refractive procedure. Minimization of astigmatism is especially important when implanting multifocal lenses, which have a low tolerance for this aberration. When the expected visual outcome is not achieved, topography can uncover corneal irregularities that may not be evident on slit lamp examination.[2] Adjustment and removal of corneal sutures, though often not of visual importance, is also aided by topography.[18]

So is corneal topography necessary for the modern cataract surgeon, and is the added expense worth the cost? For the majority of routine cataract patients, corneal topography is probably not necessary and would not alter the surgical plan or management. However, there is a small, but rapidly growing, group of patients who would benefit from this additional information. Postrefractive surgery patients are certainly the majority of these patients.[13] Patient selection is a critical factor for success with multifocal IOLs.[19] Topography may provide additional guidance in determining who may benefit from a multifocal lens, and who should avoid them. Additionally, it can identify the patient who might need astigmatic keratectomy at the time of cataract removal to optimize multifocal lens performance. It is also essential in planning subsequent refractive procedures such as LASIK or even conductive keratoplasty that might be needed to enhance the refractive error following a multifocal IOL.[20] In addressing their refractive as well as visual outcome, corneal topography is an integral part of the total premium package of services that the refractive IOL patient has come to expect.

References

1. Hardten DR. The importance of the refractive aspects of cataract surgery. *Am J Ophthalmol.* 2005;139:906-907.
2. Corbett MC, Rosen ES, O'Brart DPS. *Corneal Topography: Principles and Applications.* London: BMJ Books; 1999.
3. Mejia-Barbosa Y, Malacara-Hernandez D. A review of methods for measuring corneal topography. *Optom Vis Sci.* 2001;78:240-253.
4. McQueen BR, Martinez CE, Klyce SD. Corneal topography in cataract surgery. *Curr Opin Ophthalmol.* 1997;8:22-28.
5. Ermis SS, Inan UU, Ozturk F. Surgically induced astigmatism after superotemporal and superonasal clear corneal incisions in phacoemulsification. *J Cataract Refract Surg.* 2004;30:1316-1319.
6. Roberto Zaldivar JCG. Pseudophakic sequential bioptics. *Cataract Refract Surg Today Eur.* 2006;Sept/Oct:16-17.
7. Lovisolo CF, Reinstein DZ. Phakic intraocular lenses. *Surv Ophthalmol.* 2005;50:549-587.
8. Pop M, Payette Y, Amyot M, Clear lens extraction with intraocular lens followed by photorefractive keratectomy or laser in situ keratomileusis. *Ophthalmology.* 2001;108:104-111.
9. Alimisi S, Miltsakakis D, Klyce S. Corneal topography for intraocular lens power calculations. *J Refract Surg.* 1996;12:S309-S311.
10. Odenthal MT, Eggink CA, Melles G, Pameyer JH, Geerards AJM, Beekhuis WH. Clinical and theoretical results of intraocular lens power calculation for cataract surgery after photorefractive keratectomy for myopia. *Arch Ophthalmol.* 2002;120:431-438.
11. Gelender H. Orbscan II-assisted intraocular lens power calculation for cataract surgery following myopic laser in situ keratomileusis (an American Ophthalmological Society thesis). *Trans Am Ophthalmol Soc.* 2006;104:402-413.
12. Stakheev AA. Intraocular lens calculation for cataract after previous radial keratotomy. *Ophthalmic Physiol Opt.* 2002;22:289-295.
13. Hamilton DR, Hardten DR. Cataract surgery in patients with prior refractive surgery. *Curr Opin Ophthalmol.* 2003;14:44-53.
14. Wang L, Booth MA, Koch DD. Comparison of intraocular lens power calculation methods in eyes that have undergone LASIK. *Ophthalmology.* 2004;111:1825-1831.
15. Holladay JT, Belin MW, Chayet AS, Maus M, Vinciguerra P. Next-generation technology for the cataract & refractive surgeon. *Cataract Refract Surg Today Suppl.* 2005:1-11.
16. Ben Simon GJ, Desatnik H. Correction of pre-existing astigmatism during cataract surgery: comparison between the effects of opposite clear corneal incisions and a single clear corneal incision. *Graefes Arch Clin Exp Ophthalmol.* 2005;243:321-326.
17. Morlet N, Minassian D, Dart J. Astigmatism and the analysis of its surgical correction. *Br J Ophthalmol.* 2002;86:1458-1459.
18. Black EH, Cohen KL, Tripoli NK. Corneal topography after cataract surgery using a clear corneal incision closed with one radial suture. *Ophthalmic Surg Lasers.* 1998;29:896-903.
19. Slagsvold JE. 3M diffractive multifocal intraocular lens: eight year follow-up. *J Cataract Refract Surg.* 2000;26:402-407.
20. Claramonte PJ, Alio JL, Ramzy MI. Conductive keratoplasty to correct residual hyperopia after cataract surgery. *J Cataract Refract Surg.* 2006;32:1445-1451.

CORNEAL TOPOGRAPHY AND REFRACTIVE IOLs—WHAT TO LOOK FOR

Ming Wang, MD, PhD, and Tracy Swartz, OD, MS, FAAO

The advent of presbyopia-correcting (Pr-C) intraocular lenses (IOLs) (accommodative and multifocal) has increased the demand for precision and accuracy of anterior segment imaging technologies such as corneal topography. Proper use of corneal topography can improve the clinical outcomes obtained with these lens technologies. Here we review basic corneal topography interpretation, and describe the common clinical applications of corneal topography as they apply to refractive IOL implantation.

The Basics of Corneal Topography Interpretation

Most topographers use Placido disk images projected on the cornea to measure corneal curvature. Placido disk systems do an excellent job of measuring irregularities in corneal curvature, and elevation data are calculated from the curvature data using arc step algorithms. They are not able to measure the posterior surface, however.

Topographic systems, which take 2-dimensional images and create 3-dimensional models of corneal shape, directly measure corneal elevation and calculate the curvature. Both anterior and posterior surfaces are evaluated by systems such as the Pentacam (Oculus, Inc., Lynwood, WA). The Orbscan (Bausch & Lomb, Rochester, New York) combines slit-scanning tomography with a Placido disk to directly measure both curvature and elevation.

SCALES

When looking at topographical maps, changing the scale, or the steps used to signify a change, can easily make "nothing" look like "something" (Figure 1). A step scale of 1.0 D for curvature and power maps, and 5-μm steps for elevation maps, are generally recommended. Too large a step size can minimize the appearance of abnormalities, whereas too small a step can exaggerate a small, and possibly insignificant, change. When comparing maps between different visits, the scale should be checked to ensure that the same step size was used. Axial maps with a 1.5-D step size are typically recommended for identifying corneal irregularity in clinical practice.

MAPS

The type of map used should also be considered, as most systems can display a variety of maps. The most common is the power map, which may be axial or tangential. The values of each point in an axial map represent the power associated to a sphere, having the same slant as the cornea. Thus, a refracting ray of light would behave in the same manner as if projected through the point. The assumed 1.3375 index used is similar to that of keratometry. The axial map is a descriptor of corneal optics rather than shape.

Tangential maps represent the local curvature of the cornea at each point. Tangential maps are sometimes referred to as "local" or "instantaneous curvature." Because the axis of reference is different for each point, there is a higher degree of variability from point to point. Tangential maps tend to show more focal irregularities, with less smoothing than the axial map, and are preferred by contact lens fitters for this reason.

Elevation maps show the difference in surface height based on a reference sphere. These can be most beneficial for patients following refractive surgery where the elevation has been purposely altered to correct the vision. An example of each of these maps in the same eye can be seen in Figure 2.

New Differentiating Features of Presbyopia-Correcting IOLs

Accommodative and multifocal IOLs differ from conventional monofocal IOLs in several ways. First, the visual outcome is more dependent on lens centration in the y plane. For standard monofocal lenses, visual outcome is less sensitive to IOL decentration until it becomes quite significant.

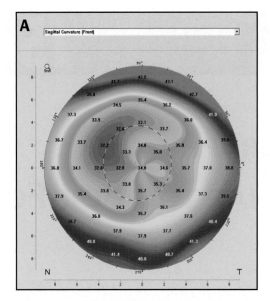

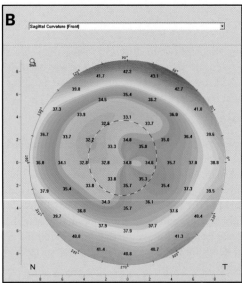

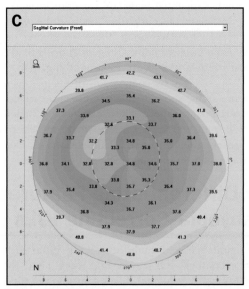

Figure 1. Manipulating the scale used can exaggerate normal findings making it appear pathological. The same eye as seen using a 0.25 D step size (A), 0.50 D step size (B) and 1.00 D step size (C).

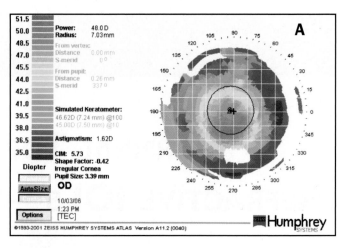

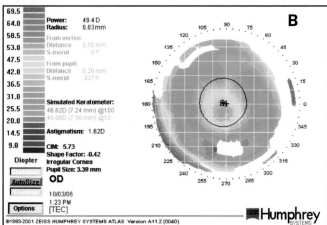

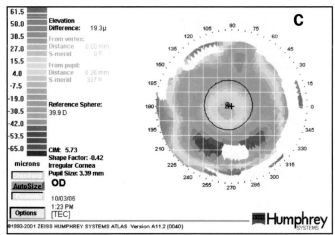

Figure 2. Central islands as viewed using an axial map (A), tangential map (B), and elevation map (C).

Using monofocal lenses, a reasonable visual outcome can still be expected when a capsular complication causes the IOL to be slightly decentered. However, if the capsular bag is torn, implantation of a multifocal lens is generally not advised because of the need for excellent centration.

In addition to needing proper centration in the y plane, the visual performance of multifocal lenses is also more dependent on their axial location. Traditional monofocal lenses may undergo a slight effective power change if the z-axis location

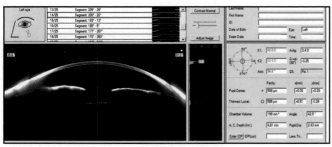

Figure 3. Scheimpflug imaging showing a deep anterior chamber. Increased AC depth will decrease the number of rings effectively used in a multifocal lens. This AC depth was measured to be 4.61 mm.

is incorrect. With a Pr-C IOL, the z-axis location not only affects its effective refractive power, but also its depth of focus. Because the depth of focus is the main advantage of Pr-C IOLs, this is important for functional success.

Finally, the size of the functional optical zone of the Pr-C IOL is important. With a traditional monofocal lens, visual function is largely independent of the size of the functional optical zone. In contrast, accommodative and multifocal lenses incorporate precise architectural features such as concentric diffractive rings. The size of the functional optical zone of the lens therefore becomes a much more important issue, as it affects both the refractive power and depth of focus.

Corneal Topographic Considerations in the Context of the New Presbyopia-Correcting IOLs

Because overall visual function depends upon each optical component along the visual axis, corneal topographic characteristics can significantly affect the visual performance of Pr-C lenses. As we will see in the following sections, the unique architectural features of the accommodative and multifocal lenses require closer alignment between the IOL and cornea. As a result, surgeons must pay closer attention to corneal topography.

Because the centration of Pr-C IOLs is extremely important for proper function, any meridional asymmetry on corneal topography can cause an effective decentration of the new IOLs. Etiologies of meridional asymmetry include significant coma associated with decentered excimer laser ablation, inferior corneal ectasia, significant corneal astigmatism, or a decentered corneal apex on the anterior or posterior surface. The effective decentration caused by such meridional asymmetry decreases the visual performance of these IOLs. Hence, surgical planning should include examination of corneal topography preoperatively to rule out corneal irregularities. If identified, corneal treatment may be required, or a traditional monofocal IOL should be used.

Modern corneal tomographers, such as the Pentacam and Orbscan, measure anterior chamber (AC) depth. The AC

depth can help predict the eventual axial location of the IOL along the z-axis (Figure 3). Deep ACs should produce a different effective lens position and refractive result compared to that of an eye with a shallow chamber depth.

Various corneal structural factors identified by corneal topography may affect the size of the functional zone. For example, a cornea following excimer laser treatment for significant refractive error has a small optical zone. This can lead to an effective reduction of the functional optical zone of the Pr-C IOL. Because the number of concentric rings recruited by diffractive multifocal lenses determines not only the lens' refractive power, but more importantly, its depth of focus, any corneal factors that change the effective functional zone can make a big difference in performance. Other corneal topography–related factors that can significantly influence the size of the functional optical zone of accommodative and multifocal lenses include excessively steep or flat keratometry and variations in AC depth. The steeper the cornea, the smaller the functional optical zone size of a Pr-C IOL is. Similarly, the greater the AC depth, the smaller the area of recruited concentric rings is. Proper consideration of these factors can improve the predictability of visual performance when using Pr-C lenses.

Corneal Ectasia and Irregular Astigmatism

Corneal ectasia and other corneal shape irregularities decrease contrast sensitivity, and cause misalignment of the optical centers of the lens and cornea. Although standard monofocal IOLs are not as sensitive to positional errors in the y plane, the same cannot be said of the complex optical architecture of Pr-C IOLs. Such misalignment may decrease contrast sensitivity enough to cause visual dysfunction and patient complaints.

Irregular corneal astigmatism may occur with a stable cornea, such as with corneal scarring (Figure 4), a decentered excimer laser ablation (Figure 5), and central islands (see Figure 2). It can also occur on an unstable, structurally weak cornea such as in keratoectasia (Figure 6) or pellucid marginal degeneration (Figure 7). For Pr-C IOLs, spatial structural variations on the cornea in the y plane, such as irregular astigmatism, can adversely affect visual performance, and should be identified and treated prior to IOL implantation.

With regard to the identification of forme fruste keratoconus (FFKC), classification programs on corneal topographers may assist in differentiating between keratoconus suspects, corneal distortion, and even patients having undergone refractive surgery from normal variations of corneal topography. Examples include the Tomey Smolek/Klyce Keratoconus program (Tomey, Inc., New York, NY), the Humphrey Pathfinder (Carl Zeiss Meditech, Jena, Germany), and the NIDEK Magellan Navigator (Nidek, Inc., Gamagori Japan). The latter program can differentiate between keratoconus, keratoconus suspect, pellucid marginal degeneration, and several other corneal conditions.

Figure 4. Corneal scarring can create irregular astigmatism. This patient suffered from recurrent herpes simplex virus keratitis.

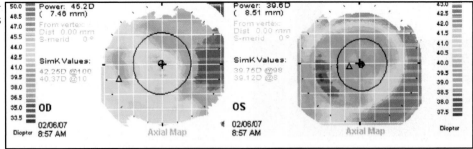

Figure 5. Decentered excimer laser ablation as seen on axial (left) and elevation (right) maps.

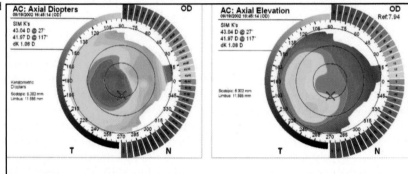

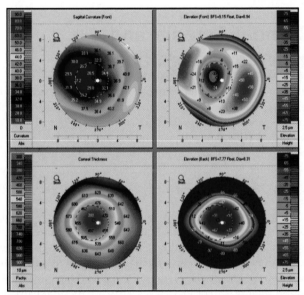

Figure 6. Keratoectasia following laser in situ keratomileusis (LASIK) for 12.50 D of myopia.

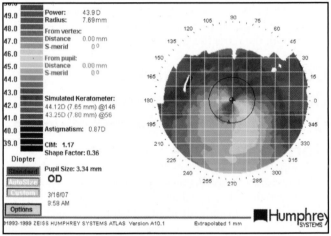

Figure 7. Early pellucid marginal degeneration.

Treating Corneas Prior to the Implantation of the New Presbyopia-Correcting Lenses

Corneal pathologies that can significantly affect the performance of Pr-C IOLs should be adequately treated before using these implants. The response to treatment may determine whether to proceed with the implantation of an accommodative or multifocal lens, a traditional monofocal lens, or to defer intraocular surgery completely.

Irregular astigmatism may be addressed in several ways. Mild corneal irregularities in patients with dry eyes respond well to increased lubrication. We typically use punctual plugs to increase tear volume, Restasis ophthalmic emulsion (Allergan, Irvine, CA) to increase tear production, and treat any lid disease such as meibomian gland dysfunction to assist in smoothing the corneal surface.

It may be difficult to discern if an irregularity is causing a decrease in vision in patients with cataracts. A gas-permeable contact lens over-refraction can be invaluable. A subjective improvement in vision using a rigid contact lens suggests that the corneal irregularities are negatively impacting vision.

For astigmatism occurring in stable corneas, therapeutic excimer laser procedures may be considered to correct corneal topographic problems, such as in corneas that are status post keratorefractive surgery. A decentered excimer laser ablation may need to be treated using techniques such as CustomCorneal Ablation Pattern (C-CAP) or custom wavefront when the wavefront-generated refraction agrees with that of manifest refraction. For astigmatism occurring in

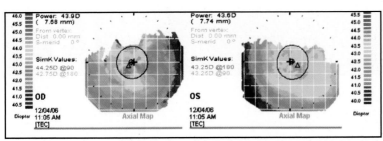

Figure 8. Central irregularities caused severe subjective vision loss following implantation of ReSTOR lens. Gas-permeable contact lens fitting was required for satisfactory vision.

unstable corneas such those with pellucid marginal degeneration, Intacs (Additions Technology, Des Plaines, IL) or ultraviolet (UV) cross-linking should be considered.

If the above approaches successfully resolve the corneal irregularity, one can consider implantation of an accommodative or multifocal lens. If the corneal pathology is likely to impair the visual function of the Pr-C IOL, such as with an ecstatic cornea following Intacs implantation or corneal scarring and irregularities not corrected by phototherapeutic keratectomy, a monofocal IOL may be a better choice.

Clinical Case

A patient presents for evaluation of visual problems following ReSTOR lens implantation OD 4 months prior. He suffers from poor visual quality, glare, "spider webs," and blurred vision not correctable with glasses. His uncorrected vision is 20/30, and manifest refraction of −0.75+0.50 × 65 improves his vision to 20/25. The refraction fails to resolve the "blur" and spider-webs the patient notes subjectively. Topography revealed central irregularities OD as shown in Figure 8.

We commenced aggressive dry eye treatment in an attempt to maximize the quality of the ocular surface and to aid the natural smoothing of the epithelium. This included punctual plugs, artificial tears 4 times per day, and Restasis 2 times per day. Dry eye treatment did improve the topographic irregularities slightly, but the quality of vision remained below the patient's expectations. We then performed a rigid contact lens over-refraction, which enabled him to see 20/20 OD. Subjectively, he reported the visual quality to be greatly improved, and spider webs significantly decreased. We suggested that he continue to wear a gas-permable contact lens to improve the visual quality.

Conclusion

Modern accommodative and multifocal lenses require precise placement within the eye to ensure proper alignment and visual success. Abnormal corneas undermine the optics of this system, creating visual problems and unhappy patients. Identification of corneal problems, such as irregular astigmatism, abnormal corneal curvature, anterior chamber depth, or functional optical zone size, using anterior segment imaging prior to the implantation of Pr-C IOLs can improve clinical outcomes.

CHAPTER 155

CORNEAL TOPOGRAPHY AND REFRACTIVE IOLS—WHAT TO LOOK FOR

David R. Hardten, MD

Patients undergoing premium intraocular lenses (IOLs) such as presbyopia-correcting (Pr-C) IOLs have very high expectations. The optics of the lenses are quite demanding, and the surgical outcome therefore deserves to be optimized. A major refracting component of the eye, even after IOL surgery, is still the corneal surface. In most of our standard IOL patients, we typically ignore the contribution of the cornea to their vision, except for measuring keratometry for our IOL calculation before the surgery. The cornea tends to be the same in power after the cataract surgery and as it is relatively constant and is not affected in a large way by the surgery. Additionally, small irregularities of the cornea do not have a major impact on the selection of IOLs, except to choose a less prolate aspheric IOL in patients that have a significant prolate shape to their cornea, such as after hyperopic laser in situ keratomileusis (LASIK) or photorefractive keratectomy (PRK) or in keratoconus.

In contrast, anything that causes light scatter in the Pr-C IOL patient can be of concern. In addition, astigmatism management is an important part of achieving high quality outcomes with Pr-C IOLs, and the topography helps us understand the best course of astigmatic management for a particular patient.

I perform topography in all my patients that are to scheduled to undergo Pr-C IOL surgery. Either placido-based topography, or slit- or Scheimpflug-based topography is helpful. I prefer that patients stay out of soft contact lenses for 2 weeks and rigid gas permeable lenses for three weeks prior to testing.

We look at several items when analyzing the topography results. The topography can serve to double check and confirm the manual keratometry or IOLMaster (Carl Zeiss Meditec, Jena, Germany) keratometry readings. In general the simulated K readings are relatively close to the readings obtained by IOLMaster or manual keratometry. If these values vary significantly, then it is worth repeating the measurements to make sure that one is not erroneous.

Analysis of the topography should be done to rule out contact lens warpage in patients that had previously worn contact lenses (Figure 1). Contact lens warpage typically is resolved within a few weeks, but in long-term polymethylmethacrylate (PMMA) lens wearers, it may take several months for the topography to stabilize.

Detection of corneal disorders can be aided by the topography. Evaluating the patient for signs of asymmetry consistent with keratoconus can be helpful in ruling out high amounts of irregular astigmatism that can be difficult to improve postoperatively and that may interfere with proper IOL function. If patients have a significant amount of inferior steepening, then they are already multifocal, and the effect of the addition of multifocality of the lens to the optical system can be unpredictable (Figure 2). Even though the IOL surgery is typically done in older patients, where keratoconus is unlikely to progress, significant irregular astigmatism is helpful to know about before surgery. If patients have only mild inferior steepening, then I still would find it acceptable to perform a Pr-C IOL (Figure 3). With significant keratoconus, however, I would choose a monofocal IOL, and typically one that is not aspheric/modified prolate, because of the significant prolate shape to the cornea (Figure 4). In patients with keratoconus, my preference is not to perform relaxing incisions, as they are not as predictable as in a normal eye. Some surgeons do use limbal relaxing incisions (LRIs) to manage astigmatism in these eyes. I prefer to perform custom PRK in the patient with mild inferior steepening if astigmatism management is needed following IOL surgery, although capturing a wavefront may be more difficult through a refractive multifocal IOL, or in cases where the capsulorrhexis is small.

Detection of irregular astigmatism from anterior basement membrane dystrophy (ABMD) is also aided by corneal topography. ABMD is more common in older patients, and can be a significant source of irregular astigmatism that can sometimes be difficult to detect on slit lamp examination (Figure 5). Again, the addition of irregular astigmatism from the ABMD to a multifocal optic may lead to dissatisfaction for the Pr-C IOL patient. ABMD, however, may often be improved by phototherapeutic keratectomy. Therefore, these patients may

Figure 1. Patient with contact lens molding. There is superior flattening. Removing contact lenses for approximately 2 weeks for soft, 3 weeks for gas permeable, and even longer if the patient has been in PMMA lenses is useful to reduce the effect of contact lenses on corneal power.

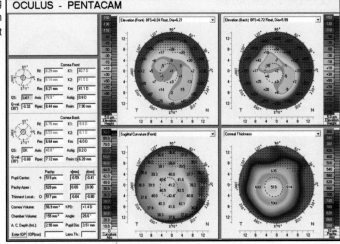

Figure 2. Patient with cataract and also post-LASIK ectasia. In this patient, because the cornea is very multifocal, addition of a multifocal IOL would lead to unpredictable results.

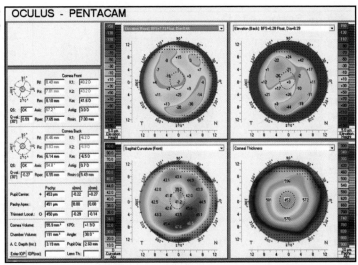

Figure 3. Patient with mild inferior steepening. In this degree of irregular astigmatism, the results may still be acceptable with a multifocal IOL.

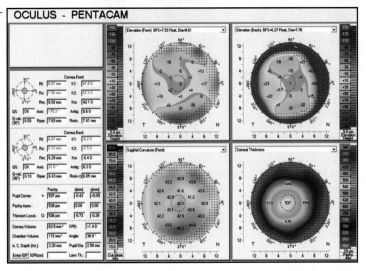

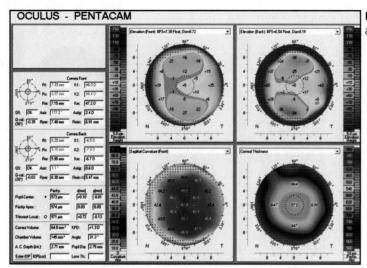

Figure 4. Patient with a very prolate cornea that would likely have less final spherical aberration with a standard IOL as opposed to a modified prolate IOL.

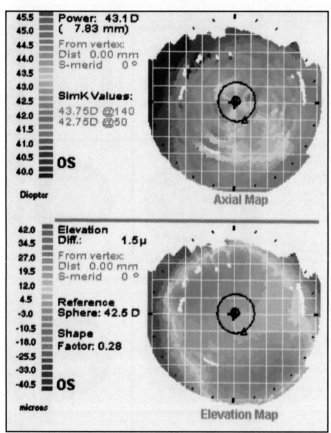

Figure 5. Patient with ABMD. Missing data are found on the topography where focal areas of elevation prevent interpretation of the curvature information on placido topography with the Humphrey Atlas (Carl Zeiss Meditec, Jena, Germany).

eventually do well with Pr-C IOLs, although the entire surgical process is more difficult for these patients.

The major clinical use of topography is for astigmatism and wound management. Analysis should be performed to see if the anterior corneal astigmatism is similar to the refractive astigmatism. In these eyes, intraoperative LRIs or astigmatic keratotomy can be performed. There are multiple techniques and nomograms used by many surgeons. My preferred technique is to use a 9-mm optical zone (approximately 1 mm in from the limbus) (Figure 6). I prefer to use arcs no longer than 60 degrees in length (2 clock hours). Incisions longer than this may lead to more irregular astigmatism and are less stable. I use a 600-micron pre-set knife. The pachymetry and regional pachymetry can be analyzed to make sure there are not areas that would be at risk of perforation with this depth (Figure 7). If the bowtie and elevation is slightly asymmetric, then the arc could be longer on one side than the other. Most surgeons operate temporally, so in cases of with the rule astigmatism, the astigmatism is increased by the cataract wound, and the relaxing incisions would need to incorporate this wound induced astigmatism into the total astigmatism to be corrected. The typical cataract wound of 3 mm causes 0.25 to 0.5 D of reduction of astigmatism in that meridian.

In some eyes, the refractive astigmatism and the anterior corneal astigmatism will be significantly disparate (Figure 8). In these eyes either posterior corneal or lenticular astigmatism (internal astigmatism) is the likely cause of difference in the refractive astigmatism. In these cases, if the astigmatism is lenticular, it would be resolved by removing the cataract. Posterior corneal astigmatism, however, would remain. Posterior corneal mapping such as with the Orbscan (Bausch & Lomb, Rochester, NY) or Pentacam (Oculus, Inc., Lynwood, WA) has some potential to identify the toricity of the back surface of the cornea, yet to date I have not found it extremely reliable. The ray tracing system by Tracey can measure internal astigmatism by comparing the corneal and total wavefront, but does not differentiate whether it is lenticular or posterior corneal. Because of this, if the topographic and refractive astigmatism is significantly different, I prefer to leave the astigmatism alone at the time of the cataract surgery, and then if needed treat it with laser vision correction a few months after the IOL surgery.

Patients with premium IOLs are more likely to desire secondary correction and enhancement of their refractive error after the initial IOL surgery, and because of this I discuss this possibility with these patients before their IOL surgery. PRK and LASIK have relatively different recovery times. I attempt to identify, before the IOL surgery, whether I would use PRK or LASIK for an enhancement if needed later. Sometimes the situation changes, and you may not use what you originally planned for the enhancement. Nonetheless, it may help patient acceptance to be able to warn them of a longer recovery if

Figure 6. One of many nomograms available for limbal relaxing incisions or large optical zone astigmatic keratotomy. The incisions are placed on the steep meridian (warmer colors on the axial or sagittal curvature maps).

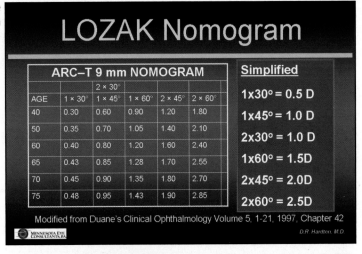

Figure 7. This patient has significant variation in corneal thickness with a peripheral thickness due to corneal scarring that would likely be unsafe and unpredictable to treat with limbal relaxing incisions or astigmatic keratotomy.

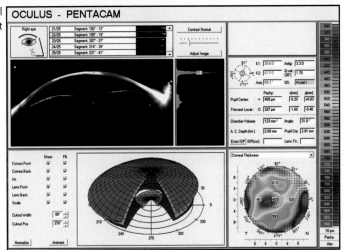

Figure 8. Patient with significant lenticular astigmatism. The patient demonstrates 2 D of astigmatism on refraction and wavefront testing. The Pentacam topography in the left eye demonstrates 0.4 D of anterior corneal astigmatism, and 0.1 D of posterior corneal astigmatism. This patient had minimal astigmatism after cataract surgery.

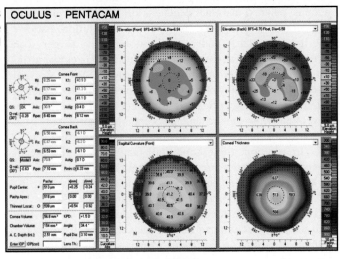

you plan on using PRK because of ABMD or unusual corneal topography.

Corneal topography is a very useful tool in the preoperative planning of premium IOL patients for presbyopia correction. It aids in assessing the resolution of contact lens warpage. It is useful for identifying significant amounts of irregular astigmatism where you may not want to perform a Pr-C IOL because of the concern of superimposing the optical effects of irregular corneal astigmatism onto the optics of the multifocal IOL. Additionally, it is useful for planning intraoperative and postoperative astigmatism management.

CHAPTER 156

CORNEAL TOPOGRAPHY AND REFRACTIVE IOLs—CASE STUDIES

William Trattler, MD and Carlos Buznego, MD

Optimal results for refractive intraocular lens (IOL) procedures require preoperative screening of corneal topography. Most cataract surgeons have not routinely performed preoperative topography prior to standard cataract surgery. However, with the high expectations of patients undergoing refractive IOL procedures as well as the performance demands of these specialty lenses, having a healthy optical system is critical to achieving the expected visual results. Although the majority of patients have normal corneal shapes, it can be surprising to the cataract surgeon that a significant portion of their patients have corneal abnormalities detectable on topography. These conditions include keratoconus, pellucid marginal degeneration (PMD), forme-fruste keratoconus, and irregular astigmatism. In addition, patients who have previously undergone keratorefractive surgery can have corneal shape abnormalities, ranging from irregular astigmatism to post–laser in situ keratomileusis (LASIK) corneal ectasia. Identification of these conditions prior to refractive IOL procedures is critical, as these corneal conditions can prevent patients from achieving acceptable uncorrected visual acuity following placement of a presbyopia-correcting (Pr-C) IOL. In addition, these conditions may prevent the use of procedures to reduce pre-existing astigmatism, such as arcuate keratotomies (AK), limbal relaxing incisions (LRIs), LASIK, and potentially even photorefractive keratectomy (PRK).

The importance of preoperative topography in assisting with patient selection can be seen in a number of cases. For example, the 68-year-old female patient with the topography seen in Figure 1 was interested in a Pr-C IOL. Because of some mild to moderate irregularities seen in the preoperative topography, a Crystalens (Eyeonics, Inc., Aliso Viejo, CA) was 'chosen. The expectation was that this patient might have a slight reduction in visual quality. However, the patient reported extreme dissatisfaction with her vision following bilateral Crystalens implantation. The patient underwent yttrium-aluminum-garnet (YAG) capsulotomy procedures for mild posterior capsular opacities with little improvement. Two months following a YAG capsulotomy, a wavefront-guided

surface ablation procedure was performed OD to reduce the residual refractive error. However, the patient was still dissatisfied with her vision (Figure 2). Although the laser vision correction slightly improved her uncorrected visual acuity (UCVA), she still reported reduced quality of vision. Her corneal topography reveals the continuing presence of irregular astigmatism (Figure 3). This case illustrates how important it is to identify even mild corneal irregularities prior to surgery and discuss the potential impact of these abnormalities with the patient. Otherwise, the patient's expectations have not been properly managed, and the patient may harbor a significant degree of disappointment.

Another interesting case emphasizes the importance of preoperative topography, as shown in Figure 4. This 72-year-old female with visually significant cataracts was interested in a Pr-C IOL OS. Preoperative topography revealed mild irregular astigmatism and best corrected visual acuity (BCVA) of 20/80 OS, with potential visual acuity (PAM) of 20/20. Note that the right eye of this patient had significant corneal surface irregularity and was suspicious for forme-fruste PMD. Following uncomplicated cataract surgery OS, the patient was only able to be refracted to 20/80 despite having a clear posterior capsule and a perfectly normal optical coherence tomography (OCT) of the macula. Potential visual acuity testing remained at 20/20. The reduced visual acuity was therefore entirely related to the irregular corneal shape (Figure 5), and the patient ended up requiring a rigid gas permeable (RGP) contact lens. For her second eye, the patient has chosen to proceed with a monofocal implant.

The preoperative topography of patients who have previously undergone LASIK requires close scrutiny. In Figure 6, a 58-year-old female provided her pre-LASIK corneal topography from 1998. Her pre-LASIK refraction in her left eye was −9.50 −5.50 × 165. The patient came to our center in 2007 for cataract surgery. The surgeon calculated the IOL carefully by using the Holladay IOL consultant and the clinical history method for adjusting the K values. The patient underwent uncomplicated cataract surgery in February 2008, but ended

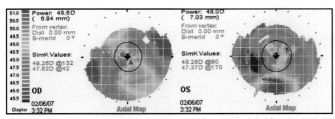

Figure 1. Preoperative topography of a 68-year-old female scheduled for a Pr-C IOL OU. Note the irregular astigmatism OU.

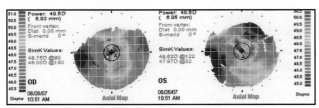

Figure 2. Postoperative topographies of a 68-year-old female after bilateral Crystalens insertion through a 2.8-mm temporal clear corneal incision. Note that both eyes have irregular astigmatism.

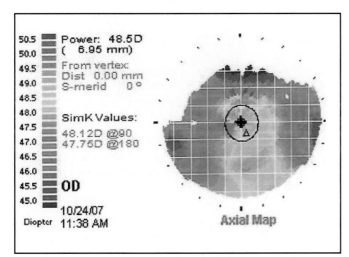

Figure 3. Topography following surface ablation OD in a 68-year-old female. The patient continued to complain of poor quality of vision OD. Irregular astigmatism is present.

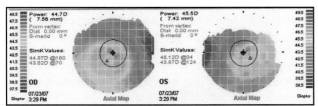

Figure 4. Preoperative topography of a 72-year-old female whose husband was extremely happy following Pr-C IOL surgery. Note the early Pellucid pattern of the topography OD and the irregular astigmatism OS.

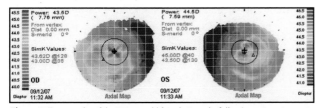

Figure 5. Topography of the 72-year-old female 6 weeks following cataract surgery OS. Irregular astigmatism is present OS, which has reduced the best-corrected vision.

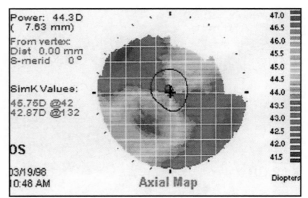

Figure 6. Pre-LASIK topography of a patient with a high refractive error of −9.50 −5.50 × 165. LASIK was performed in 1998.

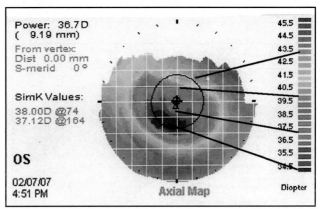

Figure 7. Topography of the patient 9 years after LASIK. A significant gradient of astigmatism is noted in the papillary axis. The patient underwent cataract surgery and ended up with a BCVA of 20/50 due to the irregular astigmatism present.

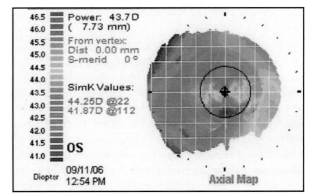

Figure 8. Preoperative topography OS. Note that this patient's contralateral eye (Figure 9) has PMD.

up with best-corrected vision of 20/60. Careful analysis of the topography OS reveals a significant gradient in the astigmatism, reaching almost 9 diopters (Figure 7). With this degree of irregular astigmatism, contact lens fitting was attempted. With a RGP contact lens, the vision improved to 20/25.

Patients undergoing refractive IOL surgery often require treatment of their astigmatism. Corneal topography is a critical preoperative test for determining whether or not to perform incisional refractive surgery to reduce astigmatism at the time of cataract surgery. In one case, a cataract surgeon performed preoperative corneal topography (Figure 8), and decided to

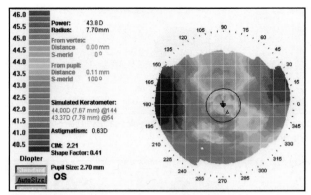

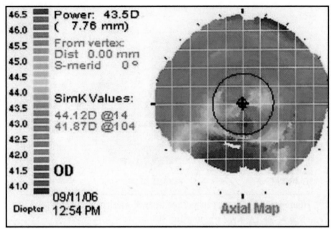

Figure 9. Topographic map of the contralateral eye (OD), which reveals Pellucid Marginal Degeneration.

Figure 11. Four weeks after placement and LRIs placed at 3 and 9 o'clock. Note the irregular astigmatism with superior steepening and a shifting axis of astigmatism compared to the topography taken 2 weeks earlier (Figure 10).

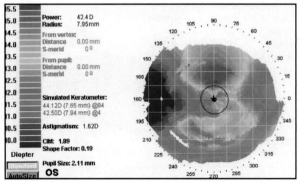

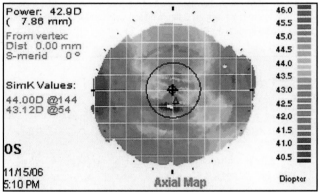

Figure 10. Two weeks after cataract surgery with ReSTOR IOL placement and LRIs placed at 3 and 9 o'clock. Note the significant overcorrection of the astigmatism, along with the area of superior steepening.

Figure 12. Six weeks following LRIs. Note the superior steepening along with the area of horizontal astigmatism, which reflects a significant shift compared to just 2 weeks earlier (Figure 11).

proceed with LRI at the time of ReSTOR implantation to reduce the 2.5 diopters of horizontal astigmatism. Of note, the contralateral eye was suspicious for early PMD (Figure 9). Analysis of the eye undergoing cataract surgery with LRI revealed slight suspicion of early Pellucid as well. Following the procedure, the patient was very dissatisfied with her vision. Corneal topography performed 2 weeks after the procedure revealed a significant overcorrection in the degree of astigmatism, along with the development of irregular astigmatism (Figure 10). The topography at 1 month (Figure 11) and 6 weeks (Figure 12) revealed that the cornea was having a significant shift in shape. The resulting shape of the cornea demonstrated a return of horizontal astigmatism, along with the development of irregular astigmatism. The patient's BCVA ended up at 20/40.

Preoperative corneal topography, in our opinion, should be a routine procedure prior to providing refractive IOL procedures, just as it is standard prior to refractive laser surgery. Analysis of preoperative topography can help determine whether or not the patient is an appropriate candidate for a refractive IOL procedure. In addition, preoperative corneal topography is critical in determining whether a patient is eligible for incisional refractive surgery to reduce astigmatism. Obviously, patients with forme-fruste keratoconus, frank keratoconus, or PMD are not eligible for LASIK due to the increased risk of post-LASIK ectasia. With the information obtained from corneal topography, appropriate counseling of the refractive IOL patient can be provided. If abnormalities are identified, the patient can therefore be advised of his or her corneal condition prior to surgery, so that surprises for both the patient and surgeon can be avoided.

CHAPTER 157

OPTIMIZING THE
OCULAR SURFACE PREOPERATIVELY

Sherman W. Reeves, MD, MPH and Richard L. Lindstrom, MD

Careful evaluation of the ocular surface is a critical but often overlooked component of the preoperative examination for a premium intraocular lens (IOL). As the first refractive plane of the eye, a smooth and healthy ocular surface must be achieved if optimal ocular optics are to be obtained. However, a variety of pathological factors may degrade this delicate region of the eye, compromising the prospects of excellent postoperative vision and disappointing the high expectations of these patients. As such, a systematic preoperative assessment of the interrelated components of the ocular surface, including the eyelids, tear film, conjunctiva, and corneal surface, can help identify and address sources of current or potential postoperative ocular surface pathology.

The Eyelids

Beyond ensuring that proper mechanical lid function is present, the preoperative examination of the eyelids should identify the presence of any anterior and/or posterior blepharitis. As these conditions can markedly degrade ocular surface quality through inflammation and increase the risk of postoperative infection, they should be identified early and treated aggressively prior to surgery.

The presence of blepharitis increases the risk of antibiotic-resistant bacteria on the ocular surface and the overall risk of postoperative endophthalmitis after lens implant surgery.[1,2] *Staphylococcus* anterior blepharitis, with its associated madarosis and collaretting of the lashes, is a common form of blepharitis[3] that typically responds to lid hygiene measures and antibiotic ointments. Likewise, seborrheic anterior blepharitis, with its greasy scales in the lashes, brows and scalp, may result in ocular surface inflammation as well as meibomian gland dysfunction on the posterior lid. This condition can also be addressed preoperatively with lid hygiene, although the addition of Nizarol (ketoconazole) shampoo (Janssen Pharmaceutica, Antwerp, Belgium) to the lid scrubs may be helpful in severe cases.

Posterior blepharitis may be less obvious than anterior forms, but may also cause significant ocular surface morbidity. The meibomian gland secretions should be examined closely for turbidity and inspissation, and meibomian orifices for clogging or, in chronic cases, obliteration. Inflammatory signs such as hyperemia and telangectasias are typically present on the posterior margin (Figure 1). Rosacea is often present, although its signs may be subtle. Thus, posterior blepharitis should also prompt a close examination of the cheek and nose skin for the tell-tale telangectasias, flushing, or pustules of rosacea. Like anterior blepharitis, lid hygiene is a mainstay of posterior blepharitis treatment, although the clinician should have a low threshold for the addition of oral doxycycline, which can markedly improve the signs and symptoms of meibomian gland dysfunction.[4] Omega-3 fatty acid supplementation may also favorably alter meibomian gland secretions[5] and may improve the symptoms of co-existing dry eye.[6,7] Topical cyclosporine 0.05% (Restasis, Allergan, Irvine, CA) has also recently been shown to improve the ocular surface in the setting of meibomian gland disease.[8] Combined anterior *staphylococcal* anterior blepharitis and posterior lid disease can often effectively be addressed with a short course of a topical antibiotic/steroid combination. The application of metronidazole 1% cream (Noritate, Dermik Laboratories, Bridgewater, NJ) to the lids may also improve the posterior blepharitis symptoms of rosacea (Table 1).

The Tear Film

In the face of an otherwise flawless surgical outcome, a compromised tear film can negate refractive gains from a premium IOL, plaguing both the patient and surgeon with chronic suboptimal visual quality. Although the complaint of dry eye symptoms may alert the surgeon to frank pre-existing dryness (Table 2), an effort should be made to also identify and treat those with marginal tear films that may decompensate postoperatively.

Clinical evaluation of the tear film is straightforward and includes a simple set of readily available tools such as the slit

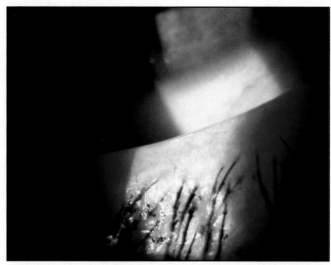

Figure 1. Posterior blepharitis with hyperemia and telangectasias of the lid margin.

Table 1

CLINICAL MANAGEMENT OF ANTERIOR/POSTERIOR BLEPHARITIS

- Lid hygiene (heat and massage)
- Systemic doxycycline (start 50 to 100 mg bid for 1 to 2 months, then consider 20 mg tablets for chronic treatment)
- Antibiotic ointments (erythromycin, bacitracin)
- Antibiotic/steroid combinations
- Cyclosporine A 0.05% (Restasis)
- Metronidazole 1% cream (Noritate) for acne rosacea
- Ketoconazole (Nizoral) shampoo for seborrheic blepharitis
- Omega-3 fatty acid supplementation [HydroEye (ScienceBased Health, Carson City, NV), BioTears (Biosyntrx, Lexington, SC), TheraTears (Advanced Vision Research, Woburn, MA) supplements, flax seed, fish oil]

Table 2

DRY EYE SYMPTOMS

- Ocular discomfort (heavy lids, burning, foreign body sensation, photophobia, tearing)
- Itching (consider concomitant seasonal/perennial allergic conjunctivitis, especially if localized to the caruncle)
- Worse in p.m., winter, low humidity, dry environment
- Increased environmental irritant sensitivity
- Increased mucous/matter (consider concomitant lid disease)

Table 3

DRY EYE SIGNS

- Conjunctival erythema
- Decreased tear strip (<0.2 mm)
- Decreased tear break-up time (<10 sec)
- Conjunctivalchalasis
- Punctate epithelial erosion (PEE)(only see with stain)

lamp and the vital dyes fluorescein and lissamine green (Table 3). Categorization of dry eye into either aqueous deficiency states or evaporative loss is helpful when planning a treatment approach, although dryness frequently occurs as a combination of the two (Table 4).

Recent evidence has elucidated inflammation as both a key consequence and cause of dry eye ocular surface disease.[9] The classical approach to dry eye therapy has started with topical lubricants and added more aggressive therapy, such as punctual plugs, incrementally. This strategy, however, fails to address inflammation in the pathophysiology of dry eye and thus often leads to low patient satisfaction, poor patient compliance, and, commonly, treatment failure. Thus, a more aggressive initial treatment regimen is required—especially in the high stakes premium IOL patient—aimed at breaking the cycle of inflammation, restoring a normal tear film, and preventing evaporative loss. Combination therapy with anti-evaporative tear supplements, lid hygiene, and anti-inflammatories should be employed to control dryness and inflammation preoperatively. Concurrent lid disease, which can exacerbate ocular surface inflammation, should also be aggressively addressed. Punctal plugs should be considered only after ocular surface inflammation has been controlled (Table 5). In patients where full restoration cannot be achieved preoperatively, a full discussion of the prospect of dryness-associated compromise of postoperative visual quality needs to occur.

Post-surgery, therapy should be continued in dry eye patients, although it may be tapered to a maintenance dose. Relapses will occur and require re-institution of more aggressive therapy. As such, patients should be well-educated as to the chronic nature of their dry eye disease.

The Corneal Surface

As a final component to ocular surface preparation for premium IOL surgery, the health of the anterior cornea should be carefully evaluated. Specifically, the surface should be closely inspected for pathology, including such conditions as pterygia, anterior basement membrane dystrophy (ABMD), Salmann degeneration, or other subepithelial pathology.

ABMD is a common and often under-recognized corneal surface condition, occurring in 5% to 18% of the population.[10] Although mild forms of ABMD are usually inconsequential, the presence of any ABMD may predispose the cornea to intraoperative and postoperative epithelial defects, and thus should be noted. More advanced stages of the disease, however, may cause significant irregular astigmatism, compromising the intended refractive outcome (Figure 2). Pterygia and Salzmann nodules likewise can result in significant induced corneal irregular astigmatism. Topography should be obtained in moderate to advanced cases of ABMD and in all cases of pterygia and Salzmann degeneration, to ensure that irregular astigmatism is not present from these conditions prior to proceeding with premium IOL surgery.

Table 4

DRY EYE CLASSIFICATION

I. Tear deficient dry eye
  A. Sjogren syndrome
    1. Primary
    2. Secondary (typically related to collagen vascular disease: rheumatoid arthritis, systemic lupuserythmatosus, systemic sclerosis, primary biliary cirrhosis, Wegener's, and others)
  B. Non-Sjogren syndrome
    1. Lacrimal disease
      a. Primary (congenital alacrima, acquired primary lacrimal disease)
      b. Secondary (sarcoidosis, HIV, graft vs. host disease, xerophthalmia, post-excimer ablation)
    2. Lacrimal obstruction (trachoma, cicatricial pemphigoid, erythema multiforme, burns)
    3. Reflex hyposecretion (neuroparalytic keratitis, chronic contact lens wear, proximal seventh nerve palsy)
II. Evaporative dry eye
  A. Oil deficient
    1. Primary (absence of lacrimal glands, distichiasis)
    2. Secondary (anterior/posterior blepharitis, obstructive meibomian gland disease)
  B. Lid related (blink disorders, aperture abnormalities, lid surface incongruity)
  C. Surface change (xerophthalmia)
  D. Contact lens or post-surgical
III. Combined tear deficient and evaporative dry eye

Table 5

CLINICAL MANAGEMENT OF DRY EYE AND ASSOCIATED OCULAR SURFACE INFLAMMATION

1. Ocular surface hydration with tear supplements (Lower tear film osmolarity, reduce shear force and mechanical trauma, dilute and wash out inflammatory cells and mediators.)
2. Corticosteroids (Reduce T-lymphocytes, reduce vascular permeability, cytokine and matrix metalloproteinase production.)
3. Cyclosporine A 0.05% (Reduce T lymphocytes, cytokine and matrix metalloproteinase production, and reduce apoptosis.)
4. Tetracycline, Doxycycline, Minocycline (Inhibit keratinization, suppress leukocyte migration, inhibit matrix metalloproteinase, bacteriostatic, suppress bacterial lipase that initiate fatty acid and diglyceride release.)
5. Lid hygiene (Control spillover inflammation from lids.)
6. Omega-3 fatty acid supplements (Alter meibomian lipid profiles, control inflammatory lipid precursors.)
7. Combination therapy
8. Punctal plugs—only after surface inflammation has been controlled

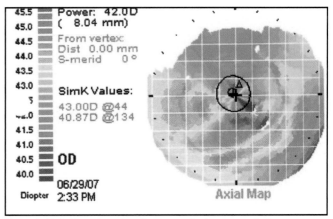

Figure 2. Marked irregular astigmatism as a result of severe anterior basement membrane dystrophy.

Mild forms of ABMD can either be observed or treated with sodium chloride ointment at bedtime prior to surgery. For more advanced forms with resultant irregular astigmatism or in patients with a history of recurrent erosion, consideration should be given to phototherapeutic keratectomy (PTK) prior to cataract surgery. Although a uniform removal of 5 microns or less during PTK would not be expected to impact the IOL calculations markedly, corneal measurements and calculations should be repeated, and if necessary, using postrefractive surgery IOL calculation methods to ensure the proper power IOL is placed after PTK is performed. Superficial keratectomy may be required in the case of Salzmanns degeneration, and removal of advancing or astigmatism-inducing pterygia should be performed prior to premium IOL placement. Keratometry measurements and IOL calculations should then be repeated after any ocular surface surgery is performed.

Conclusion

A healthy ocular surface is a key component to achieving a successful outcome with the premium IOL patient. Careful preoperative identification and aggressive treatment of surface pathology is essential prior to entering the operative suite, as is maintenance therapy for these conditions in the postoperative period.

References

1. Miño de Kaspar H, Shriver EM, Nguyen EV, Egbert PR, Singh K, Blumenkranz MS, Ta CN. Risk factors for antibiotic-resistant conjunctival bacterial flora in patients undergoing intraocular surgery. *Graefes Arch Clin Exp Ophthalmol.* 2003;241(9):730-733.
2. Scott IU, Flynn HW Jr, Feuer W. Endophthalmitis after secondary intraocular lens implantation. A case-report study. *Ophthalmology.* 1995;102(12):1925-1931.
3. Dougherty JM, McCulley JP. Comparative bacteriology of chronic blepharitis. *Br J Ophthalmol.* 1984;68(8):524-528.
4. Yoo SE, Lee DC, Chang MH. The effect of low-dose doxycycline therapy in chronic meibomian gland dysfunction. *Korean J Ophthalmol.* 2005;19(4):258-263.
5. Sullivan RM et al. Correlations between nutrient intake and the polar lipid profiles of meibomian gland secretions in women with Sjogren's Syndrome. Third International Conference on the Lacirmal Gland, Tear Film and Dry Eye Syndromes: Basic Science and Clinical Relevance. Maui, Hawaii, November 15-18, 2000.
6. Creuzot C, Passemard M, Viau S, Joffre C, Pouliquen P, Elena PP, Bron A, Brignole F. Improvement of dry eye symptoms with polyunsaturated fatty acids. *J Fr Ophtalmol.* 2006;29(8):868-873.
7. Miljanovic B, Trivedi KA, Dana MR, Gilbard JP, Buring JE, Schaumberg DA. Relation between dietary n-3 and n-6 fatty acids and clinically diagnosed dry eye syndrome in women. *Am J Clin Nutr.* 2005;82(4):887-893.
8. Rubin M, Rao SN. Efficacy of topical cyclosporin 0.05% in the treatment of posterior blepharitis. *J Ocul Pharmacol Ther.* 2006;22(1):47-53.
9. Stern ME, Pflugfelder SC. Inflammation in dry eye. *Ocul Surf.* 2004;2(2):124-130.
10. Laibson PR. Microcystic corneal dystrophy. *Trans Am Ophthalmol Soc.* 1976;74:488-531.

CHAPTER 158

RETINA ASSESSMENT FOR REFRACTIVE IOL PATIENTS—WHAT DO I DO?

*David F. Chang, MD; Jay S. Pepose, MD, PhD; Olga Konykhov, MD;
Warren E. Hill, MD, FACS; Kerry D. Solomon, MD; Luis E. Fernández de Castro, MD;
and Helga P. Sandoval, MD, MSCR*

David F. Chang, MD

If you implant refractive intraocular lenses (IOLs) in enough cataract patients, sooner or later you will be surprised to discover that you missed a patient's macular pathology preoperatively. A subtle epiretinal membrane, slight diabetic macular edema, or an old vascular occlusion that has left the macula looking morphologically normal may be difficult to detect in the presence of a significant cataract. Undiagnosed maculopathy is disappointing for the patient who, after paying for a premium IOL, may not see well with glasses, let alone without them. It is frustrating for the surgeon who, despite accurate biometry and flawless surgery, has failed in the mind of that patient.

This situation underscores what is different about doing cataract surgery, versus refractive IOL surgery, in a patient with maculopathy. In general, a significant cataract would still be removed whether the macula is perfect or not. If undiagnosed maculopathy was present, the patient's expectations may not have been met postoperatively. However, assuming that a monofocal IOL was implanted, the decision of whether and how to perform surgery would probably not have been any different. In contrast, preoperative detection of any maculopathy would certainly have altered the patient's candidacy for a multifocal IOL. Not only would that patient read poorly without glasses, but the decrease in contrast sensitivity with a multifocal IOL might reduce his or her visual function as compared to a monofocal IOL.

Optical coherence tomography (OCT) testing has revolutionized our ability to image macular details in a rapid, non-invasive fashion (Figure 1). Given its ability to examine both the macula and the peripapillary nerve fiber layer, this technology is becoming increasingly popular among non-retina specialists. Because of the added importance of screening multifocal or accommodating IOL candidates for macular pathology through cloudy media, I now utilize the newly available spectral domain OCT (Cirrus, Carl Zeiss Meditec, Jena, Germany) in my own practice. This technology is expensive,

however, and there are several simple clinical tests that can help in the preoperative assessment of macular function.

Near and Potential Vision Testing

Best corrected near vision testing is a valuable indicator of macular health in the presence of a cataract. Until they are very advanced, pure nuclear cataracts will typically depress distance acuity while having little effect on reading ability. Patients complaining of glare with 20/50 nuclear sclerosis should still be able to read J1 or J2 if the macula is healthy. If that same patient can only read J8, then other pathology should be suspected. For this reason, my optometrist, in working up cataract patients, will test best corrected near acuity prior to shining any bright lights at the eye.

Several potential acuity measuring technologies have been developed with the goal of predicting visual outcomes in eyes with media opacity.[1-4] The Guyton-Minkowski Potential Acuity Meter (PAM; Mentor, Inc., Norwell, MA), laser interferometer, and scanning laser ophthalmoscope (SLO) all work by having an operator project test images onto the macula through relatively clear regions of the lens.[1] These tests are most accurate when patients with mild to moderate cataracts and normal macular function are tested. They are least reliable when denser cataracts coexist with macular pathology—the very situation when they are most needed.[2] Other tests, such as the illuminated near card (INC) and potential acuity pinhole, test the ability of the patient to read a brightly illuminated near card through a trial frame that combines their near spectacle correction with a pinhole.[3-5] These tests appear to be of equal or greater reliability than the more expensive aforementioned technologies.

"Super Pinhole" Test

If I notice that the near acuity is reduced, I have found the monocular "super pinhole" test, as devised by Norman Ballin,

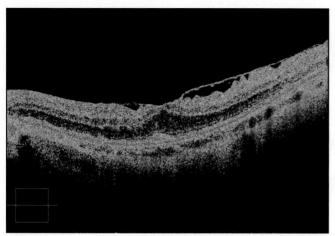

Figure 1. Macular epiretinal membrane imaged with spectral domain OCT (Cirrus, Zeiss).

Macular Examination

Media opacities certainly undermine our ability to visualize macular detail. Amsler Grid testing, however, can uncover metamorphopsia resulting from an epiretinal membrane or macular edema. This simple screening test should be done if a presbyopia-correcting IOL is being considered. Slit lamp biomicroscopy with a Goldman contact lens improves our view in several ways. In addition to the magnification and improved optics, the contact lens steadies the globe and keeps the lids apart. Finally, the patient can be referred for OCT testing if the macular status is still in question.

Occasionally, you will be uncertain as to the macular health in a patient who very much wants to receive a presbyopia-correcting IOL. The risk with a multifocal IOL is that of producing contrast sensitivity reduction without the benefit of good uncorrected near function. The risk of monofocal monovision is that the designated near eye may not read well, and that binocular function with reading glasses may be compromised by the anisometropia. In these situations, the Crystalens (Eyeonics, Inc., Aliso Valejo, CA) represents a reasonable do-no-harm option.

References

1. Cuzzani OE, Ellant JP, Young PW, et al. Potential acuity meter versus scanning laser ophthalmoscope to predict visual acuity in cataract patients. *J Cataract Refract Surg.* 1998;24:263-269.
2. Lasa MS, Datiles MB, 3rd, Freidlin V. Potential vision tests in patients with cataracts. *Ophthalmology.* 1995;102:1007-1011.
3. Hofeldt AJ, Weiss MJ. Illuminated near card assessment of potential acuity in eyes with cataract. *Ophthalmology.* 1998;105:1531-1536.
4. Chang MA, Airiani S, Miele D, Braunstein RE. A comparison of the potential acuity meter (PAM) and the illuminated near card (INC) in patients undergoing phacoemulsification. *Eye.* 2006;20:1345-1351.
5. Melki SA, Safar A, Martin J, et al. Potential acuity pinhole: a simple method to measure potential visual acuity in patients with cataracts, comparison to potential acuity meter. *Ophthalmology.* 1999;106:1262-1267.

to be an excellent clinical test of macular function. It is simple and requires no special equipment. Following pupil dilation, I place the patient's reading correction in a trial frame along with a pinhole paddle. With bright illumination of a high contrast reading card, the patient is asked to "pick one of the holes" to read the smallest paragraph they can see. Placing an array of pinholes before the dilated pupil allows the patient to choose the aperture that is least obstructed by media opacity. A brightly illuminated, glossy black-on-white reading card better compensates for contrast sensitivity lost through the pinhole and cataract. Most importantly, I can listen to the patient's reading speed. A patient with amblyopia can still read single small numbers that are presented one at a time. If the patient reads the J1 or J2 paragraph with reasonable speed, however, his or her monocular macular function must be good. It is important to perform this evaluation before the retina has been photostressed by slit lamp biomicroscopy or indirect ophthalmoscopy.

Jay S. Pepose, MD, PhD, and
Olga Konykhov, MD

Patients considering a premium intraocular lens (IOL) implant have high expectations for achieving excellent uncorrected acuity at more than one focal plane. The substantial out-of-pocket expense incurred by the patient for the services associated with the deluxe lens implant "raises the bar" considerably with respect to the results of surgery. This makes it particularly important to be able to assess retinal function preoperatively and to identify patients with associated comorbid posterior segment pathology, such as premacular fibrosis and epiretinal membranes, macular degeneration, diabetic retinopathy, glaucoma, or optic neuropathies, that can negatively impact the visual outcome of premium channel cataract surgery.

This valuable information allows the surgeon to provide a more accurate informed consent about the planned procedure, risks, benefits, and likely outcome. Patients with significant comorbid retinal or optic nerve pathology may not be ideal candidates for multifocal IOLs, which may decrease contrast sensitivity compared to aspheric monofocal IOLs. This could be particularly troublesome in patients whose optic nerve or macular function is already compromised. In addition, there has been a report of impaired stereopsis for the vitreoretinal surgeon after implanting an acrylic multifocal IOL in a patient undergoing epiretinal membrane peeling despite a clear view of the macula.[1] There have also been earlier reports of difficulty in performing vitreoretinal surgery through an Array (Advanced Medical Optics, Santa Ana, CA) silicone multifocal IOL.[2] Although there would be less concern about surgeon stereopsis or decreased contrast sensitivity after implanting an accommodating IOL, these silicone IOLs may be relatively contraindicated in patients with retinal pathology who may in the future require vitreoretinal surgery. This is because silicone IOLs may compromise intraoperative visualization due to the fogging that may occur following air-fluid exchange or with the use of silicone oil.

There is no substitute for a detailed history and retinal examination of the patient, including assessment of the macula and optic nerve with a 90- or 78-diopter (D) lens. One should

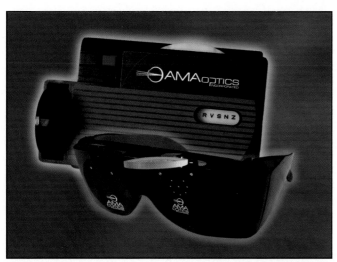

Figure 1. Preoperative assessment of the patient's potential acuity with devices such as the AMA Optics Retinal Acuity Meter may help to identify patients with comorbid retinal or optic nerve disorders that can compromise the postoperative visual outcome.

specifically look for signs of macular pathology or optic neuropathy. A careful examination of the peripheral retina should be performed, especially in high myopes who are at higher risk for retinal detachment. Optical coherence tomography (OCT) or fluorescein angiography and referral to a retinal specialist may be appropriate in patients where pathology is identified. However, many times the anatomic appearance of the lesion does not directly correspond with retinal function. For example, a gossamer-thin epiretinal membrane seen on ophthalmoscopy, confirmed by OCT with no fluorescein findings, could still have a negative impact on visual function postoperatively in a patient implanted with a multifocal or accommodating IOL. On the other hand, a patient with what appears to be severe diabetic retinopathy might have greater visual potential than was anticipated based upon the retinal appearance alone.

Several tests have evolved over the years in the attempt to predict postoperative visual acuity of the eye. The pinhole, although useful in practice by placing the eye at an almost universal depth of focus and reducing optical aberrations, has a disadvantage of light reduction due to its small aperture, thereby limiting retinal illumination, particularly in the presence of media opacities.

Clinical interferometry is based upon interference patterns forming a series of black and white lines on the retina. The distance between these lines is used to define potential visual acuity. Unfortunately, there is a tendency to overestimate retinal potential using interferometry in eyes with concurrent cataract and maculopathy, because the large grating targets (in contrast to Snellen letters) can be effectively discerned by portions of the retina outside of the macula.

The Potential Acuity Meter (PAM) (Marco Instruments; Jacksonville, FL) projects a Snellen chart in a small beam of light through the less opaque area of the lens onto the retina. It is more effective than a pinhole or interferometer due to its lack of reduced retinal illumination and the use of Snellen letters, respectively. However, its use is often cumbersome because it involves a doctor or technician having to align the letters and adjust the patient's head position. The predictabil-

ity of the PAM has been erratic in cases of dense media opacity, maculopathy, or advanced glaucoma.[2-6]

In our practice, we utilize the AMA Retinal Acuity Meter (RAM) (AMA Optics Inc., Miami Beach, FL) to provide a preoperative assessment of the patient's potential visual function. In addition to estimating retinal acuity in patients with observable retinal lesions or optic nerve pathology, it also helps to identify patients with occult comorbid retinopathy or optic neuropathy that may not have been detected by history and inspection alone. This is especially true in patients with cloudy media. The RAM unit (Figure 1) consists of an illuminated reading card and a 16-inch retractable tape measure, ensuring that the card is held exactly 16 inches from the patient so that the appropriate number of degrees of arc on the retina will be subtended by the target letters. The patient then wears a trial frame over his or her distance correction or his or her glasses, which allows insertion of an opaque disc with 8 pinholes, and a flip down +2.5-D lens available for reading add. The illuminated viewing window in the device displays single lines and the target can be rotated to present optotypes corresponding to between 20/200 and 20/20 visual acuity.

The effectiveness of RAM is based on 3 optical principles: (1) visual angle calibrated to testing at a fixed reading distance; (2) bright illumination (16 times the brightness of a standard reading card); and (3) the pinhole effect, which decreases ocular aberrations and enlarges depth of field by obscuring out of focus rays of light. Evaluation of the image through all 8 pinholes allows the patient to select his or her optimal visual axis. To do so, the patient must align the image, a pinhole, a relatively clear portion of his or her lens and cornea, and the best region of the retina, thereby optimizing the assessment of potential retinal acuity. This is different from the PAM where the examiner, rather than the patient, aligns the image and chooses the ocular axis, which appears to allow the target beam to project through the least dense lenticular opacity. A number of studies have demonstrated greater predictive accuracy with the RAM compared to the PAM device, but the predictability of all of these tests may vary in specific forms of macular comorbidity.[5-7]

Although no test of retinal function, including the RAM, has 100% specificity and sensitivity, we have favored this device over others for a number of practical reasons aside from its increased accuracy. First, the test is easy to administer for both the patient and the technician. Unlike the PAM unit, chinrest-eye alignment is not necessary, making it easier for patients with neck or back disease. The patient's head is not moving up and down on the chinrest when he or she is vocalizing responses, which can be problematic and affect test accuracy. The RAM unit is small, lightweight, and battery operated with a calibrated light source. It may be carried by technicians or doctors in a lab coat pocket, making it readily available for use in any room or examining lane without special setup and can be performed in less than 1 minute.[3]

Overall, we find RAM to be the most accurate and practical device currently available for assessment of retinal function and potential postoperative visual performance in patients with 20/100 or better preoperative visual acuity. It is not reliable for patients with best spectacle-corrected visual acuity of 20/200 or worse. It gives a measure of macular function to correlate with structural observations and helps identify patients with occult comorbid posterior segment pathology. This provides important information that assists in surgical counseling and choice of IOL, contributing to better care of our cataract patients.

REFERENCES

1. Luttrull JK, Dougherty PJ. Acrylic multifocal IOLs. *J Refract Surg.* 2007;23:329-330.
2. Mainster MA, Reichel E, Warren KA, Harrington PC. Ophthalmoscopy and vitreoretinal surgery in patients with an Array refractive multifocal lens implant. *Ophthalm Surg Lasers.* 2002;33:74-76.
3. Asbell PA, Chiang B, Amin A, Podos SM. Retinal acuity evaluation with the potential acuity meter in glaucoma patients. *Ophthalmology.* 1985;92:765-767.
4. Le Sage C, Bazalgette C, Arnaud B, Schmitt-Bernard C-F. Accuracy of IRAS GT interferometer and potential acuity meter prediction of visual acuity after phacoemulsification. *J Cataract Refract Surg.* 2002;28:131-138.
5. Chang MA, Airiani S, Miele D, Braunstein RE. A comparison of the Potential Acuity Meter (PAM) and the Illuminated Near Card (INC) in patients undergoing phacoemulsification. *Eye.* 2006;20:1345-1350.
6. Vianya-Estopa M, Douthwaite WA, Noble BA, Elliott DB. Capabilities of potential vision test measurements. Clinical evaluation in the presence of cataract or macular disease. *J Cataract Refract Surg.* 2006;32:111-160.
7. Hofeldt AJ, Weiss MJ. Illuminated near card assessment of potential acuity in eyes with cataract. *Ophthalmology.* 1998;105:1531-1536.

Warren E. Hill, MD, FACS

Because presbyopia-correcting (Pr-C) intraocular lenses (IOLs) require normal macular function for the best visual result, assessing the retina prior to proceeding with implantation of this type of IOL is very important. Experience has shown that even a relatively minor abnormality of macular function can impact on patient satisfaction with a Pr-C IOL.

Our preoperative retinal assessment begins with a careful history. A history of any abnormality that would impact on central acuity, reduce contrast sensitivity, or interfere with the central processing of vision would normally constitute a reason for exclusion.

A partial checklist for exclusion from the implantation of a Pr-C IOL is listed below. If there is a history of any of the following, or if any of these conditions are noted on examination, we will counsel the patient to consider an aspheric monofocal IOL, the type of which would be selected based on a measurement of anterior corneal spherical aberration.

Partial List of Exclusion Criteria

* Abnormalities of retinal anatomy: Epiretinal membrane, macular hole, prior central serous retinopathy
* Abnormalities of retinal function: Age-related macular degeneration, any of the hereditary macular dystrophies, prior macula off retinal detachment, any form of acquired macular disease
* Retinal vascular abnormalities: Diabetic retinopathy, history of macular edema in the operative or fellow eye, prior branch retinal vein or artery occlusion
* Abnormalities of central visual field: Glaucoma with central visual field defects, prior AION or GCA
* Central problems with the processing of vision: Prior stroke or cerebral trauma affecting the visual pathway, amblyopia, Alzheimer's disease
* History of ocular inflammation: Prior iritis with a history of recurrence

Our examination begins with a careful assessment of the retina, including 66-D biomicroscopy. Although it is by no means considered a standard, we also will perform a macular optical coherence tomography (OCT) as a preoperative baseline. If visual acuity is decreased in the immediate postoperative period, the macular OCT is repeated, looking for evidence of pseudophakic cystoid macular edema.

Kerry D. Solomon, MD;
Luis E. Fernández de Castro, MD;
and Helga P. Sandoval, MD, MSCR

A successful outcome for cataract surgery is largely dependent on patient expectations. Patient expectations continue to rise and most patients receiving a presbyopia-correcting intraocular lens (IOL) believe they will be without correction postoperatively. When this does not occur, often an explanation is sought and most commonly the source turns out to be pre-existing retinal pathology that was undiagnosed by clinical exam alone. A very useful modality employed for retinal examination is optical coherence tomography (OCT). Since its introduction in 1991,[1]

OCT has become more sensitive with increased resolution. OCT is a noninvasive, noncontact, transpupillary imaging technique that can analyze retina in cross-section with 8- to 10-µm resolution, which additionally allows quantification of macular thickness and mapping of the retinal damage.[2] It has been most clinically useful in monitoring patients with macular edema, macular holes, and epiretinal membrane (ERM).[3] For this reason, many anterior segment surgeons have begun to employ OCT as a preoperative tool to diagnose subtle changes missed in the dilated retinal exam.

We conducted a study to compare detection sensitivity of common macular diagnosis by clinical exam or OCT in the preoperative cataract patient. A retrospective review of patients that underwent routine cataract extraction with posterior chamber IOL placement from January to December 2006 at Storm Eye Institute was performed. Subjects included in the analysis were those with OCT exams done preoperatively and postoperatively. Clinical exam impression and OCT findings were compared preoperatively and approximately 1 month postoperatively. Additionally, macular thickness and best-corrected visual acuity were also evaluated.

A total of 238 of 1014 eyes (24%) had OCT preoperatively. The mean age of the patients was 68.9 ±10.1 years old. When comparing slit lamp examination to OCT exams, 7% (16 of 238) and 8% (19 of 238) of eyes had an abnormal exam, respectively. Of those eyes with abnormal findings, 1% (3 of 238) had cystoid macular edema (CME) evident at both slit lamp examination and OCT examination. ERM was evident in 1% (3 of 238) using slit lamp examination and in 4% (9 of 238) using OCT exam. One eye (0.4%) had a macular pseudohole by OCT exam, which was not evident by slit lamp examination. However, 2% (4 of 238) of eyes were found to have a macular hole by both slit lamp and OCT examinations.

The mean macular thickness found by OCT of all eyes was 187 ± 37 μm (range, 107 to 312 μm). Patients with macular thickness greater than or equal to 230 μm (11%, 26 of 238) had worse visual acuity postoperatively than those patients with macular thickness less than 230 μm.

When comparing the slit lamp examination with OCT findings in the eyes with macular thickness greater than or equal to 230 μm (11% [3 of 26] of eyes with slit lamp examination), an abnormal exam was evidenced, compared to 35% (9 of 26) of eyes using OCT. Additionally, 4% (1 of 26) of eyes were found to have ERM when performing slit lamp examination compared to 23% (6 of 26) using OCT exam. No differences between slit lamp and OCT exam were noticed when reporting CME and macular holes 4% (1 of 26).

Overall, our findings suggest that OCT exam is superior to slit lamp examination in detecting ERM prior to cataract surgery, especially in patients found to have a macular thickness greater than or equal to 230 μm. However, there are no differences between slit lamp and OCT exam when detecting CME or macular holes. Therefore, while OCT is certainly clinically useful in evaluating patients, it should not replace a thorough clinical examination.

Conclusion

A good thorough dilated retinal exam must be performed to ensure the health of the retina. Attention must be given to the macula to ensure minimal, if any, changes are present. If any subtle ERM is picked up by OCT, patients may be excluded from refractive IOL technology given the high incidence of CME and ocular and visual distortion. All candidates for premium IOLs (multifocal, accommodative, and toric) should have an OCT as part of their preoperative examination. While measured macular thickness by itself may not carry much predictive information regarding postoperative outcomes, the presence of an ERM could. Additionally, use of nonsteroidal anti-inflammatory drugs and steroids preoperatively and postoperatively may be indicated to minimize the development of CME. Finally, a retinal consult may be of benefit.

Acknowledgments

Supported in part by NIH/NEI EY-014793 (vision core) and an unrestricted grant to MUSC-SEI from Research to Prevent Blindness, New York, NY.

References

1. Huang D, Swanson EA, Lin CP, et al. Optical coherence tomography. *Science.* 1991;254:1178-1181.

2. Perente I, Utine CA, Ozturker C, et al. Evaluation of macular changes after uncomplicated phacoemulsification surgery by optical coherence tomography. *Curr Eye Res.* 2007;32:241-247.

3. Puliafito CA, Hee MR, Lin CP, et al. Imaging of macular diseases with optical coherence tomography. *Ophthalmology.* 1995;102:217-229.

SECTION X

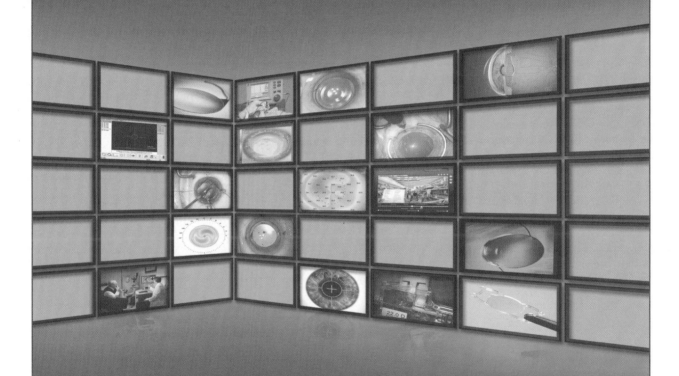

Managing Astigmatism

CHAPTER 159

MEASURING ASTIGMATISM

Noel Alpins, FRANZCO, FRCOphth, FACS and George Stamatelatos, BSc Optom

"Keratometry, topography, and refraction are fundamental determinants of astigmatic status, and disagreement in magnitude and/or axis is prevalent."—N. Alpins

Corneal shape and refractive power are the basic means to measure astigmatism. Each measurement can be utilized in incisional surgery (ie, cataract, astigmatic keratotomy, limbal relaxing incisions), refractive laser procedures, and postkeratoplasty for suture removal or intraocular lens (IOL) power calculations. Accurate measurement of the magnitude and orientation of astigmatism may improve visual outcomes and patient satisfaction through more effective treatment.

Astigmatism can be measured in the consulting room using one of several methods, including corneal topography, manual or automated keratometry, manifest refraction, and wavefront refraction.

Corneal Topography

This measurement provides qualitative and quantitative evaluations of the corneal curvature. Most topographers evaluate 8000 to 10,000 specific points over the entire cornea and center the acquisition on the corneal apex. This method of measuring astigmatism identifies multiple steep and flat meridians at 3-, 5-, and 7-mm optical zones. Topographers incorporating scanning slit photography also measure the power and the astigmatism of the posterior corneal surface, which may improve correlation with the refractive astigmatism. Topography values are imperative for IOL power calculations following previous corneal surgery, and are also useful when postsurgically examining the cornea for signs of irregularity.

Manual Keratometry

In contrast to topography measurements, manual keratometry only has 4 data points within 3 to 4 mm of the central anterior surface of the cornea. The reading does not provide data from the central or peripheral cornea, and therefore conditions such as keratoconus or pellucid marginal degeneration (PMD) may not be detectable. The measurements, like topography, are obtained by centering the cross-hairs on the corneal apex. In cases of irregular astigmatism, manual keratometry measurements may be quite difficult due to the distorted appearance of the mires that do not allow for accurate superimposition. In such cases, the contours of topography are more meaningful than the mild variations shown between the orthogonal steep and flat meridia in keratometry. Naturally occurring lenticular astigmatism, astigmatism of the corneal posterior surface, or tilted IOL is not taken into account. Despite this, keratometers are more readily available in most consulting suites and provide a quick, reliable means of gauging corneal astigmatism magnitude and its meridian with an experienced observer. Automated keratometers can be a useful screening device, although not as sensitive with low magnitudes of astigmatism for accuracy of axis.

Manifest Refraction

Subjectively measuring astigmatism extending from the anterior cornea to the perceptual levels at the visual cortex, manifest refraction considers the total amount of astigmatism the patient accepts or rejects, despite what has been measured objectively on the cornea or by wavefront aberrometry. Refraction can identify only one steep and one flat refractive axis orthogonal to each other (ie, regular astigmatism).

An experienced observer is the key to accuracy. For moderate to high astigmatism, retinoscopy may be a useful starting point for manifest refraction and as a crosscheck against the refraction.

Wavefront Refraction

These measurements are done by centering the mires on the middle of the pupil. It measures the aberrations within the optical system and does not deal with the nonoptical com-

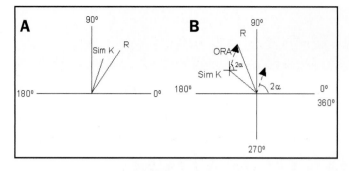

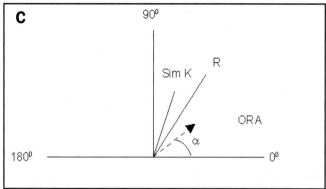

Figure 1. Calculation of ORA. (A) The polar diagram represents the corneal and refractive astigmatism as they appear on the eye. (B) The DAVD shows these same parameters with the angles doubled and the magnitudes the same; the ORA is the vectorial difference between the refractive and corneal astigmatism. It is also shown in its translocated position at the origin. (C) This displays the ORA calculated as it would appear on the eye.

ponent of refractive astigmatism (ie, cerebral integration of visual images). The second-order astigmatism magnitude and axis must be within a certain range of that measured by manifest refraction to be acceptable for use as treatment. Advising patients not to read in the waiting area and leaving them in a dark room for approximately 10 minutes before the aberrometry measurement may improve the accuracy of a wavefront refraction. Obtaining at least 3 captures of each eye is recommended for consistency.

Furthermore, it is a very useful exercise to cross-check the manifest refraction obtained with the wavefront refraction, particularly for the cylinder magnitude and axis. If they differ, repeat manifest refraction may be in order. Using the same instruments pre- and postoperatively and similar lighting conditions, where possible, adds to the accuracy of any postsurgical outcome analyses.

Astigmatic Discrepancy

The treatment of astigmatism would be considerably simpler if refractive and corneal astigmatism always coincided in magnitude and axis. Variance between manifest or wavefront refraction and keratometry or topography is widely prevalent, however, and the consequence is that an inevitable amount of astigmatism remains in the eye after treatment.

Refractive laser surgery conventionally relies on manifest refraction. Incorporating corneal and refractive parameters

into this treatment plan using vector planning may potentially improve visual outcomes,[2,3] principally by reducing the amount of remaining corneal astigmatism. During cataract surgery, preferential reliance is on keratometry or topography. Subjective refraction information is inaccurate because of the cataract and its subsequent removal. Incisional surgery including astigmatic keratotomy (AK) or limbal relaxing incisions (LRIs) to correct pre- or postoperative astigmatism may be based upon keratometry, topography, refraction, or a combination of corneal and refractive parameters using vector planning. Keratometry, refraction, and topography parameters can guide suture removal or laser surgery retreatment following penetrating keratoplasty.

To quantify the discrepancy between corneal and refractive astigmatism measurements, calculate the vectorial difference between the refractive cylinder (ie, measured by wavefront or manifest refraction) and the corneal astigmatism (ie, measured by topography or keratometry). This vectorial difference is known as the ocular residual astigmatism (ORA), and is expressed in diopters (D).[2,3] The greater its magnitude, (1) the greater the astigmatic difference between the refractive and corneal astigmatism in magnitude and/or axis, and (2) the more postoperative astigmatism will remain. Eyes with irregular astigmatism (ie, keratoconus, keratoglobus, PMD) generally have a poorer correlation between corneal and refractive values. Hence, they have a higher ORA than a normal astigmatic eye. Studies have shown that ORA in healthy astigmatic eyes is between 0.73 and 0.81 D.[2,3] In keratoconic eyes, it has been calculated to be 1.34 D—derived from a series of 45 eyes with myopic astigmatism treated using photoastigmatic refractive keratectomy (PARK) in an ongoing study at NewVision Clinics.[4] The ORA has also been referred to as intraocular, lenticular, and noncorneal astigmatism.

CALCULATING OCULAR RESIDUAL ASTIGMATISM

Figure 1A displays (1) refractive astigmatism measured by manifest or wavefront refraction and (2) simulated keratometry measured by topography. To calculate the difference between these two parameters, the axes are doubled and the magnitudes remain unchanged (Figure 1B). The ORA, which has a direction from the simulated keratometric reading (SimK) to the refractive astigmatism, is then calculated using basic trigonometric principles, and the ORA vector is transferred to the origin (x = 0, y = 0) and halved to simulate how it would exist within the eye (Figure 1C).

TOPOGRAPHIC DISPARITY

Topographic disparity (TD) is a precise vectorial measure of corneal irregularity. The greater the topographic disparity, the greater the ORA.[4] The TD quantifies both the nonorthogonal and asymmetrical component of corneal irregularity as a single number with an axis. It is a precise, convenient way of assessing the variable of irregularity. The TD is calculated as the dioptric distance between the displays of superior and inferior topographical values on a 720-degree double-angle vector diagram (DAVD).

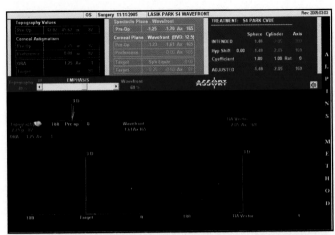

Figure 2. The treatment screen of the ASSORT outcomes analysis software program displays the wavefront refraction in the middle (gray) column and the simulated keratometry from topography on the left column. The emphasis bar determines what proportion of the ORA will be left on the cornea compared with the refraction.

Astigmatic Treatments and Correction

REFRACTIVE LASER SURGERY

Treatment of astigmatism using excimer laser surgery optimally incorporates both corneal and refractive parameters and leaves the minimum amount of astigmatism in the eye. Including the topography data reduces the amount of astigmatism remaining on the cornea. This has the potential for improving best-corrected visual acuity (BCVA) and reducing higher-order aberrations. Vector planning is used for the optimized astigmatism treatment.

Figure 2 displays a wavefront refraction of –1.25 DS/–1.70 DC × 165 at the spectacle plane and a simulated keratometry of 42.87/45.62 at 82 from topography. The ORA has been calculated as 1.25 D × 1. The best that can be done for this patient is to leave 1.25 D entirely on the (1) cornea, (2) spectacle refraction, or (3) apportioned between the two in varying amounts ranging from 1% topography/99% refraction to 99% topography/1% refraction, as indicated by the emphasis bar. It is important to note that the corneal target is 90 degrees away from the ORA axis to neutralize the vectorally calculated amount of astigmatism within the eye's optical system. In this example, the emphasis to correct the residual astigmatism (ORA) was set at 40% topography/60% refraction. Instead of treating –1.23 DS/–1.61 DC × 165 by using refractive parameters alone, the laser treatment (ie, –1.48 DS/–2.05 DC × 169) was derived from the combined refractive and corneal parameters.

The maximum correction of astigmatism is achieved with this method of treatment, and the corneal plus refractive astigmatism values remaining are at the minimum, whatever the emphasis value is between 0% and 100%. However, the most desirable result should be achieved by optimizing the emphasis to reduce corneal astigmatism to a minimum in this way.

CATARACT SURGERY AND REFRACTIVE LENS EXCHANGE

Employing incisions to minimize postoperative astigmatism is effective in cataract surgery. Application of the incision at varying points around the limbus will reduce the amount of remaining astigmatism, provided that an accurate keratometry measurement determining the steepest meridian is performed. Patients with previous corneal surgery require a more detailed topography measurement to accurately calculate the IOL power. The use of astigmatism data from manifest refraction is limited here, apart from gauging the BCVA, as it represents a combination of lenticular and corneal astigmatism as well as other components of the optical pathway and nonoptical psychophysical components of subjective astigmatism. If these measurements do not match up, then the first parameter to be removed from consideration is the refraction. The steepest meridian becomes the most effective site for the incision. This is measured by keratometry and topography and leaves the smallest amount of resultant astigmatism and rotates the target astigmatism meridian to the most favorable orientation toward 90 degrees (ie, with-the-rule).

INCISIONAL SURGERY

AK and LRIs are also effective at reducing the preoperative astigmatism. In the postoperative cataract eye, it is important to know what astigmatic effect the major incision and paracentesis had on the corneal astigmatism and to plan the corrective incisional surgery on the resultant shifted magnitude and axis. When planning the treatment, consideration of the keratometry, topography, and refraction is invaluable in these cases. This is particularly important for surgeons who perform LRIs simultaneous to cataract surgery. Accurate postoperative astigmatism measurements using manifest refraction, keratometry, and topography will give reliable outcome analysis, ie, the amount of flattening and torque produced by the incisions[6] (Figure 3) with rotation and reduction of the existing astigmatism. These analyses can then be used to refine future incision nomograms for further enhanced satisfaction.

Having measured the astigmatism of these 3 modalities using pre- and postoperative values, a more accurate analysis and parallel comparison of astigmatism changes by refraction, keratometry, and topography is enabled. This can be done using the target induced astigmatism vector (TIA), which quantifies the intended astigmatism treatment at the corneal plane and is the key to enabling an integrated analysis to be performed by any modality of astigmatism measurement—corneal or refractive. It is important to note that the preoperatively calculated TIA can be based on refractive, corneal, or a combination of both parameters as determined by the surgeon.

Over- or undercorrection of the incision effect (AK or LRI) can be calculated using the correction index (CI), which is the ratio of the surgically induced astigmatism vector (SIA) to the TIA. The CI is preferably 1.0. It is greater than 1.0 if an overcorrection occurs, and less than 1.0 if there is an undercorrection.

Determining whether the incision was on- or off-axis is calculated using the angle of error (AE), which is the angle

Figure 3. Mean flattening via keratometry of cornea by incisions at various meridia (OD). The numerics located at each meridian indicate the number of eyes and the amount of flattening in diopters is shown in the table on the left.

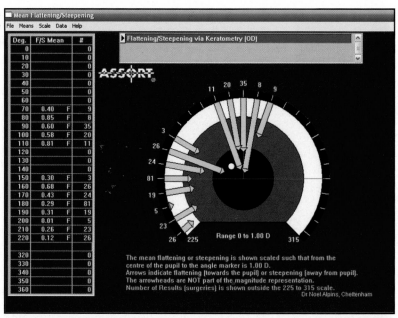

Figure 4. Astigmatic analysis showing correction index (CI) of 0.91 and angle of error (AE) of 4 degrees in CW direction.

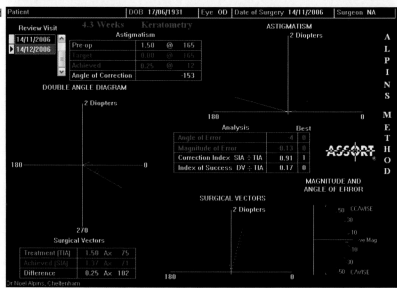

described by the vectors of the achieved correction (SIA) versus the intended correction (TIA). The AE is positive if the achieved correction is counterclockwise (CCW) to the intended angle, and negative if it is clockwise (CW) to its intended axis.

Using an example, Figure 4 shows a case with preoperative corneal astigmatism as measured by keratometry of 1.50 D at 165. LRIs were performed at meridian 165/345 degrees to reduce the astigmatism and 1-month postoperative keratometry readings showed 0.25 D at 12. The SIA, calculated using the vectorial difference between the post- and preoperative values, was 1.37 D × 71 (Figure 4, "Double Angle Diagram"). The CI determined by the SIA to TIA ratio = 1.37/1.50 = 0.91, showing an undercorrection of 9%. The AE can also be calculated using basic trigonometry as −4 degrees, which is in a CW direction from the TIA (Figure 4, "Analysis"). These calculations can be performed to obtain means on multiple cases of the CI and AE to further refine outcomes.

POSTKERATOPLASTY ASTIGMATISM

Keratometry, corneal topography, and manifest refraction are used to determine the steep meridian for postoperative suture removal. Agreement in these measurements indicates a good visual prognosis, whereas disagreement may result in a greater chance of a decrease in visual acuity.[7,8] Refraction and keratometry are inaccurate in keratoplasty patients who have irregular astigmatism (ie, nonorthogonal and asymmetrical), because they only evaluate the astigmatism as one steep and one flat meridian. Topography allows for more information about the corneal shape in separate parts of the cornea and assists in selective suture removal. Corneal topography can also quantify the amount of nonorthogonal asymmetrical irregularity using the vector parameter of TD.[4]

When planning an excimer laser retreatment, it is useful to compare the outcomes of the first treatment by all 3 modalities—refraction, keratometry, and topography. This enables quantification of over- or undercorrection of astigmatism and adjusting the amount of the second treatment according to the effect achieved by the first surgery.

These 3 measures, keratometry, topography, and refraction, all provide useful information regarding the astigmatic status of patients. When the astigmatism measured by these tools is not in agreement in (1) magnitude, (2) orientation, or (3) both, then the surgeon needs to decide where to place more emphasis—either on the corneal or refractive astigmatism, depending on what procedure is being planned.

Accurate interpretation of astigmatism change is dependant on the type of surgical procedure being investigated. Systematic or surgical technique errors can be revealed by aggregate analysis using the CI and AE. The TIA is the key to enabling an integrated and more precise analysis to be performed by all refractive or corneal astigmatism measurement modes.

References

1. Prissant O, Hoang-Xuan T, Proano C, et al. Vector summation of anterior and posterior corneal topographical astigmatism. *J Cataract Refract Surg.* 2002;28:1636-1643.

2. Alpins NA. New method of targeting vectors to treat astigmatism. *J Cataract Refract Surg.* 1997;23:65-75.

3. Alpins NA. Astigmatism analysis by the Alpins method. *J Cataract Refract Surg.* 2001;27:31-49.

4. Alpins NA. Treatment of irregular astigmatism. *J Cataract Refract Surg.* 1998;24:634-646.

5. Alpins NA, Stamatelatos G. Customized PARK treatment of myopia and astigmatism in forme fruste and mild keratoconus using combined topographic and refractive data. *J Cataract Refract Surg.* 2007;33:591-602.

6. Alpins NA. Vector analysis of astigmatism changes by flattening, steepening, and torque. *J Cataract Refract Surg.* 1997;23:1503-1514.

7. Sebai Sarhan AR, Dua HS, Beach M. Effect of disagreement between refractive, keratometric, and topographic determination of astigmatic axis on suture removal after penetrating keratoplasty. *Br J Ophthalmol.* 2000;84:837-841.

8. Harris DJ, Waring GO, Burk LB. Keratography as a guide to selective suture removal for the reduction of astigmatism after penetrating keratoplasty. *Ophthalmology.* 1989;96:1597-1607.

CHAPTER 160

LRIs—How Do I Get Started?

Jonathan B. Rubenstein, MD and Vanee Virash, MD

You have now decided to try to manage astigmatism in your cataract patients. This chapter will help you to take the necessary steps to get started with limbal relaxing incisions (LRIs) or what should actually be called peripheral corneal relaxing incisions (PCRIs).

The first step in managing astigmatism is to develop a consciousness for recognizing and thinking about astigmatism in your cataract patients. Often, cataract surgeons think of keratometry measurements only as a value to help calculate intraocular lens (IOL) power in their IOL formula. Thinking about the amount, axis, and cause of astigmatism is the first step toward correcting it.

LRIs can be considered in any patient that has ≤1 diopter (D) of astigmatism. Either toric IOLs or LRIs can be utilized if the cylinder ranges from 1.0 to 2.5 D. Toric IOLs can currently correct up to 2.5 D of cylinder, whereas an LRI can correct up to 4 D, depending upon the age of the patient. Currently, when greater than 2.5 D exists, an LRI must be employed until newer toric IOLs are introduced. LRIs can also be utilized in addition to a toric IOL for an additive effect. Because current toric IOLs can only be put into an intact capsular bag, the use of a toric IOL must be aborted if there is loss of capsular integrity during surgery. These patients can still have an LRI performed on a firm eye at the end of surgery even with a sulcus fixated nontoric IOL.

The next step is learning the technique. Several options are available, including direct observation of an experienced teacher, reviewing literature or videos from experts, or courses at any of the major ophthalmologic meetings. Ideally, utilizing multiple resources and learning about different techniques and instrumentation will help learning surgeons choose what ultimately will work best for them.

Preoperative evaluation should include a complete ophthalmologic examination and a careful slit-lamp examination. Special attention should be paid to the peripheral cornea where the incisions are to be made. Look for any scars or vascularization that may complicate or alter results and pay particular attention to any corneal thinning that may increase the chance of perforation. A good refraction should be done,

noting the location and magnitude of the cylinder. Be sure to also include standard keratometry and topography. These tools are helpful to determine the axis of astigmatism and whether the astigmatism is irregular or asymmetric. Pachymetry should be performed, particularly at the planned incision sites to look for any abnormal thinning. Elevation mapping using an Orbscan or Pentacam can be useful to show topography as well as pachymetry over the entire surface of the cornea. Finally, IOL measurements are performed in the same manner as for any cataract surgery.

Patient selection begins with the initial refraction and astigmatic management is first considered if he or she has greater than 1 D of astigmatism. The astigmatic procedure can then be explained to the patient and if he or she is interested, further testing can be continued. Keratometry and topography will help determine the magnitude and the axis of astigmatism. Comparison of the keratometry and topography with the refractive cylinder can also help determine if the astigmatism is corneal or lenticular. Planning for the correction of astigmatism should be based on corneal astigmatism. Keratometry and topography can also determine the regularity of the astigmatism (regular versus irregular/nonorthogonal). LRIs may not be as successful with irregular astigmatism. Keep in mind that the effect of LRIs increases with age. Finally, get a feel for patient expectations. LRIs often will not completely neutralize all of the patient's astigmatism and, like any surgical procedure, has its risks. Furthermore, the patient may or may not be willing to pay the extra premium cost for an LRI.

Published nomograms serve as guidelines for determining the length of the LRIs based upon the patient's age and the amount of astigmatism. Several published nomograms are available such as the Gills/Fenzel, Nichamin, or Koch nomograms. After studying results from many cases, it will be possible to develop your own nomogram or produce a modification of existing nomograms.

Prior to surgery, devise a surgical plan. Know the planned location, length, and depth of LRI incisions. Know and take into account the astigmatic effect of your corneal cataract incision. Then bring that plan to the operating room so that you can refer to it when you begin surgery.

Basic equipment needed for LRIs is listed here:

* LRI blades
  * Many types, many manufacturers—preset or adjustable
  * Expensive diamonds versus cheaper black diamonds
* Astigmatic markers with combined astigmatic dial and corneal marks
* Simple markers
  * Corneal markers with degrees or mm marks
* Astigmatic dials or rulers
  * Method for marking the steep axis of astigmatism

Deciding on instrumentation may be difficult given the multitude of types and manufacturers available. However, only 2 main tools are necessary: an LRI blade and an astigmatic corneal marker. Several types of blades are available, including diamond blades, which are more expensive, and the less expensive black diamond blades. Be sure that the blade is double cutting so that the blade can be pushed or pulled in either direction to make the incision. In addition, some blades come with a preset depth and others are adjustable. Astigmatic dials or rulers are available and are used for marking the steep axis of astigmatism. Corneal markers vary from simple markers with either degree or millimeter marks, to combined astigmatic dials with corneal marks.

Once the preoperative plan is in place, the surgical procedure begins. The first step is to mark the cornea with the patient still awake and sitting up to avoid cyclotorsion of the eye. The patient should be looking straight ahead with both eyes open and the limbal area is marked at the 6-o'clock position with a marking pen. Once positioned and prepped, a paracentesis is made and the anterior chamber filled with vis-coelastic. The eye is then marked using an astigmatic marker by aligning the 6-o'clock position with the 90-degree mark on an astigmatic dial. The preplanned incisions are made according to the markings and then the usual technique for cataract surgery can follow.

There are several nuances to note. First, you should know the astigmatic effect of your temporal cataract incision. This should be taken into account in the preoperative planning. Furthermore, the location of the LRI in relation to the cataract incision as well as the paracentesis must be considered. In the case of a temporal LRI, limit the initial incision to 3 mm. Make the clear corneal temporal incision within the LRI and, if necessary, lengthen the LRI after the IOL has been placed and the chamber is reformed. In a case of with-the rule astigmatism, avoid crossing the LRI with the paracentesis. Make the paracentesis either peripheral or central to the LRI. If a perforation is noted intraoperatively and leakage is seen through the LRI, suture the incision.

Postoperative foreign body sensation is common in the first 12 to 24 hours and the patient should be forewarned. Rarely, wound leaks may also occur and the incisions must either be sutured or glued until the leak ceases. Imperfect results can be due to several things, including undercorrection or overcorrection with a flipped axis. With overcorrection, the LRI may need to be sutured closed. If undercorrection is the problem, the LRI can be lengthened. Residual refractive error can always be managed with glasses, contact lenses, or further refractive surgery once the refraction is stable for at least 1 month postoperatively.

You have now had a basic introduction to LRIs and hopefully you will feel more comfortable offering this effective surgical modality to your cataract patients with significant amounts of corneal astigmatism.

CHAPTER 161

LRIs and Refractive IOLs—My Way

Louis D. "Skip" Nichamin, MD

In recent years, interest in refractive cataract surgery has steadily increased, reaching an almost urgent state with the approval of the latest generation of presbyopia-correcting intraocular lenses (IOLs) and changes in reimbursement for these devices. As such, the need to manage preexisting astigmatism has become a requisite aspect of modern phaco surgery. Experience with keratorefractive surgery has proven that astigmatism of as little as 0.75 D may leave a patient symptomatic with visual blur, ghosting, and halos. The dedicated implant surgeon must now aspire to a level of refractive accuracy that one would equate with corneal-based refractive surgery. For astigmatism, the most popular approach to achieve this goal is through the use of corneal, and specifically, limbal relaxing incisions (LRIs).

Limbal Relaxing Incisions

The notion of treating preexisting astigmatism at the time of cataract surgery dates back to the mid-1980s when pioneering surgeons such as Dr. Robert Osher first suggested performing concomitant astigmatic keratotomy with the cataract procedure.[1,2] Over time, a number of authors began to recognize the benefit of moving these incisions out to a more peripheral, limbal location.[3-5] Indeed, experience has shown us that LRIs hold several advantages over astigmatic keratotomy incisions placed at a more central optical zone. These include less tendency to cause a shift in the resultant cylinder axis and less likelihood of inducing irregular astigmatism. These incisions are easier to create and overall are simply more forgiving. Another important advantage gained by moving out to the limbus involves the "coupling ratio," which describes the amount of flattening that occurs in the incised meridian relative to the amount of steepening that results 90 degrees away; paired LRIs (when kept at or under 90 degrees of arc length) exhibit a very consistent 1:1 ratio, and therefore elicit little change in spheroequivalent, obviating the need to make any change in implant power.

Developing a Plan

Perhaps the most challenging aspect of astigmatism surgery involves determining the quantity and exact location of the cylinder that is to be corrected, and thereby formulating a surgical plan. Unfortunately, preoperative measurements—keratometry, refraction, and corneal topography—do not always correlate. Lenticular astigmatism may account for some of this disparity, particularly in cases where there is a wide variance between refraction and corneal measurements; however, some discrepancies are likely due to the inherent shortcomings of traditional measurements of astigmatism. Standard keratometry, for example, measures only two points in each meridian at a single optical zone of approximately 3 mm.

When confounding measurements do arise, one may compromise and average the disparate readings; for example, if refraction shows 2 D of astigmatism and keratometry reveals only 1 D, it would be reasonable to correct for 1.5 D. Alternatively, if preoperative calculations vary widely, one may defer placing the relaxing incisions until a stable refraction postimplantation is obtained, and then correct the astigmatism. LRIs lend themselves nicely to in-office use either as a primary procedure or as an enhancement technique. Corneal topography can be very helpful when refraction and keratometry do not agree, and it is increasingly becoming the overall guiding measurement upon which the surgical plan is based. Topography is also helpful in detecting subtle corneal pathology such as keratoconus fruste, which would likely negate the benefit of LRIs, or subtle irregular astigmatism such as that caused by epithelial basement membrane dystrophy.

Nomograms

Once the amount of astigmatism to be corrected has been determined, a nomogram must be consulted to determine the appropriate arc length of the incisions. A number of popular nomograms are currently available.[6] Our nomogram of choice originated from the work of Dr. Stephen Hollis and incorporates concepts taught by Spencer Thornton, MD, particularly his age modifiers.[7] As seen in Table 1, astigmatism is considered to be with-the-rule if the steep axis (plus cylinder) is between 45 and 135 degrees. Against-the-rule astigmatism is considered to fall between 0 and 44 and 136 and 180 degrees. One aligns the patient's age with the amount of preoperative cylinder to be corrected and finds the suggested arc length that the incisions should subtend.

An empiric blade depth setting is commonly used when performing LRIs, typically at 600 microns. This would seem to be a reasonable practice when treating cataract patients; however, in the setting of refractive lens exchange surgery or when employing presbyopia-correcting IOLs—where ultimate precision is required—it is our preference to perform pachymetry and utilize adjusted blade depth settings. Pachymetry may be performed either preoperatively or at the time of surgery. Readings are taken over the entire arc length of the intended incision, and an adjustable micrometer diamond blade is then set to approximately 90% of the thinnest reading obtained. Refinements to the blade depth setting as well as nomogram adjustments may be necessary depending upon individual surgeon technique, the instruments used, and, in particular, the style of the blade. It should also be noted that in eyes that have previously undergone radial keratotomy, the length of the incisions should be reduced by approximately 50%, and in eyes that have undergone "significant" prior keratotomy surgery, it may be best to avoid additional incisional surgery and employ a toric IOL or laser technology instead.

Technical Pearls

In most cases, the relaxing incisions are placed at the outset of surgery in order to minimize epithelial disruption. The one exception to this rule occurs when the phaco incision intersects or is encompassed within an LRI of greater than 40 degrees of arc; if it is extended to its full arc length at the start of surgery, significant gaping and edema may result secondary to intraoperative wound manipulation. In this setting, the phaco incision is first made by creating a shortened LRI whose arc length corresponds to the width of the phaco and IOL incision. This amounts to a 2-plane grooved phaco incision whose depth is either 600 microns or has been determined by pachymetry as described above. Following IOL implantation and prior to viscoelastic removal, while the globe is still firm, the relaxing incision is extended to its full arc length as dictated by the nomogram. When an LRI is superimposed upon the phaco tunnel, the keratome entry is accomplished by pressing the bottom surface of the keratome blade downward upon the outer or posterior edge of the LRI. The keratome is then advanced into the LRI at an iris-parallel plane. This angulation will promote a dissection that takes place at mid-stromal depth, which will help assure adequate tunnel length and a self-sealing closure.

Proper centration of the incisions over the steep corneal meridian is of utmost importance. According to Euler's theorem, an axis deviation of 5, 10, or 15 degrees will result in 17%, 33%, and 50% reduction, respectively, in refractive effect.[8] This reduction in effect holds true for both relaxing incisions and toric IOLs. Also, increasing evidence supports the notion that significant cyclotorsion may occur when the patient assumes a supine position.[9] For this reason, most surgeons advocate placing an orientation mark at the 12:00 or 6:00 limbus while the patient is in an upright position. This is particularly important when employing injection anesthesia wherein unpredictable ocular rotation may occur. An additional measure that may be used to help center the relaxing incisions is to identify the steep meridian (plus cylinder axis) intraoperatively using some form of keratoscopy. The steep meridian over which the incisions are to be placed corresponds to the shorter axis of the reflected corneal mire. Another common way in which the steep meridian is marked utilizes a Mendez ring or similar degree gauge, which is aligned with the previously placed limbal orientation mark, and then locating the cylinder axis on the 360-degree gauge.

The LRI should be placed at the most peripheral extent of clear corneal tissue, just inside of the true surgical limbus. This holds true irrespective of the presence of pannus. If bleeding does occur, it may be ignored and will cease spontaneously. One must avoid placing the incisions further out at the true surgical limbus because a significant reduction of effect will likely occur due to both increased tissue thickness and a variation in tissue composition; these incisions are, therefore, really intralimbal in nature. In creating the incision, it is important to hold the knife perpendicular to the corneal surface in order to achieve consistent depth and effect, and will help to avoid gaping of the incision. Good hand and wrist support is important, and the blade ought to be held as if one were throwing a dart such that the instrument may be rotated between thumb and index finger as it is being advanced, thus leading to smooth arcuate incisions. Typically, the right hand is used to create incisions on the right side of the globe, and the left hand for incisions on the left side. In most cases, it is more efficient to pull the blade toward oneself, as opposed to pushing it away.

Complications

LRIs have without question become a very safe and effective way of managing astigmatism at the time of cataract surgery. Nonetheless, as with any surgical technique, potential complications exist, and several are listed in Table 2. Of these, the most likely to be encountered is the placement of incisions upon the wrong axis. When this occurs, it typically takes the form of a 90-degree error with positioning upon the opposite, flat meridian. This, of course, results in an increase and likely doubling of the patient's preexisting cylinder. Compulsive attention is required in this regard. The surgeon ought to consider employing safety checks to prevent this frustrating complication from occurring, such as having a written plan that is brought into the operating room and is kept visible and properly oriented. Incisions are always placed upon the plus (+) cylinder axis, and opposite to the minus (−) cylinder axis.

Although very rare, corneal perforation is possible. This may be due to improper setting of the blade depth, or as a result of a defect in the micrometer mechanism. This latter problem may arise after repeated autoclaving and many sterilization runs. Periodic inspection and calibration is therefore warranted, even with preset single-depth knives. When

THE "NAPA" NOMOGRAM

Nichamin Age- and Pachymetry-Adjusted Intralimbal Arcuate Astigmatic Nomogram

Louis D. "Skip" Nichamin, MD ~ The Laurel Eye Clinic, Brookville, PA

Table 1

WITH-THE-RULE (Steep Axis 45°-135°)

PREOP CYLINDER (Diopters)	Paired Incisions in Degrees of Arc					
	20-30 yo	31-40 yo	41-50 yo	51-60 yo	61-70 yo	71-80 yo
0.75	40	35	35	30	30	
1.00	45	40	40	35	35	30
1.25	55	50	45	40	35	35
1.50	60	55	50	45	40	40
1.75	65	60	55	50	45	45
2.00	70	65	60	55	50	45
2.25	75	70	65	60	55	50
2.50	80	75	70	65	60	55
2.75	85	80	75	70	65	60
3.00	90	90	85	80	70	65

AGAINST-THE-RULE (Steep Axis 0-44°/136-180°)

PREOP CYLINDER (Diopters)	Paired Incisions in Degrees of Arc					
	20-30 yo	31-40 yo	41-50 yo	51-60 yo	61-70 yo	71-80 yo
0.75	45	40	40	35	35	30
1.00	50	45	45	40	40	35
1.25	55	55	50	45	40	35
1.50	60	60	55	50	45	40
1.75	65	65	60	55	50	45
2.00	70	70	65	60	55	50
2.25	75	75	70	65	60	55
2.50	80	80	75	70	65	60
2.75	85	85	80	75	70	65
3.00	90	90	85	80	75	70

Blade depth setting is at 90% of the thinnest pachymetry.

Reprinted with permission from Nichamin L. Management of astigmatism in conjunction with clear corneal phaco surgery. In: Gills JP, ed. *Complete Surgical Guide for Correcting Astigmatism: An Ophthalmic Manifesto*. Thorofare, NJ: SLACK Incorporated; 2003.

Table 2
POTENTIAL PROBLEMS
• Infection
• Weakening of the globe
• Perforation
• Decreased corneal sensation
• Induced irregular astigmatism
• Misalignment/axis shift
• Wound gape and discomfort
• Operating upon the wrong (opposite) axis

encountered, unlike radial microperforations, these circumferential perforations will rarely self-seal and will likely require placement of temporary sutures.

Conclusion

Refinement of the refractive outcome may arguably be the single most pressing challenge faced by today's cataract surgeon. Along with spherical error, preexisting astigmatism may now be safely and effectively reduced at the time of cataract surgery. Astigmatic relaxing incisions are the most common method used to accomplish this goal. By moving these incisions out to an intralimbal location, the complications and difficulties associated with astigmatic keratotomy have been greatly reduced.

References

1. Osher RH. Combining phacoemulsification with corneal relaxing incisions for reduction of preexisting astigmatism. Paper presented at the annual meeting of the American Intraocular Implant Society; 1984; Los Angeles, CA.

2. Maloney WF. Refractive cataract replacement: a comprehensive approach to maximize the refractive benefits of cataract extraction. Paper presented at the annual meeting of the American Society of Cataract and Refractive Surgery; 1986; Los Angeles, CA.

3. Budak K, Friedman NF, Koch DD. Limbal relaxing incisions with cataract surgery. *J Cataract Refract Surg.* 1998;24:503-508.

4. Muller-Jensen K, Fischer P, Siepe U. Limbal relaxing incisions to correct astigmatism in clear corneal cataract surgery. *J Refract Surg.* 1999;15:586-589.

5. Nichamin LD. Changing approach to astigmatism management during phacoemulsification: peripheral arcuate astigmatic relaxing incisions. Paper presented at the annual meeting of the American Society of Cataract and Refractive Surgery; May 20, 2000; Boston, MA.

6. Gills JP. *A Complete Guide to Astigmatism Management.* Thorofare, NJ: SLACK Incorporated; 2003.

7. Thornton SP. *Radial and Astigmatic Keratotomy: The American System of Precise, Predictable Refractive Surgery.* Thorofare, NJ: SLACK, Incorporated; 1994.

8. Abrams D. Ophthalmic optics and refraction. In: Duke-Elder SS, ed. *System of Ophthalmology.* St. Louis: Mosby; 1970:671-674.

9. Swami AU, Steinert RF, Osborne W, et al. Rotational malposition during laser in situ keratomileusis. *Am J Ophthalmol* 2002;133:561-562.

CHAPTER 162

LRIs and Refractive IOLs—My Way

James P. Gills, MD and Pit Gills, MD

When performing cataract surgery with Crystalens (Eyeonics, Inc., Aniso Viejo, CA), we have the opportunity to provide our patients with functional vision and minimal dependence on glasses. In order to achieve these excellent visual results, the surgeon must pay attention to every factor that could affect postoperative vision, including both preexisting, surgically induced astigmatism and the coupling effect. Minimizing postoperative astigmatism is achieved by managing the cataract incision, using relaxing incisions, and customizing surgical strategies with corneal topography.

The last 2 decades have seen a number of major advances that have dramatically impacted astigmatism management. These advances include:

1. Foldable lens technology along with a rise in phacoemulsification use that spurred the development of small incision surgery

2. Sutureless incision architecture, which eliminates distortion caused by sutures

3. Side incision surgery, which can control or reduce against-the-rule astigmatism

4. SLiC (scleral-limbal-corneal) cataract incisions, which represent the ultimate in minimally invasive cataract surgery

5. Improvement in relaxing incision techniques that can reduce or eliminate preexisting astigmatism with fewer overcorrections

6. Development and use of corneal topography for cataract patients to identify preexisting astigmatism, irregular and nonorthogonal patterns, keratoconus, and other corneal pathologies, and monitor wound healing postoperatively

These advances address 2 issues involved with astigmatism management. First, today's cataract incisions provide excellent control of surgically induced astigmatism, either by virtually eliminating induced astigmatism (so-called "astigmatism neutral" surgery), or by using induced astigmatism at the steep axis to counteract low levels of preexisting astigmatism. Second, improved techniques for correcting astigmatism allow many patients with preexisting astigmatism to have better vision postoperatively than they have ever had.

Astigmatism in Three Dimensions

In order to reduce unwanted astigmatism, the surgeon must lead the way in his or her practice to develop a systematic approach to surgical correction. Reducing astigmatism begins with effective preoperative assessment. Most cataract surgeons depend on trained technicians to perform preoperative astigmatism measurements, which include refraction, keratometry, and videokeratography or corneal topography. Unfortunately, most technicians do not think about astigmatism in 3 dimensions because these measurements generate numbers or 2-dimensional color maps. For technicians and surgeons to be effective in astigmatism control, it is helpful to understand and visualize astigmatism, especially corneal astigmatism, in 3 dimensions. Such terms as the "flat axis," the "steep axis," and "coupling" become easier to grasp when thinking of corneal shapes rather than numbers or colors.

To help your staff understand astigmatism in 3 dimensions, try using the football mnemonic to describe astigmatism.[1] The steep meridian of the eye (axis of the plus cylinder) corresponds with the laces of the football. The flat meridian of the eye (axis of minus cylinder) corresponds with the tip (Figure 1). Relaxing incisions are placed along the steep axis to flatten the cornea, or "loosen the laces." Applying this concept further, imagine that the football is lying on its side (Figure 2). This represents with-the-rule astigmatism, whereas standing the football on end represents against-the-rule astigmatism (Figure 3).

With this fundamental understanding of what the term "regular astigmatism" means, all members of the team will find astigmatism correction easier to understand.

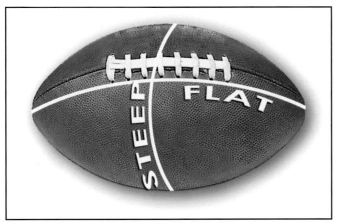

Figure 1. The flat curve of a football corresponds with the tip, the steep curve corresponds with the laces.

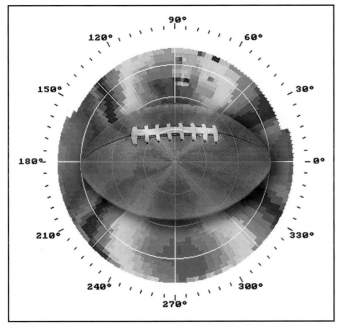

Figure 2. With-the-rule astigmatism is represented by a football lying on its side.

Options for Correcting Astigmatism Along With Presbyopia-Correcting Intraocular Lenses

Both limbal and corneal relaxing incisions have advantages and disadvantages, and can be applied depending on the individual circumstances, amount of astigmatism, and desired coupling effect.

Limbal relaxing incisions (LRIs) are simple to perform and cause little if any discomfort.[2] Following LRI, the corneal topography is smoother and more homogenous than with CRIs, and there is less risk of irregularity. LRIs are quite effective for low to moderate astigmats (≥3 diopters [D]) and are more forgiving because the longer length means precise "on-axis" placement is not as critical. The incision depth is important to consider, but does not require pachymetry pre-

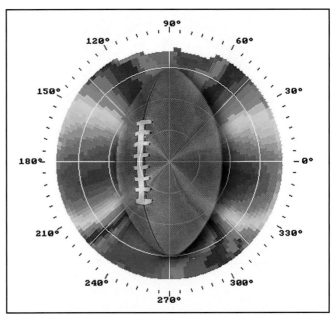

Figure 3. Against-the-rule astigmatism is represented by a football standing on end.

operatively. Refractions stabilize more quickly, and overcorrections are rare and simple to correct. The disadvantage of LRIs is that a longer incision is required. The longer incision, particularly if only one is performed, results in a higher coupling ratio. This is a very important consideration, because a higher coupling ratio can produce a hyperopic shift in the postoperative spherical equivalent.

CRIs, on the other hand, are more powerful. Because of this, a shorter incision can be used to achieve a greater effect. The shorter length and placement in a smaller optical zone produce a lower coupling ratio. They also produce a "multifocal cornea" effect, which improves the patient's depth of focus. The disadvantages of CRIs include a greater risk of perforation and corneal irregularity, and more discomfort postoperatively.

When learning the art of astigmatism correction, LRIs are typically the best first-line solution. It is usually best to reserve CRIs for use in conjunction with other procedures such as toric intraocular lenses (IOLs), LRIs, and strategic wound placement to treat higher levels of astigmatism.

Laser in situ keratomileusis (LASIK) affords yet another treatment option, and may be ideal for patients with 3 or more diopters of astigmatism.[3] This is an extremely accurate way to address residual astigmatism following surgery. It is important to consider the possibility of LASIK when making the preoperative plan. The patient should be prequalified for LASIK prior to receiving the Crystalens. When using LASIK to treat postoperative astigmatism, we recommend making the flap after the cataract surgery. Conductive keratoplasty (CK) is an excellent option for correcting residual hyperopic astigmatism.

Surgical Planning

The goal for astigmatism control for many has typically been for the patient to have less than 1 D of astigmatism at any axis postoperatively. With previous lens technology, this usually afforded the patient a satisfactory result. However, with the introduction of presbyopia-correcting IOLs, patients'

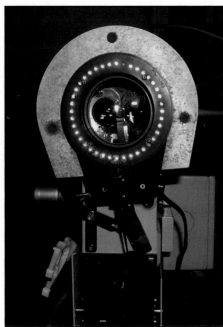

Figure 4. The Varitronics Nevyas 360-degree Fixation Light (Broomall, PA) is used to customize astigmatic keratotomy to the individual, improve accuracy, and avoid overcorrections.

expectations are even higher, and surgeons must aim for as close to a spherical result as possible.

One of the more challenging tasks the surgeon faces is deciding which astigmatic preoperative measurements should be used when planning a surgical correction. Do we depend on the amount and axis of cylinder from the refraction, manual keratometry, or corneal topography?

For phakic patients, the manifest refraction does not provide accurate measurement of the corneal curvature, because the refractive cylinder represents the combined impact of the corneal and lenticular astigmatism. In our practice, we measure astigmatism with the IOL Master (Carl Zeiss Meditec, Jena, Germany), and confirm with corneal topography. If there is any discrepancy or if the patient has any difficulty fixating, manual keratometry is used.

Dry eyes are a frequent hindrance to obtaining accurate keratometric measurements. Technicians should be trained to evaluate the patient's tear film by checking the smoothness and regularity of the reflection of the corneal rings from topography, or mires from the keratometer. If the rings or mires appear distorted, the patient should be instructed to blink, and artificial tears should be instilled if necessary. However, care should be taken when instilling artificial tears. The technician should instruct the patient to blink several times before proceeding to avoid an inaccurate measurement.

The surgical keratometer is the final arbiter for measuring astigmatism (Figure 4). It is fixed to the microscope, and should be used to assess corneal astigmatism before, during, and after astigmatic keratotomy. Although nomograms provide a general guideline for creating the surgical plan, use of the surgical keratometer allows the surgeon to "fine tune" the desired correction to the individual. This is the "art" of correcting astigmatism. When there is a question of the validity of preoperative measurements, it is safest to delay astigmatism

correction until the refraction is stable postoperatively. At that point, astigmatism correction is based on the *refractive* cylinder rather than *keratometric* cylinder.

Surgical Technique

CONSTRUCTION OF THE CATARACT INCISION

We typically perform a SLiC incision for the cataract wound.[4] The goal is to catch a "wisp of white" at the limbal scleral junction to ensure the best seal postoperatively. The exact location of the incision may vary slightly depending on anatomical variations. A 17-degree angle of incidence is desired between the keratome and endothelium to create a firm inner seal. In cases of against-the-rule astigmatism, the LRI can be incorporated into a Langerman-style cataract incision[5] by lengthening the outer edge of the initial groove of the cataract incision.

INCISION TECHNIQUE

When performing astigmatic keratotomy, we use a predetermined blade setting of 600 microns to create 4- to 8-mm relaxing incisions, 0.5 to 0.6 mm in depth at the periphery of the cornea, just anterior to the limbus. The relaxing incision is placed at the steep meridian.

When performing LRIs alone, the initial plan for the number and length is determined according to the nomogram described below. The surgical keratometer is used to confirm the result.

Although the nomogram provides a good guideline for the amount of surgery to perform, customizing the surgical plan based on topography and using a surgical keratometer are essential for accommodating individual variation and increasing the predictability and accuracy of the procedure. The surgical keratometer can gauge the actual response to treatment and allow the surgeon to enhance the surgical plan during surgery. This ability to adapt the surgery to individual variation on the spot is especially important when attempting to correct larger amounts of cylinder. By starting conservatively and increasing the amount of surgery if the surgical keratometer measurements warrant, large over- and undercorrections can be avoided.

The Gills' nomogram for correcting astigmatism with LRIs is shown in Table 1. This nomogram, which titrates surgery by length and number of LRIs, should be considered a starting point. The length and placement of incisions can vary based on topography and other factors. The goal is to reduce cylinder power and absolutely avoid overcorrecting with-the-rule cases, because we want to minimize against-the-rule astigmatism. In cases with ≤0.5 D of cylinder, only an astigmatically neutral cataract incision is used.

Patients with low (<1.5 D) against-the-rule astigmatism (180 degrees) typically receive a single LRI in the steep meridian, placed opposite to the cataract incision. However, if astigmatism is greater than 1.5 D, a pair of LRIs must be used. In against-the-rule cases, one of the pair of LRIs can be incorporated into a modified Langerman hinge incision by elongating the first plane of the hinge (Figure 5). The length of the LRI is

Table 1

GILLS LRI NOMOGRAM FOR THE TYPICAL 73-YEAR-OLD PATIENT

Amount of Astigmatism	Number of Incisions	Length of Incisions
1 D	1	6 mm
2 D	2	6 mm
3 D	2	7 mm
4 D	2	8 mm
	*CRIs based on correction desired over 4 D	2 mm for every D over 4 D at the 8-mm optical zone

*CRIs may be utilized rather than LRIs even in lower amounts of astigmatism where the desired effect is to alter the coupling ratio to minimize corneal flattening. A 2-mm incision made at the 8-mm optical zone corrects approximately 1 D of corneal cylinder.

not affected by the presence of the cataract incision.

In low with-the-rule cases, a single 6.0-mm LRI is made at 90 degrees, 0.6 mm in depth. The LRI is independent of the cataract incision in with-the-rule cases.

A 6-mm relaxing incision generally corrects about 1 D of astigmatism for the 73-year-old patient. For more astigmatism, paired LRIs may be used. If the patient has 2 to 3 D, the pair of LRIs can extend up to 8 mm. If the astigmatism measures 4 D or more, consider combining LRIs with corneal relaxing incisions.

UNDERSTANDING THE PRINCIPLE OF COUPLING

When performing astigmatic keratotomy, one must understand the principle of corneal coupling and the impact on the patient's postoperative spherical equivalent. Coupling describes the relationship between the change in corneal power at the incision site versus the change in corneal power 90 degrees away.[6] The coupling ratio is defined as the amount of flattening at the incision site over the amount of flattening or steepening 90 degrees away. Therefore, if an incision induces twice as much flattening as steepening, the coupling ratio is 2:1. Flattening produces a hyperopic shift, steepening produces a myopic shift. Creating incisions that are within a 15- to 20-degree arc produces less of a hyperopic shift. The effect of corneal coupling can be manipulated by altering the surgical plan (Table 2).

Relaxing incisions can flatten the cornea, affecting the postoperative spherical equivalent. A coupling ratio of 1:1 means the flattening induced by the incision is equivalent to steepening in the meridian 90 degrees away. The corneal power is not affected by a 1:1 coupling ratio. In general, shorter incisions produce greater coupling, whereas longer incisions produce less.

The length, location, and type of incision performed all impact the postoperative spherical equivalent, and should be considered when selecting the IOL power. If the coupling ratio

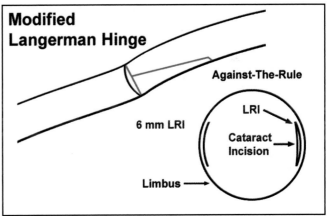

Figure 5. Schematic diagram of the cataract incision and LRI. Note that the LRI can be incorporated into the top plane of a Langerman-style hinge incision.

is not expected to be 1:1, the power of the IOL may need to be adjusted accordingly. For example, a single, long limbal incision produces the highest coupling ratio (least coupling effect) and results in a hyperopic shift postoperatively. If this technique is used, it is important to compensate for the hyperopic shift by adding power to the IOL. For LRIs, we add 1/3 of a diopter of the corneal cylinder to the IOL power to compensate for the corneal flattening.

Conclusion

Success with presbyopia-correcting IOLs requires attention to detail. In addition to calculating the correct IOL power, astigmatism reduction is an extremely important portion of providing the patient with the best uncorrected acuity possible. Reducing astigmatism requires a systematic approach with the cataract incision and by the surgeon who is committed to correcting presurgical astigmatism over 0.75-D. LRIs are an important addition to our surgical approach to refractive cataract surgery.

Table 2

CORNEAL COUPLING CAN BE MANIPULATED BY CHANGING THE FEATURES OF THE SURGICAL PLAN

Incision Characteristics	High Coupling Ratio	Low Coupling Ratio
Length	Long incisions	Short (1- to 2-mm) incisions
Type	Transverse (arcuate) incisions	Radial incisions
Number/symmetry	Asymmetrical incisions (eg, single long LRI)	Symmetrical paired incisions (eg, short pairs of CRIs)
Optical zone	Large optical zones	Small optical zones

By sharing our nomogram, we've provided a starting point; however, the art of correcting astigmatism involves using many different techniques, all dependent on the individual and planned procedure. By paying attention to seemingly small details, we can ensure our patients have the best possible outcome.

References

1. Gills JP. Football mnemonic for correction of preoperative astigmatism. *J Am Intraocul Implant Soc.* 1983;9:57.
2. Gills JP, Wallace RB, Miller K, et al. Reducing pre-existing astigmatism with limbal relaxing incisions. In: Gills, J, ed. *A Complete Surgical Guide for Correcting Astigmatism.* Thorofare, NJ: SLACK Incorporated; 2003:99-119.
3. Norouzi H, Rahmati-Kamel M. Laser in situ keratomileusis for correction of induced astigmatism from cataract surgery. *J Refract Surg.* 2003;19:416-424.
4. Grabow HB, Gills JP, Fish JR, et al. Advanced cataract incisions. In: Gills, J, ed. *Cataract Surgery: The State of the Art.* Thorofare, NJ: SLACK Incorporated; 1998:29-51.
5. Langerman, DW. Architectural design of a self-sealing corneal tunnel, single-hinge incision. *J Cataract Refractive Surg.* 1994;20:84-88.
6. Gills JP, Rowsey JJ. Managing coupling in secondary astigmatic keratotomy. In: Fine IH, Packer M, Hoffman RS, eds. *A Complete Surgical Guide for Correcting Astigmatism.* Thorofare, NJ: SLACK Incorporated; 2003:131-140.

CHAPTER 163

PERIPHERAL CORNEAL RELAXING INCISIONS AND REFRACTIVE IOLs— MY WAY

Kevin M. Miller, MD

I have gained considerable experience implanting multifocal intraocular lens (IOL) implants since they were approved by the US Food and Drug administration in April 2005. These IOLs markedly enhance the lifestyles of patients who opt for them. All ophthalmologists know that patients implanted with multifocals have problems occasionally, but those patients are the minority. It is important for cataract surgeons to know who is eligible for deluxe lenses and who is not.

Who Is Eligible for a Multifocal Lens Implant?

Only 40% of my cataract surgery patients are eligible for a multifocal lens. How do I arrive at this percentage? Let's look at everyone who comes to the preoperative visit. A flow chart of the various patient categories is shown in Figure 1. Ten percent of potential patients are excluded because they are pseudophakic in one eye already, having been implanted with a monofocal lens. I do not believe in mixing different types of presbyopia-correcting lenses. Another 40% of potential patients have vision-limiting ocular comorbidity such as macular degeneration, an epiretinal membrane, diabetic retinopathy, dry eyes, and a host of other problems. Another 10% have moderate to high astigmatism, greater than 1.5 to 2 diopters (D). After these patients are excluded, only 40% remain who are eligible for a multifocal lens. I usually describe the pros and cons of monofocal versus multifocal lenses to my eligible patients, and then leave it to them to decide which one they will receive. Fifty percent of eligible patients choose a multifocal; the other 50% choose a monofocal. That means 20% of all my cataract surgery patients choose a multifocal.

After patients with ocular comorbidity are removed from the mix, it is up to the surgeon to achieve excellent refractive outcomes so that the patients who choose multifocal IOLs will benefit from them without needing to wear glasses, contact lenses, or undergo postoperative refractive surgery. Preoperative biometry must be excellent. At the Jules Stein

Eye Institute, we use partial coherence interferometry and immersion A-scan techniques only. On many occasions we will perform both measurements on the same eye and compare results.

It is important to reduce preexisting corneal astigmatism to 1 D or less. Because toric multifocal lens implants are not yet available, preexisting astigmatism must be corrected by incisions at this time.

My Peripheral Corneal Relaxing Incisions Nomogram

I developed a simple nomogram for peripheral corneal relaxing incisions (PCRIs). The nomogram works well only for patients who are in typical cataract age range, ie, from the early 60s onward. Deeper and/or longer incisions are needed for younger patients. To use the nomogram, the surgeon must first examine the corneal topography map and decide whether the astigmatic bowtie is symmetric or asymmetric. In symmetric bowtie astigmatism, the cornea shows equal steepness on both sides of the pupil and the axis of astigmatism remains constant as one moves from point to point across the entrance pupil. Asymmetric bowties come in 2 varieties. In the first type, the axis remains constant from point to point but the cornea shows a greater steepness on one side than the other. In the second type, the axis changes from point to point across the pupil and the bowtie centerline looks curvilinear. Although patients with asymmetric bowtie astigmatism can often be helped by PCRIs, their treatment is more complex. Pre- and postoperative corneal topography maps from one patient with a "floppy" bowtie are shown in Figure 2.

For regular symmetric bowtie corneal astigmatism, I make paired peripheral corneal incisions that are as long in clock hours as the cornea is steep in diopters. The incisions are made in the steep corneal axis and the phacoemulsification tunnel is placed inside the most convenient peripheral corneal relaxing incision (PCRI). The PCRI can be likened to the vertical

Figure 1. This flow diagram shows that 40% of patients coming in for cataract surgery in my practice are eligible for a multifocal IOL. The ReSTOR is my multifocal IOL of choice. Of those eligible, 50% choose to receive a ReSTOR and 50% decline.

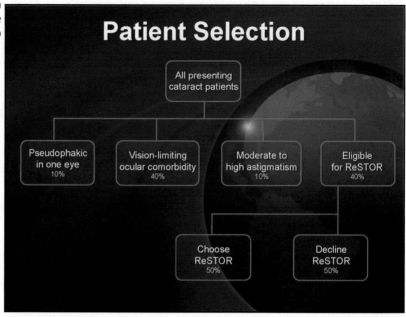

Figure 2. PCRIs can be used to treat asymmetric corneal astigmatism such as this example of a floppy bowtie on corneal topography.

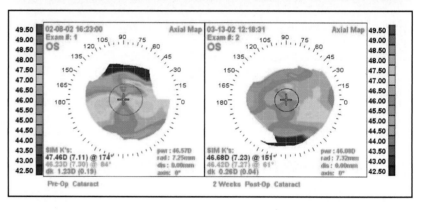

groove of a 2-step phacoemulsification incision. Figures 3 through 5 show the topography maps from illustrative patients before and after surgery.

I like to make my PCRIs at the beginning of surgery using a Mastel single-footplate diamond knife. The blade extends anywhere from 450 to 650 μm. I get consistent globe pressure and achieve consistent incision depth by making the incisions at the beginning of surgery. Some surgeons prefer to make their incisions at the end of surgery in the event they experience a full-thickness perforation. This is an uncommon complication.

Once a multifocal lens is implanted in the capsular bag, I like to position it just a little nasal to center. I do this because the pupil is anatomically a little nasal to the center of the bag, and I want the rings on the multifocal to be concentric with the pupil. If a lens is off center 0.5 to 1 mm after surgery, it will not affect the visual outcome, but if it is off by more than that, the patient may experience a degradation of vision and require IOL repositioning.

What I Have Learned

I have learned that refractive results are very important for making patients implanted with multifocal IOLs happy. The spherical power must be within 0.5 D of intended and the postoperative astigmatism must be <1 D. Visual acuity drops off faster with multifocal lenses as a function of spherical or astigmatic defocus than it does with monofocal IOLs.

There must be no vision-limiting comorbidity. Included in the list are amblyopia, dry eye, anterior basement membrane dystrophy, prominent amiodarone corneal deposits, posterior capsule opacification, cystoid macular edema, epiretinal membranes, diabetic retinopathy, and macular degeneration.

If patients express dissatisfaction with the near vision results after surgery, I hold −3-D lenses in front of their eyes to simulate what it would be like to have a multifocal for monofocal IOL exchange. This simple exercise usually helps patients appreciate the benefits of their multifocal IOLs.

Surgeons must expect to spend more time talking to patients *after* surgery. I find that the amount of time I spend before surgery is almost the same for monofocal and multifocal patients. When all goes well, chair time after surgery is also similar. When things don't go well, however, I expect to spend considerably more time hand holding and dealing with the visual complaints of the multifocal patients. Out-of-pocket money raises the level of expectation of these patients considerably.

I let patients know that both eyes must be implanted before their best reading vision will be achieved. I encourage them

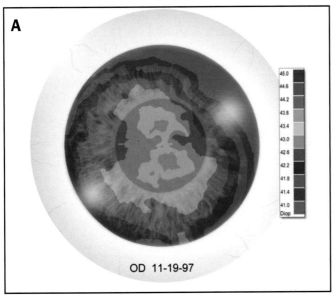

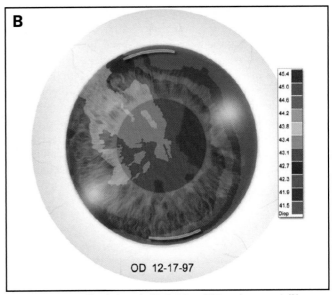

Figure 3. This patient had 1 D of vertically oriented symmetric bowtie topographic astigmatism (A). It was corrected by placing paired 1-clock-hour PCRIs on the steep axis (B).

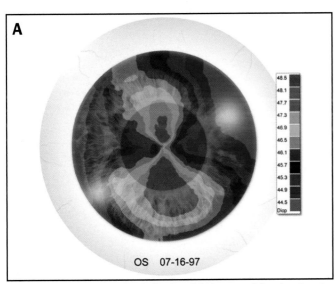

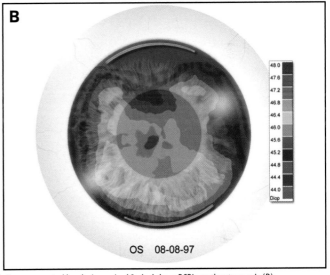

Figure 4. This patient had 2 D of vertically oriented, fairly symmetric bowtie astigmatism (A). It was corrected by placing paired 2-clock-hour PCRIs on the steep axis (B).

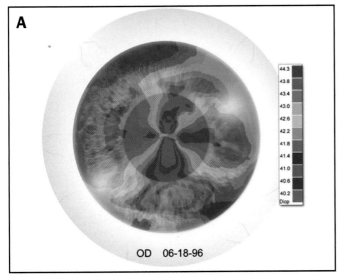

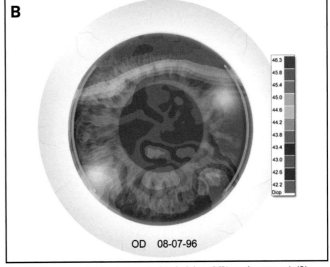

Figure 5. This patient had 3 D of horizontally oriented symmetric bowtie topographic astigmatism (A). It was corrected by placing paired 3-clock-hour PCRIs on the steep axis (B).

to delay judging their reading acuity until their second eye is implanted. I believe the best results are achieved when both eyes are focused to the same point in space; therefore, I do not mix presbyopia-correcting lens implant styles.

Most of the patients I have implanted with multifocal IOLs are not bothered by halos around lights at night. Many patients do not even see them. Although most multifocal patients notice halos, I usually hear they can ignore them without difficulty.

At the time of this writing, IOL power calculations are inaccurate for patients with a history of radial keratotomy, photorefractive keratectomy, or laser in situ keratomileusis. Virtually every patient who has ever had corneal refractive surgery wants a multifocal lens implant. My advice at this time is, "Don't do it!" If corneal power measurements and IOL formulas improve in the future, it may be reasonable to implant multifocal IOLs in these patients at that time.

It is exciting to be able to practice in the era of presbyopia-correcting IOLs. The technology is interesting, the results are impressive, and the patients are generally very happy with their outcomes.

CHAPTER 164

LRIs AND REFRACTIVE IOLs—MY WAY

Eric Donnenfeld, MD, and Renée Solomon, MD

The single most important aspect of being able to provide good surgical outcomes for patients with refractive intraocular lenses (IOLs) is the ability to treat residual corneal astigmatism. Astigmatism decreases visual acuity through meridional blur; one axis of the cornea is steeper than the other, causing the cornea to distort images (Figure 1). Astigmatism of a value as small as 0.50 diopter (D) may result in glare, symptomatic blur, ghosting, and halos.[1] There are several types of regular astigmatism, including where the angle between the steep meridian and flat meridian is 90 degrees. Examples of regular astigmatism include with-the-rule astigmatism (Figure 2A), against-the-rule astigmatism (Figure 2B), and oblique astigmatism (Figure 2C). In general, irregular astigmatism (Figure 2D) should not be treated with limbal relaxing incisions (LRIs). There are several different options for treating astigmatism, including excimer laser photoablation and conductive keratoplasty. However, not all of these options are available to the cataract surgeon. Furthermore, the ability to reduce corneal astigmatism with LRIs is more cost-effective and convenient than other techniques. A common misconception is that presbyopia-correcting (Pr-C) IOL patients will tolerate small refractive errors, but nothing could be further from the truth. Pr-C IOL patients are incredibly sensitive to even minor refractive errors, and refractive IOL surgeons must be willing and able to treat small postoperative astigmatism in order to achieve happy postoperative patients.

LRIs are corneal incisions placed adjacent to the limbus that are used to relax the steep axis of regular corneal astigmatism while steepening the flat axis. The procedure allows the eye to heal into a more spherical shape (Figure 3). There are several advantages of LRIs over astigmatic keratotomy, which is a similar incisional procedure that is performed more centrally towards the visual axis. These advantages include a reduced tendency to cause axis shift, less irregular astigmatism, a 1:1 coupling ratio, and a reduced likelihood of perforation.

For 0.5 D of cylinder up to 1.5 D of cylinder, LRIs work very well. Once a patient has more than 1.5 D of astigmatism, LRIs may be considered but there is an increased risk of irregular astigmatism. For these patients, a LRI may be performed to "debulk" the astigmatism and an excimer laser photoablation can be performed after IOL implantation for residual refractive error. Excimer laser photoablation may also be performed for less than 1.5 D, and certainly for less than 1 D of cylinder. LRIs, however, are extremely helpful for these patients and are certainly cost-effective.

With 1 or 2 LRIs, it is very easy to fix up to 1.5 D of cylinder. LRIs can easily be performed in the operating room for preexisting astigmatism (Figure 4). Postoperatively, most of my minor adjustments for astigmatism are performed at the slit lamp (Figure 5), although they can certainly be performed under an operating room or excimer laser microscope.

There are a number of LRI nomograms for correcting small amounts of cylinder and many studies evaluating LRIs have been performed.[1-16] One study on the effectiveness of LRIs showed that there is a 60% average reduction of cylinder,[17] with 79% of patients corrected to less than 1 D of cylinder, and 59% corrected to less than 0.5 D of cylinder. The 60% reduction in cylinder compares favorably with the results achieved using toric IOLs, which result in 58.4% mean reduction in cylinder.[18] Correction of preexisting corneal astigmatism is not a covered benefit of Medicare or most insurance plans. Therefore, patients must pay out-of-pocket for LRIs, or they can be bundled in with your Pr-C IOLs. In general, it is best to practice the techniques of LRIs and develop your own nomogram to achieve consistent results.

Many LRI nomograms are adjusted for age and cylinder axis, making them detailed and complex, and giving the impression that the procedure is extremely precise and unforgiving. However, in my opinion this simply isn't the case. LRIs are as much an art as a science. For this reason, we have developed a very simple nomogram that works extremely well (Table 1) and is ideal for the novice LRI surgeon. The Donnenfeld nomogram (DONO) is available on the Internet at www.lricalculator.com (Figure 6). The online LRI calculator uses vector analysis to calculate where to make LRIs based on preoperative patient keratometry and the surgeon's induced

Figure 1. Normal cornea (left) shaped like a basketball in which both axes are equal and astigmatic cornea (right) shaped like a football in which one axis is steeper than the other.

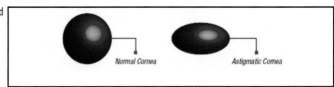

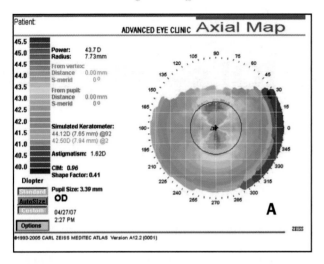

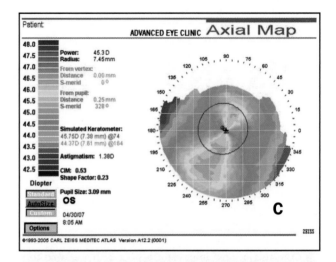

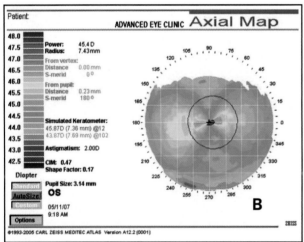

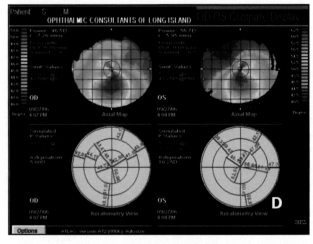

Figure 2. Three types of regular astigmatism based on which axis is steepest (A—with the rule, B—against the rule and C—oblique astigmatism) and irregular astigmatism (D).

astigmatism. The LRI calculator employs the Donnenfeld nomogram and provides a visual map of the axis and length of incisions that should be performed. A printout of the LRI calculator can be brought to the operating room and used as a guide when marking the cornea and performing LRIs.

The operating room is the best place to start doing LRIs and they can be done with routine cataract surgery. In the beginning, peribulbar anesthesia and conventional monofocal IOLs might further facilitate the procedure. LRIs should be done at the beginning of the cataract surgery while the eye is firm, and when the cornea has not been thinned by dehydration under the operating microscope. A preset diamond knife is employed, and the arc is made in clear cornea 0.5 mm central to the limbus and centered on the axis as determined by vector analysis of residual cylinder. There are several companies that make preset diamond knives. I prefer to use a preset depth of 0.6 mm. While in the operating room, the LRI calculator printout or the preoperative corneal topography can be used to locate the axis of the intended LRI incisions. The topogra-

phy may be turned upside down, and held near the patient's eye. When the topography is held upside down, the top of the topography correlates with 12 o'clock on the patient's eye. The episclera is grasped at the limbus with a 0.12-caliber forceps, 180 degrees away from the incision's intended site. An incision is made into clear cornea 0.5 mm from the limbus with the diamond knife held perpendicular to the cornea. Once the diamond knife has been placed into the cornea, it is held in position for a full second before advancing to make sure that the full depth of the blade is achieved. The incision is then extended to its desired length. We prefer to draw the diamond knife towards the surgeon to increase control. For most patients, a preset diamond knife with a depth of 0.6 mm is used for the LRIs. For 0.75 D of cylinder or less, I do not mark the cornea. For larger cylindrical errors, an astigmatism marker can be placed on the cornea and the cornea can be marked (Figure 7). One of the most common mistakes novice LRI surgeons make is to not press the LRI blade firmly against the cornea, which results in a shallow, ineffective incision.

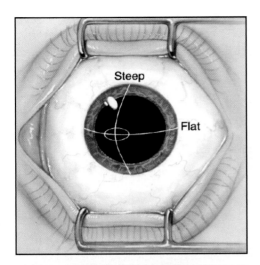

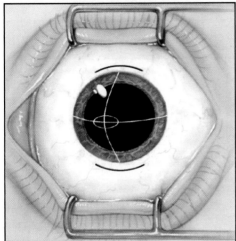

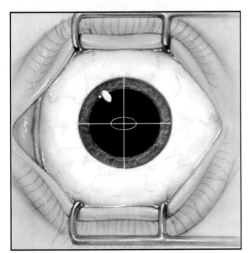

Figure 3. LRIs relax the steep axis of the astigmatism and allow the eye to heal into a more spherical shape.

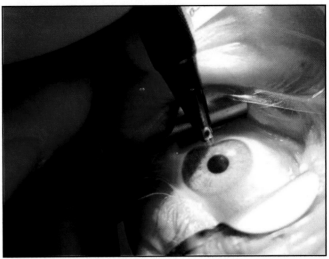

Figure 4. LRIs can easily be performed in the operating room for preexisting astigmatism.

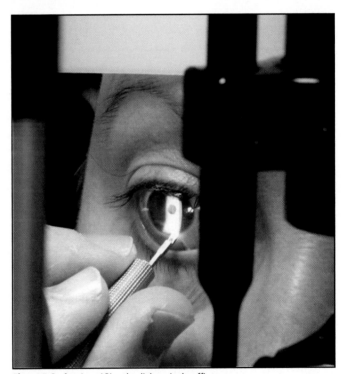

Figure 5. Performing a LRI at the slit lamp in the office.

A LRI is performed on all patients who, judging from their topography and surgical incision, are likely to end up with 0.50 D or more of residual cylinder. For example, surgeons who make their incisions superiorly, need to be aware that additional against-the-rule cylinder will be induced. For a patient who has against-the-rule cylinder of 0.5 D it would be appropriate to perform a limbal relaxing incision at 180 degrees preopera-

tively. On the other hand, for a patient who has preexisting 0.5 D of cylinder with-the-rule, this astigmatism will be corrected by the surgical technique of a superior incision. For oblique astigmatism, a vector analysis of the preoperative astigmatism and incision will yield the correct axis and magnitude of cylinder to be corrected.

There is another myth about LRIs, which is certainly not true, and that is that surgeons are not comfortable performing LRIs. Actually most surgeons are probably comfortable performing this procedure, but don't use it as often as is needed because they don't have access to an operating microscope in their offices. For these surgeons, there is a very simple solution, and that is to perform LRIs at the slit lamp. For this procedure, lidocaine gel is used to anesthetize the

Table 1

NOMOGRAM FOR LIMBAL RELAXING INCISIONS

Astigmatism (in diopters)	Incision
0.50 D	1 incision, 1.5 clock hours (45 degrees each)
0.75 D	2 incisions, 1 clock hour (30 degrees each)
1.50 D	2 incisions, 2 clock hours (60 degrees each)
3.00 D	2 incisions, 3 clock hours (90 degrees each)

- Use 5 degrees more for against-the-rule astigmatism.
- Use 5 degrees more for younger patients.
- Use 5 degrees less for older patients.

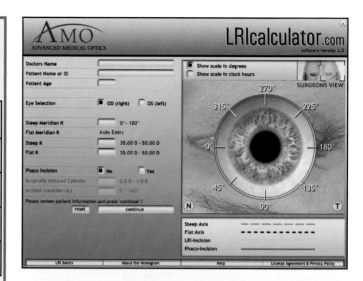

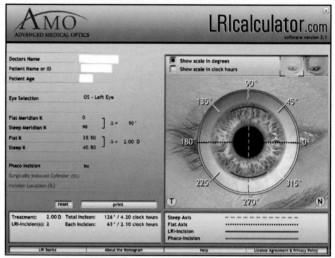

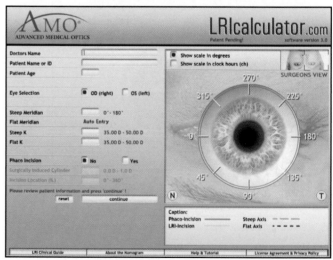

Figure 6. The Donnenfeld nomogram is available at www.lricalculator.com.

eye. For the slit lamp procedure, a phoropter is used to locate the incision axis and the phoropter is placed adjacent to the patient's eye, with the cylinder stripe aligned on the steep axis of astigmatism. The incisions are made on this axis exactly as they would be under an operating microscope. This can be done in the office with a diamond knife. For LRIs performed at the slit lamp, I prefer an angle diamond knife. It is important to make certain that the patient's head is forward against the headband of the slit lamp, as the surgeon comes from the side. Slit lamp LRIs are a 30-second procedure, and patients walk away seeing better that day. The same antibiotic and anti-inflammatory agent that is used with the surgeon's standard cataract procedure can be prescribed 4 times daily for 5 days following the LRI.

As with any surgical procedure, there are potential complications associated with LRIs, but most are either temporary or correctable. The procedure is generally not associated with glare or starburst, as may be seen with radial keratotomy or astigmatic keratotomy. The possible problems with LRIs include overcorrection, undercorrection, infection, perforation of the cornea, decreased corneal sensation, induced irregular astigmatism, and discomfort. For patients with significant remaining astigmatism, it may be necessary to retreat by redeepening or extending the LRI. For overcorrections, we recommend waiting and then later cleaning out the wound with a Sinskey hook and then suturing the wound with 10-0 nylon if necessary. For smaller overcorrections, an excimer laser photoablation may be employed. We never recommend placing LRIs perpendicular to the original LRIs for consecutive cylinder, as this may induce irregular astigmatism. If the cornea is perforated, it may be self-sealing or a suture may be needed. To reduce postoperative discomfort, a topical nonsteroidal anti-inflammatory drug (NSAID) can be prescribed.

When a surgeon transitions from cataract to refractive IOL surgery, it is important to pay attention to detail. One of the

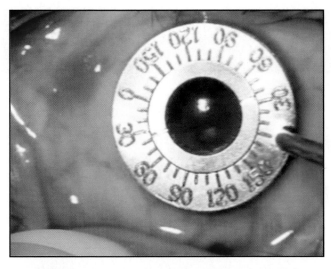

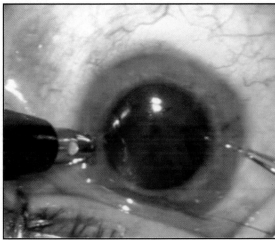

Figure 7. An astigmatism marker can be used and the cornea can be marked.

most important concepts is to treat small residual refractive errors. Learning to perform LRIs is a major step that many surgeons will take to become good refractive cataract surgeons and the good news is that it is an easy step to make.

References

1. Nichamin LD. Nomogram for limbal relaxing incisions. *J Cataract Refract Surg.* 2006;32:1048.

2. Nichamin LD. Astigmatism control. *Ophthalmol Clin North Am.* 2006;19:485-493.

3. Wang L, Misra M, Koch DD. Peripheral corneal relaxing incisions combined with cataract surgery. *J Cataract Refract Surg.* 2003;29:712-722.

4. Budak K, Friedman NJ, Koch DD: Limbal relaxing incisions with cataract surgery. *J Cataract Refract Surg.* 1998;24:503.

5. Gills JP. Treating astigmatism at the time of cataract surgery. *Curr Opin Ophthalmol.* 2002;13:2-6.

6. Oshika T, Shimazaki J, Yoshitomi F, et al. Arcuate keratometry to treat corneal astigmatism after cataract surgery: a prospective evaluation of predictability and effectiveness. *Ophthalmology.* 1998;105:2012.

7. Maloney WF, Grindle L, Sanders D, et al. Astigmatism control for the cataract surgeon: a comprehensive review of surgically tailored astigmatism reduction (STAR). *J Cataract Refract Surg.* 1989;15:45.

8. Price FW, Greene RB, Marks RG, et al. Astigmatism reduction clinical trial: a multicenter prospective evaluation of the predictability of arcuate keratotomy. *Arch Ophthalmol.* 1995;113:277.

9. Devgan U. Corneal correction of astigmatism during cataract surgery. *Cataract Refract Surg Today.* 2006;7:41-44.

10. Tejedor J, Murube J. Choosing the location of corneal incision based onpreexisting astigmatism in phacoemulsification. *Am J Ophthalmol.* 2005;139:767-776.

11. Kaufmann C, Peter J, Ooi K, Phipps S, Cooper P, Goggin M; The Queen Elizabeth Astigmatism Study Group. Limbal relaxing incisions versus on-axis incisions to reduce corneal astigmatism at the time of cataract surgery. *J Cataract Refract Surg.* 2005;31:2261-2265.

12. Muller-Jensen K, Fischer P, Siepe U. Limbal relaxing incisions to correct astigmatism in clear corneal cataract surgery. *J Refract Surg.* 1999;15:586-589.

13. Akura J, Matsuura K, Hatta S, Otsuka K, Kaneda S. A new concept for the correction of astigmatism: full-arc, depth-dependent astigmatic keratotomy. *Ophthalmology.* 2000;107:95-104.

14. Faktorovich EG, Maloney RK, Price FW Jr. Effect of astigmatic keratotomy on spherical equivalent: results of the Astigmatism Reduction Clinical Trial. *Am J Ophthalmol.* 1999;127:260-269.

15. Price FW, Grene RB, Marks RG, Gonzales JS. Astigmatism reduction clinical trial: a multicenter prospective evaluation of the predictability of arcuate keratotomy. Evaluation of surgical nomogram predictability. ARC-T Study Group. *Arch Ophthalmol.* 1995;113:277-282. Erratum in *Arch Ophthalmol.* 1995;113:577.

16. Oshika T, Shimazaki J, Yoshitomi F, Oki K, Sakabe I, Matsuda S, Shiwa T, Fukuyama M, Hara Y. Arcuate keratotomy to treat corneal astigmatism after cataract surgery: a prospective evaluation of predictability and effectiveness. *Ophthalmology.* 1998;105:2012-2016.

17. Bradley MJ, Coombs J, Olson RJ. Analysis of an approach to astigmatism correction during cataract surgery. *Ophthalmologica.* 2006;220:311-316.

18. Package Insert. Acrysof ToricTM SA60T4IOL, Alcon Laboratories, Inc.

CHAPTER 165

CRIs AND THE
TERRY-SCHANZLIN ASTIGMATOME

Allan M. Robbins, MD, FACS

Over the past 35 years, cataract surgery has evolved from merely removal of the cloudy lens of the eye to physiological replacement with optical improvements. As cataract surgery has evolved from large-incision intracapsular and extracapsular surgery to small-incision phacoemulsification, our concept of astigmatism control has undergone a paradigm shift of major proportions. With the advent of clear corneal incisions (CCIs), phacoemulsification, and foldable intraocular lenses (IOLs), merely not introducing additional astigmatism into the equation is no longer sufficient. Instead, we are now expected by our peers and patients to reduce or eliminate preexisting astigmatism. In the past decade, patient expectations after cataract surgery have increased to the point where they demand spectacle-independent near and distance vision, combined with a quick visual rehabilitation. This requirement to reduce or eliminate preexisting astigmatism has become even more acute with the introduction of premium IOLs. The potential benefits of wavefront-adjusted, multifocal, or accommodative implants cannot be achieved without careful attention to corneal toricity. Limbal relaxing incisions (LRIs) and the corneal relaxing incisions (CRIs) produced with the Terry-Schanzlin Astigmatome (OASIS Medical, Inc., Glendora, CA) provide 2 approaches to remedy astigmatism at the plane where the optical error is being introduced. By converting the cornea into its spherical equivalent, problems introduced by the potential rotation of a toric IOL are avoided. Incisional keratotomies are a quick, safe, and cost-effective alternative. By using corneal incisions either combined with cataract surgery or as part of an enhancement at a later date, from .5 to 5.0 diopters (D) of astigmatism can be treated. Corneal incision can also be used in conjunction with toric IOLs to extend the therapeutic range.

Options for Altering Corneal Toricity

Russian ophthalmologist Svyatoslav Fyodorov is the father of all modern weakening incisions to alter corneal curvature.

Although radial keratotomy (RK) has been supplanted by the excimer laser, relaxing incisions to flatten the steep axis still have applications to modern phacoemulsification and refractive lens exchange (RLE).

What we have learned from our RK experience is that to achieve predictable permanent results, the incision depth must be at least 90% of corneal thickness. Longer incisions provide greater effect and moving away from the optical center provides less both in terms of desired outcome and side effects. Arcuate incisions that follow the corneal curvature produce coupling, whereby proportionate steepening of the orthogonal axis is achieved. The goal of incisional keratotomies is a full correction or slight undercorrection of the existing cylinder. Undercorrections are well-tolerated and can be readily enhanced if necessary. In contrast, overcorrections or shifts in the axis are not well-tolerated by patients and are more difficult to rectify. Therefore, a conservative approach is always preferable even if it ultimately results in a somewhat higher enhancement rate.

CLEAR CORNEAL INCISIONS

Modifying the cataract incision to coincide with the steep corneal axis can affect to some degree the astigmatic outcome. In general, a well-constructed CCI will introduce .25 to .50 D of flattening as would be expected from essentially a mini-LRI. By rotating the incision to the steepest meridian, the surgeon can either produce a decrease in the preexisting astigmatism for small errors or augment the effect of arcuate incisions.

LIMBAL RELAXING INCISIONS

CRIs were introduced in the late 1970s to treat preexisting astigmatism in patients undergoing RK. These arcuate incisions were produced with a diamond blade and usually placed 7 to 8 mm from the optical center (Figure 1). Although they represented a powerful tool for correcting higher degrees of astigmatism, the results were highly surgeon-dependent. CRIs required perfect arcs of perfect lengths that were uniformly the proper depth. This is extremely difficult to produce free-

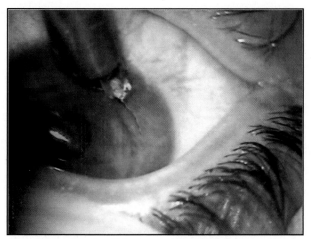

Figure 1. Freehand astigmatic keratotomy with diamond blade.

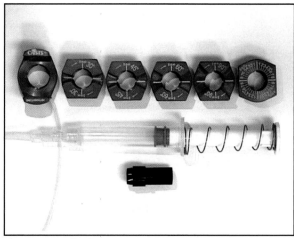

Figure 2. Terry-Schanzlin Astigmatome Kit.

hand, even for the experienced RK surgeon. LRI is somewhat of a misnomer for a corneal relaxing incision moved out toward the limbus, usually at 10 mm, somewhat dependent on the white-to-white (WTW) measurement. LRIs are much easier to perform than classical CRIs and much more forgiving. The advantages of moving the treatment further from the optical center is that placement "on-axis" is not as critical and overcorrections are rare. However, LRIs are much less effective for a given length because they are further from the optical center. As a result, they must be quite large to significantly alter the corneal curvature. Large incisions of greater than 120 degrees weaken the cornea in the event of blunt trauma and may delay wound healing. When they are placed nasally or temporally, they interrupt the corneal innervation and can often exacerbate an underlying dry eye, much like those seen with superiorly hinged LASIK flaps.

For the above-mentioned reasons, I find that LRIs are quite effective for low and moderate astigmats ≤2 D. Like RK, the effectiveness of all corneal incisions tends to be age-dependent, with more surgery required for younger patients. Therefore, my cut-off for relying on CRIs with devices such as the Terry-Schanzlin Astigmatome is lower in younger patients under the age of 45.

THE TERRY-SCHANZLIN ASTIGMATOME

The Terry-Schanzlin Astigmatome is a disposable microsurgical cutting instrument designed to make arcuate CRIs of a controlled length and depth with extremely accurate axis alignment. By consistently controlling these factors, the Terry-Schanzlin Astigmatome allows the average cataract or refractive surgeon to achieve results previously only obtainable by the RK masters. By creating the arcuate incisions much closer to the optical zone (OZ) at 8 mm, the Terry-Schanzlin Astigmatome is a powerful tool for eliminating astigmatism with much smaller incisions. In my hands, up to 5 D of corneal astigmatism can be addressed in a predictable fashion. This has vastly increased the pool of potential candidates for RLEs or presbyopia correction with multifocal or accommodative IOLs.

The Terry-Schanzlin Astigmatome consists of essentially 4 parts that are assembled in a customized fashion to address the unique needs of the surgery at hand (Figure 2).

1. Vacuum Alignment Speculum. This provides both fixation to the globe and lid separation. It also is the receptacle for the templates. The use of a separate lid speculum with the astigmatome is optional.

2. Spring-Loaded Vacuum Syringe. A disposable vacuum syringe provides suction to adhere the vacuum speculum to the cornea.

3. Arc Templates. Interchangeable templates fit into the vacuum speculum to allow for precise arcs in set lengths determined in degrees. Five cutting templates are available (0 to 360, 30, 45, 60, 90 degrees).

4. Astigmatome Blades. A variety of blades are available with preset OZs and depth. Blade length options are 500, 550, 600, 650, and 700 microns for arcuate cuts at the 8-mm OZ and 550, 600, 650, and 700 microns at the 10-mm OZ. There are also 6.0-mm OZ blades specifically used for post–penetrating keratoplasty (PKP) patients available in 500-, 550-, and 600-micron depths. Double- or single-blade designs are available, but for almost all cases the double blades are utilized. Using topography as the guide, nonorthogonal asymmetric corrections can be created with the single astigmatome blades.

Preoperative Assessment

Biometry is performed in the usual manner, either with immersion or the IOLMaster (Carl Zeiss Meditec, Jena, Germany). In this day and age, topography is mandatory to determine that the astigmatism is regular and not being caused by some underlying pathology such as keratoconus or pellucid marginal degeneration (PMD). No incisional surgery of any type should be utilized to treat irregular astigmatism. Both the Orbscan (Bausch & Lomb, Rochester, NY) and Pentacam (Oculus, Inc., Lynwood, WA) are very useful to identify and confirm the steepest meridian, determine amount of corneal astigmatism, measure corneal thickness at the anticipated surgical sites, and rule out underlying pathology. Alternatively, ultrasonic pachymetry can be utilized to determine thickness at the proposed treatment sites to determine blade settings.

Figure 3. The Terry-Schanzlin Astigmatome Surgical Worksheet. (Courtesy of OASIS Medical, Inc.)

A S T I G M A T O M E

8mm Terry/Schanzlin ASTIGMATOME™ Surgical Worksheet

Date_____

Patient Name _____ Age _____ Sex _____

Consent Obtained _____ Map Obtained _____ Preop Meds Given _____

Operative Eye: OD OS   Lens Type: Phakic Pseudophakic

Preop VA   cc   20/ _____   Pachymetry: OD OS

20/ _____

sc   20/ _____

20/ _____

Preop Rx: _____ @ _____ 20/ _____

Preop K's: _____ @ _____

_____ @ _____

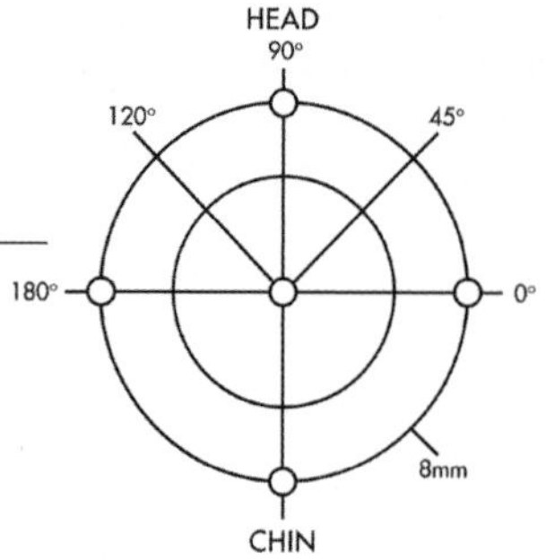

HEAD
90°
120°   45°
180°   0°
8mm
CHIN

Use plus cylinder notation measurements taken along the intended blade path (8mm).

Surgical Goal: _____ diopters Limbal Diameter: _____ mm

Optical Zone:_____ Template Selection/Degrees of ARC: _____

Selected Depth of Blade(s):_____

Blade Lot No.: _____ Blade Reference No.: _____

Postop K's: _____ @ _____ Notes: _____

Postop Meds: _____ (Postop eye only)

Follow-up: 1 day   1 week   1 month

When using manual pachymetry, measurements are taken centrally and at the superior, inferior, nasal, and temporal quadrants 1.5 to 2 mm in from the limbus. Although we have become very reliant on the Pentacam for our refractive surgery evaluations, I still find the older EyeSys (Houston, TX) unit with the Holladay analysis a very useful tool both for identifying the steep meridian and uncovering irregular astigmatism.

Surgical Plan

When first beginning to introduce LRIs or CRIs to the surgical armamentarium, it is helpful to use a separate surgical worksheet. The Terry-Schanzlin Astigmatome Surgical Worksheet provided by OASIS Medical was designed for CRIs but can also be adapted for use in planning LRIs (Figure 3). Thinking in plus cylinder avoids confusion and insures that the cuts are placed correctly at the steepest meridian. I currently do my surgical planning on the EyeSys Axial Map, which highlights the corneal astigmatism. I print the axial map for each eye separately and transfer on the margin the pertinent information such as refraction, pachymetry, age, and any discrepancies between refractive and topographic cylinder. It is not uncommon to find that the axis varies as much as 15 degrees when comparing refraction, automated K readings, Pentacam, and the EyeSys. When there is a question, I tend to find the patient's old spectacle correction a helpful guide; however, it is important to recognize that the corneal cylinder is what should be eliminated as opposed to the refractive cylinder

ASTIGMATOME NOMOGRAM

Terry Schanzlin

To provide eye surgeons with a starting point when performing astigmatic corrective surgery, Dr. Terry and Dr. Schanzlin have each developed nomograms. While both of their nomograms provide a starting point, every surgeon will need to adjust them based on their achieved results. Both the Terry and the Schanzlin nomograms assume blade depth settings between 95%–100% of corneal thickness, but never to exceed 100%.

The Terry Nomogram

Against the Rule 10mm

Diopter	65-85 years*
2	60°
3	80°
4	100°

With the Rule 8mm

Diopter	65-85 years*
2	70°
3	80°
4+	90°

* Surgeons should adjust incision length for patients under 65 years old.

OASIS

514 S. Vermont Ave., Glendora, CA 91741
800.528.9786 • 800.631.7210 Fax
www.oasismedical.com

The Schanzlin Nomogram 8mm*

Against the Rule (0°-45° & 135°-180°)		Age					
		21-30	31-40	41-50	51-60	61-70	71-80
Diopters	2.5 to 3.0	90°	60°				
	3.0 to 3.5	90°	60°	60°			
	3.5 to 4.0	90°	90°	60°	60°	45°	45°
	4.0 to 4.5		90°	90°	60°	60°	45°
	4.5 to 5.0				60°	60°	60°
	5.0 to 5.5				60°	60°	60°
With the Rule (45°-135°)		Age					
		21-30	31-40	41-50	51-60	61-70	71-80
Diopters	1.0 to 1.5	60°	60°				
	1.5 to 2.0	90°	60°	60°			
	2.0 to 2.5	90°	90°	60°	60°	45°	45°
	2.5 to 3.0		90°	90°	60°	60°	45°
	3.0 to 3.5				90°	60°	60°
	3.5 to 4.0				90°	60°	60°

The Schanzlin Nomogram 10mm*

Against the Rule (0°-45° & 135°-180°)		Age					
		21-30	31-40	41-50	51-60	61-70	71-80
Diopters	0.5 to 1.0	45°	30°	30°	30°	30°	30°
	1.0 to 1.5	60°	45°	45°	45°	30°	30°
	1.5 to 2.0	90°	60°	60°	45°	45°	45°
	2.0 to 2.5	90°	90°	60°	60°	45°	45°
	2.5 to 3.0			90°	90°	60°	60°
	3.0 to 3.5				90°	90°	60°
With the Rule (45°-135°)		Age					
		21-30	31-40	41-50	51-60	61-70	71-80
Diopters	1.0 to 1.5			90°	90°	60°	60°
	1.5 to 2.0				90°	90°	60°

* All 8mm and 10mm treatments are paired incisions in degrees at optical zone indicated.

OASIS

Providing the highest quality products to the eye care professional

Figure 4. Schanzlin nomogram for the Terry/Schanzlin Astigmatome. (Courtesy of OASIS Medical, Inc.)

in a patient undergoing simultaneous lens removal. I mark on the topographic map my surgical plan as determined by consulting with the Schanzlin Nomogram for the Terry-Schanzlin Astigmatome (Figure 4) or the James P. Gills Nomogram for LRIs. In eyes with WTW measurements greater than 11.5 mm, I use the Terry-Schanzlin Astigmatome with the 10-mm template to create arcuate incisions that are in essence equivalent to LRIs in smaller eyes.

I overlay the proposed surgery on the topographic map and write on the borders the pertinent information such as blade depth, arc length, and OZ. I bring this map into the operating room with me to consult immediately prior to the surgery.

Surgical Technique: Terry-Schanzlin Astigmatome

In the OR suite, I mark the surgical eye with the patient sitting up on the stretcher. We have learned from our LASIK experience that cyclotorsion of the eye can exceed 20 degrees in some individuals. Particularly when working closer to the OZ with the astigmatome, errors of even 5 to 10 degrees can result in incomplete corrections. I utilize the Mendez marker and either create a spot with a sterile marking pen at the exact steep meridian or the 180-degree axis, depending on the level of patient cooperation and accessibility. The patient is then prepped and draped in the usual sterile fashion. At this juncture, I apply additional 1% Lidocaine PF (1% Lidocaine HCL inj. USP 10mg/ml Preservative Free, Hoispira, Inc., Lake Forest, Il) and then dry the corneal surface. If the 180-degree axis was marked, I now place marks at the limbus identifying the steep axis after consulting again with my topographic map. A central corneal mark is made with an inked Sinsky hook and the surface rewetted either with the 1% Lidocaine or balanced salt solution (BSS).

I make my arcuate incisions, be they with the Terry-Schanzlin Astigmatome or LRIs, before entering the eye for cataract surgery or RLE. This provides a firm eye in which to

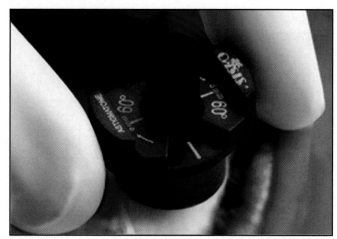

Figure 5. Vacuum alignment speculum on the eye.

perform arcuate incisions and makes it easy to identify the rare perforation. Another advantage is that the eye is usually the most anesthetized at the very start of the procedure and any oral or intravenous (IV) sedation provided is also at its peak performance. I perform the arcuate incisions or LRIs under the lowest powers of the microscope with coaxial illumination.

The vacuum alignment speculum is attached to the eye with the aid of the vacuum syringe in a manner to coincide with the steep corneal meridian (Figure 5). The alignment speculum must be not only aligned with the steep axis but also centered on the cornea. Vacuum is applied by releasing the syringe piston and centration is verified by observing the limbus at the four notches in the barrel. Utilizing the surgical plan and Schanzlin Nomograms, a template of between 30 and 90 degrees is selected and placed in the alignment speculum. Centration is then confirmed by viewing the central corneal mark. Adequate suction should be established by noting the eye and alignment speculum move in unison and no conjunctival tissue is trapped under the footplate.

The Terry-Schanzlin Astigmatome blade is then inserted based on the preoperative thickness values at the site of the incisions corresponding to 100% of the corneal thickness. Because the goal is incisions of at least 90% depth but not perforation, the pachymetry readings are rounded downward to the nearest available astigmatome blade. For example, if the readings were 631 and 618 microns, I would select a 600-micron blade. The decision as to whether a single or double blade is indicated is again determined by consulting with the Schanzlin Nomogram and the topographic map.

Although quality control seems to be excellent, it is always a good idea to inspect the blades under the microscope. With the blade guard extended, the Terry-Schanzlin Astigmatome blade is placed into the template. The indicator tabs on the blade barrel should be oriented with the starting point of the intended arc. The design of the Terry-Schanzlin Astigmatome blade is such that it will only cut in a clockwise direction, so the incision is initiated with the indicator tabs against the most counterclockwise walls of the template. Prior to making the actual incision, it is important to rock the Terry-Schanzlin Astigmatome blades into the cornea to insure penetration to the preset depth. Before beginning, verify that vacuum is maintained and that centration has not been altered. Maintaining

equal pressure on both blades, a single sweeping motion is made clockwise to the endpoint stop of the template. It is tempting to roll the blade between the forefinger and thumb, but best results are obtained by moving your arm and hand together in a sweeping motion. Once the end point is reached, vacuum in the syringe is released by the assistant and the devices removed from the eye. I then confirm that the incisions are of uniform depth the entire length with a Sinskey hook.

Guidelines for Beginning

I place the CCI at the steep meridian for all patients who are undergoing multifocal or accommodative IOLs. Although CCIs induce very little cylinder, adding .25 to .50 D of astigmatism to someone who already had .50 to .75 D to begin with can be a recipe for a poor outcome. My experience has been that even small degrees of residual astigmatism can result in problems with patients who have chosen multifocal IOLs. A CCI placed at the steep meridian may be all the treatment required for a patient with .50 to .75 D of astigmatism.

LRIs are useful if the patient has between .75 and 1.50 D of astigmatism. If the patient is older than 65 years of age, I move the upper limit to 2.0 D of astigmatism. This can be predictably managed with a combination of CCI placement and LRIs without significant corneal weakening or drying.

Beyond 2 D of corneal toricity, I find the Terry-Schanzlin Astigmatome to be most useful. The ideal first candidates should have less than 3 D of regular against-the-rule astigmatism. Patients with a nice symmetrical bowtie on topography tend to respond the best and are excellent early cases. In general, with-the-rule astigmatism is more difficult to treat, with slightly less reproducibility. Healthy corneas without any significant dry eye syndromes are preferable particularly for the first cases.

For patients with greater than 3 D of corneal astigmatism, the surgeon may alternatively choose to utilize a toric IOL combined with LRI or CCI.

Medications

The introduction of nonsteroidal anti-inflammatory drugs (NSAIDs) into the IOL regimen has made it much easier to manage these patients both intra- and postoperatively. Since adding an NSAID to the drop regimen, the patients are remarkably comfortable even on the day of surgery. This has made a huge difference in how well patients accept astigmatism treatment as part of their routine cataract surgery. I start all of my patients on a fluoroquinolone and NSAID 3 times per day 3 days prior to surgery. Following surgery, a steroid is added to the regimen and continued for 3 weeks. The NSAID is continued for 6 weeks and even longer in patients at high risk for cystoid macular edema (CME).

Enhancements

The goal of incisional keratotomies is to eliminate or reduce astigmatism without producing overcorrections. The Terry-Schanzlin Nomograms are somewhat conservative and designed with slight undercorrections in mind. Usually if an enhancement is required, the finding is that the spherical equivalent of the residual refractive error is the intended target, but the cylinder has not been sufficiently treated. The refractions tend to stabilize at the 4- to 6-week period, at which point the incisions can be lengthened in the office to achieve the desired effect. In the rare case of an overcorrection or spherical error, it is best to wait 2 to 3 months before performing LASIK to remedy the situation.

CHAPTER 166

LRIs: An Alternative to Free-Hand Incisions

Randall J. Olson, MD

Over the years, many surgeons have resisted learning to perform limbal relaxing incisions (LRIs). The system that has evolved for me is one based upon the KISS principle ("keep it simple, stupid") where simplicity is the *primary* ingredient. I have tried to look at all the reasons why surgeons have resisted doing LRIs and have formulated an approach that has been published[1] and is one that we have found to be very successful in treating underlying astigmatism.

This system is based upon the concept that making a free-hand arcuate keratotomy incision is not something that many ophthalmologists are comfortable doing.

The system uses a guide (Figure 1) that also can determine the relaxing incision length. This guide has machined marks every 10 degrees, with prominent black marks at each 90-degree orientation and small black dots at the 45-degree intervals. This functions as a simple Mendez ring without the numbers, providing the ability to orient the primary meridian. Once the steep meridian centerline is marked, the black marks are centered over this. The surgeon simply needs to "cut by the numbers" on each side to the appropriate length according to the nomogram being employed.

Earlier versions of my system aimed for an 11-mm optical zone. After more than 10 years of experience, I have now readjusted the nomogram to a 10-mm optical zone, which is controlled by the ring guide diameter and the integrated diamond/footplate offset.

A special ultrathin diamond blade (Figure 2), which cuts a 600-μm depth incision, is run along the edge of the guide by means of a specially curved footplate, creating a perfect arc perpendicular to the corneal surface. The blade is sharp enough so that only light pressure on the cornea is needed (which minimizes epithelial drag) to complete the deep incisions required to achieve consistent outcomes with minimal regression.

In most cases, I use the IOLMaster (Carl Zeiss Meditec, Jena, Germany) as my topographer; however, if there is any doubt about the information, additional corneal topography is obtained. Generally, I have found the IOLMaster results to be as good as any other reported and they are the basis of the publication listed.

Once we have determined the cylinder axis, the formula is very simple and based upon both our own experience and a presentation by Kevin Miller, MD, at the Utah Ophthalmology Society many years ago.

Basically, the approach is to incise 1 clock hour (30 degrees) for every 0.5 D of cylinder correction. The maximum incision size allowed is 6 clock hours of correction, with no more than 3 clock hours (90 degrees) on either side of the axis mark. This provides a total astigmatic correction of approximately 3 D. Our results, looking at patients over the age of 60, did not show a significant difference with respect to age. Because my cataract incisions are temporal, for those that are with-the-wound (against-the-rule in this particular case), 0.2 D is subtracted and for those that are against-the-wound (with-the-rule), then 0.2 D is added to the results in coming up with the final amount to be corrected. This is a function of coupling.

Other modifications are that I perform a full 90-degree arcuate incision either under the lid (because this is an area that seems to irritate the patients least) or nasally in that temporal relaxing incisions sometimes make clear corneal incisions less stable. Additional incisions are added only after a full 90 degrees is placed. I determine the 180-degree meridian as best I can while the supine patient opens both eyes and looks straight ahead (Figure 3). The steep axis is determined from this using the guide instrument (Figure 4). Next, the number of degrees intended for the incision as determined from the guide is marked with methylene blue dye (Figure 5). The metal guide is then held in place to make sure that the entire incision will be in the peripheral cornea. These truly are intended to be peripheral clear corneal incisions because their effect is more consistent compared to limbal incisions. The incision is extended from mark to mark by following the guide with the diamond blade (Figure 6).

The process rarely takes more than 60 to 90 seconds and it, therefore, adds very little additional time to the procedure. The results as we have published them have been very effec-

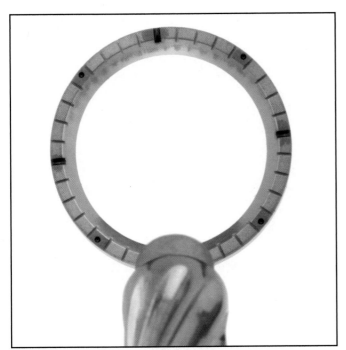

Figure 1. Olson ring guide.

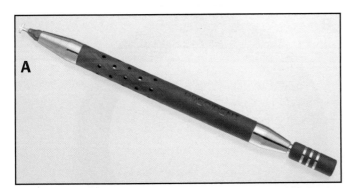

A

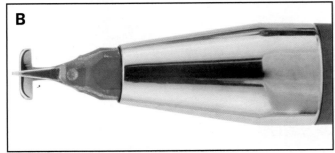

B

Figure 2. Nichamin classic 600-µm preset scalpel.

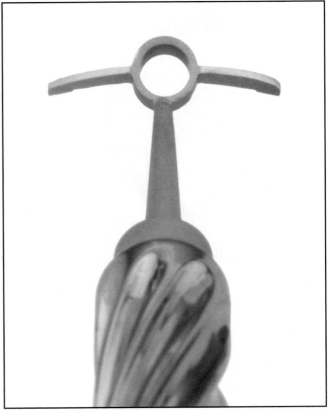

Figure 3. Bores two ray meridian marker.

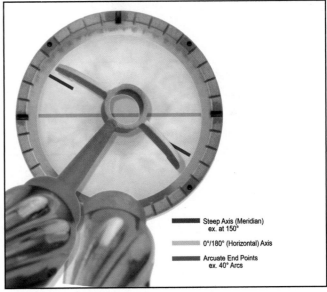

Steep Axis (Meridian)
ex. at 150°

0°/180° (Horizontal) Axis

Arcuate End Points
ex. 40° Arcs

Figure 4. Olson ring guide marking steep meridian.

tive in eliminating approximately 60% of the patient's astigmatism through a range of about 4.0 D.

Some things we have learned from our study are that patients with less than 1.0 D of cylinder either by IOLMaster or topography often did not have an accurate axis, which gave poor predictability of results. I, therefore, like to see axis consistency with both the IOLMaster and topography before I will work on patients with less than 1.0 D of cylinder. We have also found that we are less likely to have the desired effect with oblique astigmatism. Because of this, I suggest to such patients that I do not expect that we will get as good of a result, but we often can still improve their cylinder. Our work to date suggests this is likely due to lid position affecting how these wounds gape.

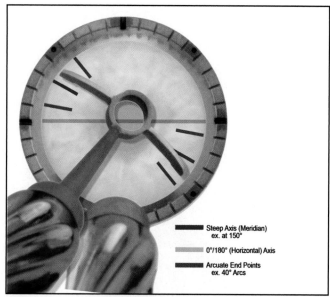

Figure 5. Olson ring guide marking arcuate end points.

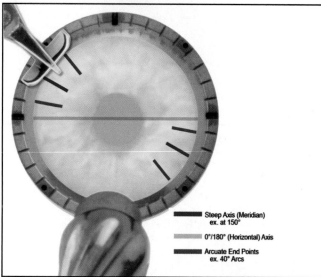

Figure 6. Olson ring guide and Nichamin classic 600-μm preset scalpel.

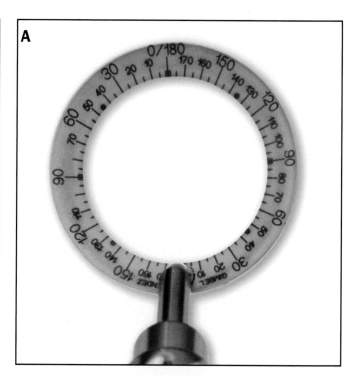

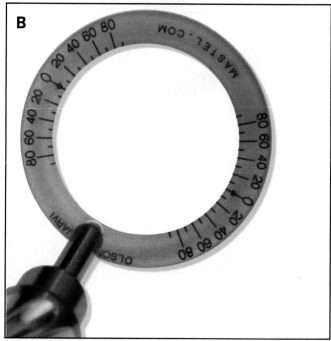

Figure 7. (A) Gimbel Mendez ring and (B) Jarvi Olson ring.

Some newer guides have been developed that list the degrees for those uncomfortable with counting the marks (Figure 7).

In those patients for whom the preoperative keratometric measures are not consistent or who have less than 1.0 D, a separate procedure is later performed in the minor operating room postsurgery, which is based on a stable postoperative refraction.

No one should feel uncomfortable with this particular approach because the system is very simple. The special blade guide makes the keratotomy results easy, reproducible, accurate, and consistent every time. Doug Mastel has been kind enough to work with me in developing the system.

Reference

1. Bradley M, Coombs J, Olson RF. Analysis of an approach to astigmatism correction during cataract surgery. *Ophthalmologica.* 2006;220(6):311-316.

CHAPTER 167

LRI PEARLS

R. Bruce Wallace, III, MD; Jonathan B. Rubenstein, MD; and Steven J. Dell, MD

R. Bruce Wallace, III, MD

Limbal relaxing incisions (LRIs) are probably the friendliest and most cost-effective refractive procedures we can offer our patients. There's no expensive laser, no central cornea or intraocular trauma, and perforations are rare in healthy corneas. So why is it that many cataract surgeons are not yet using LRIs? Some of us are not convinced that they are reliable, especially if after purchasing the instruments the results were disappointing. For many, just the awkwardness of incisional corneal surgery along with an uncomfortable change in routine for surgeon and staff have placed LRIs in a negative light. Yet judging by the swell in attendance at teaching events like Skip Nichamin's LRI wet labs at the last few American Academy of Ophthalmology (AAO) and American Society of Cataract and Refractive Surgery (ASCRS) meetings, the popularity of LRIs is growing rapidly.

We owe a great deal of thanks to early pioneers who promoted the benefits of combining astigmatic keratotomy with cataract surgery many years ago. A partial list would include Drs. Gills, Hollis, Osher, Maloney, Shepherd, Koch, Thornton, Gayton, Davison, and Lindstrom. Dr. Robert Osher has advocated peripheral relaxing keratotomy at the time of cataract surgery since 1983, learning the principles of the technique from Dr. George Tate.[1]

I have had the pleasure of teaching LRI techniques with Drs. Nichamin, Maloney, Dillman, and many others for over 10 years. During these training sessions, I have learned the steps necessary to convince cataract surgeons that LRIs can be an important part of refractive cataract surgery. Before a cataract surgeon transitions to the routine use of LRIs, he or she must understand the benefits, be confident in the "system" of treatment, and be confident with his or her technique.

Treatment Systems

A systematic approach to LRI use improves results. A number of LRI nomograms have been developed by Gills, Lindstrom, Nichamin, and myself. I first used Dr. Nichamin's excellent nomogram and then modified it to slant more toward one incision for lower levels of cylinder. Because we make our LRI incisions so far in the corneal periphery, paired incisions were not found to be as important for postoperative corneal regularity as traditional astigmatic keratotomy made at the 7-mm optical zone (OZ). An advantage of Nichamin nomograms and their modification is that treatment is planned in degrees of arc rather than cord length. With corneal diameters varying and the fact that we make arcs not straight-line incisions, degree measurements are universally more accurate.

For lower levels of astigmatism (less than 2.0 diopters [D]), selecting the axis of cylinder can be challenging.[2] I look at all axis measurements but usually select the ones from computerized corneal topography. Sometimes, especially with smaller cylinder corrections, there is poor correlation of axis with refraction, K readings, and topography. Many times when I encounter this situation with first eyes for cataract surgery, I will postpone the LRI and measure the postop cylinder.[3] If there is visually disturbing postoperative astigmatism, I will perform LRI centered on the axis of the postoperative refraction the same day the patient returns for cataract surgery in the fellow eye.

Some surgeons concerned about cyclotropia will mark the 6 and 3 or 9 o'clock limbal axis at the slit lamp prior to surgery. For lower levels of astigmatism, this may offer little benefit. Yet for higher levels (over 3.0 D), marking the limbus prior to surgery may be worthwhile. An instrument to mark the horizontal axis while the patient is sitting up in the preop area, the

Bakewell Marker (Mastel Inc., Rapid City, SD), may be more convenient than marking at the slit lamp.

Questions often arise concerning intraocular lens (IOL) power modifications with LRIs. With low to moderate levels of cylinder (0.50 to 2.75 D), corneal "coupling" equalizes the central cornea power so there is less chance the IOL power selection will be inaccurate. Longer LRI incisions for higher cylinder (>3.0 D) may create a radial keratotomy (RK) effect and produce unwanted postoperative hyperopia. Increasing the IOL power 0.5 to 1.0 D may be necessary in these cases.

Instrumentation

Simplification of instruments and techniques improves efficiency and comfort with the procedure. There are many excellent LRI instrument sets available from Mastel, Rhein, Katena, ASICO, and others. I designed the "Wallace LRI Kit" (Duckworth & Kent USA Ltd., St. Louis, MO; no financial interest) with Duckworth and Kent and Storz. This kit includes:

* Preset single foot plate trifacet diamond knife (600 microns)
* Mendez axis marker
* 0.12-caliber forceps

The trifacet diamond is less likely to chip. The Mendez marker has actual numbers on the dial to help guide the surgeon to the proper axis mark. (This orientation guide is valuable because the biggest fear besides a perforation is placing the incision in the wrong axis.) All of these instruments are made of titanium to increase longevity.

Patient Counseling

Similar to preoperative discussion of the new refractive IOLs, informing patients about the option of surgical treatment for astigmatism has become a common event in many cataract practices. We start by describing the optical disadvantages of astigmatism and the relative effectiveness and low risk surrounding LRIs. In the United States, when charging Medicare patients for an additional out-of-pocket fee for LRIs, an Advanced Beneficiary Notice (ABN) should be filed.

Technique

A surgeon's LRI technique will vary depending on the instruments used for the procedure. The routine I use with the D&K instruments is:

* Do LRI before phaco after wetting the cornea
* Mark the axis of astigmatism (Mendez ring and 0.12 forceps)
* Mark the incision borders (Mendez ring and 0.12 forceps)
* Fixate the globe (0.12 forceps)
* Advance the knife toward fixation (usually toward the surgeon)

Try to insert the knife into the peripheral corneal dome (approximately 1.5 mm from the actual limbus) as perpendicular as possible. Maintain this blade orientation and with moderate pressure complete the LRI by "connecting the dots" on the cornea and twirling the knife handle to make an arcuate incision using the limbus as a template.

Postoperative Care

For many years, we added a topical nonsteroidal anti-inflammatory drug (NSAID) (Acular, Allergan, Irvine, CA) to our postoperative cataract surgery regimen to improve corneal analgesia. We now use an NSAID (Acular LS) routinely for all cataract surgery patients, pre- and postoperatively, mainly to help reduce inflammation and the incidence of cystoid macular edema. A topical fourth generation fluoroquinolone (Zymar, Allergan) and steroid (PredForte, Allergan) are routinely prescribed for cataract surgery. We do not patch the eye after LRIs but do apply Betadine 5% on the cornea preoperatively and immediately postoperatively.

Measuring Results

A number of methods are available to measure our results with LRIs. Newer computer software such as the Holladay II S.O.A.P. includes postoperative astigmatic analysis. Surgically induced refractive change (SIRC) and vector analysis are often used to demonstrate astigmatic change. A simpler way to follow results is just to measure the amount of postoperative cylinder at any axis. If a patient has ≤0.75 D of postoperative astigmatism, he or she is likely to be happy with the result.

The Future of Limbal Relaxing Incisions

Like phacoemulsification, LRI instruments and techniques will continue to evolve. As we follow LRI results with imaging such as more sophisticated corneal topography and wavefront aberrometry, modifications such as adjustments in blade depth and OZ diameter will help us improve. Competition with toric IOLs and combinations of bioptics with corneal laser and light adjustable IOLs may reduce LRI popularity. Regardless, any improvement in methods to reduce unwanted astigmatism will continue to be an important part of successful refractive cataract surgery.

References

1. Osher RH. Consultations in refractive surgery. J Refract Surg. 1987;3:240.
2. Wallace RB. On-axis cataract incisions: where is the axis? In 1995 ASCRS Symposium of Cataract, IOL and Refractive Surgery Best Papers of Sessions. 1995:67-72.
3. Wallace RB. Reducing astigmatism. In: Wallace RB, ed. Refractive Cataract Surgery and Multifocal IOLs. Thorofare, NJ; SLACK Incorporated; 2001:167-172.

Jonathan B. Rubenstein, MD

Control of astigmatism is essential in order to produce a satisfied patient when using premium or refractive IOLs. Patients receiving presbyopia-correcting IOLs (Pr-C IOLs) expect excellent uncorrected visual acuity postoperatively. These patients are usually very intelligent, informed, and often demanding and have heard a lot of "hype" touting the incredible spectacle independence that occurs with these IOLs. On top of that, they have paid a premium to the hospital, surgical center, and surgeon for these lenses. Therefore, astigmatism must be minimized postoperatively for these patents to realize a satisfactory result and relative spectacle independence. As of now, Pr-C IOLs do not correct for astigmatism. Therefore, astigmatism must be controlled either postoperatively or intraoperatively with the use of limbal relaxing incisions (LRIs). This short chapter will give the reader some "pearls" to help master the technique of intraoperative LRIs.

Although LRIs are the only intraoperative technique for managing astigmatism with Pr-C IOLs, conventional IOL patients with astigmatism can be managed with either LRIs or toric IOLs. Why chose an LRI over a toric IOL? Toric IOLs are often preferred by surgeons who have never made corneal incisions. These IOLs behave similarly to standard IOLs; therefore, the surgeon does not need to learn new surgical techniques to use these lenses. Careful attention to the astigmatic alignment of these IOLs is critically important. Also, careful preoperative assessment of the patient's astigmatism leading to the choice of the proper toric IOL is essential. However, there are also some clear indications when LRIs are preferable to toric IOLs. As of now, toric IOLs only can correct up to 2.5 D of cylinder, while LRIs can correct up to 4 D in some patients. Also, LRIs can be used in conjunction with toric IOLs in those patients with greater than 4 D of astigmatism. LRIs can also be used in patients that have an unexpected break in their posterior capsule that negates the possible use of a toric IOL. In these cases, the LRI can be made when the globe is firm after a standard IOL is placed in the ciliary sulcus. Lastly, LRIs produce a reliable correction of the axis of astigmatism when performed correctly. Toric IOLs have the potential to rotate postoperatively, while an LRI will not move. Every degree of rotation of these IOLs reduces the intended astigmatic effect by 3.3%. Conversely, LRI use removes the possibility of changing astigmatic correction in the postoperative period once the incisions have healed.

Choice of a proper astigmatic blade is very important to astigmatic surgery. Choose a double-cutting diamond blade. This allows the surgeon the option of pushing or pulling the blade in either direction to make the incision. Rehearse the incision before cutting to feel if pushing or pulling the blade feels more comfortable. Choose a blade with a single foot plate that allows the surgeon to visualize the entire blade during the incision. This allows the surgeon to assess the depth of the incisions while making them and also alerts the surgeon immediately to a perforation when one is produced. Finally, consider the reliability, sharpness, and cost of the blade. Diamond blades can vary in cost from ~$500.00 to $3000.00. Anticipate how carefully your operating room (OR) staff will handle your blade and avoid a very expensive blade if you anticipate a high risk of damage in the cleaning and sterilization process.

Create all of your surgical plans preoperatively. Perform a careful preoperative exam and come to the OR with a complete written surgical plan. Examine the cornea thoroughly and look specifically at the peripheral cornea for areas of thinning, scarring, or vascularization at the intended sites of the LRIs. Analyze the refractive, keratometric, and topographic cylinders before creating your surgical plan. Understand the location and amount of astigmatism your average clear corneal cataract incision produces and factor this information into your surgical plans. Lastly, anticipate the location of your LRIs relative to the location of your temporal clear corneal cataract incision and paracentesis incisions. Limit your LRI incision on the temporal side to 3mm when it is incorporated into the cataract wound. Produce the cataract incision within the temporal LRI and only extend the LRI after the IOL is in place with the eye still firm and filled with viscoelastic. This avoids the lateral tearing of the LRI cuts that can occur when a long incision is subjected to the forces of the phaco handpiece. Likewise, avoid intersecting the paracentesis with a LRI cut at 90 degrees. Make the paracentesis more peripheral and the LRI slightly more central to avoid crossing them.

Make sure to differentiate corneal from lenticular astigmatism. Remember that the refractive cylinder consists of both the corneal and lenticular astigmatism. Since the lenticular astigmatism will be removed with the cataract, base your LRI surgical planning on the corneal astigmatism as measured by keratometry and topography. The refractive cylinder can help guide the assessment of the axis of the cylinder but not the magnitude of the cylinder. Finally, the spherical equivalent or the overall corneal power of the eye will not change with LRIs due to the coupling effect of these incisions. For every 1 D of corneal flattening in the axis of the cut, there is 1 D of corneal steepening 90 degrees, away leaving the overall corneal power the same. Therefore, you do not have to change the IOL power when performing LRI incisions.

Hopefully, these LRI pearls will help you feel more comfortable planning and performing this astigmatic technique. LRIs are a very valuable and powerful surgical tool, especially when combined with the use of Pr-C IOLs.

Steven J. Dell, MD

Perhaps the most important pearl I can think of relating to LRIs is to optimize the ocular surface before any measurements are even taken for surgical planning. The most important day in the life of a cornea is the day it is measured for surgical planning, and vigorous steps should be followed to improve epithelial health. The quality of the reflection from the convex mirror of the ocular surface is the basis for several important measurements in surgical planning,

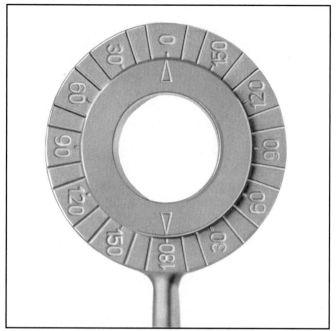

Figure 1. Dell Astigmatism Marker, top view. The astigmatic pattern is automatically rotated to the correct orientation when the instrument is set to the desired axis. Photo courtesy of Rhein Medical.

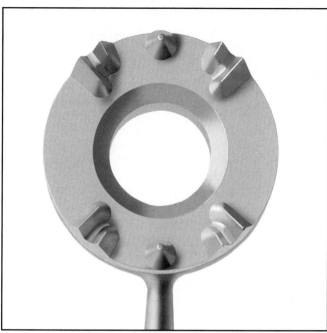

Figure 2 . Dell Astigmatism Marker, bottom view. The marker is available for both cord-length and degree-of-arc based nomograms. Photo courtesy of Rhein Medical.

and so treatment of even subclinical dry eye is helpful. In my practice, this almost always involves the use of artificial tears, and oral omega-3 fatty acid supplementation. Higher risk patients will benefit from topical cyclosporine, steroids, and/or punctual occlusion. I have a very low threshold for inserting punctual plugs in higher risk patients.

It is easy to forget posteroperatively that LRIs will render the cornea partially neurotrophic, so dry eye management will be critical after surgery as well. This is particularly true of paired incisions. In many ways, these patients react similarly to many of our older laser in situ keratomileusis (LASIK) patients, with inferior epithelial breakdown.

I always obtain multiple topographical images of both eyes prior to any surgical intervention. In fact, I would be very uncomfortable operating on an eye without at least 2 different, good quality topographical images of that eye. The contralateral eye should always be imaged as well to screen for occult structural abnormalities that might produce an unpredictable result. Unpredictable outcomes may occur in cases of forme fruste keratoconus or pellucid marginal degeneration. On the other hand, several surgeons have achieved good results with LRIs in patients with mild inferior steepening on topography. Also beware of corneal verticillata seen in patients taking amiodarone. This can alter the astigmatic pattern seen on topography, with possibly unpredictable results. Map-dot-

fingerprint dystrophy patients can be challenging for similar reasons.

Overcorrections should be handled conservatively. Resist the tendency to chase the astigmatism around the eye. I observe overcorrections for several months, and if they persist, I will reopen and suture the original incision, aiming for an overcorrection 90 degrees away. Patients with prior radial keratotomy may achieve much more effect with a limbal relaxing incision, so caution is advised. Fuchs dystrophy patients may also achieve overcorrections owing to prolonged corneal swelling and gaping of the LRI.

Undercorrections can be addressed with reopening and deepening or lengthening of the original incisions, depending on the clinical situation. Information on the peripheral corneal thickness from a device such as the Pentacam can be especially helpful in these cases. If the original incision is very peripheral, vigorous healing and regression may occur. In this case, a new incision central to the original one may be preferred.

The biggest error commonly seen in limbal relaxing surgery is placement of the incision in the incorrect axis. This can be a serious error since the astigmatism is doubled as opposed to eliminated. Several instruments have been designed to avoid this error, such as the Dell astigmatism marker (Figures 1 and 2) from Rhein Medical Inc (Tampa, FL). This instrument automatically rotates the desired astigmatism pattern to the correct meridian.

CHAPTER 168

LASER ENHANCEMENT FOR ASTIGMATISM—BIOPTICS

Johnny L. Gayton, MD

With the recent convergence of cataract and refractive surgery and the introduction of premium intraocular lenses (IOLs), such as multifocal and toric implants, cataract patients are expecting even better uncorrected vision. To provide these optimal outcomes, it is imperative that surgeons manage astigmatism effectively.

Correcting astigmatism in patients undergoing lens surgery is both challenging and rewarding. We are now able to achieve better uncorrected vision after refractive lens surgery than was ever thought possible in my early years in ophthalmology. In fact, I thought I was doing something very advanced when in 1985 I proposed routinely performing cataract surgery on patients with against-the-rule or no astigmatism from a temporal approach. The concept was in such disfavor that my first talk on the subject was given to a near empty room on the last day of a major meeting. Now, we not only adjust the position and construction of the wound, but we also have the options of limbal relaxing incisions (LRIs), toric lenses, and bioptics. These options can be used separately or in combination with one another. For example, I frequently combine LRIs with toric lenses and perform laser vision correction on patients who have had LRIs with their lens surgery. Today, many lens patients are considering presbyopia-correcting implants. These implants generally do not work well when the patient has astigmatism. However, if you withhold this technology from patients with astigmatism, you are significantly reducing the number of people in your practice who can have these lenses. You are also preventing potentially great candidates from benefiting from presbyopia correction.

Like many surgeons, I have converted to using a temporal self-sealing wound almost 100% of the time. In conjunction with this wound, I use the following guidelines for reducing astigmatism in my cataract and lensectomy patients:

* For patients with against-the-rule astigmatism of 0.5 diopter (D) or less, I make a temporal wound and use aspheric monofocal or multifocal IOLs.

* For patients with against-the-rule and with-the-rule astigmatism of 0.5 to 2 D, I perform LRIs if the patient is having a multifocal or aspheric IOL implanted; otherwise, I recommend a toric IOL.

* Patients with corneal astigmatism of more than 2 D should undergo laser vision correction postoperatively, receive a toric IOL, or undergo a combination of 2 or more astigmatism correction methods.

It is imperative to make patients understand that astigmatism surgery and lens surgery are 2 separate procedures. This helps justify the additional surgical fee and lets them know that they are having a more complicated procedure. Also, I stress that LRIs are meant to reduce astigmatism, but not necessarily eliminate it. LRIs are somewhat unpredictable, with some patients getting very little response. Consequently, I tell patients that the surgery may keep them from having to undergo a laser procedure, but if it doesn't, it will at least reduce the amount of laser correction needed. If the patient wants to have only one procedure to correct the astigmatism, I encourage them to consider either laser vision correction or the toric IOL.

My approach to the bioptics patient is as follows. Whatever IOL is chosen, I plan to have a myopic result unless the patient has a very flat cornea. I prefer doing a myopic ablation because visual recovery is generally faster. For example, if a patient has 3 D of corneal astigmatism, I try to achieve a post lens refraction of $-0.5-3.0 \times$ at whatever axis. We have an inventory of loaner glasses to get the patient through the approximately 6 weeks that must transpire between the lens surgery and the laser vision correction. In patients with very flat corneas, such as post–radial keratotomy (RK) patients, I actually prefer to steepen the cornea a bit by doing a hyperopic ablation. Consequently, we try to target the patient near plano or with a slightly hyperopic spherical equivalent. If the patient has preexisting dry eyes, I usually start Restasis (Allergan, Irvine, CA) and/or insert punctal plugs. I also encourage the use of omega 3 and flaxseed oil capsules. Patients are also told to take 1000 mg of vitamin C per day for 6 months in order to reduce haze.

I prefer surface laser treatment to laser in situ keratomileusis (LASIK) for many reasons, and I think it is especially advantageous in multifocal patients. As we all know, a dry eye is detrimental to quality of vision in patients with multifocal lenses, and LASIK certainly causes more long-term dry eye than surface ablation.[1,2] I am especially concerned about the strategy of cutting a LASIK flap on patients prior to lens surgery. We know that lens removal causes temporary surface problems due to medications, irrigation, and severing of a few corneal nerves. These surface problems are magnified in the dry eye patient, and creating a preoperative LASIK flap causes an immediate dry eye. The flap also turns out to be unnecessary in some patients.

With surface ablation, corneal innervation and tear production generally return to prelaser levels in 6 to 12 months.[3-6] This is especially beneficial to the elderly patient with reduced tear production and the multifocal patient.

Because there are no absolutes in the surgical management of astigmatism, I would like to present some case studies to show how they were managed.

Toric Intraocular Lens With a Limbal Relaxing Incision

A 77-year-old woman presented with a cataract and astigmatism in her right eye. She experienced glare during the day and at night, and she was unable to drive at night secondary to poor vision. Preoperatively, her uncorrected distance visual acuity was 20/200, and her manifest refraction was +2.00+3.75 × 010 = 20/25. Keratometry readings were 43.37 × 100 degrees/46.37 × 010 degrees. She underwent phaco with AcrySof Toric IOL (SN60T5) (Alcon, Fort Worth, TX) implantation and LRIs. The placement of the 2 LRIs was as follows: one at 40 degrees of arc at 010 degree and one at 40 degrees of arc at 190 degrees. Postoperatively, her uncorrected distance visual acuity improved to 20/60. Manifest refraction was −1.00 sphere = 20/20. Keratometry was 44.2 × 088/45.75 × 178.

Laser Vision Correction After Lens Surgery

A 42-year-old woman had a history of lensectomy with AcrySof ReSTOR IOL implantation in both eyes. Residual astigmatism would be treated with surface laser ablation after lensectomy. Target refraction was −1.15 D in the right eye and −0.96 D in the left eye.

Before laser vision correction, her uncorrected distance visual acuity was 20/40 in the right eye and 20/60 in the left eye, and her uncorrected near visual acuity was 20/30 OD and 20/50 OS. Manifest refraction was −1.50+1.50 × 100 = 20/20 in the right eye and −1.75+2.25 × 090 = 20/20 in the left eye. Keratometry was 43.50 × 001/45.25 × 091 in the right eye and 43.25 × 176/46.12 × 086 in the left eye.

She underwent surface laser ablation in both eyes to treat residual astigmatism. One-year postoperative lensectomy and surface laser ablation, her uncorrected distance visual acuity was 20/25 in the right eye and 20/20 in the left eye. Uncorrected near visual acuity was 20/20 in the right eye and 20/25 in the left eye. Manifest refraction was +0.50 sphere = 20/20 in the right eye and −0.25+0.25 × 090 = 20/20 in the left eye.

Toric Intraocular Lens, Mild Astigmatism

A 78-year-old man had a cataract and astigmatism in his right eye. He complained of problems with glare during the day and at night, and he also experienced decreased distance and near vision. Preoperatively, his uncorrected distance visual acuity was 20/50, and his uncorrected near visual acuity was 20/40.

Manifest refraction was −1.50+1.50 × 010 = 20/40. With +2.50 add, he was 20/20. Keratometry was 44.25 × 095/45.50 × 005.

He underwent phacoemulsification and AcrySof Toric IOL (SN60T3) implantation. Postoperatively, his uncorrected distance visual acuity was 20/20, and his uncorrected near visual acuity was 20/200.

His manifest refraction was plano.

Laser Vision Correction After Lens Surgery on Preexisting Radial Keratotomy

A 50-year-old woman had a history of RK and phacoemulsification with IOL implantation in her right eye. Her uncorrected distance visual acuity was 20/40, and manifest refraction was +0.50+0.50 × 031 = 20/25. Keratometry was 35.50 × 118/36.00 × 028.

She then underwent surface laser ablation. Postoperatively, her uncorrected distance visual acuity was 20/30. Manifest refraction was −0.50 sphere = 20/25.

Toric Lens Surgery on Preexisting Radial/Astigmatic Keratotomy and Penetrating Keratoplasty

A 50-year-old man had a history of extensive RK/astigmatic keratotomy (AK) in his left eye and penetrating keratoplasty (PKP) due to severe visual fluctuation and corneal scarring. He then developed a cataract. Before cataract surgery, his uncorrected distance visual acuity was 20/400. Manifest refraction was −10.00+3.50 × 005 = 20/30, and keratometry was 43.87 × 079/46.25 × 169.

The patient underwent phacoemulsification and AcrySof Toric IOL (SN60T5) implantation. Postoperatively, his uncorrected distance visual acuity was 20/200, and his uncorrected near visual acuity was 20/20. Manifest refraction was −2.50+0.75 × 092 = 20/25, and keratometry was 44.75 × 069/45.50 × 159.

Toric Lens Surgery on Preexisting Radial Keratotomy and Laser In Situ Keratomileusis

A 60-year-old man had a history of RK and LASIK in his right eye. He complained of decreased vision and problems with glare during the day and at night. He had also developed a cataract in his right eye.

Before cataract surgery, his uncorrected distance visual acuity was 20/50. Manifest refraction was $-2.00+1.00 \times 003 = 20/30$, and keratometry was $46.23 \times 083/47.20 \times 173$.

He underwent phacoemulsification and AcrySof Toric IOL (SN60T3) implantation. Postoperatively, his uncorrected distance visual acuity was 20/20 +2, with a manifest refraction of plano.

Conclusion

The introduction of premium IOLs and the convergence of cataract and refractive surgery have raised the bar with respect to patient expectations. To achieve the best outcomes for patients, proper management and reduction of astigmatism is critical. The first tool in effectively managing astigmatism is the cataract incision itself. Surgeons must understand how much surgically induced astigmatism is produced by the incision and become comfortable with moving its location in order to maximize or utilize its effect. They must also understand the use of incisional and pseudophakic methods of correcting astigmatism, such as LRIs or AK, lasers, and toric IOLs, individually and in combination, to achieve the best outcomes for patients.

References

1. Charters L. Numerous risk factors found for corneal ectasia after LASIK. *Ophthalmol Times.* 2006;31:1, 42.

2. Trattler W. Known risk factors for ectasia. *Cataract Refract Surg Today.* 2005:109-113.

3. Erie JC, McLaren JW, Hodge DO, Bourne WM. Recovery of corneal subbasal nerve density after PRK and LASIK. *Am J Ophthalmol.* 2005;140:1059-1064.

4. Duteille F, Petry D, Dautel G, et al. A comparison between clinical results and electromyographic analysis after median or ulnar nerve injuries in children's wrists. *Ann Plastic Surg.* 2001;46:382-386.

5. Perez-Gomez I, Efron N. Change to corneal morphology after refractive surgery as viewed with a confocal microscope. *Optom Vis Sci.* 2003;80:690-697.

6. Lee SJ, Kim KJ, Seo KY, et al. Comparison of corneal nerve regeneration and sensitivity between LASIK and laser epithelial keratomileusis (LASEK). *Am J Ophthalmol.* 2006;141:1009-1015.

CHAPTER 169

TORIC IOLS—
HOW DO I GET STARTED?

Jeffrey D. Horn, MD

Rapid improvements in both cataract surgical techniques and technologies have, combined with the success of laser vision correction, elevated our patients' demands and expectations to an all-time high. This is often reflected in our patients' desire to be spectacle independent following surgery. This, in turn, often requires that preexisting astigmatism be corrected at the time of cataract surgery. It has been reported that 15% to 20% of patients undergoing cataract surgery have at least 1.5 diopters (D) of preexisting corneal astigmatism.[1]

Options for treating preexisting corneal astigmatism at the time of cataract surgery include toric lens implants and incisional techniques, such as limbal relaxing incisions (LRI) or astigmatic keratotomy (AK). Laser vision correction (laser in situ keratomileusis [LASIK] or photorefractive keratectomy [PRK]) performed after cataract surgery may also be used.

Historically, most surgeons who treated astigmatism in cataract patients tended to rely on corneal incision–based surgery. Although effective, these techniques are limited by the amount of correction possible. In addition, there may be potentially unpredictable outcomes with under- or overcorrections due to variations in technique and variability in patient healing. Finally, incisional keratotomy introduces the possibility of complications such as wound gape or perforation. LASIK requires an additional procedure, and may be cost prohibitive to both the patient and surgeon.

My preferred approach for these patients, therefore, is to implant a toric intraocular lens (IOL) at the time of surgery. This is assuming the patient does not desire presbyopia correction with a multifocal or accommodative IOL. In patients with corneal cylinder of significant magnitude, I may combine the toric lens with LRIs, but this is beyond the scope of this chapter. Currently, there are 2 toric implants available in the United States: the STAAR Toric IOL (STAAR Surgical, Monrovia, CA) and the Acrysof Toric IOL (Alcon, Fort Worth, TX). The Acrysof lens is based on the SN60AT design, a one-piece hydrophobic acrylic lens with a yellow chromophore. The lens comes in cylindrical powers of 1.50 (T3), 2.25 (T4), and 3.00 (T5) D. This corresponds to 1.03, 1.55, and 2.06 D of correction at the spectacle plane. It is available in a spherical range of 6 to 30 D. Because of rotational stability problems with the STAAR lens, my toric lens of choice in virtually all cases is the Acrysof.[2,3]

As with any surgical procedure, the most important determinant of a good outcome, in addition to good surgical technique (and excellent biometry in the case of lens-based surgery) is proper patient selection. This is especially important for those surgeons who are just adding toric IOLs to their armamentarium. The cataract patient must have astigmatism, and desire relative spectacle independence, at least for distance (remember, these are monofocal implants) in order to qualify for consideration. Surgeons typically have many questions prior to using toric IOLs for the first time. How much astigmatism is necessary in order to use this strategy, and how much is too much (at least for a surgeon's first cases)? What type of astigmatism does the patient have and why does this matter? What other anatomical factors should be considered for the first few cases, until the surgeon is comfortable with using these IOLs? Last, but not least, are the financial considerations, because toric lenses are more costly. They require a greater amount of preoperative testing, and slightly increased surgical times with a few extra surgical maneuvers.

The first point to address, of course, is determining how much of the patient's astigmatism actually requires correction. In other words, astigmatism for this discussion can be defined as either *refractive* (that amount found in the patient's refraction or glasses) or *corneal* (that amount on the cornea as measured with keratometry or topography). Because the patient is undergoing cataract removal, only corneal astigmatism should be considered when determining the need for a toric IOL. A patient may have several diopters of cylinder in his or her glasses, but minimal corneal cylinder. This patient requires cataract surgery with a non-toric lens. Likewise, the patient may have little or no cylindrical correction in his or her refraction, but may be left with a significant amount postoperatively if a toric lens is not used, because he or she had significant corneal astigmatism that was in effect negated, or masked, by the human crystalline lens. Both the magnitude and direction of astigmatism need to be accurately measured. I would suggest a manual keratometer for the determination of both the magnitude and particularly the axis of astigmatism. Also, because most cataract incisions are not entirely astigmatically neutral, it is important for the surgeon to know how his or her incision impacts corneal curvature. This will have an effect on the residual corneal cylinder, which is the ultimate factor in determining which power toric IOL (if any) is indicated, and at what axis it should be aligned. The online Alcon Toric Calculator (www.acrysoftoriccalculator.com) takes the effect of the incision into account in order to determine both the power of the cylindrical portion of the lens (T3, T4, or T5) and the proper axis of final lens orientation. The surgeon first calculates the spherical lens power using his or her preferred IOL formula, and then inputs this into the calculator. For purposes of those surgeons new to this technology, I would recommend starting with a patient who would fall into the T4 or T5 category, if for no other reason than you will have increased gratification when you correct a significant amount of astigmatism, and can then understand how well this technology works. I personally use the T3 lens frequently, as even these patients realize significant benefit.

Not only is it important to determine corneal astigmatism accurately, but it is also important to determine the nature of the astigmatism. These lenses were specifically designed to correct regular astigmatism, and it is for these eyes that the lens works best. Although some may advocate using these lenses in more complicated situations, such as in patients with keratoconus or other causes of irregular astigmatism, I would not suggest using these toric IOLs for these patients. Therefore, corneal topography is essential in determining one's candidacy for a toric lens implant.

If the patient meets the necessary criteria based upon the preoperative data, the next pearl I would offer to the beginning toric implant surgeon would be to check pupil size. Because the marks on the lens denoting its axis are at the periphery, inadequately dilated or miotic pupils can make positioning the lens difficult at best. The only potentially new surgical techniques include marking the eye pre- and intraoperatively, and careful rotation of the lens to align it with the marks found on the lens optic near the haptics. Marking the eye is a 2-step process. I first mark the eye in the operative suite (or in the preoperative area) at the 3- and 9-o'clock limbi with a gentian violet marker. This can either be done freehand or with a commercially available marker. This should be performed with the patient seated upright as cyclotorsion of the eye is not uncommon in the supine position. These marks can be reinforced at the start of surgery. After removal of the cataract and reinflation of the capsule with viscoelastic, the surgeon then marks the eye with an astigmatic marker aligned with the previously placed reference marks, and set to the axis of final lens position determined by the toric calculator. I use a Dell Marker (Rhein

Medical, Inc., Tampa, FL) for this step. My technique for toric IOL alignment is to completely remove the viscoelastic with the lens approximately 10 degrees underrotated, and then use the silicone sleeve irrigation and aspiration (I&A) tip on foot position 1 to rotate the lens into the proper position. I would suggest practicing this maneuver on non-toric Acrysof lenses first, to become accustomed to the technique, because these implants are sticky (which is why they have such excellent rotational stability). It is not a hard procedure to master. One note of caution is to make certain the proper axis has been marked. One can perform beautiful surgery only to place the lens at the wrong axis. I print the page that is provided by the calculator showing in diagrammatic form the proper axis of implantation and hang it on the operating microscope to help prevent this from occurring.

The only other variable in the surgical procedure itself is the incision size and location. These lenses go through a 2.2- to 3-mm incision using the Monarch II injector with the C cartridge. Although the individual surgeon can make the incision at any meridian (eg, operating on the steep axis), I would suggest using the online calculator to calculate surgically induced astigmatism as discussed previously, and make the incision where he or she normally would. In other words, change as little as possible.

Because toric implants are designed to reduce preexisting corneal astigmatism, the best measurements of success are uncorrected distance vision and ultimately spectacle independence. If these are not achieved as expected, then pupil dilation needs to be performed to make certain the lens is at the appropriate axis. However, I would suggest that the beginning toric implant surgeon dilate the eye early on (1 day and or 1 week) just to be certain of the lens placement and position. The excellent outcomes achieved with the Acrysof toric can be attributed to its rotational stability. I have never seen this lens rotate, dating back to the clinical trial.

In summary, on the basis of increased patient expectations, the prevalence of preexisting astigmatism, which could affect post cataract surgery outcomes, and improvements in lens technology, I would strongly suggest that those surgeons not currently offering toric IOLs to their patients get started. There is no time like the present! I think both you and your patients will be glad you did.

References

1. Hoffer KJ. Biometry of 7500 cataractous eyes. *Am J Ophthalmol.* 1980;90:360-368.
2. Till JS, Yoder PR Jr, Wilcox TK, Spielman JL. Toric intraocular lens implantation: 100 consecutive cases. *J Cataract Refract Surg.* 2002; 28:295-301.
3. Horn JD. Status of toric intraocular lenses. *Curr Opin Ophthalmol.* 2007;18:58-61.

CHAPTER 170

STAAR Toric IOLs

Stephen Bylsma, MD

Until recently, the only toric intraocular lens (IOL) available in the United States was the STAAR Toric IOL (S-TIOL; Monrovia, CA). Accordingly, this IOL has been extensively studied and numerous reports document its efficacy and safety since its approval by the Food and Drug Administration (FDA) in 1998.[1-13] Other lens designs were found to be inappropriate as a toric platform because they underwent counter-clockwise rotation months after implantation as the capsule contracted around the IOL.[14-16] In contrast, the S-TIOL was observed to be stable against long-term malrotations. However, the same plate-haptic design that stabilizes the S-TIOL against late rotations was observed to be infrequently associated with very early postoperative off-axis rotation, including occasional clinically significant rotations requiring correction through secondary surgical intervention. Now, with the recent availability of the Alcon Toric IOL (A-TIOL; Fort Worth, TX) with its unique "one-piece" haptic design and acrylic material that together may stabilize the IOL against both early- and late-postoperative rotations, studies are underway to evaluate its short- and long-term efficacy and safety. The aim of this chapter is to review the current status of the S-TIOL and to provide an understanding of the technique and results associated with what has been to date the standard of care with respect to toric IOL implantation in the United States.

The STAAR Toric IOL: Design

The S-TIOL is a posterior-chamber foldable IOL made of first-generation silicone with a plate-haptic design (Figure 1). The S-TIOL is available from STAAR Surgical in 2 models that differ in their overall length. Model AA4203-TF, available in a spherical equivalent power of 21.5 D to 28.5 D is 10.8 mm in length. Model AA4203-TL, available from 9.5 D to 23.5 D spherical equivalent power, is 11.2 mm in overall length. Both S-TIOL models sport a 6.0-mm optic with two 1.5-mm fenestration holes in the haptics to promote fibrosis of the capsule and promote stability within the capsular bag. The longer -TL

model is made in the lower diopter range to increase stability against off-axis rotation in the larger capsules of myopic eyes.

The S-TIOL is manufactured as a plus-cylinder lens. Two hash-marks at the peripheral optic junction designate the axis of the toric power and are to be aligned along the steep keratometric axis as for any plus-cylinder lens. There are also 2 toric powers for correcting differing magnitudes of astigmatism: the +2.0 D toric power corrects 1.2 to 1.4 D of keratometric astigmatism, whereas the +3.5 D toric power corrects 2.2 to 2.4 D of astigmatism. The S-TIOL is packaged with the toric power facing upward. The manufacturer's labeling calls for the anterior, toric surface to be implanted facing the anterior capsule. Alternatively, the S-TIOL may be implanted in a "reversed" configuration to promote early rotational stability.[12,13]

The surgeon's usual IOL formulas and nomograms are used when choosing the spherical equivalent power of the S-TIOL power and model to implant. The keratometric cylinder determines which of the 2 toric powers to use. Corneas with less than 1.2 D of corneal cylinder should not receive the S-TIOL to avoid "flipping" of the refractive astigmatic axis. For eyes with between 1.4 to 2.3 D of corneal astigmatism, the manufacturer calls for the +2.5 D toric power, and the +3.5 D power is chosen for corneal astigmatism over 2.3 D. However, the author recommends choosing the toric power based on the modified "reversed" nomogram to promote early rotational stability: for keratometric asymmetry of 1.2 D to 2.1 D, use the +2.0 D toric power in the "reversed" optic position, and for corneal astigmatism over 2.2 D, the +3.5 D TIOL in the "reversed" position is used. The "reversed" position is attained by loading the S-TIOL upside down in the cartridge so the toric, anterior surface of the optic faces the posterior capsule. Using this "reversed" nomogram reduces the frequency of early off-axis rotations.[12,13]

The S-TIOL should be aligned as would any plus cylinder lens to neutralize the keratometric astigmatism. The intended axis of implantation is typically based on preoperative keratometric data to determine the steep corneal axis, or the axis may be determined intraoperatively by qualitative

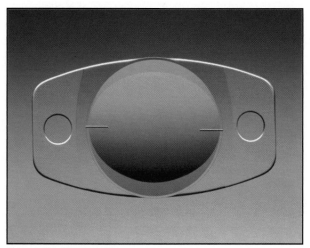

Figure 1. The STAAR Toric IOL.

keratometry. Irregular corneal astigmatism will not be appropriately corrected by the S-TIOL.

Implanting the S-TIOL is similar to implanting other plate-haptic IOLs and should not be implanted with a compromised capsular bag. The cartridge and injector design allows easy delivery through a 3.0-mm clear cornea incision into a viscoelastic-filled capsule using a "pumping" action of the plunger to avoid capture of the trailing haptic. The S-TIOL is then oriented into the desired axis with the I/A tip or other second instrument. An important step to prevent early off-axis rotation of the S-TIOL is to ensure that viscoelastic is removed from between the IOL and the posterior capsule. As opposed to the new A-TIOL, the S-TIOL may be rotated in either direction within the capsular bag to achieve its final orientation along the desired axis. Some surgeons suggest leaving the eye slightly soft to encourage stabilization of the S-TIOL.

Clinical Results With the STAAR Toric IOL

Both S-TIOL models (-TF and -TL) have been widely evaluated and convincingly demonstrate a predictable improvement in uncorrected visual acuity (UCVA), although the results vary as to the incidence of early off-axis rotation.[4-13] Likewise, numerous studies have confirmed the reliability, safety, and efficacy of the S-TIOL in improving postoperative UCVA compared to other IOLs; without enumerating those studies in detail, the best way of summing up the clinical results is to say that the S-TIOL provides outstanding correction of corneal astigmatism and is infrequently found to rotate off-axis only in the early postoperative period and not later. This early malposition is felt to be due to a mismatch between the size of the capsular bag and the plate-haptic design of the IOL in some eyes. Two important findings have significantly reduced the frequency of the off-axis rotations: the manufacturing of the longer -TL model,[11] and the technique of implanting the S-TIOL in a "reversed" configuration whereby the anterior (toric) surface of the IOL is positioned against the posterior capsule.[12,13]

The variability in the frequency and severity of these early off-axis malrotations can be accounted for by several factors.

Chief among them is that the older studies utilized only the shorter -TF model and that viscoelastic removal from behind the IOL was not consistently achieved. Today, with recommendations of employing the longer -TL model whenever possible, directing attention toward removal of viscoelastic from behind the IOL, and using the technique of intentionally implanting the S-TIOL in the "reversed" configuration, the author finds off-axis deviations to be rare and the need for secondary surgical intervention occurs in less than 2% of S-TIOL cases.

In those rare cases of off-axis deviation that require surgical intervention, the recommended time for repositioning of the S-TIOL is between 1 to 2 weeks postoperatively. If repositioned earlier, there may be a recurrence of the malposition; if attempted later, fibrosis may prevent repositioning of the S-TIOL.

STAAR Toric IOL in the Future

The current S-TIOL has demonstrated excellent clinical reliability as noted earlier, yet there are 2 main reasons for its limited acceptance among some surgeons: the older lens design and the occasional off-axis rotation in the early postoperative period (day 1). To address these issues, the manufacturer plans a release of a new toric IOL (CC4203-TL) using its proprietary Collamer material, which should provide many benefits. First, the Collamer material is a unique hydrophobic polyhema copolymer containing highly purified collagen, which possesses outstanding optical and biocompatibility characteristics. Also, the currently available Collamer IOL (CC4203-BF) with its "Indigo" injector, on which the new toric version is based, provides highly controlled and atraumatic IOL delivery with implantation through a 2.6-mm incision. Most importantly, the Collamer IOL shows excellent rotational stability within the capsule. Thus, this new platform is expected to provide further significant improvements over the currently available S-TIOL.

Conclusion

The recent availability of the Alcon Toric IOL has renewed enthusiasm for correcting astigmatism optically. The only previous toric IOL available in the United States was the S-TIOL, and excellent results have been routinely obtained with this lens. So far, limited studies have directly compared these 2 toric platforms, and such studies are now underway. As new data becomes available on the long-term results obtained with the A-TIOL, comparison may be made in both prospective- and retrospective-analysis against the extensive data accumulated previously on the S-TIOL. With future improvements expected in both the A-TIOL and S-TIOL platforms, including the addition of aspheric designs and new materials, both surgeon and patient may continue to demand more accurate and complication-free results.

References

1. Sanders DR, Grabow HB, Shepherd J. The toric IOL. In: Grills JP, Martin RG, Sanders DR, eds. *Sutureless Cataract Surgery.* Thorofare, NJ: Slack Inc; 1992:183-197.

2. Gills JP, Martin RG, Thornton SP, Sanders DR, eds. *Surgical Treatment of Astigmatism*. Thorofare, NJ: Slack Inc; 1994:159-164.

3. Grabow HB. Early results with foldable toric IOL implantation. Eur J Implant Refract Surg. 1994;6:177-178.

4. Grabow HB. Toric intraocular lens report. *Ann Ophthalmol*. 1997 (29);161-163.

5. Sun XY, Vicary D, Montgomery P, Griffiths M. Toric intraocular lenses for correcting astigmatism in 130 eyes. *Ophthalmology*. 2000;107(9):1776-1781.

6. Kershner RM. Toric intraocular lenses for correcting astigmatism in 130 eyes (Discussion). *Ophthalmology*. 2000;107(9):1781-1782.

7. Rushwurm I, Scholz U, Zehetmayer M, Hanselmeyer G, Vass C, Skorpik C. Astigmatism correction with a foldable toric intraocular lens in cataract patients. *J Cataract Refract Surg*. 2000 Jul;26(7):1022-1027.

8. Leyland M, Zinicola E, Bloom P, Lee N. Prospective evaluation of a plate haptic toric intraocular lens. *Eye*. 2001 Apr;15(Pt 2):202-205.

9. Nguyen TM, Miller KM. Digital overlay technique for documenting toric intraocular lens axis orientation. *J Cataract Refract Surg*. 2000 Oct;26(10):1496-1504.

10. Till JS, Yoder PR, Wilcox TK, et al. Toric intraocular lens implantation: 100 consecutive cases. *J Catarct Refract Surg*. 2002;28:295-301.

11. Chang DF. Early rotational stability of the longer Staar toric intraocular lens: fifty consecutive cases. *J Cataract Refract Surg*. 2003;29:935-940.

12. Bylsma S. Toric intraocular lenses. In: Roy FH, Arzabe CW, eds. *Master Techniques in Cataract and Refractive Surgery*. Thorofare, NJ: Slack, Inc; 2004.

13. Bylsma S. STAAR Toric IOL. In: Fine, IH, Packard, M, Hoffman, RS, eds. *Refractive Lens Surgery*. Springer, Inc; 2005.

14. Shimizu K, Misawa A, Suzuki Y. Toric intraocular lenses: correcting astigmatism while controlling axis shift. *J Cataract Refract Surg*. 1994;20:523-526.

15. Patel CK, Ormonde S, Rosen PH, Bron AJ. Postoperative intraocular lens rotation: a randomized comparison of plate and loop haptic implants. *Ophthalmology*. 1999 Nov;106(11):2190-2195; discussion 2196.

16. Hwang IP, Clinch TE, Moshifar M, et al. Decentration of 3 piece versus plate-haptic silicone intraocular lenses. *J Cataract Refract Surg*. 1998;24:1505-1508.

CHAPTER 171

TORIC IOLS—
STAAR VERSUS ACRYSOF

David F. Chang, MD

Toric intraocular lenses (IOLs) are highly effective as a means for reducing pre-existing astigmatism in patients undergoing cataract surgery. They are particularly useful in younger cataract patients, in whom incisional keratotomy is much less effective, and in patients with higher degrees of astigmatism for whom astigmatic keratotomy is less predictable. In the latter instance, it may be necessary to combine astigmatic keratotomy with a toric IOL to maximize the cylindrical correction. There are three important prerequisites for success with toric IOLs. First, the surgeon must be able to perform astigmatically neutral surgery so that the IOL's cylindrical power and axis can be selected based on the preoperative keratometry measurements. Second, the axis of the toric IOL must be properly aligned during surgery. Finally, the lens must not rotate out of alignment postoperatively.

Misalignment of the toric IOL axis reduces the amount of astigmatism corrected and shifts its axis (Figure 1). With 10 degrees of axis deviation, approximately one-third of the astigmatic correcting effect is lost. With 20 degrees of axis deviation, approximately two-thirds of the effect is lost. Lens misalignment greater than 30 degrees produces an overall increase in astigmatism. Fortunately, significant late rotation of toric lenses has not been reported with any toric design. Therefore, the key to success with toric IOLs is to avoid early postoperative rotation of the lens. Once the capsular bag has contracted, it appears that the IOL is no longer mobile. There are currently two Food and Drug Administration (FDA)–approved toric IOLs available in the United States.

STAAR Toric IOL

The STAAR silicone plate haptic toric IOL (AA4203; STAAR Surgical, Monrovia, CA) was approved in November 1998. Several earlier studies found that the plate haptic design provided excellent long-term rotational stability. Using serial digital photographs Patel demonstrated that late, delayed postoperative rotation (>10 degrees) was unusual with plate haptic lenses (14%), but more frequent with 3-piece designs (37%).[1]

Patel also found that both lens designs could rotate during the immediate postoperative period. Forty-one percent of three-piece and 38% of plate haptic lenses had rotated >10 degrees by 2 weeks. However, severe early rotation (>30 degrees) occurred more frequently with the plate haptic design (24% vs 5%). Presumably, the plate haptic IOL could rotate until enough capsular bag contraction occurred to fixate the corners of the lens. The Patel study evaluated a 10.5-mm long plate haptic IOL, which is shorter than the two toric IOL sizes (10.8 and 11.2 mm) commercially offered by STAAR (Figure 2).

The STAAR silicone toric plate haptic IOL comes in two astigmatic powers. The +2.00 toric model corrects approximately 1.50 diopters (D) at the spectacle plane, whereas the +3.50 toric add corrects approximately 2.25 D of keratometric astigmatism. The STAAR toric lens is also available in two different lengths. The "TF" model was the original FDA-studied design, and has an overall length of 10.8 mm. To improve early rotational stability, STAAR released the longer 11.2-mm "TL" model 1 year later. Because myopic eyes tend to have larger diameter capsular bags, the TL model is available for spherical powers of <23.5 D. Both toric models have large round fenestrations in the plate haptics. The rationale is that rotation may be prevented if the anterior and posterior capsules fuse together through this opening. The haptics of the longer lens also have a matte finish to make them less slippery.

In the US FDA study data, 24% of the STAAR plate haptic toric IOLs ended up >10 degrees off axis (12% were >20 degrees off, 8% were >30 degrees off, and 5% were >45 degrees off axis). The FDA study only evaluated the shorter 10.8-mm toric size.

Alcon AcrySof Toric IOL

Approved in 2006, the Alcon toric lens (Alcon, Fort Worth, TX) utilizes the identical single-piece AcrySof platform as the SA60 model series, with the toric correction placed on the posterior side of the optic (Figure 3). This hydrophobic acrylic

Figure 1. Correction of cylinder as a function of axis deviation with the STAAR toric IOL. (Courtesy STAAR Surgical.)

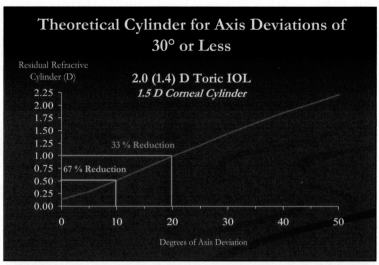

Figure 2. STAAR toric TF (10.8 mm) and TL (11.2 mm) IOLs next to standard non-toric STAAR plate haptic IOL (10.5 mm). (Courtesy STAAR Surgical.)

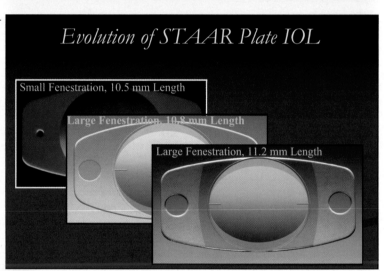

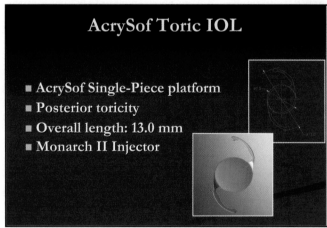

Figure 3. AcrySof Toric IOL. (Courtesy Alcon.)

lens has an overall 13.0-mm length and is available in three different astigmatic correcting powers. The SN60T3 has 1.5 D of cylinder at the IOL plane, which corrects approximately 1 D of corneal astigmatism. The SN60T4 has 2.25 D of cylinder at the IOL plane and corrects approximately 1.5 D of corneal astigmatism. Finally, the SN60T5 has 3.0 D of cylinder at the IOL plane, which corrects approximately 2.0 D of corneal

astigmatism.

In the US FDA clinical trial, the mean rotation for all 3 AcrySof toric IOL models was 4 degrees, and 97.6% of the IOLs rotated 15 degrees or less.

Personal Learning Curve— First 6 Consecutive Cases With STAAR TF Toric Lens

In February 1999, I implanted my first six STAAR TF (10.8 mm) toric IOLs in four different patients. At that time, only the shorter TF model was available. I used Viscoat (Alcon) in these uncomplicated cases, which were performed under topical anesthesia. In three eyes, the toric IOL axis remained within +15 degrees of the targeted axis postoperatively. However, one patient had IOL axis misalignments of 70 degrees and 85 degrees in each of her two eyes by the first postoperative day (POD 1). In each instance, proper initial surgical IOL alignment was confirmed by reviewing the operative video, indicating that rotation had occurred during the first day. Each time, the IOL was immediately repositioned because the doubling of her astigmatism was intolerable. Both lenses have remained perfectly aligned since then.

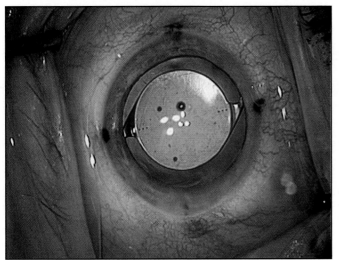

Figure 4. AcrySof SN60T5 toric IOL. Surgeon is sitting at the temporal side and two ink spots denote the 3 and 9 o'clock positions. Two additional ink spots mark the 100 degree (+) axis of corneal astigmatism. The hash marks on the toric IOL have been aligned with the astigmatic axis.

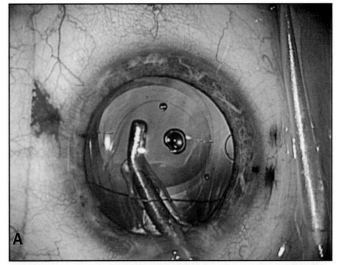

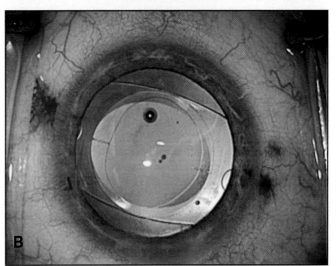

Figure 5. STAAR AA4203 TL toric IOL. OVD is removed with I-A tip positioned behind the optic (A). The hash marks are then aligned with the two ink spots marking the 75 degree (+) axis of corneal astigmatism (B).

A third IOL was 30 degrees misaligned by the first postoperative day, and I waited the recommended 2 weeks to surgically realign the lens. At surgery, I discovered that the anterior capsule was already becoming fibrotic and the anterior and posterior capsules had already fused peripheral to the IOL. Aggressive use of a spatula and viscodissection were needed to reopen the capsular bag to allow the plate haptic IOL to be rotated. The lens did not move easily, but proper and stable alignment was eventually achieved.

STAAR made the longer TL (11.2 mm) model available in the United States in March 1999. In addition to slightly modifying my surgical technique, I subsequently used only the longer 11.2-mm "TL" IOLs (except for powers over 23.5 D). Only 3 of the next 90 consecutive STAAR toric IOLs that I implanted required repositioning. Eighty were the longer TL IOLs, and 10 were TF IOLs in powers >24.0 D.

Preoperative Planning and Counseling

Regardless of which toric IOL model is used, the preoperative planning is identical. The spherical power of the toric IOL is calculated in the same way as for a conventional IOL. Next, after performing keratometry and identifying the (+) axis of astigmatism, the cylindrical power is selected without having to adjust the spherical power. Hash marks on both toric IOL models allow the cylindrical power to be surgically aligned with the steeper "plus" axis of astigmatism (Figures 4 and 5). Alcon offers an online calculation program to help select the power, the axis, and the correct model toric IOL www.acrysoftoriccalculator.com. For the STAAR toric series, always use the longer TL IOL if it is available in the desired power (<23.5 D). To avoid any potential influence of lenticular astigmatism, one should use the keratometric reading, rather than the refraction, for determining the toric power and axis of the IOL. Corneal topography is also useful to assess the regularity and symmetry of corneal astigmatism. Rigid contact lens wear should be discontinued for at least 1 to 2 weeks in order to increase the accuracy of keratometry and topography measurements. These patients should also understand that rigid contact lenses will no longer be an option to correct any residual refractive error in the future.

With respect to informed consent, the patient should understand the potential for unwanted lens rotation that might rarely require surgical repositioning. One must be careful to emphasize that the toric IOL may not eliminate all astigmatism and does not fully replace the need for spectacle correction. Finally, certain intraoperative circumstances (eg, torn capsulorrhexis or posterior capsule) may preclude implantation of a toric lens.

Toric IOL Surgical Technique

I routinely employ topical anesthesia without postoperative patching or shields. With the patient sitting upright just prior to surgery, the 3 and 9 o'clock limbus is dotted with a

---

Table 1

SELECTED DATA FROM PUBLISHED STUDIES OF THE STAAR TORIC TF IOL*

- FDA   12% (1%) > 20 degrees
- Sun   25% (1%) > 20 degrees
- Rumsworth   19% (11%) > 10 degrees
- Leyland   18% (1%) > 30 degrees
- Till   14% (3%) > 15 degrees

* Data from the Chang series using the STAAR toric TL IOL are highlighted in parentheses.

Table 2

PATIENT CHARACTERISTICS FROM TWO CONSECUTIVE SERIES OF TORIC IOLs

	STAAR Toric n=50	AcrySof Toric n=100
< 65 yo	42%	50%
> 24.5 mm AL	70%	60%
< 19.0 D IOL	78%	70%

---

skin-marking pen. Once under the microscope, a degree gauge (eg, Dell astigmatism marker, Rhein Medical, Inc., Tampa, FL) is used to orient two limbal ink marks that identify the desired axis (see Figure 4). Once the IOL is implanted, its axis marks can be aligned with these ink marks, and double-checked against the preoperative notes or chart (see Figures 4 and 5).

My surgical technique for either toric IOL employs the following guidelines:

* Use an astigmatically neutral, temporal clear corneal incision.

* The capsulorrhexis should be round and should circumferentially overlap the optic edge so as to avoid asymmetric capsular contractile forces that could decenter the optic.

* Use a cohesive ophthalmic viscosurgical device (OVD), such as Healon (Advanced Medical Optics, Santa Ana, CA), Provisc (Alcon), Amvisc or Amvisc Plus (Bausch & Lomb, Rochester, NY). Dispersive OVDs tend to coat and lubricate the IOL surface, making it more slippery and prone to rotation.

* For the STAAR silicone IOL, remove any OVD trapped behind the IOL with irrigation-aspiration to maximize contact between the IOL and the posterior capsule (see Figure 5a). I do not find this to be necessary with the AcrySof toric IOL.

* At the conclusion of surgery, do not overinflate the eye, which will tend to inflate the capsular bag as well. Because the silicone STAAR lens is more slippery when wet, leaving the eye somewhat "softer" than usual permits the flaccid capsular bag to collapse around the plate haptic IOL more quickly.

* Neither single-piece acrylic nor silicone plate haptic IOLs should ever be implanted in the ciliary sulcus. The presence of a torn capsulorrhexis or posterior capsule is a contraindication to implanting a silicone plate haptic IOL, and a single-piece AcrySof lens should not be implanted in these situations unless the surgeon is confident in the positional and rotational stability of the lens.

Postoperatively, I perform a dilated exam on postoperative day one (POD 1) to check the IOL axis. Any rotation tends to occur between the time of surgery and the first postoperative morning. I have yet to record any significant change from the POD 1 axis with either the STAAR or AcrySof toric lenses. With a silicone IOL, capsular contraction and fibrosis occur quite quickly. Based on my experience with three badly misaligned STAAR toric IOLs, I would recommend that any repositioning of a misaligned plate haptic IOL be performed within the first postoperative week, if possible. Once the capsular bag fully contracts (eg, by 2 weeks with my third case), more force is required to rotate the STAAR toric IOL, and this might increase the chance of tearing the capsular bag or zonules.

Clinical Results With the STAAR Toric Lens

Early studies with the STAAR TF toric IOL reported a fairly high rate of rotational instability and of IOL repositioning (Table 1). In the FDA clinical trial of the shorter TF model, 24% of patients had >10 degrees of rotation, 12% had >20 degrees of rotation, and 8% had >30 degrees of rotation from the intended axis. In a series of 130 TF toric IOLs reported by Sun, 25% of patients had >20 degrees of rotation and 7% had >40 degrees of rotation.[2] A repositioning procedure was performed in 9.2% of the eyes. Smaller clinical series of TF toric lenses reported rotation of 19% >10 degrees (Rumsworth) and 18% >30 degrees (Leyland).[3,4] Till reported 14% of patients with >15 degrees of rotation in the first clinical series to include the longer TL model, which accounted for 37% of the mixed series of TF and TL toric IOLs.[5] Nine percent of patients would have required IOL repositioning, but four patients returned too late to undergo reoperation.

In 2003 I published the first prospective series of the longer TL STAAR toric lens, in which none of the first 50 patients required lens repositioning.[6] Forty-two percent of the implants were used in patients younger than 65 years old, consistent with my preference for using toric IOLs to correct astigmatism in younger cataract patients (Table 2). The majority of the patients receiving the TL toric IOL were myopic, with 70% having axial lengths >24.5 mm and 78% receiving spherical powers <19.0 D. The mean preoperative refractive cylinder was 3.68 D (+1.38 D).

The series was eventually extended to 90 consecutive cases.[7] All 90 implants were of the higher +3.50 D toric power. Aside from 11 IOLs that were >23.5 D and therefore only available in the TF model, the remaining 79 toric IOLs were the longer TL model. Excellent rotational stability was

Table 3

ALIGNMENT DATA FROM TWO CONSECUTIVE SERIES OF TORIC IOLs

Position of IOL	STAAR Toric n=90	AcrySof Toric n=100
< 5 degrees	66 (73%)	90 (90%)
< 10 degrees	82 (91%)	99 (99%)
< 15 degrees	87 (97%)	100 (100%)

achieved, which was superior to prior studies of the shorter TF model. Seventy-three percent were within 5 degrees of target axis; 91% were within 10 degrees of target axis; 97% were within 15 degrees of target axis (Table 3). This is a significant improvement over the FDA data (see Table 1) and data from previous series,[2-5] in which the shorter TF IOL was used. My repositioning rate was 3.3% (3/90) with the longer TL IOL. For the first 50 cases, the mean decrease in refractive cylinder was 2.76 D (+1.2 D).

Clinical Results with the AcrySof Toric Lens

Starting with its availability in 2006, I prospectively implanted 100 consecutive AcrySof toric IOLs with the same surgical method used in my series of 90 STAAR toric IOLs. Fifty percent of the implants were used in patients younger than 65 years old. The majority of the patients receiving the AcrySof toric IOL were myopic, with 60% having axial lengths >24.5 mm and 70% receiving spherical powers <19.0 D (see Table 2). The mean preoperative refractive cylinder was 2.46 D (+0.95 D). The rotational stability was even better than that achieved with the STAAR toric platform (90% were within 5 degrees of target axis; 99% were within 10 degrees of target axis; 100% were within 15 degrees of target axis) (see Table 3). Furthermore, none of the AcrySof toric IOLs has required repositioning.

Clinical Comparison

Due to the slippery nature of silicone, the STAAR toric IOL spins much more easily within the capsular bag during surgery, making adequate overall length extremely critical to its rotational stability. In contrast, the tacky surface of the AcrySof hydrophilic acrylic material tends to adhere to the posterior capsule upon contact. This feature, the ease of injection, and the greater familiarity of the single-piece acrylic platform make the AcrySof lens my current toric design of choice.

One important difference between the two toric IOL platforms is the incidence and management of secondary membrane. Without a truncated posterior edge, secondary posterior capsule opacification is more frequent with the STAAR plate haptic IOL. Anterior capsule contraction and fibrosis are also much greater with silicone IOLs, and this poses the possibility of late malposition if either the capsulorrhexis or the IOL are too small. Finally, one must be careful to make a rounded and smaller opening when performing Nd: yttrium-aluminum-garnet (YAG) laser posterior capsulotomy with a plate haptic IOL. Larger capsulotomy openings with stellate edges have been associated with posterior dislocation of plate haptic IOLs into the vitreous.

Conclusion

Toric IOLs are an excellent complement or alternative to astigmatic keratotomy, and are particularly useful in those cases where limbal corneal relaxing incisions are not powerful or predictable enough. With the STAAR plate haptic toric lens, proper IOL sizing is critical for initial rotational stability. Until the capsular bag begins to contract within the first day or so, a slippery silicone plate haptic IOL that is too small for the bag can rotate. Rotational stability of the AcrySof toric lens is excellent, thanks to the surface tackiness of the hydrophobic acrylic material that clings and adheres to the posterior capsule. Its ease of implantation and the widespread popularity and familiarity of the single-piece acrylic IOL platform have made the AcrySof toric lens the preference of most surgeons.

References

1. Patel CK, Ormonde S, Rosen PH, Bron AJ. Postoperative intraocular lens rotation: a randomized comparison of plate and loop haptic implants. *Ophthalmology.* 1999; 106:2190-2196

2. Sun XY, Vicary D, Montgomery P, Griffiths, M. Toric intraocular lenses for correcting astigmatism in 130 eyes. *Ophthalmology.* 2000;107:1776-1781; discussion by RM Kershner, 1781-1782.

3. Ruhswurm I, Scholz U, Zehetmayer M, et al. Astigmatism correction with foldable toric intraocular lens in cataract patients. *J Cataract Refract Surg.* 2000;26:1022-1027.

4. Leyland M, Zinicola P, Bloom P, Lee N. Prospective evaluation of a plate haptic toric intraocular lens. *Eye.* 2001;15:202-205.

5. Till JS, Yoder PR, Wilcox TK, Spielman JL. Toric intraocular lens implantation: 100 consecutive cases. *J Cataract Refract Surg.* 2002;28:295-301.

6. Chang DF. Early rotational stability of the longer STAAR toric IOL—50 consecutive (TL) IOLs. *J Cataract Refract Surg.* 2003;29:935-940.

7. Chang, DF. Chapter 15: The STAAR toric intraocular lens: indications and pearls. P. 169 – 177. In: Gills J, ed. *A Complete Surgical Guide for Correcting Astigmatism.* Thorofare, NJ: SLACK Incorporated; 2003.

CHAPTER 172

AcrySof Toric
IOL Technique

Edward Holland, MD

The AcrySof Toric intraocular lens (IOL) (Alcon, Fort Worth, TX) allows surgeons to precisely correct astigmatism and predictably achieve distance spectacle freedom for their patients. With only minor modifications to their routine cataract procedure, cataract surgeons can quickly become comfortable implanting this lens because they already have the skill set needed for successful implantation.

The AcrySof Toric Lens

The AcrySof Toric IOL is based on the AcrySof natural single-piece platform and is a foldable lens with a fully functional 6.0-mm toric optic (Figure 1). The lens' acrylic material is highly biocompatible and has adhesive properties that, along with the haptic design, help to prevent rotation of the IOL after implantation in the capsular bag. The posterior surface of the IOL has added cylinder power and axis markings to assist the surgeon with IOL alignment following implantation into the capsular bag. The AcrySof Toric IOL is available in various models to provide a wide range of astigmatism correction.

To determine the required spherical lens power for a particular patient, surgeons should use their preferred method and formulae. Surgeons should then use the online AcrySof Toric IOL Calculator (located at http://www.acrysoftoriccalculator.com) to assist in selecting the correct model and optimal axis location within the capsular bag. The calculator is unique in that it compensates for the effect of surgically induced astigmatism in the calculation of both IOL cylinder power and axis location, thus increasing overall precision.

To achieve the desired level of precision in the calculations, it is important for surgeons to customize their surgically induced astigmatism (SIA) factor by using their own clinical data.

Surgical Technique

The initial step in my surgical technique is to make reference marks at the 3, 6, and 9 o'clock meridians. This is done in the preinduction area with the patient sitting in the upright position in order to avoid the effect of cyclorotation of the eye that occurs when the patient moves to the supine position for the cataract procedure. I then perform my standard capsulorrhexis, hydrodissection, and phacoemulsification in preparation for implantation of the lens.

Following implantation of the IOL, it is critical to precisely align the IOL with the predetermined axis of placement. This is accomplished through a 3-step process of gross alignment, viscoelastic removal, and final alignment.

Gross alignment of the IOL is achieved following implantation and prior to the IOL fully unfolding in the capsular bag. The IOL should be rotated to a point that is 10 to 15 degrees counterclockwise from the final position of the lens. I use a second instrument (Sinskey hook or cyclodialysis spatula) to hold the lens in place while the viscoelastic is carefully removed from behind the lens and then finally anterior to the lens. I then use the same second instrument to carefully nudge the IOL clockwise into the final axis alignment. In rare cases where the lens over-rotates, the surgeon will need to refill the capsular bag with viscoelastic and repeat the IOL alignment process as described above.

Surgical Outcomes

Two factors are critical to visual outcomes with the AcrySof Toric IOL: on-axis placement of the IOL and the lens remaining rotationally stable within the capsular bag to maintain visual performance.

An unpublished randomized, prospective, multicenter study included 494 patients and 11 clinical investigators and compared the AcrySof Toric IOL with the monofocal AcrySof Model SA60AT as a control.[1] Follow-up data at 6 months included unilateral implantation of 211 AcrySof Toric IOL eyes and 210 control eyes. The AcrySof Toric IOL demonstrated excellent rotational stability with an average rotation of less than 4 degrees from initial placement through 6 months postoperatively.

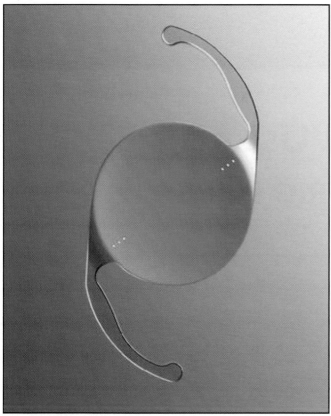

Figure 1. AcrySof toric IOL.

Additionally, the AcrySof Toric IOL was significantly more successful at providing spectacle freedom for distance vision compared to the control. In the clinical study, 60% of patients who received unilateral AcrySof Toric IOL implantation achieved spectacle freedom for distance vision. In the same study, a subset of patients implanted bilaterally achieved 97% spectacle freedom for distance vision.

These lenses are a tremendous benefit to patients with astigmatism, and cataract surgeons will become comfortable implanting them after only a few procedures. With minimal modification to your surgical technique, excellent results can be achieved, allowing most patients to achieve distance vision spectacle freedom.

Reference

1. Lane SS. The AcrySof Toric IOL's FDA Trial Results: A look at the clinical data. *Cataract & Refractive Surgery Today.* May 2006;66-68.

CHAPTER 173

WHEN DO I USE LRIs VERSUS TORIC IOLs?

David F. Chang, MD

Corneal Relaxing Incisions— Pros and Cons

As reported by many other surgeons, I have found "limbal" corneal relaxing incisions (LRIs) to be very effective for reducing low to moderate amounts of astigmatism (<2.00 D). The majority of cataract surgical patients with astigmatism fall into this category. I use a preset 600-micron blade (Accutome, Malvern, PA) (Figure 1) and the Gills nomogram (see Chapter 162). The Dell astigmatism marker (Rhein Medical, Inc., Tampa, FL) is inked with a disposable skin-marking pen, and guides placement of the incisions (Figure 2), which are made prior to making the phaco incision.

There are several excellent astigmatic keratotomy nomograms that are presented within this textbook. These all serve as a starting point for surgeons to use, and the Gills nomogram, which specifies the chord length of each incision, was the first to be developed. Although it is theoretically more accurate to measure an arcuate incision in degrees of arc, the chord length method works well from a practical standpoint because the corneal diameter varies so little between different individuals.

Very little extra instrumentation is needed to perform LRIs and there is no significant alteration of surgical technique or postoperative management. It is a fast and simple method that does not compromise the surgical view, and it generally does not increase patient discomfort. LRIs do not require a change in intraocular lens (IOL) power calculation and the refraction stabilizes quickly. Finally, aside from the possibility of perforation, LRIs do not increase surgical risk. The main potential problem is that of overcorrecting the astigmatism and flipping the axis.

Although it is easy to learn and perform, the predictability of so simple an approach is affected by three variables. First, a preset blade depth does not adjust for individual variation in peripheral corneal thickness, resulting in a variable percentage of incisional depth achieved. Years ago, Bill Maloney did an unpublished study showing that varying blade depth according to corneal pachymetry measurements did not improve the outcomes of LRIs. A second variable is corneal diameter. Placing the incisions just anterior to the limbal vessels means that larger optical zones will result in eyes with larger diameter corneas.

The third and most important variable is the patient's age. With any incisional keratotomy, increasing patient age amplifies the effect of a given incision length. Unfortunately, this relationship is not linear. The same length of incision may be surprisingly ineffective in a 50-year-old patient and unintentionally powerful in a 90-year-old patient. Because of these three variables, the greater the amount of targeted astigmatism reduction, the more inconsistent and unpredictable the results of LRIs will be.

For these reasons, I have found LRIs to be less effective for two categories of patients. One is the younger cataract patient (<65 years) with >1.50 to 2.00 D of astigmatism, but whose younger age significantly reduces the attainable effect from incisional keratotomy. The second group consists of patients with the largest degrees of astigmatism (eg, >+2.50 D). In addition to more unpredictability, against-the-rule (ATR) astigmatism in these patients requires combining the temporal clear corneal incision with a temporal LRI. Initiating the phaco incision within a curvilinear temporal LRI often leads to a slight override of the incision edges postoperatively. This can cause significant discomfort and foreign body sensation for these patients. It is for these two groups of patients that I have found toric IOLs to be particularly helpful. I also use toric IOLs for those patients for whom LRIs are inadvisable for some reason. One example might be a patient with severe dry eyes, as LRIs can aggravate this condition by interrupting corneal nerves.

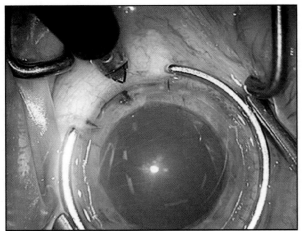

Figure 1. Single depth 600-micron diamond blade (Accutome) used for astigmatic keratotomy.

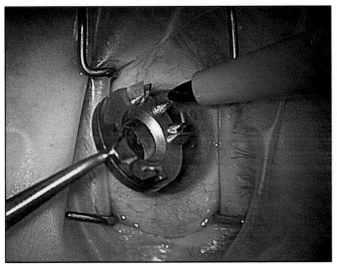

Figure 2a. After setting Dell astigmatism marker to the correct axis, a felt-tip pen is used to mark the axis and the 6-mm LRI marks.

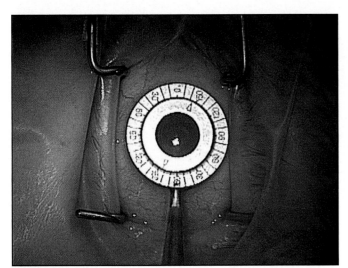

Figure 2b. Dell marker is used to mark the 155 degree axis of (+) astigmatism.

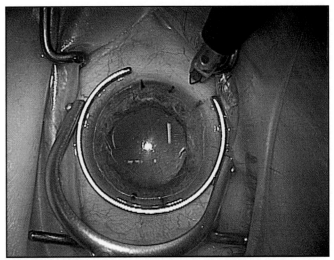

Figure 2c. The globe is fixated with a Fine-Thornton ring, and the diamond blade is held in the right hand.

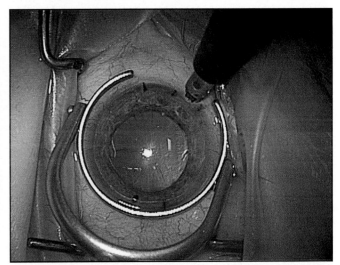

Figure 2d. The blade is seated to its full depth. After a brief pause, it is advanced just anterior to the limbal vessels.

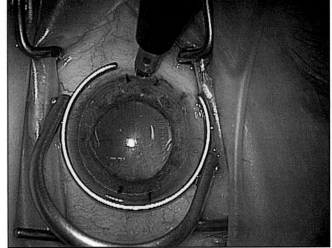

Figure 2e. A 6-mm chord length incision is completed by cutting from one mark to the other.

Toric IOLs—Pros and Cons

A potential complication of any toric IOL is that of misalignment, which can occur either because of inaccurate intraoperative positioning or postoperative rotation. Depending on the degree, toric IOL misalignment can reduce or negate the refractive benefit, or even worsen the refraction. As long as an adequately large Staar plate haptic toric IOL is selected, rotational stability with this lens platform is good.[1] The plate haptic silicone design has several disadvantages however. It can more easily slip out of alignment immediately postoperatively, and is associated with greater posterior capsular opacification and anterior capsule contraction over time. Finally, plate haptic IOLs carry the additional risk of posterior dislocation following a yttrium-aluminum-garnet (YAG) capsulotomy.

As discussed elsewhere, the Acrysof toric IOL has excellent rotational stability due to its tacky surface, which immediately adheres to the posterior capsule. Its availability in the familiar single-piece hydrophobic acrylic platform already preferred by many surgeons has already made this the most popular toric IOL in the United States. The main disadvantage of toric IOLs compared to astigmatic keratotomy is the increased cost of the lens. A second disadvantage is that there are currently no toric presbyopia-correcting IOLs available. For patients desiring presbyopia correction, astigmatism must be managed either with astigmatic keratotomy or with postoperative keratorefractive laser surgery.

Current Approach to Astigmatism Management in Cataract Patients

While placing the incision on the steep axis has some rationale, I prefer to use the same temporal, sub-3.0 mm clear corneal incision for every patient. Because of its location and small size, this is the most astigmatically neutral incision I can make. I do, however, alter the incision construction depending on the astigmatic goals. In the case of with-the-rule astigmatism, I do not want any flattening of the 180-degree axis, and I avoid making a perpendicular groove prior to the keratome entry.

With low degrees of ATR astigmatism (eg, +0.50 D ATR) that do not warrant making a LRI, I employ a Langerman-type perpendicular groove prior to the keratome entry. Depending on the patient's age, this may produce some desired flattening of the 180-degree axis.

With >0.75 diopter of astigmatism, I consider performing LRIs. For ATR astigmatism, I again employ a Langerman-style, deep perpendicular groove for the temporal phaco incision. This can be paired with a nasally placed LRI. To increase the effect, I can lengthen the temporal groove, or place it slightly more anteriorly. For fear of significant incisional discomfort, I prefer not to combine a curvilinear temporal LRI with my phaco incision.

I consider toric IOLs for younger patients (eg, <65 yo) with >1.50 to 2.00 D astigmatism. I also consider toric IOLs for any patient with astigmatism >2.50 D, regardless of age. With the reliable rotational stability of the Acrysof toric IOL, adding supplemental LRIs is an option to enhance the correction for higher targeted amounts of astigmatism. For younger patients with significant astigmatism who desire a presbyopia-correcting IOL, a bioptics approach is usually recommended. Astigmatic keratotomy can be attempted in these younger eyes, but is often surprisingly ineffective. In this case, leaving the patient more myopic will better facilitate the astigmatic laser in situ keratomileusis (LASIK) enhancement procedure.

An ideal time to correct astigmatism would be 1 to 3 weeks postoperatively. At this time, an accurate refraction can be performed, and the net effect of the phaco incision upon the astigmatism can be measured. Furthermore, the capsular bag has significantly shrunken by this time, preventing IOL rotation and movement. A light-adjustable IOL whose spherical and toric power could be modified postoperatively would be the ultimate solution for ammetropia.

Reference

1. Chang, DF. Early rotational stability of the longer Staar Toric IOL—50 consecutive (TL) IOLs. *J Cataract Refract Surg.* 2003;29:935–940.

CHAPTER 174

WHEN DO I USE LRIS VERSUS TORIC IOLS?

Richard A. Lewis, MD; Louis D. "Skip" Nichamin, MD; Edward Holland, MD;
Kerry D. Solomon, MD; and Luis E. Fernández de Castro, MD

Richard A. Lewis, MD

Technology has changed dramatically during my 24 years of practicing ophthalmology, but patients' expectations have remained the same; they want the best possible technology and outcomes.

I have approached cataract surgery very carefully. I have not recommended limbal relaxing incisions (LRIs) and have never implanted plate-haptic toric intraocular lenses (IOLs). This is contrary to the recommendation of many of the well-known cataract and refractive surgeons in this country. Despite the clinical evidence, I am not a believer. In fact, having been in practice before and after the era of radial keratotomy (RK) surgery, I have been very suspicious of LRIs. I was unable to discern how LRIs could perform differently in regard to reliability and long-term efficacy and regression as compared to RK. The plate-haptic silicone IOL has also been a big concern, especially in regard to capsular stability.

Over the years, my preferred IOL has been the single-piece acrylic AcrySof (Alcon, Fort Worth, TX). This IOL platform provides an ease of insertion with excellent centering and stability, yet remains very forgiving and predictable. I've had very good success over the years with this IOL.

The introduction of the AcrySof toric IOL into my practice seemed comfortable. There was good science supporting the data. The launch of the product was well-structured and included an online tutorial course. The most important decision was the determination of IOL power and placement and alignment of the IOL. Alcon developed a Web site to be used for determination of lens power and toricity (http://www.acrysoftoriccalculator.com/calculator.aspx). After providing information such as incision location, Ks and spherical power, the calculator specifies the necessary IOL parameters. After taking the course and speaking with some of the investigators, I realized that the cataract surgery and IOL placement are essentially no different than what I had been doing for years. The only difference was preoperatively marking the conjunctiva for the toric axis and then positioning the IOL on that axis. I recommend the AcrySof toric IOL in patients with greater than 1 diopter (D) of cylinder power on the corneal plane. Unlike multifocal lenses, there is no degradation of vision and no contraindications in patients with glaucoma or macular degeneration. I have also recommended this lens in patients who desire monovision and relative spectacle freedom.

Conclusion

The AcrySof toric IOL has provided excellent visual results for my patients. I do not feel that I am compromising corneal integrity with these lenses as compared to performing LRIs. Furthermore, the implantation of this lens is essentially the same as my nontoric IOL.

Louis D. "Skip" Nichamin, MD

The decision to use incisional surgery to correct pre-existing astigmatism, versus insertion of a toric IOL should be based upon the individual surgeon's comfort level with each of the respective techniques, along with the specifics of the particular case and clinical situation.

My personal use of astigmatic keratotomy in conjunction with cataract surgery began in 1989, and subsequently evolved to the use of LRIs in the mid 1990s. Given my experience with this technique, it remains my preferred choice to address astigmatism at the time of implant surgery except in 2 circumstances: 1) the existing astigmatism is beyond the level that I consider treatable through an incisional approach alone, or 2) there exists a contraindication to the use of LRIs.

Based upon the patient's age, I find that I am able to safely and reproducibly correct up to 3 D of astigmatism through the use of LRIs (Table 1). For levels greater than this, my prefer-

Table 1

THE NAPA NOMOGRAM:
NICHAMIN AGE AND PACHYMETRY-ADJUSTED INTRALIMBAL ARCUATE ASTIGMATIC NOMOGRAM

WITH-THE-RULE (Steep Axis 45° to 135°)

Preop Cylinder (Diopters)	Paired Incisions in Degrees of Arc					
	20 to 30 yo	31 to 40 yo	41 to 50 yo	51 to 60 yo	61 to 70 yo	71 to 80 yo
0.75	40	35	35	30	30	
1.00	45	40	40	35	35	30
1.25	55	50	45	40	35	35
1.50	60	55	50	45	40	40
1.75	65	60	55	50	45	45
2.00	70	65	60	55	50	45
2.25	75	70	65	60	55	50
2.50	80	75	70	65	60	55
2.75	85	80	75	70	65	60
3.00	90	90	85	80	70	65

AGAINST-THE-RULE (Steep Axis 0-44°/136-180°)

Preop Cylinder (Diopters)	Paired Incisions in Degrees of Arc					
	20 to 30 yo	31 to 40 yo	41 to 50 yo	51 to 60 yo	61 to 70 yo	71 to 80 yo
0.75	45	40	40	35	35	30
1.00	50	45	45	40	40	35
1.25	55	55	50	45	40	35
1.50	60	60	55	50	45	40
1.75	65	65	60	55	50	45
2.00	70	70	65	60	55	50
2.25	75	75	70	65	60	55
2.50	80	80	75	70	65	60
2.75	85	85	80	75	70	65
3.00	90	90	85	80	75	70

Blade depth setting is at 90% of the thinnest pachymetry

Reprinted with permission from Gills JP. *A Complete Surgical Guide for Correcting Astigmatism: An Ophthalmic Manifesto.* Thorofare, NJ: SLACK Incorporated; 2003.

ence is to combine the use of both modalities. As such, up to 6 D of astigmatism may be corrected with a toric implant and maximal (90 degree) peripheral intralimbal relaxing incisions. I have on several occasions combined the use of LRI, toric IOL, and excimer laser (bioptics) to successfully manage congenital astigmatism of over 9 D!

The other indication for a toric IOL in my practice would be a situation in which use of an LRI is contraindicated. This would include eyes that have previously undergone RK in that further incisional surgery may lead to corneal instability. Additional contraindications would include keratoconus, other topographic abnormalities, or known peripheral corneal disease. One should also be circumspect when dealing with patients who suffer from advanced autoimmune or rheumatoid disease that might predispose to healing problems following use of such peripheral corneal incisions (Table 2).

Table 2

RELATIVE CONTRAINDICATIONS FOR LIMBAL RELAXING INCISIONS

- Prior corneal (especially incisional) surgery
- Keratoconus, k. fruste, irregular astigmatism
- Peripheral corneal pathology
- Terrien's, gutter, or furrow degeneration
- Autoimmune or rheumatoid disease

As a final caveat, I believe that we all will become increasingly dependent upon the excimer laser to reduce residual astigmatism following "successful" implant surgery, including eyes that have received LRIs or toric IOLs. Our current goal is to leave patients with less than 0.75 D of cylinder; my prediction is that the bar will soon be raised to a level of +/- 0.25 D for both sphere and cylinder, and we will therefore be "enhancing" an increasing proportion of our patients. Let us be prepared!

Edward Holland, MD

I always prefer to use a toric IOLwhen treating astigmatism. My toric IOL of choice is the AcrySof toric IOL. I choose toric IOLs over LRIs because they are safer to use and provide more predictable outcomes. LRIs require additional corneal incisions, are less predictable, undergo regression, and are not as precise as the AcrySof Toric IOL. Additionally, treating astigmatism with a toric IOL is safer and less invasive than performing additional corneal incisions.

However, since not all patients are appropriate candidates for a toric IOL, it is sometimes necessary to employ other methods of astigmatism correction like astigmatic keratotomy (AK), LRIs, or laser corneal treatment (LCT). For example, if a patient has zonular dehiscence and there are concerns about IOL stability, you should not implant a toric lens. I would implant a monofocal lens in these cases, and perform LRIs to reduce the astigmatism.

Additionally, if a patient desires a presbyopia-correcting IOL (Pr-C IOL) and the astigmatism is not too severe (1.0 to 2.0 D), I will implant the Pr-C IOL and reduce the astigmatism by using corneal incisions.

For patients with higher levels of astigmatism (>2.5 D), I will combine an LRI with implantation of an AcrySof Toric IOL to achieve the desired level of correction. Until the higher powers of the AcrySof toric IOL are available, this is often the best alternative for these patients.

Because effective astigmatism management is so critical to a patient's visual outcomes, I find it very helpful to have each of these techniques available. However, when possible, I will always select a toric IOL because it is the safest and most precise and predictable way to treat astigmatism in patients undergoing cataract surgery.

Kerry D. Solomon, MD, and Luis E. Fernández de Castro, MD

Astigmatism treatment has been brought to the forefront of refractive cataract surgery. Surgeons today have numerous options available for the treatment of astigmatism in conjunction with cataract surgery. These options include LRIs, toric IOLs) and laser vision correction.[1] With the advent of Pr-C IOLs, it is imperative that astigmatism be treated in these patients in order to maximize the patient's visual recovery and minimize dependence on glasses for distance, intermediate, and/or near tasks. In fact, the old adage that less than 1.0 D of astigmatism was clinically acceptable has really been updated. Currently, the majority of refractive cataract surgeons are now aiming to reduce the amount of astigmatism to less than 0.5 D whenever possible.

The treatment of astigmatism as an adjunct to lens-based surgery is based on measured keratometric astigmatism. It is vital that patients be tested with corneal topography to rule out any irregular, asymmetric astigmatism prior to contemplating the use of a Pr-C lens or the management of corneal astigmatism. Regular symmetric corneal astigmatism is ideally suited for performing surgical correction. Surgeons should stay away from eyes with irregular, nonorthogonal corneal astigmatism because surgical results are less predictable and

underlying forme fruste keratoconus may be present. If a patient has more astigmatism in his or her refraction than that which is measured in his or her cornea, the assumption is that the extra astigmatism is present in the lens, which will be removed. It is, therefore, essential that surgeons focus on assessing the corneal astigmatism as well as the regularity and symmetry of that corneal astigmatism. If patients are not candidates for corneal refractive surgery (LRIs, photorefractive keratectomy [PRK], or laser in situ keratomileusis [LASIK]) due to irregular astigmatism, they are not good candidates for Pr-C lenses or refractive cataract surgery, which includes the management of astigmatism. The use of corneal topography has been incredibly helpful in the management and assessment of astigmatism. My preference is one of the newer corneal topographers such as the Pentacam (Oculus, Inc., Lynwood, WA) or Orbscan (Bausch & Lomb, Rochester, NY), which not only provide curvature data, but also elevation data of both anterior and posterior curvatures of the cornea.

For patients receiving Pr-C IOLs, refractive cataract surgeons have 2 options—LRIs or laser bioptics—for treating corneal astigmatism. I use LRIs when the amount of astigmatism is 1.25 D or less. I utilize the Nichamin nomogram as well as the Nichamin blade (Mastel Precision, Rapid City, SD), which is preset at 600 µm.[2] In my experience, LRIs are predictable and relatively easy to perform for 1.25 D or less of corneal astigmatism. These are performed at the same time as the lens surgery (cataract or refractive lens exchange [RLE]). My preference with Pr-C lens implantation is to perform the LRIs at the beginning of the lens extraction surgery.

For Pr-C IOL patients with more than 1.25 D of corneal astigmatism, I do not attempt to treat these with LRIs. Instead, patients are notified in advance that their astigmatism will be treated with laser vision correction (PRK or LASIK) following their Pr-C IOL implant.[3] My rationale for performing laser vision correction for astigmatism greater than 1.25 D is quite simple. In my hands, the reliability and accuracy of the treatment is greater with laser vision correction than it is with LRIs. Even though Dr. Nichamin has used LRIs to treat 2.0 D or more of astigmatism, and this is certainly an option if you choose to do so, I still prefer laser vision correction.

The treatment of astigmatism in patients who are not receiving Pr-C IOLs is somewhat different. Toric IOLs are another modality that can be used to treat regular, symmetric astigmatism. Currently, 2 toric IOLs are available for commercial use. The STAAR toric IOL (STAAR Surgical Company, Monrovia, CA) with cylindrical powers of 2.0 D and 3.5 D can correct 1.4 D and 2.3 D of astigmatism at the corneal plane, respectively. The AcrySof toric IOL (Alcon Laboratories, Inc., Fort Worth, TX) with cylindrical powers of 1.5, 2.25, and 3.0 D can correct 1.03, 1.55, and 2.06 D of astigmatism at the corneal plane, respectively. These toric lenses do provide very reliable and predictable treatment of preexisting astigmatism. Because of the possibility of cyclotorsional rotation, it is important to place reference marks on the eye prior to reclining the patient in the surgical suite. I prefer to mark the eye at the 12:00 position, as well as the 3:00 and 9:00 positions. I then use a degree gauge to mark the steep (+) axis of astigmatism. At the completion of the case, the toric IOL is then rotated into the position such that its astigmatic axis is aligned with the steep axis or meridian of the cornea. The STAAR Toric IOL rotates quite readily within the capsular bag. My preference is to have the patient lie flat for 30 minutes at the completion of the case and remain relatively inactive for the first 24 hours after surgery to minimize any immediate rotation of the STAAR toric IOL in the capsular bag. My experience has been that the likelihood of this lens rotating is much less after the first 24 to 48 hours.

In my experience, the AcrySof toric IOL has excellent rotational stability almost immediately from the time of implantation. My preference is to initially orient the lens to within 20 degrees of the steep axis (20 degrees counterclockwise to where the lens will finally rest). This is easily done with a second instrument prior to the unfolding of the haptics once the optic is placed into the capsular bag. With viscoelastic removal, the lens tends to rotate 10 to 20 degrees in the clockwise direction, and any final adjustments can be made with a second instrument to align the lens along the steep axis of the cornea. Once the AcrySof Toric IOL is properly aligned, the lens position is stable long term. I do not require that patients lie flat nor do I restrict their activities when I use the AcrySof toric IOL.

LRIs or laser vision correction can be combined with a toric IOL for those patients with very large amounts of astigmatism. The advantage of using toric IOLs in these eyes is the excellent clarity and quality of vision that they provide.

IOL surgeons have a variety of options and modalities available to them for the management of preexisting corneal astigmatism. Now that so many patients are expecting spectacle independence after cataract surgery, LRIs and/or toric IOLs are essential tools for maximizing patient satisfaction and achieving success.

References

1. Nichamin LD. Treating astigmatism at the time of cataract surgery. *Curr Opin Ophthalmol.* 2003;14:35-38.
2. Nichamin LD. Astigmatism control. *Ophthalmol Clin North Am.* 2006;19:485-493.
3. Zaldivar R, Davidorf JM, Oscherow S, et al. Combined posterior chamber phakics intraocular lens and laser in situ keratomileusis: bioptics for extreme myopia. *J Refract Surg.* 1999;15:299-308.

CHAPTER 175

CAN I COMBINE TORIC IOLS AND PCRIS?

Kevin M. Miller, MD

The simple answer to this question is yes! Of course, the 2 procedures can be combined. Generally, however, they are only used in combination to achieve levels of astigmatism correction that cannot be obtained with either procedure alone. This occurs at 2.5 to 3 diopters (D) or more of corneal astigmatism.

Astigmatism Management

My cataract surgery patients are offered an astigmatism management service at the time of their preoperative visit. My noncovered service waiver and the first page of a frequently asked questions sheet are shown in Figures 1 and 2. If a patient opts for this refractive service, I map out his or her corneal astigmatism using an EyeSys topographer (EyeSys Vision, Houston, TX) and Pentacam (Oculus, Lynwood, WA), decide the best treatment approach, and correct the astigmatism in the operating room using whatever technique is best suited for their eye. I offer the astigmatism management service to all of my patients, regardless of the lens they choose, as long as their visual potential is better than 20/200, but will not implant a deluxe or presbyopia-correcting lens unless they opt for it.

Stepladder Approach

The cataract and refractive lens surgeon needs to have a systematic approach for dealing with corneal astigmatism. I will present my approach here, which I think is fairly straightforward.

A clear corneal phacoemulsification tunnel incision corrects 0.35 to 0.5 D of corneal astigmatism if placed on the steep axis. A 3.2 mm wide phacoemulsification incision corrects 0.5 D of astigmatism with a confidence interval of 0.4 to 0.6 D.[1] For patients with 0.75 D or less of astigmatism, I simply perform the phacoemulsification on steep axis. I rotate my sitting and hand position to whatever axis is required. This simple approach manages the astigmatism of approximately 80% of my patients.

When the amount of corneal astigmatism reaches 1 D and the corneal topography map shows a symmetric bowtie, I add a matching peripheral corneal relaxing incision (PCRI) on the opposite side in the steep meridian. Paired 1-clock-hour incisions correct 1 D of corneal cylinder assuming the phacoemulsification tunnel incision is placed inside of one of the PCRIs.

The PCRI nomogram I use is simple. For symmetric bowtie corneal astigmatism, I make paired incisions just inside the limbus that are as long in clock hours as the cornea is steep in diopters. I think it is easier to create a mental image of clock hours than degrees or millimeters. For symmetric bowtie astigmatism of 1, 2, or 3 D, I make paired incisions that are 1, 2, or 3 clock hours in length. Figure 3 shows the nomogram in table form for 1-, 2-, and 3-D corrections. Figure 4 shows before and after corneal topography maps from a patient whose symmetric bowtie astigmatism was corrected using this nomogram.

Between 1 and 2.5 D of corneal astigmatism, both PCRIs and the currently available toric intraocular lens (IOL) implants work nicely. Alcon (Fort Worth, TX) manufacturers 3 toric lenses with IOL-plane toric powers of 1.5, 2.25, and 3.0 D as shown in Figure 5. These powers vertex to approximately 1, 1.5, and 2 D of correction in the corneal plane. STAAR Surgical (Monrovia, CA) manufactures 2 toric lenses as shown in Figure 6. STAAR lenses have 2 and 3.5 D of cylinder correction in the IOL plane. In the corneal plane, these powers vertex to 1.4 and 2.3 D of correction.

I have gained considerable experience implanting both companies' lenses. Because STAAR Surgical toric lenses are made from silicone, they are slippery and somewhat difficult to align accurately in the capsular bag. The shorter AA4203TF model has a propensity to rotate after surgery as demonstrated in Figure 7. I had to reposition 7 STAAR toric lenses early in my experience, including the one shown in the illustration.[2] The Alcon toric lens has more power choices and does not rotate after implantation. The Alcon toric lens is, therefore, my current toric lens of choice.

Astigmatism Management
(Non-covered Service Waiver)

Dr. Miller routinely measures and corrects for corneal astigmatism at the time of cataract and other eye surgeries. This is often called **refractive cataract surgery** or, alternatively, **refractive eye surgery**. It is a combination of the techniques of cataract, lens implant, and refractive surgery. The purpose of astigmatism management is to reduce dependence on eyeglasses for best vision after surgery. Medicare and most health insurance plans will not pay for astigmatism management. Refractive surgery performed solely to reduce a patient's dependence on eyeglasses or contact lenses is considered cosmetic and is excluded from coverage according to Medicare (Social Security Act, Title XVIII, Section 1862 [7] and [10]). The Medicare Coverage Issues Manual (CIM) contains specific instructions about non-coverage of refractive keratoplasty in Section 35–54. Most health insurance plans comply with Medicare reimbursement rules.

The fee for astigmatism management in this office is $950 for surgery on one eye, and $1,700 for surgery on both eyes. These fees are the patient's responsibility.

YES

I authorize Dr. Miller to proceed with astigmatism management at the time of my cataract or other eye surgery. Dr. Miller or one of his staff has informed me that Medicare and most private health insurance plans do not cover astigmatism management. I agree to be personally and fully responsible for payment. Additionally, I acknowledge that I have read and initialed each page of the accompanying document, "Frequently Asked Questions About Astigmatism Management."

_____   _____
Patient's Signature   Date

NO

I do not authorize Dr. Miller to proceed with astigmatism management. Dr. Miller or one of his staff has informed me that Medicare and most other health insurance plans do not cover astigmatism management. I understand that my astigmatism may stay the same or worsen during surgery as a result of not treating it. Additionally, I acknowledge that I have read and initialed each page of the accompanying document, "Frequently Asked Questions About Astigmatism Management."

_____   _____
Patient's Signature   Date

Figure 1. Kevin M. Miller's astigmatism management noncovered service waiver.

Frequently Asked Questions About Astigmatism Management

What is astigmatism?
It is an abnormality in which the optical surfaces of the eye are shaped like a football (oval) rather than a baseball or basketball (round). Astigmatism is the most common optical problem after myopia (nearsightedness) and hyperopia (farsightedness).

How does astigmatism affect vision?
When it is uncorrected, astigmatism blurs vision at all distances, near and far.

Is astigmatism correction something new?
No. We have been correcting astigmatism at the time of cataract surgery (and other eye operations) for years. Medicare and private health insurance plans do not cover it.

How do I know if I have astigmatism?
There is no way of knowing without specific testing. Overall astigmatism is approximately the sum of what is in the cornea and what is in the lens. Cataract surgery eliminates the lens component of astigmatism. Any amount remaining in the cornea will contribute to reduced image quality without glasses following surgery. Some people have no astigmatism in their eyeglass measurements, yet they have astigmatism in their corneas. The only way of knowing if corneal astigmatism is present is to test for it.

What if I have no astigmatism or only a small amount?
Knowing there is little or no corneal astigmatism is just as important as knowing there is a lot because it determines how and where we make the incision.

How is astigmatism corrected?
There are three methods. The first involves placing one or more incisions in the steep axis of the peripheral cornea. The second involves modifying the length, depth or number of incisions. The third involves implanting a special intraocular lens, called a toric lens. The latter two approaches can be combined to achieve high amounts of astigmatism correction, if necessary.

What if I don't have it corrected?
If you have residual astigmatism after surgery, there is a greater chance you will need glasses or contact lenses to see clearly. Your astigmatism can easily worsen after surgery if it is not measured before surgery and managed appropriately during surgery.

Are there other options?
The only other option is to perform your eye surgery without astigmatism correction and evaluate your astigmatism afterwards. Astigmatism can be corrected secondarily if you don't like the initial result. However, this will require a second trip to the operating room, which will not be covered by Medicare or other health insurance. In this case, the cost

Kevin M. Miller, MD   Patient's initials: _____
Page 1 of 4   Date: _____

continued

Figure 2. Kevin M. Miller's astigmatism management service list of frequently asked questions.

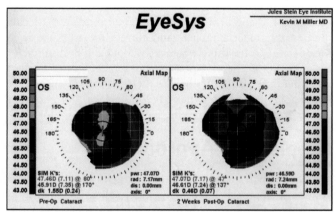

Figure 3. Kevin M. Miller's nomogram for PCRIs based on clock hours of corneal incision length. For symmetric topographic bowtie astigmatism, two PCRIs are placed in the steep axis. Each incision is as long in clock hours as the cornea is steep in diopters.

Figure 4. This patient had 1.55 D of preoperative corneal astigmatism (left map). It was reduced to 0.46 D after surgery by placing symmetric 1-clock-hour incisions in the 85-degree meridian (right map). The phacoemulsification tunnel was placed inside the superior PCRI.

At this time I perform PCRIs for up to 1.5 D of corneal cylinder and implant toric IOLs for 1.5 to 2.5 D of corneal cylinder. I prefer to place the phacoemulsification incision on steep axis whenever I implant a toric lens to reduce the corneal cylinder component. That way, I can use the lowest possible power in the toric lens.

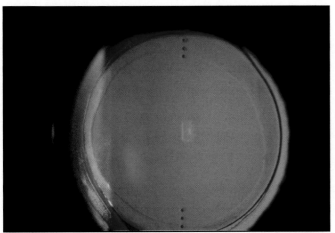

Figure 5. This slit lamp photo shows an Alcon toric IOL in retroillumination view. The axis of the correcting plus cylinder in the 90-degree meridian is marked with 3 dots.

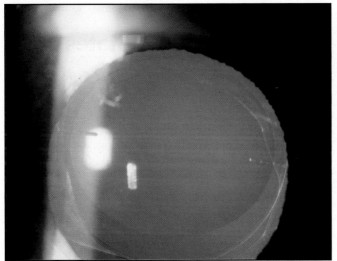

Figure 6. This slit lamp photo shows a Staar Surgical toric IOL in retroillumination view. The axis of the correcting plus cylinder in the 167-degree meridian is marked with linear tic marks.

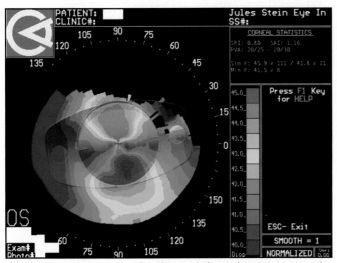

Figure 7. This shows how a Staar toric IOL rotated after implantation as compared to preoperative topography.

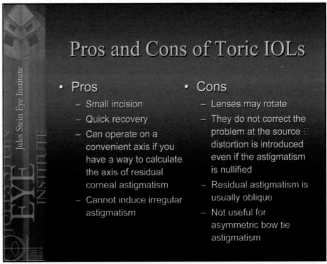

Figure 8. Pros and cons of toric IOLs.

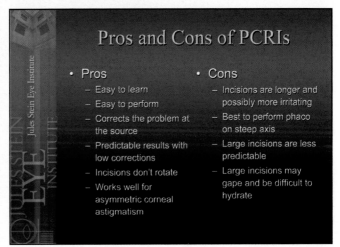

Figure 9. Pros and cons of LRIs.

Pros and Cons of Toric IOLs Versus Peripheral Corneal Relaxing Incisions

Toric IOLs and PCRIs have advantages and disadvantages. These are summarized in Figures 8 and 9. The chief advantages of PCRIs are that they correct astigmatism at the source, they are simple and cheap to perform, and they do not rotate. The chief advantages of toric lens implants are greater precision, a smaller incision, and a more predictable outcome.

In an Ideal World

If a patient with high corneal astigmatism has that astigmatism fully compensated by a toric lens in the IOL plane, such that the net spectacle-plane astigmatism is 0 D, and the patient has no spherical refractive error, will the patient then have no optical aberration? Not really. One toric lens placed in front of another toric lens introduces distortion. In an ideal world, a better way to treat the astigmatism would be to neutralize it at the source—the cornea. It would be better to have a spherical

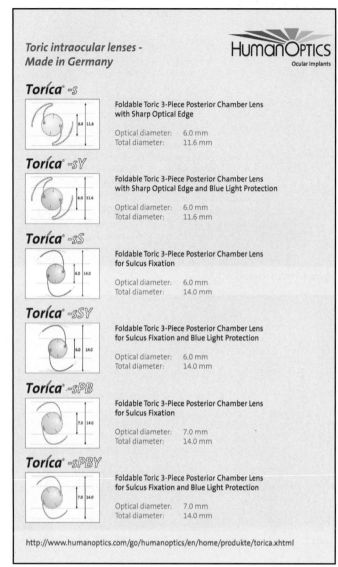

Figure 10. HumanOptics manufactures toric IOLs that correct up to 12 D of astigmatism in the IOL plane. This page is copied from their Web site.

cornea in front of a spherical IOL than to have a toric cornea in front of a compensating toric IOL. Because of the distortion effect, I prefer to correct high amounts of corneal astigmatism to the extent that I am able to with PCRIs, and then add a toric lens to correct the portion that cannot be compensated by the PCRIs.

For Greater Than 3 Diopters

Few patients have greater than 3 D of corneal astigmatism, but these patients are the ones we really want to help. So what happens when a patient's corneal astigmatism is higher than 3 D? The answer to this question depends on where in the world you live. If you live in the United States, the highest available toric lens is the STAAR Surgical lens at 3.5 D of cylinder correction in the IOL plane. As mentioned previously, this lens achieves 2.3 D of correction in the corneal plane. If an on-axis phacoemulsification incision is performed, that adds 0.5 D of additional effect for a total correction of 2.8 D.

The most effect one can reasonably hope to achieve with PCRIs is 3.0 D, and doing so requires paired 3-clock-hour incisions. After each side of a cornea has been cut 3 clock hours, half the cornea has been incised. Cutting any further risks a neurotrophic state and corneal decompensation.

To correct greater than 3 D of corneal astigmatism in the United States at this time (2008), it is necessary to combine toric IOLs and PCRIs. If we assume that the maximum reasonable correction that can be achieved with a toric lens is in the 2 to 2.5 D range and the maximum reasonable correction that can be achieved with PCRIs is in the 2.5- to 3-D range, then the maximum amount of overall astigmatic compensation that can be reasonably achieved is about 5 D. Patients with this amount of corneal cylinder do not come along very often, but they exist. I have had a number of them in my practice and the combined approach has produced satisfactory results.

Outside the United States

For surgeons who live outside the United States and have access to IOLs on the international market, there is an alternative to combining toric lenses and PCRIs. HumanOptics AG (Erlangen, Germany) manufactures a series of high-powered toric lens implants designed for capsular bag (Torica–s and Torica–sY), sulcus (Torica–sS), or piggyback (Torica–sPB) implantation. Figure 10 shows a page from the HumanOptics Web site. HumanOptics Torica lenses correct from 2 to 12 D of corneal astigmatism in 1-D increments in the regular series, and from 1 to 6 D of regular astigmatism in 1-D steps in the piggyback series. If a surgeon in the United States wants to use one of these lenses, it is possible to obtain an individual compassionate use exemption from the US Food and Drug Administration.

Alcon plans to roll out toric lens implants in higher powers. They will extend the IOL-plane correction of their SN60TT series to 5 D in the SN60T9 model. This lens will compensate for approximately 4 D of corneal cylinder. If and when this lens becomes available, the number of patients who will need both a toric IOL and PCRIs will drop dramatically.

It is possible to improve our patients' unaided visual acuities dramatically by reducing or eliminating their corneal astigmatism. Patients who have worn glasses since childhood are amazed at the results, particularly if they can achieve spectacle independence.

References

1. Gross RH, Miller KM. Corneal astigmatism after phacoemulsification and lens implantation through unsutured scleral and corneal tunnel incisions. *Am J Ophthalmol.* 1996;121:57-64.

2. Nguyen TM, Miller KM. Digital overlay technique for documenting toric intraocular lens axis orientation. *J Cataract Refract Surg.* 2000;26:1496-1504.

SECTION XI

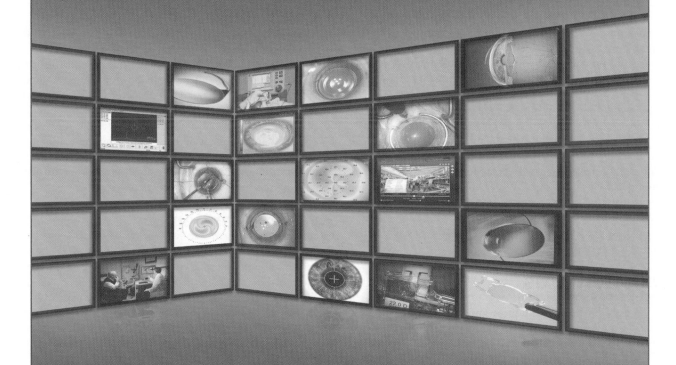

Premium Cataract Surgery

CHAPTER 176

PEARLS FOR IMPROVING YOUR CATARACT SURGICAL SKILLS

David F. Chang, MD

Implanting presbyopia-correcting intraocular lenses (IOLs) raises the cataract surgical stakes and places greater pressure on the surgeon's surgical skills. Refractive success requires far more than advanced IOL technology alone, and leaves the ophthalmologist with little surgical margin for error. In addition to requiring accurate biometry and IOL calculation, the IOL must be centered within an intact capsular bag with a symmetrically overlapping capsulorrhexis. There must be thorough cortical cleanup and the incision must be astigmatically neutral. A clear postoperative day 1 cornea is a prerequisite for creating a "WOW" factor. Finally, posterior capsular rupture usually carries the added disappointment of aborting implantation of the intended IOL. With flawless surgery at a premium, here are several pearls for each of the major surgical steps.

Capsulorrhexis

The capsulorrhexis is the most important step of cataract surgery. Circumferential anterior capsular overlap of the optic edge is important for reducing posterior capsule opacification (PCO) and for achieving consistent axial IOL position. When we customize our A-constant, effective lens position (ELP) is one of the most significant variables that differ from one surgeon to another for this reason. Reducing PCO and attaining a consistent ELP are especially important when implanting multifocal IOLs. In addition, the capsulorrhexis size impacts the ability of accommodating IOLs, such as the Eyeonics, Inc. Crystalens (Aliso Viejo, CA) or the Visiogen, Inc. Synchrony (Irvine, CA), to move. Correctly centering and sizing the capsulorrhexis diameter is difficult, however, because of individual variability in pupil and corneal diameter, corneal magnification, and the effects of parallax as the globe moves and tilts.

The best solution for consistently achieving a perfect capsulorrhexis size and shape is to err on making the diameter initially smaller than desired. After the IOL is implanted, the capsulorrhexis diameter can be secondarily enlarged if necessary by making an oblique snip in the edge with microscissors,

and re-tearing it. I discuss and illustrate this technique further in Chapter 182.

When there is difficulty controlling the capsulorrhexis flap for reasons of visibility, chamber shallowing, patient cooperation, or weak zonules, making the diameter smaller reduces the risk of a radial tear. This is critical in the case of accommodating IOLs where implantation must be aborted in the event of a peripheral anterior capsule tear. Mastering the technique of secondary enlargement permits us to "play it safe" by making a smaller primary capsulorrhexis if we encounter difficulty controlling the flap.

Hydrodissection

Hydrodissection is the most underrated step of cataract surgery. Without rotation we cannot otherwise safely access subincisional nucleus and epinucleus, and overly adherent subincisional cortex carries added risk of a capsular tear. Therefore, successful hydrodissection improves our efficiency, reduces the risk of posterior capsular rupture, and by cleaving the cortical attachments, reduces the rate of posterior capsule opacification.

Using an ophthalmic viscosurgical device (OVD) to deepen the anterior chamber (AC) and to flatten the anterior capsular convexity makes it much easier to control the developing capsulorrhexis tear. However, by exerting downward pressure against the nucleus, overfilling the AC with an OVD increases the resistance that the posteriorly directed hydrodissection wave must overcome. It is therefore advisable to burp out some OVD immediately prior to initiating hydrodissection. Partially emptying the AC will permit the nucleus to rise anteriorly away from the posterior capsule upon separation.

The hydrodissection wave frequently fails to travel completely across the posterior capsule. Given the importance of preferentially loosening the sub-incisional cortex, it is therefore logical to initiate the hydrodissection wave from the subincisional anterior capsular rim. A partially incomplete wave that started from the contra-incisional fornix will leave the sub-incisional cortex maximally adherent. I advocate a

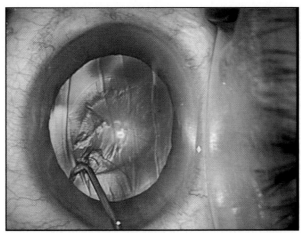

Figure 1A. Chang right angle hydrodissection cannula (Katena) hooks the subincisional capsulorrhexis edge.

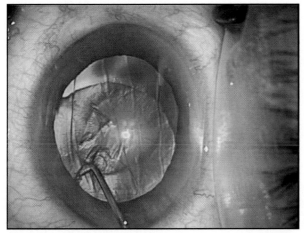

Figure 1B. Initial hydrodissection wave hugs the posterior capsule, and preferentially loosens the subincisional cortex.

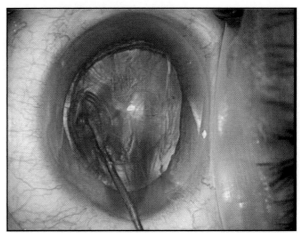

Figure 1C. Angling the tip slightly internally creates a hydrodelineation wave that cleaves the epinucleus from the endonucleus.

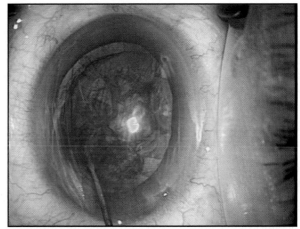

Figure 1D. The blunt point on the tip is used to rotate the nucleus with circular raking motions.

right-angle hydrodissection cannula tip (Chang hydrodissection cannula, Katena, ASICO, Rhein Medical) because, like a right-angle I&A tip, this configuration can access the proximal 180 degrees of capsular rim (Figure 1). I prefer to sever the last remaining capsular attachments by using the blunt point of the cannula tip to rotate the nucleus within the bag prior to phaco. The short, right angle tip works well at engaging the peripheral anterior nuclear surface and rotating it with circular raking motions (see Figure 1d).

Use a Micro Phaco Tip

Going from a 19-gauge to a 20-gauge phaco tip is one strategy that all surgeons can use to enhance safety regardless of their brand of phaco machine. This single modification reduces surge lessens the chance of accidentally aspirating iris or capsule, and makes it easier to pluck thin or crumbling nuclear fragments from the capsular fornices. The latter advantage stems from the fact that the smaller tip occludes without having to penetrate too deeply into the nucleus. The larger the tip surface area, the more deeply the entire tip must be embedded to create a vacuum seal with a peristaltic pump. If one is trying to elevate a thin, crumbling segment of nucleus out of the peripheral bag, one may need to penetrate dangerously close

to the capsule to occlude the tip. The narrower tip lumen restricts flow, reduces surge, and prevents material from rushing in as fast as through a standard diameter needle shaft. Like using a smaller I-A tip opening, a micro phaco tip also provides greater control over which tissue is or is not aspirated. Slowing things down in this way helps when one wants to guard against snagging the capsule, such as when aspirating epinucleus or thin nuclear pieces abutting the peripheral capsular bag.

Counterbalancing these advantages are several tradeoffs. Micro phaco tips tend to increase nuclear chatter because of the smaller "mouth." They take longer to evacuate a bulky nucleus—like drinking a milkshake through a small straw. Finally, the smaller surface area of the tip's opening reduces the effective holding power for any given vacuum level. Fortunately, we can solve the chatter/followability problem with hyperpulse phaco modulation, with torsional (non-longitudinal) phaco, and by chopping the nucleus into smaller pieces. Improved pump technology enables us to safely use higher aspiration flow and vacuum to compensate for the other factors. This makes it possible to reap the benefits of a smaller phaco tip regardless of whether one performs coaxial or bi-axial phaco, and this is the most overlooked safety modification that surgeons can make.

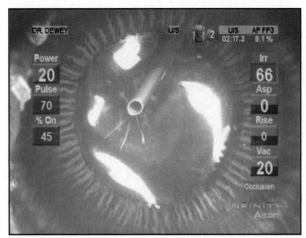

Figure 2. Miyake-Apple view of Dewey radius phaco tip aspirating cadaver posterior capsule without cutting it. (Photo courtesy of Steven Dewey.)

The Dewey Radius phaco needle (Microsurgical Technologies, Redmond WA) is another tip option that can reduce the risk of a tear should the posterior capsule be aspirated (Figure 2). Surprisingly, brunescent nuclei can be effectively emulsified despite rounding the sharp edge contour of the standard phaco needle.

Sequentially Changing Memory Settings

Another important strategy is that of customizing machine memory settings for each sequential stage of the procedure. Although it is tempting to seek the simplicity of one set of parameters that can be used for every type of nucleus and for each step of the case, doing so sacrifices control. The fluidic imize cutting efficiency so as to avoid pushing the lens against the bag), chops (maximize holding power to fixate, separate, and then elevate chopped segments), or removes loose fragments (maximize followability, reduce chatter and turbulence, and avoid any momentary surge once the posterior capsule is exposed).

For this reason, one should pre-program ultrasound and vacuum parameters that best prioritize the specific objectives of each step in nuclear emulsification. For example, memory settings with different "packages" of parameters could be set up for sculpting, for chopping, for fragment removal, and for epinucleus aspiration. As a general principle, higher aspiration flow and vacuum are desirable early on to optimize holding power for chopping, separating, and aspirating the initial fragments, when enough remaining nucleus obscures or blocks the posterior capsule. However, high flow and vacuum later become a liability as the final pieces are removed and the posterior capsule is exposed to the phaco tip. Flow and vacuum should be significantly reduced to avoid surge at this stage of the case.

Inserting the IOL Cartridge Tip Bevel Up

Proper IOL implantation technique allows for insertion through as small a clear corneal opening as possible, while avoiding excessive stretching or tearing of the edges of the incision. Both the bevel up and bevel down orientations work, but there are three reasons that I introduce the IOL cartridge tip into the clear corneal incision bevel up (Figure 3):

* The proximal edge of the bevel cannot drag debris from the conjunctiva into the anterior chamber. If the tip is inserted bevel down, the proximal edge can scrape surface mucous or debris off of the conjunctiva, which will then be deposited behind the center of the IOL optic inside the capsular bag.

* Just as the heel is the most difficult part of the foot to squeeze into a leather boot, the proximal edge of the beveled opening is the last part of the cartridge tip to pass through a tight clear corneal incision. With a leather boot, one grips the back of the boot opening (closest to the heel) to facilitate this tight passage. Likewise, if the tip enters bevel up we can use toothed forceps to lift the anterior incision lip closest to the proximal bevel.

* The forceps should merely evert the anterior lip of the clear corneal incision to facilitate guiding the cartridge tip into the incision (see Figures 3A and 3B). It is important not to pull on the anterior lip of the clear corneal incision with the forceps as a means to apply counter traction. Doing so risks tearing off a piece of the thin roof of the corneal tunnel. Instead, as the bevel up cartridge tip encounters resistance, use it to push the globe posteriorly toward the orbital apex (see Figure 3C). This produces the necessary counter fixation to advance the cartridge tip further through the incision. The surgeon can view when at least half of the beveled opening has cleared Descemet's membrane. At this point, the tip, having encountered more resistance, can be twisted into the anterior chamber without a tendency for it to back out (see Figure 3D). The bevel is rotated posteriorly so that the lead haptic is introduced through the capsulorrhexis and into the capsular bag (see Figure 3E).

Centering a Diffractive Multifocal IOL

As soon as you start implanting a diffractive multifocal IOL such as the ReSTOR, you realize that the pupil and the center of the capsular bag are usually not aligned, with the constricted pupil being nasally off center. Paolo Vinceguerra's chapter (Chapter 184) nicely explains the optical desirability of centering the diffractive optic with the pupil. Based on his recommendation, I orient the haptics of the Acrysof ReSTOR

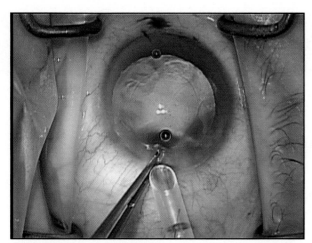

Figure 3A. Forceps evert the corneal lip.

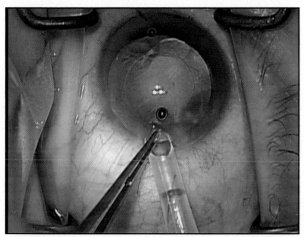

Figure 3B. Cartridge is introduced bevel up until Descemet's membrane bisects the oval top opening.

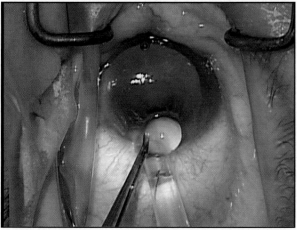

Figure 3C. When resistance is encountered, the back of the cartridge tip is used to depress the globe into the orbit. This creates sufficient counter pressure without having to use the forceps to pull on the incision lip.

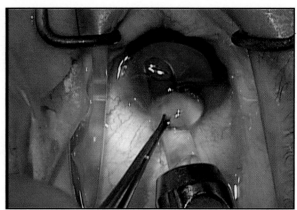

Figure 3D. The cartridge tip is twisted to advance it into the anterior chamber.

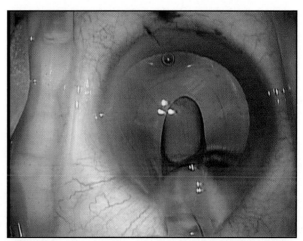

Figure 3E. The bevel is rotated posteriorly to direct the lead haptic into the capsular bag.

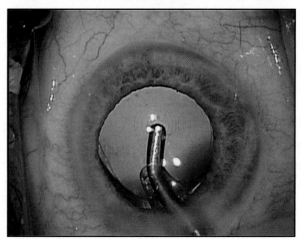

Figure 4. ReSTOR optic is first oriented with haptics along the 6 to 12 o'clock vertical axis. The optic is then nudged slightly nasally by the irrigation-aspiration tip (entering through the temporal incision).

vertically from 6 to 12 o'clock, and then nudge the optic nasally as the OVD is removed with the IA handpiece (Figure 4). The tacky hydrophobic acrylic material causes the lens to remain where it is left, and this simple technique is surprisingly consistent at aligning the IOL with the pupil without the need to constrict the pupil intraoperatively.

CHAPTER 177

PEARLS FOR IMPROVING YOUR CATARACT SURGICAL SKILLS

Uday Devgan, MD, FACS

The sun is setting on the old mindset of cataract surgery. The old paradigm is that of elderly patients with dense cataracts who do not mind wearing glasses after surgery. The new age of cataract surgery involves younger patients with milder cataracts who have an expectation of freedom from glasses for most activities.

Every year our technology and surgical techniques get better and better. Compare the phacoemulsification machines from a decade ago to the modern marvels we use now. The same applies for our intraocular lens (IOL) technology. Within the next 10 years or less, we will have IOLs that provide a much larger amplitude of accommodation, superb image quality, and highly accurate refractive results.

To perform premium IOL surgery we need to embrace the concept that cataract surgery is refractive surgery. We must provide excellent refractive results and treat our patients like luxury consumers. Improving our cataract surgical skills is crucial and I offer the following pearls.

Pearl 1: Achieve Postoperative Refractive Accuracy

Precise IOL calculations are the foundation for improved refractive accuracy. Every effort should be taken to use optical methods of axial length determination. For cases where an optical measurement is difficult or impossible, immersion A-scan ultrasonography should be employed. The traditional method of applanation ultrasonography can be highly inaccurate and is operator dependent. An error of just 0.3 mm can result in a 1-D refractive surprise postoperatively.

Using the most precise technology to measure the axial length is not enough. We must also personalize our A-constants to achieve consistency. Keeping track of postoperative refractive results and then comparing the expected outcome versus the actual outcome will help us to hone our lens calculations. In calculating the IOL power, it is critical to use a newer-generation theoretical formula (Hoffer Q, SRK-T, Holladay I and II, Haigis) and not a regression formula. There is evidence that a specific IOL formula may be more accurate for a subset of eyes. There are also multivariable formulas, such as the Holladay II and Haigis, which may produce more accurate results once personalization is achieved (Figure 1).

The determination of the true keratometric value is usually straightforward, but it can be more difficult in postcorneal refractive surgery eyes. In these patients, dozens of methods to estimate the corneal power have been described, which means that none of these methods is perfect. It is typically best in these eyes to err on the side of myopia and to make sure that the patient understands the high probability of ametropia and the possible need for an enhancement to achieve the desired postoperative refractive goal.

The cataract surgeon needs to have a method of fixing postoperative refractive surprises. For most small degrees of ametropia, corneal excimer laser refractive surgery is the best option because it is accurate, less invasive, and can be performed in the clinic. Other options include the use of piggyback IOLs or even IOL exchange. For cataract surgeons who do not currently perform corneal refractive surgery, it may be wise to pair up with a corneal refractive surgeon.

Pearl 2: Reduce Pre-Existing Corneal Astigmatism

Every incision made into the cornea has the potential of affecting the astigmatism. For your routine cataract surgery, what is the effect of your incision? For most surgeons using a 2.5- to 3.0-mm self-sealing corneal incision, there is a flattening effect of about 0.25 to 0.50 D at the axis of the incision.[1] If the patient has a small amount of pre-existing corneal astigmatism at the site of your planned incision, it will work out well. However, a considerable percentage of patients will have significant corneal astigmatism that needs to be specifically addressed.[2]

Learning to use limbal relaxing incisions (LRIs) at the time of cataract surgery is an effective way to reduce the

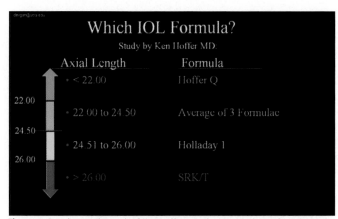

Figure 1. Based upon the work of Ken Hoffer MD, the IOL calculation formula can be customized to the axial length of the eye.

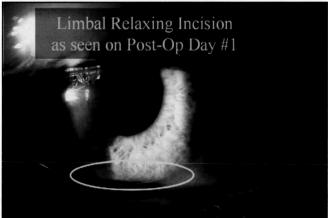

Figure 2. Slit lamp photo of a limbal relaxing incision at the 90 degree meridian.

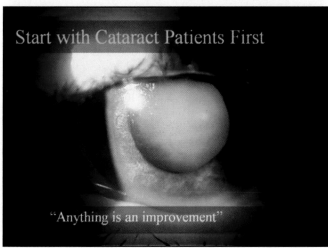

Figure 3. Patients with dense cataracts are more tolerant of residual refractive errors of dysphotopsias since their pre-operative vision is so poor. They often say that "Anything is an improvement."

pre-existing corneal astigmatism and achieve postoperative emmetropia (Figure 2). Topography is the most effective way to properly understand the extent of the corneal astigmatism and will make your LRI planning more accurate. Excellent nomograms and instructions are available from some of the pioneers of LRIs, including Louis D. "Skip" Nichamin, MD,[3] Doug D. Koch, MD,[4] and Jim P. Gills, MD[5], among others.

Because correction of preexisting corneal astigmatism is not a covered benefit of Medicare and most insurance plans, patients pay out of pocket for LRIs and similar procedures. Practicing the technique of LRIs as well as honing your own LRI nomogram will help you deliver consistent results.

Pearl 3: Fix Postoperative Refractive Surprises

It is not always possible to achieve postoperative emmetropia. There are variations in lens calculations, lens labeling, lens position, and patient healing. In these patients, it is helpful to have methods to address postoperative refractive surprises. For small spherical residual refractive errors, implanting a piggy-back IOL into the ciliary sulcus is an easy option for most cataract surgeons.

Corneal refractive surgery can be a very accurate way to correct residual refractive errors. For postoperative hyperopic surprises, use of conductive keratoplasty (CK; Refractec, Irvine, CA) is a viable option that is well within the skill set of most general ophthalmologists. For those with access to an excimer laser, surface ablation or laser in situ keratomileusis (LASIK) is very accurate. For surgeons without excimer access, I suggest teaming up with a local refractive surgeon.

Pearl 4: Start With Cataract Patients First

For your first few refractive IOL patients, start with patients that have very significant cataracts (Figure 3). When the patient's preoperative vision is 20/100 or worse, they tend to be happy by just clearing their visual axis. As one patient put it, "Anything is an improvement!" These patients already have problems with acuity, contrast, glare, halos, and color perception, so that even a complicated surgery by a first-year resident would likely result in an improvement in vision.

Once you feel that you have honed your refractive results, consider performing refractive lens exchange on precataract patients. These patients already have vision that is correctable to 20/20 or close to it, and as such, they will be far more demanding of precise postoperative results.

Pearl 5: Choose the Right Initial Patients

To further stack the odds in your favor, choose initial patients who are hyperopic with low amounts of corneal astigmatism. These hyperopes are reliant on glasses for all distances preoperatively and elimination of spectacles for even part of their visual needs is a huge improvement for them.

Patient personality is also a factor. A perfectionist mentality is fine for the surgeon, but is best avoided in the patient. I tell patients that these IOLs are not the fountain of youth and that no surgery can make them see like teenagers again. Having an easy-going mindset goes a long way towards achieving postoperative satisfaction for both the patient and the surgeon.

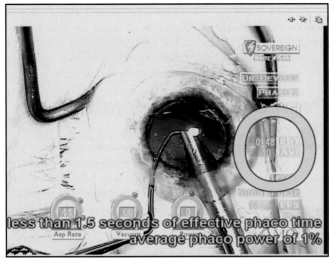

Figure 4. Using phaco power modulations, the total ultrasonic energy used to remove even a dense cataract can be reduced dramatically.

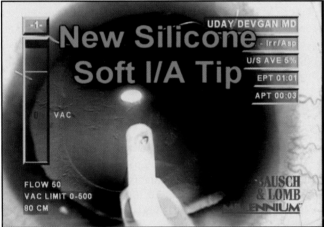

Figure 5. The silicone-coated soft I/A tips prevent metal-to-capsule contact and may decrease the incidence of posterior capsule rupture during cortex removal.

Pearl 6: Deliver Clear Corneas

Refractive surgery patients want clear vision, and that requires clear corneas. It is just not acceptable to routinely induce corneal edema, Descemet's folds, and massive inflammation from surgery. Techniques to protect the corneal endothelium and minimize the phaco energy must be employed (Figure 4). Good-quality viscoelastics, mechanical nucleus disassembly via phaco chop, and phaco power modulations are all helpful in achieving consistently clear corneas immediately after surgery.

Pearl 7: Minimize Complications—Soft Irrigation and Aspiration

If you perform exactingly accurate IOL calculations, reduce the corneal astigmatism, remove the cataract with minimal phaco energy, but then break the capsular bag during cortex

clean up, the refractive result has been jeopardized. One of the most important new innovations in cataract surgery has been the development of the silicone-coated soft irrigation and aspiration (I&A) tip (MicroSurgical Technologies, Redmond, WA) (Figure 5), which prevents any metal to capsule contact. The silicone tip is far gentler to the posterior capsule than steel, and in my hands this tip has not damaged a single capsule in hundreds of cases.

Pearl 8: Prevent Cystoid Macular Edema—Nonsteroidal Anti-Inflammatory Drugs

There are now multiple published studies that conclusively show that the perioperative use of topical nonsteroidal anti-inflammatory drugs (NSAIDs) is important for the prevention and treatment of cystoid macular edema (CME).[6] The selection of one brand of NSAID over another is the subject for another article, but you should clearly be using your choice of NSAID for all cataract and lens surgery patients.

It is hard to explain to patients why they don't see well, even though you chose the optimum IOL, you eliminated their astigmatism, and you performed excellent surgery. Preventing CME is as important as preventing intraoperative complications.

Pearl 9: Choose the Right IOL

There are currently three refractive IOLs that address presbyopia that are approved by the Food and Drug Administration (FDA). They are the ReZoom from Advanced Medical Optics (Santa Ana, CA), the Crystalens from Eyeonics (Aliso Viejo, CA), and the ReSTOR from Alcon (Fort Worth, TX). Each of these IOLs addresses presbyopia differently and they work in different ways. The surgeon must understand these differences and evaluate patients to determine if they are appropriate candidates for each IOL option. I have found that patients truly do need time to adapt to these new IOLs and that the period of neuroadaptation may take months.

Pearl 10: Underpromise and Overdeliver

Our goal for any refractive surgery is primarily to meet or exceed the patient's expectations. Making sure that patients have a realistic expectation of the limits of refractive IOL surgery is important, as no surgery is perfect. A 65-year-old patient does not expect a plastic surgeon to make her look 25 years old again; rather she expects to look better. Similarly, we need to help our 65-year-old patient understand that she will not be able to see as she did when she was 25 years old; rather we will help her see better.

References

1. Borasio E, Mehta JS, Maurino V. Torque and flattening effects of clear corneal temporal and on-axis incisions for phacoemulsification. *J Cataract Refract Surg.* 2006;32:2030-2038.

2. Kaufmann C, Peter J, Ooi K, Phipps S, Cooper P, Goggin M. Limbal relaxing incisions versus on-axis incisions to reduce corneal astigmatism at the time of cataract surgery. *J Cataract Refract Surg.* 2005;31:2261-2265.

3. Nichamin LD. Nomogram for limbal relaxing incisions. *J Cataract Refract Surg.* 2006;32:1408.

4. Wang L, Misra M, Koch DD. Peripheral corneal relaxing incisions combined with cataract surgery. *J Cataract Refract Surg.* 2003;29:712-722.

5. Gills JP. Treating astigmatism at the time of cataract surgery. *Curr Opin Ophthalmol.* 2002;13:2-6.

6. O'Brien TP. Emerging guidelines for use of NSAID therapy to optimize cataract surgery patient care. *Curr Med Res Opin.* 2005;21:1131-1137.

PEARLS FOR IMPROVING YOUR CATARACT SURGICAL SKILLS

Brian Little, FRCS, FRCOphth, FHEA

The steady migration toward earlier and safer cataract surgery over recent years has coincided and combined with the availability of presbyopia-correcting intraocular lenses (IOLs) to reach its logical conclusion: the development of refractive lens exchange (RLE).

By pursuing and promoting this exciting development, we have unwittingly created a rod for own back in that we now have to work in a much more exacting and less forgiving environment with lower margins for error at every level.

We are all well aware that there is, as yet, no synthetic substitute that comes even close to the crystalline lens of our youth. All current options are a compromise. As a consequence, we need to be alert to the paramount importance of careful patient selection, comprehensive counseling, accurate biometry, and choice of appropriate IOL in our obligation to under-sell and over-deliver when it comes to our patients' expectations. We need to develop our skills in the emerging subspecialty of psycho-ophthalmology.

On the "over-delivering" side of the equation we need to pay particular and meticulous attention to our surgical technique in order to minimize the risk of the heart-sinking disappointment that comes from a suboptimal outcome.

I present my 5 surgical "pearls" that are born out of experience gained from my tentative venture into this potential minefield.

Stable Watertight Incision

It makes clear sense to stick to the easy cases that have near-spherical corneas. In order to maintain this sphericity and induce no significant corneal astigmatism, I much prefer to use a scleral incision placed fairly anteriorly. This can be either grooved or uniplanar (Figure 1). A scleral tunnel incision requires minimal additional time to perform because of the need for a small peritomy and hemostasis. However, being more elastic than a corneal incision due to the random fiber arrangement, scleral tunnel incisions not only easily accommodate the IOL injector but also self-seal beautifully without the need for stromal hydration. Their ability to rapidly self-

seal also contributes to improved chamber stability during surgery by avoiding chamber collapse, particularly as the phaco tip is removed. This may seem a little obsessive but with RLE, we are often dealing with a younger group of patients with healthy eyes who may not yet have a posterior vitreous detachment (PVD). I believe that anything we can do to minimize any forward movement of the vitreous body during surgery may reduce the effects of vitreomacular and vitreoretinal traction with their inherent risks. The feel of the surgery is a little different than it is through a corneal incision because the angle of approach is flatter. However, if you remain reasonably anterior with the external entry site, then it just takes a little getting used to, but it is well worth the effort.

Correctly Sized Capsulorrhexis

The continuous curvilinear capsulorrhexis also needs to be central, circular, and the correct size, particularly when implanting premium IOLs. This is easier said than done. What exactly is the correct size? We now know for certain that it needs to overlap the edge of the optic all the way around. This helps to maintain good centration of the implant and retains the optic in the correct plane. The shrink-wrap effect together with a continuous and sharp square edge to the optic also minimizes the risk of future lens epithelial cell migration and proliferation behind the optic leading to posterior capsular opacification (PCO).[1]

The diameter of the capsulorrhexis needs to be about 1 mm less that the diameter of the optic of the implant. This means that the capsulorrhexis needs to be around 5 mm for a 6-mm optic, giving an anterior capsule overlap of 0.5 mm all the way around the optic.

A smaller 4-mm capsulorrhexis will overlap the same 6-mm optic by 1 mm all the way around. You do not really want the capsulorrhexis to go below about 4-mm diameter. The reduction in surface area from a 5-mm to a 4-mm capsulorrhexis is a surprising 33%, and the difference in surface area between a 5-mm and 3-mm capsulorrhexis is a staggering 66%. You start getting into tiger country below 4 mm for 2 reasons. The

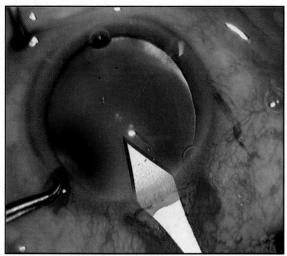

Figure 1. 2.85-mm single-plane scleral tunnel.

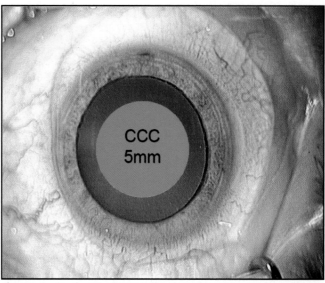

Figure 2. Overlay of a circle of 5 mm, half the vertical corneal diameter, for gauging the capsulorrhexis "freehand."

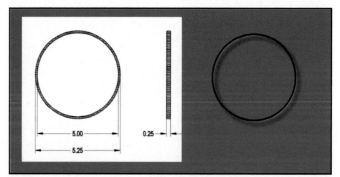

Figure 3. Type 5 blue PMMA caliper ring for accurately sizing the capsulorrhexis (placeholder).

first is the increased surgical risks of capsular block, anterior capsular tear, and postoperative anterior capsular phimosis. The second problem is unique to the multifocal IOLs. With the ReSTOR lens (Alcon, Fort Worth, TX), for example, the functional central diffractive zone of the optic, which balances the distribution of light between near and distance as a function of pupil size, is 3.6-mm wide. The 5 concentric refractive zones in the ReZoom lens (Advanced Medical Optics, Santa Ana, CA) extend out to 5 mm of the 6-mm optic.

How can you reliably and accurately produce a capsulorrhexis that is consistently between 4 and 5 mm in diameter? Well, it mostly boils down to practice and experience, which needs to be combined with a sprinkling of manual dexterity. From a pragmatic approach, you can use the pupil as a reference for circularity and centration but not for size. For size, you can use the vertical corneal diameter as a gauge by recognizing that it is fairly consistently 10.50 mm. You can then project a circle that is half of this diameter (ie, the corneal radius) onto the center of the capsule. Think of it as a 0.5 cup/disc ratio (Figure 2).

Unfortunately, there is no equivalent of a plug-cutter or intraocular trephine that will do the job for you. However, there have been some ingenious attempts to make a more accurate result easier to achieve. Recently, Professor Marie-José Tassignon has developed a simple "Ring Caliper" made of blue polymethylmethacrylate (PMMA) (Morcher GmbH, Stuttgart, Germany). It acts as a template that is placed temporarily on the anterior capsule (Figure 3). Internal diameters of 5 mm or 6 mm are available to produce a capsulorrhexis of approximately 4.75 mm and 5.75 mm, respectively. In my experience this device works very well indeed and is also an excellent tool for resident training.[2]

There are also capsulorrhexis forceps available with calibrated shafts for reference. Although these can be useful early on in a surgeons career to get some idea of scale and size, they are not a fixed reference as the shafts move around with the movements of the forceps.

You should practice in the wet-lab as much as you can and judge the result compared to the known diameter of an implant optic. Remember that practice merely makes permanent and only perfect practice makes perfect (well almost).

Stabilize the Chamber: Take Out the Second Instrument

My third pearl is definitely nonintuitive—in fact it is frankly counter-intuitive, as well as undeniably controversial. I probably risk being ostracized by the broad community of ophthalmologists as a heretic. However, it is based on unshakable logic and I can assure you that it works very reliably to stabilize the chamber during removal of the nuclear fragments. It even has some evidence and data to support it, although it has been said that most physicians use statistics much like a drunk uses a lamp-post; more for support than illumination. So, deep breath in and here goes.

When you are ready to phaco the nuclear fragments from the capsular bag, you should withdraw your second instrument from the eye. That is it! Pure and simple. Any takers? I know it sounds insane but bear with me while I try to convince you.

The first observation is that the commonest time for a posterior chamber (PC) tear in the course of phaco is during removal of the final fragment. This is due to the presence of an empty capsular bag that allows the posterior capsule to flop forwards in the presence of chamber instability. For this reason, traditionally we tend to advocate the use of a blunt second instrument placed behind the phaco tip to "protect"

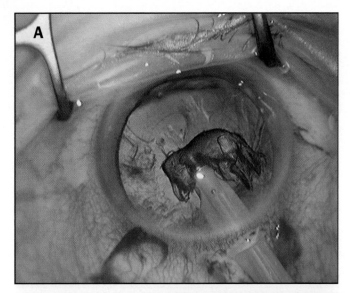

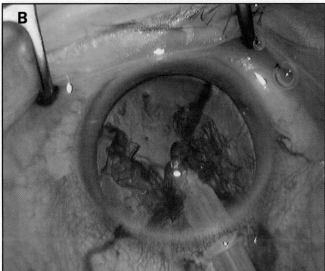

Figure 4. (A) Single-handed removal of final nuclear fragment in iris plane. Posterior cortical fibers defocused, as capsular bag remains fully inflated. (B) Single-handed iris plane phaco, removal of first nuclear fragment.

removed during segment removal (p<0.005).[3] As a result, I tried withdrawing the second instrument from the eye during removal of the final fragment. Much to my delight the chamber became rock solid and was much more secure than with the second instrument in situ (Figure 4A). I then just extended the principle, which should apply equally to the first segment as much as to the last, and so began to withdraw the second instrument at the beginning of segment removal (Figure 4B). Not surprisingly, the result was a more stable chamber throughout segment removal. Most of our junior residents now use this technique out of choice because they feel a lot safer with greater chamber stability. The only down side is that with harder nuclei you can get a little more "chatter & scatter" and lollipopping of the fragments despite the excellent fluidics and power modulations now available. However, you can always reintroduce your second instrument when needed and then withdraw it again.

It is definitely counterintuitive, but it really does work. It improves chamber stability during segment removal and is particularly effective during removal of the final fragment by keeping the bag inflated and the posterior capsule out of harms way. Try it for yourself.

Anterior Capsule Polishing

Anterior capsule polishing is an added enhancement of the surgical procedure that has passed in and out of favor over the years. However, it is now established that capsular fibrosis results from metaplasia of anterior lens epithelial cells (LEC) into myofibroblasts with consequent contraction and collagen deposition. It stands to reason, therefore, that removing as much of the population of these cells as possible from the anterior capsule is likely to reduce the risk of subsequent anterior capsule fibrosis, phimosis, and PCO. This indeed has been shown to be the case.[4] Its detractors often suggest that it is too time-consuming to perform but in reality it takes only a couple of minutes at the most. It is best performed after implantation of the lens as the capsule is then under tension and the implant protects the posterior capsule. You need to use high magnification and to position the eye to obtain an optimal red reflex. The layer of LECs is then clearly visible and gives a mottled geographic appearance to the anterior capsule rim (Figure 5). The contrast between polished and unpolished areas is readily seen as the "dust layer" of cells is aspirated (Figure 6). I personally prefer to use bimanual IA as the standard, which allows a full 360 degrees of access (180 degrees from either sideport). A word of warning about the standard of finish on the edge of the aspiration port of many disposable bimanual handpieces. Most are sharp edged and can easily capture and tear the capsule, the posterior being more vulnerable than the anterior. Reusable handpieces generally have a polished or chamfered edge to the port so the capsule can be safely incarcerated without tearing (Figure 7). My personal preference is Duckworth & Kent's (Hertforshire, England) 23-gauge aspiration cannula (8-657) and 23-gauge open-ended irrigation cannula (8-652-2).

When using coaxial IA it is difficult even with an angulated tip to gain safe or easy access to the subincisional sector of anterior capsule so that in practice the polishing is a little more limited to around 270 degrees. In either case, it is impossible

the posterior capsule. However, it dawned on me that when the second instrument is in the eye during phaco, the only thing that it is actually doing for over 90% of the time is causing a leak through the sideport. In theory, the presence of a second instrument may well be contributing to chamber instability and paradoxically endangering rather than protecting the posterior capsule when it is kept in the eye.

We tested this theory by taking some simple measurements and recently demonstrated that even with precisely dimensioned incisions matched to instruments, incisional leakage actually accounted for a staggering two-thirds (67%) of the total volume of irrigating fluid used during surgery. This means that only one-third (33%) of the total fluid that is used is removed through the phaco tip or aspiration port during IA, and the remaining two-thirds is lost through incisional leakage (main incision plus sideports). We also found that there was a significant reduction in fluid loss between those cases where the second instrument was left in situ and when it was

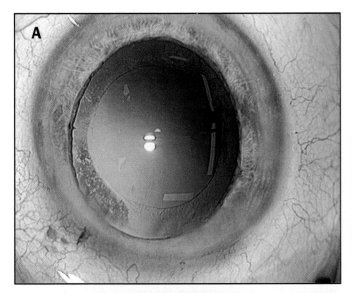

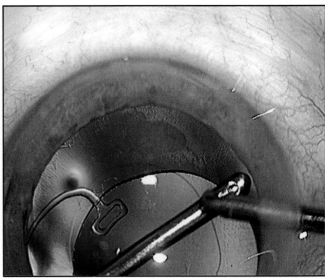

Figure 6. Anterior capsule polishing. Contrast between adjacent polished and unpolished areas.

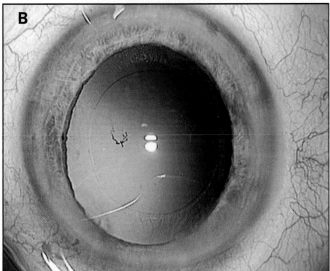

Figure 5. (A) LECs before anterior capsule polishing, empty bag. (B) LECs removed. Clear anterior capsule after polishing, empty bag.

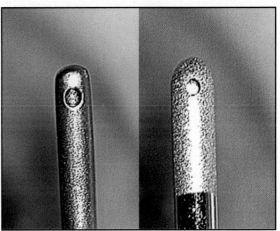

Figure 7. Ports of bimanual aspiration cannulae; right is disposable with sharp internal edge; left is reusable with chamfered polished internal edge.

to remove all the cells but the majority can be gently aspirated from the undersurface of the anterior capsule without any difficulty, and this will reduce the downstream incidence of capsular fibrosis and PCO.

Centralize the IOL: Use a Capsular Tension Ring

Late decentration of any IOL can be problematic but this is particularly so with the multifocal IOLs such as the ReZoom and ReSTOR. Care has to be taken to ensure that the lens implant sits centrally within the capsular bag at the time of surgery, so make sure as a final act that it is well centered on the operating room table after all the ophthalmic viscosurgical device (OVD) has been removed. We also know that it needs to remain in this position postoperatively for the lifetime of the patient. The lens can decenter for many reasons. Firstly, there may be a size mismatch between the implant and the capsular

bag, with the implant being relatively small. This occurs most commonly in large highly myopic eyes, but many lens manufacturers now offer lenses of larger overall diameter suitable for such cases.

The other causes of decentration involve capsular fibrosis and contraction. These phenomena occur more prolifically with older silicone plate lenses.

However, decentration can still occur with modern acrylic lenses of current designs. Unexpected capsular contraction can occur as a result of diffuse zonular weakness and laxity and is also stimulated by early postoperative intraocular inflammation.

There is nothing more persuasive than personal experience and having had to deal with the problems associated with multifocal lens decentration from contraction of the bag I have become acutely aware of the need to keep these newer premium lenses well centered. In order to maximize the chances of doing so, I have developed a preference for inserting a capsular tension ring (CTR) in all cases involving multifocals

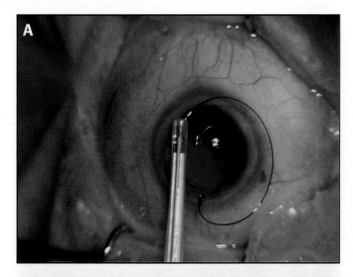

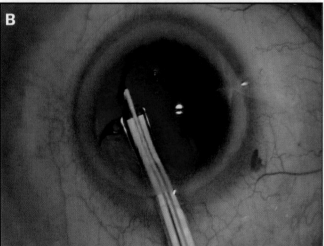

Figure 8. (A) Morcher CTR Type 13 with soft curved leading shoulder. (B) Injection of Morcher CTR Type 13 using EyeJet injector with transparent nozzle.

lenses. I do this when the bag is empty and after fully inflating it with OVD. The Morcher CTR type 13 has been designed with a curved leading shoulder specifically for insertion into an empty bag without snagging (Figure 8A). It is delivered into the empty bag with ease using their new EyeJet injector (Figure 8B). Other rings may work equally well but some models are less flexible than others so they can be more difficult to insert into an empty bag without snagging.

This may seem to many an excessive "belt and braces" approach, but the insertion of a CTR gives some welcomed added security in such cases, bearing in mind that we are practicing an inexact science in a highly exacting environment and we need all the help that is available.

References

1. Nishi O, Nishi K, Wickstrom K. Preventing lens epithelial cell migration using intraocular lenses with sharp rectangular edges. *J Cataract Refract Surg.* 2000;26:1543-1549.

2. Tassignon M, Rozema J, Gobin L. Ring-shaped caliper for better anterior capsulorrhexis sizing and centration. *J Cataract Refract Surg.* 2006;32(8):1253-1255.

3. Liyanage S, Angunawela RI, Wong SC, Little BC. There's a hole in my bucket: incisional leakage and chamber instability in coaxial phacoemulsification. Electronic poster presented at ESCRS XXV; 2007; Stockholm, Sweden.

4. Sacu S, Menapace R, Wirtitsch M, Buehl W, Rainer G, Findl O. Effect of anterior capsule polishing on fibrotic capsule opacification: three-year results. *J Cataract Refract Surg.* 2004;30(11):2322-2327.

PEARLS FOR IMPROVING YOUR CATARACT SURGICAL SKILLS

Rosa Braga-Mele, MEd, MD, FRCSC

Cataract surgical techniques and technology have changed dramatically over the past few years. At the same time, there has been a trend toward refractive cataract surgery with premium intraocular lens (IOL) insertion and higher patient expectations.

In order to maximize visual outcomes and minimize complications, it is important to refine our cataract surgical skills. In addition it is important to select patients appropriately and marry the correct IOL to the correct patient personality profile. One must also perform accurate biometry and K readings. Preoperative treatment with topical medications can make the intraoperative and postoperative course more stable. Topical non-steroidal anti-inflammatory (NSAID) agents help to maintain intraoperative mydriasis. They also help control postoperative inflammation thereby reducing the need for long-term topical steroid usage. NSAIDs have also been proven to reduce the risk chronic macular edema.[1] The use of preoperative antibiotics, such as the fourth generation fluoroquinolones, may also reduce the risk of postoperative infections.

Incision Placement and Astigmatism Correction

It is important to ensure proper wound construction with a shelved incision that is secure at the end of the procedure. Typically, temporal incision placement will induce the least amount of astigmatism. However, surgeons should measure the amount of astigmatism that their incisions induce or reduce prior to commencing premium IOL surgery. It is also important to reduce any pre-existing corneal astigmatism with limbal relaxing incisions to <0.50 D, as higher amounts of residual cylinder will degrade visual acuity and intensify any dysphotopsias.

Theoretically, smaller incisions, such as those used when performing with biaxial microincisional cataract surgery (1.5 mm or less) or coaxial microincisional cataract surgery (1.8 mm

to 2.2 mm), may induce less astigmatism, increase chamber and incision stability, and reduce the risk of endophthalmitis.

Capsulorrhexis

Creating a centered and properly sized capsulorrhexis is another essential step. Good capsulorrhexis centration will in turn maximize IOL centration and stability. The ideal capsulorrhexis diameter is between 4.5 and 5.0 mm. This will ensure IOL stability and maximize the optical function of a multifocal or accommodating IOL.

If there is any zonular laxity, one should rethink implantation of a premium IOL. Ideally, the anterior and posterior capsules should remain intact. If the posterior capsule breaks but the anterior capsule is still intact, one can implant a 3-piece multifocal IOL in the sulcus with the optic captured and fixated through the anterior capsulorrhexis, as described by Howard Gimbel. Do not implant an accommodating IOL or a single-piece IOL in the sulcus or in the bag if the posterior capsule is ruptured.

Viscoelastic

During these procedures, it is important to protect the corneal endothelium with a dispersive viscoelastic such as Viscoat (Alcon, Fort Worth, TX) or Vitrax II (Advanced Medical Optics, Santa Ana, CA). This should minimize endothelial cell trauma and maximize rapid visual recovery. Steven Arshinoff's soft shell technique[2] is my preference, utilizing the dispersive viscoelastic as an adjunct to help in coating the corneal endothelium. With Arshinoff's technique, the dispersive viscoelastic is injected initially to fill about half of the anterior chamber, followed by a cohesive viscoelastic that will force the dispersive agent up against the cornea. If the eye has a shallow anterior chamber or small pupil, consider one of the newer viscoadaptive agents (Healon 5, Advanced Medical Optics). Their ability to occupy space makes them ideal for deepening the anterior chamber and stretching the pupil.

Phacoemulsification Technology

There have been many technological advancements over the past decade that have enhanced not only surgical technique but surgical outcomes. It is important to become familiar with these new technologies to optimize the patient's visual outcomes. The driving force behind new phacoemulsification techniques and technology is the goal of reducing ultrasound power and energy utilized within the eye. Reducing phaco power diminishes potential damage to the endothelium, trabecular meshwork, and other intraocular structures.

Recent refinements in power modulations have improved nuclear segment followability and holdability. In essence, this translates into reduced fluid usage and turbulence within the eye, lower ultrasound use, and, ultimately, clearer corneas and better postoperative visual acuities.

Some of these advancements include hyperpulse and microburst technologies with variance of the duty cycle. If the surgeon wants to modulate phaco power based on the number of distinct shots of ultrasound energy per second, each shot is usually called a pulse. The length of the "off" time between pulses, or the interval, varies depending on the duty cycle selected. In pulse mode duty cycle represents the percentage of each second of ultrasound mode that the surgeon wants power delivered.

Alternatively, the surgeon can modulate power by varying the relative lengths of "on" and "off" time. In this case, the shots of ultrasound energy are called bursts or microbursts. The duty cycle is the ratio between burst length and the cycle time (burst duration + rest interval). If the surgeon chooses a mode that varies the duty cycle based on foot pedal position, cycle time will also vary as the pedal moves.

Due to the shorter bursts of phaco power followed by quiet intervals during which only vacuum is removing the fragment, these modalities definitely minimize ultrasound energy and maximize the hold on the nuclear fragment.

Torsional phacoemulsification is another modality that will help to minimize ultrasound energy utilized. Torsional ultrasound improves followability by reducing the repulsive properties of longitudinal phaco because the ultrasound needle oscillates from side to side, rather than back and forth.

One should match and optimize power modulations and fluidic parameters to the specific phaco technique being used in order to maximize efficiencies and provide better overall outcomes.

Phacoemulsification Technique

Recent refinements in power modulations have led most surgeons to use techniques that utilize less phacoemulsification energy and thus reduce thermal energy delivery and injury to the eye.[3,4] This is carried out by using mechanical forces to disassemble the nucleus, by using higher vacuum levels to aspirate the nucleus, or a combination of both. It is important when dealing with any challenging case to be aware of what one is confronting and to have a game plan to facilitate the surgery. Although most surgeons excel at using their primary technique, it is essential to be flexible and able to vary the phaco technique depending on the situation.

For the soft nucleus, one can either perform a hydrochop technique or flip the nucleus into the anterior chamber. For the hydrochop technique,[5] the hydrodissection cannula is used to create a central groove within the nucleus. Irrigation occurs through the cannula as it moves back and forth to create the groove, so as not to impale the nucleus. The groove is extended for the length of the diameter of the capsulorrhexis to a depth of one half to two thirds of the nucleus. The irrigation delivered through the cannula cleaves the nucleus in half through the central plane.

For the moderate/dense nucleus a quick chop technique is more efficient. In performing quick chop, complete hydrodissection is essential. I find that it is valuable to "burp" out a little of the viscoelastic prior to hydrodissection to allow a little bit more space in the anterior chamber. This way a fluid wave can be more easily created. Next, I get my efficient fluid wave with cortical cleavage hydrodissection as described by I. Howard Fine.[6] It is important to make sure that the lens is fully mobile in the bag, by rotating it 30 to 60, or, even 90 degrees. If you are doing coaxial phacoemulsification, it is important to expose more of the phacoemulsification needle tip to allow better purchase of the nucleus.

With this in mind, winding the sleeve down on the tip, I will enter the eye bevel down and approach the nucleus slightly more proximal than centrally. I next take a Koch chopper (Storz, Bausch & Lomb, Rochester, NY), and do a chop with a vertical technique. I then take my chopper just a bit distal to the phacoemulsification needle tip and embed it into the nucleus. Double-handed action is then needed. The chopper will push down into the nucleus and pull down and to the left. My phacoemulsification needle now having good purchase in the nucleus pulls up and to the right. With that we create the initial crack. If the nuclear crack does not go through the posterior plate, one will not get a clean split and this will create future problems.

It is important to re-coat the corneal endothelium with viscoelastic when using either a flip technique or when dealing with a dense nucleus.

One must also do a thorough cortical clean-up to ensure low posterior capsule opacification (PCO) rates, because any amount of PCO will degrade vision and promote visual dysphotopsias in the premium IOL population.

Conclusion

Although surgical technique and technology are important, one must take the whole patient into account. As stated previously, proper patient evaluation and selection and setting appropriate patient expectations are important steps for achieving good results.

References

1. McColgin AZ, Heier JS. Control of intraocular inflammation associated with cataract. *Curr Op Ophthalmol.* 2000;11(1):3-6.

2. Arshinoff SA. Dispersive-cohesive viscoelastic soft shell technique. *J Cataract Refract Surg.* 1999;25:167-173.

3. Fine IH, Packer M, Hoffman R. New phacoemulsification technologies. *J Cataract Refract Surg.* 2002;28:1054-1060.

4. Fine IH, Packer M, Hoffman R. Use of power modulations in phacoemulsification—Choo-choo chop and flip phacoemulsification. *J Cataract Refract Surg.* 2001;27:188-197.

5. Khan B., Braga-Mele R. HydroChop technique. *J Cataract Refract Surg.* 2006;32:18-20.

6. Fine IH. Cortical cleaving hydrodissection. *J Cataract Refract Surg.* 1992;18:508-512.

PEARLS FOR IMPROVING YOUR CATARACT SURGICAL SKILLS

William J. Fishkind, MD, FACS

Premium intraocular lens (IOLs), either aspheric or multifocal, require consistently excellent surgery for their best performance. This demand for high-quality surgery is created by heightened patient expectations for outstanding visual outcomes. To meet these expectations, preoperative antibiotic prophylaxis for infection and nonsteroidal prophylaxis for cystoid macular edema (CME) are mandatory. The wound must induce reproducibly low amounts of astigmatism. Astigmatism is managed with limbal relaxing incisions. The capsulorrhexis must be centered, round, and sized appropriately. Hydrodissection and hydrodelineation must be performed impeccably. Hydrodissection allows for gentle and zonular friendly phaco and irrigation and aspiration (I&A). Hydrodelineation allows for lens disassembly that minimizes the risk of a torn posterior capsule. Phaco must be gentle so as not to damage the capsular bag or the zonules. Placement of the IOL requires flawless centration without tilt. Finally, at the end of the procedure, the anterior segment must be reinflated to an adequate pressure and must remain stable in order to prevent IOL decentration and wound leak with potential of IOL movement or endophthalmitis.

Preoperative Prophylaxis

All patients are started on Zymar (gatifloxacin) 0.3% (Allergan, Irvine, CA) and Acular LS (ketorolac) 0.4% (Allergan) 4 times per day for 3 days prior to surgery.[1] They are continued on these drops with the addition of Pred Forte 1% (prednisilone acetate) (Allergan) for 1 week after surgery.

At the time of instillation of topical anesthesia, or peribulbar block, povidone-iodine 5% is instilled in the cul-de-sac and over the lid margin.

Postoperatively, if CME becomes clinically significant (usually 2 to 3 weeks after surgery), a subconjunctival injection of Kenalog (triamcinolone) 20 mg is administered. This is mixed by adding 0.5 cc of Kenalog 40 mg/cc and 0.2 cc of 1% xylocaine plain, in a TB syringe. A pledget of proparicane is placed in the inferior cul-de-sac. After waiting a few minutes, the pledget is removed and the injection is performed inferiorly through the anesthetized conjunctiva. This injection is usually painless and is often successful in resolving the CME.

Incision

The incision location[2] is almost always temporal. A Mastel Stealth Diamond Trapezoidal blade (Mastel, Rapid City, SD) is used. This blade is 100 µm thick and enables a uniplanar incision with effective wound stability. The width of the wound is 2.8 mm and the radial length 1.75 mm. This provides tight wound apposition around the phaco tip, allows injection of a silicone or acrylic IOL without enlarging or stretching the incision, and permits an excellent watertight closure of the wound with stromal hydration (Table 1). The against-the-wound astigmatic shift at 3 months following surgery reliably averages 0.25 D.

Astigmatism is managed by limbal relaxing incisions or toric IOL implantation.

Smaller phaco tip/sleeve combinations and injectors will soon allow for even smaller incisions.

Limbal Relaxing Incisions

These are performed when there is more than 0.75 D of corneal astigmatism as measured with the IOL Master (Carl Zeiss Meditec, Jena, Germany).

The horizontal axis is marked on the sclera with the patient sitting upright prior to the surgical prep. Prior to the cataract surgery a Mendez degree marker is used to mark the steepest axis obtained by keratometry. A predetermined arc of treatment is then marked. A Mastel Olsen Diamond (Mastel) with a fixed pre set 600-µm blade, is then used to cut the arc at the limbus. A Nichamin nomogram is used to determine the arc length based on patient age, and the axis and quantity of cylinder.

Table 1

PREMIUM IOL: CONSIDERATIONS FOR SUCCESS

- Prohylaxis for endophthalmitis and CME
- Incision constriction
  ○ Reproducible generation of cylinder
- Limbal relaxing incisions
- Capsulorrhexis size and centration
- Cortical cleaving hydrodissection
- Phacoemulsification
  ○ No zonular or capsular damage
- Watertight wound closure

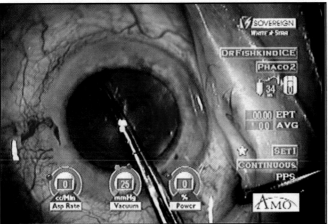

Figure 1. The modified Masket-Utrata Forcep has a 5-mm mark simplifying the construction of a centered and correctly sized CCC.

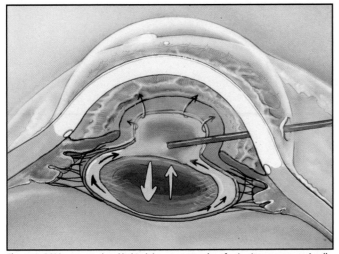

Figure 2. BSS has accumulated behind the cataractous lens forcing it to move anteriorly. Gentle pressure with the cannula pushes the nucleus posteriorly, forcing fluid trapped behind the nucleus around the equator causing lysis of the cortical-capsular bonds. (Reprinted with permission from Fishkind W. *Complications in Phacoemulsification.* New York, NY: Thieme Publishers; 2002:57.)

Capsulorrhexis

The capsulorrhexis must be round, centered, and smaller than the IOL optic. Centration and size can be assisted by utilizing one of the instruments with measuring marks at 5 mm, 5.5 mm, etc. I use one designed by Rhein Instruments (Tampa, FL) (Figure 1). With it, a 5-mm capsulorrhexis can be centered in the pupil. This will minimize the chance of IOL decentration secondary to later contraction of the capsular bag.

The capsulorrhexis diameter must be smaller than that of the optic of the IOL. This will produce a posterior capsular bend that will block posterior migration of lens epithelial cells, which might cause early capsular opacification. Presbyopia-correcting IOLs are exquisitely sensitive to opacification of the posterior capsule and patients will sometimes demand early YAG capsulotomy while the surgeon perceives only mild capsular opacification.

Finally, should an IOL require removal and replacement, viscodissection to reopen the capsular bag is immeasurably simplified when the IOL has prevented the anterior and posterior capsule from fusing.

Hydrosteps

There is a definite advantage to have a nucleus that is freely movable within the capsular bag. To achieve this, it is necessary to hydrodissect the cortex from the capsule, and to hydrodelineate the epinucleus from the endonucleus. After the continuous curvilinear capsulorrhexis (CCC), a 27-gauge Akahoshi cannula with a 1.6-mm tip bent at a 50-degree angle is placed under the edge of the CCC and passed toward the periphery without irrigation. When the cannula is in the proper position, gentle but firm irrigation is employed to produce a fluid wave to the opposite side. The end point of this irrigation is the anterior movement of the nucleus. This movement occurs when fluid amasses between posterior capsule and cataract pushing the nucleus anteriorly. The cannula is then used to press the lens posteriorly, which forces fluid out from behind the lens along the equator. This step will lysing the corticocapsular adhesions (Figure 2). The cannula is then repositioned at the opposite side where irrigation is repeated, so that the nucleus can then be rotated freely within the capsular bag. This is mandatory in order to minimize zonular stress during phaco and cortical clean up.

Hydrodelineation is performed by placing the cannula into the periphery of the nucleus at the CCC edge. With irrigation into the nucleus, the balanced salt solution will find the cleavage plane between the endonucleus and epinucleus. This allows the surgeon to emulsify the endonucleus within the confines of a surrounding epinuclear shell, protecting the posterior capsule.

Phacoemulsification

Any type of phaco procedure is acceptable. Phacoemulsification and cortical aspiration must not damage the zonules or the capsular bag. The posterior capsule must be polished to remove lens epithelial cells. A Terry squeegee (Alcon, Fort Worth, TX) is the perfect instrument for this. There should be no residual cortex and lens epithelial cells should be adequately removed to minimize early chances of posterior capsular opacification (PCO).

Wound Closure

The wound must be watertight.[3] The increased risk of endophthalmitis with poor wound integrity has been clearly demonstrated. Further, wound leaks may also lead to undesired shifts in IOL position. Fine, Packer, and Hoffman[3] recently published data indicating that stromal hydration has a 24-hour duration of action. Therefore, all wounds should be stromally hydrated to assure watertight closure.

References

1. Mah, Francis S. For how long should topical antibiotics and non-steroidal anti-inflammatory drugs be used before and after cataract surgery? In: Chang D, ed. *Curbside Consultation in Cataract Surgery.* Thorofare, NJ: SLACK Incorporated; 2007:65-68.

2. Nichamin LD, Chang DF, Johnson SH, et al. American Society of Cataract and Refractive Surgery Cataract Clinical Committee. ASCRS White Paper: What is the association between clear corneal cataract incisions and postoperative endophthalmitis? *J Cataract Refract Surg.* 2006;32:1556-1559.

3. Fine IH, Hoffman RS, Packer M. Profile of clear corneal cataract incisions demonstrated by Ocular coherence tomography. *J Cataract Refract Surg.* 2007;33(1): 94-97.

PEARLS FOR IMPROVING YOUR CATARACT SURGICAL SKILLS

Lisa Brothers Arbisser, MD

Every surgery and patient deserves our highest level of skill. With the exception of monocular patients, the stakes are rarely higher than for those who have opted for premium intraocular lenses (IOLs). Expectations for perfection are high: great uncorrected acuity, rapid recovery, and predictable outcomes. The technology itself demands surgical perfection because multifocals divide light energy between simultaneous images, which in turn reduces contrast sensitivity. Therefore, concomitant imperfections are not just additive but logarithmically decrease image quality and visual function. Accommodating lenses require thorough cortical cleanup and a perfect capsulorrhexis overlapping the hinge but not the optic for optimal function. I offer these 5 pearls for more consistent surgery.

Snug Unstretched Incisions

The size of the main incision should be snug but not tight, permitting insertion of the silicone sleeved instruments with minimal leak. An oversized, leaking incision results in greater fluid turbulence, an unstable environment and excess balanced salt solution (BSS) flow through the anterior chamber. An undersized incision restricts irrigation inflow causing more surge. It may also compromise the internal Descemet's valve integrity, requiring more hydration for closure, and providing a less secure barrier to inflow in the early postoperative period—a risk for endophthalmitis. I incise with a diamond trapezoidal blade, Arbisser-Fine Triamond blade from Mastel (Rapid City, SD) (the author has no financial interest). This can fashion any size incision and is least likely to cause a Descemet's detachment. I firm the eye with ophthalmic viscosurgical device (OVD) through the sideport for a predictable entry. Whenever I introduce an instrument into the incision, I employ a second instrument through the sideport for counter traction. I enter into an OVD filled environment on foot position 0 rather than enter on foot position 1 where the flow of BSS precludes a view of Descemet's. I do not often hydrate the stroma on completion of surgery but find that if I irrigate

the incision to eliminate any residual material between the lips of the internal valve, a secure seal is formed. In eyes with very thin or rigid tissue the roof and sides of the incision may require plumping to their original shape without whitening to achieve a dry gutter at normal intraocular pressure: my goal in every case.

Remember the importance of the paracentesis size. Classically we were encouraged to make a 1-mm sideport opening often with a 15-degree metal blade. If there is only one pearl of wound construction, it would be to make the paracentesis as small as possible. I make a 0.3- to 0.5-mm incision with at least a 1-mm-length tunnel with my Triamond blade to admit my Rosen Splitter, which functions well for every nucleus density. That means my blade goes in and out with no sideways motion. This snug incision prevents my having to chase fragments to the sideport during phaco and improves the stability of the chamber. My average case requires only 50 to 75 cc of BSS. Richard Mackool once measured 22 cc per minute of BSS lost through a 1-mm sideport, which can be correlated with endothelial trauma. This incision should also be ascertained to be watertight at the end of surgery (Figure 1).

Perfectly Sized and Proportioned Capsulorrhexis

A symmetric capsulorrhexis (CCC) appropriately sized to the lens optic promotes lens centration and a stable and predictable refractive error. Although these benefits extend to every IOL, they are particularly critical for toric implants. Covering a truncated edge may improve long-term dysphotopsia risk as well as reducing posterior capsule opacity. A perfect CCC reduces intraoperative complications. Because of variations in white-to-white diameter and pupil dilation, an independent reference must be used. I prefer not to mark the cornea as pristine epithelium leads to faster visual recovery. I simply hover above the cornea with calipers centered on the pupil set to 5 mm (for 6 mm optics and 6 for Crystalens [Eyeonics, Inc., Aliso Viejo,

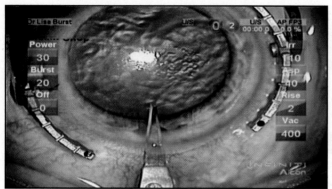

Figure 1. Arbisser-Fine Triamond diamond trapezoidal blade (Mastel) makes any size incisions.

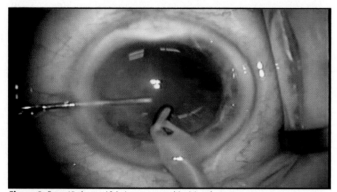

Figure 2. Bent 45-degree I&A tip accesses subincisional cortex.

CA]). I notice how far the edge of the rhexis will need to be from the edge of the pupil. I begin with a cystotome to raise a flap of capsule and then proceed to maneuver this flap with forceps. I have learned from experience what the initial radius of curvature must feel like to set the stage for a 5- to 5.5-mm capsulorrhexis and I am further guided by my mental image of how close to come to the pupil margin from the caliper placement a moment before. Once I establish this first quadrant radius, and assuming the pupil is symmetrically dilated, I can follow the pupil edge for completion. With an asymmetric pupil, I continue to focus on the symmetry of the radius for each quadrant, and not on the capsulorrhexis diameter. With topical anesthesia, I can enlist the patient's help to stay central and planar with the microscope by asking them to "stand their ground and not be dragged away from the light of the microscope." Regrasping every time my vector is not optimal (about once per quadrant) has this advantage—if the patient were to move I would not tear out to the periphery. I always err on the small side, as it is easy to enlarge the CCC with a tangential cut and a spiraling forceps motion once the lens is implanted to perfect the shape and size of the capsulorrhexis, with the optic under it as a template.

Endothelial Protection All Through Phacoemulsification

There is zero tolerance for corneal edema. The best way to prevent it is to maintain a dispersive OVD barrier throughout

the case. The Arshinoff soft shell technique helps us establish our first barrier. I use Duovisc (Alcon, Fort Worth, TX) so I can use the cohesive and dispersive viscoelastics to their highest purpose. Reducing turbulence and ultrasound time with a noncontinuous phaco strategy along with torsional ultrasound to improve followability and reduce chatter is helpful. If there is a brunescent lens, I use circumferential vertical chop to debulk the endonucleus using almost all the energy at or below the iris plane before elevating the nucleofied epinucleus for completion. If at any point I sense that the endothelial barrier has dissipated, I stop, leaving the phaco tip in place, I exchange the chopper for the Viscoat cannula (Alcon) and instill the OVD through the sideport with the foot pedal in position 0 until the chamber is entirely full. One must first establish flow in foot position 2 before reengaging phaco power to avoid wound burn.

I avoid chamber shallowing by instilling BSS through the sideport while removing the phaco or irrigation and aspiration (I&A) handpiece routinely. I irrigate the incision while OVD is in place after IOL insertion so when I complete OVD removal and exit, the chamber won't shallow and risk endothelial lens touch.

Total Cortex Removal

Thorough cortical removal leads to faster recovery, better centration, less cystoid macular edema and a lower Nd-YAG capsulotomy rate. It is worth the trouble. I prefer a 45-degree bent tip and a silicone sleeve that lets me take care of subincisional cortex without a bimanual approach. I always remove the subincisional cortex first while the "shoe tree" represented by the cortex is there to maintain the shoe's (capsular bag's) shape. Taking a sequential and systematic approach going from subincisional clockwise half way and then subincisional counterclockwise back towards the nasal quadrant avoids missing any hidden sector of cortex. Residual wisps sometimes remain where the 2 end points meet nasally. This is the easiest place to access on a capsule vacuum (lower flow lower vacuum setting). This capsule vacuum mode can be used anytime fishing for wisps or residual cortical capsular fibrotic remnants under the CCC edge is necessary, especially in hypermature and intumescent cases. Always removing cortex from the anterior leaf rather than the posterior leaves the cleanest capsule (Figure 2).

Remove All Ophthalmic Viscosurgical Devices from Posterior Chamber

The "rock and roll" technique of OVD removal often doesn't work. If we want to ensure stability of lens position, anterior, posterior, as well as laterally, and we want to avoid rotation of a toric lens we must empty the bag of OVD. There is a safe and simple technique to reliably clear the posterior chamber. While the chamber is controlled with viscoelastic after lens insertion, the I&A tip is insinuated under the edge of the optic, nudging it to the side if necessary and lifting it up

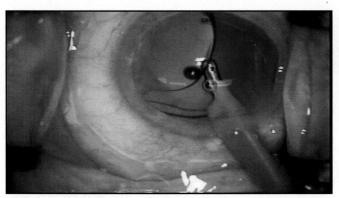

Figure 3. The I&A tip lifts the lens optic, gaining access to the posterior chamber for complete OVD evacuation.

while in foot position 0. The port is more up than down but mainly sideways oriented so as neither to be tamponaded by the optic nor to engage posterior capsule. Foot position 2 is then engaged allowing all OVD to be evacuated from under the IOL. The lens is then allowed to fall backward into the bag and now the anterior chamber is evacuated. This works in every case and for every model lens so long as the posterior capsule is intact. The maneuver can be repeated if a pocket of residual OVD is visualized behind the lens (Figure 3).

Attention to these details and the pursuit of perfection increase the likelihood of fulfilling the high visual expectations of our patients.

CHAPTER 182

SIZING THE CAPSULORRHEXIS

David F. Chang, MD; Steven Dewey, MD; Richard Tipperman, MD;
and Barry S. Seibel, MD

David F. Chang, MD

The capsulorrhexis is generally considered the most important step in cataract surgery. A continuous curvilinear capsulorrhexis (CCC) provides numerous surgical advantages.[1] A continuous curvilinear capsular edge reduces the chance of a capsular tear occurring during surgery. Like an elastic waistband, the capsulorrhexis will stretch in response to surgical forces, rather than tear. A continuous edge is necessary to perform cortical cleaving hydrodissection, and it facilitates cortical cleanup and placement of both haptics into the capsular bag. It also converts the anterior capsule into a contingency platform for intraocular lens (IOL) support should the posterior capsule tear.

The postoperative advantages of a properly sized capsulorrhexis are equally important. As the capsular bag contracts, it prevents pea-podding or escape of either haptic.[2,3] Asymmetric capsular forces resulting from an eccentric CCC can cause delayed optic decentration. Continuous circumferential overlap of the IOL optic edge will produce a capsular shrink-wrap effect whereby the posterior capsule is kinked by the optic edge—a major factor in the prevention of posterior capsule opacification.[4,5] It will also lessen any edge dysphotopsias as it opacifies over time. Finally, such continuous overlap of the optic edge is the only way to attain consistency in the axial IOL position from case to case. Being able to accurately predict this effective lens position is a critical factor in calculating the proper IOL power for emmetropia. Achieving these advantages is all the more critical for multifocal and presbyopia-correcting IOLs.

It follows that a capsulorrhexis whose diameter extends beyond the optic edge in some or all areas loses these advantages. Posterior lens epithelial cell (LEC) migration will occur in any region where the posterior capsule is not kinked by the optic edge.[5] Slight optic decentration may result from asymmetric capsular contractile forces over time. Finally, as the posterior capsule tenses postoperatively, it may displace the optic slightly more anteriorly wherever it is not restrained by a taut capsulorrhexis edge, resulting in a myopic shift.

What are the disadvantages of a capsulorrhexis with too small a diameter? In addition to impeding surgical steps such as the removal of subincisional cortex, a small-diameter CCC may create postoperative problems as well. The increased load of LECs on the back of the anterior capsule can increase inflammation and cause anterior capsular fibrosis and opacification, and excessive contraction of the capsulorrhexis and capsular bag.[6-8] This can lead to zonular damage or dehiscence and optic decentration.[9,10] With sufficiently weakened zonules, visually significant capsulophimosis or subluxation of the bag-IOL complex can occur.[7,11] Finally, excessive anterior capsular opacification can impair visualization of the peripheral retina.

Given the importance of attaining a proper capsulorrhexis diameter, it is ironic that this is one of the only cataract surgical steps that have not been improved by new technology. We continue to use the "low tech" method of a manual tear performed with a needle and/or forceps whose intended diameter is estimated visually. Individual variability in corneal magnification and in anterior segment and pupil diameter makes it difficult to precisely size the capsulorrhexis. Parallax occurring with movement of the globe makes it difficult to judge the symmetry and centration of the evolving capsulotomy.

My personal solution is to plan on performing a 2-stage capsulorrhexis when necessary (Figure 1). As I make the primary capsulorrhexis, I try to err on the small side because the diameter can always be enlarged, but not reduced. I take a moment to assess the appropriateness of the CCC diameter after implantation of the IOL. Frequently, the size and centration are fine, but it is surprising how often the CCC is slightly eccentric to the center of the optic (see Figure 1A). Sometimes, a perfectly round CCC becomes ovoid following implantation of the IOL, due to the directional stretch of the stiff 3-piece haptics. This is a sign of zonular laxity and insufficient centrifugal tension in the areas perpendicular to the haptic axis.

In either of these situations, or if the overall diameter is too small, I enlarge the capsulorrhexis by first making an oblique cut with scissors, and grasping the resulting flap with capsule forceps (see Figure 1B,C). The cut should be oblique, rather than radial, to better incline the resulting flap to tear in a

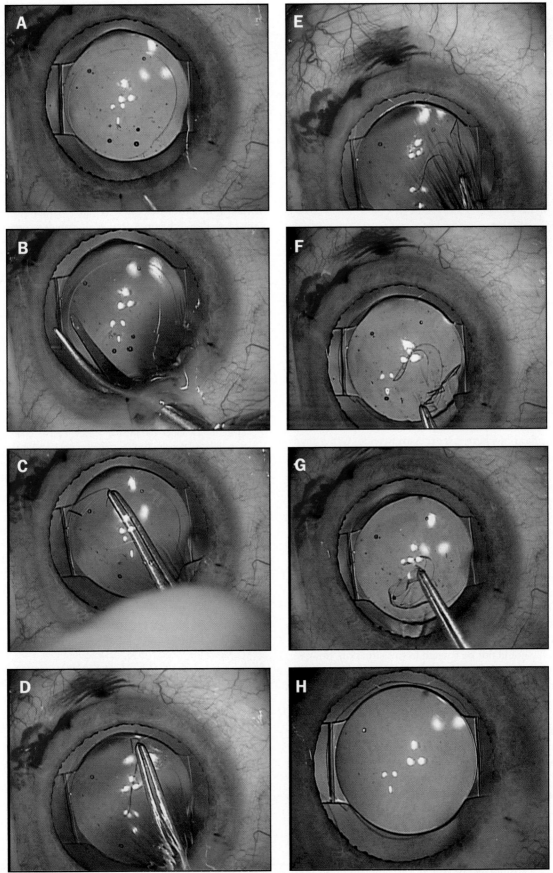

Figure 1. (A-H) Small-diameter capsulorrhexis is enlarged with forceps after creating a new flap with an oblique microscissor cut. For the Crystalens Five-0 (Eyeonics, Inc., Aliso Viejo, CA), the goal is to make a capsulorrhexis that is larger than the optic.

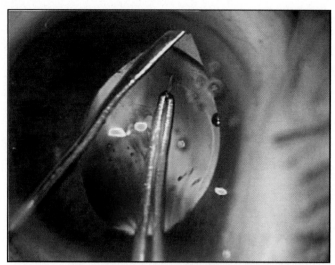

Figure 2. Lester hook is used to retract the iris to better view the IOL optic edge.

variability in CCC diameter will have a greater effect on ELP for a hinged IOL design. With dynamic accommodating designs, such as the Visiogen Synchrony IOL (Irvine, CA), too large a CCC diameter may allow the anterior optic to partially protrude through the capsulotomy. Too small an opening may cause capsulophimosis or excessive capsular fibrosis that can strain the zonules, stiffen the bag, and incapacitate the accommodative mechanism. Initially erring on the small side, with the option to enlarge it when and where necessary, is the only 100% reliable way I have to consistently attain a perfect sized capsulorrhexis diameter.

Finally, comfort with this maneuver is important if one is having difficulty steering the flap during the primary capsulorrhexis. Whether the cause is poor visibility, patient movement, a shallow chamber, or weak zonules, one can make a smaller diameter opening in order to increase control and to better avoid a peripheral extension. The diameter can be secondarily enlarged after the IOL has been implanted.

References

Gimbel HV, Neuhann T. Development, advantages, and methods of the continuous circular capsulorrhexis technique. *J Cataract Refract Surg.* 1990;16:31-37.

Assia EI, Legler UF, Merrill C, et al. Clinicopathologic study of the effect of radial tears and loop fixation on intraocular lens decentration. *Ophthalmology.* 1993;100:153-158.

Ram J, Apple DJ, Peng Q, et al. Update on fixation of rigid and foldable posterior chamber intraocular lenses. Part I: Elimination of fixation-induced decentration to achieve precise optical correction and visual rehabilitation. *Ophthalmology.* 1999;106:883-890.

Ram J, Pandey SK, Apple DJ, et al. Effect of in-the-bag intraocular lens fixation on the prevention of posterior capsule opacification. *J Cataract Refract Surg.* 2001;27:367-370.

Nishi O, Nishi K, Wickstrom K. Preventing lens epithelial cell migration using intraocular lenses with sharp rectangular edges. *J Cataract Refract Surg.* 2000;26:1543-1549.

Hansen SO, Crandall AS, Olson RJ. Progressive constriction of the anterior capsular opening following intact capsulorrhexis. *J Cataract Refract Surg.* 1993;19:77-82.

Davison JA. Capsule contraction syndrome. *J Cataract Refract Surg.* 1993;19:582-589 .

Joo CK, Shin JA, Kim JH. Capsular opening contraction after continuous curvilinear capsulorrhexis and intraocular lens implantation. *J Cataract Refract Surg.* 1996;22:585-590.

Hayashi K, Hayashi H, Nakao F, Hayashi F. Anterior capsule contraction and intraocular lens decentration and tilt after hydrogel lens implantation. *Br J Ophthalmol.* 2001;85:1294-1297.

Hayashi H, Hayashi K, Nakao F, Hayashi F. Anterior capsule contraction and intraocular lens dislocation in eyes with pseudoexfoliation syndrome. *Br J Ophthalmol.* 1998;82:1429-1432.

Jahan FS, Mamalis N, Crandall AS. Spontaneous late dislocation of intraocular lens within the capsular bag in psuedoexfoliation patients. *Ophthalmology.* 2001;108:1727-1731.

circumferential direction. The flap is then maneuvered with capsule forceps under a generous amount of ophthalmic viscosurgical device (OVD). Curved Uthoff-Gills capsulotomy scissors with blunt tips (Katena K4-5126) have the perfect shape for creating an initial curved cut to either side of the phaco incision (see Figure 1B). If the pupil is small enough to conceal the optic edge, it can be locally retracted with a Lester hook (Figure 2). In some cases, I only trim a part of the remaining anterior capsular rim where it is excessively wide. Other times, I may retear the entire 360-degree circumference of the opening (see Figure 1).

Executing the second-stage enlargement may be easier than the primary capsulotomy for several reasons. Following removal of the cataract, the red reflex is improved, and there is no convexity to the anterior capsule to promote radial extension of the tear. The optic provides a perfect visual template for resizing the CCC diameter. Finally, in cases of weak zonules, the presence of the 3-piece haptics or a capsular tension ring increases outward tension on the capsular bag, which improves control over the direction of the tear. It is reassuring that, should the tear escape peripherally, there should be no subsequent surgical steps that would extend the tear posteriorly. The IOL should not be rotated in this situation, however, for this reason.

Although in most cases, enlargement of a small diameter capsulorrhexis is not absolutely necessary, I would encourage the mastery of this technique. With multifocal IOLs, achieving a symmetric capsulorrhexis that completely overlaps the optic edge is particularly important. There is even less margin for CCC diameter error with accommodating IOLs, such as the Eyeonics Crystalens (Eyeonics, Aliso Viejo, CA). Excessive

Steven Dewey, MD

No single feature of a refractive lens exchange carries as much importance as a properly sized, centered, and intact capsulorrhexis. A poor incision can be sutured. Residual astigmatism can be corrected with an excimer laser. Even the visual impact of vitreous loss due to a posterior capsule rupture can be minimized if the capsulorrhexis is centered and properly sized.

In routine cases, overlapping the edge of the optic by .5 to 1 mm will result in a consistent lens position from case to case, and has the benefit of driving the sharp posterior edge of an intraocular lens (IOL) into the posterior capsule and reducing the potential for posterior capsular opacification (PCO). In a less-than-routine case, having an intact capsulorrhexis allows for optic capture to secure the IOL, even if the posterior capsule is completely absent.

Sizing the capsulorrhexis can be a challenge. The variability of pupil dilation and corneal diameters can make it difficult to consistently create the proper opening. The easiest method is the most direct. Prior to loading the IOL in the insertion device, simply hold the IOL over the surgical field and mentally establish the relative size of the optic to the size of the eye. This can also help center the capsulorrhexis over the visual axis.

Several techniques have been developed to gauge the size of the capsulorrhexis. Dr. Bruce Wallace has used an optical zone marker to effectively provide a size guide. Dr. Barry Seibel has created capsulorrhexis forceps with a millimeter marker on the shaft as an intraocular gauge. This product is manufactured by MST and can easily work with either a standard or bimanual incision.

Instrumentation inherently creates different size openings, and this appears to be related to the tangential forces applied as the capsule is torn. A bent needle holds the flap closer to the tear, and creates a smaller capsular opening. Forceps grasp the capsule further from the tear, and generally will create a larger one.

Preserving the capsulorrhexis is just as important. Early in the case, a radial tear might result in a dropped nucleus. Although a radial tear later in the case does not prevent in-the-bag IOL placement, the IOL may become significantly decentered in the absence of uniform capsule contraction. In most cases, tears occur because of inappropriate contact of the capsule with a sharp instrument, or occasionally because the capsule is pinched between 2 instruments, sharp or not. Keeping an awareness of the edge of the anterior capsule throughout the case and maintaining a deep anterior chamber with appropriate viscoelastic and balanced salt solution (BSS) infusion pressure can avoid these mistakes. Recognizing that things can and will happen, my most effective primary defense is to avoid all sharp instruments in the eye during surgery. The rounded edges of the Dewey Radius Tip from MST can effectively remove even the densest cataract, but, unlike standard sharp phaco needles, are very forgiving if incidental contact with the capsulorrhexis edge or posterior capsule does occur.

Although I prefer a 0.5- to 1-mm overlap of the anterior capsule on the optic, more overlap is not a problem as long as the surgical technique can deal with removing the nucleus and cortex through a smaller opening. To keep my capsulorrhexis size smaller, I generally prefer a dispersive viscoelastic to flatten the capsule, and I use a bent needle. In cases of poor visualization or loose zonules, the forceps provide an extra degree of control. Of course, a larger capsulorrhexis is appropriate when the situation warrants, such as when dealing with a very dense cataract, or in cases of zonular laxity where an endocapsular approach should be abandoned.

Richard Tipperman, MD

Creating an appropriately sized capsulorrhexis is critical to achieving excellent clinical results with presbyopia-correcting intraocular lenses (IOLs). Regardless of the IOL, having a consistent size to the capsulorrhexis will improve predictability in the implant power calculation. For accommodating IOLs, a specific capsulorrhexis size will be ideal for maximizing optic exposure, centration, and movement. For a true multifocal (simultaneous vision) IOL, if the capsulorrhexis is too small, it will limit the amount of light that can travel through the peripheral portion of the IOL and thereby limit the light energy transmitted from this portion of the lens.

A variety of techniques have been described to try and create a specific sized capsulorrhexis. The following is an approach that has worked well in my clinical practice.

At the start of surgery, I have the patient fixate on the microscope light and I try to center a 6-mm radial keratotomy (RK) optical zone marker on the reflection from the microscope light. This gives me a 6-mm circular indentation on the patient's cornea, which is roughly centered on their visual axis. I then begin the tear of my capsulorrhexis and bring it out until it is in line with the inner edge of the mark from the optical zone marker.

At this point, if the pupil is round and symmetric, I no longer need to shift my focus between the anterior capsule and the corneal dome where the optical zone marker is visible. I simply mentally note the distance between the capsulorrhexis edge and the iris sphincter. I then complete the tear for the full 360 degrees while trying to maintain this constant distance for the entire capsulotomy.

This is a simple technique using readily available instrumentation that provides for a consistent capsulorrhexis size. Surgeons often find that shifting their fixation from the corneal dome to the anterior capsule while trying to bring the tear around can be cumbersome at best. At worst, this will lead to unpredictable sizing or difficulty with completing the capsulorrhexis. Using the corneal marker to create a landmark for the peripheral border of the tear and then completing the capsulorrhexis with a different constant landmark in the anterior capsule plane (ie, pupillary margin) makes consistent sizing of the capsulorrhexis much simpler.

Barry S. Seibel, MD

The continuous curvilinear capsulorrhexis (CCC), as pioneered by Thomas Neuhann and Howard Gimbel, is unquestionably one of the fundamental components of modern phacoemulsification surgery. The additional strength of this type of capsulotomy, as compared to the older canopener technique, has resulted in fewer posterior capsule ruptures via anterior capsulotomy extensions, as well as fewer displaced intraocular lenses (IOLs). The prior state of the art involved an approximation of a desired capsulotomy diameter. However, the demands of refractive cataract surgery have placed additional importance on the precision of this measurment.

For example, work by Drs. David Apple and Okihiro Nishi has underscored the importance of a complete overlap of the lens optic by the CCC to achieve optimal posterior capsule opacification (PCO) inhibition by a posterior square edge design. Without such an overlap, the anterior and posterior capsule can fuse, and the fibrotic fusion can migrate centrally under the posterior edge of the optic. Such a fusion can also lead to a lens tilt as well as a shift in the overall anterior-posterior Effective Lens Position, with a corresponding degradation in predictability of the target refraction postoperatively. A complete CCC overlap of the anterior optic also augments the function of a posterior square edge lens design by pressing this edge into the posterior capsule for more effective inhibition of centripetal lens epithelial cell migration.

Notwithstanding the preceding benefits of a complete optic overlap of the capsulorhexis, too small a CCC diameter can compromise the optics of the newer multifocal IOLs. For example, the ReSTOR (Alcon, Fort Worth, TX)gives a progressively better distance image with less glare as the pupil enlarges to expose more of the distance dominant peripheral optics; however, this design will be ineffective if too small a fibrotic anterior capsule is overlapping the optic periphery. Other multifocal designs are similarly compromised if the CCC diameter is also smaller than the physiologic pupil, especially in mesopic conditions. A notable exception to this rule is the Crystalens, which many surgeons feel benefits from a

6-mm CCC diameter (larger than the optic) to better facilitate pseudoaccomodative flexing.

In order to address the need for CCC sizing, the Seibel Rhexis Ruler was developed with MicroSurgical Technology (Redmond, WA) to facilitate measuring a desired distance on the surface of the capsule, thereby avoiding magnification errors caused by estimating capsulotomy size from corneal markings. The numbers and registration marks are smoothly laser etched on to the surface to avoid traumatizing or peeling Descemet's membrane as the instrument is manipulated through a corneal incision. Furthermore, the bottom of each number represents the 0.5-mm point between the 1-mm hash marks for added precision. The instrument is initially placed as shown with the jaws closed to establish a visual "gap" to be present between the pupil edge and the desired CCC, shown in Figure 1 by purple double-head arrows for a desired 5-mm CCC. Having established this visual gap, the surgeon incises the capsule in the center and then tears peripherally until the gap is reached at point G, and this gap is maintained throughout the CCC; note point I and green dashed arrow in lower Figure 2. Of course, the surgeon must visually compensate for the relative gap with irregularly dilated or otherwise eccentric pupils. Using the Rhexis Ruler in this fashion can greatly enhance reproducibility of a desired CCC diameter, with corresponding benefits as mentioned previously.

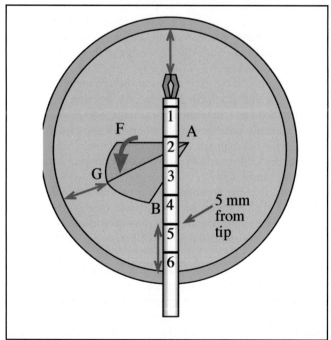

Figure 1. The instrument is initially placed as shown with the jaws closed to establish a visual "gap" to be present between the pupil edge and the desired CCC. (Reprinted with permission from Seibel BS. *Phacodynamics: Mastering the Tools and Techniques of Phacoemulsification Surgery, Fourth Edition*. Thorofare, NJ: SLACK Incorporated; 2005.)

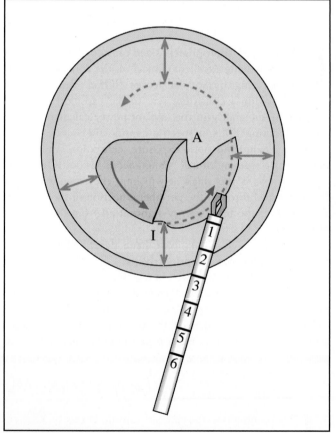

Figure 2. The surgeon incises the capsule in the center and then tears peripherally until the gap is reached at point G, and this gap is maintained throughout the CCC (note point I and green dashed arrow). (Reprinted with permission from Seibel BS. *Phacodynamics: Mastering the Tools and Techniques of Phacoemulsification Surgery, Fourth Edition*. Thorofare, NJ: SLACK Incorporated; 2005.)

CHAPTER 183

IMPROVING THE CORNEAL INCISION SEAL

Michael Y. Wong, MD

Some premium intraocular lenses (IOLs) require precise placement and seating in the capsular bag. This places a greater emphasis on making clear corneal incisions absolutely water-tight in order to stabilize the anterior chamber in the early postoperative period. Other accommodating IOLs require a slightly larger entry wound. Enhancing the seal of a corneal incision becomes ever more important. Beyond that, the increasing popularity of clear corneal incisions in cataract surgery has been accompanied by a worrisome suggestion that the incidence of bacterial endophthalmitis[1] and toxic anterior segment syndrome is also on the rise.[2] These complications would be devastating in the era of premium IOLs and refractive lens exchange. This article describes a simple, quick, inexpensive technique to tightly appose both lips of the incision and thus secure and prolong the seal.

Technique

Prior to creating the clear corneal incision, I make a supraincisional stromal pocket 0.5 mm anterior to the intended entrance. With a simple stab of a diamond or metal keratome, I create a 2-mm pocket that resembles an equilateral triangle, with its base toward the limbus. The pocket's depth can be anywhere from one-third to two-thirds stromal thickness.

I hydrate the stroma through this pocket with balanced salt solution at the end of the case, thus creating a bulge that exerts an inward pressure on the external lip of the clear corneal incision. The internal lip is pressed outward by the intraocular pressure (IOP). The combined pressure makes for a tight apposition of both lips of the incision and thus prevents the egress or ingress of fluid through the wound for a period of 24 hours. By that time, the ciliary body is producing aqueous, and the endothelial pump has brought the lamellae of the stroma tightly together. The seal is firm enough to withstand fluctuations in IOP, whether high or low.

One may create 2 pockets instead of a single pocket if desired, and I have found that there is tremendous latitude in the dimensions of the pocket(s) without impairing the effect

(Figures 1 and 2). There are no significant complications with this technique. The technique, formally described as *stromal hydration of a supraincisional pocket*, is colloquially called the *Wong Way*.

Increased Margin of Safety

A perfectly constructed, square or nearly square clear corneal incision created with a diamond knife is safe and secure.[3,4] The outward forces of the IOP press up on the internal aspect of the corneal lip to provide a sufficient seal until the endothelial pump dries the internal channel of the incision. In practice, however, conditions are less than perfect. Many surgeons employ a metal knife, the incision's edges are not as clean or long as desired, its lips shrink because of heat from the phaco tip or become stretched by the IOL's insertion, or the limbal structures are weakened by a limbal relaxing incision. The Wong Way can provide a margin of safety in these instances.

Effective Seal Through Vulnerable Period of Hypotony

The structural weakness of a standard clear corneal incision can be exposed in the postoperative period when additional biomechanical stress occurs with blinking, rubbing of the eye, ocular movement, and hypotony from a relative shutdown of the ciliary body. In vitro, hypotony in a cadaveric eye results in an inflow of India ink placed on the ocular surface.[5] In vivo, the release of aqueous through a clear corneal incision to manage a postoperative pressure spike can result in temporary hypotony with a subsequent superficial inflow of fluorescein placed in the tear film.[6] The resilience of the sclera causes the globe to expand from a relatively collapsed state in hypotony to produce a vacuum action. This situation may be one cause of toxic anterior segment syndrome.

In contrast, the Wong Way incision remains watertight in the presence of hypotony as evident upon hydrating the

Figure 1. The surgeon begins by creating a stromal pocket that is 1.5- to 2.0-mm wide. If using 2 stab incisions, the surgeon places them side by side so that the incision resembles an upside down W (A). A side view shows the pocket to be just anterior to and above the usual entry into the anterior chamber (B).

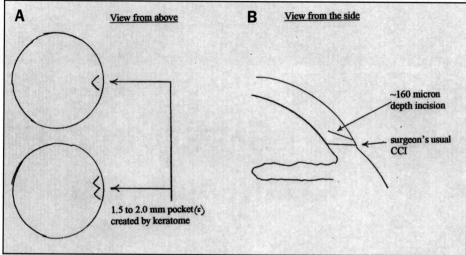

Figure 2. At the conclusion of the case, the surgeon uses a 30-gauge cannula to hydrate the tip and edges of the supraincisional stromal pocket with balanced salt solution (A). The reformed anterior chamber pushes upward on the internal aspect of the corneal lip, while the stromal hydration pushes downward on the wound (B).

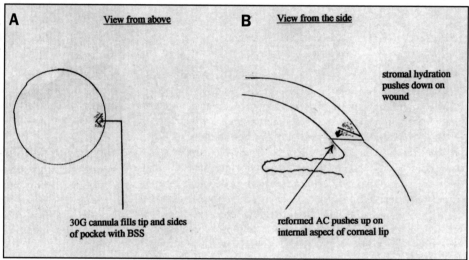

pocket at the end of a cataract operation without reforming the anterior chamber and exerting external pressure with a cellulose sponge. The IOP is low, and the incision does not leak. In the estimated 20% of patients who experience postoperative hypotony,[7] the eye would thus be protected from a superficial influx of fluid that might contain bacteria or other toxic substances.

More Effective Location Of Stromal Hydration

The stromal hydration of the sides and superior roof of the clear corneal incision can create the impression that the wound is watertight while the patient is on the operating table. This fluid, however, is often reabsorbed during the first few hours after surgery because it is relatively close to the endothelial pump. Further, my experience with laser in situ keratomileusis (LASIK) surgery has shown that apposing stromal lamellae are more adherent when desiccated. Stromal hydration within the channel of the clear corneal incision works in opposition to this concept.

On the other hand, stromal hydration in a separate and distinct stromal pocket that is external and anterior to the clear corneal incision typically lasts for 24 to 36 hours. The inward pressure remains beyond the time period of ciliary shutdown and hypotony. Further, because this supraincisional pocket of fluid is distal to the clear corneal incision with regard to the endothelium, the stromal lamellae within the channel of the clear corneal incision are desiccated and secure before the endothelium reabsorbs the supraincisional fluid.

Alternatives

Concern over leakage and a possible association with endophthalmitis[1] with clear corneal incisions has prompted some surgeons to switch back to scleral tunnels. However, relying on a thin layer of conjunctiva that often retracts with blinking is an unreliable defense. Other surgeons suggest sealing the clear corneal incision with a fibrin adhesive, but doing so adds time, expense, and potential toxicity[8] and may interfere with the desiccation of the stromal lamellae within the channel. Of course, if there is remaining doubt about the seal of a wound, a suture can be placed.

Uses

I prefer to hydrate a supraincisional pocket with every main clear corneal incision for cataract surgery even though I recognize that a perfectly constructed square wound is self-sealing. It is like being a safe driver but still wearing a seat belt. Other surgeons use the technique only when the seal of the wound is tenuous at the end of a case or in situations when anterior chamber stability is of the utmost importance during the early postoperative period. For instance, when using a fixed optic, flexible haptic design IOL such as the Crystalens (Eyeonics, Inc., Aliso Viejo, CA), Akkommodative 1CU (Human Optics, Erlangen, Germany), or Kellan Tetraflex IOL (Lenstec, St. Petersburg, FL), a momentary wound leak on the day of surgery could lead to IOL vault or the Z-syndrome. Accommodating intraocular lenses such as the Synchrony IOL (Visiogen, Inc., Irvine, CA) or Sarfarazi Twin-Optic IOL (Bausch & Lomb, Rochester, NY) require a larger wound, which increases the risk of a leak. This technique provides a greater margin of safety. I also find that the technique is useful for a paracentesis of questionable competence and when the corneal structure is less rigid than usual. That occurs when the clear corneal incision is within a limbal relaxing incision or with a young patient.

Conclusion

The Wong Way aids in sealing a clear corneal incision quickly, easily, and intuitively, and it entails no additional expense. Practically speaking, this technique is complication free. The best thing I can say about the Wong Way is that the worst thing that can happen is nothing.

References

1. Taban M, Behrens A, Newcomb RL, et al. Acute endophthalmitis following cataract surgery. *Arch Ophthalmol.* 2005;123:613-620.

2. Mamalis N, Edelhauser H, Dawson D, et al. Toxic anterior segment syndrome. *J Cataract Refract Surg.* 2006;32:324-333.

3. Ernest P, Kiessling LA, Lavery KT. Relative strength of cataract incisions in cadaver eyes. *J Cataract Refract Surg.* 1991;17:668-671.

4. Masket S, Belani S. Proper wound construction to prevent short-term ocular hypotony after clear corneal incision cataract surgery. *J Cataract Refract Surg.* 2007;33:383-386.

5. Mc Donnell PJ, Taban M, Sarayba M, et al. Dynamic morphology of clear corneal cataract incisions. *Ophthalmology.* 2003;110:2342-2348.

6. Chawdhary S, Anand A. Early post-phacoemulsification hypotony as a risk factor for intraocular contamination: in vivo model. *J Cataract Refract Surg.* 2006;32:609-613.

7. Shingleton B, Wadhwani R, O'Donoghue M, et al. Evaluation of intraocular pressure in the immediate period after phacoemulsification. *J Cataract Refract Surg.* 2001;27:524-527.

8. Realini T. Wound construction key to avoiding endophthalmitis. *EyeWorld.* 2007;February:64-66.

CHAPTER 184

DIFFRACTIVE MULTIFOCAL IOL CENTRATION

Paolo Vinciguerra, MD and Fabrizio I. Camesasca, MD

The introduction of multifocal intraocular lenses (IOLs) opened up a whole new horizon of possibilities in presbyopia correction with cataract surgery. With multifocal IOLs, simultaneous distance and near images fall on the retina, with one focused, and the other highly defocused and typically ignored. Presently available multifocal IOLs can be divided into 2 groups: refractive and diffractive. Refractive multifocal IOLs feature multiple concentric zones of alternating refractive power. Different powers are created by varying curvature of anterior or posterior surface. The refractive zones can be spherical or aspherical, with each acting mostly as an independent refractive lens. Junctions between the different refractive zones create discontinuities diffracting the passing light. This uncontrolled diffraction reduces image quality and induces visual disturbances, which are usually influenced by pupil dimension. When the pupil is dilated, glare or halos are thus increased, contrast sensitivity is decreased, and rings around point light sources can be experienced at night.

A different optical solution is offered by diffractive IOLs (ReSTOR, Alcon, Fort Worth, TX; Tecnis Multifocal, Advanced Medical Optics, Santa Ana, CA). These multifocal IOLs use the diffractive principle. The optic features concentric diffractive steps, which diffract light in smaller waves. Waves interfering in a positive way generate a focused image, whereas waves interfering in a negative way will eliminate each other. Diffractive steps introduce phase delays of light at zone boundaries. In summary, in a refractive IOL, each optical zone will create a single focus, whereas in a diffractive IOL each diffractive step will create several focal points.

The ReSTOR IOL is a particularly interesting option.[1-4] It is an apodized diffractive multifocal IOL, and the distance between the peripheral rings is spaced so as to direct more light to the center for distance correction when the pupil enlarges (Figure 1). Furthermore, there is a precise reduction in diffractive step heights moving from the center to the periphery of the 3.6-mm-diameter diffractive region. Steps reduce in height from 1.3 to 0.2 µm.

Emmetropia to minimal hyperopia is the best refractive endpoint for ReSTOR.[1] Surgeons must be aware that at night patients will perceive halos around point sources of light, and that neural adaptation will diminish the perception of this problem with time, particularly when the IOL is bilaterally implanted.

In our experience, ReSTOR is an outstanding IOL, providing excellent distance visual acuity, good near vision without correction, and a better optical wavefront than standard spherical monofocal IOLs. A cautious and organized approach, however, is mandatory in order to obtain the best results. There are several pearls for success, such as not implanting ReSTOR when astigmatism is greater than 0.50 D, performing accurate biometry selecting patients carefully and performing impeccable surgery. Most importantly, but often overlooked, perfect IOL centration is mandatory.[5,6]

Decentration

A decentered ReSTOR will obviously impair optical performance compared to a well-centered one, in which all of the diffractive steps align and work with the visual axis (Figure 2). Residual refractive abnormalities may be induced by imperfect centration, and these are generally poorly tolerated by patients with diffractive multifocal IOLs.

Similarly to what happens in excimer laser refractive surgery with centration of an ablation, it is important to remember that the center of the pupil and the line connecting it with the fixating object (line of sight [LOS]) are not always coincident with the visual axis (the line connecting the fovea with the fixation object) or with the geometrical corneal center (optical axis). Indeed, the mean distance between the center of the pupil (LOS) and the visual axis of the eye (angle kappa) is 2.6 degrees horizontally and 0.6 degree vertically. Furthermore, the center of the pupil shifts during miosis or mydriasis.

Thus, centering a multifocal IOL in the capsular bag in a fully dilated eye does not mean centering it on the pupil, and the pupil center may not be coincident with the visual axis.

Figure 3 presents a Nidek OPD (Nidek, Gamagori, Aichi, Japan) aberrometer wavefront evaluation of an eye with a

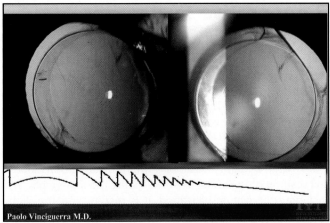

Figure 1. ReSTOR IOL. Note the difference in height and distance between the peripheral rings of the optic.

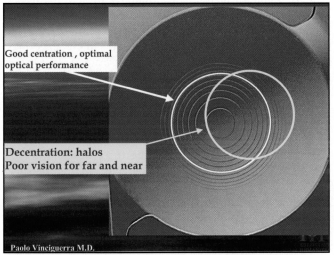

Figure 2. A decentered ReSTOR will induce residual refractive defects.

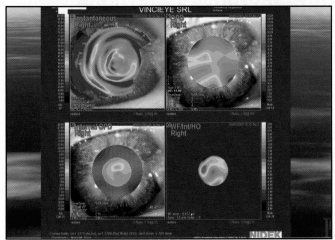

Figure 3. OPD evaluation of an eye with a decentered ReSTOR. Total aberrations (above right) are remarkable. Internal high-order aberrations (HO, below, right) are elevated and coma is the main component (below, left).

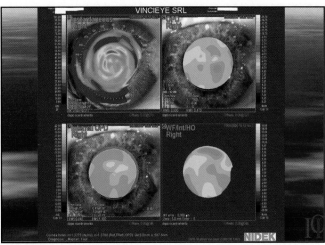

Figure 4. Same eye of Figure 3 after ReSTOR repeated centration. Total, internal, and HO aberrations are markedly reduced.

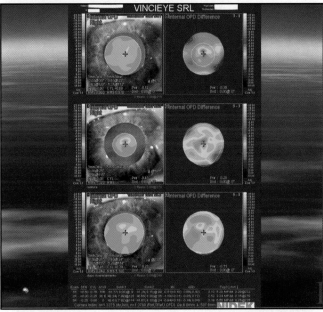

Figure 5. Difference between internal aberrations preoperatively (above, left), immediate postoperatively with IOL decentration (middle, left), and after recentration (below, left). Differential map (above, right) between pre- and immediate postoperative situations clearly shows induction of coma by imperfectly centered IOL. Note how preoperative and final internal aberration maps are similar.

decentered ReSTOR. This patient complained of poor vision and ghost images. Nidek OPD mapping of total aberrations (above, right) showed a considerable amount of aberration. Internal higher-order aberrations (HO, below, right) were elevated and coma was the main component (below, left).

Figure 4 presents the same eye after surgical recentration of the ReSTOR IOL. Total, internal and HO aberrations were markedly reduced. Figure 5 displays the difference between internal wavefront aberrations preoperatively (above, left), immediate postoperatively with IOL decentration (middle, left), and after recentration (below, left). The differential internal aberrations map (above, right) clearly shows induction of coma by an imperfectly centered IOL. Note how the preoperative (above, left) and final (after recentration) (below, left) internal aberration maps are similar. Following recentration, this patient's vision improved and he no longer had ghosting of images. We have now recentered 4 out of 56 implanted IOLs (7.1%).

To provide the best possible centration of the ReSTOR multifocal IOL, we recommend the following.

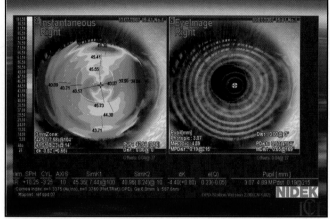

Figure 6. An eye with a pupil centered on the cornea, but a visual axis decentered inferonasally.

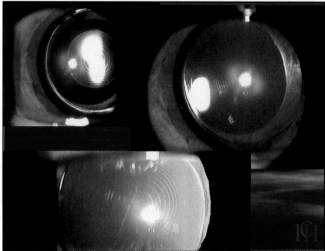

Figure 7. A well-centered ReSTOR.

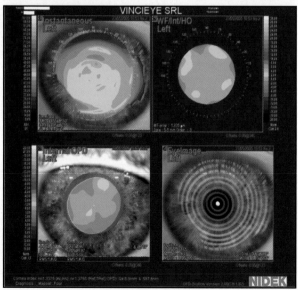

Figure 8. OPD evaluation of an eye with good ReSTOR centration, showing low internal total and HO aberrations (below, left, and above, right, respectively).

Preoperative Evaluation

Ideally, the visual axis, pupil center, and the center of the IOL should be coincident. We therefore presently exclude patients with a very disparate visual axis and pupil center, as well as those whose pupillary centers differ significantly between miosis and mydriasis. This can be verified pre-operatively with a combined topographer-aberrometer (ie, Nidek OPD). This also provides important information about total—internal and corneal—ocular aberration. This examination—based on patient fixation—will provide information on the position of the visual axis. Evaluating the topography and excluding the map visualization, it is easy to visualize if the pupil is centered with the topography rings, and thus with the visual axis. Furthermore, the wavefront examination provides information pertaining pupil centration on the cornea (optical axis). Pupil diameter and centration with both miosis and mydriasis is also measured. Figure 6 shows an eye with a pupil centered on the cornea, but a visual axis decentered inferonasally. The patient fixates on the center of the topography rings: thus the visual axis (line between the fovea and the fixation object) is not coincident with the center of the pupil.

Performing biometry with IOL Master (Carl Zeiss, Meditec, Jena, Germany) is also extremely important. Because it measures to the fovea of the fixating patient, this device provides precise determination of the axial length along the visual axis, and also reduces operator error due to corneal indentation characteristic of contact ultrasonography. In our personal experience, however, we integrate the IOL Master keratometry measurements with topography-derived K readings, (ie, the mean pupillary power derived from 4000 topography measurements points). In our opinion, estimating corneal curvature on the basis of only 6 points is not accurate enough.

Intraoperative Centration

Given how unforgiving it is of misalignment, surgical centration of the ReSTOR is particularly important. Ideally, the IOL must be centered on the visual axis, which cannot be determined intraoperatively. Once we know from the preoperative examination that the visual axis is almost coincident with the center of the pupil and thus with the line of sight, the miotic pupil becomes the reference guide for centration. The ideal capsulorrhexis has a symmetric and well-centered, 5-mm-diameter opening, and obviously posterior capsule rupture must be avoided. The surgeon must accurately center the IOL in the bag, remove the viscoelastic, check the centration again, and finally inject a miotic.

When pupil constricts to 3 to 4 mm, the surgeon should align the diffractive rings with the miotic pupil. In cases of even minimal decentration on day 1, the IOL should be immediately recentered with the miotic pupil. Usually, despite physiological postoperative fibrosis, the haptics will keep the IOL in this final position (Figure 7). Nidek OPD aberrometric evaluation of an eye with good ReSTOR centration (Figure 8) shows low internal total and HO aberrations (below, left, and above, right, respectively).

The Acrysof (Alcon, Fort Worth, TX) optic and haptics are tacky enough to increase in-the-bag stability and prevent decentration. If recentration becomes necessary, this must be accomplished by IOL rotation, and not simply by shifting or tilting the optic. Postoperative dilation of a ReSTOR IOL properly centered with the constricted pupil may reveal IOL decentration within the capsular bag (see Figure 1).

Conclusion

Diffractive multifocal IOLs produce excellent patient satisfaction if precise pupil centration is achieved. In addition, accurate biometry and topography-based keratometry should be adopted, and tight exclusion criteria should be respected. A well-centered ReSTOR, in particular, will provide excellent distance and good near vision without correction, and an ocular wavefront that is superior to that with standard spherical monofocal IOLs.

References

1. Blaylock JF, Si Z, Vickers C. Visual and refractive status at different focal distances after implantation of the ReSTOR multifocal intraocular lens. *J Cataract Refract Surg.* 2006;32:1464-1473.

2. Chiam PJ, Chan JH, Aggarwal RK, Kasaby S. ReSTOR intraocular lens implantation in cataract surgery: quality of vision. *J Cataract Refract Surg.* 2006;32:1459-1463.

3. Alfonso JF, Fernandez-Vega L, Baamonde MB, Montes-Mico R. Prospective visual evaluation of apodized diffractive intraocular lenses. *J Cataract Refract Surg.* 2007;33:1235-1243.

4. Vingolo Em, Grenga P, Iacobelli L, Grenga R. Visual acuity and contrast sensitività: AcrySof ReSTOR apodized diffractive versus AcrySof SA60AT monofocal intraocular lenses. *J Cataract Refract Surg.* 2007;33:1244-1247.

5. Baumeister M, Neidhardt B, Strobel J, Kohnen T. Tilt and decentration of three-piece foldable high-refractive silicone and hydrophobic acrylic intraocular lenses with 6-mm optics in an intraindividual comparison. *Am J Ophthalmol.* 2005;140:1051-1058.

6. Negishi K, Ohnuma K, Ikeda T, Noda T. Visual simulation of retinal images through a decentered monofocal and a refractive multifocal intraocular lens. *Jpn J Ophthalmol.* 2005;49:281-286.

CHAPTER 185

WHY USE TOPICAL NSAIDs?

John R. Wittpenn, MD

The availability of multifocal intraocular lenses (IOLs) has raised patient expectations regarding surgical outcomes and thus also raises the bar for ophthalmic surgeons performing refractive lens implantation procedures. Today, most patients opting for multifocal lenses pay all or part of the cost of these lenses themselves without insurance reimbursement. Perhaps because of this large personal financial (and often emotional) investment, many patients expect a rapid and uneventful postoperative recovery with the immediate return of excellent, spectacle-free, near and far vision. These outcomes may be particularly important for younger, healthier patients who elect to undergo refractive lens exchange prior to the development of cataracts. They have excellent-quality vision going into the procedure and consequently, will have very low tolerance for complications or any degradation of visual function. As a result, we must do everything possible to maintain both visual acuity and visual function in these patients.

Importance of Avoiding Cystoid Macular Edema

Multifocal IOL implantation frequently causes some degradation of contrast sensitivity.[1-4] Therefore, it is critical to take steps to prevent any further loss of contrast sensitivity, such as might occur with cystoid macular edema (CME). CME is thought to be mediated by inflammatory processes stimulating prostaglandin synthesis. Although CME frequently occurs after complicated intraocular procedures, it can occur after surgeries with no obvious complications and in patients without known risk factors. Patients with clinical CME present with blurred or decreased central visual acuity. CME can be subclinical or asymptomatic and may be detectable only through fluorescein angiography and/or optical coherence tomography (OCT) (Figures 1 and 2). The degree of retinal thickening required to compromise vision is not known, but recent studies suggest that an increase in thickening of as little as 15 μm may reduce contrast sensitivity.[5,6]

Ophthalmic NSAIDs to Prevent and Manage Cystoid Macular Edema

Nonsteroidal anti-inflammatory drugs (NSAIDs) specifically and irreversibly inhibit prostaglandin synthesis by interfering with the activity of cyclooxygenases (COX-1 and COX-2). One such NSAID, ketorolac, has been shown to be an effective treatment for acute and chronic CME in combination with steroids[7] and also prevents postoperative CME.[8,9] Other NSAIDs, such as indomethacin and diclofenac, may offer benefits as well but have not been studied as extensively.[10,11]

Several recent studies provided important information with regard to the use of ketorolac 0.4% to prevent CME in low-risk patients undergoing multifocal IOL procedures.[6,12] In the ACME (Acular LS for the Prevention of CME) study, in which this author was an investigator, low-risk patients undergoing cataract surgery were prospectively randomized into 2 groups: Group 1 received ketorolac 0.4% 4 times per day for 3 days prior to surgery plus 4 doses immediately preoperatively. They continued to use ketorolac 4 times per day postoperatively, with the addition of prednisolone acetate 1% (Pred Forte, Allergan, Inc.; Irvine, CA) QID. Group 2 received ketorolac 0.4% for only 4 doses immediately preoperatively and used prednisolone acetate 1% 4 times per day postoperatively without additional ketorolac. OCT was performed preoperatively and at 1 week and 4 weeks postoperatively. The OCT scans were evaluated by a masked retina specialist.[6,12]

The ACME investigators found that patients in group 1 (ketorolac 0.4% + steroid) were significantly less likely to have definite, probable, or possible CME compared to patients in group 2 (steroid only).[6,12] Mean retinal thickening was also significantly less in group 1 compared to group 2 (3.9 versus 9.6 μm, respectively; $P = .003$).[6] Furthermore, increasing retinal thickening was shown to be associated with decreasing contrast sensitivity.[6] The combination of ketorolac 0.4% and

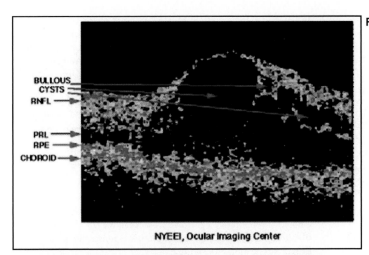

Figure 1. Cystoid macular edema.

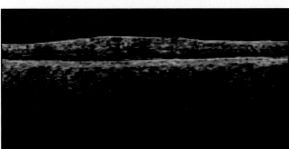

Figure 2. Cystoid macular edema.

steroid appeared to improve visual acuity compared to steroid treatment alone. Patients in group 2 were more likely to have suboptimal visual outcomes (ie, <20/40) 1 month postoperatively than patients in group 1 (2.5% and 1.3%, respectively; $P = .360$).[12]

These findings suggest that even the small amounts of retinal thickening reduced visual function especially contrast sensitivity following even uncomplicated cataract surgery. Patients who pay a premium for a multifocal IOL procedure expect better outcomes than a best-corrected visual acuity (BCVA) of 20/40 or even 20/30 at 4 weeks after surgery.

Many patients in the ACME study eventually regained 20/20 vision but experienced a permanent loss of contrast sensitivity. For example, one of my patients who participated in the study had 20/40 vision at 4 weeks. Although she regained her 20/20 vision, she never considered her vision very good in the surgical eye. When we tested her contrast sensitivity, we found it to be abnormal at all points despite the 20/20 BCVA. Her other eye still has a cataract, but she has delayed the second surgery because of the disappointing results with her first eye. This case illustrates the potential negative long-term consequences of CME, even if visual acuity ultimately returns to 20/20.

Two other recent investigations support these findings. Donnenfeld and coworkers evaluated the effects of ketorolac 0.4% in 26 patients undergoing cataract surgery with a bilaterally implanted multifocal IOL.[13] Ketorolac 0.4% was instilled 4 times per day for 3 days preoperatively and 3 weeks postoperatively in one eye. The second eye received ketorolac 0.4% for 3 doses only, every 15 minutes beginning 1 hour prior to surgery. Uncorrected visual acuity (UCVA), BCVA, and mesopic and photopic contrast sensitivities under high-contrast and low-contrast illumination were measured unilaterally at 2 weeks following lens implantation in each eye. Two weeks after the second implantation, the eyes that received pre- and postoperative ketorolac 0.4% had significantly improved contrast sensitivity compared to eyes not receiving the NSAID. There was also a trend toward improved UCVA and BCVA in the eyes treated with ketorolac 0.4%, as well as significant patient preference for the ketorolac-treated eye.[13]

In a study by Roberts, 200 patients undergoing phacoemulsification were randomized to receive steroids plus antibiotic alone or steroids plus antibiotic plus ketorolac 0.4%.[14] Roberts's findings were similar to the ACME and Donnenfeld et al studies: Patients who received ketorolac 0.4% showed average retinal thickening of 4.2 μm compared to 10.4 μm in the patients who received only steroids. Patients receiving pre- and postoperative ketorolac 0.4% also had a statistically significantly lower decrease in contrast sensitivity compared to the steroid-only group.

Conclusion

Despite their ability to provide excellent visual acuity with both near and far spectacle-free vision, multifocal IOLs have been shown to produce some degradation of contrast sensitivity. It is therefore imperative that patients undergoing multifocal IOL procedures avoid the development of any retinal thickening with its potential for permanent loss of contrast sensitivity and possibly decreased final visual acuity. We now have good evidence that the preoperative and postoperative use of ketorolac tromethamine 0.4%, the most extensively studied ocular NSAID in this setting, can significantly improve visual outcomes in patients implanted with multifocal IOLs. Thus, ketorolac should become the standard of care for optimizing visual outcomes and patient satisfaction. We anxiously await further studies of the other available NSAIDs before concluding they provide similar protection.

KEY POINTS

- Multifocal IOL implantation will result in some degradation of contrast sensitivity.
- Patients undergoing multifocal IOL procedures must avoid the development of even subclinical CME, which can result in retinal thickening and additional, often permanent loss of contrast sensitivity.
- Pre- and postoperative use of ketorolac tromethamine 0.4% has been shown to significantly reduce the incidence of both CME and subclinical CME and improve visual outcomes in low-risk patients.
- Ketorolac tromethamine 0.4%, the most extensively studied ocular NSAID, represents an important tool for optimizing visual outcomes and patient satisfaction with refractive lens implantations.

References

1. Ravalico G, Baccara F, Rinaldi G. Contrast sensitivity in multifocal intraocular lenses. *J Cataract Refract Surg.* 1993;19:22-25.
2. Williamson W, Poirier L, Coulon P. Compared optical performances of multifocal and monofocal intraocular lenses (contrast sensitivity and dynamic visual acuity) *Br J Ophthalmol.* 1994;78:249-251.
3. Pearce JL. Multifocal intraocular lenses. *Curr Opin Ophthalmol.* 1996;7:2-10.
4. Leyland M, Pringle E. Multifocal versus monofocal intraocular lenses after cataract extraction. *Cochrane Database Syst Rev.* 2006;18:CD003169.
5. Ball JL, Barrett GD. Prospective randomized controlled trial of the effect of intracameral vancomycin and gentamicin on macular retinal thickness and visual function following cataract surgery. *J Cataract Refract Surg.* 2006;32:789-794.
6. Wittpenn JR, Silverstein S, Hunkeler J, et al, for the Acular Cystoid Macular Edema (ACME) Study Group. Subclinical cystoid macular edema (CME) reduces contrast sensitivity and final visual acuity in low-risk cataract patients. Poster presented at the Annual Meeting of the Association for Research in Vision and Ophthalmology (ARVO), May 6-10, 2007, Fort Lauderdale, FL.
7. Heier JS, Topping TM, Baumann W, Dirks MS, Chern S. Ketorolac versus prednisolone versus combination therapy in the treatment of acute pseudophakic cystoid macular edema. *Ophthalmology.* 2000;107:2034-2038.
8. Flach AJ, Stegman RC, Graham J, Kruger LP. Prophylaxis of aphakic cystoid macular edema without corticosteroids. A paired-comparison, placebo-controlled double-masked study. *Ophthalmology.* 1990;97:1253-1258.
9. Donnenfeld ED, Perry HD, Wittpenn JR, Solomon R, Nattis A, Chou T. Preoperative ketorolac tromethamine 0.4% in phacoemulsification outcomes: pharmacokinetic-response curve. *J Cataract Refract Surg.* 2006;32:1474-1482.
10. Shimura M, Nakazawa T, Yasuda K, Nishida K. Diclofenac prevents an early event of macular thickening after cataract surgery in patients with diabetes. *J Ocul Pharmacol Ther.* 2007;23:284-291.
11. Yavas GF, Oztürk F, Küsbeci T. Preoperative topical indomethacin to prevent pseudophakic cystoid macular edema. *J Cataract Refract Surg.* 2007;33:804-807.
12. Wittpenn JR, Silverstein S, Heier J, et al, for the Acular Cystoid Macular Edema (ACME) Study Group. A masked comparison of topical ketorolac 0.4% plus steroid vs. steroid alone for the prevention of macular thickening following cataract surgery. Poster presented at the American Academy of Ophthalmology (AAO), Nov 11-14, 2006, Las Vegas, NV.
13. Donnenfeld, E, Solomon, K, Chu R, et al. the effect of a topical NSAID on quality of vision with a multifocal IOL. Poster presented at the Annual Meeting of the Association for Research in Vision and Ophthalmology (ARVO), April 30-May 4, 2006, Fort Lauderdale, FL.
14. Roberts CW. Improving quality of vision with nonsteroidal agents. Oral presentation at The American Society of Cataract and Refractive Surgery (ASCRS), March 17-22, 2006, San Francisco, CA.

CHAPTER 186

MAINTAINING PATIENT SATISFACTION POSTOPERATIVELY

Richard Tipperman, MD

In the Food and Drug Administration (FDA) core studies of the various presbyopia-correcting (Pr-C) platforms, overall patient satisfaction was reportedly very high. One of the reasons for this is that the patients enrolled in FDA studies tend to be "cherry picked" as being among the best possible candidates for that particular intraocular lens (IOL). Just as important, and often overlooked, is the fact that by being in the "core study," the patients have an incredible emotional investment in the outcome. They rightfully consider their enrollment to be at least partially altruistic and truly view the surgeon as their advocate and ally. As a result they tend to focus on and overreport positive findings while minimizing or downplaying any potential problems.

Clearly then, one of the most important aspects of the postoperative management of Pr-C IOL patients is maintaining a strong therapeutic relationship between the patient and the physician. This helps to keep the patient emotionally invested with a positive outlook. Although the vast majority of your Pr-C IOL patients will be happy with their results, there will certainly be some patients who are not satisfied. A similar phenomenon occurs with monofocal IOLs as well but for a number of factors, including the fact that patients with Pr-C IOLs have more of an emotional and financial involvement in their results, they can require more support than monofocal IOL patients.

One of the most important concepts to understand in evaluating postoperative patients is the difference between a patient's "complaints" and their "observations." As ophthalmologists we are acutely aware of all the nuances and changes that can occur in the postoperative cataract surgery period for our patients. It is easy to forget that for our patients, the entire experience is novel and none of it is familiar or intuitive. As a result, patients will often report a variety of symptoms to their physician not because they are "complaining," but because they are observing different phenomena that they are not sure are normal or not and they want reassurance.

A classic example of this is the patient who undergoes cataract surgery and then reports to their surgeon "my eye feels scratchy." In this instance, the patient is not really complaining (though most ophthalmologists will internalize the situation this way), but instead they are noting an observation and want reassurance from their surgeon that this is normal. Once they learn "the scratchiness is normal, don't worry," the patient is reassured and relieved. If the surgeon instead perceives this as a "complaint," they may communicate their frustration back to the patient with either verbal or nonverbal cues. This reduces the quality of the physician-patient relationship and creates a situation where the "complaint" exists "between the physician and the patient." If the surgeon instead realizes that the patient is making an observation and explains the treatment rationale or cause for the symptom, then their position as the patient's advocate or ally is strengthened because they "are on the same side" as the patient as far as the symptom is concerned.

A very similar phenomenon occurs with multifocal IOL patients. They will often report a variety of visual observations not because they are "complaining" about them, but because they want to know if the symptoms they are experiencing are normal or not. If the surgeons becomes defensive or does not respond to these observations in a positive manner, then the therapeutic relationship between the patient and physician is weakened. It again creates a situation where the patient is "on one side of the problem" and the physician is "on the other side." If instead, the physician validates the patient's concern and either addresses them as normal or discusses a management strategy, then the physician and the patient will be "on the same side" of the problem and the therapeutic relationship will be strengthened.

Patients who do not feel their doctor is listening to them or responding to their problems are likely to become increasingly anxious and more demanding. Patients who feel their doctor is their advocate in addressing their problems will be reassured and more relaxed. The former patients will tend to accentuate and dwell on negative aspects of their postoperative experience whereas the latter patients will, like the core study patients, tend to focus on the positive aspects of their postoperative experience.

Statements by the surgeon that demonstrate the surgeon is not concerned or validating the patient's problems will create a chasm between the patient and the surgeon by putting the "problem" in between them. Examples of such statements by the surgeon include the following:

"I don't know why you're not happy."
or
"You should be happy."
or
"You're doing great."
or
"You're crazy."

Surgeons need to be aware of the nonverbal messages they can send to a patient who is unhappy. Gestures, facial expressions, and body language can all send a message to the patient that the concerns they are voicing are not being taken seriously. This can significantly undermine the therapeutic relationship between physician and patient and create a more difficult postoperative experience.

Statements by the surgeon that can strengthen the therapeutic relationship and put the patient more at ease include the following:

"I know you are frustrated and so am I."
or
"I want to get the best possible result for you that we can possible achieve."
or
"I will stick with you through thick and thin."

Despite a strong therapeutic physician-patient relationship, there will still be Pr-C IOL patients with problems in the postoperative period. The most common significant problem patients will describe is poor vision. Without question the vast majority of these "problems" will be related to a residual refractive error. With Pr-C IOLs, some patients will have poor quality distance and/or near vision with a residual spherical error of as little as 0.5 D. Astigmatic refractive errors are often even more significant especially if they are at an oblique axis.

Even patients with 20/25 to 20/40 vision will at times report dissatisfaction with their vision. Many times when these patients are refracted by a superb technician, a notation will be made in the chart: "no improvement with manifest refraction." In these instances, it is critical that the physician perform a careful refraction typically with retinoscopy—in many instances a small residual cylinder or spherical error is detected. When this is placed in trial lenses, the patient will normally report complete resolution of their symptoms.

This is an important step because if a Pr-C IOL patient is dissatisfied with their surgical results, then at some point, nearly all these patients begin imagining that their IOL must be "defective." By demonstrating and explaining to the patient that their vision improves by correcting the residual refractive error, the patient realizes that their IOL is working properly but just needs to be "better focused." The approach to enhancements of residual refractive errors in multifocal IOL patients is discussed elsewhere in this book.

There are definitely patients who have had multifocal IOLs implanted who are reading and functioning well at near and yet are not satisfied with their results. In these instances, it is often not that the patients are "high maintenance" or "difficult," but rather that they do not have a frame of reference with which to compare their visual function. Although they may have heard and understood during their preoperative counseling that their "functional near vision would be much better than a monofocal IOL and that they still might wear glasses from time to time," they may not remember this concept during the postoperative period.

In these instances, the −3.00-D lens test is invaluable. I inform the patient that I will hold a lens up in front of their Pr-C IOL eye, which will make the lens function like a conventional implant. This will allow me to see if the new lens "is providing any assistance with near vision and also allow them to see what their vision would be like if a monofocal IOL had been implanted." It is not uncommon when performing this test for the patient to look up with a stunned expression and remark "You mean that is what my vision would have been like if I had a regular lens? I can't see anything up close! This new lens must really be working well for me!" Without performing this test, patients really have no way of knowing how much better they are because they do not have a "yardstick" for comparison.

This test is an important educational tool in the postoperative period and should be demonstrated even for very happy patients. The rationale for this is as follows: at some point even after successful bilateral surgery, a happy patient is likely to suffer "buyer's remorse." They often do not realize why or how they are better than a "regular" cataract patient. They may meet a friend who had conventional cataract surgery who is happy with their visual results with a monofocal IOL. By showing the "happy" or "perfect" Pr-C IOL patient the −3.00-D lens test, the patient can see first hand how much better they are than if they had chosen a monofocal IOL.

Another significant postoperative problem is dysphotopsia. Although this phenomenon has been reported with all IOL platforms, it does appear to have an increased frequency with Pr-C IOLs and particularly multifocal IOLs, which create simultaneous vision. This is one area where preoperatively counseling and discussion make postoperative management much easier.

Personally, I inform each patient preoperatively that although serious or bothersome glare and halo are rare following multifocal IOL implantation, they are a real concern because we cannot predict ahead of time which patients will be bothered by them and which will not. I then explain that if the patient does notice the glare and halo postoperatively, they will often improve over time. In the rare instances where the symptoms are truly troubling and do not resolve, I have preoperatively discussed with patients that their procedure is "reversible" in that the multifocal IOL can be replaced with a monofocal IOL.

Pharmacologic therapy can be helpful for some patients with Pr-C IOLs. With both the ReZoom (Advanced Medical Optics, Santa Ana, CA) and Crystalens (Eyeonics, Inc., Aliso Viejo, CA), agents such as pilocarpine or brimonidine can constrict the pupil and limit nighttime dysphotopsias. With the ReSTOR lens (Alcon, Fort Worth, TX), 0.5% tropicamide can dilate the pupil and allow more of the light energy to travel through the peripheral pure refractive portion of the IOL, thereby weighing more of the incoming light energy to the distance image and minimizing nighttime dysphotopsias.

Conclusion

Transitioning surgeons should have confidence that there is a resolution for almost all postoperative problems. In addition to the resources provided by this book, the companies that provide Pr-C IOLs have clinical specialists who can offer advice to surgeons who may have a question regarding a particular issue with a Pr-C IOL patient.

In many instances, the company may be able to have a more experienced surgeon contact you to review any specific clinical concerns you might encounter. This, along with the detailed information found throughout this book, is a powerful resource to the surgeon starting Pr-C IOLs.

Surgeons should remember that despite all the technological resources they have in their armamentarium to help their patients, still the greatest asset they have is related to the quality of the physician-patient relationship they establish. Even in the face of difficulties, showing and expressing a genuine concern for the patient's issues with a Pr-C IOL goes a long way in helping alleviate their anxiety and dissatisfaction.

PREMIUM IOL SURGERY PEARLS FOR POSTOPERATIVE MANAGEMENT

Kevin L. Waltz, OD, MD

Postoperative management begins with preoperative counseling. It is imperative that the patient understand what is likely to happen after the surgery and what is reasonably possible. This is the essence of informed consent. When the patient is informed of the preferred outcome after surgery and the alternative outcomes after surgery, the postoperative course will be less frightening to the patient.

In most cases, the postoperative management of a patient should be predictable to the surgeon, the staff, and the patient prior to the surgery. For instance, what is the follow-up schedule for exams after surgery? It is helpful for both you and the patient to schedule these preoperatively to optimize time management. This is especially true of younger patients with busy work schedules who receive premium intraocular lenses (IOLs). It is inconsiderate, as well as a little scary, to "surprise" them with a routine follow-up appointment with a few days notice when they could have been told what to anticipate preoperatively.

Many of the patient's postoperative concerns can be anticipated. It is very helpful to prepare them for these symptoms preoperatively, which will reduce their concern when it actually happens (eg, telling them that increased floaters and an increased sensitivity to light for several months after lens surgery are expected).

When you tell a patient to expect something postoperatively and he or she experiences it, you have predicted the future for them. This is a very powerful way to increase patient confidence and confers great positive benefits to both you and the patient. It encourages them to believe you when you tell them something else and to be reassured by what they have noticed.

The most powerful postoperative management tool is "tough love." You tell the patient what to expect after the surgery during the preoperative consult. When your predictions come true, you support the patient emotionally and remind the patient that what they are experiencing is normal and expected. This is the type of tough love we give our family, and our patients understand this concept and respond to it very well. Be frank and honest with the patient. If you use a monofocal IOL and aim for a plano refractive endpoint, tell the patient he or she will need reading glasses after the surgery. Do not apologize for it. If you think it is appropriate, tell the patient he or she will experience halos after the surgery. When he or she experiences them, do not apologize for it. You should confirm that the patient was advised about these preoperatively, you should support them emotionally, and you should move on.

CHAPTER 187

MAINTAINING PATIENT SATISFACTION POSTOPERATIVELY

Uday Devgan, MD, FACS

Patients who elect to receive presbyopia-addressing refractive intraocular lenses (IOLs) tend to be younger with milder cataracts and they may be paying a premium for their surgery. These patients have higher expectations and they want to quickly recover sharp vision at a variety of distances without complications.

The postoperative management of these patients actually begins before surgery, during the preoperative consultation when the patients must be educated and their expectations understood. If the postoperative course and visual recovery are discussed in detail with the patients prior to the surgery, they will be more satisfied and more realistic in their expectations.

Timeline of Healing and Visual Recovery

It is helpful to provide the patients with an approximate timeline of their anticipated visual recovery. They may not realize that they need time to adapt to pseudophakic vision, particularly when multifocal or accommodating IOLs are used. Although the patient may recover reasonably good vision the day after surgery, a total of 4 to 6 weeks is needed to achieve capsular contraction and refractive stability.

Even though, as ophthalmologists, we went to medical school, completed an internship, and learned full-body anatomy, how many of us know the timeline of healing after arthroscopic knee surgery? Can you walk and put pressure on the leg after 1 week? 3 weeks? 3 months? When will the brace be removed? When can you resume exercise? These simple questions would seem too basic to an orthopedic surgeon, but to the patient, they are important and the answers are unknown.

Similarly for our patients, we need to tell them when their vision will stabilize, when they will be able to read well, how much light they will need to optimize near vision, and when they can resume activities.

The initial recovery of vision is usually very rapid, with most patients seeing relatively well the same day or the day after the surgery. In cases of a dense cataract, where more phaco energy is used and some corneal edema is anticipated, explaining the need for a week or two to recover initial vision is crucial.

With multifocal IOLs, there is a period of neuroadaptation where the brain and visual system needs to adapt to the new way of seeing—intraocular image rivalry, with 2 or more distinct images from different focal points focused on the retina at once. As the neuroadaptation progresses, patients become more comfortable with their new vision and their perception of side effects, such as glare, halos, and dysphotopsias, tends to diminish.

With accommodative IOLs, there is also a period of adaptation as the eye and ciliary muscle complex become functionally able to move the IOL in response to an accommodative stimulus. This process may take weeks to months.

Minimize Complications

In order to achieve optimal visual results, we need to minimize the potential postoperative complications. This includes the prevention of subclinical cystoid macular edema (CME), which has been shown to occur in a significant percentage of routine cataract surgeries. The development of CME in the postoperative period will cause decreased visual acuity and a reduction in contrast sensitivity and the quality of vision. In patients with multifocal IOLs, where there is already a compromise in their contrast sensitivity, even mild CME can be severely detrimental to their vision. Use of topical nonsteroidal anti-inflammatory drugs (NSAIDs) in the postoperative period has been shown to decrease the incidence of subclinical CME. For this reason, many surgeons use NSAIDs routinely for all patients undergoing cataract or refractive lens surgery.

The most common complication after routine cataract surgery is the development of posterior capsule opacification (PCO). With refractive IOLs, even mild amounts of PCO are detrimental to the visual performance of the lens implant. Multifocal IOLs split the light going into the eye, which results in decreased contrast sensitivity. Adding any opacity to the posterior capsule makes this even worse. For accommodating IOLs, care must be taken to ensure that the capsular contraction does not cause a misalignment or shift in the position of the IOL. In addition to performing a capsulotomy to treat any PCO, there may be a need to perform anterior capsule relaxing incisions with the yttrium-aluminum-garnet (YAG) laser to prevent capsular phimosis.

Postoperative Refractive Status

Determining the perfect IOL power for a specific patient is not always easy, particularly if the patient has had prior corneal refractive surgery. In these cases, there may be a need in the postoperative period to fine-tune the refractive result of the eye. Patients should be aware of the potential need for a second surgery or enhancement to achieve a specific refrac-tive goal. This may be in the form of further corneal refractive surgery, a piggy-back IOL, or perhaps even an IOL exchange. Refractive IOLs require optimal refractive results, and this may mean an additional surgical procedure.

Encouragement and Feedback for Patients

Finally, we need to spend time giving the patient feedback and encouragement during the postoperative period. With accommodating IOLs, the near vision requires effort from the ciliary muscle. For most patients, the ciliary muscle has not been used to focus their crystalline lens for decades. Therefore, when it is called upon to focus the new IOL, there is often a feeling of fatigue. This fatigue resolves with time and the near vision improves as the ciliary muscle regains strength. When certain visual milestones are reached, patients should be congratulated on their new vision.

CHAPTER 188

CREATING A PREMIUM REFRACTIVE PATIENT ENVIRONMENT

James D. Dawes, MHA, CMPE, COE

When the Centers for Medicare & Medicaid Services established the opportunity for patient-shared billing in the summer of 2006, ophthalmologists were given an opportunity to prove that patients would pay additional fees for medical technology that provided differentially better visual outcomes. The Centers for Medicare and Medicaid Services ruling also allowed our practice to demonstrate that patients are more inclined to make the choice for an "upgrade" in technology if the environment and the total patient experience were at a premium level of service. As early adopters of the accommodating and multifocal intraocular lens (IOL) technology, our surgeons quickly recognized the lifestyle benefits and satisfaction experienced by our patients after undergoing a refractive IOL procedure. In this chapter, I routinely reference accommodating and multifocal IOLs as premium lenses and refractive IOLs.

Patient Selection

Assuming that a patient is considered a candidate for a refractive IOL based on appropriate clinical criteria, it is imperative to give him the opportunity to learn about the lifestyle benefits of all refractive IOLs after cataract surgery. The vast majority of our patients arrive at their cataract evaluation or comprehensive eye examination unaware of the latest advancements in IOL technology. We educate and advise these patients about the risks, benefits, and fees associated with the premium lens procedure. During the counseling session conducted by nonclinical patient care counselors, the patient's willingness to tolerate the visual adaptation to the refractive IOL technology is assessed. Next, it is determined if the patient has a strong emotional connection to the lifestyle benefits of improved vision that results from the procedure.

The use of a lifestyle questionnaire is helpful to the counselors, the technicians, and the surgical team to assess the patient's visual needs as they relate to lifestyle. For example, a patient who enjoys needlepoint and e-mailing her grandchildren may have slightly different visual needs than another patient with different lifestyle interests. These specific visual needs are helpful in selecting the best refractive IOL so as to maximize the patient's satisfaction. In addition, the premium lens procedure creates a strong emotional connection relating to the patient's desire for the procedure, which can be used in conversations with the patient to reaffirm the buying decision.

We have learned the importance of withholding our judgment regarding a patient's willingness to pay for the premium lens upgrade until he clearly understands the benefits. In many cases, patients who do not seem to have the financial means to afford a premium lens procedure will gladly pay for the upgrade in order to achieve spectacle independence. With a qualifying cataract, the fees for the procedure are similar to what patients might pay for a refractive procedure such as laser in situ keratomileusis (LASIK). As with other elective procedures, more than 25% of our patients choose to finance the cost with either no interest or extended monthly payment plans. Today, over one third of our IOL procedures are performed with a refractive IOL.

Creating an Experience

As with most purchases, the patient evaluates the cost of a premium lens procedure in the context of other flexible spending. In order for a patient to choose to spend discretionary income on an elective surgery, the overall experience itself must be differentially better than the average nonelective medical care experience. This begins with the first phone call from a patient to the practice, and continues through all aspects of the premium lens procedure and postoperative follow-up care. In order to create this quality experience, we first had to assess our environment. In most cases, health care delivery in the United States is a far cry from a luxurious, relaxing, and choreographed experience that one might find in a 5-star hotel or fine restaurant. Our practice is fortunate in that our founding surgeon has an overriding commitment to patient satisfaction and superior customer service. Therefore, modifying our practice to achieve the desired patient experience was not as difficult as it might be in some surgeons' offices. The following information outlines the assessment areas and key points.

ENVIRONMENTAL ASSESSMENT

When we examined the ambiance in our office, we started by walking through the front door. Upon entering the practice, the atmosphere must be professional, courteous, relaxing, and informative. Flowing through the practice and the surgery center, each hallway, examination room, counseling room, and diagnostic area must convey those same characteristics. We had to tweak our space plan to accommodate these requirements. Most challenging is creating an environment that is both relaxing and informative. Careful placement of internal marketing and patient education materials must be balanced with tasteful décor that allows the patient to learn while soothing anxieties he may have about seeing a surgeon. In addition to the physical surroundings, it is equally or more important to assess the atmosphere created on the telephone lines. Patients must be able to speak to a person as soon as possible without waiting on hold, and they must be able to get answers to questions generated by the practice's marketing messages.

While examining the environment it is also important to look for underutilized space. Often additional space for counseling rooms or educational areas can be created from the existing floor plan. To ensure that the revenue-producing exam lanes are maximally utilized, patient counseling and education can occur in the exam lanes if they are not otherwise in use. However, in a busy practice where room turnover is critical for ensuring return on the capital investment of an exam lane, patient counseling should occur in space not otherwise being used for revenue generation. By handling the counseling and education in a space that would otherwise be non–revenue-generating, the practice throughput is not decreased and the revenue generated per square foot should actually increase.

MARKETING AND MESSAGE ASSESSMENT

Due to the lack of public knowledge about the latest IOL technology, the practice must introduce educational information well before the patient is sitting in front of the surgeon. This educational process starts before the individual walks in the door. The referring physician must have materials that can be provided to the patient prior to the consultation. The practice's Web site should provide a comprehensive overview of the technology as well as lifestyle benefits associated with the procedure. Patients must have an opportunity to speak with a counselor prior to the examination in order to have general questions answered and to understand exactly what will happen on the day of his visit to the practice. All of this information must be carefully coordinated and scripted to relate to the public relations and awareness campaign being created through advertisements, direct mailings, and seminars.

The appropriate use of technology in the practice can also be very helpful in educating patients about refractive IOLs, as well as cataracts, the treatment of astigmatism, and the visual benefits of the premium lens procedure. Software programs can be purchased or DVDs may be provided by lens manufacturers to assist in the educational process. In our experience, we have found that allowing patients to view educational DVDs or software animations reduces the number of questions that the patient may have for the clinical staff, counselors, or surgeon and may help to reduce some of the anxiety that exists around any new technology.

PERSONNEL ASSESSMENT

The most important part of any organization is the human element. It is the staff who make or break all other investments in the office environment or marketing. In order for the staff to deliver a better experience, they must understand what that experience should be. In addition to constantly assessing the staff's customer service performance and providing continual training, the staff must understand the technology, lifestyle benefits, and pricing of the procedure. We have created talking points and word tracks for all personnel to help create harmonious communication. The front desk staff, technicians, counselors, surgeons, clinical assistants, and the check-out staff must not only inform patients but also reaffirm their choice to move forward with the premium lens procedure. Role playing and constant monitoring of the staff's ability to communicate the appropriate messages must be performed on a routine basis. The human element is the most difficult piece of the puzzle to manage; however, it produces the greatest return on investment. We also provide incentives to our staff based on the demonstration of superior customer service and achieving our practice goals.

MONITORING SUCCESS

Refractive laser vision correction practices have created several key reporting metrics that can be applied to a cataract and refractive IOL facility. The following list is a sampling of the important metrics our practice tracks and reports on a weekly or monthly basis:
* Telephone calls converted to appointments
* Media and referral sources
* Marketing cost per lead
* Marketing cost per surgical procedure
* Conversion of IOLs to premium
* Postoperative patient satisfaction

Conclusion

Continual monitoring of the practice's performance is a key element of success. However, more important is the process of sharing the data with the staff and surgeons in order to allow for constant reinvention of the practice's marketing messages, patient flow protocols, and office environment to ensure that you are exceeding your patient's expectations and meeting your practice goals for refractive IOLs. Remember the human element; investment in the staff will reap the greatest return.

CHAPTER 189

THE PREMIUM PATIENT EXPERIENCE

Darrell E. White, MD

In one of the first chapters of this book we introduced the importance of the concept of patient experience in the premium IOL (intraocular lens) world. What was once simply a solution to a medical problem (eg, I can't see because I have cataracts) is now also a solution to a lifestyle problem (eg, I don't want to wear glasses). Patients are now paying, and paying handsomely, for the choice of spending a lifetime relatively free of glasses. Because they are paying with their own money and not simply using an insurance policy, they are now behaving more like luxury consumers in addition to being patients. We have reengineered our practices to provide a premium experience to these patients as we deliver a premium product. But what does this mean to our patient? What constitutes a premium experience in *their* eyes (pun most definitely intended)?

In order to answer these questions, we must not only return to the thought experiment of placing our patient in the middle of a blank white piece of paper, but we must also take a moment and leave the arena of medicine entirely to learn the importance of customer experience in a pure consumer setting. Let us choose to examine the experience of purchasing a luxury automobile because there are so many parallel processes involved that are similar to the premium IOL world. Every customer has the option of choosing products that vary from the purely functional to the absolute epitome of luxury or speed or versatility. The choice is ultimately theirs.

Our driver could choose the most economical option, opting for transportation at the lowest cost (any number of cars applies here). She could choose a BMW, a high-performance vehicle that asks a little more of the driver and gives much back to one who will make the effort (kind of like the Crystalens [Eyeonics, Inc., Aliso Viejo, CA]). She might choose to go for the most widely chosen option like a Mercedes for the quality of the ride and the comfort and safety (perhaps reminding one of ReSTOR [Alcon, Fort Worth, TX]). Finally she may opt for an Infinity, which offers dazzling technology but has a smaller following (à la Tecnis [Advanced Medical Optics, Santa Ana, CA]). For any given product, the customer can choose among multiple dealerships, all of which will sell them the same vehicle but each of which will provide them with a slightly different experience along the way. Sound familiar?

There are three components to a consumer experience in the luxury or premium market, and these are magnified when we add a component of technology that is beyond the casual grasp of the consumer. The first is *trust*, the assumption that the seller of the product or the provider of the service is competent in managing the technology involved in the product. Next is the *experience* of buying the product or receiving the service itself. This is a significant step for each consumer (or patient) and she wants to enjoy every part of it as much as possible. She also wants to feel at every step along the way that she is making the right decision. The third component of the experience is actually *using* the product or enjoying the benefit of the experience. The pleasure of making the purchase would extend into the enjoyment of using the product, which should remind her of how much she enjoyed the process of buying it. Let us look at each one of these components in turn.

When we buy a luxury automobile, we assume that everything will work as it should. We do not consider the possibility that the car will not move forward as expected when we engage the clutch and stomp on the gas. We know that the ABS system will stop the car if necessary, and we expect that our driving experience will be trouble-free. The vast majority of this book is concerned with the technology involved in making, choosing, and implanting Premium IOLs. This is the equivalent of what happens at the automobile factory and in the garage, and this is the technology that our patient takes for granted. She assumes, and is perfectly correct in doing so, that you as the surgeon have handled this technical part as well as the wizards building and selling luxury automobiles. *You cannot differentiate yourself here!* This is the table stake, the ante that you must put up simply to be in the game. Most of this book deals with doing just this. Accurate preoperative measurements, safe and repeatable surgery, and predictable outcomes are our versions of building, outfitting, and tuning a luxury car. They are mandatory because your patient assumes that they are there.

So the patient asks, "Are you a premium practice?" With this question she is comparing your practice with a luxury car dealership, a luxury hotel, buying shoes in a boutique or Nordstrom's, or all of the above. In order to understand what your patient is expecting, think back to the last time you personally had any of these experiences and think about what they all had in common. Each one is a highly personalized experience with multiple points of interaction occurring in an atmosphere designed to make one feel comfortable, valued, and ready to make the decision to go forward. Each experience involves maximizing the amount of interaction that occurs between the business and the consumer and minimizing the amount of time that the consumer is left unattended. This is the experience our patient should have, too.

The lobby is the entry to the premium practice and it should extend right into the home of the patient. The initial telephone conversation is the first opportunity to let her know that this is an experience unlike anything she has ever encountered in medicine. This "extended lobby" experience includes any information sent to the patient prior to actually entering the office. Anyone who is even remotely a candidate for a premium IOL can receive information about this exciting opportunity before she reaches the front door of the practice. In addition to information sent through the mail it is very possible to invite patients to visit your cyber office, your Web site. Companies like Eyemaginations (Towson, MD) and others have incredible products in the pipeline to enable us to introduce these IOLs to our patients through e-mail and other Web applications.

Once the patient has actually entered the office and steps onto the "Premium Express" the "personal touch" kicks in. It is probably more important to know how often and for how long your premium patient is *unattended* than it is to know how long she spends with each or your staff members along her journey. Being attended means having a value-added experience, but not necessarily having a staff member or doctor in attendance. If there are forms that must be filled out they can include introductory information about the special premium services provided in your practice. During the brief wait in your lobby, at which time she is surrounded by reminders of your services and your successes, perhaps she can view a video or visit your Web site. While waiting for a doctor or while dilating, there should be some activity that will provide more information and will help her decide whether to choose a premium option. The visit should involve a seamless flow of information and experiences that encourage her to stay on the "Premium Express," attempting to fill as much "empty airtime" as possible.

If all goes according to plan and she has opted to go with a premium IOL, you have chosen the best lens for her and counseled her about the particulars of this IOL choice, and you have done impeccable, precise, and safe surgery. Now it is time to help your patient enjoy her choice. Just like most luxury automobiles, all of our appropriately chosen premium IOLs work just the way they are supposed to work. Did you ever wonder why your dealer has you come back a couple of weeks after you purchase your luxury automobile for a check, even though it's doing just what it's meant to do? Your premium IOL patient should come back for all of the postoperative checks that we know so well, but she should also come back so that she can be reminded that it was YOUR premium practice that gave her this wonderful lifestyle solution. The excitement of using her new vision is part of the pleasure involved in making the decision to have the surgery and choose the premium IOL. You and your practice are part of the reason your patient is now less dependent on spectacles and every time she comes in, everyone in the practice should celebrate right along with her.

We have entered a new era in eye care—the era of the patient experience, driven by the development of Premium IOLs. We are not only solving medical problems, but we are now solving lifestyle problems as well. In order to thrive in this new world, it is helpful to examine it through the eyes of our patients, as they are comparing our new premium practices with other high-end consumer goods and services. How do they see this new world? Spend some time shopping for shoes, test driving cars, or comparing steak houses. From whom did you want to buy that car? Who made you want to return for your next meal or to purchase your next pair of dress shoes? What made you feel that way? *That's* the experience you need to provide to your premium IOL patient!

Doctors, start your engines...

SECTION XII

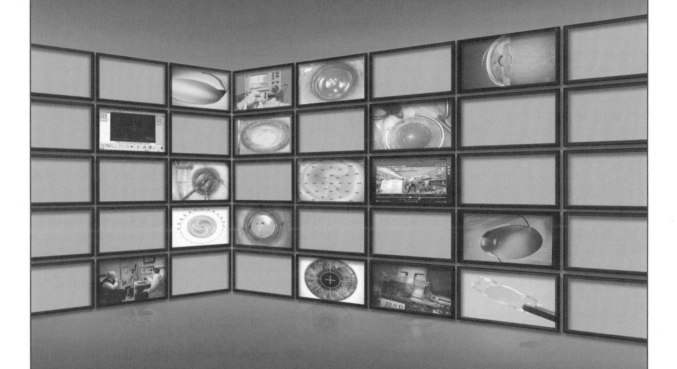

Refractive Lens Exchange

CHAPTER 190

THE PRELEX STORY

R. Bruce Wallace, III, MD, FACS

We Need a Name

Today we are witnessing a significant era in lens refractive surgery, whether that be for cataract or pre-cataract eyes. This presbyopia-correcting surgery journey of 20 years (or 58 years if you start with Sir Harold Ridley) has finally begun to go mainstream. However, only if patients know that this procedure exists will we see it capture the international attention it deserves.

A Brief Personal History

My first experience with multifocal intraocular lenses (IOLs) dates back to 1988. I had approached Dr. John Sheets about designing a multifocal IOL on his 3M (St. Paul, MN) monofocal platform. To my surprise, he shared with me that a multifocal IOL project had just been launched, thanks to a diffractive optic design recommended by an engineer at 3M, Dr. William Isaacson.

Later, with Dr. Richard Lindstrom as medical monitor, I was invited to participate in the 3M multifocal IOL Food and Drug Administration (FDA) study. In 1992, after jumping through the many hoops and hurdles of an FDA clinical trial, including a complex driving simulation substudy, the 3M multifocal IOL was recommended for premarket approval. Unfortunately, the full FDA membership did not accept this recommendation and Alcon (Fort Worth, TX) bought this multifocal IOL patent and began research on how to improve the optic with the guidance of a former 3M optical physicist, Dr. Michael Simpson. Meanwhile, Allergan (Irvine, CA) continued to study a refractive multifocal IOL designed by Dr. Val Portney. I was also part of this Allergan multifocal IOL clinical trial, which eventually led to FDA approval of the Array multifocal IOL in 1997.

Because we had been implanting multifocal IOLs for almost a decade (including investigating 2 other multifocal IOLs), implementing the Array IOL into our cataract practice did not take long. We encountered a few patients that were bothered with halos at night, but the vast majority, to this day, have enjoyed excellent uncorrected multifocal vision. However, many practices did not warm up to the Array. Allergan knew that any multifocal IOL required extra work for the surgeons and their staffs and launched Array "familiarity seminars." When teaching one of these sessions I met Dr. Michael Orr, an experienced cataract and corneal refractive surgeon from Indianapolis. Dr. Orr was very interested in, and even concerned about, the Array because he was about to implant this IOL into the eyes of his partner, Dr. Kevin Waltz. I encouraged Dr. Orr to proceed, and fortunately, Dr. Waltz had a great result. To my knowledge, Dr. Waltz was the first ophthalmologist to have bilateral implantation of a multifocal IOL.

At the 1998 American Academy of Ophthalmology meeting, Dr. Waltz joined Drs. Hampton Roy, Jack Holladay, and me as faculty for an instruction course on multifocal IOLs. For the first time, one of our colleagues could explain what Array multifocal vision was really like. With time many skeptics began to see the value of multifocal IOLs and adoption began to increase, albeit slower than Allergan anticipated.

The Origin of PRELEX

Dr. Waltz and I began to correspond on a regular basis along with 2 important drivers for the Array IOL at Allergan, Mike Judy and Chris Calcaterra. We all knew where we were going with the Array—beyond cataract surgery to pure refractive procedures for unhappy presbyopes. Dr. Waltz and I came to the realization that potential patients were simply not aware that a surgical procedure to reduce their dependency on bifocals even existed. By this time, laser in situ keratomileusis (LASIK) was a household word. Like LASIK, we strongly felt that a universal name for presbyopia-correcting IOL implantation would greatly improve credibility and popularity of corrective lens surgery. Dr. Waltz called me soon after and asked, "What about presbyopic lens exchange being shortened to PRELEX"? I liked PRELEX immediately.

After making certain that the name PRELEX was not already patented for other purposes, we organized a series of international seminars, the first being held on March 1, 2001 in Indianapolis. Because this concept was considered "off-label" and not FDA approved, Allergan decided to not directly endorse our PRELEX seminars. We also developed a PRELEX Web site and even designed PRELEX polo shirts for attendees. Dr. Waltz and I hoped we would see PRELEX begin to be used universally for all lens surgery intended to restore multifocal vision, regardless of which multifocal or accommodating IOL was used. To date, for various reasons, this has not occurred in the United States. However, in Europe PRELEX is widely utilized and continues to be a popular way for patients to tell their friends how they were able to acquire their new vision.

A Procedure, Not an IOL

A major advantage of having a name for lens refractive surgery is that patients do not fixate on one aspect of the ingredients to success, that is, the presbyopia-correcting IOL.

When patients are told they are a candidate for the procedure "PRELEX" they begin to regard the entire preoperative, intra-operative, and postoperative elements that play important roles in achieving the desired result. Consequently, if visual disturbances occur postoperatively due to problems not related to the IOL, such as dry eye, posterior capsular opacification, or a refractive error, patients are not as likely to assume their problem is because of their presbyopia-correcting IOL.

Conclusion

Because LASIK has become a household name for corneal refractive surgery, patients tend to believe in the procedure. They know what this procedure can provide and tend to discuss LASIK with their friends. If lens refractive surgeons adopt a name like LASIK that has international usage, patient awareness and acceptance of lens-based refractive procedures are likely to grow more rapidly.

CHAPTER 191

PATIENT AND SURGEON MINDSET— WHAT IS DIFFERENT?

Avery Alexander, MD

With the growing consumer interest in presbyopia-correcting intraocular lens (Pr-C IOL) surgery, many cataract surgeons are now transitioning or expanding their practices to offer Pr-C IOL surgery. Based on my years of experience in performing these procedures, I would like to share my thoughts and insights on making the transition from cataract surgeon to "complete refractive surgeon." This I define as a surgeon who not only performs laser vision correction but who can go inside the eye and perform phakic IOL and Pr-C IOL surgery. The transformation to complete refractive surgeon is built on the foundation of the cataract surgeon's highly refined skills combined with the unique mindset of a refractive surgeon.

Many leaders in the refractive field now believe that the future of refractive surgery will move inside the eye. To be a surgeon who performs only laser vision correction would restrict one from the vast growth potential in the field of Pr-C surgery and the immensely gratifying rewards associated with helping presbyopic patients see both in the distance and up close.

Intangible Attributes of a Complete Refractive Surgeon

All success begins with a proper state of mind. Intangible attributes are often the most important ones in achieving success in this subspecialty as in life itself. The mindset of a complete refractive surgeon must be steeped in an unquestioning belief in the procedure and its benefits for patients. One needs to believe that great outcomes are obtainable through study, effort, and practice, and that one will be able to significantly improve the patient's quality of life. The value of the Pr-C IOL procedure to the patient will far outweigh the monetary return to the surgeon.

It is important to understand that your patients will not believe in you or these procedures unless you first have an unquestionable belief in yourself and in the surgery. If you

lack this, it may be best to mentor or consult with other experienced surgeons first to build the unshakable confidence you need to succeed.

As eye surgeons, we have honed certain skills and abilities. In addition to these skills themselves, each of us must have faith not only in those abilities but also in the effectiveness of the procedures we perform. This faith must be there, even when there is no apparent solution immediately available. This is what gives you the tenacious persistence to continue when challenges arise, as they always will. One way to build this faith is to talk with colleagues, thought leaders in the field and, of course, successful and grateful patients. Their experiences can often provide the energy and enthusiasm to renew and strengthen one's faith.

Enthusiasm is another key attribute needed for the transition to Pr-C IOL surgeon. Enthusiasm has the power to shift your perspective on the work, changing it from labor to a labor of love. Being enthusiastic about the positive impact you will make on patients' lives will allow you to deeply enjoy what you are doing. It will open the door to continual personal growth in your practice and it will spread and infect both your patients and your staff.

Yet another mindset characteristic to help your transition is commitment. The margin for error in refractive IOL surgery is extremely small, because patient expectations and demands are much higher than those of cataract patients. Because they are usually "fee for service" patients, they demand an extremely high value for their expenditure. To meet these expectations, the surgeon must have a strong commitment to the procedure.

An effective way to meet these demands is to communicate to patients and staff that this surgery is part of a process of moving toward perfection, not just a single surgical event. Patients need to understand through consultation and communications that you as the surgeon are going to "optimize" the conditions of their eyes in order for the refractive IOL to obtain the best possible distance and near visual acuity. This may require patience on their part, and persistence and commitment on the part of the surgeon.

Another aspect of this commitment to the procedure is the willingness to invest in the best possible technology to deliver the highest level of care and best possible outcome. It will take research and patience to evaluate technology options and find the best, but this attitude of excellence and commitment to a higher standard of care will permeate your practice. Patients will recognize and understand your commitment to their best interests.

Staff training also reflects your commitment. Our staff spends more time with the patient than we do, and we must continually educate them and be vigilant about their attitude within the practice. From in-house training programs, to outside speakers, to travel to meetings and group reviews of books, staff training pays tremendous dividends. The enthusiasm and excitement it generates in your staff will filter down to your patients. Your staff's belief in you and in the procedures you perform is an integral part of your success.

Having an open mind on all subjects is critical to the growth of one's skill set and knowledge base. It can be difficult at times to keep an open mind, but I have found that, more often than not, it is when I have humbled myself that the greatest learning and quantum levels of improvement occur. Especially in this field, one needs to be ever aware that even the slightest improvement in the surgeon's skill or the technology can translate into a profound improvement in outcomes.

Technical Skills of a Refractive IOL Surgeon

The technical skill set necessary to be a complete refractive IOL surgeon includes:

* All the abilities and skills of an accomplished anterior segment surgeon
* The understanding of incisional keratotomy as it relates to limbal relaxing incision and astigmatic keratotomy to reduce and eliminate corneal astigmatism
* A complete understanding of and comfort with all aspects of laser vision correction procedures

In regard to anterior segment surgery, you need to advance your comfort level from operating on cataract patients with 20/40 or worse vision to having the confidence to operate on demanding 20/20 patients with no ocular pathology. For many surgeons, this may simple entail a mental shift in perspective.

One may need to use state-of-the-art small incision cataract techniques to meet the demands of these patients for fast visual recovery at both distance and near vision without complications. Many of these techniques are covered in other areas of this book. Of particular importance, however, is the polishing of the posterior capsule and the evacuation of all viscoelastic agents around the implant. Multifocal and accommodating IOLs are particularly sensitive to posterior capsule opacification (PCO) and the loss of light transmission. Evacuation of viscoelastics from behind the IOL is critical to developing a consistent, effective lens position that leads to greater accuracy with your IOL power calculations.

It is important to use an advanced IOL power calculation formula such as the Holladay consultant program. This is a complete program that allows you to track and optimize outcomes. The program factors in a range of variables, including 1) date of birth, 2) target RX, 3) refraction, 4) best corrected distance vision (BCVA), 5) uncorrected visual acuity (UCVA), 6) vertex, 7) K values, 8) horizontal white to white, 9) axial length, 10) A-scan type: IOLMaster (Carl Zeiss Meditec, Jena, Germany), 11) phakic ACD, and 12) lens thickness. The utilization of this type of regression analysis formula will help to ensure continual and ongoing optimization of your patient outcomes.

Selection of the appropriate IOL is another key consideration—one that can present a stumbling block in making the transition to Pr-C IOL surgery. There is no value to waiting for the "perfect" Pr-C IOL. The time to get started is the present, while this field is still in its infancy. In order to proceed with confidence, you must understand and accept that each of the currently available lenses involve compromises when compared to the human lens. The surgeon must fully understand the strengths and weakness of every lens option and what is needed to maximize the outcome with each particular lens. In addition, the surgeon must be able to manage each patient's expectations according to the lens type selected and its performance characteristics. Again, it may be best for the transitioning surgeon to mentor with an experienced refractive Pr-C IOL surgeon to gain this understanding and confidence.

Developing the skill set for incisional keratotomy takes time and practice as well. Although limbal relaxing incisions (LRI) and AK may not be as technically challenging as intraocular surgery, they require an understanding of the fundamentals and being methodical in order to achieve consistent success. One may start with a published nomogram and optimize it according to your own technique. Accurate topography, corneal thickness data, and knowledge of the diamond blade's true calibration are all keys to successful LRI surgery.

Laser Vision Correction Skill Set

The complete refractive Pr-C IOL surgeon must have the skill set of a competent laser vision correction surgeon. Attaining these skills is absolutely necessary in order to provide a complete and comprehensive approach for Pr-C IOL patients. The expectations of today's patients are for 20/20 distance vision and at least J2 near visual acuity. Anything less than that will lead to patient dissatisfaction and your continual frustration as a surgeon.

The ability to fine tune a patient's outcome with laser in situ keratomileusis (LASIK) or photorefractive keratectomy (PRK) is critical for the success of Pr-C IOL surgery. Pr-C IOL lenses simply do not have the latitude to tolerate very much residual refractive error. Even with optimized IOL formula calculations, I would recommend ownership of laser vision correction facilities. Ownership of or proximity to such a facility provides a clear competitive advantage. What's more, it demonstrates to your patients your willingness to do whatever is necessary to achieve the best possible outcome.

There are numerous manufacturer courses and wet labs available to allow those new to the laser vision correction (LVC) field to get started and achieve a comfort level with the procedure. One must have the skills to treat small amounts of refractive error post IOL surgery and should be able to care for all of the complications involved with LVC. A complication with LVC surgery for a minor refractive error after Pr-C IOL placement would be devastating for both the surgeon and the patient.

Postoperative Patient Management

The goal of Pr-C IOL surgery is to create a situation where patients are independent of glasses or contact lenses for both distance and near activities. For most patients it takes a DVA of 20/20 and a NVA of J2. Inevitably there will be some postoperative deviation from your expected outcomes that will require additional work on your part to make the patients happy.

In my opinion, the refractive endpoint in each eye should be plano ±0.25 with a cylinder correction of less than 0.75 D. This may not be immediately possible on all patients, and the surgeon will need to employ LVC to obtain this goal. Unfortunately, most of the complaints that a surgeon will hear will be due to these residual refractive errors. Undesirable visual aberrations increase the larger the residual refractive error is. Again, the confidence of the surgeon in an action plan to improve the patient's situation goes a very long way toward alleviating their fears and anxiety. Patience is a virtue for both the surgeon and the patient so as not to perform enhancements too soon.

During the postoperative period the ability to obtain and repeat accurate and reliable refractions is absolutely necessary for all LASIK and Pr-C IOL patients. For that reason, it is important to continually train and improve the skill set of those performing these refractions because even a small refractive error can have a profound impact on post LASIK enhancements after Pr-C IOLs.

As part of postoperative management, laser vision correction enhancement healing needs to be controlled and dry eye complaints need to be addressed with aggressive therapy. The purpose of this therapy is to obtain consistent and reliable refractions and vision. A stable refraction is absolutely mandatory before any additional enhancements are performed. In our practice a minimum of two refractions separated by at least 8 weeks is necessary to document stability. Our experience has shown refractive variability up to at least 4 months postoperatively, especially when large LRIs are performed or with patients that have significant dry eye conditions. Although halos and glare are discussed preoperatively with patients, they often arise again as postoperative complaints. It is essential to realize, understand, and communicate to your patient that these symptoms will significantly decrease over time as emmetropia is achieved and corneal astigmatism is reduced to below 1 D through the process of neuroadaptation.

Patient Selection and Education

At the heart of your successful Pr-C IOL surgery practice is a combination of sound patient selection and continual patient education. One of the first concepts I need to hear my patients articulate is that they realize they are truly presbyopic. Patients need to understand that even with adequate distance correction they lack the ability to accommodate or see up close. This is different from the mildly myopic patient who states, "I can see up close if I just take off my glasses." That myope does not truly understand the concept of presbyopia.

A full discussion with each patient about their expectations after the procedure is critical to their satisfaction and to your ability to treat them. It is important that the expectations they have match what you are able to deliver with the IOLs you use. If this is not the case it is necessary to reshape their expectations to match what you believe will be the expected outcome. Revising their expectations to what you can deliver is very necessary if they are to have reasonable goals, and to be able to accept possible side effects. Continual enthusiasm and general encouragement on the part of the surgeon and the staff will assist patients and help influence each person's perception of their outcome. As a result, many of the most challenging patients eventually become the best goodwill ambassadors for your practice and will aggressively recruit new patients for your clinic.

Conclusion

It is obvious that the complete refractive surgeon must possess tangible skills including excellent phacoemulsification techniques, incisional keratotomy techniques, and competency in laser vision correction techniques. Your skill set as a cataract surgeon forms the foundation for this transition. However, it is the intangible attributes of the surgeon that truly make the difference in one's success.

In contrast to most cataract patients, Pr-C IOL patients are a very demanding group, expecting 20/20 distance and near vision—all without glasses. It takes a mindset built on commitment and belief in the good one is doing; a strong desire to meet the demands of every patient despite costs; and a dedication to delivering the appropriate level of care to achieve the best possible outcome. The personal rewards of meeting these expectations, however, can be tremendous. These patients are sincerely grateful for the improvement in their vision. Moreover, presbyopia correction is one of the most exciting fields in anterior segment ophthalmology today, and I find it both personally and professionally rewarding to be a part of this movement.

CHAPTER 192

PRESBYOPIC REFRACTIVE PATIENTS—
LVC OR IOL?

Y. Ralph Chu, MD, and Dan Davis, OD

For a presbyopic refractive patient, the main factor in deciding whether we perform laser vision correction or select an intraocular lens (IOL) is the presence of a cataract. When the patient comes in for a refractive evaluation in the presbyopic age range, it is important to probe more deeply in the history to elicit any potential signs of early cataract change. Complaints, such as needing more light to read or having increasing difficulty while night driving, may be early clues to precataractous change or increasing spherical aberration of the naturally aging lens. If these symptoms are ignored, they may lead to a potentially unhappy patient if laser vision correction is performed.

For these patients, a thorough discussion of the findings is important. The appropriate decision may then be made by both the patient and the surgeon with respect to proceeding with any surgery at all, or to consider a refractive procedure based on lens exchange. Objective findings on slit lamp examination can help confirm suspicions elicited during the history, as these patients may still exhibit 20/20 Snellen acuity. The patients who come in for a refractive evaluation with more obvious signs of cataract change, such as decreased best-corrected visual acuity due to lenticular changes, have a more straightforward discussion. Other techniques for objectively assessing subtle lenticular changes are the Scheimpflug imaging capabilities of the Pentacam (Oculus, Inc., Lynwood, WA) and evaluating the spherical aberration value on wavescan.

It is important to discuss with the patients the objective criteria set forth by insurance companies for cataract evaluation. This may help clarify for the patient why their procedure would not be covered and would be considered a refractive lens exchange versus a cataract extraction. If the patient does not meet the criteria for coverage, no submission to insurance is done.

Another discussion to have with patients considering refractive surgery is what would be the most appropriate method of correction based upon their unique refractive error. These patients include the higher hyperopes as well as the more controversial higher myopes. Some of the benefits we discuss with patients when performing refractive lens exchange for higher degrees of correction are not only the improved quality of vision patients may achieve but also the possibility of choosing an implant that will offer them the ability to see distance, intermediate, and near.

Other scenarios where we favor refractive lens exchange over laser vision correction are patients with severe dry eye or ocular surface disease and thin corneas. Dry eye as a potential complication appears to be less of a problem with small incision cataract surgery compared to laser vision correction of the cornea. Although these patients may be considered better candidates for lens implant surgery, it is still critical to assess the quality of the ocular surface. One should attempt to rehabilitate any surface abnormalities prior to considering any type of refractive IOL surgery. It is important to remember that the ocular surface is the most important refracting surface of the eye in determining the quality of vision postoperatively. It is difficult to arbitrarily and exactly establish a safe cutoff for corneal pachymetry measurements when considering laser vision correction. We think it is the relationship between the amount of refractive error and the corneal pachymetry that will determine the safety of the procedure.

The purest group of refractive lens exchange patients is the individual in the presbyopic age group seeking refractive surgery with no sign of cataracts and no history of lens-induced aberrations. We think every patient in this age group deserves to know that there are lens implants available and approved for treating cataracts, which would potentially offer a wider range of focus than is attainable with laser vision correction. Patients that choose these lens implants for refractive lens exchanges need to be informed that this would be an off label use of these approved lenses. The lenses that are currently available in the United States are the ReZoom (Advanced Medical Optics, Santa Ana, CA), ReSTOR (Alcon, Fort Worth, TX), and Crystalens (Eyeonics, Inc., Aliso Viejo, CA).

Knowing if the patient has previously tried and tolerated monovision is important. With this knowledge, the surgeon is able to properly plan the surgical procedure, the lens implant type, and the target refraction for patients. A happy monovision patient may simply need the same amount of residual myopia targeted postoperatively. If the patient tolerated a small amount of monovision, the surgeon may target the nondominant eye with a little myopia to achieve a comfortable result. A preoperative contact lens trial may enhance patient understanding of a targeted outcome.

We think all patients who are considering refractive lens exchange need to be worked up preoperatively as thoroughly as a laser vision correction patient. The preoperative examination should include a pupil measurement, which will help in determining if a premium presbyopia-correcting lens may help. This may influence the decision of whether to perform laser vision correction or consider a presbyopia correction IOL. We currently do not offer presbyopia-correcting refractive lens exchange for patients with form fruste keratoconus or abnormal topography. We feel that it is important for these patients to have healthy corneas with normal topography and pachymetry. This allows an enhancement with laser vision correction for small amounts of residual refractive error if they need it. Also, patients who have preoperative refractions in the low-myopic group (−2.00 or less) may not be good candidates for a presbyopia-correcting lens exchange. The currently available lens technology cannot match the quality of near vision that these patients may already have preoperatively.

Exciting new presbyopia-correcting lens technologies have increased the options patients have in choosing refractive surgical options. Listening to your patients needs and understanding the demands of their lifestyles will help you match the proper procedure and lens technology for that patient. As patient expectations and demands increasingly grow, it is important that they are thoroughly educated about all of their options, whether they are corneal-based or lens-based refractive surgery.

CHAPTER 193

PRESBYOPIC REFRACTIVE PATIENTS— LVC OR IOL?

Sheraz M. Daya, MD, FACP, FACS, FRCS(Ed), FRCOphth

A presbyopic patient desires vision correction. What should the solution be—laser vision correction (LVC) or a presbyopia-correcting intraocular lens (IOL)? Obviously there is no simple answer! Whenever there are choices, decisions are made based on a number of different factors that are bound to change as available products improve. In addition, the choice will be influenced by better surgical techniques and by successful experiences as one pushes his or her personal boundaries. This chapter will attempt to provide a personal perspective based on my evolving experience and baked by evidence where available.

As a corneal surgeon, practicing refractive surgery since 1992, the concept of refractive lensectomy during the mid-1990s seemed rather aggressive. Especially when I started performing laser in situ keratomileusis (LASIK) in 1995, most refractive errors could be treated fairly successfully. Then every so often I had the patient in their mid-50s who was very disappointed with the loss of near vision postoperatively. Even worse, some of them developed lens changes requiring cataract surgery roughly 5 years later. I became reluctant to deal with patients in this age group, especially if there were any lens changes in terms of discoloration and if a high refractive correction was required (–8.00 and above or +3.50 and above). Furthermore, the increased incidence of persistent dry eye in the middle-aged female hyperope made me think twice about LVC in this group of patients. The numbers of patients being turned down for LASIK continued to increase, resulting in disappointment for both those patients and our practice. Part of this has been the result of changing demographics, with baby boomers now moving well into the presbyopic age group. This group, however, is also increasingly seeking vision correction now that they have more disposable income with all debts paid off and children off their hands. They are also paying more attention to their health and lifestyle, and seek greater visual freedom.

Several additional events increased my interest in refractive lens exchange (RLE) or "early cataract surgery." Siganos and Pallikaris[1,2] presented data on the success of RLE in hyperopia, in which they highlighted problems in the quality of vision following LVC. In particular, night vision disturbances were becoming an issue in patients with high refractive errors—especially in presbyopic myopes. Wavefront procedures became available in late 2000 and thanks to using wavefront analyzers, aberrations were quantified in different age groups. Spherical aberration was demonstrated to increase with age,[3,4] as a result of increased sphericity of the cornea and changes in the crystalline lens. Myopic ablative surgery on the cornea further contributed to spherical aberration, resulting in a marked reduction in contrast.[5,6] It was obvious that an alternative approach to this age group was required.

I then decided to take a look at RLE in those presbyopic patients with mild lens changes. Although I was able to correct these patients spherically and astigmatically, there was no other significant benefit, except that in time there would be no need for further cataract surgery. Additionally spherical aberration induced by IOLs has been recognized since the late 1980s[7] and in spite of newer designs, IOL spherical aberration was still an issue in the early 2000s. Development of newer designs such as the Tecnis aspheric IOL (Advanced Medical Optics, Santa Ana, CA) were underway and promised better visual quality, but at the time evidence was still being gathered. In terms of "added value," the option of presbyopia correction afforded by the Array IOL (Advanced Medical Optics) was attractive and had its supporters. However, because I frequently saw refractive patients who were referred to me with severe night vision issues, I was reluctant to embark on this option. The Crystalens (Eyeonics, Inc., Aliso Viejo, CA) was also becoming available and following a number of conversations with users, I decided to try the lens out. Essentially I had nothing to lose. At worst patients would get good distance vision, while having to use readers. At best they would get the benefit of near, middle and distance vision. My experience with Crystalens was very good. However, several patients experienced lens shift and the subsequent refractive change led to some disappointment. In addition, in 35% of my cases, functional near vision was not achieved. Capsular fibrosis resulting in a change in refraction

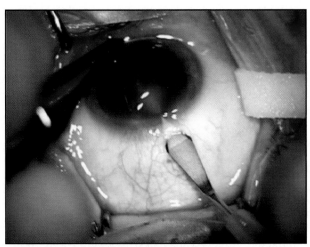

Figure 1. Transconjunctival superior scleral stab incision.

or posterior capsule opacification requiring a ytrrium-aluminum-garnet (YAG) capsulotomy occurred in 11.7% of my patients. Although the problems could be rectified, this was an issue for patients who had not been counselled about this possibility before the procedure.

To my amazement, the introduction of Crystalens as a refractive option resulted in a significant increase in the volume of lens based procedures in my practice. In constant pursuit of improvement, I next introduced the ReSTOR (Alcon, Fort Worth, TX) multifocal IOL. Being initially skeptical of reported results and wary of side effects, such as halos and rings at night, I approached this option cautiously. I tried to select the most suitable patients, such as hyperopes with no astigmatism, and I counseled them very carefully about issues of intermediate vision and night vision. The outcomes with ReSTOR were surprisingly good and in time, with the confidence of being able to treat residual refractive error using laser vision correction, I started pushing the boundaries of combining refractive IOL surgery with limbal relaxing incisions (LRIs). Residual astigmatism could be treated by repeating the LRIs at the slit lamp or by performing surface ablation laser vision correction at 3 months postoperatively. In reality, the percentage of those presbyopia-correcting IOL patients requiring laser surgery enhancement has been only 1% over the last 2 years. The inability to read in dim light conditions such as in an aircraft has probably been the biggest complaint amongst my ReSTOR patient population, many of whom are business executives. Alternative lenses, including the Acri.LISA (Acri.Tec, Henningsdorf, Germany) and Tecnis multifocal IOL, are better overall in terms reading in dim light. Although these multifocal IOLs are not apodized, they do not appear to cause any greater problems with night vision or halos.

Strikingly, the patient conversion rate to refractive lensectomy with a premium lens has been very high and in many ways has been more easily accomplished than laser vision correction. The main reason for this is probably the fact that, unlike laser vision correction, reading vision is addressed along with distance correction. This added value comes with little additional cost. The fact that this option might involve 2 procedures on separate dates and carries a slightly higher degree of risk does not seem to be a major barrier for this age group. Good counseling and patient education have been

important factors in contributing to a high acceptance rate. In a refractive practice, administrators, nurses, and technicians are very accustomed to providing the higher level of counseling required by these patients. This counseling process has been further enhanced by providing manufacturer brochures, and using patient education videos such as the IOL Counsellor (Patient Education Concepts, Houston, TX) and those from Eyemaginations (Towson, MD). Although the number of laser vision correction procedures has remained relatively flat, our volume of RLE has grown and now approaches 35% of all vision correction procedures performed at our center.

Making the Choice Among Vision Correction Procedures

In the presbyopic age group, choices for vision correction procedures are not simply between laser vision correction and refractive lensectomy. Phakic implants, are another worthy consideration, but posterior chamber lenses such as the implantable contact lens (ICL) are probably best avoided in patients over 50 years old because of a possible increased risk of cataract. The Artisan (Ophtec BV, Groningen, Netherlands) (including the Toric) and Artiflex (Ophtec BV) are probably better suited in this age group and in very high myopes.

So how should this decision be made? Like many such decisions in medicine, there are no hard and fast rules and much depends on a variety of factors. These include the patient's lifestyle, desires, expectations, refraction, risks, and ocular health balanced with what technology is available to meet the expectations of both the patient and surgeon.

RISK

The question of risk is a good place to start. What concerns me the most about RLE is the long-term risk of retinal detachment. This is reportedly higher in myopes and some believe that the risk increases with time following lensectomy.[8] The retinal detachment risk with refractive lensectomy is much lower in hyperopia.[9] The other important risk is endophthalmitis, which, before the era of intracameral prophylaxis, ranged in incidence between 0.1%[9] and up to 0.5%.[10,11] Corneal incisions have been associated with a higher incidence of endophthalmitis compared to scleral incisions and temporal location appears to carry more risk than superior incisions.[12,13] The introduction of intracameral cefuroxime has resulted in a major reduction in the incidence of endophthalmitis.[12-14] Having tried all approaches, my own personal approach for the last 10 years or more has been to perform a transconjunctival stab scleral incision superiorly for all IOL surgery (Figure 1). To avoid ballooning of conjunctiva, I create tangential conjunctival incisions after the stab incision (Figure 2). I also use intracameral cefuroxime (1 mg) in all cases where there is not an allergic contraindication. Although there has been controversy over the findings of the European Society of Cataract and Refractive Surgeons study,[12] one cannot ignore the dramatic reduction of endophthalmitis using intracameral cefuroxime in Tanzania to zero in over 21,000 cases where the incidence was previously as high as 0.24% at a single unit.[14]

Intraoperative complications are another important risk, but can be minimized with highly competent cataract surgeons.

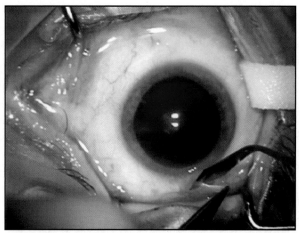

Figure 2. Tangential conjunctival incisions enlarges conjunctival opening to prevent undesirable conjunctival ballooning during phacoemulsification.

Problematic symptoms from multifocals including "halos" and "rings around lights" are significant (bothersome) in 8% of our patients. Appropriate patient selection is vital and preoperative counseling must stress this possibility to avoid "surprising" the patient postoperatively. I have not personally had to exchange a multifocal IOL because of patient dissatisfaction. The patient's occupation and lifestyle are probably the most important factors to consider. Implantation of a multifocal lens is probably inadvisable in a chauffeur or an airline pilot. The importance of intermediate vision must be considered, such as with a patient who spends a great deal of time in front of a computer screen. I have not used a mixing approach for these patients and am presently reluctant to do so, with an inherent bias against zonal refractive lenses used to provide intermediate vision. Preoperative astigmatism is also an important consideration, but I have not felt this to be a significant contraindication as it is usually correctable. The advent of toric implants has been particularly helpful for patients with higher amounts of astigmatism. Toric multifocals are now becoming available in Europe (Acri.Tec, Acri.LISA Toric) and about to be investigated.

Many methods to evaluate patient suitability have been described and the questionnaire by Steven J. Dell15 is an excellent way to evaluate patients' personalities and expectations. We developed our own questionnaire, which provides a thumbnail view of the patient and is more concise. This is supplemented by a face-to-face conversation with myself at the time of consultation.

BENEFIT

The benefit of RLE over laser vision correction in the presbyopic age group is obviously the ability to provide more depth of focus. The better optics that characterize aspheric and aberration-free IOLs are an additional benefit. In Europe, the Tecnis Multifocal and Acri.LISA are both aspheric multifocal IOLs and we now have the ReSTOR IQ. Deciding which IOL to choose requires preoperative topography to evaluate the spherical aberration Q value. This can be done with a number of newer topographers including the Pentacam (Oculus). Determination of Q values are also possible using the Orbscan (Bausch & Lomb, San Dimas, CA) in association with

the "K Q calculator" available at special request from Bausch & Lomb. This software was previously used to calculate Zyoptix aspheric treatments. Patients with corneas with a 0 or positive Q value will benefit from the use of an aspheric IOL and will hopefully attain mildly negative postoperative Q values, which are felt to be optimal in terms of minimizing spherical aberration.

How Do We Make a Decision With All of the Preceding Considerations?

In our practice, our patients are evaluated as though they are refractive surgery candidates In addition to a full ophthalmic evaluation and refraction, they also undergo contrast sensitivity testing, brightness acuity testing, pupil size measurements under mesopic conditions, Orbscan tomography, screening aberrometry with the Zywave, and biometry with the IOL Master (Carl Zeiss, Oberkochen, Germany) using the Holladay 2 formula for "outliers" (eg, deep anterior chambers, short or very long axial lengths, and large corneas). We evaluate the tear film, ocular surface, and lid status, as these are just as important considerations for multifocal IOL patients as they are for laser vision correction candidates because of the potential for reduced visual quality and contrast sensitivity issues. This process is time consuming but eventually faster diagnostic devices will become available.

With this information in hand, we next go through a mental checklist of parameters and the IOL is selected. These cases will demonstrate the art behind this IOL selection process.

Checklist

AGE

>65	RLE
60-65	RLE, LVC only if low level of correction
55-60	RLE, possible LVC if low level of correction (myopes and hyperopes)
50-55	RLE (hyperopes), LVC
45-50	LVC

REFRACTION

Hyperopia

* RLE if >3.00 D, otherwise LVC
* If post LVC K readings greater than 49.00 D, no LVC and possible RLE
* Female >50, RLE more likely (concern about dry eye)

Myopia

* LVC if possible (corneal thickness and optic zone size permitting)
* RLE if lens changes or myopia greater than 5.00 D and age >55

Astigmatism

>3.00 D	Special emphasis on possible need for supplementary LVC at counseling or consider monofocal toric or now Acri.LISA Toric
<3.00 D	All multifocals with LRI

PUPIL SIZE

>5.0 mm	Tecnis MF or Acri.LISA
4.0-5.0 mm	ReSTOR, Tecnis MF, or Acri.LISA
<3 mm	Tecnis MF or Acri.LISA

PATIENT OCCUPATION

* Required to drive at night or high-risk profession (eg, Pilot): Monofocal or Crystalens
* If reading in dim light required: Tecnis MF or Acrilisa

PATIENT EDUCATION AND EXPECTATIONS

* Educated and well researched: RLE or LVC
* Motivated to correct presbyopia: RLE with multifocal
* RLE only if: Understands and prepared to take the risk of intraocular surgery

Q VALUE

Positive:	Tecnis Multifocal or Acrilisa
Negative:	ReSTOR or Acri.LISA if pupil small and required to read in dim light

DRY EYE

* RLE

POOR TEAR FILM

* Improve prior to surgery—consider monofocal or Crystalens

The above factors are some objective parameters; however, there are a number of "shades of grey" and the final decision is made between myself and the patient based on my understanding of their expectations, psyche, as well as their understanding of the risks and benefits along with level of motivation.

I do feel it is necessary to put a "time stamp" on this chapter, as this is the current state of my thinking and approach to whether to "lensectomy or not" in August 2007. In time, as we push back boundaries along further understanding of optical systems, ocular physiology, patient response, and availability of newer treatment modalities, this is likely to change and it is quite possible that a good portion of what has been stated above will find its way into obsolescence!

I hope that this personal thought process and internal debate in how I deal with the presbyopic patient has been useful to you the reader.

REFERENCES

1. Siganos DS, Pallikaris IG. Clear lensectomy and intraocular lens implantation for hyperopia for +7 to +14 dipoters. *J Refract Surg.* 1998;14:105-113.
2. Siganos DS, Siganos CS, Pallikaris IG. Clear lens extraction and intraocular lens implantation in normally sighted hyperopic eyes. *J Refract Corneal Surg.* 1994;10:117-121; discussion 122-124.
3. Guirao A, Redondo M, Artal P. Optical aberrations of the human cornea as a function of age. *Opt Soc Am A Opt Image Sci Vis.* 2000;17:1697-1702.
4. Artal P, Berrio E, Guirao A, Piers P. Contribution of the cornea and internal surfaces to the change of ocular aberrations with age. *J Opt Soc Am A Opt Image Sci Vis.* 2002;19:137-143.
5. Marcos S. Are changes in ocular aberrations with age a significant problem for refractive surgery? [Review.] *J Refract Surg.* 2002;18: S572-S578.
6. Hersh PS, Fry K, Blaker JW. Spherical aberration after laser in situ keratomileusis and photorefractive keratectomy. Clinical results and theoretical models of etiology. *J Cataract Refract Surg.* 2003;29:2096-2104.
7. Smith G, Lu CW. The spherical aberration of intra-ocular lenses. *Ophthalm Physiol Opt.* 1988;8:287-294.
8. Colin J, Robinet A. Clear lensectomy and implantation of a low-power posterior chamber intraocular lens for correction of high myopia: a four-year follow-up [review]. *Ophthalmology.* 1997;104:73-77; discussion 77-78.
9. Montan P, Lundström M, Stenevi U, Thorburn W. Endophthalmitis following cataract surgery in Sweden. The 1998 national prospective survey. *Acta Ophthalmol Scand.* 2002;80:258-261.
10. Patwardhan A, Rao GP, Saha K, Craig EA. Incidence and outcomes evaluation of endophthalmitis management after phacoemulsification and 3-piece silicone intraocular lens implantation over 6 years in a single eye unit. *J Cataract Refract Surg.* 2006;32:1018-1021.
11. Khan RI, Kennedy S, Barry P. Incidence of presumed postoperative endophthalmitis in Dublin for a 5-year period (1997–2001). *J Cataract Refract Surg.* 2005;31:1575-1581.
12. Endophthalmitis Study Group, European Society of Cataract and Refractive Surgeons. Prophylaxis of postoperative endophthalmitis following cataract surgery: results of the ESCRS multicenter study and identification of risk factors. *J Cataract Refract Surg.* 2007;33:978-988.
13. Lundström M, Wejde G, Stenevi U, Thorburn W, Montan P. Endophthalmitis after cataract surgery: a nationwide prospective study evaluating incidence in relation to incision type and location. *Ophthalmology.* 2007;114:831-832.
14. Wood M, Bowman R, Daya SM. Prophylactic cefuroxime and endophthalmitis in East Africa. *J Cataract Refract Surg.* Letter accepted for publication.
15. Dell SJ. An algorithm for presbyopic IOL patients. Cataract Refract Surg Today. 2006. Available online at http://crstoday.com/ PDF%20Articles/0306/CRST0306_F6_Dell.html.

CHAPTER 194

RLE WITH MULTIFOCAL IOLS— BIOPTICS APPROACH

José F. Alfonso, MD, PhD and Robert Montés-Micó, PhD

Multifocal intraocular lenses (MIOLs) are widely used to provide pseudoaccommodation after lens removal.[1-9] One of the most important aspects of successful pseudoaccommodative IOL implantation is accurate IOL power calculation. Residual refractive error after cataract or refractive lens exchange (RLE) decreases the benefits of pseudoaccommodation by reducing visual performance at distance and near.[2] The combination of a monofocal posterior chamber IOL with a photorefractive keratectomy (PRK) or laser in situ keratomileusis (LASIK) adjustment have been previously reported.[10] Leccisotti reported the use of PRK as a secondary procedure after Array IOL implantation, showing how this procedure improves distance vision.[11] His report is the only one that uses laser vision correction after MIOL implantation to improve near vision. Laser vision correction after MIOL implantation is an interesting option to treat residual refractive error. LASIK with a mechanical microkeratome[12-14] and with a femtosecond laser[14,15] has been found to be an effective procedure for the treatment of refractive errors.

We performed a study of the efficacy, safety, predictability, and stability of 31 bilateral RLE in patients who have had implantation with the AcrySof ReSTOR IOL (Alcon, Fort Worth, TX) followed by LASIK with femtosecond laser for correction of residual refractive error in 53 eyes. Before and after LASIK surgery, patients had a complete ophthalmologic examination. Postoperative assessment was routinely performed at 1 day, 1 week, and 1, 3, and 6 months after LASIK surgery. The criteria used to treat residual refractive error after RLE was patient dissatisfaction with their uncorrected visual acuity (UCVA). All patients had a minimum of 0.50 D of residual spherical equivalent (SE) and all patients achieved improvement in their distance visual acuity without impairing their near vision using a trial frame refraction prior to femtosecond LASIK.

Femtosecond laser surgery was utilized to treat residual refractive error in all cases after the post-RLE refraction had stabilized (minimum follow-up period after the RLE surgery of 6 months). Following informed consent, surgery was performed under topical anaesthesia utilizing the IntraLase

femtosecond laser FS60 (IntraLase Corp., Irvine, CA) to create the flap and the Visx Star S4 (Santa Clara, CA) excimer laser to photoablate the cornea. This combination of lasers has recently been termed IntraLase LASIK. The femtosecond laser flaps were created with the following settings: 100 µm flap thickness, 8.0 to 9.0 mm diameter, 45-degree superior hinge angle, 70-degree side-cut angle, laser raster patterns spot/line separation of 10/10 µm and stromal energy of 1.0 µJ with a side-cut energy of 1.8 µJ. The excimer laser was programmed with the conventional Visx S4 algorithm to achieve emmetropia (software version 4.60). Treatment prerequisites were no contact lens wear for 2 weeks before the baseline preoperative examination, stable refractive error for at least 2 months before surgery, and visual acuity improvement with trial lenses of at least ≥ 1 line. Laser surgery was not performed if there were corneal irregularities or corneal thickness of <500 µm. There were no complications in any of the cases with a minimum of 6-month follow-up.

The SE, keratometry, and pachymetry measured prior to IntraLase LASIK enhancement are displayed in Table 1. Best-corrected distance visual acuity (BCDVA) in decimal acuity was essentially unchanged at 0.85 ± 0.15 preoperatively and 0.86 ± 0.16 at 6 months ($p = 0.5$). Six months postoperatively, mean uncorrected distance visual acuity (UCDVA) was 0.83 ± 0.20 ($p < .01$). The overall efficacy index (mean postoperative UCDVA/mean preoperative BCDVA) at 6 months was 0.97. The safety index (ratio of postoperative and preoperative BCDVAs) at 6 months was 1.01. With respect to safety, none of the examined eyes lost ≥2 lines of BCDVA by 6 months after surgery (Figure 1). The mean postoperative SE was 0.01 ± 0.17 D (range, −0.50 to 0.75). The deviation of the achieved SE refraction from the targeted SE refraction was calculated. By 6 months, all eyes were within ±1 D of the aimed refractive change (Figure 2) ($R = 0.96$), and 51 eyes (96.2%) were within ±0.50 D of the target refractive error. The change in mean SE over time was 0.19 D (Figure 3).

The near vision was excellent, and the best corrected near visual acuity (BCNVA) was essentially unchanged with 0.89 ±

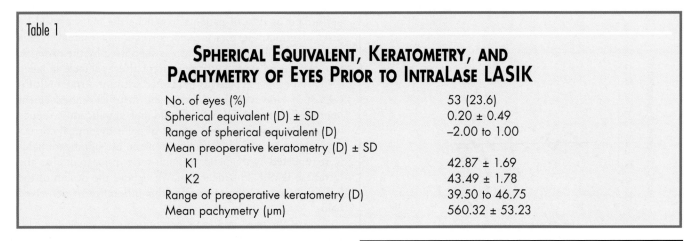

Table 1

SPHERICAL EQUIVALENT, KERATOMETRY, AND PACHYMETRY OF EYES PRIOR TO INTRALASE LASIK

No. of eyes (%)	53 (23.6)
Spherical equivalent (D) ± SD	0.20 ± 0.49
Range of spherical equivalent (D)	−2.00 to 1.00
Mean preoperative keratometry (D) ± SD	
K1	42.87 ± 1.69
K2	43.49 ± 1.78
Range of preoperative keratometry (D)	39.50 to 46.75
Mean pachymetry (µm)	560.32 ± 53.23

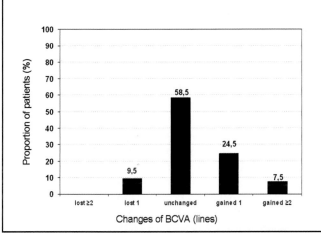

Figure 1. Changes in best spectacle-corrected distance visual acuity (BCVA) 6 months after LASIK with femtosecond laser surgery.

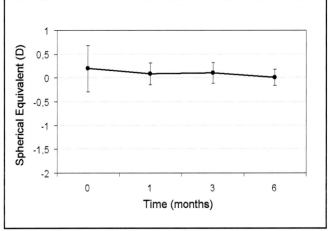

Figure 3. Time course of the spherical equivalent after LASIK with femtosecond laser surgery (stability). D = diopters.

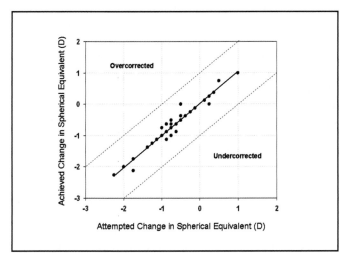

Figure 2. Attempted versus achieved correction (predictability) 6 months after femtosecond laser surgery ($R = 0.96$; $y = 1.001x − 0.006$). D = diopters.

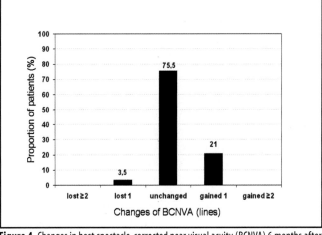

Figure 4. Changes in best spectacle-corrected near visual acuity (BCNVA) 6 months after LASIK with femtosecond laser surgery (safety).

0.14 preoperatively and 0.90 ± 0.13 at 6 months ($p = 0.4$). Six months post-IntraLase LASIK enhancement, the mean uncorrected near visual acuity (UCNVA) was 0.88 ± 0.12. The efficacy index (mean postoperative UCNVA/mean preoperative BCNVA) at 6 months was 1.03. None of the examined eyes lost ≥ 2 lines of BCVA (Figure 4). The safety index (ratio of postoperative and preoperative BCNVA) at 6 months was 0.99.

There were no complications during surgery (ie, fixation losses or epithelial displacement), and no eye required a secondary laser intervention. No potentially sight-threatening complications such as persistent corneal edema, flap dislocation, retinal detachment, or endophthalmitis occurred during the postoperative period. In addition, no eye required a Nd:yttrium-aluminum-garnet (YAG) capsulotomy at the time of the last postoperative visit. No patients complained of

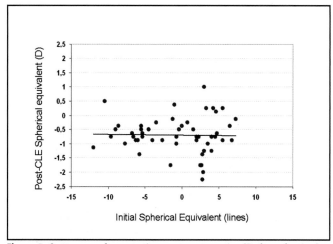

Figure 5. Scattergram of preoperative versus postoperative SE after refractive lens exchange (RLE) and multifocal intraocular lens implantation. The solid line represents the best linear fit for the data ($R = 0.01$; $y = -0.001x - 0.69$).

moderate or disturbing halos either before or after the laser enhancement surgery.

It would be useful for patient counseling to know whether the refractive error of the eye prior to RLE surgery was a predictor of postoperative residual refractive error. Based on this study, there was no significant correlation between residual SE treated by IntraLase LASIK and the original SE prior to RLE ($R = 0.01$; $p > 0.1$) (Figure 5).

Previous clinical trials evaluating clinical, functional, and quality of life outcomes after presbyopia-correcting IOL implantation have shown that these IOLs can improve near vision while providing a good level of distance vision.[1-9] The availability of new IOLs has expanded the opportunity for refractive surgeons to consider RLE with multifocal IOLs. In our experience, however, it is important to correct any residual refractive error to achieve the optimum benefit of RLE.

Our study showed an improvement in UCDVA after Intralase LASIK to enhance RLE with the AcrySof ReSTOR IOL with all eyes achieving an UCDVA of 20/30 or better at 6 months. The postoperative BCDVA was 0.86 ± 0.16, and the efficacy index (0.97) and the safety index (1.01) were both good. In our study, there was a small regression of effect of 0.19 D of SE between the first month and 6 months of follow-up (see Figure 3). None of the eyes lost ≥ 2 lines of either BCDVA or BCNVA at 6 months.

Pop et al[10] evaluated the visual outcomes achieved with PRK and LASIK enhancement after RLE with monofocal IOL implantation in 65 eyes. These authors found that both PRK and LASIK plus the initial RLE with monofocal IOL implantation resulted in the loss of no more than 1 line of BCVA by 1 month following the last procedure. By 1 year postoperatively, 87% of the eyes had UCVA within 1 line of their initial BCVA before all treatment. They concluded that RLE with monofocal IOL implantation and PRK or LASIK enhancement resulted in good refractive outcomes for the retreated eyes without clinical laser-related complications. Leccisotti[11] reported refractive outcomes in 18 eyes that had PRK for a residual refractive error after RLE with Array multifocal IOL (Advanced Medical Optics, Santa Ana, CA) implantation. He reported that PRK adjustment was

performed in 19% of patients to reduce the halos caused by residual refractive errors. Optical correction of residual myopia can alleviate photic phenomena, as supported by the observation of reduced starburst or ring effect after spectacle-induced 0.5 D hyperopia in patients implanted with the Array multifocal IOL.[16] However, the author found that PRK enhancement improved distance UCVA but did not significantly reduce halos indicating that improvement of halos by optical correction is not a benefit of PRK enhancement. No significant halos were reported by the patients in our series prior to or after the IntraLase LASIK enhancement. We believe the design of the ReSTOR optic is the reason for this difference in perceived halos.[1,2,9]

One of the most important components for successful RLE with multifocal IOLs is precise preoperative measurement of axial length and accurate IOL power calculation. Shorter or longer axial lengths increase the incidence of inaccurate measurements. Fernández-Vega et al[8] have reported minimal deviation from target refraction after RLE when using the SRK/T in myopic eyes and the Holladay II in hyperopic eyes for IOL power calculation. The residual refractive error does not depend on the initial ammetropia, and similar amounts of residual refractive error were found with different degrees of both myopia and hyperopia preoperatively.

RLE with IOL implantation accomplishes a very stable refraction without regression.[7,17,18] An IOL exchange to correct low amounts of residual myopia would significantly increase the risks of surgical complications.[18-20] Although piggyback implantation may also be considered[21,22] the risk of late interlenticular opacification exists.[10]

We have shown that IntraLase LASIK enhancement is highly predictable and safe for the correction of refractive error[13,14] after RLE with multifocal IOL implantation. With proper patient selection, RLE with multifocal IOL implantation followed by IntraLase LASIK produce good refractive outcomes without a significant risk of laser-related complications.

References

1. Montés-Micó R, Alió JL. Distance and near contrast sensitivity function after multifocal intraocular lens implantation. *J Cataract Refract Surg*. 2003;29:703-711.

2. Montés-Micó R, España E, Bueno I, et al. Visual performance with multifocal intraocular lenses: mesopic contrast sensitivity under distance and near conditions. *Ophthalmology*. 2004;111:85-96.

3. Schmidinger G, Simader C, Dejaco-Ruhswurm I, et al. Contrast sensitivity function in eyes with diffractive bifocal intraocular lenses. *J Cataract Refract Surg*. 2005;31:2076-2083.

4. Kohnen T, Allen D, Boureau C, et al. European multicenter study of the AcrySof ReSTOR apodized diffractive intraocular lens. *Ophthalmology*. 2006;113:578-584.

5. Waltz KL, Wallace RB. PRELEX: Surgery to implant multifocal intraocular lenses. *Ophthal Prac*. 2001;19:343-346.

6. Hutz WW, Eckhardt HB, Rohrig B, Grolmus R. Reading ability with 3 multifocal intraocular lens models. *J Cataract Refract Surg*. 2006;32:2015-2021.

7. Alfonso JA, Fernández-Vega L, Señaris A, Montés-Micó R. Quality of vision with the Acri.Twin asymmetric diffractive bifocal intraocular lens system. *J Cataract Refract Surg*. 2007;33:197-202.

8. Fernández-Vega L, Alfonso JF, Rodríguez PP, Montés-Micó R. Clear lens extraction with multifocal apodized diffractive intraocular lens implantation. *Ophthalmology*. 2007;114:1491-1498.

9. Alfonso JF, Fernández-Vega L, Baamonde B, Montés-Micó R. Prospective visual evaluation of apodized diffractive intraocular lenses. *J Cataract Refract Surg.* 2007;33:1235-1243.

10. Pop M, Payette I, Amyot M. Clear lens extraction with intraocular lens followed by photorefractive keratectomy or laser in situ keratomileusis. *Ophthalmology.* 2001;108:104-111.

11. Leccisotti A. Secondary procedures after presbyopic lens exchange. *J Cataract Refract Surg.* 2004;30:1461-1465.

12. Alió JL, Montés-Micó R. Wavefront-guided versus standard LASIK enhancement for residual refractive errors. *Ophthalmology.* 2006;113: 191-197.

13. Ghanem RC, Napoli JD, Tobaigy FM, Ang LP, Azar DT. LASIK in the presbyopic age group safety, efficacy, and predictability in 40- to 69-year-old patients. *Ophthalmology.* 2007;114:1303-1310.

14. Montés-Micó R, Alió JL, Rodríguez-Galietero A. Femtosecond laser versus mechanical keratome LASIK for myopia. *Ophthalmology.* 2007;114:62-68.

15. Montés-Micó R, Rodríguez-Galietero A, Alió JL, Cerviño A. Contrast sensitivity after femtosecond laser flap creation for laser in situ keratomileusis. *J Refract Surg.* 2007;23:188-192.

16. Hunkeler JD, Coffman TM, Paugh J, et al. Characterization of visual phenomena with the Array multifocal intraocular lens. *J Cataract Refract Surg.* 2002;28:1195-1204.

17. Fernandez-Vega L, Alfonso JF, Villacampa T. Clear lens extraction for the correction of high myopia. *Ophthalmology.* 2003;110:2349-2354.

18. Siganos DS, Pallikaris IG. Clear lensectomy and intraocular lens implantation for hyperopia from +7 to +14 diopters. *J Refract Surg.* 198;14:105-113.

19. Colin J, Robinet A, Cochener B. Retinal detachment after clear lens extraction for high myopia. Seven-year follow-up. *Ophthalmology.* 1999;106:2281.

20. Horgan N, Codon PI, Beatty S. Refractive lens exchange in high myopia: long term follow up. *Br J Ophthalmol.* 2005;89:670-672.

21. Alfonso JF, Fernández-Vega L, Baamonde MB. Secondary diffractive bifocal piggyback intraocular lens implantation. *J Cataract Refract Surg.* 2006;32:1938-1944.

22. Akaishi L, Tzelikis PF. Primary piggyback implantation using the ReSTOR intraocular lens: case series. *J Cataract Refract Surg.* 2007;33:791-795.

CHAPTER 195

RLE—Lens Removal: What Is Different?

I. Howard Fine, MD; Richard S. Hoffman, MD; and Mark Packer, MD, FACS

The notion of removing the crystalline lens through 2 microincisions is not a new concept and has been attempted with varying degrees of success and failure since the 1970s.[1-7] With the development of new phacoemulsification technology and power modulations,[8] we are now able to disassemble and emulsify lens material without the generation of significant thermal energy. Thus removal of the cooling irrigation sleeve and separation of infusion and emulsification/aspiration through separate incisions is now a viable alternative to traditional coaxial phacoemulsification. Machines such as the Whitestar Sovereign and Signature (Advanced Medical Optics, Santa Ana, CA), the STAAR Sonic Wave (STAAR Surgical, Monrovia, CA), the Infiniti with torsional phaco (Alcon, Forth Worth, TX), and the Millennium and Stellaris (with pulse shaping) (Bausch & Lomb, Rochester, NY) offer the potential of relatively "cold" lens removal capabilities and the capacity for biaxial lens surgery.[9-12]

With advances in multifocal and accommodative lens technology, removal of the crystalline lens as a form of refractive surgery (refractive lens exchange) will become a more popular procedure. We believe bimanual microincision phacoemulsification has several independent advantages that make it a procedure of choice for refractive lens exchange. The following is our current technique for refractive lens exchange utilizing bimanual microincision phacoemulsification.

Technique

The procedure is performed under topical anesthesia after appropriate informed consent, preoperative measurements for intraocular lens (IOL) determination, and preoperative dilation and antibiotics. A 1.1 to 1.3 mm 3D diamond knife from Rhein Medical (Tampa, FL) or a Fine Paratrap diamond keratome (Mastel Precision Surgical Instruments, Rapid City, SD) is utilized to create two 1.1-mm clear corneal incisions 30 to 45 degrees from the temporal limbus (60 to 90 degrees from each other) (Figure 1). One half cubic centimeter of nonpreserved lidocaine 1% is instilled into the anterior chamber, followed by complete expansion of the anterior chamber with Viscoat (Alcon). A straight 25-gauge needle is then inserted through the right-handed microincision to perforate the central anterior lens capsule while simultaneously lifting a flap edge to begin a capsulorrhexis (Figure 2). Needles routinely bent at the tip for conventional capsulorrhexis initiation have been found to lacerate the roof of the microincision during withdrawal of the needle. The straight unaltered 25-gauge needle is less likely to result in this complication. After removal of the needle, a Fine-Hoffman capsulorrhexis forceps (catalog no. DFH-0002; MicroSurgical Technology, Redmond, WA), specially designed to fit and function through a 1-mm incision, is inserted through the incision and used to complete a 5- to 6-mm rhexis (Figure 3). Alternatively, the capsulorrhexis can be initiated by pinching the central anterior capsule with the capsulorrhexis forceps to capture a knuckle of capsule, and then begin the rhexis by pulling the knuckle to create a tear (Figure 4).

Cortical cleaving hydrodissection[13] with decompression is then performed in 2 separate distal quadrants followed by a third round of hydrodissection to prolapse the entire lens or at least one half of the lens out of the capsular bag. The microincision irrigating handpiece (Figure 5) is placed in the left-hand incision and the unsleeved phaco needle is inserted through the right-hand incision. Lens extraction is then performed in most cases without phaco power, utilizing high levels of vacuum while carouselling the relatively soft lens in the plane of the iris until it is consumed (Figure 6). Small amounts of ultrasound energy can be utilized when needed. Care should be taken to avoid directing the infusion flow towards the phaco needle tip so as to prevent dislodging nuclear material from the tip. While maintaining infusion with the irrigating handpiece, the phaco needle is removed and the aspiration handpiece is inserted to remove residual cortex and polish the posterior capsule. If subincisional cortex is difficult to extract, the irrigation and aspiration (I&A) handpieces can be alternated between the 2 incisions in order to gain easier access to the subincisional capsular fornix (Figure 7).

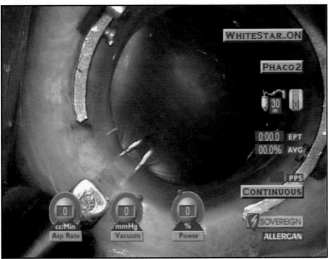

Figure 1. Left-handed 1.1-mm clear corneal microincision placed 45 degrees from the temporal limbus utilizing a Mastel Paratrap diamond knife.

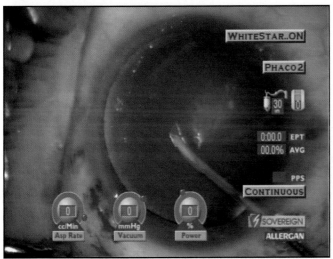

Figure 2. A straight 25-gauge needle begins the capsulorrhexis by perforating the central anterior lens capsule while simultaneously lifting a flap edge.

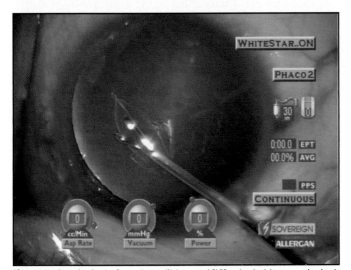

Figure 3. Capsulorrhexis formation utilizing an ASICO microincision capsulorrhexis forceps.

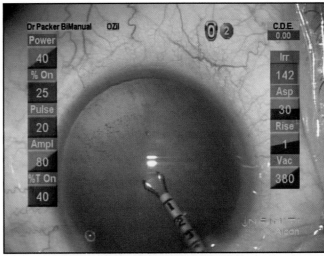

Figure 4. The tips of the microforceps are touched to the anterior capsule surface with just enough pressure to cause slight dimpling; squeezing the handle tines then pinches the capsule and initiates the tear.

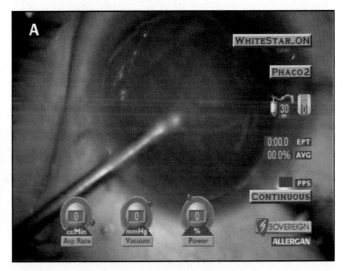

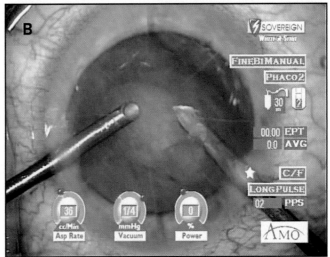

Figure 5. (A) The Duet System (MicroSurgical Technology) beveled irrigating handpiece within the left-handed microincision. (B) Bimanual microincision phacoemulsification of a cataract between RK incisions.

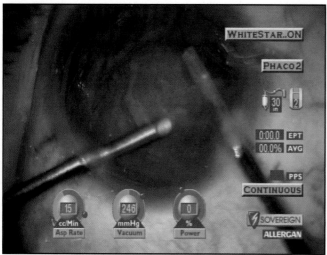

Figure 6. The soft lens is carouselled in the iris plane and consumed utilizing high vacuum levels. Forward movement of the lens is prevented with the irrigating handpiece.

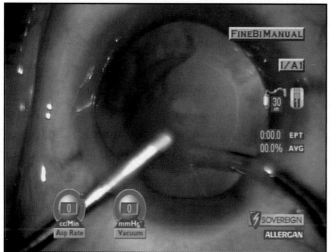

Figure 7. Subincisional cortex is easily removed using the Duet System bimanual irrigation and aspiration handpieces. (Note the effective phaco time [EPT] = 0 and average percent phaco power [AVG] = 0 following lens removal.)

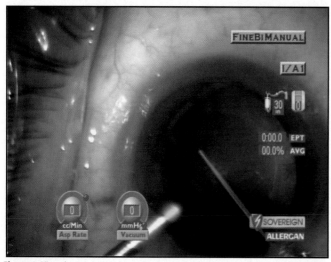

Figure 8. Viscoelastic is injected into the capsular bag while maintaining infusion with the irrigating handpiece.

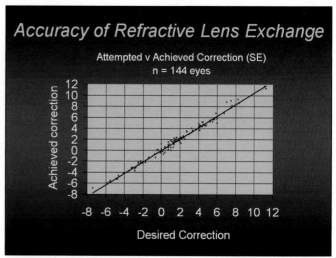

Figure 9. Attempted versus achieved spherical equivalent correction for the Array multifocal IOL.

Once all cortex has been removed, the aspiration handpiece is removed and viscoelastic is injected into the capsular bag and anterior chamber while withdrawing the irrigating handpiece (Figure 8). Following this, the viscoelastic cannula is removed from the eye and a new 2.5-mm clear corneal incision is placed between the 2 microincisions for IOL insertion. After IOL insertion, stromal hydration of the 2.5-mm incision is performed to assist in its self-sealing. Bimanual I&A is performed to remove all viscoelastic. The aspiration handpiece is then removed and irrigation of the anterior chamber maintained. Stromal hydration of the empty incision is performed to assist in closure of the microincision. The irrigation handpiece is then removed, followed by stromal hydration of that incision. In this manner, the eye is fully formed and pressurized throughout the procedure, avoiding hypotony, shallowing of the anterior chamber, and trampolining of the vitreous face during the surgery. Cataractous lenses removed for refractive lens exchange are disassembled in the usual bimanual microincision technique, with the use of an irrigating chopper in the left hand for endolenticular disassembly, and mobilization from the eye with low phaco power and high vacuum, or torsional phaco with low power and low vacuum.

Results

We achieved excellent results utilizing the Array (Advanced Medical Optics) multifocal foldable IOL. Almost all of our achieved spherical equivalents were within 0.5 D of our target spherical equivalent values (Figure 9). Our visual acuity results were also very good with approximately 44% of our patients achieving almost complete spectacle independence and a second 44% receiving near spectacle independence, with some exceptions, most notably prolonged reading or driving at night[14] (Figure 10).

The early results that we achieved with the Eyeonics, Inc (Aliso Viejo, CA) Crystalens AT-45 are seen in Figures 11 and 12. We see that 73% of the patients achieved distance, near, and intermediate visual acuities of 20/25 or better and that corresponds extremely well with the percentage of patients

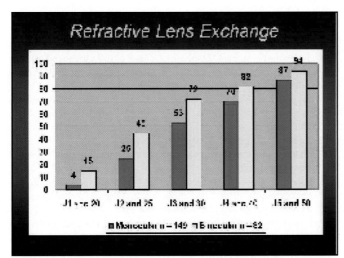

Figure 10. Refractive lens exchange results using the Array multifocal IOL.

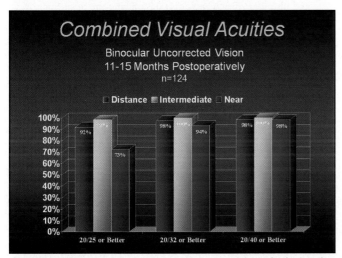

Figure 11. Combined visual acuity results in refractive lens exchange for the Crystalens accommodative IOL.

Bilateral Satisfaction (n=130)

Do not wear spectacles	25.8 %
Wear almost none of the time	47.7
	73.5%
Wear some of the time	15.6
Wear most of the time	6.3
Wear almost all the time	4.7

Figure 12. Quality of life data for Crystalens refractive lens exchange patients.

who believe themselves to be totally spectacle independent (see Figure 12). Our experience with both the Array and Crystalens incline us to believe that what is necessary for spectacle independence is an uncorrected visual acuity of 20/25 at all distances.

With the ReSTOR (Alcon) and the ReZoom (Advanced Medical Optics) multifocal IOLs, we achieve approximately 75% spectacle independence. When we use multifocal IOLs, we customize the choice of lens based on patients' needs and previous experience with refractive error, and we do a considerable amount of mixing and matching. If the patient is happy and satisfied with the first IOL implanted, we will use that lens in the second eye. If the patient is not happy, we address the compromises in the first eye with either minimonovision, using the same IOL in the second eye, or a different IOL in the second eye that compensates for the compromises in the IOL in the first eye. We have found that spectacle independence and patient satisfaction depend on minimizing compromises.

Discussion

Bimanual microincision phacoemulsification offers advantages over current traditional phacoemulsification techniques for both routine cataract extraction and refractive lens exchanges. Although it is true that coaxial phaco is an excellent procedure with low amounts of induced astigmatism,[15] bimanual phaco offers the potential for truly astigmatic neutral incisions. In addition, these microincisions should behave similar to a paracentesis incision with less likelihood for leakage and, theoretically, a lower incidence of endophthalmitis.

The major advantage we have seen from bimanual microincisions has been an improvement in control of most of the steps involved in endocapsular surgery. Because viscoelastics do not leave the eye easily through these small incisions, the anterior chamber is more stable during capsulorrhexis construction and there is much less likelihood for an errant rhexis to develop. Hydrodelineation and hydrodissection can be performed more efficiently by virtue of a higher level of pressure building in the anterior chamber prior to eventual prolapse of viscoelastic through the microincisions. In addition, separation of irrigation from the aspirating phaco needle allows for improved followability by avoiding competing currents at the tip of the needle. In some instances, the irrigation flow from the second handpiece can be used as an adjunctive surgical device—flushing nuclear pieces from the angle or loosening epinuclear or cortical material from the capsular bag. Perhaps the greatest advantage of the bimanual technique lies in its ability to switch hands, both during phacoemulsification and removing subincisional cortex, without difficulty. As originally described by Brauweiler,[16] switching handpieces between 2 microincisions, 360 degrees of the capsular fornices are easily reached.

The minor disadvantages of bimanual phacoemulsification are real but easy to overcome. Maneuvering through incisions, 1.1mm internally and 1.3 mm externally, can be awkward early in the learning curve. Also, additional equipment is necessary in the form of small incision keratomes, rhexis forceps, irrigating choppers (for denser nuclei), and bimanual I&A handpieces. All of the major instrument companies are currently working on irrigating choppers and other microincision adjunctive devices for microincision surgery. For refractive lens exchanges, irrigation can be accomplished with the bimanual irrigation handpiece that can also function as the second "side-port" instrument negating the need for an irrigating chopper.

The greatest criticism of bimanual phaco lies in the fluidics and the current limitations in intraocular lens technology that could be utilized through these microincisions. By nature of the size of these incisions, less fluid flows into the eye than occurs with coaxial techniques. Most current irrigating choppers integrate a 20-gauge lumen that limits fluid inflow. This can result in significant chamber instability when high vacuum levels are utilized and occlusion from nuclear material at the phaco tip is cleared. Thus, infusion needs to be maximized by placing the infusion bottle on a separate intravenous pole that is set as high as possible. Also, vacuum levels usually need to be lowered below 350 mm Hg to avoid significant surge flow.

At the conclusion of bimanual phaco, perhaps the greatest disappointment is the need to place a relatively large 2.5-mm incision between the 2 microincisions in order to implant a foldable IOL. An analogy to the days when phaco was performed through 3.0-mm incisions that required widening to 6.0-mm for polymethylmethacrylate (PMMA) IOL implantation is clear. It was not until the development of foldable IOLs that we could truly take full advantage of small incision phaco. Similarly, we believe the advantages of bimanual phaco will prompt many surgeons to try this technique, with the realization that microincision lenses will ultimately catch up with technique. Although these lenses are currently not available in the United States, many microincision IOLs are in use or under development in other parts of the world.[17-21]

Utilization of bimanual microphacoemulsification as we have described for refractive lens exchange and routine cataract surgery offers an enormous advantage of maintaining a more stable intraocular environment during lens removal. This may be especially important in high myopes who are at a greater risk for retinal detachment following lens extraction.[22-24] By maintaining a formed and pressurized anterior chamber throughout the procedure, there should be less tendency for anterior movement of the vitreous body with a theoretical lower incidence of posterior vitreous detachment occurring from intraoperative manipulations. Future studies will need to be performed in order to document a significant reduction in posterior segment morbidity utilizing this method of lens removal.

We have found this technique to be simple, efficacious, and safe because most of the lens extraction is occurring in the plane of the iris, away from the posterior capsule and the corneal endothelium.

References

1. Girard LJ. Ultrasonic fragmentation for cataract extraction and cataract complications. *Adv Ophthalmol.* 1978;37:127-135.
2. Shock JP. Removal of cataracts with ultrasonic fragmentation and continuous irrigation. *Trans Pac Coast Otoophthalmol Soc Annual Meet.* 1972;53:139-144.
3. Shearing SP, Relyea RL, Loaiza A, Shearing RL. Routine phacoemulsification through a one-millimeter non-sutured incision. *Cataract.* 1985;2:6-10.
4. Hara T, Hara T. Endocapsular phacoemulsification and aspiration (ECPEA)—recent surgical technique and clinical results. *Ophthalmic Surgery.* 1989;20(7):469-475.
5. Tsuneoka H, Shiba T, Takahashi Y. Feasibility of ultrasound cataract surgery with a 1.4 mm incision. *J Cataract Refract Surg.* 2001;27:934-940.
6. Tsuneoka H, Shiba T, Takahashi Y. Ultrasonic phacoemulsification using a 1.4 mm incision: Clinical results. *J Cataract Refract Surg.* 2002;28:81-86.
7. Agarwal A, Agarwal A, Agarwal S, Narang P, Narang S. Phakonit: phacoemulsification through a 0.9 mm corneal incision. *J Cataract Refract Surg.* 2001;27:1548-1552.
8. Fine IH, Packer M, Hoffman RS. The use of power modulations in phacoemulsification: Choo choo chop and flip phacoemulsification. *J Cataract Refract Surg.* 2001;27:188-197.
9. Soscia W, Howard JG, Olson RJ. Microphacoemulsification with WhiteStar. A wound temperature study. *J Cataract Refract Surg.* 2002;28:1044-1046.
10. Hoffman RS, Fine IH, Packer M, Brown LK. Comparison of sonic and ultrasonic phacoemulsification utilizing the Staar Sonic Wave phacoemulsification system. *J Cataract Refract Surg.* 2002;28:1581-1584.
11. Fine IH, Packer M, Hoffman RS. New phacoemulsification technology. *J Cataract Refract Surg.* 2002;28:1054-1060.
12. Alzner E, Grabner G. Dodick laser photolysis: thermal effects. *J Cataract Refract Surg.* 1999;25:800-803.
13. Fine IH. Cortical cleaving hydrodissection. *J Cataract Refract Surg.* 1992;18:508-512.
14. Fine IH, Packer M, Hoffman RS. Power modulations in new technology: Improved outcomes. *J Cataract Refract Surg.* 2004;30:1014-1019.
15. Masket S, Tennen DG. Astigmatic stabilization of 3.0 mm temporal clear corneal cataract incisions. *J Cataract Refract Surg.* 1996;22:1451-1455.
16. Brauweiler P. Bimanual irrigation/aspiration. *J Cataract Refract Surg.* 1996;22:1013-1016.
17. Kreiner C. The Acri-Smart IOL (Acri.Tec GmbH). In: Agarwal A, ed. *Bimanual Phaco: Mastering the Phakonit/MICS Technique.* Thorofare, NJ: SLACK Incorporated; 2005:215-222.
18. Agarwal S. Bimanual phaco with the Acri.Tec GmbH) IOL. In: Agarwal A, ed. *Bimanual Phaco: Mastering the Phakonit/MICS Technique.* Thorofare, NJ: SLACK Incorporated; 2005:223-228.
19. Centurion V, Lacava AC, Caballero JC. Bimanual phaco with the ThinOptX Rollable IOL. In: Agarwal A, ed. *Bimanual Phaco: Mastering the Phakonit/MICS Technique.* Thorofare, NJ: SLACK Incorporated; 2005:229-238.
20. Agarwal A. Corneal topography after bimanual phaco with a 5.0mm optic rollable IOL. In: Agarwal A, ed. *Bimanual Phaco: Mastering the Phakonit/MICS Technique.* Thorofare, NJ: SLACK Incorporated; 2005:239-244.
21. Pandey SK, Werner L, Mamalis N, Olson R. Ultrasmall incision IOLs: Experimental studies and clinical applications. In: Agarwal A, ed. *Bimanual Phaco: Mastering the Phakonit/MICS Technique.* Thorofare, NJ: SLACK Incorporated; 2005:251-256.
22. Rodriguez A, Gutierrez E, Alvira G. Complications of clear lens extraction in axial myopia. *Arch Ophthalmol.* 1987;105:1522-1523.
23. Ripandelli G, Billi B, Fedeli R, Stirpe M. Retinal detachment after clear lens extraction in 41 eyes with axial myopia. *Retina.* 1996;16:3-6.
24. Colin J, Robinet A, Cochener B. Retinal detachment after clear lens extraction for high myopia: seven-year follow-up. *Ophthalmology.* 1999;106:2281-2284.

CHAPTER 196

RLE—Lens Removal: What Is Different?

Steven Dewey, MD

After reading the other chapters on refractive lens exchange (RLE), it becomes critical to understand the fundamental differences in operative procedure between RLE and cataract surgery. These differences are absolutely paramount in delivering the utmost quality of vision to our RLE patients and helping to bridge the potential gap between the patient's expectations and our surgical results.

For those of you who now have even the tiniest amount of suspense at the surgical secrets to be unveiled here, here's the spoiler: There are no differences between RLE and cataract surgery that can be distinguished in the operating room. The expectations of our patients do not differ, whether they have a simple desire to rid themselves of coke-bottle spectacles or somehow got to 20/70 without symptoms and then failed the Department of Motor Vehicle test. Thinking from our perspective: how many patients have stated preoperatively they do not mind wearing glasses, only to reveal postoperatively their disappointment that they did not expect to need any after the surgery?

Some Rules You Already Know

* Any surgical technique is an interdependent amalgam of experience, instrumentation, and available technology.

* Some patients pay specifically for RLE. All patients expect the result.

* Videotapes do not lie.

* Your mother was right: Never play with sharp instruments around the eye.

* Any capsule can break at any time.

* The knowledge base surrounding state-of-the-art RLE surgery has a shelf life only a tad longer than the milk in the refrigerator.

* Like that refrigerator, every now and then it helps to take everything out of a surgical procedure, examine each component, throw out what's outdated, and put it back together again.

* In true RLE, I am not removing the patient's cataract. I am creating it.

* Under promise and over deliver.

Applying Those Rules

I would have to say that conquering a new technique or procedure is one of the greatest professional joys we can experience. But I do not know how many anecdotal reports I have heard about a surgeon giving up on a potential significant advance because of a single misstep. Although the consequences for an individual patient may have been significant, the problem may not have been as simple as the new instrument, device or technique itself. Rather, many times the problem is the interdependence of individual steps, and how changing one created other changes that were not fully anticipated.

Videotape Everything

Yes, everything. "Conceptualizing" a new step or technique can be quite effective, but when it was performed, did it work out exactly as expected?

Nothing hides from video. Even the most basic camera attached to an old VHS unit will allow a surgeon to quickly learn which aspects of the technique are effective, and which aspects are simply painful to watch. Of course, if the video is to be watched by others, the better the system, the easier it is to see the details. Attaching the same camera to the inputs of the family digital video camera will improve the clarity of capture immensely. Moving to a 3-chip camera and a digital videotape deck is usually the next step, and this combination produces outstanding video quality.

Do not skimp on the microscope adapter. This is probably the one overlooked item that can make a very expensive camera produce cheap-looking video.

The advantage of reviewing video is the objectivity that can be achieved once the emotional immediacy of the surgery is completed. Obviously, complication management

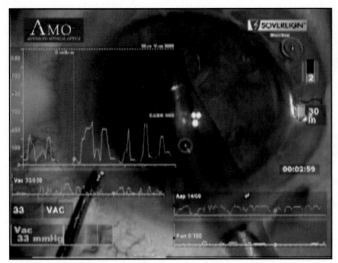

Figure 1. The overlay of the Surgical Media Center from AMO shows real-time graphs demonstrating the changes of vacuum, aspiration, and power.

benefits from review, but surprisingly, much can be learned from watching routine cases. Is the capsulorrhexis creation appropriate for the intraocular lens (IOL) and nuclear removal technique? Was the side port in proper position relative to the primary incision? Some of these details can significantly affect the consistency of surgery.

Beyond a camera and taping source, a video overlay is exceptionally helpful at finding the cause of a successful or unsuccessful event. Overlays are available for the 3 major phaco unit platforms, and display a number of useful items such as vacuum, power, aspiration, foot pedal position, bottle height, etc., at the time of the capture of the video frame. The only problem with the standard overlay is that the information is relatively static—it only provides a snapshot of that brief moment in the case.

The leading edge of surgical video capture is found in the Surgical Media Center (SMC) from Advanced Medical Optics (Santa Ana, CA). This software program captures the video from the S-video output of the camera directly to the hard drive of a laptop computer. First and foremost, the absence of videotape makes the files 1) immediately available for review and 2) exceptionally easy to store on a hard drive.

More to the point of teaching with the SMC is the real-time graphic display of the case as it is seen in the video. Although the older overlays provide a snapshot, these graph displays of the SMC show the changes in power, vacuum, and aspiration that occurred before, during, and after a particular point on the video (Figure 1). The advantage of being able to fully evaluate the moment in surgery has tremendous potential to refine techniques and further reduce complications. The graphs can also be moved on the video, such that if the activity of the case is down and to the left, the graphs can be moved to the right, out of the way of the action.

Technology

Really, is the same phaco unit that was new in 1995 sufficient for patients expecting nothing short of perfection in the 21st century?

My summary answer to this is that "good enough" does not come close to meeting the goals of a surgeon performing RLE or the patient paying for the procedure. All 3 of the major ophthalmic surgical manufacturers have innovative phaco platforms for the delivery of state-of-the art care. These include technologies to reduce phaco power,[1-3] decrease turbulence and chatter, reduce postocclusion chamber surge, eliminate incision burns, and make it easier for the staff to turnover the operating room (OR) to boot.

Remembering rule number 1, do not purchase the first new phaco unit that you get the chance to test drive. If your platform is over 5 years of age, it is likely that any of the units will seem quite impressive by comparison. Rather, try as many of the machines as is reasonable to truly evaluate the features to see which will help you advance your technique to the next level.

Taking the Procedure Apart

Asking why a particular surgeon performs a particular step is sometimes answered with one of these choices: cost, old habit, and "that's the way I learned it in residency." In re-evaluating the components of the technique, this is the time to start correlating the events of the procedure with the desired postoperative result, as opposed to the events of the procedure that simply allow the surgeon to be done with that case. The best thing about losing the limitations of an old phaco unit is the ability to explore the limits of one's own procedure, and begin a transition to more advanced techniques as one becomes comfortable.

An example: With my older phaco unit, postocclusion surge was a particular problem. My second instrument did not stray from the proximity of the sharp phaco needle, usually holding the posterior capsule back from the lumen of the needle. We upgraded the phaco unit to a new model, and within a few months, my second instrument was helping guide the nuclear fragments toward the tip, and was almost never needed to prevent chamber surge. It was only through reviewing and comparing videotaped cases that I could see this difference.

Another example: With the new phaco unit, I was able to try sleeveless biaxial cataract surgery.[2] I found the technique to be very intriguing—I had never removed a cataract through a pair of such tiny incisions—and potentially better.[3-7] But when I reviewed my particular efficiencies in the OR, I decided I preferred coaxial surgery. Despite returning to coaxial phaco, I did keep the use of the microvitreoretinal (MVR) blade for a much more precise sideport creation over the 30-degree supersharp blade I was using. The MVR blade creates an incision exactly where I place the tip, and is the exact configuration every time for an outstanding watertight seal.

The Phaco Needle

What is an optimum vitrectomy rate? Zero is a number that I do not believe is currently attainable. Then what then is an acceptable vitrectomy rate?

For the last 3 years, I have used the Dewey radius tip (MicroSurgical Technologies, Redmond, WA) nearly exclusively for cataract surgery and refractive lens exchange. This is exactly the needle I was using before, except the sharp edges

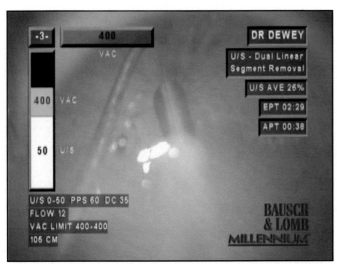

Figure 2. The rounded edges of the Dewey radius tip have demonstrated significant improvements in safety. In this cadaver eye specimen, the phaco power is at 50% and the vacuum at 400 mm Hg, with the capsule still intact. This capsule had survived numerous combinations of power and vacuum until it finally broke soon after this image was taken, but only after 38 cumulative seconds of phaco power had been delivered.

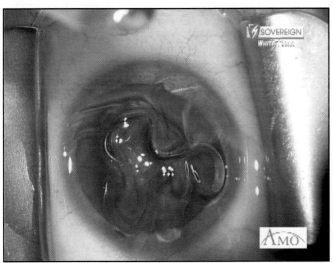

Figure 3. Dispersive viscoelastic and BSS are mixed on the cornea to create a clear layer that does not require frequent irrigation to maintain visualization. The layers of viscoelastic will merge within a few seconds and remain in place for at least 10 minutes.

along the inner and outer rims of the distal tip are completely rounded. It is surprisingly efficient at removing even the densest cataracts. For RLE, where phaco power and cutting with a sharp edge are unnecessary, it is perhaps even more efficient than a sharp needle by allowing a safer freedom of movement in the anterior chamber.

The best thing about the needle is that its use does not require any other changes—same techniques, same settings, etc. The surgeon can simply choose the configuration and gauge to which they are accustomed and get to work as normal. The rounded edge is intrinsically safer for incidental contact—no sharp edge to cut the iris or capsule, or especially the edge of the capsulorrhexis.

Somewhat surprising is that the refinement of the rounded edge has had an unexpected effect—it does not cut the capsule with the same ease as a sharp edge even with the ultrasound on. In cadaver eye studies, it was somewhat routine to see power at 10% to 20%, and even up to 50%, with vacuums from 100 to 400 mmHg applied to the capsule for several seconds before the capsules would rupture (Figure 2).[4]

Although we all accept a given complication rate with standard cataract surgery, the RLE patient does not have the same understanding that a fundamental impairment of vision has forced them to the operating room. Rather, they have taken a leap of faith that the procedure will be performed under the safest conditions possible. The Dewey radius tip is absolutely indispensable for RLE, or for providing an additional margin of safety when attempting new cataract removal techniques.

A Clear View

Think how annoyed you would be if someone squirted you in the face with water every few seconds. A simple solution to irrigating the cornea frequently is to place a small amount of dispersive viscoelastic on the cornea at the beginning of the case (Figure 3). It is important to do this in the presence of dripping balanced salt saline (BSS) as a dispersive viscoelastic on a dry cornea is a very good method of epithelial removal.

Once the viscoelastic is in place, it will take a few seconds to achieve good clarity and will provide just a bit of magnification. This will allow for good visualization for 10 minutes on a consistent basis and can be reapplied at any time during the surgery to improve visualization.

The Incision

From my perspective, all of the arguments for the use of a diamond blade are just as valid for using a steel blade. The absolutely most important facet of the incision is that it does not require stromal hydration to seal even in the face of pressure applied to the region of the posterior lip of the incision. Stromal hydration can provide just enough of a fluid imbalance as the incision seals to induce unexpected astigmatism. The creation of a self-sealing incision speaks more to the craft of the surgeon than an empirical advantage of one blade material over another.

Of course, where the incision is placed is just as important. In the debate between clear corneal and scleral, I am a bit surprised that more surgeons do not create the incision at the limbus, just anterior to the insertion of the conjunctiva. The limbus-based incisions have the significant advantage of fibrovascular healing, and unlike clear corneal incisions, only rarely induce a late against-the-incision astigmatism.

In my experience, 3-plane stepped incisions provide much greater control during their creation compared to single-plane stab incisions, and take only a few seconds longer to create.

Lastly, using a bent phaco needle will allow better access for endocapsular procedures if one wants to make a longer tunnel incision. The straight needles are more likely to create striae and oar locking through longer tunnels as one works to remove material below the iris plane.

The Capsulorrhexis and the Capsule Surgeon

Manfred Tetz, MD, of Berlin, Germany, made a very nice observation at an European Society of Cataract and Refractive Surgeons meeting a couple of years ago: When we remove a lens before it has become a cataract, and then the patient develops posterior capsular opacification (PCO), we have then created the patient's primary cataract. Or, if you want to look at it from a slightly different perspective still, with RLE, we have become capsule surgeons, not cataract surgeons.

A properly sized capsulorrhexis is an absolute must for standardizing the results of cataract surgery. In routine cases, overlapping the edge of the optic by 0.5 to 1 mm will result in a consistent lens position from case to case, and has the benefit of driving the sharp posterior edge of an IOL into the posterior capsule and reducing the potential for PCO. In a less-than-routine case, having an intact capsulorrhexis allows for optic capture to secure the IOL, even if the posterior capsule is completely absent.

Sizing the capsulorrhexis can be a challenge. The variability of pupil dilation and corneal diameters can make it difficult to consistently create the proper opening. The easiest method is the most direct. Prior to loading the IOL in the insertion device, simply hold the IOL over the surgical field and mentally establish the relative size of the optic to the size of the eye.

Several techniques have been developed to gauge the size of the capsulorrhexis. Dr. Bruce Wallace has used an optical zone marker to effectively provide a size guide. Dr. Barry Seibel has created capsulorrhexis forceps with a millimeter marker on the shaft as an intraocular gauge. This product is manufactured by MicroSurgical Technologies and can easily work with either a standard or bimanual incision.

Instrumentation inherently creates different size openings, and this appears to be related to the tangential forces applied as the capsule is torn. A bent needle holds the flap closer to the tear, and creates a smaller capsular opening, especially when using cohesive viscoelastics. Forceps grasp the capsule further from the tear, and generally will create a larger one.

Although I prefer the 0.5- to 1-mm overlap of the anterior capsule on the optic, more overlap is not a problem as long as the surgical technique can deal with removing the nucleus and cortex through a smaller opening. Of course, a larger capsulorrhexis is appropriate when the situation warrants, such as when dealing with a very dense cataract, or in cases of zonular laxity where an endocapsular phaco approach should be abandoned.

And one last observation regarding the importance of the capsulorrhexis (perhaps this one comes from the crystal ball.): I believe that one of the future advancements in IOL surgery will be the ability to exchange an old encapsulated IOL for current technology IOLs, even restoring some of the flexibility of the capsule. For this to work, techniques involving sealed-capsule irrigation[5] will need to fit securely within the confines of a capsulorrhexis created some years ago. The capsule cannot be too fibrotic, and cannot have had a yttrium-aluminum-garnet (YAG) capsulotomy. The sealed-capsule irrigation can then deliver an agent to target the adherence of the

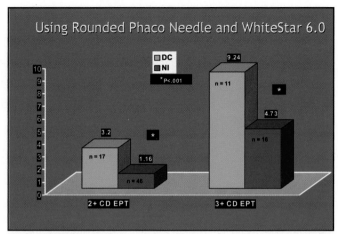

Figure 4. The difference in estimated phaco time using the Dewey radius tip comparing divide and conquer and a horizontal chop.

regenerating cortex and potentially restore a capsule to accept any one of the accommodating IOLs.

Nucleus Removal

In theory, RLE patients don't have nuclear sclerosis, but in reality we know they do have some. The emphasis should be the least amount of phaco power in the eye. Trenching is inherently inefficient at removing nuclear material, as the power is delivered without the stability provided by vacuum occlusion (Figure 4). Flipping or chopping provides much more efficient ways to occlude the lumen of the needle with a vertical face of the lens material. For flipping, a slightly larger capsulorrhexis is always important to avoid tearing the edge of the rhexis by stretching or manipulation.

Chopping, either vertical or horizontal, creates a vertical face for occlusion with mechanical energy only. Although vertical chopping has the benefit of good visualization of all the instruments in the center of the surgical field, the softer lenses of RLE will not have the rigidity to cleanly split, and the sharp instrument for vertical chopping can be a problem itself if it improperly contacts the capsule. Horizontal chopping is my preferred technique. It uses blunt instruments only, and can cleave any density nucleus. Sometimes, if the lens is soft enough, it simply mechanically "mashes" things a bit for easier aspiration.

If one finds that they must trench, turn the maximum power on the phaco unit to an exceptionally low level, say 10%. Combining this with a Dewey radius tip will make it very difficult to break the capsule, and avoids the inadvertent delivery of excessive power.

Phaco Needle Bend, Bevel, and Gauge

First, use smaller gauge needles for smaller pupil cases, 20-gauge or smaller.

Second, think bent needles for efficiency of lens material removal, or for longer, more astigmatically stable incisions (see "The Incision" on p. 715).

Third, larger-gauge needles can reduce power delivery in the eye by removing larger portions at a time, and are more difficult to truly occlude. The efficiency of a larger-gauge needle can probably be undone if the surgeon chooses to chop the nucleus into 8 segments instead of 4 or 6. The 8-segment cleavage creates wedges that can be too small to effectively occlude the lumen of a 19-gauge needle.

Microphaco coaxial phaco needles may provide an advantage with incision size, but may decrease the efficiency of the procedure due to the altered fluidics. The surgeon will have to make the decision regarding the benefit of the trade-off.

Cortical Removal

Here I have another weapon—a J-cannula for irrigating cortex rather than aspirating it.[6] This technique has the advantage of displacing cortex from the equator of the lens, many times simply out of the eye. From my perspective, this is the most efficient way to ensure the most thorough removal of cortical fibers from the periphery of the lens. When properly performed, the likelihood of capsule rupture is reduced significantly as aspiration in areas of poor visualization is avoided.

About the same time J-cannula irrigation started working efficiently in my hands, Dr. Charles Kelman was working on a steerable irrigation and aspiration (I&A) hand piece for removing subincisional cortex. Although the steerable I&A is no longer with us, the silicone-tipped I&A hand piece thankfully still is. This innovation has proven invaluable at preserving the capsule by avoiding sharp metal-to-capsule contact with the aspiration port.[7] The silicone-tipped I&A can be used to polish the underside of the capsule.

IOL Implantation

All IOL implantation techniques are dependent on a distended capsule, and a cohesive viscoelastic serves this purpose best.[8,9] First, it is readily removable after IOL implantation, and second, it does not impede the implantation itself. The singular problem of using only a cohesive viscoelastic for the IOL is the tendency for the viscoelastic to displace itself out of the incision as the incision is opened. This can result in a significant shallowing of the anterior chamber and capsule, and can potentially compromise the insertion process.

To avoid the displacement, I use a small "blob" of dispersive viscoelastic trailing from the center of the capsulorrhexis to the incision. This additional barrier keeps the chamber fully deep and the capsule safely back as the IOL is going in (even with forceps).

Viscoelastic Removal

To remove the cohesive viscoelastic, I simply prefer to lift the edge of the IOL in the capsule and irrigate directly. Once the capsule is visibly clear, I then irrigate the chamber angle directly. I find it assists in aspirating the viscoelastic from the rest of the chamber, and removes any mechanical blockage of the trabecular meshwork. Without intracameral lidocaine, the patient may feel this step under topical anesthetic.

Refilling the Globe

Only reinflate the globe via the sideport incision. Avoid manipulating or hydrating the primary incision as this may result in the creation of unexpected astigmatism. Finally, apply the first drop of fourth-generation fluroquinolone in the OR while the patient is still on the table. Although the preoperative dosing is paramount, antibiotic prophylaxis should be initiated in a timely fashion,[10] and administering the first postoperative dose in the OR avoids issues of patient compliance.

Conclusion

Every patient having a clear or cloudy lens removed desires a RLE. For a surgeon to think otherwise is simply a failure to understand the expectations of the 21st century patient. The differences between cataract surgery and RLE outside of the operating room are inconsequential to the operative procedure. Thus, RLE has become a process more than a procedure. This pragmatic approach to the final goal of the surgical outcome shares more with cataract surgery than differs from it. Rather, the differences we as surgeons perceive between RLE and cataract surgery represent the steps we all must take in the evolution of our surgical technique to achieve the highest standard of care for our patients.

References

1. Fishkind W, Bakewell B, Donnenfeld ED, Rose AD, Watkins LA, Olson RJ. Comparative clinical trial of ultrasound phacoemulsification with and without the WhiteStar system. *J Cataract Refract Surg.* 2006;32:45-49.
2. Fine IH, Hoffman RS, Packer M. Optimizing refractive lens exchange with bimanual microincision phacoemulsification. *J Cataract Refract Surg.* 2004;30:550-554.
3. Kurz S, Krummenauer F, Gabriel P, Pfeiffer N, Dick HB. Biaxial microincision versus coaxial small-incision clear cornea cataract surgery. *Ophthalmology.* 2006;113:1818-1826.
4. Dewey SH. Ultrasonic polishing of the posterior capsule with the Dewey radius tip. *Tech Ophthalmol.* 2006;4:139-148.
5. Maloof A, Neilson G, Milverton EJ, Pandey SK. Selective and specific targeting of lens epithelial cells during cataract surgery using sealed-capsule irrigation. *J Cataract Refract Surg.* 2003;29:1566-1568.
6. Dewey SH. Cortical removal simplified by J-cannula irrigation. *J Cataract Refract Surg.* 2002;28:11-14.
7. Blomquist PH, Pluenneke AC. Decrease in complications during cataract surgery with the use of a silicone-tipped irrigation/aspiration instrument. *J Cataract Refract Surg.* 2005;31:1194-1197.
8. Arshinoff S. Ultimate soft-shell technique and AcrySof Monarch injector cartridges. *J Cataract Refract Surg.* 2004;30:1809-1810.
9. Dewey SH. Forceps insertion with incisional anesthesia for Sensar intraocular lenses. *J Cataract Refract Surg.* 2002;28:1097-1104.
10. van Kasteren ME, Manniën J, Ott A, Kullberg BJ, de Boer AS, Gyssens IC. Antibiotic prophylaxis and the risk of surgical site infections following total hip arthroplasty: timely administration is the most important factor. *Clin Infect Dis.* 2007;44:921-927.

CHAPTER 197

RLE—LENS REMOVAL: WHAT IS DIFFERENT?

Barry S. Seibel, MD

The surgical fundamentals are quite similar between refractive lens exchange (RLE)/ refractive cataract surgery and routine standard cataract surgery. However, notwithstanding a commitment to all patients to provide the safest possible procedure in all cases, there exists an additional benchmark in refractive cases. These patients do not have any pathology being addressed by the refractive procedure, and therefore it might be argued that their risk-to-benefit ratio is higher as compared to routine surgery for a visually significant cataract. In order to equilibrate the ratios, the risk should be correspondingly lowered in the refractive cases, or perhaps the perceived benefit should be greater. This idea of course is the tip of a philosophical and ethical debate that is beyond the scope of this chapter, but it does call attention to the importance of minimizing complications and adequately addressing complex surgical situations. Astigmatism management, pseudoaccommodation, or multifocality are of diminished utility if traumatic surgery and/or vitreous loss has caused cystoid macular edema (CME) with a corresponding reduced best-corrected visual acuity (BCVA).

The risk of complications increases if an excessive machine parameter (eg, ultrasound, vacuum, flow) is used for a given step in surgery. The fundamental tenant of phacodynamics[1] is to parse surgery into discrete steps, identify relevant machine parameters at that stage, and to adjust them accordingly to accomplish the clinical goal at that point in time. In earlier years of phacoemulsification, the trend was to use arbitrarily high parameter levels (first in ultrasound, then more recently in vacuum); however, for many cases these higher levels were in excess of what was required, and the excess amount presented a clinical liability without a corresponding and offsetting benefit.

As opposed to having the surgeon memorize large, unwieldy, and complex tables of various machine parameters for different surgical situations, phacodynamics looks at the 4 basic machine parameters (flow, vacuum, bottle height, and ultrasound) and analyzes which are most relevant for any given surgical step and how to best adjust them for safety and efficiency according to visual feedback through the operating microscope. For most of the basic parameters, current phaco machines offer control permutations and modulations.

For example, when using the more prevalent flow-based (ie, peristaltic) pump at a basic level, the surgeon increases or decreases flow rate as needed to provide adequate but not overly aggressive attraction of material into the aspiration port. An overly aggressive flow rate would increase the risk of attracting unwanted material into the aspiration port, such as capsule or iris. Flow rate also controls rise time, and is increased for time efficiency and decreased for more complex environments such as weak zonules or a shallow anterior chamber. On a more advanced level, the flow rate can be linearly controlled by foot pedal movement, and in a further control modulation, the level of flow or linearity may often be programmed to change once the aspiration port is occluded. For example, the surgeon may wish to use a higher flow rate to attract material to the aspiration port but then have flow rate decrease to slow the rate of vacuum buildup for additional safety if unwanted material is inadvertently attracted, such as the iris in intraoperative floppy iris syndrome (IFIS).

Vacuum functions to grip material that is occluding the aspiration port, and with the help of ultrasound as needed, to deform it sufficiently to allow aspiration and removal of the material through the phaco needle and aspiration line. The minimum vacuum level is determined by the clinical goal, and the maximum level is determined by nuclear density and safety concerns. For example, a certain minimum level of vacuum is needed for adequate grip and stability of the nucleus when using one of the various chop techniques. However, if the surgeon notes erratic aspiration of small pieces of nuclear material from an engaged quadrant or heminucleus at the needle tip (without application of ultrasound), then the vacuum is too high for that particular nuclear density and becomes counterproductive; the erratic and partial aspiration of material interrupts the vacuum seal and precludes an optimum grip and stabilization. Furthermore, the use of an excessively high vacuum level increases the risk of operative morbidity (eg, more damage of inadvertently aspirated iris or capsule) without giving any clinical advantage over a lower, more appropriate vacuum level. As with flow, many modern machines have control modulations that include linear pedal control as well as level shifts depending on the state of aspiration port occlusion. When titrating vacuum level for adequate grip of occluding lens material, always remember to first create an adequate vacuum seal, with the aspiration port adequately embedded into the nuclear material.

Throughout the history of phacoemulsification, we have decreased the magnitude of and increased our control over ultrasound power. Whereas Charlie Kelman's original technique depended mostly on high levels of ultrasound power for aspiration of lens material, the emphasis has now shifted toward utilizing higher vacuum levels to adequately deform nuclear material into and through the phaco needle and out of the eye. This is supplemented with smaller amounts and applications of ultrasound as needed. The reduced use of ultrasound provides a gentler and more stable anterior chamber environment, with correspondingly less potential damage to corneal endothelial cells. Less ultrasound also reduces the risk of an incisional burn. In addition to adjusting the level of ultrasound with linear pedal control, the surgeon may modulate power with various burst, pulse, and hyperpulse settings, the latter being popularized by Advanced Medical Optics' (Santa Ana, CA) WhiteStar platform. Hyperpulse, a phrase coined by David Chang, breaks ultrasound down into very short discrete "on" intervals separated by very short discrete "rest" or "off" intervals, the latter of which provide re-seating of nuclear material for improved followability as well as time for dissipation of incisional heat produced by the friction of the "on" interval. Many combinations of hyperpulse duration and duty cycles (on–off ratios) have been described, and while no definitive answer exists, some form of hyperpulse is recommended for virtually all applications of ultrasound. Alcon's (Fort Worth, TX) Ozil handpiece is another approach to optimizing safety and followability by producing a rotatory, non-axial needle vibration. The repulsive nature of ultrasound must of course be balanced appropriately with fluidics to ensure efficient aspiration of lens material without being its being chattered or repelled by the needle tip. Bausch & Lomb's (Rochester, NY) Dual Linear Pedal Control allows simultaneous and independent control of fluidics and ultrasound.

Relative to the harder nuclei of medically significant cataracts, the softer nuclei of RLE patients do not require as much ultrasound energy. Surgeons may be tempted to use vacuum and flow alone to evacuate these lenses. However, the use of small (eg, 10% phaco power with hyperpulse) amounts of ultrasound can significantly augment the effect of vacuum in deforming and aspirating soft nuclear material. The relationship of vacuum and ultrasound in this setting is synergistic and not simply additive. As such, one gains a greater safety margin of decreasing potentially excessive vacuum levels more than creating liability by increasing a small amount of ultrasound.

As compared with the single choice of a 19 ga uniform diameter phaco needle that came with Dr. Kelman's original phaco machine (as well as most of the machines that followed for the ensuing 2 decades), today's surgeons may choose from a variety of sizes and styles of phaco needles. Diameters may be large or small, with larger sizes providing more grip for a given level of vacuum and more time efficiency of nuclear removal. In contrast, smaller diameter needles better restrict outflow to improve control chamber stability. The best designs combine both of these sizes and benefits, such as the Bausch & Lomb MicroFlow (designed by Graham Barrett), the Alcon Flare Tip, and the Surgical Designs (Armonk, NY) Cobra Tip. Shapes may be straight (generally better for chopping) or bent (generally better for sculpting, eg, Kelman tip). Several designs enhance thermal protection of the incision, such as the MicroFlow, Flare Tip with High Infusion Sleeve, and MicroSeal.

Bottle height is adjusted to maintain adequate anterior chamber stability, understanding that an excessively high level will abnormally deepen and distort the chamber (compromising weak zonules if present) and exacerbate extraneous incisional leakage. Bottle height is an important parameter in mitigating against post-occlusion surge, which occurs when material occluding the aspiration port is suddenly broken down and aspirated, accompanied by a momentarily high rate of outflow that is in excess of steady state pedal position 2 (Figure 1). In addition to raising the irrigation bottle height to combat surge, the surgeon may also need to reduce the vacuum level. Although bottle height is typically associated with the function of "irrigation," recall that it also equates to "pressurization" when in pedal position 1. To further enhance chamber stability, surgeons should utilize the "continuous irrigation" feature on many machines, which maintains pressurization even when in pedal position 0 so as to prevent inadvertent chamber shallowing or collapse.

In addition to optimizing technology to maximize safety and reduce the risk of complications, surgeons must not neglect the optimization of technique as well. Utilizing various principles of mechanical advantage illustrated throughout Phacodynamics, stress to the eye and the potential for inadvertent damage can be minimized. In particular, many of the chopping methods utilize mechanical energy for nuclear subdivision so as to reduce the need for various machine parameters of flow, vacuum, and ultrasound as compared to what would be required with the larger nuclear pieces that must be manipulated with quadranting (Shepard), heminuclear (Gimbel Divide and Conquer), or whole nuclear (eg, Brown Phaco Flip) techniques. Interested surgeons should read David Chang's *Phaco Chop*, which includes a surgical DVD to demonstrate the various methods.[2] Needless to say, an excellent surgeon can do masterful surgery using almost any one of the various methods. Although especially effective with harder nuclei, chopping techniques can also be applied to the softer nuclei of RLE patients; an excellent example is included on the DVD in David Chang's *Phaco Chop*, showing the clean edge of a vertically chopped soft nucleus. Chopping has the advantage in these settings of providing a regular framework and consistency to the case (ie, chop, aspirate fragment, rotate, repeat) as opposed to the more random nature of simply trying to aspirate an entire softer nucleus. Remember to hydrodissect to facilitate nuclear rotation with these softer nuclei.

Hand-held instrumentation should be scrutinized for design, function, and ergonomics to further enhance not only the safety and efficiency of the surgery, but also patient comfort. Even so basic a device as the lid speculum influences the patient's perception of the procedure, and the various

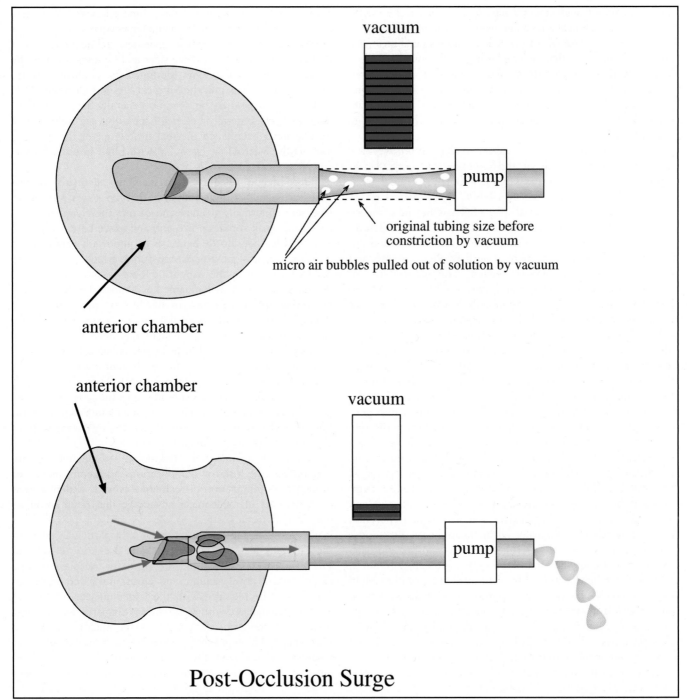

Figure 1. As vacuum builds between the pump and the cataract that is occluding the aspiration port, fluidic compliance is produced in the form of tubing constriction and air bubble production. (Reprinted with permission from Seibel BS. *Phacodynamics: Mastering the Tools and Techniques of Phacoemulsification Surgery, Fourth Edition.* Thorofare, NJ: SLACK Incorporated; 2005.)

Seibel 3-D Lid Speculums (Bausch & Lomb, Rhein) uniquely adjust their support blade angle as they open to approximate globe curvature and minimize tarsal plate distortion and pain in a setting of topical anesthesia, which does not numb the adnexae. Second-hand instruments (no, not pre-owned) should have a design that makes sense both to the method being utilized as well as surgeon ergonomics. Many surgeons like the wraparound grip of the compound curve Chang Horizontal Chopper (Katena Products, Inc., Denville, NJ), whereas others may prefer the simpler single curve of the Seibel Horizontal

Safety Chopper (Rhein Medical, Inc., Tampa, FL) for easier entry and exit through the paracentesis.

Surgeons need to understand the basis of the instruments and the desired phaco method, and correspondingly would know that neither of the aforementioned choppers would work well for vertical chopping. Vertical choppers must penetrate posteriorly into the anterior nuclear surface and should have a correspondingly smaller surface area (as viewed vertically from the operating microscope). Whereas a sharp-tipped vertical chopper allows the technique in very dense brunescent

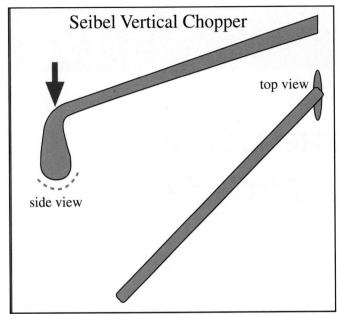

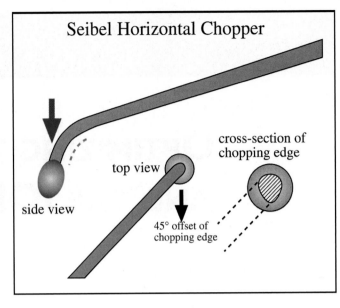

Figure 2. With breakdown of the occluding fragment, a postocclusion surge can occur with chamber shallowing or collapse caused by the additional outflow from the potential energy built up by compliance load. (Dashed green line represents location of chopping.) (Reprinted with permission from Seibel BS. *Phacodynamics: Mastering the Tools and Techniques of Phacoemulsification Surgery, Fourth Edition.* Thorofare, NJ: SLACK Incorporated; 2005.)

nuclei, the less aggressive edge profile of the Seibel Vertical Safety Chopper is designed to have less potential for capsule rupture with inadvertent contact and still works well for a majority of nuclear densities. This instrument is available as an opposite end of a double-ended instrument with both the Chang Horizontal Chopper as well as the Seibel Horizontal Safety Chopper (Figure 2).

When working with the softer lenses of RLE patients, remember the utility of both hydrodissection as well as hydrodelineation. As mentioned earlier when discussing chopping, hydro-steps are especially useful in these softer nuclei that tend to cling to epinucleus and capsule when attempting lens rotation. Hydrodelineation will also allow the creation of an artifactual epinucleus that keeps the capsular bag better formed during endonuclear removal. Howard Fine's Cortical Cleaving Hydrodissection technique facilitates removal of this epinucleus along with much of any residual cortex. The thicker cortex of RLE patients effectively occludes the aspiration port of the irrigation-aspiration (I-A) tip and usually requires only moderate vacuum and flow settings. With the stringier residual cortical fibers of denser nuclei, higher flow settings are often required to generate sufficient friction without complete port occlusion for cortical aspiration.

All lens implant patients benefit from clear capsules, and in particular David Apple's work validated the use of posterior capsule vacuuming/polishing to decrease residual lens epithelial cells and reduce the incidence of posterior capsule opacification (PCO). PCO is not an innocuous event; yttrium-aluminum-garnet (YAG) laser capsulotomy has a small but defined risk of CME and retinal detachment. Safety is enhanced at this stage with the use of a silicone I-A tip (Alcon, MST), which precludes a capsule rupture that could otherwise be caused by

a spurious burr on a metal I-A aspiration port/tip (presentation by Robert Osher, MD). When vacuuming the capsule, remember to include the posterior surface of the anterior capsule to potentially decrease the risk of postoperative capsule phimosis as well as to decrease the overall antigenic load in the anterior chamber during healing.

Conclusion

The surgical approach to refractive cataract surgery and RLE is a mirror of the vigilance and attention to detail that is employed in routine cataract surgery, with regard to enhancing safety and efficiency. Phacodynamics provides a context of reasoning to allow the gentlest procedure possible with the least likelihood of complications, by optimizing machine parameter settings as well as the usage and choice of second-hand instruments. Notwithstanding the fact that we give all of our patients our best efforts, bear in mind that RLE patients along with patients choosing premium upgrades to cataract surgery will be less tolerant of complications to achieve their elective vision enhancement as compared to patients who will better accept a small risk in exchange for removing their pathology.

References

1. Seibel BS. *Phacodynamics: Mastering the Tools and Techniques of Phacoemulsification Surgery.* 4th ed. Thorofare, NJ: SLACK Incorporated; 2005.
2. Chang D. *Phaco Chop: Mastering Techniques, Optimizing Technology, and Avoiding Complications.* Thorofare, NJ: Slack Incorporated; 2004.

CHAPTER 198

OPTIMIZING THE CORNEA AND THE **IOL** WITH **RLE**

Michael B. Brenner, MD, FICS

When considering using a premium IOL for the correction of presbyopia or combined with cataract removal, a greater attention to details that affect the entire visual system must be considered. Today's baby booming refractive surgery candidate for presbyopia correcting intraocular lenses, or PresbyIOLs, are typically more discerning about various qualitative aspects of their vision. This may not be obvious to the surgeon or even to themselves at first glance. This chapter will focus on maximizing your preparedness prior to lens surgery in order to manage various possible outcomes.

It is naïve to think that PresbyIOL surgery stops at IOL implantation. The cornea plays just as vital a role in the effects on a patient's optic axis. Regardless of the choice of lens style implanted, additional surgical modalities should be at the surgeon's disposal. The lines between refractive cataract surgery and refractive lens exchange have been blurred and indeed overlap with corneal refractive surgery. Many anterior segment surgeons find themselves performing procedures on the lens and cornea. Alternatively, a cataract/lenticular surgeon may fair well by pairing up with a corneal refractive surgeon thereby allowing a patient to be surgically co-managed by two MD's via a "team" approach.

In a Perfect World

More specifically worded: "in a perfect eye" the cornea has mid-range average K-values with natural asphericity and no toricity. This scenario combined with accurate biometry and lens calculations should and does provide the patient with a favorable quality of vision. The problem arises when corneal-pseudolenticular mismatch occurs with respect to lower or higher order aberrations. We have developed an algorithm to restore a better match between corneal and pseudolenticular optics based on corneal curvature that has resulted in significantly enhanced visual outcomes. The goal is to leave the cornea keratometrically neutral when the crystalline lens has been removed resulting in the least possible residual aberrations (Table 1).

Managing Corneal Astigmatism

In the presbyopic eye or one with only mild cataract formation, we can rely on the fact that in the majority of cases, 65 to 85% of the corneal toricity will be manifested by refraction.[1] Proper placement of paired limbal relaxing incisions will neutralize the corneal astigmatism when performed at the time of lens exchange surgery (Table 2).[2] The Nichamin system will yield great results when done correctly. To minimize the chance of regression I offer a few caveats to this surgical approach:

* Always plan the correction in advance and center the paired incisions on the steep axis. Utilize a diagram that is oriented in an identical fashion to the surgeon's view through the microscope
* Mark the 3-9 axis for against the rule astigmatism or the 6-12 axis for with the rule astigmatism with the patient upright to negate any cyclotorsion that may occur while the patient is supine.
* Verify desired depth under the microscope if using an adjustable diamond blade and periodically calibrate using a micrometer or similar device.
* Incisions should be paralimbal within the corneal vascular arcades to assure a predictable and more sustained result.
* Incisions should be performed at the start of the case so that fluid can flow into the incision for a wound-spreading effect. If needed, you can incorporate the paracentesis or Keratome sites within the arcuate incision.

When manifested cylinder in not appropriately reflected in the corneal curvature, this typically means that the astigmatism is lenticular in nature and will be alleviated, reduced and/or changed by removal of the crystalline lens. In these cases, relaxing incisions at the time of surgery is not indicated. Another scenario yielding suboptimal results occurs when the keratometry or topography does not correlate with the refracted cylinder power and axis. Our approach to this situation is to

Table 1

ALGORITHM FOR STAGING PROCEDURES BASED ON CORNEAL CURVATURE

Average K-Value	Biometry Offset	Planned Staging
Average K <43.00 D	Dioptric subtraction	Second staged CK
Average K 43.00 to 46.00 D	No adjustment to biometry	LRI at time of surgery
Average K >46.00 D	Dioptric addition	Second staged LVC

Table 2

STARTING NOMOGRAMS FOR THE PLACEMENT OF LIMBAL RELAXING INCISIONS AT THE TIME OF IOL IMPLANTATION

Against-the-Rule Astigmatism

Steep Axis 0-30 degrees/150-180 degrees   Degrees of arc to be incised

Preop cylinder	30-40 yo	41-50 yo	51-60 yo	61-70 yo	71-80 yo	81-90 yo	>90 yo
+0.75 arrow +1.25 nasal limbal arc only Paired limbal arcs on steep axis	55	50	45	40	35	35	
+1.50 arrow +2.00 paired limbal arcs on steep axis	70	65	60	55	45	40	35
+2.25 arriw +2.75 Paired limbal arcson steep axis	90	80	70	60	50	45	40
+3.00 arrow +3.75 Paired limbal arcs on steep axis	(down arrow) o.z. to 8 mm 90 deg	(down arrrow) o.z. to 8 mm 90 deg	85	70	60	50	45

With-the-Rule Astigmatism

Steep Axis 45-145 degrees   Degrees of arc to be incised

Preop cylinder	30-40 yo	41-50 yo	51-60 yo	61-70 yo	71-80 yo	81-90 yo	>90 yo
+1.00 arrow +1.50 Paired limbal arcs on steep axis	50	45	40	35	30		
+1.75 arrow +2.25 paired limbal arcs on steep axis	60	55	50	45	40	35	30
+2.50 arriw +3.00 Paired limbal arcson steep axis	70	65	60	55	50	45	40
+3.25 arrow +3.75 paired limbal arcs on steep axis	80	75	70	65	60	55	45

Adapted from L.D. "Skip" Nichamin.

Table 3

STARTING NOMOGRAM TO DETERMINE ARCUATE LENGTH FOR CUSTOMIZED MICROKERATOTOMY

Age	18-25	26-35	36-49	50-80	>80
1.0	30 x 2*	30 x 2*	30 x 2*		
1.5	60 x 1	30 x 2*	30 x 2*	30 x 2*	
2.0	45 x 2**	45 x 2**	45 x 2**	30 x 2*	30 x 2*
2.5	60 x 2	45 x 2**	45 x 2**	30 x 2*	30 x 2*
3.0	60 x 2	60 x 2	45 x 2**	45 x 2**	30 x 2*
3.5	90 x 2	60 x 2	60 x 2	45 x 2**	30 x 2*
4.0	90 x 2	90 x 2	60 x 2	60 x 2	45 x 2**
4.5		90 x 2	60 x 2	60 x 2	45 x 2**
5.0		90 x 2	90 x 2	60 x 2	45 x 2**
5.5			90 x 2	90 x 2	45 x 2**
6.0				90 x 2	60 x 2
6.5				90 x 2	60 x 2
7.0					90 x 2

*30 degrees X 2 = 45 degrees X 1
**45 degrees X 2 = 90 degrees X 1

Adapted from Charles Casebeer for the correction of astigmatism after IOL implantation.

place paralimbal incisions or perform arcuate keratotomy on a subsequent date typically one month following temporal clear corneal surgery.

Utilizing nomograms for arcuate keratotomy at the 7.0 mm optical zone for the correction of residual astigmatism can be a very effective tool when the spherical equivalent is near plano[3] or even slightly hyperopic to account for corneal coupling (Table 3).[4] It is important for the reader to always bear in mind that all nomograms become more accurate when adjustments are made based on careful outcomes analysis.

Another situation is topographical astigmatism that is either asymmetric and/or nonorthagonal representing more complex forms of corneal toricity. Even when such astigmatism is not detected by or does not fully correlate with the refraction, applying customized microkeratotomy (CMK) can significantly improve postoperative acuity regardless of the type of implant used.[5] This dictates varying the arcuate lengths according to the asymmetry on topography and placing the incisions at 2 different hemi-meridians to accommodate nonorthogonality (Figure 1). Applying CMK to corneas with regular irregularities can result in significant qualitative visual improvement in near plano eyes. Ongoing work with comparative aberrometry is showing that, unlike standard arcuate keratotomy, CMK can actually reduce coma and secondary astigmatism resulting in a diminution of ghosting and shadowing that may be seen after implantation of multifocal IOLs.

Managing the Flat Cornea

Just as the world functions better round than flat, the human eye was not designed to function at its best with a flat cornea. Whether a patient's cornea is naturally flat (Average K less than 43.00 D) or has been flattened via previous refractive surgery, it has been shown that there is a greater likelihood of dysphotopsias following IOL surgery. Aberration reducing IOLs have merit in reducing this by offsetting the residual negative spherical aberration that would normally exist in a standard pseudophakic eye.[6] However, when utilizing PresbyIOLs that do not adjust the overall net spherical aberration within the confines of the pupil, the logical approach focuses on adjusting corneal curvature especially when the mean keratometry value is in the flat range.

Early on we found and others reported that a hyperopic outcome following Crystalens implantation, could be effectively managed by steepening the paracentral cornea using conductive keratoplasty (CK)[7] with LightTouch technology (Refractec, Irvine, CA).[8] Anecdotally we discovered that these were some of our happiest patients. Further retrospective review in our practice showed that of those patients who had flatter corneas prior to surgery, a subgroup that had staged CK after IOL implantation with adjusted biometry, had less higher-order aberrations and fared better on subjective numerical grading to visual ranking questionnaires.

This approach to managing the optics in the face of flatter corneas is simple using planned bioptics. In so doing, the key

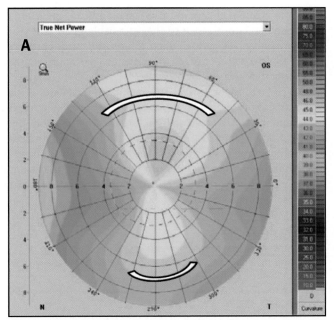 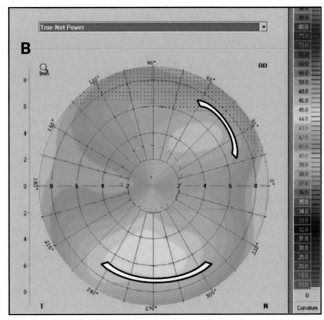

Figure 1. Tangential topography demonstrating CMK at the 7.0-mm optical zone with asymmetric corneal toricity (A) and with nonorthagonal astigmatism (B). In each case, the arcuate sum of the incisions is equivalent to nomogram-determined paired incisions (see Table 3).

Table 4

STARTING NOMOGRAM FOR CONDUCTIVE KERATOPLASTY UTILIZING LIGHTTOUCH TECHNIQUE

Desired Correction*	Number of 8-Spot Rings	Optical Zone
+1.00 D	1	8 mm
+1.75 D	1	7 mm
+2.50 D	2	7 mm and 8 mm

*Range of ±0.25 diopters.

Adapted from H. L. "Rick" Milne.

---

is to utilize a spherical offset in the IOL calculations that will be corrected with the 2nd stage of CK. For example, lets look at the patient who has an average K of 41.5 diopters. For best optical performance, the eye would fare better with a corneal curvature between 43 and 45 diopters. To achieve this would require at least 1.5 diopters of corneal steepening, which would be the planned target for the second stage of the bioptics procedure. Looking at the Light Touch CK nomogram implemented by Dr. Milne (Table 4), we see that we would plan to perform a single ring of 8 spots at the 7.0 mm optical zone. Prior to this we would offset our biometric lens calculations diopter for diopter by subtracting 1.5 diopters from the final lens calculation to allow for the planned increase in corneal power. This technique is ideally suited for Crystalens (Eyeonics, Inc, Aliso Viejo, CA) implantation because of the combination of increased depth of field resulting from posterior IOL vaulting as well as anterior corneal steepening, but may also be applied, however, to eyes implanted with the ReSTOR (Alcon, Fort Worth, TX) or ReZoom (Advanced Medical Optics, Santa Ana, CA) as long as there is minimal preoperative corneal toricity.

When combining crystalens implantation with conductive keratoplasty in eyes with flat and/or oblate corneas, the visual system also benefits from a significant reduction in higher order aberrations. This is the result of the hyperprolate shape caused by "belt-like" tightening of the mid-peripheral corneal stroma.

For most patients, stability of their postoperative refractive error should occur within a month, which is important in allowing patients and surgeons to plan their schedules accordingly. The question of cost typically arises when performing bioptics on any surgery candidate. It has been our practice to charge a nominal amount in advance for the 2nd stage to cover the hard costs and time involved to perform that procedure.

Managing the Steep Cornea

When planning PresbyIOL surgery in a patient with steep (Average K>45.00 diopters) or highly toric (>2.50 diopters change on keratometric map) corneas, laser vision correction (LVC) works best. If the steepness of the cornea correlates with biometry and pachymetry reveals sufficient thickness, utilizing planned bioptics can yield superior results. The reported 3-stage technique of fabricating a femtosecond laser flap without lifting, followed by lens implantation, and finishing with an initial flap lift and excimer laser ablation has yielded the best outcomes. This "forgiving" approach not only affords the correction of induced myopia as well as simple or compound myopic astigmatism, but affords the neutralization of any residual lower and higher order aberrations. If a femtosecond laser is not available and flap creation cannot be performed prior to lens implantation, it is advisable to wait 3 months prior to performing the staged ablation via LASIK using a microkeratome in order to assure IOL stability within the capsular bag complex.

As previously described, one must reduce the calculated IOL power by the spherical equivalent of the planned ablation. An example would be patient scheduled for refractive lens exchange with topography revealing 46.00/47.50 @ 90 degrees. The average keratometric value is 46.75 diopters which is 1.75 diopters greater than that required to be at the upper limit of our ideal range of corneal power of 45.00 diopters. This amount would, therefore, be added to the dioptric lens power calculation in order to offset the staged ablation. This calculation offset methodology is applicable to various types of LASIK or other flap based procedures as well as surface ablation.

Staging for Success

Whether accomplished in 1, 2, or 3 stages, preparing the presbyopic refractive surgery candidate will likely result in a positive experience for both you and your patient. Patients are more involved when proceeding along this stepwise approach to vision correction and appreciate the staged improvement in visual function at each stage. Our role as surgeons is to stress the positive changes at each step and to clearly impart knowledge and confidence so that attainable goals and visual milestones may be clearly defined. This fosters the appropriate "team" approach and engages the patient to participate in their own refractive surgical journey.

Staged treatment strives to maintain the natural corneal aspherocity as much as possible when we embrace the paradigm shift of refractive IOL surgery. In this case, once a patient is determined to be a good candidate for refractive lens exchange or desires to upgrade to a PresbyIOL technology while having cataract surgery, the next emphasis should be evaluating the cornea for effective planning of the desired end- result optical system.

References

1. Milder B, Rubin ML. *Astigmatism. The Fine Art of Prescribing Glasses.* Gainesville, FL: Triad; 1974: 76-85.

2. Nichamin LD. Astigmatism control. *Ophthalmol Clin North Am.* 2006; 19(4):485-493.

3. Waring GO, Casebeer JC, Dru RM. One-year results of a prospective multicenter study of the Casebeer system of refractive keratotomy. Casebeer Chiron Study Group. *Ophthalmology.* 1996; 103(9):1337-1347.

4. Gills JP, Rowsey JJ. Managing coupling in secondary astigmatic keratotomy. *Int Ophthalmol Clin.* 2003;43(3):29-41.

5. Brenner MB. Enhanced outcomes using adjuvant treatment modalities following presbyopic lens exchange. *Ophthalmic Practice.* 2002; 20(9):330-336.

6. Beiko GHH. Personalized correction of spherical aberration in cataract surgery. *J Cataract Refractive Surg.* 2007;33(8):1455-60

7. Claramonte PJ, Alió JL, Ramzy MI. Conductive keratoplasty to correct residual hyperopia after cataract surgery. *J Cataract Refract Surg.* 2006;32(9):1445-51.

8. Milne HL. *Light Touch Conductive Keratoplasty. Conductive Keratoplasty: A Primer.* Thorofare, NJ: SLACK Incorporated; 2005:79-84.

CHAPTER 199

RETINAL DETACHMENT RISK IN MYOPES

Barry S. Seibel, MD

The risks of refractive lens exchange (RLE) include all of the same risks for cataract surgery, and as such, should be carefully discussed with potential RLE candidates. RLE is a potential option for patients desiring reduced dependence on glasses or contact lenses but who are 1) outside the ideal range of laser vision correction in terms of excessive hyperopia or myopia, or 2) presbyopic and monovision intolerant, and therefore potential candidates for a presbyopia-correcting IOL. Relative to the optics of a lens implant, higher power laser vision correction is more likely to lead to suboptimal visual quality.[1] Therefore, highly myopic and hyperopic patients, whose quality of life is poorest due to their absolute dependence on thick spectacles or contact lenses, are often not ideal candidates for corneal refractive surgery. With current technology, RLE offers the best potential optics for the presbyopic patient who is intolerant of monovision.

General risks for cataract and RLE surgery are discussed in Chapter 121 by Dr. Salz. Ophthalmic Mutual Insurance Company (OMIC) consent forms mention the risks of infection, corneal edema/scarring (which could possibly require a penetrating keratoplasty), possible equipment malfunction, retinal detachment, hemorrhage, retinal vein or artery occlusion, blindness, and loss of the eye.[2] The RLE consent includes the risk of an IOL power miscalculation, a malpositioned IOL, and cystoid macular edema. Although the latter is listed only with refractive lens exchange, its actual rate is extremely low.[3] However, the potential risk of retinal detachment must be discussed with each patient relative to any additional risk factors that they may have in order to determine the existence of an adequate risk to benefit ratio.

Retinal Detachment Risk and Cataract Surgery

A recent population-based study has substantiated the risk of retinal detachment (RD) in routine cataract surgery even in the absence of risk factors. Jay Erie utilized the Rochester Epidemiology Project database to look at 10,256 cataract surgeries over a 2-year period from 1980 through 2004, with calculated probabilities being adjusted for the period of follow-up.[4,5] A progressively increasing cumulative probability of RD with cataract surgery was found up to 20 years following the cataract surgery, culminating in a 1.79% overall risk at 20 years. This represented a 4-fold increased risk over age-matched controls who did not have cataract surgery. As 29% of the RD's in this study occurred ≥5 years after cataract surgery, Erie points out that studies with less than 5 years of follow-up may be missing important outcomes data.

RLE and Myopia

RD is perhaps the most worrisome risk for one key RLE demographic group in particular—myopes in whom the vitreous has excessive liquifaction (synchisis) at younger ages. Goldberg reviewed the literature in 1987 and concluded that any possible optical benefits of RLE with axial myopia were usually outweighed by the visual severity of the risks, looking not only at the rate of RD but also the visual outcomes of retinal reattachment surgery.[6] Rosen revisits the subject as of 2006, and while he finds improved results in studies subsequent to Goldberg's paper, he still points out that many questions remain unanswered and that prospective patients should be apprised of the potentially increased risk of RD.[7]

Assessment of the risk is difficult, however, because the various studies differ greatly with regard to their inclusion scopes, criteria, and follow-up durations. For example, Tuft looked at 63,298 cataract procedures performed between August 1994 and March 2003 and found a 3-fold increased risk of RD with axial lengths >23 mm.[8] Guell et al examined 44 eyes with a mean correction of −15.77 D for 4 years and found a 0% retinal detachment rate.[9] Fernandez-Vega et al examined 190 eyes with a 26- to 39-mm axial length for 5 years and found a 2.1% rate of retinal detachment.[10] Pucci examined 25 eyes with corrections of greater than −12.00D for 43 months and found a 4% incidence of retinal detachment.[11] Arne studied 36 eyes with −17.00 D manifest refractions and 28-mm axial lengths for 4 years and found a 5.5% incidence of retinal detachment (in 2 eyes, both of which received PMMA IOLs and underwent a yttrium-aluminum-garnet [YAG] posterior capsulotomy.[12] Fritch examined 481 eyes with axial lengths greater than 26-mm for 7 years and found only a 0.4% incidence of retinal detachment, one-tenth the rate of Pucci's study.[13] Alio looked at 439 eyes with ≥6 D myopia or axial length ≥26 mm and mean follow-up of 5 years, and found a 2.7% incidence of RD.[14] Ripandelli observed an RD rate of 8.0% as compared with 1.2% of control eyes in a study of 930 eyes with myopia between –15 and –30 D over a follow-up of 36 months.[15] The highest rate of retinal detachment (8.1%) was found by Colin et al, who examined 52 eyes that were treated with RLE for more than 12.00 D of myopia for 7 years.[16]

Colin's reported RD rate is almost double the 4.8% incidence which would be predicted by the natural history of myopia as reported by Perkins based on Moorfield's data.[17] The difference between the baseline rate and the higher study rate represents the incremental risk, which is perhaps the most pertinent for informed consent for these prospective patients. Compare these rates to the risk of RD in the general population of 0.01%.[18]

Sanders' Analysis

In order to sort through this somewhat perplexing range of outcomes from differently designed studies, Don Sanders performed an extensive literature review of 14 studies of refractive lens exchange with a PCIOL.[3] These studies included a total of 1372 myopic eyes (range, –6.00D to –33.75D) of mostly young patients in their 30s and 40s. All but 46 surgeries were performed with phacoemulsification, and the follow up ranged from 15 to 45.9 months. Of all eyes, only 14 developed retinal detachments, for an incidence of 1%. Sanders also examined the rate of cystoid macular edema in this literature review and found it to be only 0.1%. Although some of the studies were somewhat limited in their length of follow up, the Sanders review is commendable for attempting to apply some homogeneity to this area of study.

Like Goldberg, this paper is significant for looking beyond the simple incidence of retinal detachment and considering the visual sequelae of this event. Sanders noted that retinal reattachment rates averaged 85%, with some series quoting success rates as high as 98%. However, the final visual acuity after reattachment varied, with 60% of patients achieving 20/40 or better, 20% achieving 20/50 to 20/100, and 20% being worse than 20/100. By combining these visual outcomes data with a conservative estimate of 4% incremental risk of RD, Sanders determined an overall long-term incremental risk of moderate-to-severe vision loss with myopic refractive lens exchange of 4%. This represents a conservative estimate in that the inclusion of a 4% incremental risk of RD is even higher than the 3.3% observed by Colin's study (8.1% observed in study minus the 4.8% predicted by Perkins baseline incidence of RD in myopes).

RD Risk Factor of YAG Capsulotomy

Reports are mixed with regard to YAG laser posterior capsulotomy as a risk factor for RD. Dr. Colin's study mirrored the Perkins baseline RD data of 2% at the 4-year follow-up, but then increased quickly to 8.1% within 2 years of YAG posterior capsulotomy performed on 3 eyes. Arne's paper also had an association of increased RD risk with YAG capsulotomy. Javitt's study of 57,103 patients revealed a 3.9-fold increased risk of RD following YAG capsulotomy.[19] Olsen and Olson originally reported an increased incidence of RD following YAG capsulotomy, but after changing their method to one with lower energy and a smaller treatment area, they reported no RD or cystoid macular edema (CME) in phacoemulsification patients with 6.5 years of follow-up.[20] Additionally, no increased risk of RD with YAG capsulotomy was noted by the large studies from Erie, Tuft, Russell, and Alio, with the first three studying cataract surgery in general and Alio looking specifically at myopes.[5,8,21,14]

RD Risk Factors of Age and Gender

Independent of myopia, additional factors may predispose RLE and cataract surgery patients to RD. Erie found a 6-fold increase in risk of RD in patients younger than 60 years old as compared to those 60 and older. Similar results were found by Russell's 10 year retrospective review of 1793 patients, in which 5.17% of patients younger than 50 years had RD after phacoemulsification as compared to only a 0.64% rate for patients older than 70.[21] In addition to younger age, male gender is a predisposing risk factor for RD with cataract surgery. Shwu-Jiuan's study of 9388 Taiwanese patients found a cumulative 6-year RD rate of 1.90% in the male subgroup, and a 0.56% rate in the female subgroup.[22] Tuft found males to have a risk that was 2.2 times that of females, and Erie found a similarly increased rate of males being 2.9 times more at risk than females. Erie points out that risk factors are nonlinearly additive, with a young male myope having a 5-fold increased risk of RD as compared to a patient without any risk factors. Bear in mind that in his study this would represent a risk of 8.95% at 20 years postoperatively (5 × 1.79%) for such patients, who would represent a substantial portion of the potential RLE demographic.

Mechanisms of RD With Lens-Based Surgery

A number of related mechanisms may be etiologic in RD following lens-based surgery. Most relate to either causing or exacerbating a posterior vitreous detachment (PVD). Sheard found an increased incidence of PVD in pseudophakic eyes as compared to phakic eyes.[23] One would hypothesize that anterior shifting of the vitreous results from evacuation of the space formerly occupied by the crystalline lens, and such shifting can conceivably produce peripheral and posterior retinal traction that leads to breaks. Although this anterior vitreous shift is reduced post-operatively by a properly placed PCIOL with posterior angulated haptics, it can still occur intraoperatively prior to IOL placement. Wilkinson and Rice cite several studies that indicate little or no difference in new PVD rate between phakic and aphakic patients following cataract surgery.[24] Retinal traction may also occur as a result of the inertial destabilization of vitreous intraoperatively. Prior to such stabilization by an IOL with posteriorly angulated haptics, variable anterior chamber pressures and turbulence along with globe manipulation may proportionately and adversely mobilize the vitreous; therefore, attention to phacodynamic settings and proper instrument manipulation may be helpful in reducing vitreous movement.[25] These vitreous dynamics could conceivable play a role in phakic IOL implantation in which anterior chamber pressures also vary with attendant changes in anterior chamber depth and potential retinal traction.

The mechanism of YAG-induced retinal detachment is thought to be that the laser's energy and resultant shock waves destabilize the hyaluronic acid matrix that supports the vitreous cortex structure. This in turn leads to synchesis (liquifaction) and syneresis (collapse). When such vitreous changes occur due to normal aging, they do so in tandem with normal age-related reduction of vitreoretinal adhesions. However, when associated with cataract surgery and younger age, synchesis and syneresis can lead to an anomalous posterior vitreous detachment, which in turn leads to a retinal detachment due to inertial vitreous destabilization and traction in association with strong vitreoretinal adhesions.[26] Another theory predicts that the YAG energy disrupts the anterior hyaloid face, decreasing the concentration of hyaluronic acid (HA) in the vitreous. The HA serves to maintain vitreous clarity via a supporting structure that keeps collagen fibrils separated by at least one wavelength of incident light. Decreased HA concentration therefore results in syneresis (collapse) of the vitreous cortex, leading to an anomalous posterior vitreous detachment, which in turn leads to retinal detachment.[27] These structural changes can produce a new PVD or alternatively cause pathologic progression of an existing PVD.[23]

Additional considerations come into play when postulating the mechanism of retinal detachment in young myopes, in whom early synchesis increases the chance for syneresis and posterior vitreous detachment. The latter produces an inertial destabilization of the vitreous that creates traction on the anterior attached retina. These same forces do not typically result in a retinal tear in a naturally occurring PVD in an older patient due to the associated weaker vitreoretinal adhesions. However, an anomalous posterior vitreous detachment occurs in young myopes prior to normal age-related vitreoretinal dehiscence; therefore, a break is more likely due to inertial vitreal traction being more directly transmitted to the retina. Furthermore, the young myope will have synchesis as described earlier, which is more likely to dissect through a break as opposed to formed vitreous; this dissection typically results in retinal detachment.[26] Note that the foregoing discussions of the mechanism of an anomalous posterior vitreous detachment are consistent with the findings of Erie and Tuft

with regard to younger age being a general risk factor for RD with cataract surgery.[5,8]

Present and Future Guidelines

Given the aforementioned risk factors for RD with cataract surgery and refractive lens exchange, what should ophthalmologists do now and in the future? Patients should be informed of the disparity in the literature. With regard to myopic patients, some papers state an unchanged or even reduced risk of retinal detachment relative to a myope's natural history. More conservative estimates include Sanders stating a 4% incremental risk of moderate-to-severe visual loss with retinal lens exchange and Colin et al suggesting a 3% incremental risk of retinal detachment. The numbers might be explained to patients as being relatively small at low single digits, but simultaneously representing an approximately twofold increase in risk compared to no cataract or lens surgery. Additional risk factors of age and gender should be mentioned even in the absence of myopia.

A retinal specialist might evaluate these patients preoperatively and consider retinal detachment prophylaxis such as laser or cryoretinopexy for suspicious areas. However, Goldberg found equivocal benefits of retinal detachment prophylaxis, and noted retinal breaks in or away from areas of prophylactic treatment. Inflammation from prophylactic treatment could also induce other sequelae such as an epiretinal membrane, posterior vitreous detachment, or retinal detachment.[6] Similar findings were noted by Wilkinson.[28] Rosen points out a potential error in logic of having such retinal pretreatment; to the extent that PVD formation or progression is the inciting event of a RD after cataract surgery (presumably by creating a new retinal break), then treatment of other areas that may have been suspicious pre-operatively may have no effect on the PVD-etiologic tear that will appear in an indeterminate area as a result of PVD formation or progression.[7]

Moving into the future with myopic, hyperopic, and presbyopic refractive lens exchange, a new, large database of age-matched controls should be established for the natural history of patients with varying levels of axial length and refractive error to verify the baseline incidence of retinal detachment. The Perkins data are limited and 25 years old, and yet form the benchmark for judging the incremental risk of retinal detachment. While the large population based studies of Erie and Tuft are significant steps in the right direction, a large, prospective, multicenter, study of refractive lens exchange as well as cataract surgery should be organized with standardization of modern small-incision techniques and technology, notwithstanding the inevitable change in these factors with the rapid advances in this area of ophthalmology. The study should also span 10 or more years, given the late occurrences of retinal detachment in the Colin and Erie studies. Also for the future, more studies are needed to validate the role of retinal detachment prophylaxis preoperatively given the doubts cast by Goldberg and Wilkinson. Objective evaluation modalities of the vitreous should be developed as preoperative predictors of retinal detachment risk with myopic refractive lens exchange, such as dynamic light scattering or 3-D B-scan ultrasonography.[27] Further evaluation is also needed on the potential role of pharmacologic vitreolysis to reduce the retinal detachment risk especially in the face of myopia and/or younger age that predisposes to anomalous PVD.

Conclusion

RD is one of the most significant risks of lens-based surgery, including both cataract surgery and refractive lens exchange. There is considerable variation in the literature regarding the risk of RD and the significance of myopia and YAG laser posterior capsulotomy. The literature is also inconsistent in establishing the success rate of retinal reattachment surgery, with regard to both anatomical cure and preservation of vision. Younger age and male gender seem to be significant risk factors for RD with cataract surgery. However, with proper and reasonable informed consent for the patient, along with meticulous attention to surgical technique (to minimize vitreous disturbance and reduce the likelihood of posterior capsule opacification requiring YAG posterior capsulotomy), RLE and cataract surgery remain viable procedures with very high overall success rates that can significantly enhance the quality of life for millions of patients.

References

1. Schallhorn SC. Pupil size and quality of vision after LASIK. *Ophthalmology.* 2003; 110; 1606-1614.

2. Ophthalmic Mutual Insurance Company. Risk Management Forms. San Francisco, California.

3. Sanders, DR. Actual and theoretical risks for visual loss following use of the implantable contact lens for moderate to high myopia. *J Cataract Refractive Surg.* 2003;29:1323-1332.

4. Erie JC. Risk of retinal detachment after cataract extraction, 1980-2004. *Ophthalmology.* 2006;113(11):2026-2032.

5. Erie JC. Risk of retinal detachment after cataract extraction, 1980-2004. *Trans Am Ophthalmol Soc.* 2006;104:167-175.

6. Goldberg MF. Clear lens extraction for axial myopia. *Ophthalmology.* 1987;94(5):571-582.

7. Rosen E. Risk management for rhegmatogenous retinal detachment following refractive lens exchange and phakic IOL implantation in myopic eyes. *J Cataract Refract Surg.* 2006;32:697-701.

8. Tuft SJ. Risk Factors for Retinal Detachment after Cataract Surgery. *Ophthalmology.* 2006;113(4):650-656.

9. Guell JL, Rodriguez-Arenas AF, Gris O. Phacoemulsification of the crystalline lens and implantation of an intraocular lens for the correction of moderate and high myopia: four-year follow-up. *J Cataract Refract Surg.* 2003;29:34-38.

10. Fernandez-Vega L, Alfonso JF, Villacampa T. Clear lens extraction for the correction of high myopia. *Ophthalmology.* 2003;110:2349-2354.

11. Pucci V. Clear lens phacoemulsification for correction of high myopia. *J Cataract Refract Surg.* 2001;27:896-900.

12. Arne JL. Phakic intraocular lens implantation versus clear lens extraction in highly myopic eyes of 30- to 50-year-old patients. *J Cataract Refract Surg.* 2004;30:2092-2096.

13. Fritch CD. Risk of retinal detachment in myopic eyes after intraocular lens implantation: a 7-year study. *J Cataract Refract Surg.* 1998;24:1357-1360.

14. Alio JL et al. The risk of retinal detachment in high myopia after small incision coaxial phacoemulsification. *AJO.* 2007;144:93-98.

15. Ripandelli G. Cataract surgery as a risk factor for retinal detachment in very highly myopic eyes. *Ophthalmology.* 2003;110(12):2355-2361.

16. Colin J et al ,Rabinet A, and Cochener B. Retinal detachment after clear lens extraction for high myopia: seven-year follow-up. *Ophthalmology.* 1999;106:2281-2284.

17. Perkins ES. Morbidity from myopia. *Sight Saving Review.* 1979 Spring;49:11-19.

18. Jaffee NS. Retinal detachment in aphakia and pseudophakia. In: Klein EA, ed. *Cataract Surgery and Its Complications.* 5th ed. St. Louis: C.V. Mosby; 1990:653-665.

19. Javitt JC. National outcomes of cataract extraction—Increased risk of retinal complications associated with Nd:YAG laser capsulotomy. *Ophthalmology* 1002;99:1487-1498.

20. Olsen G, and Olson, RJ. Update on a long-term, prospective study of capsulotomy and retinal detachment rates after cataract surgery. *J Cataracat Refract Surg.* 2000;26:1017-1021.

21. Russell M. Pseudophakic retinal detachment after phacoemulsification cataract surgery. *J Cataract Refract Surg.* 2006;32:442-445.

22. Shwu-Jiuan S, Luo_Ping G, Jane-Fang C. Male sex as a risk factor for pseudophakic retinal detachment after cataract extraction in Taiwanese adults. *Ophthalmology.* 2007;14(10):1898-1903.

23. Sheard RM. Posterior vitreous detachment after neodymium:YAG laser posterior capsulotomy. *J Cataract Refract Surg.* 2003;29:930-934.

24. Wilkinson CP, Rice TA. *Michels Retinal Detachment.* 2nd Ed. St. Louis: Mosby; 1997:180.

25. Seibel BS. Chapter 2 In: *Phacodynamics.* 4th ed. Thorofare, NJ: Slack, Inc.; 2005:154-167.

26. Sebag J. *Stucture, function, and age-related changes of the human vitreous.* New York, NY: Springer-Verlag; 1987.

27. Sebag J. *Vitreous from Biochemistry to Clinical Relevance.* Vol 1. Duanes; 1998;28.

28. Wilkinson CP. Evidence-based analysis of prophylactic treatment of asymptomatic retinal breaks and lattice degeneration. *Ophthalmology.* 2000;10:12-16.

CHAPTER 200

RETINAL DETACHMENT RISK IN MYOPES

Jorge L. Alió, MD, PhD and Mohamed H. Shabayek, MD, PhD

A frequent point of debate between refractive and retinal surgeons is the risk of pseudophakic retinal detachment (RD) in highly myopic eyes, which can be defined as eyes with an axial length greater than 26 mm (sometimes even exceeding 34 mm) and spherical equivalent ≤ −6.00 diopters (D). This degree of myopia is mostly associated with degenerative changes that involve the sclera, choroid, retina, and vitreous. However, it is important to determine the risk of RD after both lens exchange (LE) (whether cataractous or a clear lens), and phakic intraocular lenses (Ph-IOLs) (whether anterior or posterior chamber), especially in highly myopic eyes.

The risk of RD in highly myopic patients is mainly due to 2 possible causes: a higher incidence of predisposing retinal lesions in myopic eyes compared to general population and the hypothesis that LE and Ph-IOL might induce several iatrogenic factors that will increase the incidence of retinal tears.

The main issue to be addressed in this chapter is whether the incidence and the risk of RD increases in highly myopic patients after LE and Ph-IOL, taking into account the preexisting risk factors in highly myopic eyes.

The Risk of Retinal Detachment in Unoperated Highly Myopic Eyes

Previous studies have reported a higher incidence of RD in unoperated highly myopic eyes compared to nonmyopic eyes (whether emmetropic or hypermetropic).[1,2] These studies reported a risk of RD that ranged between 0.71% and 3.2%.[1,2] Previously published reports studied highly myopic eyes with a spherical equivalent (SE) > −6.0 D and included 1000 eyes.[2] The annual incidence was 0.015% in eyes with myopia ≤4.75 D, 0.07% in myopic eyes ranging between −5.0 and −9.75 D, and 0.075% in eyes with myopia >10 D.[3] In myopes of up to −15 D, the risk of developing a RD increases 15 fold com-

pared to the general population. This risk increases 110 fold in highly myopic patients > −15 D when compared to the general population. Burton[4] reported that high myopes > −5.0 D with retinal degeneration are prone to an extraordinary risk of developing RD, especially with long life expectancy. The risk of developing RD during the second, third, or fourth decade of life is very high in such patients, mainly due to atrophic retinal holes. However, Burton did not provide results on severe myopia due to high axial length.

The Risk of Retinal Detachment in Highly Myopic Eyes After Phakic IOLs

RD development after Ph-IOL implantation has been reported by several authors,[5-10] but with high variability. Our group analyzed 12 eyes that developed RD out of 294 consecutive highly myopic eyes after Ph-IOL implantation (incidence of 4.08%).[11] We analyzed the cumulative risk by Kaplan-Maier analysis, which demonstrated a cumulative risk of RD after Ph-IOL implantation of 1.36% at 5 months, 2.6% at 17 months, 3.61% at 27 months, and 5.63% at 52 months.[11] Recently, we conducted another retrospective study to evaluate RD development in 522 consecutive highly myopic eyes after Ph-IOL implantation.[12] We reported 15 eyes that developed RD with an incidence of 2.87%. We found a cumulative risk of RD development (Kaplan-Maier analysis) of 0.57% at 3 months, 1.64% at 12 months, 2.73% at 36 months, and 4.06% at 92 to 145 months.[12]

We compared the annual incidence of RD of unoperated high myopia (mean SE = −10 D) (0.075%)[3] to our results after Ph-IOL implantation and observed a higher incidence after Ph-IOL (2.87%), which is similar to that of severe myopic patients (3.2%), but with higher annual risk. Therefore we concluded that the development of RD is higher in our cohort of myopic eyes corrected with Ph-IOL than in the unoperated highly myopic population. Longer follow-up for these patients might reveal a greater incidence of RD. However, the mean SE of our study was –18.00 D, which is significantly higher than the –10.0 D mean SE of the RD study of unoperated myopes,[3] which can be a factor contributing to this higher incidence of RD in addition to the surgical intervention. In other words, because of the differing severity of myopia (mean SE and axial length), it is hard to make a valid comparison between our Ph-IOL group and the previously published study of RD in unoperated high myopes.[3] Incisions larger than 4 mm with attendant shallowing of the anterior chamber can predispose to vitreous instability and eventually vitreous detachment in young myopes receiving a large incision Ph-IOL.

When reviewing the incidence of RD in highly myopic eyes after small-incision Ph-IOLs, such as the Kelman-Duet (Tekia Inc., Irvine, CA), Artiflex (Ophtec BV, Groningen, The Netherlands), and the STAAR ICL (STAAR Surgical, Monrovia, CA),[13,14] the incidence of RD was lower when compared to larger-incision surgeries. However, most of the reported studies are of limited value due to lack of sufficient postoperative follow-up and the small number of cases included. The theory that small-incision (under 3 mm) Ph-IOL implantation is less likely to result in RD cannot be proven from the reported studies, but these studies are suggestive of a reduced risk of RD[13] in highly myopic eyes compared to the large incision (over 5 mm) required for implanting previous models of Ph-IOL. Zaldivar and colleagues[10] reported a very low incidence of RD of 0.8% after mean follow-up of 11 months in 124 highly myopic eyes.

In conclusion, Ph-IOL implantation seems to be related to an increased risk of RD in the high myope when an incision larger than 5 mm is used. Small-incision (<3.5 mm) Ph-IOLs do not seem to be associated with as high a risk of RD. Further studies with longer follow-up and a larger number of cases are mandatory to confirm the relationship between incision size and increased risk of RD.

The Risk of Retinal Detachment in Highly Myopic Eyes After Lens Removal

Analyzing previous reports studying the incidence of RD after lens removal in highly myopic patients is difficult. Previous studies have reported on differing populations using differing surgical techniques (extracapsular cataract extraction [ECCE] and phacoemulsification), whereas others compared the incidence after clear and cataractous lens extraction. Significantly, the mean follow-up, mean SE, and mean age varied highly in these published reports.[15-24]

Previous studies have reported an incidence of 2.10% in 190 myopic eyes after clear lens exchange (CLE) "phacoemulsification" after a mean follow-up of 4.78 years.[25] Other studies reported an incidence of 4.0% in 25 highly myopic eyes (>12.0 D),[16] and 3.2% in 62 eyes.[18] However, a study that included 930 highly myopic eyes with SE ranging from –30.0 to –15.0 D reported an incidence of 8%, with mean age of 62.5 years and mean follow-up of 36 months.[19] In another study with longer mean follow-up of 62.3 months and mean axial length of 30.22 mm, the reported incidence of RD was 1.3%, but this study involved a smaller cohort (73 eyes).[20] Other authors have reported a RD incidence of 6.1%,[22] 7.3%,[23] and 8.1%.[24]

Colin and colleagues[24] suggests that the risk of RD after CLE in highly myopic patients can increase with the time, and this may explain why studies with less than 4 years of follow-up demonstrate much lower rates of RD. Surprisingly, they reported RD incidence of 0% after 12 months,[26] 1.9% after 48 months,[25] and 8.1% after 84 months[24] of follow-up.

We cannot compare RD incidence after CLE to cataract extraction in highly myopes (as the incidence is lower after cataract extraction). In young patients, especially with long life expectancies, CLE can induce vitreous changes and increasing traction on the retina—changes that would not expected to occur in elderly patients after cataract extraction.[21]

We conducted a retrospective study[27] in which we analyzed RD incidence in 439 highly myopic eyes of 274 patients after lens surgery (CLE and cataract), with a mean age of 62.2 ± 11.7 years (range, 21 to 90 years), and a mean follow-up of 61.5 ± 29.6 months (range, 2 to 147 months) with different surgeons. All highly myopic eyes with axial length of over 26 mm and spherical equivalent ≥ –6.00 D were included. Eyes previously operated on for RD or other intraocular surgeries (3 eyes) were excluded from this study. Mean outcome measures were the occurrence of RD, age, axial length, operative complications (vitreous loss), PCO, and Nd:YAG capsulotomy, in addition to postoperative best spectacle-corrected visual acuity (BSCVA) and SE. Patients were divided into 2 groups according to their age at the time of surgery. group 1: patients 50 years or younger (82 eyes); group 2: patients 50 years or older (357 eyes). Eyes were also divided according to axial length (≤28.00 mm = 274 eyes; >28 mm = 165 eyes) for analyzing the risk of RD over time (Kaplan-Meier analysis).

RD occurred in 2.7% of eyes. The mean age of the patients affected by RD was 56.16 ± 9.96 years (range, 38 to 70 years). The mean axial length in RD eyes was 27.85 ± 1.83 mm (range, 26.00 to 31.34 mm), and the mean spherical equivalent –13.4 ± 5.8 (range, –28.00 to –6.50 D). In group 1 the incidence of RD was 3.65% (3 out of 82 eyes), whereas in group 2 it was 2.52% (9 out of 357 eyes). Eyes with relatively longer axial lengths demonstrated a higher incidence of RD. In eyes with axial lengths ≤ 28.0 mm, RD occurred in 2.18% (6 out of 274 eyes), compared to 3.36% in eyes with axial length > 28.0 mm (6 out of 165 eyes).

Kaplan-Meier analysis was performed to evaluate the cumulative risk of RD with time. The cumulative risk among all 439 eyes (Figure 1) was 0.47% at 3 months, 0.71% at 6 months, 1.71% at 15 months, 2.59% at 48 months, and 3.28% at 63 through 105 months. In group 1 the risk increased to 1.23% at 3 months and 4.46% at 63 through 147 months. In group 2 the risk was 0.58 % at 6 months, 1.83% at 15 months, 2.56% at 48 months, and 2.96% at 52 through 118 months (Figure 2). The cumulative risk of onset of RD in eyes with axial length ≤ 28.0 mm was 0.40%, 1.64%, 2.12%, and 2.62% for 6, 15, 48, and 52 through 147 months, respectively. In eyes with axial length >28.0 mm, the cumulative risk was 1.22%, 1.87%, 3.35%, and 4.42% for 4, 14, 42, and 63 through 117 months, respectively (Figure 3).[27]

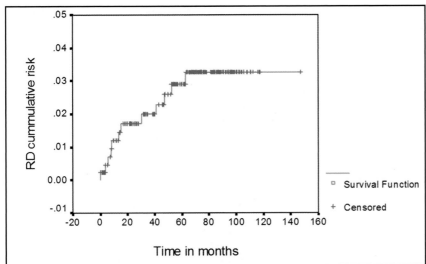

Figure 1. Kaplan-Maier analysis for the risk of RD. All eyes *n* = 439.

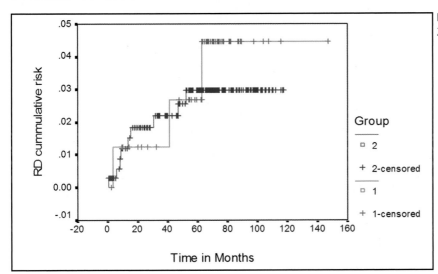

Figure 2. Kaplan-Maier analysis for the risk of RD. 1 = ≤ 50 years. 2 = > 50 years.

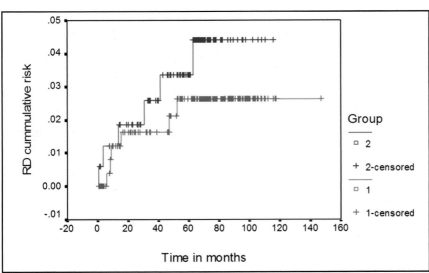

Figure 3. Kaplan-Maier analysis for the risk of RD. 1 = ≤ 28 mm. 2 = > 28 mm.

A trend was found indicating an association between age at surgery of less than 50 years and an increased risk of RD. Assuming that the risk of RD for group 1 (< 50 years) was 4.46% at 146 months compared to 2.96% at 118 months for group 2 (> 50 years), it would be necessary to include 1066 eyes in each group, making a total of 2132 eyes in the study to achieve statistical significance. Similarly, for the axial length categories, assuming that the cumulative risk of RD was 2.62% at 147 months for eyes with axial length ≤ 28.0 mm and 4.42% at 117 months for eyes with axial length >28.0 mm, it would be necessary to include 680 eyes in each group, totaling 1360 eyes in the study to achieve statistical significance with respect to axial length measurement.[27]

Other important factors when analyzing RD development after lens surgery are intraoperative capsular tear with vitreous loss and Nd:YAG laser capsulotomy.

Previous studies have demonstrated significant differences in the incidence of PCO after lens surgery. Fernandez-Vega reported an incidence of 77.89%,[15] Horgan 61%,[28] our study 34.6%,[27] Gabric 30.5%,[29] Tosi 16.4%,[20] and Colin 61.2% with 7 year follow-up.[24] However, such data are difficult to analyze due to variable follow-up periods, differing age groups (the younger the age, the greater the incidence of PCO), and the varying types of IOLs used. As such, reliable conclusions regarding the influence of Nd:YAG capsulotomy on the development of RD are difficult.

Conclusion

After an extensive analysis of the literature, including our latest case series (439 eyes), we could not define any particular risk factors related to the development of RD in the high myope following lens removal, although a trend, albeit not statistically significant, toward a higher incidence in patients with high axial length (> 28.0 mm) and age younger than 50 years was observed. A large multicenter collaborative study is recommended to gather a larger number of cases to ascertain conclusively which risk factors might lead to the occurrence of RD in highly myopic eyes and to determine the real risk of this complication. The findings will have important implications for the indications of lens removal.

References

1. Kaluzny J. Myopia and retinal detachment. *Polish Med J.* 1970;9:1544-1549.
2. Schepens CL, Marden D. Data on the natural history of retinal detachment: further characterization of certain unilateral nontraumatic cases. *Am J Ophthalmol.* 1966;61:213-226.
3. Michels RG, Wilkinson CD, Rice TA. *Retinal Detachment.* St. Louis, MO: Mosby; 1990:83-84.
4. Burton TC. The influence of refractive errors and lattice degeneration on the incidence of retinal detachment. *Trans Am Ophthalmol Soc.* 1990;87:143-155.
5. Alió JL, Ruiz-Moreno JM, Artola A. Retinal detachment as a potential hazard in surgical correction of severe myopia with phakic anterior chamber lenses. *Am J Ophthalmol.* 1993;115:145-148.
6. Ruiz-Moreno JM, Alió JL, Pérez-Santonja JJ, et al. Retinal detachment in phakic eyes with anterior chamber intraocular lenses to correct severe myopia. *Am J Ophthamol.* 1999;127:270-275.
7. Panozzo G, Parolini B. Relationships between vitreoretinal and refractive surgery. *Ophthalmology.* 2001;108:1663-1670.
8. Fechner PU, Strobel J, Wicchmann W. Correction of myopia by implantation of a concave Worst-iris claw lens into phakic eyes. *Refract Corneal Surg.* 1991;7:286-298.
9. Pesando PM, Ghiringhello MP, Tagliavacche P. Posterior chamber collamer phakic intraocular lens for myopia and hyperopia. *J Refract Surg.* 1999;5:415-423.
10. Zaldivar R, Davidorf JM, Oscherow S. Posterior chamber phakic intraocular lenses for myopia of −8 to −19. *J Refract Surg.* 1998;14:294-305.
11. Ruiz-Moreno JM, Alió JL. Incidence of retinal diseases following refractive surgery in 9,239 eyes. *J Refract Surg.* 2003;19:534-547.
12. Ruiz-Moreno JM, Montero J, de la Vega C, Alio JL, Zapater P. Retinal detachment in myopic eyes after phakic intraocular lens implantation. *J Refract Surg.* 2006;22:247-252.
13. Sanders DR. Actual and theoretical risks for visual loss following use of the implantable contact lens for moderate to high myopia. *J Cataract Refract Surg.* 2003; 29:1323-1332.
14. Alio JL, Piñero D, Bernabeu G, et al. The Kelman Duet phakic intraocular lens: 1-year results. *J Refract Surg.* 2007; 23:868-79..
15. Fernandez-Vega L, Alfonso JF, Villacampa T. Clear lens extraction for the correction of high myopia. *Ophthalmology.* 2003;110:2349-2354.
16. Pucci V, Morselli S, Romanelli F, et al. Clear lens phacoemulsification for correction of high myopia. *J Cataract Refract Surg.* 2001; 27:896-900.
17. Fan DS, Lam DS, Li KK. Retinal complications after cataract extraction in patients with high myopia. *Ophthalmology.* 1999;106:688-691.
18. Horgan N, Condon PI, Beatty S. Refractive lens exchange in high myopia: long term follow up. *Br J Ophthalmol.* 2005;89:670-672.
19. Ripandelli G, Scassa C, Parisi V, et al. Cataract surgery as a risk factor for retinal detachment in very highly myopic eyes. *Ophthalmology.* 2003;110:2355-2361.
20. Tosi GM, Casprini F, Malandrini A, et al. Phacoemulsification without intraocular lens implantation in patients with high myopia: long-term results. *J Cataract Refract Surg.* 2003;29:1127-1131.
21. Ravalico G, Michieli C, Vattovani O, et al. Retinal detachment after cataract extraction and refractive lens exchange in highly myopic patients. *J Cataract Refract Surg.* 2003;29:39-44.
22. Chastang P, Ruellan YM, Rozembaum JP, et al. Phakoémulsification à visée réfractive sur cristallin clair; a propos de 33 yeux myopes fortes. *J Fr Ophthalmol.* 1998;21:560-566.
23. Barraquer C, Cavelier C, Mejía LF. Incidence of retinal detachment following clear-lens extraction in myopic patient; retrospective analysis. *Arch Ophthalmol.* 1994;112:336-339.
24. Colin J, Robinet A, Cochener B. Retinal detachment after clear lens extraction for high myopia: seven-year follow-up. *Ophthalmology.* 1999;106:2281-2285.
25. Colin J, Robinet A. Clear lensectomy and implantation of a low-power posterior chamber intraocular lens for the correction of high myopia. *Ophthalmology.* 1994;101:107-112.
26. Colin J, Robinet A. Clear lensectomy and implantation of a low-power posterior chamber intraocular lens for the correction of high myopia: four-year follow-up. *Ophthalmology.* 1997;104:73-77.
27. Alió JL, Ruiz-Moreno JM, Shabayek MH, et al. The risk of retinal detachment in high myopia after small incision coaxial phacoemulsification. *Am J Ophthalmol.* 2007;144:93-98.
28. Horgan N, Condon PI, Beatty S. Refractive lens exchange in high myopia: long term follow up. *Br J Ophthalmol.* 2005;89:670-672.
29. Gabric N, Dekaris I, Karaman Z. Refractive lens exchange for correction of high myopia. *Eur J Ophthalmol.* 2002;12:384-387.

CHAPTER 201

RETINAL DETACHMENT RISK IN MYOPES

Kerry D. Solomon, MD and Luis E. Fernández de Castro, MD

Over the past 30 years, there have been few published population-based studies on the incidence of retinal detachment (RD). Most of those studies were done before 1982, and had multiple limitations because of variations in inclusion criteria and methods of data collection. Increasing age[1] and axial length of 25.00 mm or more[2] are known to be associated with an increase risk of RD. The overall risk of RD after cataract surgery increases to as high as 2% to 7% in eyes with high myopia.[3] In a large population-based case-control study, Tielch and colleagues[4] found that cataract surgery in patients with axial lengths of 26.00 mm or more were associated with an 8-fold higher risk of developing RD as compared with patients with axial lengths of 22.00 mm or less.

Modern cataract surgery is very successful in treating the visually significant cataract. The development of phacoemulsification and foldable intraocular lenses (IOLs) have allowed for smaller incisions and an overall safer procedure for the eye, including a decreased risk of RD. A recent review by Lois and Wong[2] compared RD rates described in the literature for intracapsular (ICCE), extracapsular (ECCE), and phacoemulsification techniques for cataract removal. Reviewed series showed RD rates of 1.0% to 6.7% for ICCE, 0.0% to 7.5% for ECCE, and 0.0% to 3.6% for phacoemulsification. Considering phacoemulsification after 1980, this RD rate drops to 0.0% to 0.9%.[2]

Numerous studies have presented combined results after ECCE and phacoemulsification. In general, their estimated risk for RD following cataract surgery are based on data from large databases, which have the advantage of providing sufficient power to study infrequent events in a specified population that is covered by that data source. However, the assessment and interpretation of incidence rates from such data sources are limited by their inability to take account of the influence of factors that are possible confounders—for example high myopia predisposing to RD. This may partially explain why some studies show a significant risk of RD following cataract surgery. Additionally, specific risk factors such as intraoperative events cannot be fully assessed because this type of information is not routinely collected in these databases unless a specific intervention has been performed that is related to the primary procedure. Additionally, some of the findings relate to clinical practices from more than 2 decades ago during a period characterized by changing surgical technique and technological advances in IOL design and development. An example is the study by Javitt and coauthors,[5] who reported 338,141 Medicare beneficiaries older than 65 years of age who underwent cataract extraction in 1984. The RD incidence over a 4-year evaluation was 1.55% for ICCE, 0.9% after ECCE, and 1.17% after phacoemulsification. This article does not differentiate between known high-risk factors associated with RDs, such as degree of myopia, axial lengths, and the presence or absence of peripheral retinal degeneration. Moreover, the article does not provide information relevant to intraoperative issues such as surgical technique, type of IOL inserted, surgical time, degree of anterior chamber collapse, vitreous manipulation, and the presence of a capsular tear.

The interest in refractive surgery, principally laser in situ keratomileusis (LASIK) and photorefractive keratectomy (PRK), grows each year. Many individuals undergoing these procedures have mild to moderate refractive errors. Refractive lens exchange (RLE) with placement of an IOL is a viable option for correcting refractive errors (hyperopia/myopia), with a high rate of excellent uncorrected and best-corrected visual acuities (UCVA and BCVA) in this population. With the advent of presbyopia-correcting IOLs, it is likely that there will be a significant rise in the number of RLE procedures. Because of the combination of success and safety with phacoemulsification procedures, their utility has extended to the treatment of refractive errors, particularly myopia. Addressing high myopia separately, RD after RLE with an IOL is important, as axial length is one of the risk factors for an RD after cataract surgery. Several reports have indicated RD rates similar to those found in phacoemulsification for cataracts. The RD rates associated with RLE in high myopic patients based on the literature from surgeries beginning in 1990 to present is variable, and ranges from 0% to 8.1%. The highest

Table 1

STUDIES FROM WHICH A RETINAL DETACHMENT RATE WAS ESTIMATED

Author (year)	Number of Cases	Axial Length ≤25 mm Number of Cases	Follow-Up (months)	Age ≥40 Years	Myopia ≤8 D	RD (%)
		Mean (Range) Filtered Data				
Boberg-Ans et al (2003)[7]	5797	21.4 to 25.0	15 to 52	N/A	N/A	0.17%
Olsen et al (2000)[8]	1024	<24.00	12 to 96	N/A	N/A	0%

Mo: months; D: diopters; RD: retinal detachment; N/A: not available.

incidence of RD was reported by Colin and collaborators,[6] who prospectively evaluated the incidence of complications following RLE, particularly RD, after 7 years of follow-up. The incidence of RD after RLE was nearly double that estimated for persons with myopia greater than −10.0 diopters (D) who do not undergo surgery.

In order to represent the true incidence of RD following modern routine cataract surgery, known risk factors for RD, such as axial length ≥25.00 mm and myopia ≥8.0 D need to be excluded from the populations studied. We identified pertinent articles on cataract surgery and RD published from 1990 up to 2007 in the peer-reviewed journals. These articles were reviewed and RD rates following cataract surgery were compiled. We then applied filters to the studies, so that high-risk individuals (axial length ≥25.00 mm and myopia ≥8.0 D) were excluded. This allowed us to analyze the RD risk associated with pseudophakia in typical patients undergoing cataract surgery or RLE, who were not higher myopes.

For RD following phacoemulsification, 18 articles were identified, and for RD following RLE, 16 articles were identified. These articles reported an incidence of RD for both phacoemulsification and RLE that varied from 0% to 8.61%, with a follow-up range between 2 months and 12 years. Only 2 articles had qualified data once filtered parameters were applied (Table 1).[7,8] The remaining articles did not disclose axial length, had short follow-up periods, combined results of ECCE and phacoemulsification, had too small a number of cases, or did not qualify once filtered parameters were set. The 2 qualifying articles encompass approximately 6800 cases with follow-up ranging from 12 to 96 months. The incidence of RD using small-incision phacoemulsification obtained once filtered parameters were applied was approximately 1 in 1000 or less. This figure is close to the general risk for RD in phakics eyes (unoperated) of 1.2 in 1000 in a matched age group.[7] The filtered parameters could not be applied to any of the RLE articles as they all exceeded the parameters described above.

In conclusion, our findings show a lower RD rate once risk factors associated with RD have been removed, filtered parameters placed, and surgeries limited from 1990 to present. We also showed that for the average patient undergoing modern cataract surgery or RLE, the rate of RD is approximately equal to the rate of RD in an unoperate eye. This would include hyperopia and mild to moderate myopia patients undergoing cataract or RLE surgery. A thorough evaluation is recommended preoperatively in all high myopes. It is important that risks of intraocular refractive lens surgery, including RD, are discussed in detail with prospective surgical candidates. Proper patient education regarding the risk and benefits of the various refractive surgical options is essential for a prospective patient who will undergo an elective procedure to make an informed decision.

References

1. Rowe JA, Erie JC, Baratz KH, et al. Retinal detachment in Olmsted County, Minnesota, 1976 through 1995. *Ophthalmology.* 1999;106:154-159.
2. Lois N, Wong D. Pseudophakic retinal detachment. *Surv Ophthalmol.* 2003;48:467-487.
3. Lyle WA, Jin GJC. Phacoemulsification with intraocular lens implantation in high myopia. *J Cataract Refract Surg.* 1996;22:238-242.
4. Tielsch JM, Legro MW, Cassard SD et al. Risk factors for retinal detachment after cataract surgery. A population-based control study. *Ophthalmology.* 1996;103:1537-1545.
5. Javitt JC, Vitale S, Canner JK, et al. National outcomes of cataract extraction, I. Retinal detachment after inpatient surgery. *Ophthalmology.* 1991;98:895-902.
6. Colin J, Robinet A, Cochener B. Retinal detachment after clear lens extraction for high myopia. Seven year follow up. *Ophthalmology.* 1999;106:2281-2285.
7. Boberg-Ans G, Villumsen J, Henning V. Retinal detachment after phacoemulsification cataract extraction. *J Cataract Refract Surg.* 2003;29:1333-1338.
8. Olsen G, Olson RJ. Update on a long-term, prospective study of capsulotomy and retinal detachment rates after cataract surgery. *J Cataract Refract Surg.* 2000;26:1017-1021.
9. Norregaard JC, Thoning H, Andersen TF, et al. Risk of retinal detachment following cataract extraction: results from the International Cataract Surgery Outcomes Study. *Br J Ophthalmol.* 1996;80:689-693.

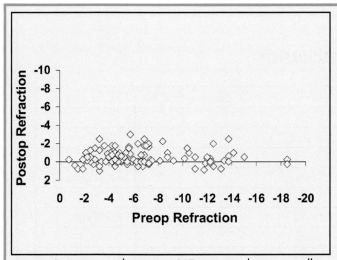

Figure 1. Patients undergoing RLE received an excellent refractive outcome, and most were within 1 D of target.

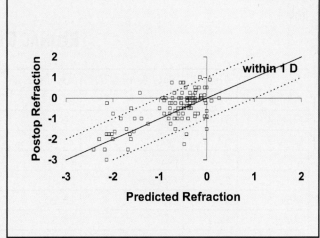

Figure 2. Patients undergoing RLE received an excellent refractive outcome, and most were within 1 D of target.

RETINAL DETACHMENT RISK IN MYOPES

James P. Gills, MD and Pit Gills, MD

When performing lens replacement surgery, retinal detachment is always a concern with high myopes. YAG capsulotomy, longer axial lengths, age, sex, and history of retinal holes are all known risk factors.

We examined a series of hyperopes and myopes who underwent refractive lens exchange (RLE) (also called clear lens replacement) to determine the retinal detachment rate and identify any other factors that could contribute to retinal detachment. Our series consisted of 452 hyperopic eyes and 438 myopic eyes.

The risk of retinal detachment is of greatest concern in myopes. Perkins[1] reports an annual risk of 0.68% for high myopes, whereas other citations in the literature range from 0% to 9.2%. Colin and colleagues[2] report an 8.1% (4 eyes) detachment rate in high myopes (> –12.0 diopters [D]) undergoing refractive lens exchange. Although it has been customary to classify myopia by refractive error, we quantify refractive error by axial length. We find this to be a more accurate indication of the myopic state of the eye, because it is not affected by corneal curvature.

Clear lens replacement was performed on patients from April 1997 to May 2005, before the availability of implantable contact lenses (ICLs). The axial lengths of these patients ranged from 19.38 to 33.37 mm. The surgeries were performed by 2 surgeons (Pit Gills, MD, and James P. Gills, MD), who used similar surgical techniques. Ninety-four percent of patients received a 2.5- to 3.0-mm limbal or corneal incision with a foldable lens. Six percent received a 5.5- to 6.0-mm incision to accommodate a polymethylmethacrylate (PMMA) lens in the required power.

Overall, patients undergoing RLE received an excellent refractive outcome, and most were within 1 D of target (Figures 1 and 2). The follow-up of our cohort ranges from 1997 to present. In the hyperopic group of 452 eyes, there were no retinal detachments. In the subset of 438 myopic eyes, the rate of retinal detachment is 1.7% (8 eyes of 6 patients).

All patients who experienced a retinal detachment received a 2.5-mm incision. There was no vitreous loss in any of the procedures performed on myopes or hyperopes. YAG capsulotomy was performed prior to the occurrence of the retinal detachment in four cases. Two patients had predisposing risk factors: one had a tear prior to the clear lens replacement procedure, and the second had a posterior vitreous detachment and a retinal hole. The range of axial lengths was 25.11 to 27.26 mm. When associated with lens removal and implant surgery, most retinal detachments occur within 4 months postoperatively. In our series, 5 of the cases occurred 2 years or later postoperatively (Table 1).

At the time the retinal detachment occurred in the patient with the prior retinal hole, the conventional teaching was to avoid prophylactic treatment. However, since our experience with this patient, we believe that prophylactic treatment is indicated in any patient with an operculum who is undergoing lens replacement surgery.

In our series, we found the risk of retinal detachment to be greatest among the moderate myopes with axial lengths ranging from 25 to 27 mm, rather than higher myopes with longer axial lengths. These moderate myopes are more likely to have lattice degeneration and are at greater risk for retinal holes. Therefore, a patient with lattice and a refractive error of –6.0 D may be at higher risk of retinal detachment than the –10-D myope. Patients in this axial length range who fall into this high-risk category should obtain clearance by a retinal specialist for prior to undergoing RLE or cataract surgery.

Lens replacement surgery is appropriate for presbyopes who are experiencing lenticular opacities; however, the availability of the ICL has afforded another treatment option for moderate to high myopes who have clear lenses. Whether performing cataract or RLE (clear lens replacement surgery), patients whose axial lengths are

Table 1

RETINAL DETACHMENTS

Sex	Age	YAG Before RD?	Axial Length	Time Between IOL Surgery and RD	Risk Factors
Female	51	Yes	25.25	3 years	
Female	51	No	25.11	1 month	
Female	62	Yes	25.39	2 years	
Male	54	No	27.26	2 years	Tear prior to CLR
Male	52	Not done	26.81	1 year	
Male	53	No	26.20	1.5 years	Hole; PVD
Male	44	Yes	25.65	1 year	
Male	44	Yes	25.74	3 years	

between 25 and 27 mm should be well informed of the risk of retinal detachment following surgery. In addition, these patients should be evaluated by a retinal specialist to determine if prophylactic treatment is required.

REFERENCES

1. Perkins ES. Morbidity from myopia. *Sight Saving Rev.* 1979;49:11-19.
2. Colin J, Robinet A, Cochener B. Retinal detachment after clear lens extraction for high myopia: seven-year follow-up. *Ophthalmology.* 1999;106(12):2281-2284.

CHAPTER 202

RETINAL DETACHMENT RISK WITH REFRACTIVE SURGERY

Yachna Ahuja, MD and Suber S. Huang, MD, MBA

Refractive Surgery and Its Complications

Refractive eye surgery has rapidly advanced over the past decade. Newer technologies, such as photorefractive keratectomy (PRK) and laser in situ keratomileusis (LASIK), have altered the types of complications as compared to older technologies such as radial keratotomy. This section serves as a brief overview of new technologies in refractive surgery and their main complications.

PRK and LASIK use the 193-nm argon fluoride excimer laser to ablate corneal stroma and thereby correct myopia. PRK involves the ablation of a disc-shaped area of corneal epithelium, which thereby changes the radius of curvature of the cornea. The most common complication of PRK is incomplete removal of the epithelium, leading to incomplete laser ablation and healing irregularities. This in turn causes postoperative corneal haze and irregular or induced astigmatism.[1-4] In contrast, LASIK involves placing a suction ring on the eye, which raises the intraocular pressure (IOP) and exposes the cornea, thereby creating a path for the microkeratome blade to create a hinged corneal flap. Laser is then used to ablate the stroma and the flap is replaced to its original position. Corneal flap abnormalities are the most common complication of LASIK, usually occurring when inadequate suction results in the creation of an irregular or thin flap, or when the corneal flap is improperly reoriented.[2-7]

Two alternatives to excimer laser corneal ablation are phakic intraocular lens (Ph-IOL) implantation and clear lens extraction (CLE). In Ph-IOL, the IOL is surgically placed at in the anterior or posterior chamber of the eye. Being an intraocular procedure, the risks include endothelial cell loss, infection, and cataract formation.[3-11] CLE involves the removal of the crystalline lens and its replacement with pseudophakic lens. Complications of this procedure include posterior capsular opacification and infection.[4-14] Retinal detachment (RD) has been noted as a rare complication of each procedure. Any type of ocular surgery can induce an inflammatory reaction that could in turn lead to retinal disease. In this article, we will focus on factors that are unique to refractive surgeries.

Mechanisms of Posterior Segments Injury Induced by Refractive Surgery

In PRK and LASIK, the impact of excimer laser shock waves on the cornea induces stress waves along the axis of the eye. As suggested by Seiler and later by Aras, these stress waves may lead to posterior segment complications particularly in eyes with preexisting vitreoretinal pathology.[5-17] However, Gobbi and colleagues demonstrated that laser photoablation-induced IOP changes in vitro and in porcine eyeballs produced no evidence of damage to the posterior segment.[6] Further experiments by Krueger and colleagues using excimer lasers on porcine and human eyeballs showed that whereas laser-induced stress waves reach maximum amplitudes of up to 100 atmospheres at the posterior lens and anterior vitreous, the wave amplitude decreases to about 10 atmospheres nearer to the retina. The authors proposed that waves of this amplitude did not pose any injury to the retinal and subretinal structures.[7,8]

A second factor posing risk to the retina during LASIK is the effect of the suction ring used to stabilize the eye. It has been postulated that the ensuing rise in IOP to pressures greater than 65 mm Hg leads to damage in the posterior segment of myopic eyes. Ozdamar and colleagues suggested that these sudden IOP changes may exert a mechanical stretch on the base of the vitreous body, which may in turn lead to RD.[9] A recent study by Davis and Evangelista involved ultrasonographically monitoring patients' eyes during LASIK. Their results showed that microkeratome suction did induce an elongation of the vitreous base; however, there was questionable significance of this finding in regards to causing

RD.[10] Other studies have shown that there are no significant changes in retinal nerve fiber layer thickness and the optic disc morphology when compared before and up to 1 year after LASIK.[11,12] The effect of traction on the vitreous base in a subset of susceptible individuals who have retinal thinning or, an abnormal vitreoretinal interface remains undetermined. Posterior vitreous detachment (PVD) rarely occurs in the typical age group for refractive surgery. However, PVD may paradoxically reduce the risk of RD by decreasing the likelihood of anterior–posterior traction on the vitreous base when stabilizing suction is applied.

Review of Reported Posterior Segment Complications Following Refractive Surgery

Previous reviews of the literature on posterior segment complications following refractive surgery have been extensive and detailed. Two excellent reviews summarize the individual case data reported in the literature on posterior segment complications following PRK, LASIK, and Ph-IOL.[13,14]

Postoperative posterior segment complications following refractive surgery that have been reported in the literature include RD, choroidal neovascularization, macular hemorrhages, macular holes, and optic neuropathy. Of these rare complications, the most frequently reported is RD. The occurrence of RD has been reported in 5 large series of LASIK patients. In 1999, Stulting and colleagues reported 1 RD out of 1062 eyes treated with LASIK (0.04%).[15] Two cases of RD were reported out of 3155 LASIK-treated eyes by Blumenkranz in 2000.[16] Arevelo and colleagues presented a case series in 2002 of 33 eyes with RD out of 38,823 LASIK-treated eyes (0.08%).[17] Ruiz-Moreno and Alio reported 11 cases out of 3009 eyes (0.36%) in 2003, whereas more recently in 2006, Lee reported 6 cases of RD out of 7065 eyes (0.08%).[18,19] Similar occurrence rates of RD following PRK have been reported in these studies. Each of these reported rates of RD is not greater than the estimated rate in myopes who have not undergone any refractive surgeries.

Comparatively higher rates of RD following Ph-IOL and CLE have been reported. For example, Ruiz-Moreno and Alio reported 7 eyes with RD out of 294 eyes that underwent anterior chamber Ph-IOL implantation (2.38%), though of note, the initial mean spherical equivalent refraction of the Ph-IOL patients was more than 5 D higher than those who underwent LASIK in the same case series reported in 2003.[18] Similarly, in a study by Fernandez-Vega and colleagues in 2003, out of 190 eyes treated with CLE with posterior-chamber IOL implantation, 4 eyes developed RD (2.10%).[4]

It is difficult to ascertain to what degree each of 2 important factors determines the risk of RDs following Ph-IOL and CLE. The first factor is the intraocular nature of these procedures, which in itself serves as an independent risk factor for RD. The second is that unlike laser corneal ablation surgeries, these procedures have the ability to correct high myopia. It follows that the majority of patients receiving Ph-IOL and CLE are generally higher myopes to begin with, which is another independent risk factor for RD.

Conclusion

Cases of posterior segment complications have been reported after most forms of refractive surgery. The incidence of these complications is exceedingly low when compared to the vast majority of refractive surgery cases that occur without subsequent posterior segment damage. To date, refractive surgery has not been directly implicated as the cause of the posterior segment pathologies in these infrequent cases.

An important issue that must be taken into consideration when discussing retinal pathologies in the patient population of refractive surgery is that the incidence of posterior segment pathologies is already significantly higher, because the majority of these patients are myopic. For this reason, there is controversy regarding whether cases of posterior segment pathologies are part of the natural process of myopic degeneration as opposed to being directly induced by the refractive surgery itself.

The identification of risk factors, if any, for post-refractive surgery retinal changes would indeed play an important role toward counseling specific groups of patients. However, it has still not been determined thus far whether those with high myopia or with preexisting posterior segment pathologies are at a higher risk for postoperative posterior segment complications.

Although Ph-IOL implantation and CLE have been associated with higher rates of postoperative retinal complications compared to excimer laser corneal ablation, it must be taken into consideration that these procedures carry the additional risk that comes with intraocular surgery. Also, patients selected for these procedures are usually significantly higher myopes than those undergoing PRK or LASIK. Thus, once again, it is difficult to determine whether the higher incidence of postoperative posterior segment pathologies is truly induced by the refractive procedure, or if it is related to the higher degree of myopia in the selected patient population.

In conclusion, though posterior segment complications have been associated with refractive surgery in many case series described in this review, the overall incidence and rate of postoperative posterior segment complications is very low. As with any other ocular surgery, prior to refractive surgery, there is always a role for a full ophthalmic examination, including dilated fundus examination to inspect the retina. When it comes to looking at the association of posterior segment complications with refractive surgeries though, it should be noted that modern refractive procedures, particularly LASIK, are widely practiced and many thousands of patients have been followed up without any ensuing posterior segment complications. Aside from standing the test of time, refractive surgery is showing steady improvement in outcomes with the advent of new technologies such as femtosecond laser-aided LASIK and wavefront-guided techniques. Techniques that do not distort the vitreous base may have a theoretic advantage in individuals at risk for development of RD.

References

1. McColin AZ, Steinert RF, Bafna S. Photorefractive keratectomy. In: Tasman W, Jaeger E, eds. *Duane's Clinical Ophthalmology*. Philadelphia: Lippincott; 2001.

2. Lui MM, Silas MA, Ugishima J. Complications of photorefractive keratectomy and laser in situ keratomileusis. *J Refract Surg*. 2003;19: S247-S249.

3. Fechner PU, Haigis W, Wichmann W. Posterior chamber myopia lenses in phakic eyes. *J Cataract Refract Surg*. 1996;22:178-182.

4. Fernandez-Vega L, Alfonso JF, Villacampa T. Clear lens extraction for the correction of high myopia. *Ophthalmology*. 2003;110:2349-2354.

5. Seiler T, McDonnell PJ. Excimer laser photorefractive kera-tectomy. *Surv Ophthamol*. 1995;40:89-118.

6. Gobbi PG, Carones F, Brancato R, et al. Acoustic transients following excimer laser ablation of the cornea. *Eur J Ophthalmol*. 1995;5:275-276.

7. Krueger RR, Krasinski JS, Radzewicz C, Stonecipher KG, Rowsey JJ. Photography of shock waves during excimer laser ablation of the cornea. *Cornea*. 1993;12:330-334.

8. Krueger RR, Seiler T, Gruchman T, Mrochen M, Berlin MS. Stress wave amplitudes during laser surgery of the cornea. *Ophthalmology*. 2001;108:1070-1074.

9. Ozdamar A, Aras G, Sener B, et al. Bilateral retinal detachment associated with giant retinal tear after laser-assisted in situ keratomileusis. *Retina*. 1998;18:176-177.

10. Davis RM, Evangelista JA. Ocular structure changes during vacuum by the Hansatome Microkeratome Suction Ring. *J Refract Surg*. 2007;23:563-566.

11. Gurses-Ozden R, Liebmann JM, Schuffner D, et al. Retinal nerve fiber thickness remains unchanged following laser-assisted in situ keratomileusis. *Am J Ophthalmol*. 2001;132:512-516.

12. Hamada N, Kaiya T, Oshika T, et al. Optic disc and retinal nerve fiber layer analysis with scanning laser tomography after LASIK. *J Refract Surg*. 2006;22:372-375.

13. Loewenstein A, Goldstein M, Lazar M. Retinal pathology occurring after laser excimer surgery or phakic intraocular lens implantation: evaluation of a possible relationship. *Surv Ophthalmol*. 2002;47:125-135.

14. Arevalo JF. Retinal complications after laser-assisted in situ keratomileusis (LASIK). *Curr Opin Ophthalmol*. 2004;15:184-191.

15. Stulting RD, Carr JD, Thompson KP, et al. Complications of laser in situ keratomileusis for the correction of myopia. *Ophthalmology*. 1999;106:13-20.

16. Blumenkranz MS. LASIK and retinal detachment: should we be concerned? [editorial]. *Retina*. 2000;5:578-581.

17. Arevalo JF, Ramirez E, Suarez E, et al. Retinal detachment in myopic eyes after laser in situ keratomileusis. *J Refract Surg*. 2002;18:708-714.

18. Ruiz-Moreno JM, Alio JL. Incidence of retinal disease following refractive surgery in 9,239 eyes. *J Refract Surg*. 2003;19:534-547.

19. Lee S-Y, Ong S-G, Yeo K-T, et al. Retinal detachment after laser refractive surgery at the Singapore National Eye Center [correspondence]. *J Cataract Refract Surg*. 2006;32:536-538.

20. Fernandez-Vega L, Alfonso JF, Villacampa T. Clear lens extraction for the correction of high myopia. *Ophthalmology*. 2003;110:2349-2354.

SECTION XIII

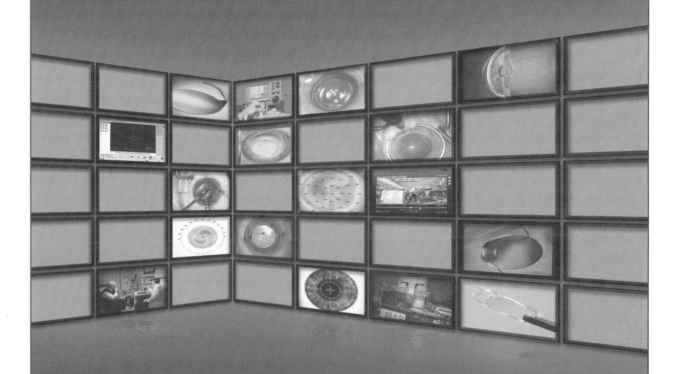

Enhancements

CHAPTER 203

APPROACHING ASTIGMATISM IN PRESBYOPIA IOL PATIENTS

Jason E. Stahl, MD

Presbyopia-correcting (Pr-C) intraocular lenses (IOLs) are a wonderful technology that we can provide to our patients. Whether used during refractive lens exchange (RLE) or cataract surgery, Pr-C IOLs require extreme precision as they treat both ametropia and presbyopia. Patients requesting Pr-C IOLs have high expectations that require the surgeon to achieve emmetropia (ie, ±0.25 diopter [D]) every time. This need for precision has renewed our attention to preoperative biometry to maximize the accuracy of IOL power calculations.

Pr-C IOLs also require surgeons to have a strategy for astigmatism correction. In my experience, as little as 0.75 D of astigmatism degrades visual quality and may leave a patient symptomatic with visual blur, ghosting, and halos. Surgical correction of astigmatism is now a necessity if one is to employ these IOLs. Because a toric Pr-C IOL platform is not yet available, surgeons must combine corneal refractive procedures (ie, limbal relaxing incisions [LRIs], laser in situ keratomileusis [LASIK], and photorefractive keratectomy [PRK]) with Pr-C IOLs to achieve the desired outcome.

Limbal Relaxing Incisions

These incisions provide a safe, effective, and practical approach for reducing ≤3.50 D of preexisting astigmatism. Paired 600-μm-deep arcuate incisions are placed in the cornea approximately 0.5 to 1 mm anterior to the limbus—on the steep meridian—at the time of lens replacement surgery. LRIs have several advantages over more centrally placed astigmatic keratotomy (AK): they are easier to perform and more forgiving than AKs; they have less tendency to induce irregular astigmatism; and there is a less likelihood of shifting in the resultant axis of cylinder. When paired LRIs are kept ≤90 degrees of arc length, they exhibit a consistent 1:1 coupling ratio (ie, the amount of flattening that occurs in the incised meridian, relative to the amount of steepening that results 90 degrees away) that elicits little change in spherical equivalence. Therefore, no alteration in the calculated lens power is needed.

Corneal topography is best used to determine the pattern, amount, and location of astigmatism. Additionally, topography can detect subtle corneal pathology that would contraindicate the use of LRIs (eg, forme fruste keratoconus). Refractive cylinder can be influenced by lenticular astigmatism, which is eliminated after removal of the crystalline lens, so surgeons should utilize topography and keratometry when treating astigmatism.

When planning the incisions, consult a nomogram that includes age modifiers (eg, Gills or Nichamin nomograms) to determine the appropriate arc length of the LRIs. Review the cylinder axis location on the corneal topography map; if there is a significant disparity between the keratometry and corneal topography (ie, ≥30 degrees), you may elect to defer the LRIs until the refraction stabilizes after lens replacement surgery. It is critical to properly center the LRIs over the steep corneal meridian because an axis deviation will result in a reduction in desired effect. Our clinic reported significant cyclotorsion when patients move from an upright to supine position.[1] Therefore, while the patient is upright, I recommend placing an orientation ink-mark at the limbus (ie, 6:00 or 12:00 position) to help identify the steep axis more accurately.

Laser Vision Enhancements

When planning Pr-C IOL surgery in a patient with a high level of preexisting astigmatism (ie, >3.00 D), a bioptics approach (ie, IOL followed by laser vision enhancement) may be needed. LRIs alone are unlikely to correct the astigmatism completely. Significant residual astigmatism in patients with Pr-C IOLs will result in suboptimal uncorrected vision. For this reason, patients will want the shortest possible interval before laser enhancement is performed.

There are several different strategies for these planned laser vision enhancements. The first is to perform the Pr-C IOL surgery followed by LASIK or PRK. LASIK surgery requires placing a suction ring on the eye that significantly increases the intraocular pressure during the flap creation. Allowing

Figure 1. Holladay II IOL Report: pre-LASIK and post-LASIK report demonstrating no change in keratometry prior to RLE surgery.

Pre-LASIK	Post-LASIK
OS Surgeon: Refraction: +5.50 -5.00 X 167 Vertex: 12.00 BCVA: 20/20 UCVA: 20/100 K1: 41.50 @170 K2: 45.75 @80 Average K: 43.63 Adjusted K: 43.63 Axial Len: 23.27 ILM Adj. AL: Hor W-t-W: 12.80 Phakic ACD: 3.41 Phakic Lens Th.: 0.00 Target Ref: 0.00 Tgt Add: 0.00	**OS** Surgeon: Refraction: +2.50 -0.50 X 10 Vertex: 12.00 BCVA: 20/20 UCVA: 20/100 K1: 43.25 @45 K2: 44.00 @135 Average K: 43.63 Adjusted K: 43.63 Axial Len: 23.20 ILM Adj. AL: Hor W-t-W: 12.80 Phakic ACD: 3.17 Phakic Lens Th.: 0.00 Target Ref: 0.00 Tgt Add: 0.00

Pre-LASIK		Post-LASIK	
Lens #2 **ReSTOR** Procedure: **Std Phaco** **MFG ACD: 5.02**		Lens #2 **ReSTOR** Procedure: **Std Phaco** **MFG ACD: 5.02**	
IOL	**Pred. Ref.**	**IOL**	**Pred. Ref.**
20.50	0.54	20.50	0.57
21.00	0.19	21.00	0.23
21.28	**0.00**	**21.32**	**-0.00**
21.50	-0.16	21.50	-0.12
22.00	-0.51	22.00	-0.48

Figure 2. Holladay II IOL Report: pre-LASIK and post-LASIK report demonstrating no significant change in change in IOL power of +21.0 D prior to RLE surgery.

phacoemulsification incisions 12 weeks to heal ensures that these incisions will not rupture during LASIK enhancement. Because PRK surgery does not use a suction ring, the PRK enhancement can be performed when the refraction has stabilized which is usually 4 to 6 weeks following IOL surgery. The second approach is to only create the LASIK flap 1 to 2 weeks before Pr-C IOL surgery, followed by lift flap LASIK enhancement 4 to 6 weeks later. This approach allows for an earlier enhancement, when the refraction stabilizes similar to the PRK option, because the LASIK flap has already been created and can simply be lifted to perform laser ablation. I prefer the third and final approach, which is to perform LASIK or PRK to reduce the astigmatism before Pr-C IOL surgery. The latter provides the patient with the best functional vision immediately following Pr-C IOL implantation. Because the preoperative data for IOL calculations is available, determining the IOL power following LASIK or PRK is not difficult. If needed, additional laser treatment could still be used to further enhance the patient's vision.

A perfect time to use the third approach, laser vision correction first followed by Pr-C IOL surgery, is when the patient has a high level of hyperopic astigmatism. A mixed astigmatism laser ablation is performed first to reduce the astigmatism without significantly changing the average keratometry. Minimal to no change in IOL power is needed when compared with pre-LASIK/PRK calculations. For example, a 64-year-old male presented with a manifest refraction OS of +5.50−5.00 × 167 = 20/20 with average keratometry of 43.63 D. Conventional LASIK was performed treating +2.50−5.00 × 167. One month postoperatively, the refraction was +2.50−0.50 × 10 = 20/20, with average keratometry unchanged at 43.63 D (Figure 1). Refractive lens exchange was performed with insertion of a +21.0 D ReSTOR IOL (Alcon Laboratories, Fort Worth, TX), which was the same power calculated prior to the LASIK (Figure 2). One month following RLE with ReSTOR, the patient's uncorrected visual acuity (UCVA)-distance was 20/20 and UCVA-near was 20/20, with refraction of +0.25−0.25 × 164.

Conclusion

Pr-C IOLs are currently the most exciting advancement in cataract and refractive surgery. Patients demand and expect great results with Pr-C IOLs. The challenges that surgeons face in meeting these expectations require extreme precision, not only when performing IOL power calculations but also when dealing with preexisting or residual astigmatism. Developing a strategy for astigmatism correction will help surgeons meet or even exceed Pr-C IOL patient expectations.

References

1. Ciccio A, Durrie D, Stahl J, Schwendeman F. Ocular cyclotorsion during customized laser ablation. *J Refract Surg.* 2006;21:S772-S774.

CHAPTER 204

APPROACHING ASTIGMATISM IN PRESBYOPIA IOL PATIENTS

Rick Milne, MD

The treatment of astigmatism at the time of cataract surgery, or post cataract surgery, has become an increasingly important part of the ophthalmic surgeon's practice. Two factors determine whether astigmatism should be addressed. The first is the patient's postoperative desires, and the second is the lens that the surgeon chooses for the patient.

The Patient's Desire

Listen to the patient: A 1-page questionnaire is very helpful as Stephen Dell and others have developed.

The starting point in making a decision of whether or not to treat astigmatism at the time of cataract surgery is the patient's preoperative assessment. It is essential for the surgeon to determine just what the patient is hoping to obtain from their postoperative outcome. If the patient has little desire to reduce dependence on eyeglasses after surgery, then astigmatism issues may be left untreated. If on the other hand the patient desires to be as free of glasses as possible, then addressing astigmatism as part of the surgical plan becomes essential.

Once it is decided that astigmatism treatment will be needed, it is wise to explain to the patient that they have 2 problems that must be corrected in order to achieve their best visual outcome. The first problem is in their lens, and it will be addressed with lens replacement during cataract surgery. I then explain astigmatism to the patient and let them know that it is possible that they may need additional fine-tuning of this problem postoperatively to give them their best opportunity for minimizing their need for glasses.

The next critical preoperative question is to determine which implant will best achieve the patient's postoperative goal. Do they want just good uncorrected distance vision postoperatively, or do they seek good near and distance vision without glasses? If they want both near and distance, then I must discern if they would (1) prefer mild-to-moderate mono-

vision with the potential need for reading glasses for fine print, or (2) if they would want premium multifocal intraocular lenses (IOLs) to try an give them binocular near and distance vision. Patients are also asked if they would have a significant problem with nighttime halos or glare, which occur much more frequently with multifocal IOLs in the presence of residual astigmatism.

It is explained that the more sophisticated the approach and the more we are trying to accomplish, the greater the potential need is for fine-tuning postoperative astigmatism or spherical refractive error. I explain the additional costs that would be incurred by the patient. I allow my staff to go over these details later.

With this background, what do I specifically do to treat corneal astigmatism in patients who need such treatment to get their best postoperative visual quality?

The Preoperative Work Up

A detailed preoperative astigmatism work up is a must and includes autorefraction, manifest refraction, checking the oldest refraction on record, K readings, Pentacam (Oculus, Inc., Lynwood, WA) testing, and corneal pachymetry. It is crucial to make sure you are not about to operate on a pathologic cornea, such as one with a corneal ectasia. It is also crucial that the patient has not worn soft contact lenses for 3 days, and hard or gas-permeable for at least 4 weeks, just like we require for laser vision correction (LVC) surgery.

It is also crucial to make determine how much of the astigmatism is corneal and how much is lenticular. If the K reading, the Pentacam testing, and the best refraction do not agree on the amount of corneal astigmatism, I do not address the astigmatism at the time of surgery. Instead, I wait to see the amount and axis of their residual astigmatism is postoperatively before planning a treatment.

Explain the Plan to the Patient

I tell the patient if we will be addressing their astigmatism as a second step after their eye has healed and what this might entail.

After listening to the patient, and reviewing their questionnaire answers, I choose the implant they will be receiving.

OPTIONS FOR THE PATIENT WANTING ONLY GOOD DISTANCE OR MONOVISION WITHOUT GLASSES

If after listening to the patient and determining that they will accept a mild monovision result, I can use either of 2 strategies. One would be to use monofocal IOLs aiming for plano in dominant eye, and –1.50 in the nondominant eye. The second option is to upgrade them to the Crystalens (Eyeonics, Aliso Viejo, CA) targeting plano in dominant eye, and –0.50 in the nondominant eye.

With these strategies, astigmatism of –0.75 or less are often as beneficial as they are detrimental. Therefore, I do not treat these lower amounts of astigmatism at the time of surgery, choosing instead to assess the patient's symptoms postoperatively.

If the patient has significant corneal astigmatism and is happy either with wearing reading glasses or targeting moderate monovision, then we have an excellent candidate for a toric IOL.

Our newest option in this category is the Alcon (Fort Worth, TX) AcrySof toric IOL. This acrylic single-piece haptic lens is available in 3 cylindrical powers: 1.5, 2.25, and 3.0 D in the IOL plane.

The acrylic material of the Acrysof toric provides excellent rotational stability. The data from the Food and Drug Administration (FDA) trial indicate that the AcrySof toric lens rarely rotates more than 5 degrees. The trial also showed that 82% of patients receiving these lenses achieved 20/20 or better postoperative vision.

PATIENTS DESIRING MULTIFOCAL INTRAOCULAR LENS OUTCOMES

If the patient chooses a premium multifocal IOL, I prefer using the ReZoom IOL (American Medical Optics, Santa Ana, CA) in the first eye. Three weeks postoperatively, I assess the refractive error, and the patient's postoperative satisfaction with the first eye. If all is well, then I recommend a ReZoom in the second eye. If their intermediate vision is good but the near vision is disappointing, then I recommend a ReSTOR (Alcon, Fort Worth, TX) in the second eye. Many in Europe are finding excellent results with the mixing the Tecnis multifocal IOL (Advanced Medical Optics) and the ReZoom.

If the patient has significant residual refractive error at 3 weeks, I often correct this before doing surgery on the second eye. Patients who are paying for premium outcomes seem to like this conservative approach.

Astigmatism Correction— Corneal Solutions

1. If I am considering astigmatic correction at the time of surgery it has become my practice to only do LRIs with a preset 600-μm blade. Once again preoperative corneal evaluation must document that the astigmatism is corneal; you do not want to treat lenticular astigmatism with LRIs. I have found Dr. Nichamin's nomograms, which specify the use of LRIs according to the type of astigmatism and the patient's age, to be invaluable. The standard Nichamin nomogram is the most conservative approach. I use this to treat 1 to 2 D of preexisting astigmatism. I do get preoperative pachymetry even for these conservative peripheral incisions to prevent any unwarranted surprises. I prefer to do these incisions at the start of the procedure before the anterior chamber has been entered.

2. Two situations will dictate delaying astigmatism correction until after cataract surgery. The first is uncertainty over the amount of astigmatism that is lenticular, whereas the second is patients with large amounts of astigmatism (eg, over 2 D). (One can be successful in treating up to 4 D with a combination of the Acrysof toric combined with LRIs.)

If the astigmatism is to be treated with a 2-stage procedure, then I tell the patient they will not achieve their final visual outcome for up to 3 or more months after their IOL surgery.

I usually treat 0.75 D of residual astigmatism or more in these patients. However, ReSTOR and ReZoom patients experience more dysphotopsias from residual astigmatism than their plano counterparts. In these instances, we may have to try to treat as little as 0.5 D of residual astigmatism.

The 3 options I choose postoperatively follow:

1. LRIs if not done previously for up to 2 D of astigmatism as discussed above. I feel comfortable doing these at 6 weeks postoperatively. These incisions have a coupling effect and there is therefore little shift in the spherical equivalent.

2. LVC

   a. Laser in situ keratomileusis (LASIK)—if the surgeon knows that there is greater than 2.5 D of astigmatism that needs to be addressed and they prefer LASIK as their LVC procedure of choice, then the flap should be cut 2 weeks preoperatively. Many surgeons are not comfortable with applying a suction ring for at least 3 months following cataract surgery. If the flap has been cut preoperatively, LASIK fine-tuning can be performed after the postoperative refraction is stable, which is usually 4 to 6 weeks after IOL surgery. If possible I use the Custom Cornea and iris registration software with the VISX (Santa Clara, CA) system.

b. Surface ablation is often preferred in these older patients and can once again be done once the refraction is stable by the 4- to 6-week postoperative time period.

3. Conductive keratoplasty (CK). This has been an excellent tool to fine tune eyes with residual astigmatism. The treatment may cause a slight myopic shift at the time of application. Two spots at 8 mm along the flattest axis will give a 1-D response, whereas 2 at the 7-mm ring position will give 2 D of flattening in most patients. CK can be used in conjunction with LRIs if the treatment is placed 90 degrees from the LRI axis. If CK spots are placed too close to the LRIs, they may cause unpredictable gaping of the relaxing incision.

Conclusion

Astigmatism does add an additional layer of complexity to the challenge of achieving the patient's desired refractive outcome. Combining proper patient selection and education with the proper astigmatic procedure can achieve excellent outcomes.

The next step forward in meeting this challenge will be the availability of a toric multifocal, and or toric accommodating, lens. Both are under development, and we await their availability with great anticipation.

CHAPTER 205

TOLERANCE OF RESIDUAL REFRACTIVE ERROR AFTER RESTOR

Luis Fernández-Vega, MD, PhD; José F. Alfonso, MD, PhD; Robert Montés-Micó, PhD

Refractive lens exchange (RLE) with a presbyopia correcting IOL is an attractive procedure to treat ametropia and presbyopia. It has the added benefit of also avoiding later cataract surgery. We have recently reported on our success with RLE while utilizing the AcrySof ReSTOR.[1] RLE with the Array multifocal IOL has been demonstrated to be a safe and effective refractive surgery modality.[2-4] Accurate biometry and IOL calculations with minimal residual refractive error are critical to optimal objective and subjective outcomes with presbyopia-correcting IOLs. Residual refractive error can usually be improved with laser vision correction,[5] IOL exchange, or piggyback IOL implantation.[6] Multifocal IOLs have a greater depth-of-focus compared to monofocal IOLs. This increased depth-of-focus would be expected to increase the patient's defocus tolerance.[6] It might also have an effect on neural adaptation to blurred images.[7,8] We will discuss our experience with patients' tolerance to defocus caused by residual refractive errors in patients who have had RLE with an AcrySof ReSTOR IOL.

We recently examined 150 eyes of 75 consecutive patients who underwent bilateral implantation of the AcrySof ReSTOR Natural IOL at the Instituto Ofthalmológico Fernández-Vega (Oviedo, Spain). Axial length and anterior chamber depth was measured with the Zeiss Humphrey IOLMaster (Carl Zeiss Meditec, Inc). The SRK/T formula was used to calculate IOL powers for myopic patients. The Holladay II formula was used for to calculate IOL powers for hyperopic patients. The targeted refraction was emmetropia in all patients. All surgeries were accomplished using a clear corneal incision of between 2.8 to 3.2-mm incision by 2 experienced surgeons (L.F.V., J.F.A.).

The AcrySof ReSTOR apodized, diffractive IOL (SN60D3 model) was implanted bilaterally, approximately 2 weeks apart. Monocular uncorrected distance visual acuity (UCDVA), best corrected distance visual acuity (BCDVA), uncorrected distance near visual acuity (UCNVA), and best distance-corrected near visual acuity (BCNVA) were recorded postoperatively at 6 m and 33 cm, respectively, in all patients.

Postoperative assessments were routinely performed at 1 week, 1, 3, and 6 months after the surgery. All patients completed 6 months of follow-up.

The data was analyzed with the method developed by Thibos and Horner[9] to represent and analyze spherocylindrical refractive errors. Using this notation, we are able to express any spherocylindrical refractive error by 3 dioptric powers: M, J0, and J45. M is a spherical lens equal to the spherical equivalent of the given refractive error. J0 and J45 two Jackson crossed cylinders equivalent to the conventional cylinder. These numbers are the coordinates of a point in a 3-dimensional dioptric space, being the power vector that originated from the origin of this space to the point (M, J0, J45). Consequently, the length of this vector is a measure of the overall blurring strength (B) of a spherocylindrical refractive error. Manifest refractions in conventional script notation [S (sphere), C (cylinder) × Φ (axis)] were converted to power vectors coordinates and B by the following formulas: $M = S + C/2$; $J0 = (-C/2) \cos (2\Phi)$; $J45 = (-C/2) \sin (2\Phi)$; $B = (M2 + J02 + J452)^{1/2}$. Trends for differences between visual acuity as a function of M value were assessed by regression analysis (we considered a $p < .01$ as statistically significant).

We have previously reported the safety, efficacy, predictability, and stability of this technique to be excellent.[1,10] A statistical summary of the distribution of the vector conversion of manifest refractive errors after RLE is shown in Tables 1 through 5, including UCDVA, BCDVA, and UCNVA. The patient demographics are listed in Table 5. There is a statistically significant improvement in UCDVA when residual refractive error was corrected both for myopic and hyperopic groups (BCDVA; $p < 0.001$). No differences were observed between UCNVA and BCNVA ($p > 0.2$). Figure 1 shows a scatter plot for the UCDVA and BCDVA versus M value for distance (top) and near (bottom) in myopic eyes. We found a significant trend toward lower visual acuity with M for UCDVA ($R = 0.77$, $p < 0.001$). In contrast, no significant trends were found for BCDVA, UCNVA and BCNVA as a function of M ($R = 0.11$, $p = 0.09$; $R = 0.07$, $p = 0.26$ and $R = 0.08$,

Table 1

SUMMARY OF RESIDUAL REFRACTIVE ERRORS AFTER RLE FOR THE MYOPIC PATIENTS

	M	J_0	J_{45}	B
Mean	−0.325	0.049	0.023	0.507
SD	0.465	0.272	0.195	0.422

Table 2

SUMMARY OF RESIDUAL REFRACTIVE ERRORS AFTER RLE FOR THE HYPEROPIC PATIENTS

	M	J_0	J_{45}	B
Mean	−0.122	0.044	−0.005	0.397
SD	0.466	0.233	0.189	0.384

Table 3

POSTOPERATIVE VISUAL ACUITIES IN DECIMAL FORM FOR THE MYOPIC PATIENTS

	UCDVA	BCDVA	UCNVA	BCNVA
Mean	0.767	0.972	0.917	0.923
SD	0.256	0.062	0.121	0.118

Table 4

THESE ARE THE POSTOPERATIVE VISUAL ACUITIES IN DECIMAL FORM FOR THE HYPEROPIC PATIENTS

	UCDVA	BCDVA	UCNVA	BCDVA
Mean	0.804	0.957	0.903	0.918
SD	0.218	0.077	0.137	0.111

Table 5

DEMOGRAPHIC CHARACTERISTICS OF PARTICIPANTS

	Myopic Group	Hyperopic Group
No. of eyes	50	100
Mean Age (yrs) ± SD	52.3 ± 4.1	51.7 ± 4.8
Range of Age (yrs)	45 to 70	45 to 70
Gender (M/F)	10/15	18/32
Mean IOL Power (D) ± SD	14.2 ± 3.0	24.2 ± 3.1
Mean Preoperative Sphere (D) ± SD	−5.43 ± 2.71	3.41 ± 2.33
Range of Preoperative Sphere (D)	−0.75 to −10	0.75 to 8
Mean Preoperative Cylinder (D) ± SD	−0.85 ± 0.56	−0.71 ± 0.74
Range of Preoperative Cylinder (D)	0 to 1.50	0 to 1.50
Mean Preoperative Keratometry (D) ± SD		
K1	43.44 ± 1.32	42.49 ± 1.53
K2	44.37 ± 1.24	43.55 ± 1.42
Range of Preoperative Keratometry (D)	40.50 to 48.00	39.00 to 47.50
Mean Axial Length (mm) ± SD	25.42 ± 1.21	22.12 ± 0.83
Range of Axial Length (mm)	23.32 to 28.77	20.26 to 24.74
Photopic pupil diameter (mm) ± SD	3.11 ± 0.56	3.14 ± 0.62

IOL = intraocular lens; SD = standard deviation

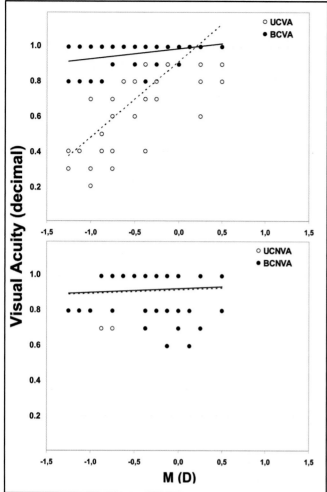

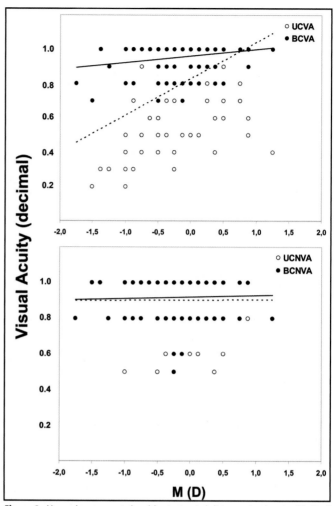

Figure 1. Monocular uncorrected and best-corrected distance visual acuity (decimal) (top) and uncorrected distance near visual acuity and best distance-corrected near visual acuity (bottom) versus spherical equivalent (M) value in diopters for previously myopic eyes. The dashed lines represent the best linear trend equation for UCDVA (y = 0.43x + 0.91; R = 0.77, p < 0.001) and UCNVA (y = 0.02x + 0.92; R = 0.07, p = 0.26). The solid lines represent the best linear trend equation for BCDVA (y = 0.06x + 0.99; R = 0.11, p = 0.09) and BCNVA (y = 0.02x + 0.92; R = 0.08, p = 0.24).

Figure 2. Monocular uncorrected and best-corrected distance visual acuity (decimal) (top) and uncorrected distance near visual acuity and best distance-corrected near visual acuity (bottom) versus spherical equivalent (M) value (D) in hyperopic pseudophakic eyes. The dashed lines represent the best linear trend equation for UCDVA (y = 0.21x + 0.82; R = 0.41, p < .001) and UCNVA (y = 0.01x + 0.90; R = 0.03, p = .31). The solid lines represent the best linear trend equation for BCVA (y = 0.04x + 0.96; R = 0.12, p = .08) and BCNVA (y = 0.01x + 0.91; R = 0.06, p = .27).

p = 0.24, respectively). There is a similar finding in the corresponding data for hyperopic eyes (Figure 2). A significant trend toward lower visual acuity with M for UCDVA was found (R = 0.41, p < 0.001). No significant trends were found for BCDVA, UCNVA, and BCNVA as a function of M (R = 0.12, p = 0.08; R = 0.06, p = 0.27, and R = 0.03, p = 0.31, respectively). Figure 3 graphs the Blur (B) versus the residual spherical equivalent in vector notation (M) for the myopic and hyperopic eyes. It demonstrates that outside of a narrow range around zero refractive error, there is a decrease in blur associated with a decrease in residual refractive error.

RLE with a multifocal IOL is an interesting refractive surgery option. Our experience suggests that the unaided visual outcome is predicted by the residual refractive error. These patients have undergone elective surgery to reduce their dependence on glasses. They are not interested in having their residual refractive error corrected by contact lenses or glasses. They readily accept laser vision correction as an enhancement to improve their uncorrected visual acuity and desire to

maximize the visual outcome of their primary refractive procedure or RLE. However, after multifocal IOL implantation some residual refractive errors may be tolerated because the large depth-of-focus associated with a multifocal IOL.

It is clear there is a significant reduction of UCDVA with increasing blur (M) whereas there is not a similar reduction in near vision. In other words, as the amount of residual spherical equivalent error increases the effective blur for distance increases. The results are similar for both previously myopic and hyperopic eyes. There is a small range around zero spherical equivalent error with associated minimal changes in blur seen in Figure 3. Otherwise, the blur increases rapidly as the refractive error increases. This is consistent with the clinical findings observed in our patients and with published data about the effect of defocus correction on visual acuity.[11] The most striking finding is to observe how both UCNVA and BCNVA show similar trends for both myopic and hyperopic eyes (see Figures 1 and 2). These results suggest that near visual acuity does not vary as much if residual distance

Figure 3. The overall blurring strength (B, diopters) versus spherical equivalent (M, diopters) values. The lines represent the best polynomial trend equation (quadratic) for myopes (solid line; y = 0.75x2 − 0.15x + 0.21) and hyperopes (dashed line; y = 0.49x2 −0.13x + 0.27).

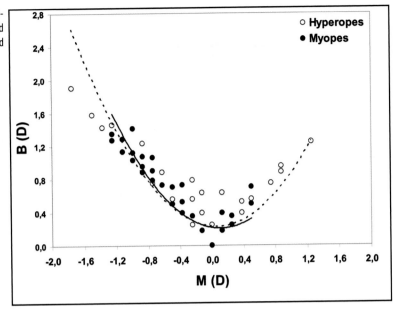

refractive error is corrected or not. It is likely that our patients are autocorrecting their refractive error at near by positioning the target to correct their effective SE at near. This strategy will work so long as there is minimal astigmatic error and the SE error is not large.

Pupil size and age need to be considered. A small pupil decreases the eye's blur circle creating a sharper retinal image.[12] The smaller the pupil, the greater the depth-of-focus is, whether in phakic eyes[13] or eyes implanted with a pseudoaccommodative IOL.[14] The relative effect on pupil size may vary depending on the optical design of the pseudoaccommodative IOL. Recently, we have reported that a larger pupil was significantly correlated with better distance visual acuity and with worse near visual acuity in patients implanted with the AcrySof ReSTOR IOL.[15]

To summarize our experience, a surgeon should strongly consider a secondary refractive procedure to optimize the visual acuity of any patient who has residual refractive error after RLE with a multifocal IOL. We have seen that the patient is relatively intolerant to defocus at distance caused by residual refractive errors in patients implanted with the ReSTOR IOL for RLE. After correcting these residual refractive errors, the blur at distance improves. There is no associated improvement in blur at near when correcting these small residual refractive errors. Near visual acuity is maintained if residual refractive error is corrected or not. We have noted similar differences in blur tolerance in patients implanted with the ReSTOR after cataract surgery.

References

1. Fernández-Vega L, Alfonso JF, Rodríguez PP, Montés-Micó R. Clear lens extraction with multifocal apodized diffractive intraocular lens implantation. *Ophthalmology.* 2007;114:1491-1498.

2. Packer M, Fine IH, Hoffman RS. Refractive lens exchange with the Array multifocal intraocular lens. *J Cataract Refract Surg.* 2002;28:421-424.

3. Dick HB, Gross S, Tehrani M, et al. Refractive lens exchange with an Array multifocal intraocular lens. *J Cataract Refract Surg.* 2002;28:509-518.

4. Waltz KL, Wallace RB. PRELEX: surgery to implant multifocal intraocular lenses ophthalmic practice. 2001;19:343-346.

5. Leccisotti A. Secondary procedures after presbyopic lens exchange. *J Cataract Refract Surg.* 2004;30:1461-1464.

6. Wang B, Ciuffreda KJ. Depth-of-focus of the human eye: theory and clinical implications. *Surv Ophthalmol.* 2006;51:75-85.

7. Webster MA, Georgeson MA, Webster SM. Neural adjustments to image blur. *Nat Neurosci.* 2002;5:839-840.

8. Montés-Micó R, Alió JL. Distance and near contrast sensitivity function after multifocal intraocular lens implantation. *J Cataract Refract Surg.* 2003;29:703-711.

9. Thibos LN, Horner DG. Power vector analysis of the optical outcome of refractive surgery. *J Cataract Refract Surg.* 2001;27:80-85.

10. Alfonso JF, Fernández-Vega L, Baamonde MB, Montés-Micó R. Prospective visual evaluation of apodized diffractive intraocular lenses. *J Cataract Refract Surg.* 2007;33:1235-1243.

11. Smith G, Jacobs RJ, Chan CD. Effect of defocus on visual acuity as measured by source and observer methods. *Optom Vis Sci.* 1989;66:430-435.

12. Montés-Micó R, España E, Bueno I, et al. Visual performance with multifocal intraocular lenses: mesopic contrast sensitivity under distance and near conditions. *Ophthalmology.* 2004;111:85-96.

13. Atchison DA, Charman WN, Woods RL. Subjective depth-of focus of the eye. *Opt Vis Sci.* 1997;74:511-520.

14. Montés-Micó R, Ferrer-Blasco T, Charman WN, Cerviño A, Alfosno JF, Fernández-Vega L. Optical quality of the eye after lens replacement by a pseudoaccommodative intraocular lens. *J Cataract Refract Surg.* In press.

15. Alfonso JF, Fernández-Vega L, Baamonde MB, Montés-Micó R. Correlation of pupil size with visual acuity and contrast sensitivity after implantation of an apodized diffractive intraocular lens. *J Cataract Refract Surg.* 2007;33:430-438.

CHAPTER 206

SHOULD I LEARN PRK/LASIK OR REFER THESE OUT?

Helen Wu, MD

As the cataract surgeon transitions to refractive intraocular lenses (IOLs), the need for enhancement of residual refractive error inevitably arises. The incidence of residual refractive error after refractive IOLs ranges from approximately 3% to 25%. This number varies greatly between surgeons and possibly between different IOLs, but is the most common reason for patient dissatisfaction after refractive IOLs. Generally speaking, greater than 0.5 diopter (D) of myopia, hyperopia, or astigmatism will cause the patient to experience some blurring of vision after surgery. IOL power predictability may be adversely affected by small inaccuracies in keratometry readings, axial length measurements, or positioning of the lens within the individual eye (especially with accommodating IOLs). Relatively small errors at each step in the process may combine to produce a more significant net refractive surprise, and the need for enhancement should be addressed as soon as refractive stability is achieved. In the case of cataract surgery after previous corneal refractive surgery, the predictability of the IOL power is compromised even further, and patients should be counseled prior to the surgery about enhancement surgery, and understand that they are more likely than the average patient who has not had refractive surgery to have an error in IOL calculation.

The factors that influence patient satisfaction after cataract surgery include visual acuity, the ability to perform activities of daily living without visual aberrations such as glare, and the experience of the surgery itself, including intraoperative and postoperative discomfort. Preoperative expectations are important in determining patient satisfaction postoperatively as well. Those individuals who undergo refractive cataract surgery, however, may have additional expectations similar to those patients who undergo refractive surgery. This may be true particularly in younger patients with incipient cataracts, or those who undergo refractive lens exchange for essentially clear lenses, especially when their preoperative refractions are near emmetropia. In refractive patients, satisfaction is directly correlated to their ability to see well without glasses, which

typically means that at least one eye is 20/20 and their refractive error is within ±0.5 D.

The timing of enhancements after refractive cataract surgery depends on the stability of the patient's refraction. Generally, eyes that receive multifocal IOLs will achieve refractive stability within a matter of several weeks, whereas those that receive accommodative IOLs will require up to several months to achieve stability, due to the variability of where the lens is positioned in these eyes.

Once refractive stability is achieved, the decision of what type of enhancement to perform is based on the type of residual refractive error the patient has. In the case of myopia with or without astigmatism, photorefractive keratectomy (PRK) and laser in situ keratomileusis (LASIK) are 2 excellent treatment modalities. In the case of mixed astigmatism, a laser vision correction procedure may be performed, but an incisional method, such as astigmatic keratotomy (AK) or limbal relaxing incisions (LRIs), may be easily performed in the appropriate individual as well. In the case of hyperopia, a laser procedure can usually treat up to 4 D of hyperopia, whereas conductive keratoplasty (CK) may be a useful alternative for up to 1.5 or 2 D of hyperopia, especially in patients with dry eyes who may experience difficulty with PRK or LASIK. Because of the relative instability of all of the corneal refractive hyperopic procedures, however, an IOL exchange or piggyback IOL may be the procedure of choice, especially when the residual hyperopia is more pronounced. IOL exchange may also be necessary in the case of marked myopia after cataract surgery, or when PRK or LASIK is not possible due to an abnormality of the cornea, such as keratoconus or a history of herpetic keratitis, among others.

Should cataract surgeons who implant presbyopia-correcting IOLs learn to perform PRK or LASIK for the purpose of enhancing patients with residual refractive error? The advantages of the cataract surgeon performing refractive surgery are many, and include knowing the patient well and understanding his or her expectations better than another surgeon might. The cataract surgeon who has the ability to do refractive enhancement surgery can keep the patient within the practice, which may be a psychological benefit for both the surgeon and the patient. In addition, the fees can be structured to include the possible enhancement afterward so that the patient or the surgeon does not have to pay a separate enhancement fee out of pocket.

The disadvantages of a cataract surgeon performing laser vision correction after IOL surgery include the not insignificant costs associated with the laser. These include the purchase and maintenance of the laser, the cost of the technical and support staff needed to perform the surgery, and the extra costs associated with the counseling and workup prior to the refractive procedure, including corneal topography, corneal pachymetry, and other associated testing. In addition, for a cataract surgeon who is adopting laser vision correction, there is a learning curve associated with PRK and LASIK, and outcomes in the initial few cases may not be as good as those of a more experienced surgeon.

The major advantage of referring a postoperative patient to a refractive surgeon for an enhancement is that an experienced refractive surgeon can choose the best refractive procedure for the patient and he or she routinely performs these types of surgeries. The refractive surgeon has the resources to perform the required ancillary testing and has the proper equipment to perform the surgery. Furthermore, if the intended refractive result is still not achieved, subsequent enhancement surgeries will typically be performed by the refractive surgeon.

The potential disadvantages of referring a patient to a different surgeon include the difficulties that any patient may experience when care is shifted to another physician or another practice. The refractive surgeon may not know the patient and his or her expectations as well as the surgeon who performed the initial cataract surgery. The patient may be anxious or angry due to what he or she perceives as a suboptimal outcome, and this can lead to an increased need for counseling with increased chair time on the part of one or both physicians. If a complication is encountered by the refractive surgeon, the patient could become correspondingly even more anxious.

From the refractive surgeon's standpoint, these patients may take a lot of time and present a different set of challenges than the standard younger LASIK patient. It may be particularly difficult to manage a patient who never was an appropriate candidate for refractive surgery in the first place. Take, for example, the case of a patient with a collagen vascular disease and severe dry eye. This patient may be a poor candidate for laser vision correction, and may be severely disappointed to find this out after undergoing cataract surgery with a presbyopia-correcting IOL if this was not discussed preoperatively. Additionally, patients in this age group generally do have a higher incidence of dry eye both before and after laser vision correction, which can make postoperative management much more challenging. If the patient is made aware of any important preoperative problems that may affect their ability to have refractive surgery, such as keratoconus, severe dry eye, or a history of herpetic keratitis, the patient will not be surprised later to learn that refractive surgery options may be more limited. It is thus important that the patient perceive that the refractive and cataract surgeons are working together to ensure a good outcome for the patient, and appropriate preoperative counseling makes this process easier.

From a business standpoint, referral of a patient to another surgeon typically requires that either the surgeon or the patient pay the refractive surgeon's fees. Many surgeons charge an initial fee that covers the cost of enhancement surgery, so that the patient does not have to pay an additional fee if additional surgery is required. Because this may reduce or eliminate the profit margin from the original surgery, an appropriate fee structure will take into account the percentage of patients requiring such surgery and still allow the cataract surgeon to make a reasonable profit. Some surgeons, however, may choose to charge the patient less for their initial refractive IOL surgery, and then make sure that the patient understands that if further refractive surgery is needed, an extra cost will be incurred. Again, management of patient expectations preoperatively allows for a smoother process postoperatively.

If, after taking these issues into consideration, the cataract surgeon decides to proceed with incorporating keratorefractive surgery into his or her practice, the most practical procedures to learn initially are PRK, CK, and some form of incisional surgery (either AK or LRIs) for astigmatism. PRK is relatively easier to learn than LASIK, and conventional procedures are generally preferred over customized ablation, because most current aberrometers are not able to obtain acceptable readings when a multifocal or accommodating IOL is present. The results from PRK and LASIK are equivalent, and PRK may even be preferable in the case of thin corneas or subtle abnormalities in corneal topography. CK may be very useful in those cases of mild hyperopia, particularly when dry eye is present, as this modality does not adversely affect the ocular surface as much as PRK and LASIK. The procedure is straightforward and quick, making for a relatively more pleasant postoperative experience than after laser vision correction. In the case of these 2 procedures, the equipment is relatively more expensive to acquire, particularly in the case of laser vision correction. Therefore, it may be more appropriate to utilize a nearby refractive surgery center and pay a user fee for their equipment rather than to purchase it outright. Mobile laser or refractive units may also be available and can provide the convenience of offering these procedures within the cataract surgeon's office.

For astigmatism without hyperopia or myopia, AK and LRIs are relatively easy to perform and require relatively little in the way of specialized equipment. Many excellent nomograms exist to treat residual astigmatism, and these procedures also do not adversely affect dry eye as much as laser vision correction procedures can. These incisional procedures may be performed either concomitantly with cataract surgery, or postoperatively to treat whatever corneal astigmatism remains. As mentioned previously, it is important to perform standard preoperative testing prior to corneal refractive procedures; thus, the surgeon and patient may be best served by incorporating corneal topography and corneal pachymetry into the workup prior to the cataract surgery, in anticipation of a potential need for refractive enhancement surgery afterward.

In summary, refractive cataract surgery is highly satisfying for both the patient and the surgeon when a good outcome is achieved. Enhancement surgery is necessary in a certain percentage of these patients to achieve the best possible refractive outcome and to ensure patient satisfaction. There are many factors that will determine what enhancement procedure will be best for any given patient, and fortunately there are now many good refractive surgical options from which to choose. The cataract surgeon has the choice of learning and offering refractive surgery him or herself, or developing a relationship with a refractive surgeon and referring the patients when necessary.

This choice should be based on (1) a realistic assessment of the current staffing and equipment that is present within the practice; (2) the possibility of obtaining the appropriate refractive equipment or utilizing a refractive surgery center; and (3) the availability of a nearby knowledgeable and helpful refractive surgeon who is willing to work together with the cataract surgeon to provide a seamless team approach for the patient.

CHAPTER 207

SHOULD I LEARN PRK/LASIK OR REFER THESE OUT?

Leonard Yuen, MD, MPH and Brian S. Boxer Wachler, MD

A 45-year-old female with a previously implanted multifocal intraocular lens came for consultation for improved vision. She had uncorrected visual acuity (UCVA) of 20/40 and manifest refraction (MRx) of −0.5 −0.25 × 132 yielding 20/25+1. Laser in situ keratomileusis (LASIK) was initially planned; however, with her low myopia, we chose to perform flap-only keratectomy (without laser). The subtlety of the procedure was to avoid overcorrection as the flap itself typically can correct 0.5 diopter (D) of myopia. The operation was successful with excellent postoperative results: UCVA was 20/20 with manifest refraction of plano −0.50 × 135. Had LASIK been performed, this patient would have likely inadvertently become hyperopic (overcorrected) and would likely be unhappy.

Understanding the nuances of refractive surgery is exciting and challenging, especially considering that photorefractive keratectomy (PRK) and laser in situ keratomileusis (LASIK) are rapidly becoming the most common ophthalmic surgical procedures performed. Many patients undergo refractive surgical enhancement after cataract surgery because their expectations are higher. Even with advanced intraocular lenses, slight postoperative refractive errors can "impair" a patient's vision and satisfaction.

The benefits of PRK and LASIK to patients' functional vision have been well documented and refractive surgery has been shown to be cost effective. Encouraging data from recently published studies shows that refractive surgery is beneficial for the older population as well. Ghanem and colleagues showed that LASIK yields positive results in the 40- to 69-year-old presbyopic population,[1] whereas Kuo and colleagues showed that laser refractive surgery is a safe, effective, and predictable for the correction of ametropia after cataract extraction (range 70 to 81 years old).[2] Despite the favorable qualitative and quantitative outcomes for refractive surgery over a wide range of patient populations, it is still important for cataract surgeons to consider various factors before deciding: "Should I learn PRK or LASIK, or refer these out?"

Factors to Consider

Patient safety is always the primary concern of the surgeon, in keeping with sound medicolegal principles.[3] Experience with patient selection and with determining the most appropriate timing of laser surgery are essential. At the same time, one should have a sufficient case volume to ensure familiarity with the equipment, and efficient interaction and communication with the laser technicians. One should have enough experience to be able to cope with the many individual variations among patients.

When LASIK and PRK were first developed, most surgeons learning these techniques were already in practice. Although refractive surgery fellowships are available after ophthalmology residencies (which provide in-depth training in LASIK and PRK), it is unrealistic to expect all surgeons who perform LASIK and PRK to have formal fellowship training in them. A recent study by McDonnell and colleagues,[4] however, revealed that after completion of their residency program, two thirds of ophthalmologists still felt that they would benefit from more subspecialty training, including refractive surgery. For young ophthalmologists who are interested in learning PRK or LASIK, further subspecialty training may therefore be desirable.

If a surgeon performs LASIK or PRK, it is prudent to be actively engaged in continuing medical education. This time commitment needs to be considered in the decision to perform LASIK or PRK. Additional sophisticated refractive procedures are swiftly evolving, each with the challenge of tackling a new set of subtleties and nuances.

Economics

From a business perspective, the economic future of refractive surgery looks favorable, with high consumer confidence at the time of this writing.[5] According to Lindstrom, adding refractive cataract surgery (presbyopia and astigmatism

> **Table 1**
>
> ## PROS AND CONS OF TREATING IN-HOUSE OR REFERRAL
>
> *Learning PRK/LASIK and Treating In-House*
>
> | Pros | Cons |
> |---|---|
> | Higher potential revenues | Time and cost for the initial set up, and maintenance of equipment and skills |
> | Favorable market for refractive surgery | Relatively higher complications rates correspond with lower procedure volume[9] |
> | Learning new skills and adding variety to a surgical practice | Time invested in attending meetings and keeping up to date with new skills |
> | Being able to personally offer refractive enhancements post cataract surgery | Proximity to a secondary center is desirable in case of complications |
> | | Potential litigation because of additional procedures performed |
>
> *Referring Out*
>
> | Pros | Cons |
> |---|---|
> | Can concentrate on building existing practice | Potential lost revenue |
> | Patient safety maximized if referred to an experienced specialist | Missed opportunity to learn and practice a new surgical skill |
> | Avoiding market competition | Potential loss of competitive edge in the market |

correction) can improve the net income of a surgeon's practice by 10% in the first year and up to 50% in the fifth year.[6] A study in 2007 by Tu and May has shown that consumers of self-pay procedures, especially in the LASIK market, rely heavily on word-of-mouth recommendations for reasons of quality concerns and the difficulty of obtaining price quotes.[7] Hence for already successful practices, the rewards can be even more attractive. Although the financial benefits appear munificent, the surgeon must keep in mind that the elective nature of surgery, high patient expectations, and the increased risk of litigation are still important considerations when deciding to perform PRK or LASIK or refer these patients to refractive specialists.

Establishing refractive surgery in one's practice requires a major investment of time and resources to learn the surgery, to market the service, and to accumulate clinical experience.[8] Often, this means having to give up a portion of an already busy, established practice to achieve this. For practices hoping to set up an in-house refractive service, the initial capital outlay and set-up costs can be high. An excimer laser costs upward of $400,000 and a microkeratome costs approximately $50,000.[8] These prices do not including usage royalties, overhead costs, maintenance fees, and the cost of training technicians and staff members.

Another option is to use "open-access" surgical centers equipped with laser instruments that are generally available for a per-procedure fee. Using such centers for a small number of cases may be time inefficient due to travel time and delays, such as waiting for other surgeons to finish their cases.

Factoring lost practice productivity, some doctors eventually decide that it may be more efficient to refer LASIK cases out.

The significant time investment does not end with the initial training period. Continuing medical education through multimedia training tools, or through courses with hands-on training and wet labs, is valuable if one is to remain proficient with the latest advances in technology.

Increased insurance and medicolegal costs should also be taken into account. Figures from 2007 show that settlements for LASIK rank third in terms of number of claims, behind cataract surgery and retinal surgery.[5]

For solo practices, ophthalmologists bringing refractive surgery "in-house" may need to consider the availability of a nearby secondary refractive surgery center in case of unforeseen operative complications. In large practices with multiple ophthalmologists, it may be possible to refer patients to colleagues who are already experienced at managing refractive surgery complications. One caveat is that prior to referral, it is important to be aware of compliancy with state laws regarding fee-splitting and anti–self-referrals.

Conclusion

The decision of whether a cataract surgeon offering refractive IOLs should now learn laser refractive surgery depends on the individual's confidence, surgical dexterity, and practice "personality." Other factors such as regional competition are also a consideration. For those who have already decided to learn keratorefractive surgery, the factors listed in Table 1 hopefully should have already been considered.

From a pragmatic perspective, learning about keratorefractive surgery may be helpful in one's daily practice. As LASIK is about to become the most common ophthalmic procedure, even if an ophthalmologist does not perform keratorefractive surgery, he or she will see patients who want to have or have had these procedures.

The technical simplicity of PRK, the consistently excellent visual outcomes of LASIK, and the relatively low complications rates of these procedures have assured the popularity and desirability of keratorefractive surgery for years to come. Meanwhile, cataract surgeons will see large increases in their volume do to the aging of our population. Cataract surgeons will increasingly be expected to manage (refer out or directly perform) a variety of post cataract refractive errors to satisfy pseudophakic patients with high expectations for their uncorrected vision. With the widening availability of refractive intraocular lenses, patient expectations will continue to increase.

References

1. Ghanem RC, de la Cruz J, Tobaigy FM, Ang LP, Azar DT. LASIK in the presbyopic age group: safety, efficacy and predictability in 40-69 year old patients. *Ophthalmology.* 2007;114:1303-1310.

2. Kuo IC, O'Brien TP, Broman AT, Ghajarnia M, Jabbur NS. Excimer laser surgery for correction of ametropia after cataract surgery. *J Cataract Refract Surg.* 2005;31:2104-2010.

3. Abbott R, Weber P. Risk management issues in refractive corneal surgery. *Ophthalmol Clin N Am.* 1997;10:473-484.

4. McDonnell PJ, Kirwan TJ, Brinton GS, et al. Perceptions of recent ophthalmology residency graduates regarding preparation for practice, 20 December 2006. *Ophthalmology.* 2007;114(2):387-391.

5. *Market Scope.* August 2007, Vol. 12, Issue 8.

6. Lindstrom R, Merging Refractive and Cataract Surgery in Your Practice, ASCRS Summer Refractive Congress (Keynote lecture), San Diego, 2 Aug 2007

7. Tu HT, May JH. Self pay markets in health care: consumer Nirvana or caveat emptor? *Health Aff (Millwood).* 2007;26:w217-w226.

8. Durrie D, Karpecki P, Aziz A, Smith B. Co-management strategies in refractive surgery. *Ophthalmol Clin N Am.* 1997;10:497-503.

9. Lin RT, Maloney RK. Flap complications associated with lamellar refractive surgery. *Am J Ophthal.* 1999;127:129-136.

CHAPTER 208

TEAMING UP WITH A LVC SURGEON

Michael T. Furlong, MD

Achieving emmetropia following cataract surgery is the usual goal with most of our patients. But when our standard monofocal intraocular lens (IOL) patients do not achieve this postoperative refractive status, it is not that disappointing to the patient, as, in general, they were expecting to wear glasses postoperatively anyway. But, when a cataract or refractive lens exchange (RLE) patient chooses a refractive IOL (multifocal, accommodating, or toric), missing emmetropia by more than 0.50 diopter (D) of sphere or cylinder can be very disappointing to the patient and surgeon alike. Being able to provide a refractive enhancement to these patients is a critical service that the operating ophthalmologists must be able to perform themselves or, alternatively, refer to a qualified refractive surgeon. Most traditional refractive surgeons have the skill set, experience, and access to an excimer laser to provide enhancements to these patients. Because not all cataract surgeons offer this service, they will have to look to outside surgeons to whom they will refer these cases. Other chapters in this book will cover nonlaser enhancements that work well in specific situations (mini-radial keratotomy [RK], astigmatic keratotomy [AK], piggyback IOL, IOL exchange), so this chapter will focus on how the cataract surgeon who does not offer laser in situ keratomileusis (LASIK) can team up with a laser vision correction surgeon in anticipation of including refractive IOLs into their practice. Specifically, this chapter will address how to work with a surgeon who can offer these appropriate post-IOL enhancement procedures: LASIK, photorefractive keratectomy (PRK), and conductive keratoplasty (CK). For the purposes of simplification, all PRK references in this chapter include all surface ablation procedures (PRK, laser epithelial keratomileusis [LASEK], epi-LASIK), as all of these avoid a stromal incision.

Refractive IOLs are not new, even in the United States. In the 1990s, the Array and STAAR (STAAR Surgical, Monrovia, CA) toric IOLs made their debut and many cataract patients received these implants in the United States and abroad. Biometry was acceptable in predicting postoperative emmetropia in the majority of cases, but because most of these patients had a cataract, the patient was not very demanding in actually achieving freedom from corrective lenses if there was significant residual refractive error. In addition, RLE was a very small percentage of the total number of primary IOL cases being done, therefore the concept of having to "enhance" an IOL patient was a foreign one. In fact, the concept of an "enhancement" was developed for the traditional refractive surgery patient. These were patients who were having keratorefractive procedures such as RK, PRK, and LASIK and were counseled about the chance of a secondary procedure should they be under- or overcorrected. What has happened over the past 3 to 5 years is a shift in thinking that was bound to happen. The ophthalmic industry's success in delivering refractive IOL technology, combined with the ability to obtain excellent biometry, has led to cataract surgery becoming 50% surgical rehabilitation of vision and 50% refractive surgery. In other words, if one performs (or intends to perform) state-of-the-art cataract surgery with the latest implant choices, one must deliver this service with the refractive surgeon's mindset. They are now refractive cataract surgeons.

Refractive surgeons have had to deal with the demanding patient all along—as the average refractive surgery patient is expecting a high level of visual function without supplemental glasses. But, it is a relatively new idea and a new expectation of our cataract patients to feel this way.

Prescreening the Potential Refractive IOL Patient—Things to Look for

It is estimated that as many 20% to 30% of our refractive IOL patients would benefit from an enhancement due to residual refractive error. It is therefore imperative that all patients about to undergo implantation of a refractive IOL also be a candidate for corneal refractive surgery. The early adopters of refractive IOL technology have guided us in choosing

Table 1
CONTRAINDICATIONS
Absolute Contraindications
• Frank keratoconus
• Other ectatic diseases like pellucid
• History of herpes simplex keratitis
• Systemic lupus erythematosus
• Rheumatoid arthritis
• Neurotrophic cornea
Relative Contraindications
• Forme Fruste keratoconus
• Dry eye
• Epithelial basement membrane dystrophy
• Other corneal dystrophies
• Sever lid disease
• Lid disorders affecting corneal health

which of our patients are ideal candidates for these lenses. Other sections of this book will cover the criteria that are usually used to select a good refractive IOL candidate (eg, 20/20 visual potential, absence of macular degeneration, amblyopia), therefore this chapter will concentrate on making sure the potential refractive IOL patient will also be a good candidate for corneal refractive touch up (LASIK, PRK, CK) should they require one.

One of the main reasons why a refractive surgeon disqualifies a potential patient from refractive surgery is keratoconus (or other ectatic disease such as pellucid marginal corneal degeneration). For this reason, corneal topography must be used before scheduling a patient for a refractive IOL surgery. This is important to avoid the scenario where the patient does not qualify for a corneal enhancement procedure *after* the IOL surgery and has residual ametropia (thereby not getting the full benefit of the refractive IOL). Forme fruste keratoconus, however, does not necessarily disqualify a patient for consideration of a refractive IOL and subsequent laser vision correction enhancement. Many refractive surgeons offer PRK to these patients with good long-term results and stability, provided that a careful informed consent with the patient be conducted, informing them of the possibility of future kerectasia.

A complete ocular history should be done to rule out prior herpes simplex keratitis, as this is an absolute contraindication for excimer laser surgery (Table 1). Autoimmune diseases such as systemic lupus erythematosus or rheumatoid arthritis are important to know about, as they can lead to corneal melting post laser vision correction.

Dry eye must be assessed and treated aggressively before considering corneal refractive surgery. Most patients with Sjögrens syndrome are poor candidates for LASIK and therefore would not qualify for a post-refractive IOL laser enhancement. In addition, these patients often have loss of best-corrected visual acuity (BCVA) due to their extreme dry eye status, and therefore wouldn't likely be a good refractive IOL candidate anyway.

Finally, patients with epithelial basement membrane dystrophy or any corneal degeneration must be carefully examined and screened, as many may not be good candidates for laser vision correction.

Which Is the Best Technique?

There are 3 excellent tools that can be used to enhance the refractive IOL patient.

LASIK and PRK are excellent techniques to enhance post–refractive IOL patients. Two decisions need to be made by the refractive surgeon that is helpful to the referring cataract surgeon to know about, so he or she can discuss these with the patient. The first is which technique is preferred in a specific case (LASIK versus PRK). The second is conventional laser versus wavefront-guided technology.

Deciding between LASIK and PRK is typically a preference choice and not one that is outcomes based. In other words, there are good data that both of these procedures work very well. LASIK has the advantage of quick recovery of vision with minimum discomfort and down time. Surface treatments have the advantage of no intraocular pressure (IOP) rise (that could theoretically open a cataract incision), no effect on inducing higher-order aberrations (because there is no stromal flap created), and less dry eye induction. The technique choice should be individualized to the patient, and the appropriate discussion between the patient and the refractive surgeon should include the risks and benefits each procedure.

In general, wavefront-guided laser procedures on virgin eyes offer significant advantages over conventional technologies. Obtaining accurate and meaningful aberrometry in a post-refractive IOL patient, however, can be challenging and sometimes impossible. Currently, there are very little data on wavefront-guided enhancements in these patients. In most patients, therefore, a conventional treatment is much more straightforward and it is not yet proven that a wavefront-guided treatment will help. A few clinical trials are underway to examine whether these are superior to conventional treatments in patients whose manifest refraction and wavefront refraction are a close match.

CK is a good technique that can reliably eliminate up to 2 D of residual hyperopia. Because CK does not involve the creation of a stromal flap, it does not induce a tear-deficiency state like LASIK, and is therefore, an excellent choice for dry eye patients.

Timing of the Enhancement

As is common in ophthalmology, there is rarely complete consensus on absolute timing of a secondary procedure. But, it is generally accepted that 2 to 3 months post IOL surgery *and* documented refractive stability be observed before considering a keratorefractive enhancement.

Aligning Yourself With A Refractive Surgeon

STEP 1: IDENTIFY THE OPHTHALMOLOGISTS IN YOUR COMMUNITY WHO PERFORM REFRACTIVE SURGERY

Refractive IOL patients appreciate excellent customer service and prompt attention. It is very important that the referral to the refractive surgeon be in close proximity to the IOL surgeon's office. The patient will appreciate the least amount of travel time to accommodate these visits.

STEP 2: CALL THE TOP 3 AND DISCUSS HOW A REFERRAL RELATIONSHIP MIGHT WORK

Do they have a clean process in place to accept these types of referrals? Do they have materials for your staff and prospective patients for education purposes? Is their office proactive in calling your patient to schedule the initial consultation? Whose office will perform the pre- and postoperative care? What is the cost to the patient for this enhancement? How do the 2 surgeons communicate to ensure quality care of the patient? When does the patient go back to the cataract surgeon? Having answers to these and other management questions up front will facilitate dealing with various patient scenarios.

STEP 3: SEND A STAFF MEMBER TO THE REFRACTIVE SURGEON'S OFFICE TO VISIT AND SEE HOW PATIENTS ARE TREATED

See for yourself or send your office manager to the refractive surgeon's office so that you have a first-hand understanding of how your patients will be treated and what kind of experience they will likely have.

STEP 4: EDUCATE YOUR PATIENT

Set your IOL patient's expectations about the probability for an enhancement *before* they have their IOL surgery. Then, go over in detail the timing, surgery types, and cost that the patient will be responsible for if they indeed pursue an enhancement. This will make the discussion after refractive IOL surgery much easier. For example, if you are implanting a ReSTOR IOL in a patient with 3 D of corneal astigmatism, there is a virtual guarantee that this patient will need a second procedure to correct this refractive error. Also, for those patients that may not be good refractive surgery candidates, an appropriate and frank discussion about the limitations of their results can take place.

STEP 5: REGULARLY MONITOR OUTCOMES AND PATIENT SATISFACTION

Call the refractive surgeon frequently for the first few patients so that everyone is on the same page regarding the patient's care and progress. This will ensure a good working relationship moving forward.

It is generally a good idea to have at least 2 refractive surgeons to whom these patients will be referred. This way, one can match personalities, styles, success rates, surgery types, promptness, customer satisfaction, etc., to the patient's needs. Also, if one of the surgeons referred doesn't work out for some reason, the referring surgeon isn't left high and dry.

Refractive IOL patients have the refractive mindset. They do not want to wait. They do not want to be inconvenienced. They do not want to be given the run around. They are typically a savvy consumer who knows what they want. Underpromising and overdelivering results is a good strategy with these patients.

KEY ISSUES TO DISCUSS

- What is the cost of the enhancement?
- Who does pre- and postenhancement care?
- Is there a solid mechanism for efficient referral and transfer of care?
- How do the 2 surgeons communicate to ensure quality care of the patient?
- When does the patient go back to the cataract surgeon?

Conclusion

In summary, refractive IOL patients today are paying a premium for superior technology and outcomes. In a significant percentage of these patients, a secondary procedure may be required to achieve emmetropia and a happy patient. If the cataract surgeon does not perform laser vision correction, he or she would benefit greatly by developing a good working relationship with a qualified refractive surgeon to achieve an excellent patient experience and happy outcome.

CHAPTER 209

DIFFERENTIATING ENHANCEMENTS FROM COMPLICATIONS

Kevin L. Waltz, OD, MD

Differentiating enhancements from complications is an important principle. Probably the single biggest difference between refractive surgery and nonrefractive surgery is the expectation that a second surgery is a normal part of the process. We have done ourselves and our refractive patients a great service by educating them from the early days of radial keratotomy (RK) through the development of laser vision correction that a second procedure is normal and potentially desirable. It allows us to fine tune the results of the initial procedure without being under a cloud of suspicion that something was done wrong. This allows us to create some margin for error with the first procedure. For instance, we can aim for a –0.25 sphere result with a prepresbyopic myope instead of a plano end result. This decreases the risk of making someone hyperopic in this situation. When we are working with micron-size precision in human tissue, it only makes sense that some patients will need fine tuning of their results. Surgeons recognized this early in the development of refractive surgery and have never looked back.

As we develop refractive lens surgery, it is important to again make the distinction between an enhancement and a complication. Cataract surgery has become refractive surgery. We have become so proficient at refractive cataract surgery that we are now applying the same skills and procedures to purely refractive lens surgery. Our patients expect to minimize their dependence on glasses after cataract surgery even with monofocal intraocular lenses (IOLs). They have even greater expectations with more advanced technologies like presbyopia-correcting (Pr-C) IOLs. For this reason, it is imperative that we develop an understanding of the difference between an enhancement and a complication with refractive IOL surgery. We do ourselves and our patients a disservice if we do not.

Broadly speaking, an enhancement is a further attempt to optimize a patient's visual outcome from the first procedure. An enhancement is a normal, expected part of any refractive surgery, including refractive lens surgery and Pr-C IOLs. An enhancement might be pharmaceutical in nature. A common example would be using pilocarpine to constrict a pupil to minimize glare after a surgery. It might be a surgical procedure

such as lifting a flap to treat residual astigmatism after LASIK. The important point is that an enhancement is expected in a certain percentage of patients to improve outcomes. An enhancement is a secondary procedure to improve the functional outcome of an initial surgery that does not involve a complication.

Enhancements must also be taken in context. There is an expected range of enhancement rates for any procedure. There are similar observations in other areas of medicine. If a general surgeon always finds a patient has appendicitis when he operates, he is probably not operating on enough patients. There is an expected percentage of negative findings when operating for appendicitis due to the inability to be certain of the diagnosis. A surgeon is expected to have at least a few enhancements after laser in situ keratomileusis (LASIK). If there are none, it is likely the surgeon is not enhancing patients that would benefit from it. Effectively, it is all but impossible for a surgeon to perform LASIK and have every patient heal in such a predictable manner that no enhancements are indicated. In the case of LASIK, we expect a certain percentage of patients will need additional surgery. This is also true for cataract surgery and refractive cataract surgery. When we do traditional cataract surgery, virtually everyone has an enhancement for residual refractive error and presbyopia. Glasses after cataract surgery are so normal that we sometimes forget what they are—an enhancement to our otherwise flawless surgery.

Needing glasses after premium IOL surgery with a Pr-C IOL is undesirable. It is still normal for a certain percentage of patients. None of the presently available IOL options have ever been suggested to eliminate glasses 100% of the time, even from the most optimistic advocate. Therefore, although it may be the goal of the surgery to eliminate the need for glasses with a Pr-C IOL, it is normal and expected for some patients to wear glasses after this type of surgery, and this is not a complication. The surgeon will also have an expected enhancement rate to minimize the number of patients who need glasses after the surgery. The laser vision enhancement rate after implanting a Pr-C IOL is between 5% and 30%. This range is consistent with the early enhancement rates after laser vision correction in the mid 1990s.

A complication is an adverse event that may cause permanent loss of function. Like an enhancement, complications have expected rates of occurrence. For instance, every surgeon has a predictable rate of posterior capsular rupture. This cannot be totally avoided, and has the potential to cause permanent loss of function. All surgeons accept that complications are a normal part of surgery. A residual refractive error after a LASIK procedure is not a complication because it does not have the potential to cause loss of function. It can be fixed with a simple enhancement such as a pair of glasses, contact lenses, or a flap lift with additional laser treatment. Similarly, a residual refractive error after refractive cataract surgery is not a complication. It can be fixed in the same fashion as residual refractive error after LASIK. It can also be fixed with an IOL exchange or a piggyback IOL.

An enhancement should never be a cause for a malpractice suit, if the patient understands that it is a normal part of the surgical process. A vision-limiting complication by itself is not sufficient cause for a malpractice suit, because all surgeries have a potential for complications. Malpractice requires a complication to be associated with a deviation from the standard of care and a loss of function. Let us evaluate a sequence of events with lens surgery to provide specific examples of enhancements versus complications. A 50-year-old male patient presents with a cataract in the right eye and no cataract in the left eye. The patient is otherwise normal and has a refractive error of −5.00 +2.00 × 180 in both eyes. The patient desires a Pr-C IOL in the right eye with the cataract. The surgery is done with an appropriately placed corneal relaxing incision and the results appear to be flawless. The patient heals normally, but is left with 1 diopter (D) of residual astigmatism. The patient is dissatisfied with his visual result. The surgeon offers an enhancement to improve the patient's outcome—glasses, contacts, or LASIK. The patient chooses LASIK. The LASIK enhancement is done without difficulty.

The patient is now plano and sees well with his right eye. He loves his vision in his right eye. He pleads to have the same surgery done on his left eye. The patient understands there is no cataract in the left eye. The procedure is elective and the patient will be responsible for payment. The surgeon implants a Pr-C IOL with a corneal relaxing incision. This time the surgeon achieves a plano end result on the first attempt.

While recovering from surgery on the second eye, the right eye develops a retinal detachment. A retinal detachment after lens surgery in a 50-year-old male is not a surprise, but it is a complication. It has the potential to decrease the patient's visual function. The patient has a scleral buckle procedure to correct the detachment. It works. The detachment is fixed, but the patient is now myopic from the buckle. This is not a complication. Myopia does not have the potential to decrease the patient's visual function.

The patient is offered an enhancement—glasses, contacts, or LASIK. The patient chooses LASIK. The LASIK is done without difficulty and the patient is again plano. Unfortunately, the patient's near vision is not satisfactory. He has a posterior capsular opacification. This is not a complication. The patient needs a yttrium-aluminum-garnet (YAG) capsulotomy—an enhancement. The YAG capsulotomy is done on the right eye and the patient develops cystoid macular edema (CME) after the procedure. The CME is a complication. It has the potential to decrease the patient's visual function. The CME is treated with intensive topical medication and resolves. The patient is satisfied with his visual outcome.

Patients must understand the difference between a complication and an enhancement. Enhancements treat problems that generally do not threaten a patient's visual function. Complications do pose a threat. Enhancements and complications are inevitable, but occur at expected rates. They do not indicate or constitute malpractice, which must be associated with a deviation from the standard of care. In most situations, low rates of enhancements and complications are normal and define the standard of care.

CHAPTER 210

INDICATIONS AND TIMING FOR LASER ENHANCEMENT

Michael Lawless, MD

Despite advanced surgical techniques and a variety of formulas, the most frequent complication following cataract surgery is residual refractive error. This assumes greater importance in multifocal intraocular lens (IOL) recipients, because they have selected the IOL, in consultation with their surgeon, because of a desire for spectacle independence.

We and others have reported on the relative safety and accuracy of laser in situ keratomileusis (LASIK) for refractive error after cataract surgery.[1,2]

In our original analysis of 112 eyes (56 patients) who received a ReSTOR multifocal IOL, the average age was 59 years. This was a younger cohort than the normal cataract population, and often the cataract surgery was performed largely for refractive reasons. The average spherical equivalent was +2.42 (SD 1.68) and cylinder 0.50 (SD 0.43) diopter (D). Spherical equivalent ranged from −1.75 to +6.75 and preoperative astigmatism from 0 to 2 D. At final follow up, 89% had unaided acuity of 20/30 or better (individual eyes) (Figure 1) and 95.6% had unaided near acuity of J2 or better (individual eyes) (Figure 2).

When binocular visual function was measured, 96% of patients were completely spectacle independent and 4% used glasses half of the time (Figure 3).

Of these 112 eyes, a secondary refractive procedure was performed in 18 (16%); 16 were treated with LASIK and 2 with secondary IOLs.

When we analyzed the quality of vision (QOV) of these patients,[3] the average score was 75.96 (SD 11.33). To put this in context using our QOV questionnaire, myopes who wear glasses and contact lenses score between 65 and 70, and normal emmetropes tend to score 90 to 95.

The longer you follow these patients, the better the QOV score obtained, and at 12 months the average for the ReSTOR group was 81.40 (SD 11.60).

For patients who have had multifocal ReSTOR IOLs and subsequent LASIK enhancement, QOV was rated at 73.63 (SD 13.74), which was not significantly different from the multifocal ReSTOR patients who had had a good result without enhancement.

The message for me is that some form of enhancement will be required in a significant minority of multifocal lens patients. Mostly this will be a laser-based treatment; either LASIK or surface ablation, but of course sometimes a secondary IOL, or indeed a lens exchange, will be needed.

I will attempt to present the decision-making process via a series of 5 actual patients.

Case 1: LASIK for a Refractive Surprise

A 56-year-old female real estate agent presented for refractive evaluation. Unaided acuity was right 20/100 and left 20/80 with a refractive error of right +2.25/−0.25 at 6 degrees and left +2.50/−0.50 at 25 degrees. Best-corrected acuity was 20/30 right and 20/30 +1 left. Dilated examination revealed cortical and nuclear sclerosis cataract in both eyes. Ocular examination was otherwise normal.

This patient was treated in early 2003, and was one of my first group of ReSTOR multifocal patients. At that stage we were using immersion A scan, and I did not have a personalized A constant for the multifocal IOL.

A decision was made to proceed with cataract and lens surgery using a multifocal IOL after a long discussion with the patient, with the understanding that she was among the first group with multifocal lenses used in my hands.

Surgery was uneventful, performed with routine phacoemulsification using a 3.2-mm incision, and the eyes were operated 1 week apart.

One month postoperatively, unaided acuity in the right was 20/60 and left 20/50. Refractive error in the right was +1.75/−0.75 at 15 degrees and left +1.25/−0.75 at 20 degrees correcting to 20/20+ in both eyes. Unaided near acuity was J3 at 35 to 40 cm.

The patient was disappointed with the quality of unaided vision for close work in particular.

Three months postoperatively, the results were identical to the 1-month readings. A decision was made to perform

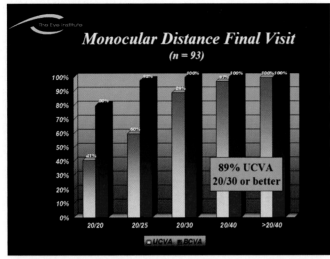

Figure 1. Final monocular distance vision.

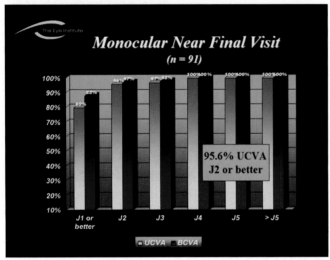

Figure 2. Final monocular near vision.

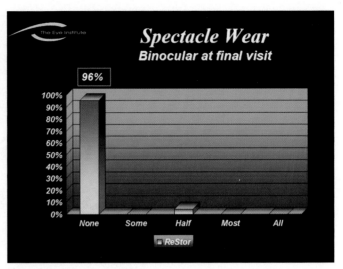

Figure 3. Final binocular spectacle requirement survey.

bilateral LASIK aiming for a plano end point in each eye.

Bilateral LASIK was performed with IntraLase (Advanced Medical Optics, Irvine, CA) and the LADARVision 4000 (ALCON, Fort Worth, TX) using a standard (nonwavefront) approach, with an optical zone to 7.00 mm and transition to 9.0 mm. There was no difficulty in tracking the dilated pupil. One month following LASIK, unaided acuity was 20/25 +1 right and 20/20 −2 left, and refractive error was right −0.25/−0.50 at 60 degrees and left −0.25/−0.25 at 120 degrees. Corrected acuity was 20/20+ in each eye.

The patient had achieved a result with which she was happy, being spectacle independent for all activities. There were minor complaints of a drop in visual quality while driving at night, but she did not feel that this was significant, and did not require distance spectacle correction. The intermediate and near unaided acuity was excellent for her working conditions, and she was J1 unaided at 30 cm.

OBSERVATIONS

Refractive surprises will still occasionally occur, but they have been reduced with the use of the IOL Master (Carl Zeiss,

Oberkochen, Germany). I do not regret operating on the second eye at 1 week, because waiting longer would have simply prolonged the overall rehabilitation. My personal experience is that I do not "learn" from the first eye in terms of IOL power selection. Others have confirmed this approach.[4]

In these patients, I pay particular attention to the tear film. Schirmer's test, and tear film break-up time were normal in this patient. These multifocal lens patients are generally older than the normal LASIK population and more likely to require intensive treatment with artificial tears and/or punctal plugs to help with tear film issues.

The minimum time I wait between cataract surgery and LASIK is 2 months, but I generally prefer to wait 3 months. I do this to be certain about the refractive result, and also the tectonic strength of the cataract incision. With modern 2.2-mm incisions, this time interval could be reduced to 6 weeks.

In this particular patient, the final result was not plano but slightly myopic. Her near range was very acceptable, and I think, somewhat luckily, she was not bothered by halos at night. These are evident in many patients with multifocal IOLs and are always more obvious if there is a residual myopic or astigmatic refractive error.

This patient represents a significant refractive surprise in my early experience with multifocal lenses, but because of the extensive preoperative discussion, and the ability to accurately and promptly resolve the refractive error, the patient has achieved her desired result.

Case 2: LASIK for Astigmatism Following Multifocal IOL Implantation

This patient was a 64-year-old woman who presented for refractive surgery; her hobbies were golf and tennis, and she had a strong desire to be spectacle independent.

Unaided acuity was 20/80 right and 20/60 left and refractive error was right +2.00/−2.00 at 98 degrees and left +1.00/−0.75 at 116 degrees. Corrected acuity was 20/25 in each eye.

Dilated examination revealed grade 1 nuclear sclerosis cataract in both eyes. Examination was otherwise unremarkable. The patient was left eye dominant and central pachymetry was 503 µm in both eyes and she had a corneal anatomy suitable for LASIK.

Because she was 64, the corneal anatomy, although suitable for LASIK, was relatively thin. Because of the desire for spectacle independence, but not monovision, the decision was made to proceed with cataract and IOL surgery using the ReSTOR multifocal lens. The surgery was straightforward using a 3.0-mm temporal incision and a standard prechop phacoemulsification technique.

One month after surgery, unaided acuity was right 20/25 with +0.50/−0.75 at 110 degrees achieving 20/20 −1, and left 20/40 with a refractive error of +0.50/−1.25 at 105 degrees achieving 20/20. Unaided near binocular acuity was J2 at 30 cm.

The patient was spectacle independent, but felt that her left eye was sensitive to glare and the vision was not as good as the right.

I waited 4 months following cataract surgery before making a decision. The symptoms persisted with suboptimal vision and glare in the left eye. The posterior capsules were clear, the anterior chambers quiet, and external examination normal.

I went ahead with left LASIK using IntraLase and the LADARVision 4000 with a 7-mm optical zone aiming for plano. The surgery was uneventful, and at 1 month following LASIK, unaided acuity was 20/20 −1, with a refractive error of left +0.25/−0.25 at 15 degrees.

The patient felt that she had a considerable improvement; the left was now the better eye both for distance and near and glare symptoms had resolved completely. She understood that the left was the dominant eye and binocularly she had excellent unaided acuity for all activities, and elected to leave the right eye alone.

OBSERVATIONS

The patient had preoperative refractive and corneal astigmatism, which did not correlate either in axis or magnitude. Presumably there was some impact from the early cataract.

As I have moved to a 2.2-mm incision for cataract surgery, I now perform astigmatically neutral cataract surgery. This was not the case, however, with incisions of 3 mm and above.

Ocular dominance was a factor in this patient's symptoms, and it was necessary to achieve an excellent refractive result in the dominant left eye.

The corneal anatomy, although thin, was adequate for LASIK, and luckily the refractive errors treated in the post-multifocal situation are generally small with minimal tissue removal.

I was concerned that the glare symptoms would not resolve, and looked carefully for any sign of posterior capsule opacification and posterior segment pathology to explain this. There was none, and glare symptoms resolved completely once the refractive error had been dealt with appropriately.

Case 3: Advanced Surface Laser Ablation Following Multifocal IOL Implantation

A 53-year-old male carpenter presented for an opinion regarding refractive surgery. Unaided acuity was 20/40 right and 20/50 left with a refractive error of right +1.00/−0.25 at 130 degrees and left +1.25/−0.25 at 90 degrees. Corrected acuity was 20/25 in each eye. Dilated examination revealed mild cortical cataract in both eyes. The central pachymetry was 480 µm right and 485 µm left with an Orbscan (Bausch & Lomb, Rochester, NY) appearance, both in corneal curvature and thickness, unsuitable for LASIK because of the risk of ectasia.

There were a number of issues to consider with this patient. The cataract was having only a minimal effect on visual quality and the patient was 53 years old. He had a corneal appearance that was not suitable for LASIK, so the options were either surface ablation or cataract and lens surgery. The patient had a strong desire for spectacle independence, and after a contact lens trial, he decided he did not want to pursue monovision. Instead, he elected to proceed with cataract and lens surgery using the ReSTOR multifocal lens.

The surgery was performed with a 2.65-mm temporal incision with a prechopping phacoemulsification technique. At 1 and 3 months post cataract surgery, the results were identical, with unaided acuity right 20/25 and left 20/40. Refractive error in the right was +0.50/−0.50 at 105 degrees achieving 20/20 and left +1.00/−1.00 at 85 degrees achieving 20/20. Unaided near acuity binocularly was J2 at 30 cm. The patient was generally happy with his visual quality, but was aware that the left eye was not as good as the right and wished to have treatment to improve this.

Because we had stable refractive and keratometric readings, and because the patient had a good tear film but a corneal anatomy unsuitable for LASIK, I performed left surface ablation 3 months after cataract and lens surgery. We used the LADARVision 6000 aiming for a plano end point with an optical zone to 7 mm and a transition to 9 mm. Two months following surface ablation to the left eye, unaided acuity was 20/20 with no measurable refractive error. The patient was happy and spectacle independent with excellent reading vision for both near and intermediate distances. He had only minimal night halos.

OBSERVATIONS

It is critical to warn such patients in advance that if a refractive error occurred after cataract surgery, then LASIK would not be possible, and that surface ablation with its slower recovery would be necessary. A contact lens trial of monovision had demonstrated that the compromise involved with monovision was not acceptable. He was therefore prepared to go through both cataract surgery and then subsequent surface excimer ablation.

As noted in case 2, most of the refractive errors dealt with post cataract surgery are relatively small and therefore suitable for either LASIK or surface ablation. I think surface ablation can be performed at around 6 weeks following cataract surgery, but this patient was happy to wait 3 months to confirm refractive stability.

Case 4: Ocular Surface Disturbance and Impact on Refractive Error

A 57-year-old female travel agent with hyperopic astigmatism presented for refractive surgery. Unaided acuity was 20/100 right and 20/70 left, and with a refractive error of right +3.00/−0.25 at 12 degrees and left +2.75/−0.75 at 150 degrees could achieve 20/25 in each eye. There was 1 D of corneal astigmatism in both eyes. Orbscan analysis was normal and dilated examination revealed bilateral cortical cataract and a left posterior subcapsular cataract.

I proceeded with cataract and lens surgery using a ReSTOR multifocal lens, with a standard prechop technique and a 3.2-mm temporal incision.

One month postoperatively, unaided acuity was 20/40 in both eyes with a refractive error of right −0.25/−1.25 at 180 degrees and left −0.50/−1.00 at 170 degrees. Corrected acuity was only 20/25 in each eye. There was no evidence of cystoid macular edema, but there was punctate staining of both corneas and an early tear film break-up time. Near acuity was J3 at 30 cm but of poor quality. The patient was advised to use +1.00 readers for computer work, and treated with intensive artificial tears and punctal plugs. Six months after cataract and lens surgery, unaided acuity was 20/20 right and 20/25 left, and refractive error was right plano/−0.50 at 5 degrees and left plano/−0.75 at 175 degrees. Corrected acuity was 20/20 in each eye. The patient was very happy and had stopped using artificial tears, but had retained the punctal plugs. She occasionally used +1.00 readers for intermediate, but was spectacle independent most of the time. She was very happy with both the comfort and the visual quality.

OBSERVATIONS

This patient had a refractive error at 1 month and also a drop in best-corrected acuity. It would have been inappropriate to intervene early because the refractive error was not accurate and she had a clinically significant tear film disturbance. Once the tear film issues were rectified with punctal plugs, and time, a truer reading of her refractive status could be obtained. It was close enough to plano so that she was content not to have any further surgery. This was a good example of not intervening too early with laser refractive surgery and recognizing when an external eye condition is the cause of the early poor-quality result.

Case 5: Monovision After Multifocal IOLs

This patient was a 62-year-old male pharmacist. He had a strong desire for spectacle independence and was a very particular and fussy patient. Unaided acuity was 20/100

right and 20/80 left, and refractive error right +2.25/−0.50 at 54 degrees and left +2.00/−0.50 at 147 degrees. Corrected acuity was 20/20 in each eye. There was no clinically significant cataract and the ocular examination was unremarkable. The left eye was dominant and the corneal anatomy was suitable for LASIK.

After considerable discussion, bilateral refractive lensectomy was performed and multifocal ReSTOR IOLs were placed. The surgical technique was again standard prechop with a 2.65-mm temporal incision.

At 3 months unaided acuity was 20/30 right and 20/25 left, and refractive error right +0.75/−0.75 at 45 degrees and left +0.25/−0.25 at 55 degrees, achieving 20/20 in each eye. Unaided acuity for near was J2 at 35 to 40 cm. The patient complained of poor-quality intermediate vision. As a pharmacist, he was often standing and holding material at arm's length, and looking at his computer on the desk while standing up. Reading vision was adequate and distance vision was very good, with no problems with night driving.

We suggested using +1.00 readers as an interim measure and waited 6 months following surgery to see what neural adaptation would do to this patient's symptoms.[5] At 6 months there was no improvement. We went through a series of contact lens trials on both eyes, demonstrating a variety of end points and got him to wear these in his work environment. In the end, it was decided that if he had a refractive error of −1.25 in the nondominant right eye, this would give a result with which he was happy. The dominant left eye would be left untreated.

I proceeded with right LASIK at 8 months following the original multifocal lens surgery using IntraLase and the LADARVision 6000 aiming for −1.25. An optical zone to 7 mm with a transition to 9 mm was used. Three months following LASIK, unaided acuity in the right eye was 20/80 and with −1.00/−0.50 at 15 degrees corrected acuity was 20/20. The patient was very happy with this result. He did not feel that his distance vision had been compromised. The near vision was still adequate for reading, but he was able to use his computer while standing and this had resulted in a significant improvement in his impression of the intermediate unaided vision.

OBSERVATIONS

Sometimes you have to individualize the result. I would not have predicted that with a multifocal ReSTOR lens I would ever aim for plano in one eye and −1.25 in the nondominant eye, but in this particular patient, this strategy was able to satisfy his visual needs. A contact lens trial was necessary to establish this, and although time consuming for both the patient and our staff, it ultimately led me to identify the correct end point for him. If we had given up and said that nothing more could be done, this patient would have been very unhappy. Therefore, exploring a somewhat unusual refractive end point was appropriate in this patient.

Conclusion

The purpose of this chapter was to explore laser refractive surgery options after multifocal intraocular lens surgery. My experience is limited to ReSTOR multifocal lenses, but the lessons learnt have application to other IOL types.

The take-home messages follow:

1. The preoperative discussion is vital. One should explain the need for subsequent refractive surgery if a refractive surprise occurs, or if it is part of a planned staged procedure. Being able to perform subsequent refractive surgery in a timely and cost-effective manner with financial informed consent makes things much easier for both the surgeon and the patient.

2. You are generally dealing with small residual refractive errors, and either LASIK or surface ablation would be applicable. Therefore, choose what would be safest given the corneal anatomy and external eye condition.

3. Only use conventional or optimized excimer laser treatments. Wavefront analysis on multifocal lenses can give unusual results, and proper algorithms have not been devised for this situation.[6] Because these are generally older patients with smaller pupils, spherical aberration does not tend to be a major issue, and the excimer laser treatment itself, because it is relatively small, is not going to induce significant spherical aberration. The recent introduction of aspheric multifocal IOLs makes wavefront-based ablation even less necessary.

4. I have never had any problems tracking with the LADARVision 4000 or LADARVision 6000 using a dilated pupil with the ReSTOR multifocal IOL.

5. These are generally older patients, so particular attention needs to be paid to the tear volume and quality. One should initiate strategies to deal with the corneal surface before problems arise.

6. With the use of IOL Master and astigmatically neutral surgery (with an incision at or below 2.2 mm), surgical planning is much more predictable now than it was even a few years ago. Toric multifocal IOLs will further help in this regard.

7. Wait an adequate time before performing corneal laser surgery after multifocal lens surgery. Enough time is needed both to document a stable refractive result, and also to be tectonically safe. Waiting an extra 4 to 6 weeks to confirm this is acceptable to most patients.

8. Even though multifocal patients are particularly sensitive to any remaining refractive error, there are some individuals who will tolerate it. Therefore, deal with the patient and not just the refractive error.

9. Sometimes you need to individualize a refractive result to suit a particular personality or work environment. Therefore, think laterally about options.

References

1. Kim P, Briganti EM, Sutton GL, Lawless MA, Rogers CM, Hodge C. Laser in situ keratomileusis for refractive error after cataract surgery. *J Cataract Refract Surg.* 2005;31:979-986.

2. Kuo IC, O'Brien TP, Broman AT, Ghajarnia M, Jabbur NS. Excimer laser surgery for correction of ametropia after cataract surgery. *J Cataract Refract Surg.* 2005;31:2104-2110.

3. Comaish I, Fraenkel G, Lawless MA, et al. Development of a questionnaire to assess subjective vision score in myopes seeking refractive surgery. *J Refract Surg.* 2004;20:10-19.

4. Jabour J, Irwig L, Macaskill P, Hennessy MP. Intraocular lens power in bilateral cataract surgery: whether adjusting for error of predicted refraction in the first eye improves prediction in the second eye. *J Cataract Refract Surg.* 2006;32:2091-2097.

5. Artal P. Neural adaptation to aberrations. *Cataract Refract Surg Today.* 2007:August;76-77.

6. Lawless MA, Hodge CB. Wavefront's role in corneal refractive surgery. *Clin Exp Ophthalmol.* 2005;33:199-209.

CHAPTER 211

LASER ENHANCEMENT— WHAT CATARACT SURGEONS SHOULD KNOW

Elizabeth A. Davis, MD, FACS, and David R. Hardten, MD, FACS

The precision of refractive outcomes of lens surgery has greatly improved in the past few decades. This revolution began in the late 1960s when Charles Kelman, MD, introduced small-incision cataract surgery using phacoemulsification. His invention not only made the surgery safer, but visual outcomes were significantly enhanced. Combined with the development of foldable intraocular lenses (IOLs), lens removal could be accomplished through an entry wound that required no sutures and could be constructed in a way that induced less than 0.50 diopter (D) of astigmatism. Our improved ability to calculate lens powers also has contributed to better results. Highly accurate biometry can now be accomplished with the use of immersion ultrasound or optical noncontact A-scans. Formulas for calculating IOL powers have also been refined to enhance the predictive accuracy. In addition to being able to achieve better refractive outcomes, the choice of IOLs for our patients has expanded. We can offer monofocal, toric, accommodative, and multifocal IOLs.

With increasing awareness of excellent outcomes, patients have greater expectations for their lens surgery. Many desire reduced dependence on glasses and contact lenses for daily activities. To achieve such results, refractive results must be highly accurate. The most desirable outcome is one in which the spherical error is within 0.50 D of intended and the astigmatic error is no more than 0.50 D.

Certainly it is not always possible to achieve exactly these results with lens surgery alone—patient may have preexisting corneal astigmatism and even with the most meticulous preoperative measurements and calculations, natural anatomic variability can lead to residual refractive errors. Therefore, additional refractive procedures are sometimes employed to achieve the targeted result. Incisional keratotomy can reduce corneal astigmatism, conductive keratoplasty can be used for hyperopia and/or astigmatism, IOL exchange or piggyback

IOLs can correct spherical errors, and laser vision correction can treat residual myopia, hyperopia, and/or astigmatism. The most precise method of all of these approaches is laser vision correction. The precision of the excimer laser is unparalleled in its ability to achieve targeted refractive outcomes.

However, not all patients are candidates for laser vision correction. Therefore, a proper screening examination is required. Some of these measurements are ideally obtained prior to the lens surgery to determine whether a laser vision-correcting procedure is even possible or safe. To begin with, refractive stability is imperative. For most small-incision lens surgeries, this occurs by 1 month postoperatively. Therefore, it is probably best to wait 1 to 3 months after lens surgery before performing a laser enhancement. At this time point, there is typically no concern for wound dehiscence with microkeratome passes for small well-constructed self-sealing incisions.

Pachymetry measurements are also important. Corneas must be of sufficient thickness to ensure adequate residual stromal bed depth. If the cornea is too thin, a surface ablation can be considered or an alternative surgical approach is required. Topography is also part of the evaluation process because it helps in identifying risk factors for postoperative ectasia.

Next, a careful ocular examination should be done. Treatment of blepharitis and lid malposition should be done prior to keratorefractive surgery to prevent dry eyes, keratitis, and exposure keratopathy. A careful slit lamp examination should be done to identify keratoconjunctivitis sicca, anterior basement membrane dystrophy (ABMD), corneal neovascularization, endothelial disease, and the clarity of the posterior capsule. Significant preoperative dry eye should be treated aggressively prior to laser surgery with artificial tears, ointments, topical cyclosporine, and/or punctal plugs. In the presence of ABMD, a surface ablation is preferred to avoid a

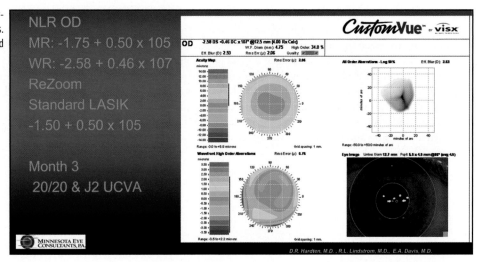

Figure 1. LASIK enhancement was performed following a ReZoom IOL implantation with excellent results. Wavefront capture was unreliable, so a standard treatment was chosen.

microkeratome-induced epithelial slough. A couple millimeters of corneal neovascularization is often not problematic, but greater amounts can lead to intraoperative bleeding. A course of preoperative steroids can sometimes improve neovascularization. Proper hinge placement, often most accurately achieved with a femtosecond laser in laser in situ keratomileusis (LASIK) can avoid cutting across these vessels. Certainly, eyes with compromised endothelium are at risk for poor flap adherence with LASIK. Posterior capsule clouding can interfere with accurate refractions and wavefront aberrometry. Hence, where indicated, yttrium-aluminum-garnet (YAG) capsulotomy should be performed prior to the enhancement. And lastly, a careful funduscopic exam should be done to exclude the presence of cystoid macular edema.

Most patients prefer bilateral simultaneous laser surgery if both eyes require enhancements. This avoids anisometropia, the inconvenience and stress of returning for 2 procedures versus 1, the need to take eye drops for a longer period of time, and the necessity of additional postoperative visits. However, in certain cases, it may be preferable to perform laser surgery on one eye at a time. The most common indication for this is a surface laser enhancement where visual recovery is slower than with a lamellar procedure. This allows for functional vision out of the nonoperated eye during the recovery period.

LASIK provides a faster visual recovery than surface ablation (PRK, laser epithelial keratomileusis [LASEK], epi-LASIK) and hence, when possible, many patients prefer this approach. However, in certain cases a surface procedure may be safer. This includes ABMD, thin corneas, and suspicious topographic patterns. Both approaches work well after lens surgery and the choice is based upon a careful evaluation, as outlined above.

When it is recognized preoperatively that a patient will require a laser vision enhancement after lens surgery, some refractive surgeons feel that it is preferable to choose a lens power targeting a myopic outcome when possible. Myopic outcomes are more tolerable for patients postoperatively during the 1 to 3 months they must wait for stability. Furthermore, some refractive surgeons believe that myopic laser surgical outcomes are more accurate and less likely to regress than hyperopic treatments, although not all would agree with this statement. In addition, some would argue that the advantage of

aiming for emmetropia is that the second laser procedure may, in fact, not be necessary after all.

Wavefront treatments are typically preferable over standard treatments, especially when reliable aberrometry measurements can be obtained. One major advantage of custom LASIK is the better result for astigmatic targeting with iris registration. Because even manifest refractions are multifocal, it is important that these patients have a pushed-plus manifest refraction to maximize accuracy of the refraction. This pushed-plus manifest refraction should match the wavefront measurement. The refraction or wavefront capture after a multifocal IOL may show results that are surprising, and it may be more difficult to capture the wavefront because of the multifocal IOL or capsular opacity (Figure 1). It is important to consider the effects of anterior capsular opacity also, as a small capsulorrhexis may preclude a 5-mm wavefront capture. Standard LASIK may be all that is possible in some eyes, and it typically provides good results. It is important that the patient's uncorrected visual acuity (UCVA) correlates with their refraction. Beware of refracting the near zones on the IOL. It does not make sense to perform a standard or custom ablation of −2.25 D for a patient who is 20/40 uncorrected.

In our experience at Minnesota Eye Consultants, in 20 eyes treated with laser vision correction after presbyopia-correcting IOLs, we felt comfortable with the wavefront capture in 20% of the eyes and were able to use custom treatments. In 80%, the wavefront capture did not adequately match the manifest refraction and UCVA, so standard treatments were used. Reduction of the astigmatism was seen from 0.98 ± 0.38 D preoperatively to 0.43 ± 0.35 D postoperatively. Reduction was obtained in the spherical equivalent (SE) from an absolute mean preoperatively of 1.08 ± 0.92 D to an average SE of −0.23 ± 0.44 D postoperatively.

Not all surgeons who perform lens surgery also perform laser vision correction. This does not mean that those surgeons cannot avail themselves of the benefits of laser vision correction. In such cases, referral to a partner or colleague in the community who is a LASIK or PRK surgeon is often possible. A financial arrangement that makes sense for the laser surgeon and the patient should be determined beforehand.

Finally, laser surgery as an enhancement procedure is best discussed at the initial visit with the patient before the lens surgery. Once the surgeon understands the refractive goals of the patient, he or she will not only be able to select the best possible lens to meet the patient's needs and desires but will have a good sense of whether secondary enhancement surgery will be required. The patient can then be counseled on the need for 2 procedures to achieve the desired visual outcome and any additional costs that might be incurred. Most patients appreciate understanding the entire process at the outset, rather than learning about it in a piecemeal fashion.

In conclusion, laser vision enhancement after lens surgery is a very accurate and successful way to achieve a precise refractive outcome. Careful preoperative screening is critical to determining appropriate candidates. Most patients are amenable to this surgical option to improve their vision but prefer to know the process and costs up front.

CHAPTER 212

LASER ENHANCEMENT—WHAT CATARACT SURGEONS SHOULD KNOW

Jose. L. Güell, MD; Javier A. Gaytan Melicoff, MD; Natalia Pelaez, MD; Merce Morral, MD; and Felicidad Manero, MD

Cataract surgery can be considered the oldest and most common refractive procedure.[4] Different techniques, equipment and formulas have been developed to obtain the most accurate IOL power for each patient. Nevertheless, unexpected postsurgical ametropia may still occur after uneventful cataract surgery.[1]

During the past 20 years, and even nowadays, postoperative refractive problems have been corrected with spectacles, contact lenses, an intraocular lens (IOL) exchange, or a piggyback procedure. The first two options are good choices if the patient agrees to wear them. An IOL exchange could increase the risk of posterior capsular rupture, iris damage, macular edema and endothelial cell loss, especially in the elderly or in cases where IOL implantation was performed years ago.[2]

As we know, laser in situ keratomileusis (LASIK) and/or surface ablation techniques (photorefractive keratectomy [PRK], laser-assisted epithelial keratomileusis [LASEK], epiLASIK) are the preferred procedures for refractive enhancement, when deemed to be feasible and safe. These are typically very effective when performed as primary procedures. Good results have also been reported for laser enhancement procedures after cataract extraction with IOL implantation.[4]

Some of the main concerns for anterior segment and refractive surgeons about performing LASIK in pseudophakic eyes are incision leakage, IOL dislocation, and increased risk of endothelial cell loss and retinal detachment. In our experience, there is no evidence of increasing these risks when the recommended safety guidelines for a refractive procedure are strictly followed.[4]

Safety Guidelines for Laser Refractive Procedures in Pseudophakic Eyes

Items to be confirmed prior to laser surgery:

* At least 3 months should have elapsed after IOL implantation or suture removal. In the event of bilateral surgery, and particularly if there is a target of monovision, we wait 3 months after the second eye procedure.
* There must be healthy epithelium around the cataract incision, especially if you are planning LASIK.
* Corneal topography showing an amount of regular astigmatism, that closely matches the subjective refraction.
* There should be no history of any other ocular surgeries beside cataract surgery and IOL implantation.
* The cornea should be clear, with no scarring. The endothelial cell count should be greater than 1,800 c/mm².
* Ultrasound, corneal topography, or anterior chamber optical coherence tomography (OCT) pachymetric evaluation should be performed.
* There should be more than two lines difference in the Snellen visual acuity between the uncorrected visual acuity (UCVA) and best spectacle corrected visual acuity (BSCVA).
* The mesopic pupil diameter should be less than 5 mm.
* The suggested treatment profile is a 6 mm ablation zone diameter for up to −5.00 D myopic, −4.00 D astigmatic and +3.00 D hyperopic correction.
* The fundus examination and intraocular pressure should be normal.

Planning Bioptics or Adjustable Refractive Surgery

There are several situations in cataract and refractive surgery where more than one procedure should be considered, because of a high spherical or astigmatic error. This will mostly depend on patient profile features such as profession, age, and visual expectations. For a patient such as a professional driver, who requires excellent distance vision, the goal will definitely be a plano target refraction. As we know, additional moderate to high astigmatism cannot be corrected by a nontoric IOL implantation at the time of cataract surgery, but could still be addressed with corneal ablational (laser) or incisional (arcuate keratotomy, limbal relaxing incisions) techniques. In other circumstances such as presbyopic patients looking for reasonable distance vision with an improvement in near vision, our approach might be a low myopic target refraction for both eyes or perhaps monovision.

In our experience, the two most important indications for a laser refractive surgery enhancement after cataract surgery follow.

HIGH AMETROPIA WITH OR WITHOUT ASTIGMATISM

In cases of myopic refractive errors, special care should be taken when evaluating the fundus. Any retinal lesion should be treated before cataract extraction and the patient should be warned about the association of high myopia with retinal detachment.[5]

In the case of high astigmatism, corneal topography is a key factor in determining whether LASIK, PRK, or arcuate incisions should be performed. Keratometry values higher than 47 D in any meridian would increase the risk of flap-related complications. PRK could be performed in such cases, to avoid microkeratome-induced complications.

We should also remember that incisional surgery at the time of cataract extraction is a highly effective approach. The major disadvantage is lower predictability when compared to laser refractive procedures performed several weeks after the cataract surgery.

When we already know before surgery that the necessary IOL power is not available, we must plan for the secondary enhancement treatment in advance.

When tailoring the ablation profile of the enhancement procedure, we must consider the optical zone, residual corneal thickness, and postoperative corneal keratometric values. Sometimes, an IOL power surprise occurs despite using the best formulas. Our strategy for IOL power calculations is always to attempt to achieve the lowest residual refractive error and then enhance with corneal surgery techniques as needed.

Some studies have reported good results in patients with high refractive errors (−17.50 to +8.50 D) prior to cataract surgery, resulting in a mean spherical equivalent as low as +0.26 D sphere, with a mean cylinder of 0.30 D, and an UCVA of 20/40 in 81.8% of the cases, after the second refractive procedure.[6]

INDUCE OR REVERSE MONOVISION

Monovision has been around for a long time and is presently gaining wider acceptance worldwide. It is a practical option for patients within the presbyopic age group. Most patients adapt to monovision without major difficulties and are satisfied with the results. Patient satisfaction begins with proper expectations and understanding of what refractive outcome can be achieved. Proper patient education is key. Patients should be told about potential fluctuations in the vision following surgery. The patient should also understand that absolutely perfect distance and near vision is unlikely and that monovision represents a compromise. Daily activities will

usually be performed comfortably without glasses but total spectacle independence is unlikely. The second key point is to explain that if the patient is unable to adapt to monovision, the myopia can potentially be reversed by a LASIK or PRK treatment.

Some presbyopic patients may be dissatisfied and disappointed with their lack of near vision after achieving bilateral emmetropia following IOL implantation. They should be given the option of monovision, with the understanding that the myopia can potentially be later reversed with additional refractive surgery. We usually recommend that patients first try monovision for this reason. If they are uncomfortable with monovision, we can later perform laser refractive surgery in one eye, to either achieve binocular near or binocular distance vision depending on the patient's preference.

When planning a monovision procedure, it is very important to determine which is the dominant eye (without using cycloplegics) in order to decide which eye should be under corrected.

In this group of patients, and especially in the elderly, it is important to consider that the older the person is, the greater the tendency will be to have a postoperative hyperopic shift, even when operating on low refractive errors. This fact could possibly be explained by a poor stromal healing response and early sub-clinical corneal edema.[4]

Unexpected Refractive Error

This is the most frequent indication for performing a refractive surgery enhancement after cataract surgery. As mentioned before, although various formulas and technologies have been developed for IOL power calculations, unexpected refractive errors may still occur.

Most of the studies have looked at this situation where correcting small to moderate residual refractive errors were shown to make a difference in patient satisfaction and lifestyle quality. In the absence of surgical complications, laser enhancement treatments have efficacy and safety results that are comparable to those of primary laser refractive treatments. One study reported achieving uncorrected vision of 20/40 or better in 91.7% of eyes with residual myopia and 20/40 or better in 90.9% of eyes with residual hyperopia.[7]

In our experience, we have found that the lower the residual refraction error is, the better the postoperative accuracy and stability are. This is the main reason we recommend using this procedure for the previously mentioned refractive ranges.

LASIK or PRK?

If you decide to perform any laser refractive procedure following cataract surgery, you should proceed as if you were approaching a virgin cornea. Surgery indications should be guided by risk factors for LASIK-related complications, such as a thin central corneal thickness, irregular axial and posterior elevations on topography, epithelial defects, corneal dystrophies, and extreme keratometry values. On the other hand, PRK should be cautiously considered when there is risk of haze related to a high amount of tissue consumption.[8]

As previously reported, and consistent with our own experience, LASIK and PRK did not show any significant difference in efficacy and safety in the setting of refractive enhancement following cataract surgery.[4]

When performing any of these procedures, you should make sure that the refraction is stabile and corneal wound healing is complete. This is the reason why some recommend waiting at least 3 months to perform LASIK or PRK, so as to prevent complications such as corneal wound leakage, or epithelial defect.[9]

Toric IOLs and Refractive Surgery

Residual refractive errors may be encountered after a toric IOL implantation as well. The first approach should always be to recheck the IOL spherical and cylindric powers as well as proper IOL cylinder axis alignment. The toric IOL should be repositioned in case of a misaligned cylindrical axis. IOL exchange could be considered if the main problem is the spherical power. The need for these surgical interventions must be ruled out before considering corneal refractive enhancement techniques. Residual spherical and astigmatic errors could be induced by other factors, such as IOL tilt or decentration. If the errors are not related to the cornea or its topography, it may be impossible to correct them by reshaping the cornea.

Aberrations and optical factors, such as point spread function (PSF) or modulation transfer function (MTF), should be considered when planning refractive enhancement after refractive IOLs, such as toric, multifocal, or accommodating lenses.

Recent studies conducted by different authors have achieved excellent results with correcting low postoperative residual refractive errors, without the need for corneal ablational techniques. This is achieved with a new technology called the LAL (light adjustable lens), where the optic of the IOL contains UVA photosensitive polymers that can be light adjusted in a way so as to alter the spherical and cylindrical power of the lens. This technology is capable of correcting spherical refractive errors of up to 3 D.[10]

Conclusion

Corneal refractive enhancement procedures can be used to improve patients' refractive outcomes, satisfaction, and quality of life. We recommend these procedures following cataract surgery, provided that the risks of technique-related complications and patient- related complications are not elevated for a given individual. Other options such as piggyback IOL implantation in pseudophakic eyes are available alternatives, but are beyond the scope of this chapter.

Besides refractive treatment, laser procedures also allow for improvement in quality of vision. In addition to low order aberrations (sphere and cylinder) correction, laser procedures can be complimented with high order aberrations (especially those spheric) refinement.

References

1. Langenbucher A, Haigis W, Seitz B. Difficult lens power calculations. *Curr Opin Ophthalmol.* 2004;15:1-9.

2. Diaz-Valle D, Benitez del Castillo Sánchez JM, Castillo A, et al. Endotelial damage with cataract surgery techniques. *J Cataract Refract Surg.* 1998;24:951-955.

3. Steinert RF, Shamik B. Surgical correction of moderate myopia. II. PRK and LASIK are the treatments of choice. *Surv Ophthalmol.* 1998;43:157-179.

4. Kuo IC, O'Brien TP, Broman AT, Ghajarnia M, Jabbur NS. Excimer laser surgery for correction of ametropia after cataract surgery. *J Cataract Refract Surg.* 2005;31:2104-2110.

5. Ravalico G, Michieli C, Vattovani O, Tognetto D. Retinal detachment after cataract extraction and refractive lens exchange in highly myopic patients. *J Cataract Refract Surg.* 2003;29:39-44.

6. Velarde JI, Anton PG, de Valentin-Gamazo L. Intraocular lens implantation and laser in situ keratomileusis (bioptics) to correct high myopia and hyperopia with astigmatism. *J Refract Surg.* 2001;17(2 Suppl):S234-S237.

7. Kim P, Briganti EM, Sutton GL, Lawless MA, Rogers CM, Hodge C. Laser in situ keratomileusis for refractive error after cataract surgery. *J Cataract Refract Surg.* 2005;31:979-986.

8. Guell JL, Gris O, de Muller A, Corcostegui B. LASIK for the correction of residual refractive errors from previous surgical procedures. *Ophthalmic Surg Lasers.* 1999;30:341-349.

9. Ayala MJ, Perez-Santonja JJ, Arola A, et al. Laser in situ keratomileusis to correct residual myopia after cataract surgery. *J Refract Surg.* 2001;17:12-16.

10. Schwartz DM. Light-adjustable lens: development of in vitro nomograms. *Trans Am Ophthalmol Soc.* 2004;102:67-72.

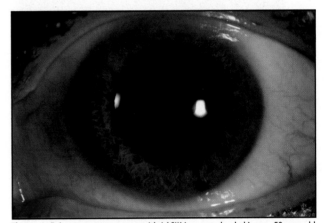

Figure 1. Enhancement treatment with LASIK in a pseudo phakic eye. 58 year-old patient with cataract extraction surgery and IOL implantation performed in both eyes. Residual, stable refraction after surgery—OD: −0.25 cyl 100 degrees, OS: −1.75 sph −1.25 cyl 80 degrees. Visual acuity on Snellen Chart—UCVA OD: 20/20, OS: 20/100; BSCVA OD: 20/20, OS: 20/20. Dominant eye—OD. Enhancement treatment with LASIK was performed on the left eye aiming for monovision, leaving an intentional 0.5 D sphere myopic undercorrection. Final refraction after OS corneal enhancement treatment: −0.5 sphere. Distance Visual Acuity—OD: UCVA and BSCVA were 20/20, OS: UCVA was 20/25, BSCVA was 20/20. The patient was comfortable with binocular distance vision as well as with binocular near vision.

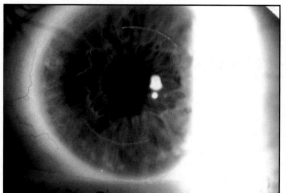

Figure 2. Arcuate keratotomies, cataract extraction, and IOL implantation (OS). A 35 year-old patient with hypermetropia and astigmatism—OD: +4.5 sph −3.0 cyl 10 degrees, OS: +3.5 sph −3.0 cyl 170 degrees. Preoperative visual acuity (Snellen)—OD UCVA 20/60 BSCVA 20/25; OS UCVA 20/40, BSCVA 20/25. Arcuate keratotomies were performed in addition to lens extraction and IOL placement. Arcuate keratotomies—OD: two separate incisions with 60-degree arc, centered at the 100-degree meridian with a 7 mm optic zone and 565 microns depth, OS: arcuate keratotomies with 60-degree arc, centered at the 80-degree meridian with a 7 mm optic zone and 565 microns depth. Postoperative refraction—OD: +0.5 sph −1.0 cyl 20 degrees, OS: +0.25 −1.25 cyl 180 degrees. Postoperative Visual Acuity (Snellen)—OD: UCVA 20/30, BSCVA 20/25; OI: UCVA 20/30, BSCVA 20/25.

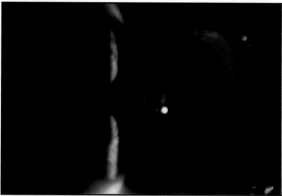

Figure 4. Arcuate keratotomies. Depth: 585 μm. Optic zone: 7 mm. Arc: 60 degrees.

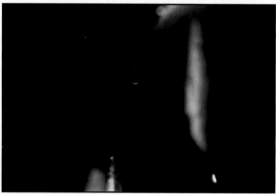

Figure 3. Arcuate keratotomy depth (585 μm).

CHAPTER 213

POST-MULTIFOCAL IOL WAVEFRONT: ARE THE READINGS RELIABLE?

Charles Campbell

When the crystalline lens is replaced with an intraocular lens (IOL), it is often found that there is a postsurgical refractive error. In this age of very successful refractive surgery, it is natural to consider removing that residual refractive error using a laser refractive surgical treatment and planning that treatment using full wavefront error information from the postsurgical eye. However, when the implanted lens is a multifocal IOL, the question arises as to whether or not the wavefront measurement of the unusual wavefront created by the multifocal IOL gives useful information for planning a refractive surgical treatment. To address this question in a more rapid and controlled fashion than would be possible in a clinical trial, it has been studied first with a theoretical treatment followed by physical testing. The theoretical treatment was done to predict the result of measuring an eye with a wavefront refractor. A physical test using a special fluid-filled test eye that allowed the IOL to act optically just as it would in a human eye and permitted it to be measured with a commercial wavefront eye refractor just as a human eye would be was then done, with the results compared to the theoretical predictions.

Theoretical Treatment

A Shack-Hartmann wavefront sensor divides the wavefront under examination into small square areas through the use of an array of lenslets, each of which is a powerful positive lens that concentrates the light from the portion of the wavefront the passes through it onto a CCD sensor. It is the position of this concentrated spot of light on the sensor that is used to find the slope of that portion of the wavefront that passed through the lenslet. The ensemble of slopes from each lenslet in the array is then used to reconstruct the wavefront. Thus a critical part of the whole Shack-Hartmann wavefront-sensing method is the character of the concentrated spot of light whose position gives the necessary wavefront slope information.

Normally a small area of a wavefront does not depart in a significant manner from a small toric surface, which is tipped with respect to the optical axis of the instrument. But in the case of a diffractive bifocal IOL, it is quite possible that one of the echelet edges, where the wavefront abruptly jumps by approximately one half of a wavelength, will pass through a lenslet. A straight forward calculation using diffraction optics principles predicts that when a half-wave phase jump occurs near the center of a lenslet, the light concentrated on the sensor splits in two, so the instead of one spot being formed one should find two. This doubling is also predicted to occur if more than one echelet edge passes through a single lenslet. In addition, if the phase jump is somewhat less than one half a wavelength, one of the 2 spots will be brighter than the other. This typically occurs because a diffractive bifocal IOL is usually designed to have half-wavelength phase jumps at a mid visible wavelength of 555 nm, whereas wavefront refractors measure, using infrared radiation, in the range of 760 to 850 nm. The question, which can only be answered by trial, is how a given wavefront eye refractor will deal with doubled spots and what its displayed measurement will show.

Some multifocal IOLs do not use a diffractive design but use a multizone refractive design where the power of the lens varies from one annular zone to its neighbors on both sides. Although there are no abrupt wavefront phase jumps in these designs, the wavefront can exhibit quite high local curvature in the transition zone between the main annular power zones, so that some lenslets will sample quite irregular portions of the wavefront. In addition, the local power and hence wavefront slope is expected to vary markedly over fairly short distances. So although the wavefront sensor will not have to deal with doubled but well-defined spots, it will have to deal with a wavefront that will appear to be highly aberrated in an overall sense.

Experimental Methods and Materials

To physically test the performance of a Shack-Hartmann wavefront eye refractor when measuring an eye with a multifocal IOL, implanted IOLs were placed in a special test eye

Figure 1. A cross-sectional view of the fluid filled model test eye configured for measurement with a wavefront eye refractor (ie, with an artificial retina inserted versus a transparent window). The IOL under test is shown suspended from its haptics in the pupil disk just as it is in human eye.

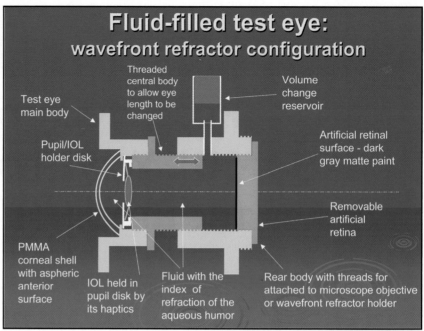

Fluid-filled test eye:
wavefront refractor configuration

that simulates quite accurately the optical conditions found in a human eye.

The only optical element in a human eye with an IOL implanted, other than the IOL itself, is the cornea. It is a highly curved meniscus shell approximately 0.5. mm thick in the center. A representative average human cornea has a central radius of curvature of 7.8 mm and is aspherical with a conic constant of −0.2. The average corneal has a posterior radius of curvature of 6.4 mm with a conic constant of −0.4. To duplicate the optical performance of this average cornea, the test eye was built with a polymethylmethacrylate (PMMA) meniscus shell as its first element. The central anterior radius of curvature of the shell was 7.8 mm. The surface was cut as an ellipse of revolution with a conic constant of −0.1. The shell was 0.5 mm thick centrally. The posterior surface was spherical with a radius of curvature of 7.22 mm. These parameters were chosen because when a collimated beam of light enters such a shell and exits into fluid with the index of refraction of a aqueous humor of the eye (1.336), the wavefront has the same central vergence and the same higher-order aberration (spherical aberration) as does a similar wavefront exiting the average cornea into the anterior chamber of the eye. Thus, if the IOL is held with respect to the artificial cornea at the same distance as it is held from the cornea in the human eye, the same optical condition exits for both situations.

In the test eye, the artificial corneal shell is attached to the main body of the eye and the inside of the test eye is filled with fluid. To provide a fluid with the correct index of refraction (1.336), sucrose was added to water to create a 2.1% solution.

Within the test eye, the IOL was held in a specially made disk that allowed the lens to be wholly supported by its haptics, thus suspending it just as it is in the human eye. The disk had a central clear aperture that simulated the pupil created by the iris in the human eye. The clear aperture chosen for testing was 5 mm. This value was chosen to insure that light only passed through optical zone of the IOLs, which had optical zone diameters of 6 mm, and none passed through the haptics

of the lenses, even it they were slightly decentered. When viewed from outside the test eye, this disk aperture size creates a visible pupil diameter of 5.75 mm. The disk is held within the body of the eye at a distance of 3.5 mm from the posterior surface of the corneal shell so that the IOL is held at the same distance from that surface as it is held from the posterior corneal surface in the human eye. This is an important consideration because if the lens is incorrectly spaced, the blurring effect of imaging objects at various viewing distances will not be similar to that found in the human eye.

The final element in the test eye is an artificial retinal surface. It is the flat surface of the plug that is screwed into and seals the rear of the test eye. This surface is painted with a flat dark gray paint that has been found to backscatter light with the same intensity as a human retina when irradiated with near infrared radiation. This allows a wavefront eye refractor to successfully measure the refractive state of the test eye just as it would measure the refractive state of a human eye.

A cross-sectional view of the model test eye is given in Figure 1.

The rear plug of the test eye is designed so that it may be replaced with a transparent window constructed of 1-mm-thick microscope slide whose internal surface is at exactly the same axial position as the artificial retinal surface. The test eye was used in this configuration during the first part of the testing so that its overall length could be adjusted to achieve the desired distance refractive error via the use of special optical apparatus. For these tests the distance refractive error of the test eye was adjusted to 0 diopter (D) (ie, an object at optical infinity).

The special optical apparatus consists of a Badal optometer illumination system having a 100-mm focal length optometer lens and a 10-μm pinhole source irradiated with a halogen lamp, a 10× microscope objective focused on the inner surface of the rear window of the test eye, a CCD (charge coupled device) camera (pixel size 5.4 x 5.4 μm) attached to the microscope objective, and a computer to display the live image created.

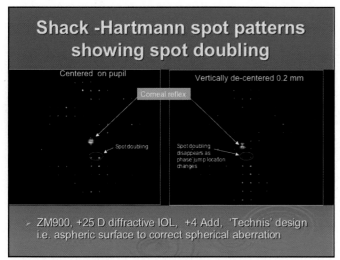

Figure 2. Shack-Hartmann spot images taken during refraction of the fluid filled test eye with a diffractive IOL inserted showing spot doubling in spots associated with some lenslets in the Shack-Hartmann array. The 2 images came from measurements taken with a different centration of the test eye pupil with respect to the refractor and the encircled spots illustrate how spot doubling is affected by the relationship of a diffractive IOL echelet to the given lenslet in the Shack-Hartmann array.

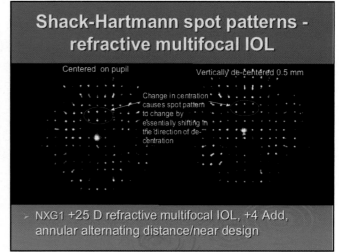

Figure 3. Shack-Hartmann spot images taken during refraction of the fluid filled test eye with a refractive multifocal alternating-zone IOL inserted. The 2 images came from measurements taken with a different centration of the test eye pupil with respect to the refractor and the encircled spots illustrate the change in the spot pattern caused by decentration of the eye with respect to the wavefront refractor. The WaveScan wavefront refractor has a lenslet pitch of 0.4 mm so the vertical decentration of 0.5 mm was a little more that 1 pitch distance and indeed it appears that the major change in the spot pattern was to shift it vertically by 1 period.

The Badal optometer was set to produce collimated light (0-D vergence) and the length of the test eye length adjusted until the best point spread was created as viewed by the microscope system. The vergence was then changed to simulate viewing a near object until a second good point spread appeared. The later step was done to ensure that the near focus of the multifocal IOL was not mistaken for the distance focus.

With the test eye properly adjusted for length, the transmission window was replaced with the artificial retinal plug and the test eye was measured with a wavefront eye refractor just as a human eye would be measured.

A number of multifocal IOLs, both diffractive and refractive, were then tested. As the general results were similar for a given type, only the results of one of each type are given here. Those lenses are the Advanced Medical Optics (Santa Ana, CA) ZM900 series (Tecnis design, with diffractive +25 D, +4 D add) and the Advanced Medical Optics NXG1 series (ReZoom design, with refractive 25 D, +4 D add).

The aberrations of the entire test eye were measured with a commercial wavefront eye refractor, the WaveScan (Advanced Medical Optics).

Results

The test eye was first measured with no IOL in place to assess the amount of higher order aberration induced by the corneal shell alone. It was found that the coefficient of the Zernike term $Z_{4,0}$ had a value of 0.20 μm with a 6-mm-diameter visible pupil. No other higher order aberrations were found to be significant.

The diffractive lens reported is a +25 D Advanced Medical Optics bifocal lens model ZM900. This lens is designed to remove 0.27 μm root-mean-square (RMS) spherical aberration error in addition to having a 4-D near point add. The Advanced Medical Optics VISX WaveScan found a residual sphere and cylinder +0.13 DS, -0.08 DC x 160 degrees. This

is, within experimental uncertainty, the vergence that the test eye was set for. The Zernike coefficients are for a 5.75-mm visible pupil diameter. This is the full-pupil diameter expected based on the 5-mm choice for the pupil disk aperture. The only significant higher order aberration found for coma ($Z_{3,1}$) where the magnitude was 0.10 μm, and for spherical aberration ($Z_{4,0}$) where the magnitude was −0.10 μm. Note that the IOL is designed to remove 0.27 μm of spherical aberration and it is known that the corneal shell alone contributed 0.20 μm of spherical aberration. Thus the measured value was quite close to the expected value of −0.07 μm. The coma found was most probably caused by a slight decentration of the lens with respect to the artificial pupil and corneal shell.

Examination of the image of Shack-Hartmann spots revealed doubled spots of unequal intensity. When the instrument was decentered with respect to the test eye by one half a lenslet period (0.2 mm), it was found that some of the doubled spots resolved into a single spot, as was expected as the half-wave phase jump was moved out of the central portion of the associated lenslet. Figure 2 shows this effect in the Shack-Hartmann images.

The refractive lens reported was a +25 D Advanced Medical Optics multifocal lens model NXG1. This lens is designed to have a near point add of 4 D. The Advanced Medical Optics VISX WaveScan system found a residual sphere and cylinder −1.27 DS, -0.07 DC x 166 degrees. This value is quite difference from the 0 DS to which the test was set. The coefficients of the higher-order aberrations reported were quite different from zero. The WaveScan system could only use spots from a visible pupil diameter of 5 mm, as the outer spots were judged to be of too low a quality to use. Figure 3 shows the effect of decentration of 0.5 mm on the spot pattern. Even though the spot pattern changed visibly with decentration, it will be noted in Table 1 that the measured higher-order aberrations did not

Table 1

MEASURED ZERNIKE COEFFICIENTS FOR BOTH TYPES OF MULTIFOCAL IOL

Lens	NXG1 +25 D Centered	NXG1 +25 D Decentered 0.5 mm Vertically	ZM900 +25 D Centered	ZM900 +25 D Decentered 0.2 mm Vertically	
Pupil diameter	5.0 mm	5.0 mm	5.75 mm	5.75 mm	
Sphere (D)	–1.27	–1.14	0.13	0.10	
Cylinder (D)	–0.07 at 166 degrees	–0.15 at 2 degrees	–0.08 at 160 degrees	–0.03 at 177	
Zernike Term	Magnitude (μm)/ Axis	Magnitude (μm)/Axis	Magnitude (μm)/ Axis	Magnitude (μm)/ Axis	Name
$Z_{3,1}$	0.19 at 264 degrees	0.26 at 334 degrees	0.10 at 348 degrees	0.09 at 335 degrees	Coma
$Z_{3,3}$	0.04 at 111 degrees	0.07 at 18 degrees	0.04 at 107 degrees	0.04 at 116 degrees	Trefoil
$Z_{4,0}$	–0.01	–0.12	–0.10	–0.10	Spherical aberration
$Z_{4,2}$	0.06 at 136 degrees	0.06 at 176 degrees	0.02 at 81 degrees	0.04 at 71 degrees	
$Z_{4,4}$	0.06 at 77 degrees	0.06 at 59 degrees	0.02 at 18 degrees	0.01 at 55 degrees	
$Z_{5,1}$	0.21 at 246 degrees	0.19 at 340 degrees	0.01 at 158 degrees	0.01 at 174 degrees	2nd coma
$Z_{5,3}$	0.02 at 91 degrees	0.02 at 107 degrees	0.01 at 30 degrees	0.01 at 37 degrees	
$Z_{5,5}$	0.09 at 20 degrees	0.04 at 4 degrees	0.02 at 36 degrees	0.01 at 43 degrees	
$Z_{6,0}$	–0.40	–0.42	0	–0.01	2nd spherical aberration
$Z_{6,2}$	0.04 at 84 degrees	0.03 at 174 degrees	0.01 at 42 degrees	0.01 at 116 degrees	
$Z_{6,4}$	0.03 at 75 degrees	0.03 at 48 degrees	0.02 at 87 degrees	0.02 at 11 degrees	
$Z6,6$	0.04 at 35 degrees	0.02 at 39 degrees	0.01 at 23 degrees	0.01 at 5 degrees	

change in a significant fashion, with the exception of coma where the magnitude changed by 0.07 μm and the axis rotated toward the vertical meridian, an expected result for a vertical decentration in the presence of a significant amount of secondary spherical aberration ($Z_{6,0}$).

The measured Zernike coefficients for both types of multifocal IOL are given in magnitude axis form[1] in the Table 1.

Conclusions and Recommendations

The wavefront refractions values found in the case of the refractive multifocal IOL are quite different from the expected values, based on the measured refractive state of the test eye using point spread images with different, known target vergences enter the test eye. The sphere and cylinder power values found were quite different from either the expected distance refractive state or the expected near refractive state for the measured add value. The higher-order aberrations were significant.

For these reasons, wavefront refraction values taken from an eye with a refractive multifocal implanted should not be used to plan refractive surgery to remove residual sphere and cylinder error. Indeed, it is most likely that if the wavefront findings were used in such cases to plan a waveguide laser refractive treatment, the multifocal effect would be removed with an uncertain outcome for sphere and cylinder. For these eyes, subjective refraction for a distance target should be used to plan a refractive treatment to remove residual post operative refractive error.

In the case of an eye with a diffractive IOL implanted, reasonable results were found that could be used to plan treatment to remove residual refractive error. However, this study was done using only one model of wavefront eye refractor and it may be that other wavefront eye refractors using the Shack-Hartmann principle, having different analysis algorithms, may be more troubled by the doubled spots than was the WaveScan. Thus, before giving a blanket recommendation to use wavefront results for eyes with these IOLs implanted, it is recommended that wavefront results be compared with refractive results found using distance-subjective refraction to ensure that the wavefront refractor in the clinic performs as well as the WaveScan did in the testing with the fluid-filled eye.

References

1. American National Standards Institute. 2004. Methods for Reporting Optical Aberrations of Eyes. *ANSI.* Z80.23:2004.

CHAPTER 214

MINI-RK:
INDICATIONS AND TECHNIQUE

Richard L. Lindstrom, MD

Myopia that occurs following cataract surgery can be reduced with radial keratotomy (RK).

Patients undergoing RK should have stable, non-progressive myopia confirmed by multiple refractions. Contact lens wear must be discontinued before consideration of RK so that any possible corneal warpage associated with contact lens use can be detected. Slit lamp examination should reveal an essentially normal cornea. Patients with ocular conditions such as glaucoma or uveitis may be poor candidates for RK because the effects of these disorders on the outcome are not well defined. Individuals with systemic conditions that might affect cornea healing, including patients with connective tissue diseases, those with herpes simplex keratitis, or patients using systemic corticosteroids, may be unsuitable candidates for RK.

RK achieves the best uncorrected visual acuity in patients who have low to moderate myopia (−1.00 to −4.00 diopters [D]). Other refractive corneal procedures are available, including excimer laser photorefractive keratectomy (PRK), laser in-situ keratomileusis (LASIK), epi-LASIK, and intrastromal corneal rings. Some patients may be better candidates for one of the other procedures if their myopia is outside the range of RK.

Surgeons must understand that although nomograms for RK are based on averages for large numbers of procedures, the outcome of surgery cannot be precisely predicted for an individual eye. Additional refractive keratotomy incisions may be needed to achieve the desired result, and spectacles or contact lenses may still be required for best visual acuity, even after surgery. Patients should be informed that contact lens fitting may be more difficult after RK because of changes in corneal topography. Candidates for RK must understand that the surgery does not alter the normal aging process of presbyopia, for which most persons require reading glasses after the age of 40 to 45 years. Some persons older than 40 may exchange dependence on distance spectacles for dependence on reading glasses after RK. In the Prospective Evaluation of Radial Keratotomy (PERK) study at 10 years, 39% of patients older than 40 years required reading glasses for near work because of presbyopia.

Patients with a specific occupational motivation must be certain that the correction of myopia by incisional keratotomy is acceptable to their employer. Some occupations or careers will exclude a person from participation because of prior RK.

Principles

There are four surgical variables that can be adjusted to achieve the desired result.

1. The diameter of the central clear zone can be adjusted between 3 and 5.5 mm. The smaller the diameter of the central clear zone, the greater the degree of flattening achieved. A review of nomograms suggests that the largest central clear zone with any efficacy is 5.5 mm. RK incisions with an optical zone of 6 mm or greater have virtually no effect on the refractive error, supporting the position that radial incisions of the midperipheral cornea are responsible for the principal mechanical effect of the procedure. Most incisional keratotomy procedures involve optical zones of 3 to 5 mm.

2. The number of incisions usually varies from two to eight. Placement of more than eight incisions is generally not warranted because these succeeding incisions have progressively less effect. Placement of four radial incisions achieves greater than 70% of the effect achieved with eight incisions. For this reason, several surgeons have recommended a staged approach to RK in an attempt to minimize overcorrection.

3. The greater the depth of the incision, the greater the degree of central flattening. Centrifugally placed incisions (American technique) incise the cornea from the optical zone outward toward the limbus. This provides greater safety with regard to unintended incisions crossing the clear optical zone; however, these incisions may have a variable depth and tend to have a beveled incision

profile at the optical zone. Incisions placed in a centripetal manner (Russian technique) incise the cornea from the limbal area toward the optical zone mark; these are deep incisions, but they carry the risk of inadvertently entering the clear optical zone. Incisions made centripetally are often not perfectly straight because of the natural tendency of the knife to stray when cutting with the vertical edge. In an effort to consistently provide deep incisions without the risk of inadvertently entering the clear optical zone, a double-pass technique has been devised that offers the benefits of both the Russian and American techniques.

4. Incisions do not need to be carried to the limbus to achieve a near maximal effect. Lindstrom has shown that the effects are similar for radial incisions from a 3-mm clear zone carried to an 8-mm optical zone (mini-RK) and for those carried to an 11-mm optical zone. In fact, a mean increase of only 7.7% was seen when incisions were extended from the 7- to 11-mm optical zone. Thus, doubling the length of the RK incision achieved an additional effect of only 7.7%. The advantage of the shorter incisions is that the structural integrity of the cornea is better maintained. This may minimize the more serious complications and side effects of RK, including persistent diurnal fluctuation, long-term refractive instability with progressive hyperopic shift, and the potential for traumatic rupture of the keratotomy scars. Thus, the use of minimally invasive RK or mini-RK may retain the benefits of RK for most low to moderate myopes while significantly reducing the risks.

The key patient variable that clearly affects the outcome is age.

❖ The greater the patient's age, the greater the effect achieved with an identical surgical technique.

Patients older than 30 years can be expected to have an increased effect of 1.5% to 2.0% per year compared with a 30-year-old, whereas patients younger than 30 years can be expected to have a lesser effect of 1.5% to 2.0% per year compared with a 30-year-old. There may be other patient characteristics that affect the results of surgery, but these are difficult to measure consistently. These variables include corneal curvature, preoperative intraocular pressure, gender, corneal thickness, corneal diameter, axial length of the globe, and ocular rigidity. Most studies show that male patients, high intraocular tension, larger corneal diameter, a thicker cornea, a flatter cornea, and a higher ocular rigidity tent to result in a greater effect. Although these minor factors usually neutralize one another, the surgeon should screen for patients at high risk of overcorrection or undercorrection. The classic overresponder is the presbyopic, ocular hypertensive man who has a large, thick, flat cornea. The classic under-responder is the very young woman with a low intraocular tension and a small, thin, steep cornea.

Surgical Planning

The key to the surgical technique is the creation of a deep, consistent incision from the central optical zone toward the periphery. Incisions should always be terminated before the

vascular arcades of the limbus. RK incisions have traditionally been carried to the peripheral cornea approximating an 11- to 12-mm optical zone; however, our preferred approach is to create consistently deep radial incisions from the desire central clear zone to the 8-mm optical zone mark.

Good candidates for RK after refractive cataract surgery can be expected, on average, to obtain a full correction with no more than a 4-incision RK. Some patients may benefit from correction of anisometropia even if full correction of the myopia is not achieved. Intense counseling is performed and proper informed consent is obtained.

The nomograms used in surgical planning for RK are shown in Tables 1 and 2 (2-, and 4-incision MRK Nomograms 1 through 4). Patients with greater than 1.00 D of astigmatism may require combined radial and astigmatic keratotomy.

Surgical Technique

The patient is prepped with a 0.5% to 1.0% povidone-iodine solution, and the eye is centered under an operating microscope. The lashes are isolated with a plastic drape or solid blade speculum. No pilocarpine drops are given because of undesired displacement of the pupil. The lids are separated with a wire speculum. Topical 0.5% proparacaine hydrochloride or its equivalent is used every 1 to 5 minutes for a total of 3 doses. The patient is asked to fixate on the filament of the operating microscope or a fixation light. The central optical zone marker is centered on the pupil. A second 8-mm marker is placed concentrically surrounding the first. The temporal paracentral corneal thickness is measured adjacent to the central optical zone marker with an ultrasonic pachymeter. The diamond micrometer blade should be calibrated with a microscope capable of calibration to the micrometer level.

The diamond micrometer knife for center-to-periphery incisions (American technique) is set at 110% of temporal paracentral pachymetry. In the periphery-to-center approach (Russian technique) and the double-pass technique (Duotrac or Genesis technique), the knife is set at 100% of paracentral pachymetry.

The knife is set at the optical zone and plunged deliberately and straight into the cornea until the footplates are firmly positioned against the cornea. The tip of the knife is pointed at the center of the crystalline lens. This is followed by a 1-second pause, and, with mild pressure (enough to keep the footplates firm on the eye), a continuous incision is made. The cornea should be slightly moist, but excess fluid should be removed from the limbal area and fornices. This enables the surgeon to immediately detect a perforation. The surgeon's goal is to maintain the blade perpendicular to the corneal surface at all times. While making the incision, the surgeon can follow the "ski tracks" made by the footplates as well as the actual incision to maintain perpendicularity. When completed, the full-depth incision should extend from the inside of the central optical zone mark to the outside of the 8-mm mark. To accomplish this with the American technique, the knife tip is set at the inside edge of the central optical zone mark, thus cutting out the peripheral mark and achieving a full-depth cut from the central optical zone at least to the 7-mm optical zone. In periphery-to-central cutting (Russian technique), the knife is

Table 1

TWO-INCISION MRK NOMOGRAM

How to Use This Nomogram

- Identify the patient's age and the diopters of refractive myopia that you wish to correct.
- Find the patient's age in the first column on the left.
- Move to the right until you reach the surgery results closest to the refractive myopia of the patient. In order to avoid overcorrection, it is suggested that you select a surgical goal somewhat less than the actual refractive myopia. The column heading then tells you which surgery is needed to achieve this result.
- Consider placing the incisions on the steeper meridian when the patient has 0.75 to 1.50 D or more of astigmatism.

Example

- A 45-year-old patient with a refractive myopia of 1.75 and 1.00 D of astigmatism on the 90-degree axis.
- Moving to the right on the Age 45 line, you see that 1.75 falls between 1.76 and 1.56. Looking at the column headings, you see that a 2 incision × 3.75-mm length will correct 1.76 D of myopia. A 2 × 4.0-mm length will correct to 1.56 D of myopia.
- The recommendation in this case is to do a 2 × 4.00-mm incision. The astigmatism should be reduced to approximately 0.50 D.

2 INCISION MRK NOMOGRAM

AGE	2 x 3.0	2 x 3.25	2 x 3.5	2 x 3.75	2 x 4.0	2 x 4.25	2 x 4.5	2 x 4.75	2 x 5.0	2 x 5.25	2 x 5.5
20	1.60	1.40	1.20	1.08	0.96	0.84	0.72	0.60	0.48	0.36	0.24
21	1.64	1.44	1.23	1.11	0.98	0.86	0.74	0.62	0.49	0.37	0.25
22	1.68	1.47	1.26	1.13	1.01	0.88	0.76	0.63	0.50	0.38	0.25
23	1.72	1.51	1.29	1.16	1.03	0.90	0.77	0.65	0.52	0.39	0.26
24	1.76	1.54	1.32	1.19	1.06	0.92	0.79	0.66	0.53	0.40	0.26
25	1.80	1.58	1.35	1.22	1.08	0.95	0.81	0.68	0.54	0.41	0.27
26	1.84	1.61	1.38	1.24	1.10	0.97	0.83	0.69	0.55	0.41	0.28
27	1.88	1.65	1.41	1.27	1.13	0.99	0.85	0.71	0.56	0.42	0.28
28	1.92	1.68	1.44	1.30	1.15	1.01	0.86	0.72	0.58	0.43	0.29
29	1.96	1.72	1.47	1.32	1.18	1.03	0.88	0.74	0.59	0.44	0.29
30	2.00	1.75	1.50	1.35	1.20	1.05	0.90	0.75	0.60	0.45	0.30
31	2.04	1.79	1.53	1.38	1.22	1.07	0.92	0.77	0.61	0.46	0.31
32	2.08	1.82	1.56	1.40	1.25	1.09	0.94	0.78	0.62	0.47	0.31
33	2.12	1.86	1.59	1.43	1.27	1.11	0.95	0.80	0.64	0.48	0.32
34	2.16	1.89	1.62	1.46	1.30	1.13	0.97	0.81	0.65	0.49	0.32
35	2.20	1.93	1.65	1.49	1.32	1.16	0.99	0.83	0.66	0.50	0.33
36	2.24	1.96	1.68	1.51	1.34	1.18	1.01	0.84	0.67	0.50	0.34
37	2.28	2.00	1.71	1.54	1.37	1.20	1.03	0.86	0.68	0.51	0.34
38	2.32	2.03	1.74	1.57	1.39	1.22	1.04	0.87	0.70	0.52	0.35
39	2.36	2.07	1.77	1.59	1.42	1.24	1.06	0.89	0.71	0.53	0.35
40	2.40	2.10	1.80	1.62	1.44	1.26	1.08	0.90	0.72	0.54	0.36
41	2.44	2.14	1.83	1.65	1.46	1.28	1.10	0.92	0.73	0.55	0.37
42	2.48	2.17	1.86	1.67	1.49	1.30	1.12	0.93	0.74	0.56	0.37
43	2.52	2.21	1.89	1.70	1.51	1.32	1.13	0.95	0.76	0.57	0.38
44	2.56	2.24	1.92	1.73	1.54	1.34	1.15	0.96	0.77	0.58	0.38
45	2.60	2.28	1.95	1.76	1.56	1.37	1.17	0.98	0.78	0.59	0.39
46	2.64	2.31	1.98	1.78	1.58	1.39	1.19	0.99	0.79	0.59	0.40
47	2.68	2.35	2.01	1.81	1.61	1.41	1.21	1.01	0.80	0.60	0.40
48	2.72	2.38	2.04	1.84	1.63	1.43	1.22	1.02	0.82	0.61	0.41
49	2.76	2.42	2.07	1.86	1.66	1.45	1.24	1.04	0.83	0.62	0.41
50	2.80	2.45	2.10	1.89	1.68	1.47	1.26	1.05	0.84	0.63	0.42
51	2.84	2.49	2.13	1.92	1.70	1.49	1.28	1.07	0.85	0.64	0.43
52	2.88	2.52	2.16	1.94	1.73	1.51	1.30	1.08	0.86	0.65	0.43
53	2.92	2.56	2.19	1.97	1.75	1.53	1.31	1.10	0.88	0.66	0.44
54	2.96	2.59	2.22	2.00	1.78	1.55	1.33	1.11	0.89	0.67	0.44
55	3.00	2.63	2.25	2.03	1.80	1.58	1.35	1.13	0.90	0.68	0.45
56	3.04	2.66	2.28	2.05	1.82	1.60	1.37	1.14	0.91	0.68	0.46
57	3.08	2.70	2.31	2.08	1.85	1.62	1.39	1.16	0.92	0.69	0.46
58	3.12	2.73	2.34	2.11	1.87	1.64	1.40	1.17	0.94	0.70	0.47
59	3.16	2.77	2.37	2.13	1.90	1.66	1.42	1.19	0.95	0.71	0.47
60	3.20	2.80	2.40	2.16	1.92	1.68	1.44	1.20	0.96	0.72	0.48
61	3.24	2.84	2.43	2.19	1.94	1.70	1.46	1.22	0.97	0.73	0.49
62	3.28	2.87	2.46	2.21	1.97	1.72	1.48	1.23	0.98	0.74	0.49
63	3.32	2.91	2.49	2.24	1.99	1.74	1.49	1.25	1.00	0.75	0.50
64	3.36	2.94	2.52	2.27	2.02	1.76	1.51	1.26	1.01	0.76	0.50
65	3.40	2.98	2.55	2.30	2.04	1.79	1.53	1.28	1.02	0.77	0.51
66	3.44	3.01	2.58	2.32	2.06	1.81	1.55	1.29	1.03	0.77	0.52
67	3.48	3.05	2.61	2.35	2.09	1.83	1.57	1.31	1.04	0.78	0.52
68	3.52	3.08	2.64	2.38	2.11	1.85	1.58	1.32	1.06	0.79	0.53
69	3.56	3.12	2.67	2.40	2.14	1.87	1.60	1.34	1.07	0.80	0.53
70	3.60	3.15	2.70	2.43	2.16	1.89	1.62	1.35	1.08	0.81	0.54
71	3.64	3.19	2.73	2.46	2.18	1.91	1.64	1.37	1.09	0.82	0.55
72	3.68	3.22	2.76	2.48	2.21	1.93	1.66	1.38	1.10	0.83	0.55
73	3.72	3.26	2.79	2.51	2.23	1.95	1.67	1.40	1.12	0.84	0.56
74	3.76	3.29	2.82	2.54	2.26	1.97	1.69	1.41	1.13	0.85	0.56
75	3.80	3.33	2.85	2.57	2.28	2.00	1.71	1.43	1.14	0.86	0.57
76	3.84	3.36	2.88	2.59	2.30	2.02	1.73	1.44	1.15	0.86	0.58
77	3.88	3.40	2.91	2.62	2.33	2.04	1.75	1.46	1.16	0.87	0.58
78	3.92	3.43	2.94	2.65	2.35	2.06	1.76	1.47	1.18	0.88	0.59
79	3.96	3.47	2.97	2.67	2.38	2.08	1.78	1.49	1.19	0.89	0.59
80	4.00	3.50	3.00	2.70	2.40	2.10	1.80	1.50	1.20	0.90	0.60
AGE	2 x 3.0	2 x 3.25	2 x 3.5	2 x 3.75	2 x 4.0	2 x 4.25	2 x 4.5	2 x 4.75	2 x 5.0	2 x 5.25	2 x 5.5

Find patient age, then move right to find result closest to refractive myopia without going over

set just outside the 8-mm optical zone marker and extended centrally until the central optical zone mark is cut out. A small rotation of the knife at the end of the incision is performed such that the tip of the blade points toward the center of the human lens. The double-pass technique combines a center-to-periphery and a periphery-to-center cut.

The double-pass technique (using the Duotrac or Genesis procedure) requires a specially designed diamond knife whose vertical facet is sharpened only on the bottom 200 to 250 μm, making it incapable of cutting beyond the end of the radial incision during deepening of the most central portion of the incision. The tips of these "two-step" knives may be pointed or square. The square tip may minimize double incisions upon the pass back to the center. The pointed tip may be less likely to cause a macro-perforation. To perform the double-cutting technique, the knife tip is set at the inside edge of the central

Table 2

Four-Incision MRK Nomogram

How to Use This Nomogram

- Identify the patient's age and the diopters of refractive myopia that you wish to correct.
- Find the patient's age in the first column on the left.
- Move to the right until you reach the surgery results closest to the refractive myopia of the patient. In order to avoid overcorrection, it is suggested that you select a surgical goal somewhat less than the actual refractive myopia. The column heading then tells you which surgery is needed to achieve this result.

Example

- A 45-year-old patient with a refractive myopia of 3.75.
- Moving to the right on the Age 45 line, you see that 3.75 falls between 3.90 and 3.25. Looking at the column headings, you see that a 4 incision × 3.25-mm length will correct to 3.90 D of myopia. A 4.0 × 3.5- mm length will correct 3.25 D of myopia.
- The recommendation in this case is to do a 4 × 3.25-mm incision.
- Consider placing the incisions on the steeper meridian when the patient has 0.75 to 1.50 D or more of astigmatism.

4 INCISION MRK NOMOGRAM
SURGICAL OPTION

AGE	4 x 3.0	4 x 3.25	4 x 3.5	4 x 3.75	4 x 4.0	4 x 4.25	4 X 4.5	4 x 4.75	4 x 5	4 x 5.25	4 x 5.5
20	2.80	2.40	2.00	1.80	1.60	1.40	1.20	1.00	0.80	0.60	0.40
21	2.87	2.46	2.05	1.85	1.64	1.44	1.23	1.03	0.82	0.62	0.41
22	2.94	2.52	2.10	1.89	1.68	1.47	1.26	1.05	0.84	0.63	0.42
23	3.01	2.58	2.15	1.94	1.72	1.51	1.29	1.08	0.86	0.65	0.43
24	3.08	2.64	2.20	1.98	1.76	1.54	1.32	1.10	0.88	0.66	0.44
25	3.15	2.70	2.25	2.03	1.80	1.58	1.35	1.13	0.90	0.68	0.45
26	3.22	2.76	2.30	2.07	1.84	1.61	1.38	1.15	0.92	0.69	0.46
27	3.29	2.82	2.35	2.12	1.88	1.65	1.41	1.18	0.94	0.71	0.47
28	3.36	2.88	2.40	2.16	1.92	1.68	1.44	1.20	0.96	0.72	0.48
29	3.43	2.94	2.45	2.21	1.96	1.72	1.47	1.23	0.98	0.74	0.49
30	3.50	3.00	2.50	2.25	2.00	1.75	1.50	1.25	1.00	0.75	0.50
31	3.57	3.06	2.55	2.30	2.04	1.79	1.53	1.28	1.02	0.77	0.51
32	3.64	3.12	2.60	2.34	2.08	1.82	1.56	1.30	1.04	0.78	0.52
33	3.71	3.18	2.65	2.39	2.12	1.86	1.59	1.33	1.06	0.80	0.53
34	3.78	3.24	2.70	2.43	2.16	1.89	1.62	1.35	1.08	0.81	0.54
35	3.85	3.30	2.75	2.48	2.20	1.93	1.65	1.38	1.10	0.83	0.55
36	3.92	3.36	2.80	2.52	2.24	1.96	1.68	1.40	1.12	0.84	0.56
37	3.99	3.42	2.85	2.57	2.28	2.00	1.71	1.43	1.14	0.86	0.57
38	4.06	3.48	2.90	2.61	2.32	2.03	1.74	1.45	1.16	0.87	0.58
39	4.13	3.54	2.95	2.66	2.36	2.07	1.77	1.48	1.18	0.89	0.59
40	4.20	3.60	3.00	2.70	2.40	2.10	1.80	1.50	1.20	0.90	0.60
41	4.27	3.66	3.05	2.75	2.44	2.14	1.83	1.53	1.22	0.92	0.61
42	4.34	3.72	3.10	2.79	2.48	2.17	1.86	1.55	1.24	0.93	0.62
43	4.41	3.78	3.15	2.84	2.52	2.21	1.89	1.58	1.26	0.95	0.63
44	4.48	3.84	3.20	2.88	2.56	2.24	1.92	1.60	1.28	0.96	0.64
45	4.55	3.90	3.25	2.93	2.60	2.28	1.95	1.63	1.30	0.98	0.65
46	4.62	3.96	3.30	2.97	2.64	2.31	1.98	1.65	1.32	0.99	0.66
47	4.69	4.02	3.35	3.02	2.68	2.35	2.01	1.68	1.34	1.01	0.67
48	4.76	4.08	3.40	3.06	2.72	2.38	2.04	1.70	1.36	1.02	0.68
49	4.83	4.14	3.45	3.11	2.76	2.42	2.07	1.73	1.38	1.04	0.69
50	4.90	4.20	3.50	3.15	2.80	2.45	2.10	1.75	1.40	1.05	0.70
51	4.97	4.26	3.55	3.20	2.84	2.49	2.13	1.78	1.42	1.07	0.71
52	5.04	4.32	3.60	3.24	2.88	2.52	2.16	1.80	1.44	1.08	0.72
53	5.11	4.38	3.65	3.29	2.92	2.56	2.19	1.83	1.46	1.10	0.73
54	5.18	4.44	3.70	3.33	2.96	2.59	2.22	1.85	1.48	1.11	0.74
55	5.25	4.50	3.75	3.38	3.00	2.63	2.25	1.88	1.50	1.13	0.75
56	5.32	4.56	3.80	3.42	3.04	2.66	2.28	1.90	1.52	1.14	0.76
57	5.39	4.62	3.85	3.47	3.08	2.70	2.31	1.93	1.54	1.16	0.77
58	5.46	4.68	3.90	3.51	3.12	2.73	2.34	1.95	1.56	1.17	0.78
59	5.53	4.74	3.95	3.56	3.16	2.77	2.37	1.98	1.58	1.19	0.79
60	5.60	4.80	4.00	3.60	3.20	2.80	2.40	2.00	1.60	1.20	0.80
61	5.67	4.86	4.05	3.65	3.24	2.84	2.43	2.03	1.62	1.22	0.81
62	5.74	4.92	4.10	3.69	3.28	2.87	2.46	2.05	1.64	1.23	0.82
63	5.81	4.98	4.15	3.74	3.32	2.91	2.49	2.08	1.66	1.25	0.83
64	5.88	5.04	4.20	3.78	3.36	2.94	2.52	2.10	1.68	1.26	0.84
65	5.95	5.10	4.25	3.83	3.40	2.98	2.55	2.13	1.70	1.28	0.85
66	6.02	5.16	4.30	3.87	3.44	3.01	2.58	2.15	1.72	1.29	0.86
67	6.09	5.22	4.35	3.92	3.48	3.05	2.61	2.18	1.74	1.31	0.87
68	6.16	5.28	4.40	3.96	3.52	3.08	2.64	2.20	1.76	1.32	0.88
69	6.23	5.34	4.45	4.01	3.56	3.12	2.67	2.23	1.78	1.34	0.89
70	6.30	5.40	4.50	4.05	3.60	3.15	2.70	2.25	1.80	1.35	0.90
71	6.37	5.46	4.55	4.10	3.64	3.19	2.73	2.28	1.82	1.37	0.91
72	6.44	5.52	4.60	4.14	3.68	3.22	2.76	2.30	1.84	1.38	0.92
73	6.51	5.58	4.65	4.19	3.72	3.26	2.79	2.33	1.86	1.40	0.93
74	6.58	5.64	4.70	4.23	3.76	3.29	2.82	2.35	1.88	1.41	0.94
75	6.65	5.70	4.75	4.28	3.80	3.33	2.85	2.38	1.90	1.43	0.95
76	6.72	5.76	4.80	4.32	3.84	3.36	2.88	2.40	1.92	1.44	0.96
77	6.79	5.82	4.85	4.37	3.88	3.40	2.91	2.43	1.94	1.46	0.97
78	6.86	5.88	4.90	4.41	3.92	3.43	2.94	2.45	1.96	1.47	0.98
79	6.93	5.94	4.95	4.46	3.96	3.47	2.97	2.48	1.98	1.49	0.99
80	7.00	6.00	5.00	4.50	4.00	3.50	3.00	2.50	2.00	1.50	1.00
AGE	4 x 3.0	4 x 3.25	4 x 3.5	4 x 3.75	4 x 4.0	4 x 4.25	4 X 4.5	4 x 4.75	4 x 5	4 x 5.25	4 x 5.5

Find patient age, then move right to find result closest to refractive myopia without going over

optical zone mark. The incision is made peripherally until the footplates cross the 8-mm optical zone mark.

The blade is then pushed centrally, deepening the incision until the blade can no longer be extended centrally. Because the vertical facet is sharpened only on the bottom 200 to 250 μm, the blunt portion restricts the blade from inadvertently entering the clear central zone while allowing the central portion of the incision to be uniformly deepened. Again, a small rotation of the knife at the end of the incision is performed, thus slightly undercutting the central optical zone.

In a 4-incision RK, 3 incisions are usually made with the dominant hand. A right-handed surgeon incises the 10:30 position first, followed by the 7:30 position and then the 1:30 position. The 4:30 incision can be completed with the left hand. When performing 4-incision RK, surgeons should strongly consider placing the incisions in an oblique orientation (Figure 1). When the pupil dilates at night, this configuration minimizes the amount of starburst or glare. If the patient squints, all of the oblique incisions will be covered by the eyelid; this may be especially helpful for night driving.

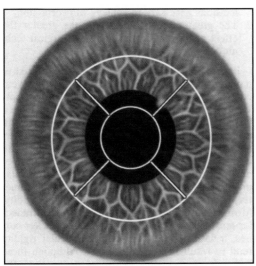

Figure 1. In mini-RK, radial incisions are placed from a clear central optical zone to an 8-mm optical zone. The incision should extend from the inside of the central optical zone mark to the outside of the 8-mm mark.

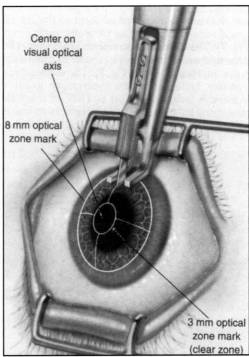

Center on visual optical axis

8 mm optical zone mark

3 mm optical zone mark (clear zone)

Figure 2. The RK incision should extend from the inside of the central optical zone mark to the outside of the 8-mm mark.

Some RK surgeons advocate that all incisions be made with the dominant hand. The eye is fixated and the incisions are made in succession, first toward the surgeon and then 135 degrees away, in an effort to exploit the natural movements of the wrist and fingers. (Figure 2) The microscope is turned successively by 45-degree intervals and the procedure repeated until all the incisions have been made. By making repeated pairs of incisions toward the surgeon and 135 degrees away, consistency of depth and pressure is better maintained. This also simplifies the procedure for the beginning RK surgeon.

Once the incision pattern is completed, no irrigation of the incision is required. Several drops of antibiotic solution, preferably fluoroquinolone, are placed on the eye. No patch or cycloplegic agents are used. Placement of one to two drops of a nonsteroidal anti-inflammatory agent such as diclofenac (Voltaren, CIBA Vision, Atlanta, GA) or ketorolac (Acular, Allergan, Irvine, CA) before and immediately after surgery decreases postoperative pain. The antibiotic-steroid drops are used by all patients for 1 week. If at the 1-week visit the patient is overcorrected more than +1.00 D, the antibiotic-steroid drops are discontinued and replaced by 5% NaCl for 4 to 8 weeks. If the patient is within ±1.00 D of the desired result, the drops are discontinued when they run out. If the patient is more than −1.00 D undercorrected, the antibiotic-steroid drops are continued 4 times daily for 4 to 8 weeks postoperatively.

Complications

OPERATIVE COMPLICATIONS: CORNEAL PERFORATION

Corneal perforation during RK may be identified as a microperforation in which a loss of one or two drops of aqueous humor is noted or as a macroperforation that is large enough to produce shallowing of the anterior chamber. Macroperforation usually requires termination of the procedure and possible closure of the perforation with a suture. The PERK study reported a 2.3% microperforation rate; however, no cases required suturing or termination of the surgery. This low perforation rate was accomplished by setting the diamond knife at 100% of the thinnest paracentral corneal thickness reading and using the American technique with center-to-limbus incisions. Most microperforations appear in the inferior and temporal cornea, where the cornea is relatively the thinnest; however, they may appear in any location of the cornea. Prolonged dehydration intraoperatively, with resultant thinning of the cornea, can increase the incidence of corneal perforation. Macroperforations occur with a frequency of 0% to 0.45%, although one report had a macroperforation rate as high as 13%.

Complications of a microperforation or macroperforation include formation of a scar at the level of Descemet's membrane, damage to the corneal endothelium, iridocorneal adhesions if the anterior chamber remains flat, and laceration of the anterior lens capsule if the incision is continued in the presence of a shallow anterior chamber after perforation.

Keratotomy incisions have been shown to cause mild injury to the corneal endothelium. Postkeratotomy endothelial cell density shows a decrease of less than 10% when measured centrally; however, a greater degree of endothelial cell injury is noted when corneal perforation occurs during RK. Studies using specular microscopy have not shown a progressive decrease in endothelial cell density or other abnormalities in endothelial cellular morphology in human eyes 1 year after RK.

POSTOPERATIVE COMPLICATIONS

Most patients experience pain, throbbing, or foreign-body sensation for 24 to 48 hours postoperatively and frequently require analgesics. Glare or starburst caused by scattering of light intraocularly occurs commonly for a few months after surgery. Glare or starburst may persist for a year or more, and in 9% of patients, it may cause diminished vision, particularly at night or on hazy, bright days.

Epithelial inclusion cysts in the incisional scars were seen in 8.6% of PERK patients after 1 year, but these do not seem to affect the visual results. In most patients, the scars tend to fade years after the surgery as collagen remodeling takes place.

A visually insignificant, brown, stellate, epithelial iron line appears in most eyes after RK. In the PERK study, 81% of eyes had a stellate epithelial iron line 6 months postoperatively. The iron line appears at the junction of the middle and inferior third of the cornea, with fingers extending from the ends of the incisions.

Anterior corneal epithelial basement membrane changes, similar to those seen in epithelial basement membrane dystrophy, are often observed after RK. These changes tend to be transient, lasting less than 3 months in most eyes. They are infrequently associated with clinical symptoms or recurrent epithelial erosion.

Endophthalmitis

Three published case reports of endophthalmitis after RK revealed a strikingly similar course. All patients developed a small hypopyon 8 to 10 days postoperatively, and *Staphylococcus epidermidis* was cultured in all cases. All patients had excellent visual outcomes several months postoperatively. Cross and Head listed nine unpublished cases of endophthalmitis that included virulent gram-negative organisms. Corneal perforation appears to be responsible for the introduction of the microorganism into the eye, either during or shortly after the surgical procedure. Thorough preoperative chemical preparation of the eye is imperative, strict adherence to sterile surgical technique is required, and postoperative antibiotics and careful follow-up are recommended. A topical 5% povidone-iodine solution has been shown to decrease the incidence of postoperative endophthalmitis, and it is recommended for the preoperative preparation of the surgical field.

Ptosis

Blepharoptosis is a reported complication of RK. Because retrobulbar injections and superior rectus bridle sutures were not used in the cases reported, the most likely cause of blepharoptosis was damage to the levator aponeurosis by the eyelid speculum. It has been suggested that a gentle wire speculum might be less likely to induce ptosis than a solid, rigid eyelid speculum.

Keratitis

Bacterial or fungal keratitis can occur in the immediate postoperative period or can be delayed several years after refractive keratotomy. The incidence seems to be higher when soft contact lenses, especially extended-wear lenses, are used after RK. Several cases of bacterial keratitis have been reported; the causative organisms included *Pseudomonas*, *Staphylococcus aureus*, and *S. epidermidis*. Prophylactic topical antibiotics are to be encouraged until re-epithelialization has occurred. Two cases of *Mycobacterium chelonei* keratitis were reported from the same surgeon's office; in these two cases, outpatient RK was performed with cold-sterilized instruments.

Traumatic Rupture of Keratotomy Incisions

Any corneal incision results in a scar that does not have the same tensile strength as the original cornea. This is true not only after incisional keratotomy but also after corneal transplantation or accidental trauma. There are several reports of traumatic rupture of keratotomy scars after blunt trauma. In a rabbit eye model, Larson and colleagues observed that the blunt force required to rupture the globe after RK within 90 days of healing was approximately half that required to rupture control eyes, which did not have surgery. In a porcine eye model, Rylander and co-workers demonstrated that ruptures occurred most frequently at the equator in normal, unoperated eyes, but they occurred through keratotomy incisions in eyes that previously underwent RK. Pinheiro and associates recently showed that, under laboratory conditions, rupture of mini-RK incisions occurs at much higher intraocular pressure than does rupture of standard RK incisions. The rupture pressures of these eyes with mini-RK incisions were no different than they were in eyes that had not had mini-RK.

REFRACTIVE COMPLICATIONS

The most frequently reported complication of RK is an inaccurate outcome. The principal complications include overcorrection, undercorrection, increased astigmatism, irregular astigmatism, a progressive postoperative shift toward hyperopia, and diurnal fluctuation of vision.

Diurnal Fluctuation

Many patients who have had RK report fluctuation of vision during the course of the day. In the PERK study, patients who complained of fluctuating vision were examined twice on the same day, before 8:00 am and after 7:00 pm. At 1 year, 42% of the eyes demonstrated a manifest refraction that changed from 0.50 to 1.25 D. At approximately 3.5 years after RK, 31% of eyes showed a change of 0.50 D or more during the course of the day. At 11 years after RK, 54% of eyes showed a change in refractive error of 0.50 D or more. Thus, diurnal fluctuation may be a permanent sequela of RK in some individuals. Keratometry and refraction demonstrated that most of the corneas underwent a gradual steepening during the course of the day, which ranged from 0.50 to 1.25 D. Therefore, patients with undercorrected vision saw best in the morning, whereas patients whose vision was overcorrected experienced an increase in visual acuity during the day.

Although the exact cause of this diurnal fluctuation is unknown, it is most likely related to structural changes induced by the keratotomy incisions and scars. Corneal edema that occurs during sleep or contact lens wear has been shown to flatten the cornea after RK. The unsutured wounds in the avascular cornea may require more than 4 to 5 years to eject the epithelial plug completely and to remodel the corneal stroma adjacent to the incisional scar. The constant pressure of the eyelids and mild epithelial and stromal edema during sleep are believed to induce a nocturnal flattening of the cornea.

Overcorrection

Consecutive hyperopia after RK may result from an initial overcorrection or from a continued effect of the procedure with time. Five-year follow-up of the PERK study showed that 22% of the eyes had a refractive change of 1.00 D or more in the hyperopic direction between 6 months and 5 years after RK. The refractive error was within 1.00 D of emmetropia for 64% of eyes in this group. However, 17% were hyperopic by more than 1.00 D. Between 6 months and 10 years after RK in the PERK study. 43% of eyes changed in the hyperopic direction by 1.00 D or more. The average rate of change was +0.21 D per year between 6 months and 2 years and +0.06 D per year between 2 and 10 years. Thus, progression toward hyperopia continues over time, with the greatest rate of change occurring in the first 2 years after RK. A progressive effect in the hyperopic direction has also been seen after 2- to 4-incision RK. In two different studies, 3.5% and 6.3% of patients were overcorrected more than 1.00 D 1 year after RK. Because of the progressive effect of RK with time, many surgeons are now intentionally leaving patients slightly myopic. Also, many RK procedures are now staged such that 2 to 4 incisions are placed initially and additional incisions are added at some point in the future should they become necessary.

Overcorrection of the refractive error after RK can be managed by spectacles or, if anisometropia is present, contact lenses. Contact lens fitting after RK has its own unique problems. The flat central cornea and the relatively steeper paracentral cornea cause the contact lens to decenter as it moves across the paracentral point. Two studies have reported only 56% and 58% success rates in fitting rigid gas-permeable contact lenses after RK. Neovascularization of perilimbal incisional scars has limited the fitting of RK patients with soft contact lenses.

Induced Astigmatism

Five-year results of the PERK study revealed that 15% of eyes had an increase of astigmatism of 1.00 D or more postoperatively. The change in refractive astigmatism ranged from a decrease of 1.50 D to an increase of 4.50 D. Although the maximum allowable astigmatism for entry into the PERK study was 1.50 D, 15% of eyes had more than 1.50 D 5 years postoperatively.

After RK, all corneas have some irregular astigmatism, which can be detected by keratoscopy. This is manifested where the regular, smooth, circular configuration of the inner mires overlying the optical clear zone contrasts with the slightly irregular configuration of the inner mires overlying the optical clear zone contrasts with the slightly irregular configuration of the outer mires overlying the incisions. Minimal irregular astigmatism appears to have little visual effect under daylight conditions, presumably because it lies outside the optical clear zone. Under dim illumination, however, when the pupil dilates, more glare and distortion result. This has been reported as a "starburst" phenomenon. Significant irregular astigmatism can occur when incisions extend too close to the visual axis in eyes with repeated operations or in eyes whose radial and transverse (or radial and circumferential) incisions intersect. Symptoms in patients with mild to moderate irregular astigmatism can be minimized by a rigid, gas-permeable contact lens.

Predictability

Five-year results of the PERK study showed that 60% of eyes had an uncorrected visual acuity of 20/20 or better and 88% had uncorrected visual acuity of 20/40 or better. Two percent had visual acuities of 20/200 or worse. Five years after surgical intervention, 64% of eyes had a refractive error between −1.00 D and +1.00 D, 19% remained myopic by more than 1.00 D, and 17% became hyperopic by more than 1.00 D. At 10 years, 38% had a refractive error within 0.50 D and 60% within 1.00 D of emmetropia. Seventy percent reported not wearing spectacles or contact lenses for distance vision at 10 years. Recent 4-incision RK studies have reported the number of eyes with overcorrections to be reduced to 3% and 6%. Also, studies show that the percentage of patients who achieve a visual acuity of 20/40 or better may be increased through the use of a second operative enhancement procedure.

Conclusion

Incisional surgical techniques have proved effective in correcting low degrees of myopia. Although technologic advances have introduced newer methods for correcting refractive error, it appears that modern incisional surgery will continue to have a role in the future of refractive surgery as a reliable method of correcting low degrees of residual myopia after refractive cataract surgery.

Bibliography

Lindstrom R. Minimally invasive radial keratotomy: mini-RK. *J Cataract Refract Surg.* 1995;21:27-34.

Spigelman AV, Williams PA, Nichols BD, Lindstrom RL. Four-incision radial keratotomy. *J Cataract Refract Surg.* 1988;14:125.

CHAPTER 215

MINI-RK:
INDICATIONS AND TECHNIQUE

Frank A. Bucci, Jr., MD

The efficient and accurate correction of residual refractive error following the implantation of presbyopia-correcting (Pr-C) intraocular lenses (IOLs) is critical for achieving high levels of both spectacle independence and patient satisfaction. One diopter of astigmatism with no spherical error corresponds to an uncorrected distance vision of 20/30. Almost all patients receiving Pr-C IOLs, but especially those paying additional fees for these premium IOLs, will consider 20/30 uncorrected distance acuity to be unacceptable. They will frequently even perceive a significant difference between 20/25 and 20/20 uncorrected distance visual acuity. Limiting your patient selection to those patients with low amounts of preoperative cornea cylinder will not eliminate your need to acquire skills for correcting residual refractive errors. Wound dynamics and other unpredictable factors inherent in IOL placement will frequently result in residual astigmatism of at least 0.75 diopter (D), even though preoperative keratotomy readings predicted that this would not occur.

My general guideline is that 0.50 D of spherical error and 0.50 D of astigmatism are consistent with acceptable uncorrected visual outcomes by the post–Pr-C IOL patient. When spherical and cylindrical postoperative refractive errors reach 0.75 D, the patient will perceive a substantial benefit when corrected.

The most frequently performed procedures for correcting residual refractive errors following use of Pr-C IOLs include (1) limbal relaxing incisions (LRIs) at the time of implantation; (2) traditional laser in situ keratomileusis (LASIK) at least a few months postoperatively; and (3) postoperative traditional surface laser ablation, such as photorefractive keratectomy (PRK), at least 1 month following implantation. In the majority of cases, I use an alternate technique, which I call micro-radial keratotomy/astigmatic keratotomy (micro-RK/AK).

What is micro-RK/AK? This technique is performed no sooner than 3 weeks postoperatively. It includes arcuate incisions in the peripheral cornea that are identical to those used in any other LRI or AK procedure. The surgeon can use his nomogram of choice for correcting astigmatism. The second component of the micro-RK/AK technique is the micro-RK. When the implant power is selected preoperatively, the target for the spherical outcome is plano to −0.50. So, in over 90% of cases, the spherical outcome is either plano or slightly myopic. Micro-RK is used to correct the small degrees of myopia in a relatively noninvasive manner.

The term "micro-RK" is used to distinguish this technique from both mini-RK and traditional RK in which optical zones as small as 3.00 mm and are frequently used. In "micro-RK" the optical zone is never smaller than 5.00 mm. Because only a very small amount of myopia is being corrected, usually only 1 or 2 micro radial incisions are necessary. The length of these incisions is always less than 2.50 mm. This is less than the thickness of 2 stacked dimes (2.75 mm). A small portion of the Lindstrom 2 incision nomogram (Figure 1) is used to select the surgical optical zone. I have been using this nomogram for 17 years and it is extremely accurate. Fluctuating vision and hyperopic shifts do not occur with radial incisions this small.

The advantages of using this technique compared to the alternative technique are numerous. The advantages of micro-RK/AK versus LRI are mostly related to accuracy, and accuracy is even more critical when dealing with demanding elective presbyopic patients. Because the micro-RK/AK is performed at least 3 weeks postoperatively, the surgeon has the advantage of knowing the exact amount of cylinder, the exact axis of the cylinder, and the exact amount of spherical error. The micro-RK component then provides you with an opportunity to fix the small amount of myopia with excellent precision. There is greater ease and precision when this procedure is performed on a "non-phaco" day because (1) the pupil is not dilated; (2) it is easier to "mark" the axis; (3) it is easier to perform pachymetry at each incision site and custom set your diamond blade; and (4) the temporal and paracentesis wounds are more stable.

The advantages of micro-RK/AK over traditional LASIK are also significant. Micro-RK/AK does not create a neurotropic cornea as does LASIK. The central 5.00 mm of the cornea is untouched. There will be no flap complications,

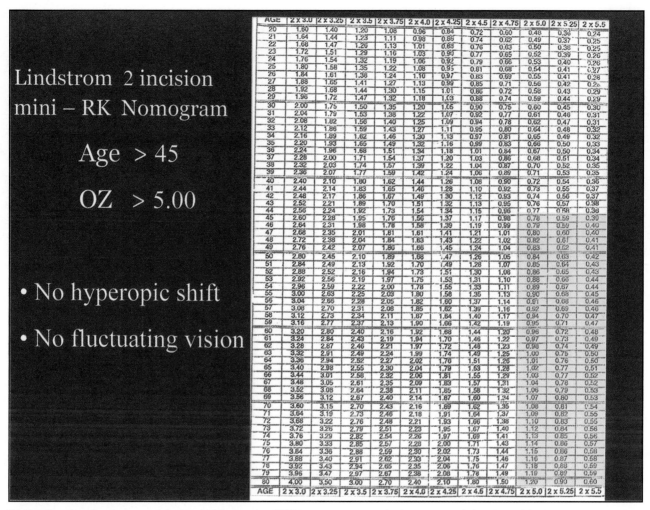

Figure 1. The astigmatic and uncorrected visual results following micro-RK/AK in 111 eyes status post clear lensectomies with the ARRAY multifocal IOL.

no diffuse lamellar keratitis (DLK), and no central epithelial defects. Patients older than 45 (especially women) are at an increased risk for dry eye and as an elective surgery patient they will be relatively demanding.

Some surgeons wait up to 3 to 6 months before performing LASIK following an implant because of concern about wound stability during creation of the flap. Micro-RK/AK can be performed with confidence much sooner. The cost of laser access (purchase or facility fee) and the procedure (procedure card and microkeratome blade) will almost always be significantly greater than this incisional technique. LASIK enhancements further complicate the patient's neurotropic dry eye and cost again becomes a factor. The small incisions of this technique produce no greater postoperative symptoms than LASIK. LASIK becomes my preferred technique when the residual cylinder or sphere increases significantly. As the residual refractive error increases, there is a relative increase in precision with laser vision correction compared to an incisional technique.

The advantages of micro-RK/AK compared to traditional PRK are also not trivial. The central 5 mm of the cornea remains untouched. There is less postoperative discomfort. Bilateral surgery is possible and the visual recovery is quicker for these demanding patients. No bandage contact lens is required, there are fewer postoperative visits, and again this incisional technique is much less costly. There is much less stress on healing of the ocular surface, especially for patients with preexisting ocular surface disorders, such as aqueous dry eye, meibomian gland dysfunction, anterior blepharitis, or delayed epithelial healing secondary to diabetes. There is frequently a subtle subepithelial haze following PRK, which is usually tolerated by the typical PRK patient. In the multifocal implant patient, who has already lost contrast sensitivity, the visual consequences of the subepithelial haze may be poorly tolerated.

I have used micro-RK/AK to correct residual refractive error following implant surgery in over 1000 cases during the past 17 years; Figures 2 and 3 summarize the results of this technique in 320 eyes after receiving multifocal IOLs. Note that the final uncorrected visual acuity of the Array eyes (*n* = 111) is slightly better because this group is exclusively younger lensectomy patients versus the ReZoom and ReSTOR eyes (*n* = 209), which are a mix of lensectomy and older cataract patients.

In conclusion, micro-RK/AK is an excellent alternative for correcting residual refractive errors following the use of Pr-C IOLs. In general, it is less costly, puts less stress on the ocular surface, is less invasive than laser vision correction, and is more accurate than intraoperative LRI.

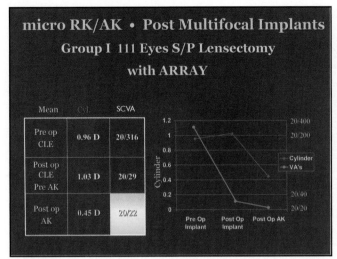

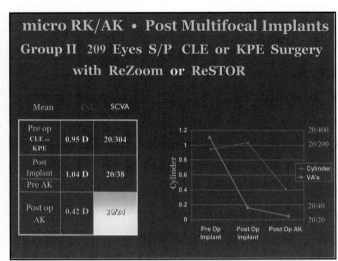

Figure 2. The astigmatic and uncorrected visual results following micro-RK/AK in 209 eyes status post either cataract surgery or clear lensectomies with the ReZoom or ReSTOR multifocal IOLs.

Figure 3. The micro-RK/AK nomogram is a subset (yellow) of the original Lindstrom 2 incision mini-RK nomogram. Small amounts of myopia are corrected using optical zones never less then 5.00 mm.

CHAPTER 216

REFRACTIVE ENHANCEMENT WITH PIGGYBACKING IOLs

Richard S. Hoffman, MD; I. Howard Fine, MD; and Mark Packer, MD, FACS

Historical Overview

Although intraocular lens (IOL) calculations following cataract surgery and refractive lens exchanges are becoming increasingly accurate, the occasional postoperative refractive surprise will necessitate a secondary procedure to refine the refractive result and achieve emmetropia. In addition to the refractive surprise, extremes of ocular axial length and current limitations in multifocal and accommodating IOL powers will require adjunctive techniques to realize a plano refraction in extremely myopic or hyperopic eyes. Piggyback IOLs, performed at the time of the primary procedure or as a secondary enhancement procedure, are a powerful method for assuring an acceptable postoperative result.

Gayton was the first to report the use of piggyback lenses in a case of microphthalmos.[1] Piggyback IOLs have quickly gained favor as one of the preferred methods to correct cases of extreme hyperopia in cataract patients, in addition to allowing for the correction of pseudophakic eyes with unacceptable under or overcorrections.[2] Initially, when primary piggyback IOLs were utilized to correct high hyperopia in cataract patients, both implants were placed within the capsular bag. Gills initially divided the lens power equally between the 2 lenses whereas other surgeons preferred to place two thirds of the lens power in the more posterior lens and one third anteriorly.[3] Our current preference is to place the maximum allowable correction in the posterior IOL to reduce the amount of optical distortion that might occur if lens decentration develops in the anterior IOL. This technique also allows for more options for refractive refinement should the anterior IOL need to be replaced with a stronger lens power.

Previous reports by Gayton and others have revealed potential complications from the technique of placing both implants within the capsular bag. Intractable interlenticular membranes, reduced visual acuity,[4] and late hyperopic shift[5] have led surgeons to recommend placement of the anterior IOL in the sulcus rather than the capsular bag. Sulcus placement of the anterior IOL will also simplify anterior lens exchange should this be necessary.

The Refractive Surprise

When presented with a refractive surprise following refractive lens exchange, the first question the surgeon should ask is why. *Did the correct patient receive the correct calculated lens?* Rarely, mix-ups can occur and everything possible should be made to discover the cause of the error and rectify any systems errors responsible for the patient receiving the wrong lens. *Was the patient's axial length extremely short or long?* These eyes are more difficult to calculate accurately and more likely to have refractive surprises. We recommend utilizing a fourth generation IOL calculation formula such as the Holladay 2 formula for all eyes and also running the Hoffer Q formula (short eyes) and the SRK/T formula (long eyes) for confirmation of the IOL power. *Were the axial lengths and keratometry measurements accurately inserted into the IOL calculation program? Did the patient have previous refractive surgery that may have affected the accuracy of the keratometry measurements?* These are all questions that should be addressed when a clinician is confronted with a refractive surprise.

The next inquiry by the surgeon should be whether the refractive error is easily reversible without a piggyback IOL or corneal refractive surgery. *Was the implant inserted properly?* The Crystalens accommodating IOL (Eyeonics, Aliso Viejo, CA) is designed in such a way that it has a grooved hinge at the haptic-optic junction, which is designed to position the IOL as far posteriorly in the capsular bag as possible. If the Crystalens is inadvertently inserted upside down, the lens will flex forward causing a myopic shift. Before considering a piggyback IOL in such a scenario, the Crystalens should be removed and repositioned correctly to maximize its function and also possibly rectify the refractive error. *Is there a capsular block syndrome?* Capsular block will also cause an IOL to rest in a more anterior position than calculated and result in a myopic shift. This can be easily rectified with either a peripheral anterior yttrium-aluminum-garnet (YAG) capsulotomy or a posterior capsulotomy. *Should an IOL exchange be performed?* Unfortunately, if the cause for the refractive surprise is unknown, there is no guarantee that exchanging the IOL for one with greater or less power will achieve emmetropia. There is also a risk/benefit factor

Table 1

NICHAMIN NOMOGRAM

Sulcus IOL: Staar AQ5010V

- Minus power = 1:1 (-2 D spherical equivalent = -2 D IOL)

- Plus power = 1:1.5 (+2 D spherical equivalent = +3 D IOL)

Table 2

PIGGYBACK IOLs FOR RESIDUAL PSEUDOPHAKIC REFRACTIVE ERRORS[3]

Secondary Piggyback Cases—Lens Placed in the Ciliary Sulcus

A. Formula: Underpowered pseudophake (hyperope)
   1. Short eye (<21 mm): Power = (1.5 × spherical equivalent) + 1
   2. Average eye (22 to 26 mm): Power = (1.4 × spherical equivalent) + 1
   3. Long eye (>27 mm): Power = (1.3 × spherical equivalent) + 1

B. Formula: Overpowered pseudophake (myope)
   1. Short eye (<21 mm): Power = (1.5 × spherical equivalent) - 1
   2. Average eye (22 to 26 mm): Power = (1.4 × spherical equivalent) - 1
   3. Long eye (>27 mm): Power = (1.3 × spherical equivalent) - 1

that must be taken into consideration when dealing with a lens that may be extremely adherent to the capsular bag secondary to acrylic lens material and/or prolonged time since the initial surgery. A capsular bag rupture during an IOL exchange could turn a relatively safe elective procedure into one requiring a host of unplanned additional procedures and costs. Especially with small residual refractive errors, the safest, most accurate, and easiest approach is to refine the power with either corneal refractive surgery or a piggyback IOL.

Piggyback IOL Calculations

Piggyback IOLs can be easily calculated as primary or secondary procedures utilizing the Holladay IOL Consultant. If the Holladay IOL Consultant is not available, there are several other nomograms and formulas that can be utilized to calculate the piggyback IOL power.

Nichamin has developed a simple nomogram that utilizes the Staar AQ5010V IOL for sulcus placement (Table 1). For myopic refractive errors, the IOL chosen is the same power as the refractive error. For hyperopic refractive errors, the IOL power is increased by 1.5 times the refractive error.

Gills has developed a more detailed nomogram based on the axial length and whether the refractive error is hyperopic or myopic. With the Gills nomogram, the spherical equivalent is multiplied by a factor of 1.3, 1.4, or 1.5 depending on whether the eye is long, average, or short. A diopter of power is then added or subtracted from this number depending on whether the patient is an underpowered pseudophake (hyperopia) or an overpowered pseudophake (myope) (Table 2).

Another quick and easy confirmation formula that can be utilized is Brown's Refractive Reasoning (Laurie Brown, COMT). Basically, 0.5 diopter (D) of IOL power will yield 0.37 D at the spectacle plane. This formula is a nice means of assuring that the IOL power calculated by the Holladay Consultant or other nomograms is on target and it can also be used to refine the calculated power when different methods give conflicting powers.

Piggyback IOL Choice

We have found the STAAR AQ2010 and AQ5010 silicone lenses (STAAR Surgical, Monrovia, CA) to be ideal for piggyback utilization secondary to their thin optic edges. The AQ 2010 is a 13.5-mm IOL with a 6.3-mm optic that is available in powers between +5 and +9 D in whole-diopter steps and +9.5 to +30 D in half-diopter steps. The AQ5010 is a 14-mm IOL with a 6.3-mm optic that is available in powers between -4 and +4 D in whole-diopter steps. Both lenses can be easily injected into the ciliary sulcus as a primary or secondary piggyback IOL.

Another option for piggyback IOL selection is the Advanced Medical Optics Clariflex (Santa Ana, CA). The Clariflex is a silicone IOL with a 6.0-mm optic. The lens has a unique OptiEdge design with a squared posterior edge and a rounded anterior edge designed to be placed in the capsular bag. Sulcus placement is an option with this lens because the rounded anterior surface will be less likely to cause pigment dispersion and secondary glaucoma that can result from IOLs with anterior square edge designs.[6,7] The Clariflex has a 13.0-mm overall length and comes in powers between -10.0 and +30.0 D in half-diopter steps. The thickened edge of the Clariflex leaves it less ideal for piggyback implantation than the thinner STAAR AQ5010.

Piggyback Implantation Technique

Piggyback IOLs can be implanted into the ciliary sulcus using folding forceps; however, the simplest means of implantation is to utilize the cartridge injector systems designed for intraocular insertion. Placing a small quantity of viscoelastic between the anterior capsule and the iris in the distal and proximal quadrants will facilitate sulcus placement. As the distal lens haptic is being ejected from the cartridge, the haptic should be oriented in such a way that it is parallel to the anterior capsule. The haptic is then placed between the iris and anterior capsule as the optic is ejected from the cartridge. Pushing the optic under the iris as it is unfolding will ensure that the lens does not flip into the wrong orientation. Once the optic has unfolded, the trailing haptic can be ejected from

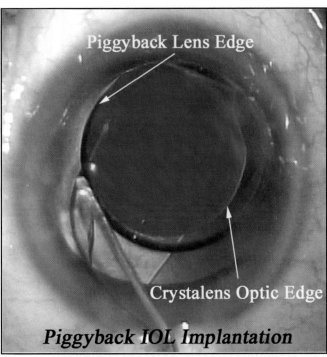

Figure 1. Low-power Clariflex IOL dialed into the ciliary sulcus over an Eyeonics Crystalens (within the capsular bag).

the cartridge and dialed into the ciliary sulcus, utilizing a blunt hook placed at the trailing haptic-optic junction (Figure 1).

Final Comments

Refractive lens exchanges with accommodating and multifocal IOLs, by virtue of their potential ability to correct extremes of hyperopia, myopia, and presbyopia, may become a dominant refractive surgery procedure in the future. As with any surgical procedure, limitations of current IOL technology, biometry, and IOL calculations may make enhancement procedures necessary to deliver the desired refractive result. Success with refractive lens exchange is a function of accuracy in technique, patient selection, and managing patient expectations. Enhancements with piggyback IOLs are a simple and accurate means of enhancing patient satisfaction with this procedure.

References

1. Gayton JL, Sanders V. Implanting two posterior chamber intraocular lenses in a case of microphthalmos. *J Cataract Refract Surg.* 1993;19:776-777.

2. Gayton JL, Sanders V, Van Der Karr M, Raanan MG. Piggybacking intraocular implants to correct pseudophakic refractive errors. *Ophthalmology.* 1999;106:56-59.

3. Gills JP, Cherchio M. Phacoemulsification in high hyperopic cataract patients. In: Lu LW, Fine IH, eds. *Phacoemulsification in Difficult and Challenging Cases.* New York: Thieme Medical Publishers; 1999:21-31.

4. Findl O, Menapace R, Rainer G, Georgopoulos M. Contact zone of piggyback acrylic intraocular lenses. *J Cataract Refract Surg.* 1999; 25:860-862.

5. Shugar JK, Schwartz T. Interpseudophakos Elschnig pearls associated with late hyperopic shift: A complication of piggyback posterior chamber intraocular lens implantation. *J Cataract Refract Surg.* 1999; 25:863-867.

6. Iwase T, Tanaka N. Elevated intraocular pressure in secondary piggyback intraocular lens implantation. *J Cataract Refract Surg.* 2005; 31:1821-1823.

7. Wintle R, Austin M. Pigment dispersion with elevated intraocular pressure after AcrySof intraocular lens implantation in the ciliary sulcus. *J Cataract Refract Surg.* 2001;27:1341-1342.

REFRACTIVE ENHANCEMENT WITH PIGGYBACKING IOLs

Warren E. Hill, MD, FACS

No one needs to be told that over the last decade patient expectations following all forms of lens-based surgery have increased dramatically. And at the end of the surgical exercise, being able to achieve the desired refractive target by the most appropriate method is no longer optional. Most commonly, when a refractive surprise occurs, the talk turns to the topic of an intraocular lens (IOL) exchange or the placement of a secondary piggyback IOL.

The four situations in which a IOL exchange, or a secondary piggyback IOL, are most commonly required are: Intolerable anisometropia; failure to achieve the refractive target, prior keratorefractive surgery with problematic IOL power calculations, and various legal issues surrounding the measurement of central corneal power, axial length, IOL power calculation, or the IOL implanted. When the refractive target remains elusive, surgeons looking to achieve the best refractive outcome must be comfortable with more than one option.

Why a Piggyback IOL?

An IOL exchange may be the best option early in the postoperative course if there is no doubt as to the reason for the refractive surprise and the power of the primary IOL is known. There may also be special circumstances where a piggyback IOL would not be a workable option.

However, there are situations in which a lens exchange may be difficult, dangerous, or ill advised. In addition, not every surgeon is comfortable with removing an IOL already in place. When this is the case, inserting a piggyback IOL into the ciliary sulcus may be the better option. One advantage of placing a piggyback IOL is that the power of the original IOL does not need to be known and the procedure is quick and relatively atraumatic.

Requirements for Success

For the placement of a piggyback IOL to be successful, the primary IOL must be completely contained within the capsular bag. If one, or both of the haptics are sitting in the ciliary sulcus, another method of correcting the refractive error must be considered such as observation and or spectacles, IOL exchange, contact lenses, or laser in situ keratomileusis (LASIK).

There must also be sufficient space between the anterior surface of the primary IOL and the posterior surface of the iris in order to place a piggyback IOL in the sulcus. One finding that is often overlooked is the geometry of the primary IOL. If the IOL within the capsular bag has a very steep anterior radius, the piggyback IOL be displaced anteriorly, or it may decenter to one side if the haptic supports do not have a large enough overall diameter.

Calculating the Power

One advantage of piggyback IOL placement over an IOL exchange is that the power calculation can be carried out in a manner that is axial length independent. If the deviation from the refractive target is less than 7.00 D myopic, or hyperopic, two simple rules of thumb may be employed.

For hyperopic refractive errors, the spherical equivalent of the spectacle refraction can be multiplied by 1.5 to arrive at the power of a secondary piggyback IOL for a plano result.

For example, let us say that Mrs. Smith underwent uncomplicated cataract surgery, with the primary IOL completely contained within the capsular bag. Her stable postoperative refractive error is +1.50 + 1.00 × 180 for a spherical equivalent of +2.00 D. For this case:

+2.00 D × 1.5 = +3.00 D

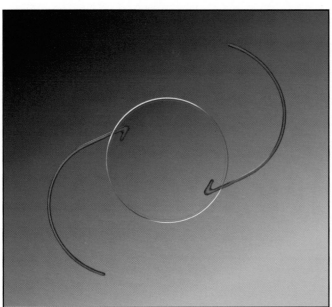

Figure 1. STAAR (Monrovia, CA) AQ-5010V 3-piece silicone IOL, a favorite of many surgeons as a secondary piggyback IOL.

A +3.00-D piggyback IOL placed in the ciliary sulcus would give a plano result.

For myopic refractive errors, the spherical equivalent of the spectacle refraction can be multiplied by 1.3 to arrive at the power of a secondary piggyback IOL for a plano result.

As another example, Mrs. Jones underwent uncomplicated cataract surgery, with the primary IOL completely contained within the capsular bag. Her stable postoperative refractive error is −3.00 + 1.25 × 180 for the spherical equivalent of −2.38 D. For this case:

$$-2.38 \text{ D} \times 1.3 = -3.09 \text{ D}$$

A −3.00-D piggyback IOL placed in the ciliary sulcus would give a plano result.

For hyperopic or myopic refractive surprises greater than 7.00 D, using the refractive vergence formula as described by Holladay[1] or the Holladay R formula, which is part of the Holladay IOL Consultant software package, would give more accurate results. For this calculation, you will need to know the manifest refraction, vertex distance, the central corneal power (an estimate will work well for the post-LASIK or radial keratotomy [RK] eye), the effective lens position and the desired target refraction.

A free Excel spreadsheet that can be used to calculate the power of a piggyback IOL based on Dr. Holladay's 1997 *JCRS*

article can be downloaded from: http://www.doctor-hill.com/physicians/download.htm.

Which Piggyback IOL?

In general, piggyback IOLs should have a low profile, smooth, rounded edges of the optic, a large optic diameter and a large overall haptic length appropriate to the size of the ciliary sulcus. A foldable optic diameter between 6.0 mm and 6.5 mm that can be inserted using an injector through the original incision gives the most satisfactory results. One lens design that has become a favorite of many surgeons is the STAAR Surgical AQ-5010V (Figure 1) in powers from −4.00 D to +4.00 D and the STAAR Surgical AQ-2010V in powers from +5.00 D upwards. This design is a 3-piece newer generation silicone IOL with a 6.3-mm optic diameter, a 13.5-mm haptic diameter, and smooth, rounded optic edges.

The placement of a 3-piece acrylic IOL may lead to problems due to thick, truncated edges, which may cause pigment dispersion and intermittent uveitis. Also, the semi-tacky nature of the acrylic material may interact with the posterior iris, which can be another source of pigment dispersion.

Single piece, large diameter PMMA IOLs with a large haptics are also a good choice, but typically require an incision size greater than 6.0 mm.

Conclusion

The placement of a piggyback IOL is generally easier than performing an IOL exchange for both the patient and the surgeon. The calculation of the optical power for a piggyback IOL can be done in a manner that is axial length independent, relying mostly on the refractive error to be corrected. There are simple rules of thumb that can be very effective for low power hyperopic and myopic refractive errors, but in general the refractive vergence formula, or the Holladay R formula, are more accurate when large deviations from the target refraction must be corrected. The surgical placement of a piggyback IOL is quick and visual rehabilitation is almost immediate. In order to avoid decentration, pigment dispersion, iris transillumination defects, secondary glaucoma and intermittent uveitis, the geometry and material of the piggyback IOL must be carefully considered.

Reference

1. Holladay JT. Standardizing constants for ultrasonic biometry, keratometry and intraocular lens power calculations. *J Cataract Refract Surg.* 1997;23:1361.

SECTION XIV

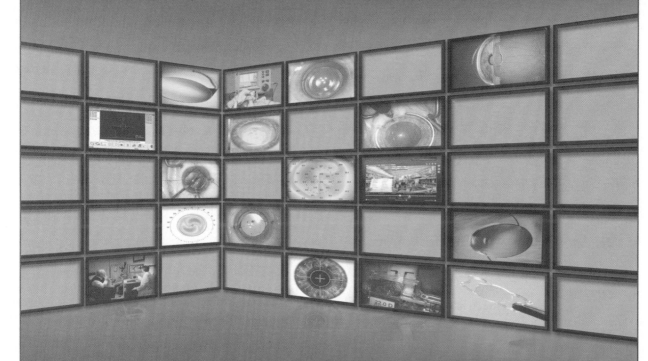

Complications—
Avoidance and
Management

CHAPTER 218

TROUBLESHOOTING SYMPTOMS AFTER REFRACTIVE IOL IMPLANTATION

Roger Steinert, MD

This chapter addresses optical complaints and complications that will occur unavoidably, even when a meticulous surgical technique has been employed. This technique is assumed to include a thorough cortical clean up, a correctly sized and well-centered capsulorrhexis, and correct intraocular lens (IOL) power selection.

Postoperative Optical Complaints

HISTORY AND EXAMINATION

When faced with postoperative visual complaints that do not have an obvious explanation, the surgeon should begin by taking a careful history. Listen closely to the patient, and ask nonleading questions in order to draw out a description of the patient's perceptions. Asking the patient to sketch how images appear can be very helpful as well as provide good documentation. The surgeon should be sure to examine the patient before as well as after dilation in order to assess IOL centration and pupil position. Measurement of the pupil size under photopic, mesopic, and scotopic lighting conditions may also be helpful. The size of the pupil is often quite different after cataract surgery than it was preoperatively, and clinical assessment should not be based upon the preoperative measurements.

Complaints about the vision not being "good" should first be divided between complaints about overall clarity as opposed to complaints about optical side effects such as halo and glare. This is followed by a careful manifest refraction using a defogging technique. With presbyopia-correcting IOLs, it is easy to "over minus" a patient on subjective refraction because the near-focus optics will be brought into focus at distance with excessive minus power refraction. Autorefractors are often erroneous with presbyopia-correcting IOLs, particularly with multifocal IOLs. Measuring corneal topography is frequently essential, in order to determine the presence of both regular and irregular corneal stigmatism or other distortions that may

impact the visual system. At the completion of this phase of the examination, the determination can be made as to whether distance vision is good or is a problem.

If the objective high-contrast distant visual acuity appears good and yet the patient perceives poor clarity, then the next step is to determine whether the issue is that the intermediate vision is good and near vision bad, or the intermediate vision is bad and the near vision good. Under either of these circumstances, many patients can be aided with the use of spectacles for specific activities, or by custom matching the IOL in the second eye. Custom matching can be accomplished by shifting the target power of the same model IOL, or by using a different model IOL.

POOR CLARITY AT BOTH DISTANCE AND NEAR

With complaints about poor clarity at distance and near that are not explained by residual refractive error, the first area to consider is the ocular surface. Lissamine green or rose Bengal dyes are useful for identifying evidence of dryness or other surface disruption. In addition, the meibomian glands need to be inspected carefully, as meibomian gland dysfunction is a frequent contributor to ocular surface disruption. The treatment is then directed by the findings, including lid hygiene, use of Restasis (topical cyclosporine A; Allergan, Irvine, CA) and/or punctual plugs, as well as non-preserved artificial tears. If the ocular surface does not appear to be a factor, then the cornea itself must be carefully examined, and evaluated using corneal topography. A definitive answer to the contribution of corneal optics is to have the patient undergo a hard contact lens overrefraction. Irregularity of the ocular surface and cornea will be optically eliminated by a hard contact lens.

If the ocular surface and cornea are normal, then the diagnosis focus shifts to the macula and optic nerve. Subtle disruptions of the macula can be difficult to see on direct examination, but optical coherence tomography (OCT) is a highly useful and straightforward manner of assessing the macula. If the macula is normal, optic nerve evaluation begins

Figure 1. The "decision tree" for the evaluation and treatment of poor clarity of distance and near vision.

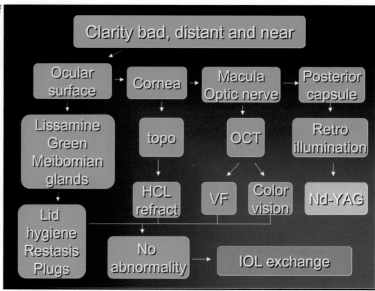

with formal visual fields and color vision testing as well as an assessment of the pupils. Neuroimaging and/or neuro-ophthalmic consultation should be considered only after performing these fundamental examinations.

The posterior capsule may prove to be the principle culprit in optical impairment. The most reliable ways of assessing the optical contribution of the posterior capsule are to visualize the red reflex on retroillumination and to view retinal details with a direct ophthalmoscope. If the posterior capsule appears to be the likeliest source of the patient's perception of lack of clarity, then Nd-YAG (neodymium:yttrium-aluminum-garnet) laser posterior capsulotomy may be necessary. Many surgeons, however, have performed posterior capsulotomies only to have the patient return with no improvement. Once the posterior capsule is open, then an IOL exchange becomes a much more challenging and potentially complicated procedure. Laser posterior capsulotomy should be reserved for cases where the surgeon is reasonably certain that an IOL exchange will not be needed.

Figure 1 shows the "decision tree" for the evaluations and treatment options described above.

Halos and Glare With Good Acuity

In this situation, a careful history and examination become very important. Be sure that the patient can accurately tell which eye is causing the troublesome symptoms. Some patients confuse symptoms originating from only one eye. If necessary, instruct the patient to cover each eye in an alternating fashion when experiencing symptoms. In addition, have the patient sketch the visual phenomenon for you. Attempt to simulate it in the office with devices such as the muscle light.

Residual uncorrected refractive error is a common culprit behind these complaints. The cornea may have uncorrected residual astigmatism and/or high-order aberrations. Here again, a careful defogging manifest refraction is critical.

Pupil size and shape are also important factors that commonly contribute to halos and glare. To identify the pupil as the source of difficulty, begin with pharmaceutical intervention such as the use of Alphagan (brimonidene; Allergan) and if that does not result in a small enough pupil, administer dilute pilocarpine, such as 0.5% solution. In some cases, a laser treatment may be helpful in correcting pupil abnormalities, either by shifting the location of the pupil slightly through photocoagulation of the mid-peripheral iris, or, in the case of an excessively small pupil, by performing laser sphincterotomies with Nd-YAG laser photodisruption. Lasers cannot make the pupil smaller, however. In some cases an experienced surgeon may be able to successfully address a pupil size problem by placing one or more cerclage sutures, but, more often, the prudent intervention is an IOL exchange.

Once again, optical irregularities of the posterior capsule can be the source of halo and glare, but laser posterior capsulectomy markedly increases the risks of IOL exchange and should be undertaken only after the surgeon has worked through all the other potential sources of halo and glare.

Figure 2 shows the "decision tree" for managing halos and glare.

Key Points

1. Allow adequate time between surgery on the first eye and the second eye to assess patient satisfaction. Although it is true that most patients do not gain the maximum benefit from cataract surgery, and especially from presbyopia correction, until the second eye has also had surgery, several weeks of experience with the first eye is very helpful for the surgeon to assess a patient's happiness with the optical function of their first eye. This provides an opportunity to "fine tune" the IOL selection and refractive target in the second eye.

2. Listen to the patient! Because visual perceptions may be subtle and the objective findings may not clearly

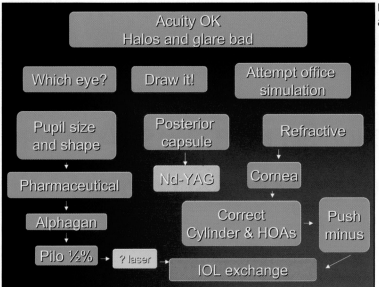

Figure 2. The "decision tree" for managing halos and glare with good Snellen acuity.

indicate the source of optical unhappiness, a patient's history can be a critical factor at arriving at the right diagnosis and treatment.

3. Be sure to convey sincere concern to the patient. The patient needs to understand that you are a partner with him or her in maximizing visual outcome.

4. Pursue the evaluation and treatment options logically and methodically.

5. An IOL exchange is the last option. This should be necessary only rarely, but, if necessary, it should be done in a manner that minimizes the risks.

6. Posterior capsulotomy limits the ability to resolve the problem by IOL exchange without further complication. Therefore, posterior capsulotomy must be reserved until thorough assessment leads the surgeon to conclude that the capsule is the most likely source of the optical complaints.

CHAPTER 219

TROUBLESHOOTING SYMPTOMS AFTER REFRACTIVE IOL IMPLANTATION

David R. Hardten, MD

Patients have very high expectations when undergoing cataract surgery, especially when a premium, presbyopia-correcting intraocular lens (IOL) has been implanted. Fortunately, most patients complete the surgical and postoperative period quite satisfied. Some have visual complains, however, and it is important to know how to manage these patients.

Patient expectations first come into play during the period between the first and the second eye operations. In addition to the type of IOL to implant, every surgeon should have a plan for the order of consecutive eye surgery. I prefer a staged approach, and typically perform surgery on the dominant eye, or the eye with the worst cataract first. I then assess patient satisfaction; as well as uncorrected visual acuity (UCVA) at distance, intermediate, and near vision at 1 to 2 weeks after surgery. I typically use a ReZoom IOL (Advanced Medical Optics, Santa Ana, CA) in the first eye. If they are satisfied with the vision at distance, intermediate, and near, then I also use a ReZoom in the opposite eye, still targeting emmetropia. If the near vision is inadequate for the patient's needs in the first eye, then I will typically aim for −0.25 to −0.75 in the second eye with the same IOL. The other option is to implant a diffractive IOL such as the ReSTOR (Alcon, Fort Worth, TX) or a Tecnis multifocal IOL (Advanced Medical Optics) in the second eye. Patients appear to tolerate either the same or different lenses in both eyes quite well.

Residual refractive error is one of the most common reasons for postoperative dissatisfaction. A careful refraction, topography, and wavefront analysis can help to determine whether this is the reason for residual complaints. This is true whether the IOL is an aspheric monofocal IOL or a multifocal or accommodating IOL. Residual sphere and cylinder affect both near and distance acuity and may result in an unhappy patient. Obviously, prevention is the best tactic if possible. Accurate biometry using the IOL Master (Carl Zeiss Meditec, Jena, Germany) or immersion ultrasound with the Prager shell (ESI, Minneapolis, MN) is important. Precise calibration of the keratometer and using the latest generation IOL power

calculation formulas are all important factors in achieving refractive accuracy and success. Still, there will likely be occasional unexpected outcomes or cases where the target refraction needs to be adjusted postoperatively based on patient feedback. In such cases, I prefer laser vision correction as the most accurate way of enhancing the outcome for most patients. For a large refractive surprise, a piggyback IOL may be useful, provided the original IOL is well positioned in the eye and there is sufficient space in the sulcus to implant a second lens. The Holladay R formula is the most appropriate power calculation formula for piggyback cases. Piggyback IOLs should probably account for fewer than 5% of total enhancements. I rely on them primarily in cases of high spherical error without much residual cylinder, although one might also consider an IOL exchange in these cases.

Astigmatism Management

I typically try to correct cylinder at the time of the original surgery with on-axis phaco incisions, limbal relaxing incisions (LRIs) or astigmatic keratotomy (AK). Although incisional techniques do not offer the same degree of predictability and accuracy as laser vision correction, doing them in the operating room at the time of surgery is convenient and can reduce the need for a second surgical procedure. I rarely do more than a pair of 45- to 60-degree arcs at a 9.0-mm optical zone (Figure 1). If there is some cylinder remaining after lens implantation and a postoperative enhancement is necessary, I always prefer to use the excimer laser. Ideally, I will do a wavefront-guided ablation with iris registration to most accurately treat the cylinder. If the capsulorrhexis is too small to get a 5.0-mm capture, or if the wavefront doesn't match the refraction or is not compatible with the uncorrected vision, then I perform a conventional treatment. I prefer laser in situ keratomileusis (LASIK) in most patients because of the quicker recovery, but if there are any corneal health issues, or if I made any LRI or AK incisions during the initial surgery, I opt for PRK. In our practice, all IOL patients are told that an enhancement may be necessary

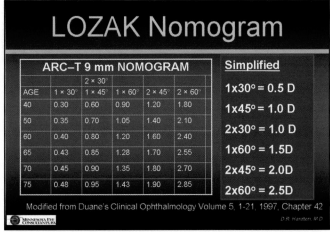

Figure 1. LOZAK nomogram. (Modified from *Duane's Clinical Ophthalmology*, Vol 5. Philadelphia, PA: Lippincott, Williams, and Wilkins; 1997:1-21.)

and that we will choose the best of several options for them should we need to do an enhancement. We still charge a fee for this, although it is less for secondary procedures than it is for patients with primary laser vision correction.

Quality of Vision Complaints

In some cases, the patient is essentially emmetropic but still unhappy. In these cases, I first take a "watch and wait" approach, because night vision symptoms and other optical complaints often improve with time. It is also important to examine the eye carefully to rule out posterior capsular opacification or striae that may be responsible for the problems. There are several nonsurgical interventions one can consider to help patients with night vision problems. Nighttime spectacles may improve their quality of vision for driving at night. If patients are bothered by halo effects from a multifocal IOL, Alphagan P (Allergan, Irvine, CA) or pilocarpine drops will cause the pupil to constrict, decreasing the effect of the outer zones of a refractive multifocal IOL.

If nonsurgical options don't solve the problem, laser vision correction may be able to resolve the unwanted symptoms due to residual refractive error. Whenever possible, I prefer to perform a wavefront-guided enhancement as this offers better astigmatic correction, especially with iris registration, and the ability to address higher-order aberrations. Typically this treatment will not sacrifice the patient's multifocality. Wavefront imaging is also helpful to ensure that the patient's subjective complaints are related to residual sphere, cylinder, or unusually high coma or spherical aberration. Often, the patient's complaints will also correlate with the appearance of the wavefront point-spread function. When planning a custom correction for a pseudophake, one should ensure that the wavefront refraction makes sense compared to the manifest refraction and UCVA. If there is any doubt about the accuracy of the wavefront, I perform a conventional ablation, making sure to push the plus and

do a careful refraction. In a recent series of eyes undergoing laser vision correction in our practice, we were only comfortable using the wavefront to guide the treatment in 19% of eyes. IOL exchange should be a last resort, which I only do if the patient is truly unhappy with multifocality, or if there is some problem with the IOL. If an exchange is necessary, I recommend placing the new IOL in the bag before removing the original IOL, if possible. This will protect the capsule during transection and removal of the IOL.

Timing of the Second Intervention

In a bilateral case, I typically wait to enhance the refraction until I have implanted IOLs in both eyes, so that we know how the optics balance. If one eye is myopic and the other close to emmetropia, for example, then the patient may be happy without any further correction. After the second eye, I generally follow the same principles I do for laser vision correction. If there is a large residual error that I know is not going to resolve itself, I will do an early enhancement. In the case of an unusual 2.0-D surprise, I may wait just a month or so for the vision to stabilize, and then perform a secondary intervention so the patient doesn't have to suffer for a long period of time. In some cases with extreme refractive errors, I may opt for a lens exchange or piggyback IOL. In most cases, however, the refractive result is within 1.0 D of the intended correction, and I generally wait 6 months before enhancing. The refraction may change again or the patient may be able to adapt to the mild residual error. During this waiting period, the capsule may contract enough to cause some change in refraction. If there is any capsular fibrosis or haze I perform a neodymium: yttrium-aluminum-garnet (Nd:YAG) capsulotomy at around 4 to 5 months postoperatively, prior to laser vision correction.

Conclusion

In summary, surgeons who implant multifocal and other premium IOLs are going to need to address problems with the result after the initial surgery. Ruling out and treating nonsurgical problems like dry eye or cystoid macular edema with lubricants, cyclosporine, or nonsteroidal drugs is helpful in some patients. Careful attention to capsular opacity, which causes more symptoms in presbyopia-correcting IOL patients, is important. Neuroadaption typically improves symptoms in patients without significant refractive error over the first year after IOL implantation. Occasionally the refractive outcome will need to be enhanced. Laser vision correction provides the most accurate method for addressing residual sphere and cylinder, and is often the best solution for quality-of-vision complaints as well. With all of the tools available to us today, we can typically provide a very satisfactory solution for patients for good uncorrected distance, intermediate, and near vision.

CHAPTER 220

MANAGING THE UNHAPPY PRESBYOPIA-CORRECTING IOL PATIENT

D. Rex Hamilton, MD, MS, FACS

On May 3, 2005, anterior segment surgery changed forever with the Centers for Medicare & Medicaid Services (CMS) ruling allowing surgeons to receive compensation for skills and services required to implant presbyopia-correcting intraocular lenses (Pr-C IOLs). Finally practices and surgeons would realize the market value of their services. This wonderful opportunity comes, of course, with added responsibilities: developing the "art" of proper preoperative screening, acquiring experience with new IOL designs, becoming proficient with corneal refractive surgery, accepting increased chair time and more labor intensive pre- and postoperative management. Even with due diligence in addressing each of these responsibilities, patients will still be unhappy in larger numbers than we were used to in the "old days." In this chapter, we will examine how to manage the unhappy Pr-C IOL patient to minimize the adverse effect such patients can have on the success of our practice.

Preoperative Screening

As a resident, the first concept we learn regarding cataract surgery is that the ease of completing each step depends on the successful completion of the previous step. This golden rule is of no less importance when applied to the management of the Pr-C IOL patient. First and foremost, we must remember that the selection of a Pr-C IOL is an *elective* choice in the strongest sense of the word. In a keratorefractive surgery practice (eg, laser in situ keratomileusis [LASIK]/ photorefractive keratectomy [PRK]), obtaining a detailed history, performing a comprehensive examination, and exercising restraint in patient selection can save the patient, and the surgeon, from adverse outcomes that may significantly impact both individuals' lives. Similarly, with the currently available Pr-C IOL technologies, it is not appropriate to place a Pr-C IOL in every patient in your practice eligible for lens surgery. Secondly, Pr-C IOL surgery carries with it significantly higher inherent expectations due to the financial outlay required by the patient. These patients, therefore, should be treated from a refractive

surgery perspective, where a premium is placed on spectacle independence. Many veteran cataract surgeons may be used to seeing their patients 2 weeks following surgery and writing a spectacle prescription for distance vision, near vision, or both. This is likely to be unacceptable for the Pr-C IOL patient who, similar to the LASIK patient, paid out of pocket for the added benefit of spectacle independence.

Taking these two most important tenets into account, the preoperative screening process plays a critical role in the success or failure of each patient, whose outcome may ultimately impact future referrals to your practice.

Setting Expectations

Clarifying postoperative expectations serves two purposes. First, it grounds the patient, bringing them back to reality with regard to what is achievable and what is not. Documentation of this communication provides a useful tool later in challenging situations where a patient may need reassurance and redirection postoperatively. Secondly, clarifying expectations can assist with the weeding-out process. Patients with very high expectations may not be accepting of what you explain as being reality. Often patients will desire a Pr-C IOL solution based on what they have read on the Internet or what they have heard from friends, family, or colleagues who rave about their results. When you define appropriate, individualized expectations based on their retina pathology, for example, they may initially show disappointment but will ultimately respect you more for your candid counsel. The Dell survey, developed by Steve Dell, MD, is a very useful one-page questionnaire designed to highlight for the patient the tradeoffs and limitations of the currently available Pr-C IOLs (see Appendix A). The survey not only forces the patient to place these limitations into an individualized context, but also includes a personality self-assessment scale. Dr. Dell has found that, contrary to conventional wisdom, the most difficult patients to satisfy seem to be those who rate themselves near the middle of the personality scale, as compared to those who rate themselves as perfectionists, possibly uncovering a "passive-aggressive" personality trait.

Setting postoperative expectations should include the following at a minimum:

1. A discussion of the chances of requiring spectacles for distance, near, and intermediate vision;

2. Financial and clinical issues associated with keratorefractive surgical enhancement to correct postoperative ametropia;

3. The need for neuroadaptation and bilateral implantation to achieve full functional performance.

4. If a multifocal IOL is under consideration, the quality of vision tradeoffs under low light conditions. (The IOL Counselor is an excellent tool to demonstrate these tradeoffs. Visit www.iolcounselor.com for details.)

Why Is a Pr-C IOL Patient Unhappy? The Top Five Reasons

SUBOPTIMAL UNAIDED NEAR VISION

Most patients, if properly counseled and screened, are satisfied with J3 unaided near vision. During the preoperative qualification process, I discuss "social near vision" as the unaided expectation that includes cell phones, menus, price tags, and magazine size print, all of which are J5 or larger. We use a near card provided by Refractec (Irvine, CA) which has small paragraphs at each Jaeger size, along with a representative "real world" example (eg, portion of a Yahoo! Webpage for J10, a Banana Republic price tag for J8). I also show the patient J1 (eg, an insert page from a medication on the Refractec card) and point out "now how often do you need to see something this small?" I also tell them "you WILL need reading glasses for this size print." I mention that threading a needle is another example of a task that the patient will need reading glasses for. When patients achieve J3 postoperatively, they are therefore, pleasantly surprised. This level of near vision is usually attainable with ReZoom (Brentwood, TN), ReSTOR (Alcon, Ft Worth, TX), and Crystalens (Eyeonics, Aliso Viejo, CA). When using the Crystalens, I prefer to start with the non-dominant eye and target −0.5 to −0.75 D, depending on the near vision requirements of the patient (mini-monovision).

Patients with the ReZoom lens may report suboptimal unaided near vision, particularly in bright light situations. This is likely due to a small photopic pupil size. Remember that the ReZoom lens has a distance-only central zone measuring 2 mm in diameter. If the photopic pupil size is less than this diameter, the patient will not have adequate near vision. Dimming the lights, if possible, can improve unaided near vision. Screening patients for small photopic pupils is crucial when considering the use of the ReZoom lens.

The Crystalens is the lens most likely to produce suboptimal unaided near vision, particularly if mini-monovision is not employed. If the patient is underwhelmed with the unaided near vision after the first Pr-C IOL, I counsel them that there will be at least a 1 line improvement following the second Pr-C

IOL implantation. This takes care of the majority of cases in this category. For the bilaterally implanted Crystalens patient who is emmetropic for distance and has suboptimal unaided near vision, conductive keratoplasty can be extremely useful for augmenting near acuity without sacrificing much at distance. One ring of 8 spots at an 8-mm optical zone will typically induce approximately 1.0 D of myopia. If the suboptimal unaided near vision is due to postoperative ametropia or other ocular co-morbidity, this should be addressed accordingly (see appropriate section later in the chapter). Notice that this category is entitled "suboptimal" unaided near vision as compared to "unrecognized" unaided near vision, which is discussed in the next section.

UNRECOGNIZED UNAIDED NEAR VISION

If you have used any of the Pr-C IOLs already, particularly the multifocal lenses, you will be familiar with the following scenario. You pick up the chart on postoperative day 1 that reveals adequate distance uncorrected visual acuity (UCVA) (eg, 20/30) and excellent near UCVA (J1 to J3). Yet, when you go in and talk with the patient, they will say "the distance is fine, doc, but I can't see up close." This is typically due to one of two reasons. First, particularly with the current version of the ReSTOR lens featuring a +3.2 D add at the spectacle plane, the near focal point is closer to the eye than patients are used to. Even though you undoubtedly pointed this out to patients during preoperative counseling, you still need to reinforce this point during the early postoperative period because, of course, old habits are hard to break. Second, neuroadaptation needs to occur with multifocal IOL optics. The brain adjusts to aberrations present in the optical system of the eye, producing perceived images that are much sharper than the aberrated retinal image. Similarly, the brain adjusts to multifocal optics, learning to suppress the near image when viewing a distant image and vice versa. The difficulty here is that adaptation takes a variable amount of time for any given patient. The good news is that nearly all patients will adapt when given enough time. Reminding the patient that this issue was discussed preoperatively and reassuring them that the near vision will improve with time (particularly once the second eye is implanted), are the mainstays of managing this early postoperative issue. The early postoperative near vision with Crystalens may also be unimpressive due to relearning to use the ciliary muscle again after many years of disuse. Word jumbles of progressively smaller letters are available from Eyeonics that help reassure patients that their near vision is improving as the early weeks pass.

SUBOPTIMAL UNAIDED INTERMEDIATE VISION

Intermediate vision is of greater importance among Baby Boomers due to the extensive use of computers throughout their daily life. Again, preoperative screening of vocational and avocational activities is crucial to identify how much a patient values unaided intermediate vision. ReSTOR is the lens most likely to provide suboptimal unaided intermediate vision due to the bifocal nature of its optics. This, of course, should be discussed during the preoperative evaluation. The first step is to make sure the patient is really making a complaint and not an observation. Richard Tipperman points out that often the ReSTOR patient complaining of intermediate vision is the same patient with outstanding distance and near acuity (20/20, J1).[1] They are simply comparing good intermediate vision with stellar distance and near vision. In this situation, reassurance will usually suffice. A patient who reports excellent near and distance vision early in the postoperative period with the ReSTOR lens implanted in the first eye is likely to be a patient who neurally adapts quickly. If this patient is really complaining of poor intermediate vision affecting their daily activities, one should consider implanting either the Crystalens or ReZoom lens in the second eye. Both options will likely boost the unaided intermediate vision. If the patient is not concerned with nighttime visual aberrations from the ReSTOR lens and does not drive at night routinely or for long periods, I would consider the ReZoom lens for the second eye. Most often in this situation, however, I would consider a Crystalens in the second eye.[2] The Crystalens will almost always provide excellent intermediate vision while the near vision will remain acceptable from the ReSTOR eye. A more difficult problem of suboptimal intermediate vision occurs in the bilaterally implanted ReSTOR patient where emmetropia was targeted in both eyes. This patient should first be managed by redirection—reminding the patient of the outstanding level of spectacle independence they undoubtedly have. The "let's look at what the ReSTOR is doing for you" strategy of putting the patient in a trial frame with −3.00 D lenses to highlight the near vision provided by the ReSTOR lens is often helpful. In addition, remind the patient that adjustments can be made to the computer (position of the monitor, screen resolution, font size, brightness levels, etc) to compensate for suboptimal intermediate vision. Make sure there is adequate ambient lighting in the patient's computer environment as the unaided near vision with the ReSTOR vision decreases under scotopic conditions due to the shunting of a larger percentage of incoming light toward formation of the distance image. Additionally, the intermediate vision does improve over time with neuroadaptation. In the case of refractory complaints, consider a keratorefractive procedure to create monovision. This should be tested first with contact lenses and undertaken only as a last resort after reminding the patient that they will be giving up some distance and near vision quality to gain intermediate. Finally, a lens exchange can be considered, but only as a last resort because there is a high chance the patient will still not be satisfied with the result. When you get to the point of considering a lens exchange, you have by definition selected a patient with very challenging expectations. The real problem is knowing what replacement lens to use—monofocal, ReZoom, Crystalens? In addition, the patient must have a clear understanding of the added risks associated with an IOL exchange procedure, and this must be carefully documented in the patient's chart.

SUBOPTIMAL UNAIDED DISTANCE VISION

During the early postoperative period with multifocal lenses, the surgeon must rule-out ametropia as a cause for suboptimal unaided distance vision. Assuming the patient is within ± 0.5 D of emmetropia with less than 0.5 D of cylinder, the most likely problem is the need for neuroadaptation. With the Crystalens, ametropia is more likely as this lens has a more variable effective lens position. In other words, the Crystalens is more sensitive to variations in capsular bag diameter. In a large, myopic eye, the lens may have a decreased posterior vault when compared to a smaller, hyperopic eye with a smaller capsular bag diameter. This variable effective lens position has become less of an issue with the newer 5.0 lens design. The lens is sturdier and appears to be more consistent in its capsular bag position. In addition, for IOL powers below 17 D, the company will automatically send the 5.2 version of the Crystalens, which features an overall length of 12.00 mm versus the 11.5-mm overall length of the 5.0 version. The rationale here is that lower lens powers are required in more myopic eyes, which are likely to have larger capsular bag diameters. This will produce a more appropriate posterior vault, reducing the chance of a myopic surprise. The non-dominant eye should be operated on first, if possible, when using the Crystalens. If the first eye ends up slightly myopic, the unaided near vision will be improved and the surgeon can make an adjustment for the unexpected effective lens position when calculating the lens power for the second, dominant eye. This way the dominant eye will be closer to emmetropia and the nondominant eye will have improved unaided near vision. In the late postoperative period, beware of subtle posterior capsular opacities, particularly with the multifocal lenses, as a cause of suboptimal unaided distance vision. There should be a very low threshold for performing a yttrium-aluminum-garnet (YAG) posterior capsulotomy in multifocal lens patients. With the Crystalens 5.0, capsular contraction can induce a myopic shift due to symmetric anterior vaulting or, in very rare circumstances, induced myopic astigmatism from asymmetric contraction. These situations are usually handled very effectively by targeted YAG capsulotomy. Of course, other ocular co-morbidities must also be ruled out in the setting of suboptimal unaided distance vision (see appropriate section later in the chapter).

SUBOPTIMAL SCOTOPIC VISUAL FUNCTION

Complaints of nighttime vision disturbances are inherent to multifocal lens designs and should not come as a surprise to patients receiving these IOLs. The IOL Counselor (http://www.iolcounselor.com) should be a mandatory part of the patient counseling process when multifocal IOLs are considered. This simulator demonstrates to patients the haloing and decreased contrast sensitivity that will occur during dim light activities with these lenses. Additionally, the Dell survey includes a question designed to determine the value a patient places on nighttime vision quality. Occupational night drivers and patients who work in dim light conditions (eg, radiologists, film editors) are not the best candidates for multifocal technology, primarily due to the reduction of contrast sensitivity. The halos and glare become less of a problem as neuroadaptation occurs. The decreased contrast sensitivity, however, does not improve with neuroadaptation as it relates directly to the amount of light used to form the retinal image. Newer lens designs, including the aspheric ReSTOR lens, should offer improved contrast sensitivity versus older designs. A patient who primarily complains of the halos/glare off lights in the early postoperative period but does not complain about difficulty seeing street signs at night will likely accept the multifocal design as neuroadaptation occurs. In this patient, the surgeon should not be dissuaded from putting another multifocal lens in the second eye. The patient whose primary complaint is of waxy night vision and difficulty seeing street signs is more of an issue. After ruling out ametropia as a cause, this is a patient to consider placing an aspheric monofocal or Crystalens in the fellow eye, depending on the need for unaided intermediate vision versus the best possible unaided distance vision. A patient who was doing well and develops suboptimal scotopic vision function in the late postoperative period should be evaluated for other ocular co-morbidities with posterior capsule opacification (PCO) at the top of the differential diagnosis.

Postoperative Ametropia

SPHERICAL AMETROPIA

Personalized A-constants along with consistent biometry and keratometry are essential to achieving emmetropia in Pr-C IOL patients. When myopia occurs in the first eye of a patient receiving the Crystalens, first ensure that your technician or optometrist is not over-minussing the patient during the manifest refraction. Make sure that the patient's unaided distance and near vision are consistent with the refraction. If the eye truly is myopic, proceed with the second eye Crystalens implantation but adjust the refractive target to account for the unexpected effective lens position that occurred in the first eye. For example, if the first eye ends up −0.75 D sphere for a target of plano, target +0.5 to +0.75 D in the second eye. Do not correct the myopia in the first eye with keratorefractive techniques or a lens exchange prior to implanting the second eye. It is more likely that a keratorefractive solution will be required in multifocal lens patients who end up myopic but the surgeon should still wait to perform an adjustment until after implanting the second eye if possible. Hyperopic ametropia can be most easily addressed using conductive keratoplasty. This minimally invasive procedure has an advantage over PRK or LASIK as there is essentially no effect on dysfunctional tear syndrome, a disorder very prevalent in the cataract patient population, particularly among post-menopausal women. The main downside to conductive keratoplasty, regression of refractive effect, is seen to a much lower degree in older patients.

ASTIGMATIC AMETROPIA

Pr-C IOL patients should be treated like refractive surgery patients. This means that topographic analysis is an essential component of the preoperative evaluation. Patients with less than 1.5 D of regular corneal astigmatism can usually be successfully treated using limbal relaxing incisions (LRI) or astigmatic keratotomy (AK) at the time of the IOL surgery. Patients with more than 1.5 D of corneal cylinder are most effectively treated with keratorefractive surgery following IOL implantation. PRK can be performed as soon as 1 month following IOL surgery. LASIK should be delayed for at least 6 weeks following IOL surgery to allow time for the clear corneal incision to heal. With the Crystalens, postoperative astigmatism of 0.75 diopters (D) or less is usually acceptable for

good function. Multifocal lenses usually require that there be 0.5 D of astigmatism or less for optimal performance. Ideally the starting Pr-C IOL surgeon should choose patients with less than 0.5 D of pre-existing corneal astigmatism.

Presbyopia-Correcting IOLs in Postrefractive Surgery Patients

Multifocal lenses are likely to produce suboptimal results in post-myopic LASIK or post-myopic PRK patients and are very likely to be suboptimal in post-radial keratotomy (RK) patients. These corneas by definition have reduced contrast sensitivity due to the oblate shape of the corneal curvature, which then adds to the decreased contrast sensitivity associated with multifocal optics. Wavefront enhancements are difficult to perform in patients with the Crystalens due to capsular opacification and the resultant degradation of wavefront data. Wavefront enhancements are usually not possible with the ReZoom lens due to corruption of the defocus portion of the wavefront by the near refractive zone. As a result, the surgeon should consider the Crystalens or aspheric, monofocal monovision as the top choices for the postrefractive surgery patient. Future aspheric versions of Pr-C IOLs should improve our results in these patients.

Other Ocular Comorbidities

DYSFUNCTIONAL TEAR SYNDROME

All refractive surgery patients must be evaluated for dysfunction tear syndrome as a possible contraindication for surgery. PrC IOL patients are no exception and are more likely to have dysfunctional tear syndrome (DTS) due to their overall older age demographic. DTS should be treated aggressively and early in patients with pre-existing dysfunction. The mainstay of treatment includes cyclosporine 0.05% (Restasis emulsion, Allergan, Inc., Irvine, CA), oral omega fatty acid supplements (eg, BioTears, Biosyntrx, Inc., Lexington, SC), punctual occlusion and lid hygiene. The role DTS plays in suboptimal results in Pr-C IOL patients cannot be overstated and should be foremost in the mind of the surgeon evaluating these patients.

POSTERIOR CAPSULAR OPACITY

Even subtle posterior capsular opacities can be clinically relevant in the Pr-C IOL patient. Particularly in the multifocal IOL patient, even a single capsular fold across the diffractive portion of the lens can decrease performance. The surgeon should have a very low threshold for performing YAG capsulotomy in these patients. The Crystalens presents the opportunity for a unique complication with regard to capsular fibrosis: capsular contraction. These patients may be doing well early on but present with decreased distance vision after several weeks. This occurs due to anterior movement of the IOL resulting from symmetric capsular contraction. This is easily treated with a small, central YAG posterior capsulotomy. Rarely, asymmetric capsular contraction can occur, leading to induced myopic astigmatism and possible reduced best corrected acuity. In this case, a targeted YAG capsulotomy focusing on the area of capsular contraction posterior to the lens haptic, together with a central capsulotomy, may be required. These patients should be treated with topical medications prophylactically for cystoid macular edema (CME) as there is a higher chance of vitreous prolapse. This asymmetric capsular contraction appears to be less common with the new 5.0 version of the Crystalens. Complete cortical clean-up at the time of the IOL surgery and somewhat longer use of postoperative topical steroids helps reduce the chance of capsular contraction.

CYSTOID MACULAR EDEMA AND EPIRETINAL MEMBRANE

Prophylaxis against cystoid macular edema is essential in all Pr-C IOL patients. Prior to the introduction of these lenses, "angiographic" CME may not have been treated as it was thought to be subclinical. Today, "angiographic" CME is now "optical coherence tomography (OCT) positive" CME and should be treated in all cases due to the inherently high patient expectations and sensitive performance characteristics of Pr-C IOLs, and multifocal IOLs in particular. Nonsteroidal anti-inflammatory drops should be started at least 2 days prior to surgery and continued for at least 4 weeks postoperatively along with topical steroids. The postoperative patient presenting with decreased BCVA should be evaluated with OCT and started promptly on NSAID/steroid combination therapy for macular thickening. Persistent CME refractory to topical therapy should be referred for retinal evaluation.

The presence of a pre-existing epiretinal membrane (ERM) should be carefully evaluated for with OCT prior to Pr-C IOL surgery. Even subtle ERMs may adversely affect the performance of a multifocal IOL. In addition, the optics of the multifocal IOL may make membrane peeling surgery more challenging for the vitreoretinal surgeon. The Crystalens may be the better Pr-C IOL choice in these patients.

AGE-RELATED MACULAR DEGENERATION AND DIABETIC RETINOPATHY

Macular dysfunction can significantly affect the performance of multifocal IOLs. Patients with pre-existing dry macular degenerations may not be the best candidates for multifocal technology. Even if the macular function is currently adequate, these patients are at somewhat higher risk of decreased macular function in the future, which may be compounded by the multifocal IOL optic. The Crystalens may be more forgiving of subtle macular dysfunction and is therefore a somewhat better choice for these patients. Similarly, patients with subtle background diabetic retinopathy likely have compromised macular function that may get worse. The Crystalens optically is a better choice than a multifocal IOL. Remember that the Crystalens is a silicone IOL, however, which may present issues in the case of advanced diabetic retinopathy requiring pars plana vitrectomy with the injection of silicone oil.

Pr-C IOLs are the lens technology of the future. We will undoubtedly be seeing further future advancements in lens design that will allow us to restore excellent unaided vision at all distances to a wider range of patients. There is also no question that we will have a higher standard of care to live up to as more and more patients receive these Pr-C IOLs. With proper preoperative assessment and attention to detail in both surgery and postoperative care, we will enjoy this amazing technology and the increased number of patients it brings to our practices for many years to come.

References

1. Tipperman R. Why I do not mix IOLs. *Cataract Refract Surg Today.* 2007;7(8):62-64.
2. Woodhams JT, Carpenter H. Mixing presbyopia-correcting IOLs: binocular + contralateral vision in Crystalens/ReSTOR IOL combination. AAO/APAO Joint Meeting (paper); November 2006; Las Vegas, NV.

CHAPTER 221

MANAGING COMPLAINTS FOLLOWING ReZOOM IOL IMPLANTATION

Tom M. Coffman, MD

As exciting as the multifocal lens experience is for most patients, a small percentage need some help to be happy. The common problems to overcome are residual refractive error, glare, decentration, and inadequate reading or distance vision. The ideal refractive result with the ReZoom IOL is −0.50 in the non-dominant eye and −0.25 in the dominant eye. The reverse of this may work just as well. The most verbalized solution to correct a +0.50 or −0.75 residual refractive error is photorefractive keratectomy (PRK) or laser in situ keratomileusis (LASIK). This works very well but, is costly and many refractive IOL surgeons are not LASIK surgeons. If the error is +1.75 or less and needs correction, conductive keratoplasty (CK) is less expensive and any eye surgeon should be able to perform it successfully. If the correction needed is for +0.50 to +1.00, surgically spinning the IOL out of the bag into the sulcus with the Coffman recentration technique will induce the proper amount of myopic shift (see Chapter 228). This strategy only works with 3-piece lenses. If the residual spherical error is −0.75 to −1.00 a single or double mini radial keratotomy (RK) incision in the plus axis or at 60 degrees and/or 120 degrees will often work quite well. Another simple solution is to piggyback a low power (− or +) IOL in the sulcus. If there is residual myopia, use a piggyback IOL of equal power to achieve the desired goal of generally −0.37. If there is residual hyperopia, a piggyback IOL with a power that is 1.5 times the hyperopic error is required.

The most common refractive enhancement needed is to correct astigmatism. Three diopters (D) or less is generally corrected by opposing limbal relaxing incisions. One hour of the clock (about a 3-mm T-marker) is the incision needed for each diopter of correction desired. This is performed over the plus axis with a 600 microns pre-set diamond blade. Make sure the corneal thickness is above 585 microns in the surgical meridian to avoid perforation. A 500 microns center thickness blade setting usually equates to over 600 microns in the periphery. At or above 3 D of astigmatism, there is some danger in creating irregular astigmatism and decreased best corrected visual acuity (BCVA) with incisional keratotomy.

Until an excimer laser custom ablation can be topographically directed this irregular astigmatism cannot be corrected, because wavefront devices cannot measure accurately through a multifocal lens. If a patient has more than 2.5 D of astigmatism preoperatively, this could be addressed by piggybacking a toric IOL during the primary procedure. The piggybacked toric lens should go into the capsular bag and be placed posterior to the multifocal with both optics centered on each other at the end of the case. Usually this is achieved with the haptics located perpendicular to each other using a toric plate haptic IOL, or with the haptics along the same axis with a 3-piece toric IOL. Both lenses may go into the bag unless they are both acrylic. When both lenses are acrylic, place one in the bag and one in the sulcus to decrease the chance of an opaque plaque forming centrally between them. It is impossible to remove these plaques. The Holladay II program is very accurate for piggyback calculations.

Another special situation would be with a refractive surprise following Crystalens (Eyeonics, Inc., Aliso Viejo, CA) implantation. If these IOLs vault too far anteriorly or posteriorly the resulting refractive shift can be about a −1.75 or +1.75, respectively. This can be nicely corrected by piggybacking a low power Array (Advanced Medical Optics, Santa Ana, CA) lens, using the aforementioned formula. These low diopter Array IOLs are still available and give the patient a very large near focus range.

Glare is always discussed in detail with patients. However, it is generally more of a worry than a real problem. Less than 0.1% of hyperopic patients are bothered by glare from a multifocal since the IOL-induced glare is less than what was seen through hyperopic glasses. Most patients will observe a halo or glare in a high contrast situation such as when viewing a single street light at night. However, only 4% of patients will be bothered by the glare. The first solution is to use a drop of Alphagan (Allergan, Irvine, CA) at sundown to prevent wide pupil dilatation. Some patients require 0.5% Pilocarpine at sundown to prevent mydriasis and a rare patent will require 1% Pilocarpine. If there is some uncorrected refractive error, wearing night-driving spectacles will also reduce the glare. Adding −0.75 D more myopic correction in the eyeglasses than the actual refraction dictates can also help reduce halos. This causes a slight decrease in visual acuity but reduces glare.

If the patient is complaining about inadequate near vision after their first ReZoom (Advanced Medical Optics) surgery, implanting a ReZoom lens in the second eye reasonably soon and aiming for −0.25 to −0.50 more myopia than with the first eye usually works. Neither eye should be left more than −0.75 myopic, however. Most importantly, it has been observed time and time again that the near vision improves weekly for 3 months and then monthly for 3 to 5 years. I suggest to all patients that they purchase over the counter reading glasses in the +1.00 to +1.75 range to use for small print or extensive reading. This makes them use the near zones of the implant and trains the brain to sort it out. A +2.00 or stronger pair of readers causes them to read through the distance zone of the ReZoom and this may impede the near adaptation process.

They will require the low power readers less and less over time.

If there is a 20/25 level of posterior capsule haze the near vision drops off quickly. With a patient complaint and glare test documentation they should have a yttrium-aluminum-garnet (YAG) capsulotomy at that time. The capsulotomy should be 4.5 to 5.0 mm in diameter to permit good near vision through the peripheral zones.

Conclusion

By employing the aforementioned strategies and solutions I have only had to explant 11 of the approximately 10,000 multifocal IOLs that I have implanted. The ReZoom IOL is not a "cure all" technology but appears to be the best lens available at this time. Often the patients tell me and their friends, "This is the best thing I have ever done for myself."

CHAPTER 222

COMMUNICATING WITH THE UNHAPPY REFRACTIVE IOL PATIENT

John W. Potter, OD, FAAO

Ideal candidates for refractive intraocular lens (IOL) surgery can now obtain simultaneous distance and near vision with less dependence on eyeglasses and/or contact lenses. This is remarkable in and of itself, and is all very good for patients.

However, if the results of refractive IOL surgery are unexpected, or if something occurs that could not have been anticipated or planned for before surgery, your patient may experience a great sense of vision loss. Some of these patients may do well, whereas others may grieve over their loss of vision.

Grieving is an important protection we humans use to deal with great loss, and I will submit to you that some patients with unexpected results from refractive IOL surgery may grieve. This can be problematic for patients and their doctors if we do not understand what is happening and what can be done about it. There are some specific stages your patients may go through in grieving, and these are outlined in Table 1.[1-3]

Disappointing results from refractive IOL surgery can be quite challenging for surgeons. Your patient may expect, or even demand, that you do something to help them surgically if their results are unexpected. However, you are not prepared to perform additional surgery that, at least for now, may not be in the patient's best interest.

You and Your Patient may Be in Shock

When your patient has a disappointing result from refractive surgery, the first response is to enter a state of shock. This stage lasts for several days but occasionally longer than a month. Shock is a good thing because it protects patients from having to deal with a difficult concept: they have not gotten from refractive surgery what they thought they would.[4]

This does not always mean that there were complications from the surgery. For example, your patient may have good distance and intermediate vision, but poorer near vision. Again, the emotion is not caused by the scope of the problem, but rather by the fact that expectations were not met. Indeed, there may even be a great sense of loss of vision. In turn, you

will probably go through some of the same emotions that your patient is experiencing.

During this period, you may also find that your patient is very accepting of the situation. Even in the worst imaginable circumstances, patients at this stage are often almost numb to the impact of their situation, and doctors mistakenly believe that everything will be just fine. As a result, you may not see your patient as frequently as you should, which often leads to some compromise in the doctor–patient relationship.

In fact, you should see your patient at least weekly for a month or so. Your purpose is to stay close to your patient because you need to be in touch as they move from this first phase to the next.

Your Patient will Express Anger and Emotion

The next phase your patient may go through will surprise you. This phase is quite predictable, so it is important to anticipate it and to be prepared. Your patient will become very emotive and highly expressive, and that almost always takes the form of anger and frustration.

My experience suggests that this phase causes doctors to step back and withdraw from their patient. This is exactly the opposite of what you should do, which is to draw yourself nearer to your patient emotionally.

Why do you back away? It is a very uncommon experience in clinical practice for a patient to yell at you or express a great deal of anger and frustration when you did not expect that level of emotion.

Your first response to this expression of emotion should be to put some distance between yourself and the patient by using the image of "going to the balcony."[5] Imagine yourself in a large auditorium. Your patient is on the stage, and you are in the last row of the balcony. This image of distance will help you maintain your poise in the face of anger, frustration, and hostility.

Table 1

GRIEVING STAGES

1. Shock
2. Expression of emotion and anger
3. Feeling depressed and alone
4. Onset of physical symptoms
5. Feelings of nearly overwhelming anxiety
6. Guilt
7. Resentment and anger
8. Resistance to returning to normal self
9. Gradually, hope returns
10. Affirmation of loss

Table 2

EXPRESSING REGRET

1. Recognition
2. Regret
3. Responsibility
4. Remedy
5. Realignment

Next, it is critical to realize that what is most important now is what the patient hears, not what you say. Too often doctors dwell on what they want to say, not what the patient needs to hear. This is a mistake because your patient will remember nearly every word you say when they are in this stage of grieving, and you need a rubric to follow to make sure what you need to say is heard. In addition, a rubric gives you a framework where you can repeat your expression of regret as many times as needed with consistency and meaning. Inconsistency and a lack of sincerity can be very damaging to the doctor–patient relationship.

There are 5 steps to making an appropriate expression of regret to your refractive IOL patient.[6] It is convenient to have a memory cue to make the flow of the apology accomplish what you intend without seeming awkward or contrived. The 5 steps are all "r-words" in this order: recognition, regret, responsibility, remedy, and realignment (Table 2).

Recognition is the first step in this process. Is this the right time to express regret? It is hard to know when, but in general it is best to do so when you are past the shock stage yourself. This may be a matter of minutes, or hours, or sometimes days, but you should express regret when you can, not when you have to do it. Second, a sincere expression of regret is needed. This is not an apology wherein you are asking for forgiveness as you would when apologizing to a loved one. As an example, "I regret that you did get the results from your surgery you expected…" Do not say that you understand what your patient is going through emotionally. This is a common, but enormous, mistake. Your patient is likely to respond to you by making it very clear that you have no idea what he or she is going through, and, in fact, you do not.

Now you can proceed to the next step, responsibility. Here, it is very important that you again be straightforward with your patient. "I am responsible for your eye and vision care and I am going to do what I can to help you." It may seem obvious you are responsible for your patients, but a dread of abandonment colors this stage of grieving, so you need to be very clear about your responsibility for your patient. Next, outline the remedy. If you know what the next steps in your patient's care should be, then say so. If you do not know, tell your patient that you do not know, but you will find out and follow up with them at a future and specific time. Because we often struggle with dealing with anger from our patients, if we are then less

than forthright with them, we are beginning to lose the doctor–patient relationship.

The final step is critical in refractive IOL surgery as this is a newer refractive procedure and there is still much to learn about it. Patients are often very concerned about the welfare of other patients in this stage of grieving. Although this may seem an odd reaction at first, it is not if you look more deeply into the emotion expressed.

Your patient has an unexpected and disappointing result from refractive surgery, and he or she is emotionally distraught and struggling to deal with the situation. The patient cannot imagine how anyone else could deal with what he or she is going through, so he or she often has a great fear that others will suffer. In my experience, patients at this stage almost always think they are handling their situation as well as they can, even though it may not appear that way to you. However, it is a very human reaction, and if you understand it, you can help your patient through it.

Your Patient Feels Depressed and Alone

Your patient may very well be feeling emotions that he or she has never had before. Such emotion becomes very confusing and often leads to a situational depressive state. It is not at all uncommon for patients to tell me or their doctors that they have thoughts of ending their own lives. I am not aware of any patient who has ever followed through with these thoughts, but it is important to realize that this expression tells you precisely where they are in dealing with their grief.

You may not hear from your patient for months, and you may be relieved. Again, this is a very common and human response, so it is perfectly acceptable to have these feelings, even if they are difficult and uncomfortable. You need to understand that your patient needs you now more than ever, but it is a difficult challenge to take the initiative to continue to try to help your patient when you are struggling yourself to deal with his or her problems.

In my experience, you either need to call or see your patient at least monthly. A call often will suffice, and it is important for you to know that you do not have to have a great deal to say when you call. Tell your patient that you were thinking of him or her and that you are concerned. You do not have to have all the remedies for the problem, but you do need to communicate your concern effectively. Your patient may say that you do not need to be concerned, or that you don't need to call, but you do.

Your Patient May Develop Physical Symptoms

This next stage of grieving over disappointing results from refractive surgery is often very alarming to the doctor.[7] As before, it is important to be able to identify the stage and understand it so you can help your patient. At this stage, it is common for your patient to say something like, "My eyes are so bad that I cannot see to do my work at all." Specifically refractive IOL patients also seem to have more eye pain and headache than photorefractive keratectomy (PRK) or laser in situ keratomileusis (LASIK) patients.

I have had patients express this emotion as back pain and other symptoms that seem unrelated to eyes or vision, but it is important to know what the emotion is telling you. Ask your patient if he or she is still working or if their eye pain or headache prevents them from going about their daily activities. Much to your surprise, your patient will often say that he or she is still working full time or is able to perform their daily activities. Your patient will often say it is difficult to do these things, but the point is that they are doing them.

You must be careful here. If you become angry with your patient because it appears that he or she is misleading you or not telling the truth, you will be making a very grave error. Instead, you should respond that you understand that activities such as working or driving at night must be difficult. If you challenge your patient on what appears to be a contradictory position, you will push him or her backward and cause a withdrawal. Your patient will believe that you simply do not understand how much he or she has suffered. This will strain the doctor–patient relationship further, and it will make it that much more difficult for your patient to progress through the other stages of grieving.

Your Patient May Become Anxious

Your patient may become anxious and think of nothing but his or her eye and vision problems. It is very common to hear the patient say, "I will go anywhere, anytime, and I will pay whatever it takes to fix my problem. This is terrible! I want this fixed now. Just tell me what to do, and I will do it."

This is the stage where refractive surgeons make their most common errors in judgment. A doctor may well be tempted to do what the patient has asked for, and an additional surgery may be performed "because the patient really wanted me to fix their problem."

Additional surgery is not a treatment for anxiety in grieving over unexpected results from refractive IOL surgery. Countless numbers of surgeons make this mistake and live with the consequences, which are almost universally not what the doctor expected. Nor are the results from doing surgery because they are anxious what the patient truly wanted, anyway. So, again, the doctor–patient relationship is strained and will often completely fracture at this stage.

Your Patient May Experience Guilt

This next phase does not last very long, but it can be quite problematic for patients and their doctors. In my experience, this phase lasts only a week or 2, but it is important to recognize it when it occurs and to be prepared for it.

Your patient may ask you if he or she made a mistake having refractive IOL surgery in the first place, and you may be at a loss for words. On one hand, you want to say that he or she did not make a mistake in having surgery, but that can be difficult because your patient has an unexpected disappointing result. On the other hand, you can't say that you think he or she made a mistake in having surgery, because he or she didn't. Both you and your patient carefully considered the options and your patient provided their informed consent to having the surgery.

There are 3 points to make that will help you and your patient. The communication skill to develop is called "feel, felt, find." First, acknowledge that the feeling your patient is having is a perfectly legitimate and reasonable concern. Doubt is a part of grieving over loss, so it is a normal human response. Second, if you have had other patients tell you something similar, or if you are aware that patients might have these feelings, it is important to tell your patient that other patients have had similar feelings as they deal with their unexpected results from refractive surgery. Third, you need to use your awareness and understanding of your patient's emotion to suggest that these feelings will diminish over the next few weeks, because they will.

Your Patient May Become Angry and Resentful

The next stage in your patient's journey can be quite difficult to understand. Your patient may develop anger and resentment over what you have done—or not done—to help him or her. The anger is almost always completely out of character for your patient, and it may be directed at family members or loved ones, too. Many times, a family member or loved one may call you and beg for your help in dealing with the patient. This can be difficult for you unless you have some sense of what is happening and why.

Your patient may begin to feel that you have forgotten how much he or she has suffered, and he or she must keep the memory of the suffering alive and well. In fact, it may become your patient's personal mission in life for months or, in some situations, years to remind you and others of how much he or she has suffered. This is most obvious on the Internet as there are several Web sites devoted to patients recounting how much they have suffered at the hands of some surgeon. Such emotion is often difficult to understand, but it is critical that you do. Otherwise, you will be of no help to your patient. I am not a great fan of this form of dealing with loss, because what your patients need are their doctors, not the Internet.

The solution is to stay close to your patient, which is often easier said than done. Unexpected disappointing results from refractive IOL surgery are not common, and grieving over vision loss is not commonly encountered in most ophthalmic practices. For this reason, staying close to your patient while they are grieving can be challenging. On the other hand, helping your patients through a difficult time during which they need you the most is also quite rewarding in the end.

Your Patient Resists Returning to His or Her Normal Self

The most complex situation you may find yourself in is one where the patient is resisting returning to his or her normal self. You may very well have a treatment or have arranged for additional surgery, but your patient will not use the treatment or won't show up for appointments. In fact, you may become quite frustrated with your patient—but it would be a mistake if you did. In fact, the harder you push, the more resistance you will encounter, even to the point of what may appear to be absurd.

You may know someone who has lost a child to illness or other tragedy, and the family keeps the child's room exactly as it was right before his or her death for years and years. They know every detail of the room, and even the slightest change is devastating. Patients suffering with unexpected results from refractive surgery may feel similarly, and you need to recognize it to deal with it effectively.

What should you do? This is difficult, but the right thing to do here is to back off completely. Tell your patient that you know having treatment or additional surgery is an important decision and that time should be taken to make sure the decision is right. Stay in touch with him or her over the next months. Do not push, but remain committed to helping when he or she is ready.

Gradually, Hope Returns

Some of the most meaningful experiences of my professional life are to have worked with patients and their doctors for several months and to then see hope return. Your patient will begin to talk about the future and not dwell on the past. Your patient may be ready to make meaningful decisions about additional surgery, and your patient may end up with better vision from additional refractive surgery. Their loss is no longer a major focus of their life. When this occurs, it is a remarkable and rewarding experience.

Your Patient Affirms the Reality of His or Her Loss

I have had patients apologize for previous behavior, which is completely unnecessary, as it is they who have suffered, not I. Additionally, I have had countless patients offer to help me by making themselves available to other patients with similar problems. Medical malpractice actions are rare when you and your patient can work together in a sphere of understanding and determination to focus on the future, and not grieve over loss.[8] Ultimately, by understanding that grieving can occur, and that we can manage it, the doctor–patient relationship is preserved. This is the best solution for everyone, especially your patients.

References

1. Kubler-Ross E. *On Death and Dying.* New York: Macmillan; 1969:37.
2. Westberg GE. *Good Grief.* Philadelphia: Fortress Press; 1962:12, 20, 64.
3. Potter J. Help refractive surgery patients cope with unexpected results. *Primary Care Optometry News.* 2006;11:23-24.
4. Hofer MA. On the nature and consequences of early loss. *Psychosom Med.* 1996;58:570-581.
5. Fisher R, Shapiro D. *Beyond Reason: Using Emotions As You Negotiate.* 1st ed. New York: Penguin Books; 2006.
6. Potter J. Learn when and how to apologize to refractive surgery patients. *Primary Care Optometry News.* 2007;12:22-24.
7. Lindemann E. Symptomatology and management of acute grief. *Am J Psychiatry.* 1944;101:141-148.
8. Coltri L. *Conflict Diagnosis and Alternative Dispute Resolution.* Vol. 1. Upper Saddle River, NJ: Pearson Education; 2004.

CHAPTER 223

LESSONS LEARNED FROM A CONSULTATION PRACTICE

Alan S. Crandall, MD

Presbyopia-correcting intraocular lenses (IOLs) have added to our armamentarium in the management of patients with cataracts and refractive errors. There are 3 Food and Drug Administration (FDA) approved presbyopia-correcting IOLs and many progressing through clinical trials. Each of the lenses uses different strategies for the correction of presbyopia and it is important to understand the optics in order to diagnose and manage the postoperative issues and complications that patients experience. In this chapter we will review the management of a number of real patients to illustrate some of these issues and our approach to the management.

When selecting IOLs for patients, it is important to understand their needs and working environment. The ReSTOR IOL (Alcon Laboratories, Fort Worth, TX) is designed for optimizing distance and near. It has a 4-D add that gives the patient effectively a +3 diopter lens so that he obtains good near vision at approximately 16 inches. The center of the lens is for near and the apodized surface sends energy to distance. Initially patients do not obtain intermediate focus although over time this improves with neuroadaptation. The amount of light that is distributed for near or distance is pupil dependent. The ReZoom lens (Advanced Medical Optics, Santa Ana, CA) uses a zonal design where the center of the lens is for distance and as the pupil enlarges more light is sent for near. The near correction is less than that of the ReSTOR but ReZoom usually gives better intermediate vision. The Crystalens (Eyeonics, Aliso Viejo, CA) is designed as an accommodating lens so that the lens moves with contraction of the ciliary body.

All of these IOLs entail compromises that are important to understand. Both the ReZoom and ReSTOR IOLs produce halos and some glare at night because of their design. These symptoms are generally tolerated and again, with time (and neuroadaptation), patients do improve. Night driving, however, can be problematic and patients may complain of waxy distance vision. The new aspheric ReSTOR does improve the quality of the vision. The Crystalens usually does not provide as much freedom from glasses as the multifocal IOLs, but the distance vision is usually quite good.

Patient 1

This patient is a 72-year-old female who presented with bilateral cataracts. Preoperatively her refraction was slightly myopic with little astigmatism, and she elected to have bilateral multifocal IOLs. After the first eye surgery she complained of poor distance and reading vision. She was told that when the second eye was done, it would be better but she elected to wait and get a second opinion.

The examination revealed the right eye to have best corrected vision of 20/30−. She had pseudoexfoliation (PXF) of the lens capsule but dilated well and had normal intraocular pressure (IOP). She had grade 2 nuclear sclerosis with water cleft changes. The optic nerve and retina were normal. The left eye was best corrected to 20/60. Her IOP was 24 and she was on Timoptic (Merck & Co., Whitehouse Station, NJ) 0.5% twice a day. Slit lamp examination revealed a clear cornea with a well-healed temporal clear corneal incision. The anterior chamber had 1+ flare and cell, as well as 1+ pigment cells. The iris had transillumination defects. The ReSTOR IOL was decentered and the haptics were in the sulcus. The posterior capsule was open. The optic nerve was healthy, but she had significant cystoid macular edema.

ASSESSMENT AND TREATMENT

A posterior capsular tear occurred at the time of the surgery and the single-piece ReSTOR was placed in the sulcus. This led to iris chaffing and pigment dispersion. The combination of iris issues and the posterior capsular rent lead to cystoid macular edema (CME) and the elevated IOP. She was started on a topical nonsteroidal anti-inflammatory drop (Acular LS) and a topical steroid (Pred Forte 1% [Allergan, Irvine, CA]). After a long discussion of the options, she preferred to have a multifocal implant. After the eye quieted down and the CME improved, she had the single-piece ReSTOR IOL explanted and replaced with a 3-piece ReSTOR placed in the sulcus. One month later, the right eye had cataract surgery with a ReSTOR

IOL placed in the bag. Postoperatively she is doing well and is happy.

CLINICAL POINTS

1. A single-piece lens is not designed for sulcus fixation and will cause iris chaffing and an increased risk of glaucoma and CME.

2. A posterior capsule tear can happen anytime (especially in patients with PXF); you need to have a back up plan in case it does.

3. Decentration of a multifocal lens can lead to significant visual issues.

Patient 2

A 68-year-old female patient was referred by her family for a second opinion. She had bilateral multifocal implants but was having trouble with both eyes and poor reading vision. Her surgeon told her the surgery was done perfectly and that in time she would improve; but after waiting 1 year, she felt her vision was still poor and not improving.

EXAMINATION

Visual acuity was 20/30 OD uncorrected, improving to 20/25 with a refraction of plano + 0.75. The left eye was 20/60 with no improvement with refraction. The uncorrected near vision was J10 OD, and J5 OS.

The IOP was normal OU.

Slit lamp examination revealed a well-centered ReZoom IOL with a clear capsule in the right eye. The left eye had a well-centered ReSTOR IOL with a grade 2 posterior capsule clouding.

The retina was normal.

I saw the patient after she had received 4 sets of dilating drops and her pupils were only 4.0 mm. The technician had made a comment that her pupils seemed small prior to instilling the dilating drops. I asked the patient to return later in the week and see me prior to any dilating drops. Her undilated pupils were 2.5 mm and only enlarged to 3.5 mm after 20 minutes in a dark room.

ASSESSMENT AND TREATMENT

The surgery was well performed but both of the multifocal IOLs used require adequate pupil function to work. In this mix-and-match setting the right has a distance-dominant multifocal IOL and the left eye has a multifocal IOL that is near dominant in the center. She essentially almost has a monovision correction, but the large add in the ReSTOR eye made her uncomfortable walking and reading as well.

The options could include laser pupilloplasty to enlarge the pupils, but this would still not improve the function of the iris in different lighting situations. One could perform a left YAG Yag laser capsulotomy to improve the near vision in this eye, but the discrepancy in vision would still exist and an open capsule would complicate the option of an IOL exchange.

After explaining the problem to her, we decided that we would exchange the ReSTOR IOL for an aspheric monofocal IOL targeted for distance. I needed to use iris hooks to aid

in the explantation, and polished the posterior capsule at the time of surgery. She now has 20/25 vision in the left eye and although she doesn't have the benefit of near function from the ReZoom in her right eye, the distance vision is good. We elected to take no action with it for now.

CLINICAL POINTS

1. Although they incorporate different optical strategies, both the ReZoom and ReSTOR IOLs require appropriate functional pupil sizes to work.

2. It is important to measure the pupil in mesopic light before dilating drops are instilled.

Patient 3

The patient is a 62-year-old male. He has cataracts, with vision best corrected to OD 20/50 and OS 20/60. Preoperatively the refraction is OD +2.50 +0.50 axis 85; OS +2.00 +1.00 axis 95. Preoperative keratometry shows OD with 44.25 × 45@90; OS with 43.75 × 43.75@95.

After being implanted with bilateral ReSTOR IOLs, the patient felt that the distance vision was not clear and he complained of double vision at near.

Vision was OD 20/25 with a refraction of −50 +1.25 × 95; OS 20/40 with a refraction of plano +1.50 × 110.

Corneal topography confirmed the astigmatism measured by refraction.

ASSESSMENT AND TREATMENT

Multifocal lenses are unforgiving of any residual astigmatism. The temporal incision generally causes approximately 0.50 D of steepening and often induces a slight axis shift. In this case, both incisions caused an increase in with-the-rule astigmatism.

The patient had bilateral limbal relaxing incisions using Doug Koch's nomogram, resulting in OD plano +0.50 × 85 20/20; OS +0.50 sphere 20/20.

CLINICAL POINTS

1. You need to know what astigmatic effect your incision will have.

2. Learn to do limbal relaxing incisions (LRIs) reproducibly.

3. An alternative to LRIs is to do a laser keratorefractive procedure for the residual refractive error.

Patient 4

A 39-year-old plumber presents with bilateral posterior subcapsular cataracts. Preoperatively, he was a −7.5 OD and −8.0 OS but had been a hard contact lens wearer for 10 years. Because his work environment included dirt, waste material, and the need for near work (in dim light frequently), we elected to use the Crystalens in him. Due to the long-term contact lens wear, we initially switched him to soft lenses and had him wait for 3 weeks to allow his corneas to resume their natural topography.

His vision preoperatively: OD 20/30, BAT 20/60 with –7.00 +2.50 × 110; OS 20/40, BAT 20/80, with –6.00 +2.75 × 080.

Slit lamp examination showed cataracts but otherwise no pathology. At the time of surgery the LRIs were performed at a depth of 600 microns using Nichamin's nomogram. Initial complaints postoperatively were poor vision at distance and near as well as severe photophobia. We waited 4 weeks post surgery and the patient still presented with +1.75 D of astigmatism. He was refractable to 20/15. We assumed that because of his youth the LRIs were less effective. We performed astigmatic keratotomy (AK) at a 9-mm optical zone and waited another 4 to 6 weeks. He also complained of severe pain and photophobia post AK. At 4 weeks post AK, the patient had a refraction of OD –1.00 +1.50 × 095 20/15; OS –0.75 +0175 × 075 20/15.

ASSESSMENT AND TREATMENT

The combination of LRI and AK was ineffective in reducing his astigmatism to allow for excellent uncorrected distance vision, and there was residual myopia. Treatment options would include attempting further surgical reduction of the astigmatism. Wearing glasses and contact lenses were not an option due to his work environment. Because of the prior AK/LRI, we elected to do laser surface ablation after 3 months to ensure corneal and refractive stability. The patient is now 20/15 distance and J5 near.

CLINICAL POINTS

1. Rigid contact lens wearers frequently manifest masked astigmatism and we must allow time for the cornea to resume its natural state. Although studies vary, most patients will stabilize by around 2 weeks. This needs to be confirmed by stable corneal topography.

2. Although LRI or AK are usually very effective, in some cases they are not (particularly young patients). A backup laser refractive treatment may be necessary.

3. It is necessary to understand the patient's work environment/lifestyle in order to choose the correct presbyopia-correcting IOL. Because this patient's work environment would involve dim lighting, a ReSTOR IOL would likely have been ineffective. This patient's job also included significant night driving, therefore the ReZoom lens would have been problematic.

Patient 5

This patient is a 52-year-old male who had laser in situ keratomileusis (LASIK) and 2 enhancements for moderate myopia (–6.50 +0.75 × 170, –1.75 +0.75 × 0.20). No data available (different state and patient actually not sure). The patient's previous LASIK was done in another state and the patient did not even remember where it was done Recently he developed central posterior subcapsular cataracts, with OD

20/60 uncorrected; 20/46 with a refraction of –2.00 +1.00 × 90. OS is 20/80 uncorrected; 20/50 with a refraction of –1.00 +0.50 × 120.

He has mild dry eyes OU (nonsymptomatic), 2+ central posterior subcapsular cataract lens, 3+ central posterior subcapsular cataract, and a normal retina.

The patient decided he would prefer a presbyopia-correcting IOL and chose a Crystalens. Calculations were done using the IOL Master (Carl Zeiss, Jena, Germany) using the Holladay formula. The American Society of Cataract and Refractive Surgery (ASCRS) Web site (utilized by members to use for postrefractive IOL powers) was used to select these IOL powers for surgery: OD 22.50 D Crystalens; OS 21.50 D Crystalens. Postoperative refraction was OD +2.75 +1.00 × 90 20/20; OS +1.25 +0.50 × 110 20/20 (determined 3 months postoperatively to ensure stability.)

MANAGEMENT OPTIONS

1. Lift old flap (LASIK was 10 years ago)

2. Piggyback implants

3. Photorefractive keratectomy (PRK)

Pachymetry suggested that there was insufficient residual corneal stromal tissue for further LASIK. He therefore underwent piggyback IOL implantation with a STAAR (STAAR Surgical Company, Monrovia, CA) AQ50IOV 2010 lens OD –3.00 and OS –1.00. Postoperative results: 1-day OD 20/20–2; 1-day OS 20/60+1 –2 PH NI; OD –3.00 lens implant in sulcus; OS –1.00 lens implant in sulcus.

CLINICAL POINTS

1. Patients who have had prior refractive surgery tend to want premium IOLs.

2. Because they have already had corneal ablation (many prewavefront), they may not be good candidates for multifocal IOLs.

3. IOL calculations post keratorefractive surgery are improving but still not perfect.

   a. Use IOL Master biometry with Holladay 2 Consultant software

   b. Use Warren Hill's Web site

   c. Use the ASCRS Web site, which includes many formulas including Masket's

4. Wait until the refraction stabilizes before making enhancements. If patients go in understanding that this is a team effort and may require an enhancement, they will be better served.

The use of presbyopia-correcting lenses is rewarding but demanding. It is important to understand the patient's needs and communicate all of the potential issues in advance.

CHAPTER 224

LESSONS LEARNED FROM A CONSULTATION PRACTICE

Sonia H. Yoo, MD; George D. Kymionis, MD, PhD; Yunhee Lee, MD; Terrence P. O'Brien, MD; and William W. Culbertson MD

Refractive lens exchange (RLE) is a new area in cataract surgery. As with every new technology in medicine, there is learning curve for both the ophthalmologist and patient.[1,2] Perhaps the best source for learning and further understanding this new technology is by evaluating the outcomes of our postrefractive intraocular lens (IOL) patients. The unhappy postrefractive IOL patients presenting to us at Bascom Palmer for second opinions or refractive IOL removal underscores the need to shorten the learning curve to avoid future similar postrefractive IOL failures.[3-8]

For surgeons (and patients) there are several critical issues to address with this new technology. Patient selection and education before the operation is crucial (perhaps more important than the operation itself), in order to have a favorable outcome.[3-8] The following are some of the essential issues that must be addressed prior to refractive lens implantation.

Patient Personality Expectations

Refractive IOL candidates are often highly demanding patients, with higher expectations typical of refractive patients compared to traditional cataract patients. It is common in a consultative practice to deal with postrefractive IOL patients that complain about their surgery outcome even though they are spectacle independent for both near and far. Patients with such unrealistic expectations of visual improvement are not good candidates for refractive IOL implantation. A detailed preoperative discussion with the patient, explaining features, benefits, and possible disadvantages of these new IOLs is mandatory in order to be sure that patient will be accepting of this technology and its limitations. It is common to encounter unhappy postrefractive IOL patients who have seen multiple ophthalmologists and who still do not have a clear explanation for their visual complaints. Before referring these patients to a psychiatrist, the ophthalmologist should understand that not all the patients are the same. Some patients expect to have

perfect vision and even small losses of contrast sensitivity may be devastating to them.

Occupational Requirements

Another issue in patient selection pertains to occupational requirements. Patients who need to drive or fly in low-light conditions cannot afford to have difficulty with these activities. They are not ideal candidates for these lenses (with the current technology) due to decreased contrast sensitivity in low-light conditions. Monofocal or aspheric IOLs would be a better option for these patients.

Bilateral Procedures

Unilateral refractive IOL implantation in patients with unilateral cataracts can cause difficulty in adapting, whereas better cortical adaptation after bilateral implantation (summation effect) has been reported. Furthermore, the combination of refractive and monofocal IOLs in the same patient may decrease the visual benefits of refractive IOLs. It seems that previously operated patients with monofocal IOLs are not the best candidates for refractive IOLs.

The Goal Is Postoperative Emmetropia

Residual refractive errors after the surgery—even small amounts of residual astigmatism or sphere—can result in increased complaints of glare and halos. Preoperative screening for corneal astigmatism with topography, accurate preoperative biometry, intraoperative management of corneal astigmatism with limbal relaxing incisions (LRIs), and good IOL centration are essential for success with these lenses. Furthermore any residual postoperative ametropia may require subsequent refractive surgery with laser in situ keratomileusis

(LASIK) or photorefractive keratectomy (PRK) to maximize patient satisfaction.

In extremely ametropic eyes (especially with high myopia), IOL calculations can be more difficult, leading to residual refractive errors. With multifocal IOLs, a portion of incoming light is focused on the retina from each image in which the patient is interested. Increased axial length can accentuate this effect on image projection, leading to further decrease in low light contrast sensitivity. These patients are not good candidates for multifocal lens implantation

Customized IOL Type Selection

The various presbyopia-correcting (Pr-C) IOLs have different design features, and the best IOL should be selected based on the patient's personal needs and lifestyle. Refractive IOLs offering better far and intermediate vision (such as ReZoom IOL [Advanced Medical Optics, Santa Ana, CA] or Crystalens accommodating IOL [Eyeonics, Aliso Viejo, CA]), may be the ideal option for patients who spend a great deal of time working with computers; patients with high demands for near vision may do better with the Acrysof ReSTOR IOL (Alcon, Fort Worth, TX).

Intraoperative Complications Management

Another source of unhappy post–Pr-C IOL patients is lens decentration and issues of pupil size. With monofocal IOLs, a small decentration will generally be well tolerated by patients. In contrast, even small amounts of decentration with refractive IOLs (especially with a multifocal) can be intolerable. It is crucial for the surgeon to evaluate intraoperatively (or preoperatively in patients with phacodonesis or pseudoexfoliation) the integrity of the capsule. In cases of weak zonules, one may need to change to a monofocal IOL to avoid the optical risk of slight decentration or tilt with a multifocal IOL postoperatively. Furthermore, pupil size is another parameter to consider

when deciding which IOL to select for the patient. It has been found that diffractive IOLs are more independent pupil size, whereas the performance of refractive multifocals are more dependent on optimum pupil size.

In conclusion, successful Pr-C IOL implantation requires understanding the patients' needs and demands and the limitations of the technology. Further improvements in the current design and technology of Pr-C IOLs hopefully will provide our patients the ultimate in visual perfection.

References

1. Olson RJ, Werner L, Mamalis N, Cionni R. New intraocular lens technology. *Am J Ophthalmol.* 2005;140:709-716.
2. Alfonso JF, Fernández-Vega L, Baamonde MB, Montés-Micó R. Prospective visual evaluation of apodized diffractive intraocular lenses. *J Cataract Refract Surg.* 2007;33:1235-1243.
3. Vingolo EM, Grenga P, Iacobelli L, Grenga R. Visual acuity and contrast sensitivity: AcrySof ReSTOR apodized diffractive versus AcrySof SA60AT monofocal intraocular lenses. *J Cataract Refract Surg.* 2007;33:1244-1247.
4. Hutz WW, Eckhardt HB, Rohrig B, Grolmus R. Reading ability with 3 multifocal intraocular lens models. *J Cataract Refract Surg.* 2006;32:2015-2021.
5. Alio JL, Tavolato M, De la Hoz F, Claramonte P, Rodriguez-Prats J-L, Galal A. Near vision restoration with refractive lens exchange and pseudoaccommodating and multifocal refractive and diffractive intraocular lenses: Comparative clinical study. *J Cataract Refract Surg.* 2004;30:2494-2503.
6. Nijkamp MD, Dolders MGT, de Brabander J, van den Borne B, Hendrikse F, Nuijts RMMA. Effectiveness of multifocal intraocular lenses to correct presbyopia after cataract surgery: a randomized controlled trial. *Ophthalmology.* 2004;111:1832-1839.
7. Baumeister M, Neidhardt B, Strobel J, Kohnen T. Tilt and decentration of three-piece foldable high-refractive silicone and hydrophobic acrylic intraocular lenses with 6-mm optics in an intraindividual comparison. *Am J Ophthalmol.* 2005;140:1051-1058.
8. Mamalis N, Davis B, Nilson CD, Hickman MS, LeBoyer RM. Complications of foldable intraocular lenses requiring explantation or secondary intervention—2003 survey update. *J Cataract Refract Surg.* 2004;30:2209-2218.

Table 1

PRESBYOPIC IOLs—LESSONS LEARNED FROM A CONSULTATION PRACTICE: OUNCE OF PREVENTION IS WORTH A POUND OF CURE.

Ounce of Prevention – Common complaints to avoid

Still spectacle-dependent:
   Near add too near
   Intermediate vision inadequate
   Distance vision blurry
	• Avoid patients with greater than 0.75 D of astigmatism or irregular astigmatism.
	• Counsel patient regarding limitations of presbyopic lenses—has to be able to accept the compromise solution.
	• Explore patient's vocation/hobbies/daily activities—help patient to select lenses that would best satisfy their visual needs.
	• Explain that small degree of ametropia can exist postoperatively—make sure that it will be possible to correct this if occurs (have to be a candidate for PRK/LASIK/LRIs—e.g., if history of herpes simplex keratitis or thin corneas, might not be able to treat)

Vision was better before:
   Night vision more difficult
   Near vision dim
	• Counsel patient regarding limitations of presbyopic lenses—has to be able to accept the compromise solution. Light is being divided between the different foci.
	• Be on the alert to recognize any patient that is exquisitely discriminating and persists in unrealistic expectations.

Cannot perform former activities/job:
   Can't drive at night/fly a plane
   Glare
   Vaseline smear
   3-D quality to vision
	• Explore patient's vocation/hobbies/daily activities—help patient to select lenses that would best satisfy their visual needs. Counsel patients away from presbyopic lenses if risk to vocation is too great.
	• Counsel patient regarding limitations of presbyopic lenses—has to be able to accept the compromise solution.
	• Be on the alert to recognize any patient that is exquisitely discriminating and persists in unrealistic expectations.
	• Avoid implanting multifocal lens if first eye already has a monofocal lens—many patients have been unable to tolerate a 3-dimentional glasses quality to their vision.

Thought vision would be better	• Avoid patients that have underlying conditions that would limit vision—patients often are hoping for restoration of vision lost to disease (ARMD/OAG).

Pound of Cure

Still spectacle-dependent:
   Near add too near
   Intermediate vision inadequate
   Distance vision blurry
	• Patient's expectation bar can be managed even after the fact with discussion/explanation.
	• Assess degree of ametropia—may be able to address residual myopia/hyperopia/astigmatism with incisional procedures (LRI, miniRK) or laser procedures (PRK, LASIK).

Vision was better before:
   Night vision more difficult
   Near vision dim
	• Patient's expectation bar can be managed even after the fact with discussion/explanation.
	  ○ Encourage using bright lamps when reading.
	  ○ Assess degree of ametropia—may be able to address residual myopia/hyperopia/astigmatism with incisional procedures (LRI, miniRK) or laser procedures (PRK, LASIK). Ametropia can affect night vision significantly.
	  ○ Patient may benefit from spectacles that are used infrequently for more extreme conditions—driving long distances at night or for reading very small print for extended periods.

Cannot perform former activities/job:
   Can't drive at night/fly a plane
   Glare
   Vaseline smear
   3-D quality to vision
	• Patient's expectation bar can be managed even after the fact with discussion/explanation.
	  ○ Disturbance of activities may be limited and may be tolerable or acceptable to patient.
	  ○ Symptoms can subside with time and with cortical adaptation
	• Assess degree of ametropia—may be able to address residual myopia/hyperopia/astigmatism and restore activity level or ability. Patient may benefit from spectacles that are used infrequently.
	• If situation not salvageable, may need to discuss IOL exchange procedure to restore activity level.

Thought vision would be better	• Wait for cortical adaptation after bilateral implantation (3 months) • Discuss possibility of IOL exchange within a timeframe that allows for "safe" lens removal (less than 1 year). • Demonstrate the loss of uncorrected near visual acuity with monofocal IOL by placing minus spectacle lenses on the patient and asking them to read.

CHAPTER 225

MANAGING CRYSTALENS COMPLICATIONS

Jeffrey Whitman, MD

Managing complications of any premium channel intraocular lens (IOL) begins in the preoperative period and extends to beyond the immediate postoperative period. However, the goal is to prevent complications.

Preoperative Management of Crystalens Patients

* Set appropriate patient expectations
  * Set refractive expectations of about 1.5 to 2.0 diopter (D) of accommodation per eye.
  * Explain that myopic target for nondominant near eye and plano for dominant eye typically results in about a 75% to 90% probability of spectacle independence.
  * Explain that about 10% to 25% of patients will wear glasses for small print or prolonged reading of small print, particularly in dim or dark lighting conditions.
* Preoperative measurements
  * Manual Ks, IOL Master Ks (Carl Zeiss, Oberkochen, Germany), immersion A-Scan, IOL Master A-Scan are performed on all patients, and multiple IOL power formulas are calculated and compared.
  * Preoperative examination includes all tests typically done for laser in situ keratomileusis (LASIK) patients, eg, Schirmer's test, pachymetry, pupil size documentation, automated topography such as Orbscan (Bausch & Lomb, Rochester, NY) testing and endothelial cell counts.
    * ❏ Tip to prevent myopic shifts: These shifts rarely occur with Crystalens Five-O (Eyeonics, Aliso Viejo, CA) (<0.1% of cases (2/7311).[1] They can be prevented with consistent and accurate IOL calculations in the preoperative period using an IOL master.

Surgical Management of Crystalens Implantation

* Surgery is performed on the nondominant eye first, with a target of −0.25 to −0.75 sphere depending on the patient's preoperative refraction and visual demands.
* Surgery on the dominant eye is targeted for plano to −0.25 sphere with modification based on the first eye refractive result.
  * Tip to prevent refractive surprises: With Crystalens patients, using this customized refractive targeting approach yields excellent results
* Make a 2.8-mm incision with a keratome, followed by 2 smaller, adjacent paracentesis incisions on either side of the main incision for use in lens manipulation.
  * Tip to prevent leaking incisions: Wong pocket incision (see Chapter 183) may also be useful in sealing the main wound at the end of the case. The paracentesis incisions are typically longer and less radial.
* Fill anterior chamber with a viscoelastic to protect the cornea. Avoid OcuCoat as it makes the lens very slippery and difficult to manipulate at the end of the case.
* Use a bent-tip cystotome to create the recommended 6.0-mm capsulorrhexis. Marking the cornea prior to surgery with a 6.0-mm optical zone marker can be a very helpful guide.
  * Tip to prevent postoperative vaulting of the lens: It is important with the Crystalens Five-O to use a 6.0-mm or larger capsulorrhexis that is round in configuration. Ideally, the anterior capsule leaflet will not be covering any part of the lens optic at the end of the case.
* Perform phacoemulsification and irrigation/aspiration.
* Clean the posterior capsule.

❖ Tip to prevent postoperative opacification: It is important to perform careful cortical clean up. If there are any posterior capsular cells, use a silicone polishing tip, and polish both the posterior capsule and the underside of the anterior capsule leaflets. I believe that it is these leftover cells combined with the smaller lens diameter that led to capsular contraction and Z-syndrome with the AT-45 lens model.

✱ Insert the lens via the injector through the 2.8- to 3.0-mm incision

❖ Tip to prevent decentration: Crystalens is a self-centering lens. The surgeon should rotate the lens to the 12 and 6 o'clock positions in every case without exception. A 12-and-6 axis orientation helps the surgeon judge vaulting and decentration more easily. This also avoids the patient noticing glare from reflection off of the lens hinge.

✱ Keep wounds well hydrated till the end of the case.

✱ The Crystalens should be left vaulted just slightly posterior to anterior capsule at the end of the case

✱ The eye should be firm but not hard. A Wong pocket incision can be helpful to this end.

✱ Instill 1 to 3 drops of cyclopentolate 1% or 1 drop of 1% Atropine prior to the patient leaving the operating room.

❖ Tip for smooth immediate postoperative period: Cycloplegia helps hold the lens steady and stable for the first few postoperative days, and helps keep the pupil dilated for the first postoperative examination.

Postoperative Management of the Crystalens Patient

✱ Examinations for distance, intermediate, and near visual acuity, intraocular pressure (IOP), and manifest refraction should be performed on postoperative day 1, 1 to 2 weeks, and 1 month.

✱ YAG capsulotomies, if needed, are ideally delayed until week 12 or after. Exceptions are if capsular fibrosis is noted. If this condition is noted, consider an early YAG procedure to prevent capsular contraction syndrome. If near vision had been doing well, but begins to fall off, check for posterior capsular haze—even slight haze will affect near vision prior to any effect on distance vision. YAG capsulotomy should be done as soon as this problem is noted.

✱ If at 3 months postoperatively, the patient presents with unchanged distance vision, but decreasing near vision (eg, from J1-J2 to J5 or J8, with or without cylinder), look for fibrotic capsular striae under slit lamp examination. This may indicate posterior vaulting of the lens. A YAG capsulotomy can be performed to release capsular tension.

There have been no reports of visual disturbances such as glare, halos or capsular contraction syndrome in the 7311 eyes implanted with Crystalens Five-O.[1] There was no effect of glare on contrast sensitivity under mesopic illumination (3 cd/m²) when the Crystalens AT-4.5 lens was compared to a standard 5.5 to 6.0 optic lens.[2] The incidence of severe and moderate halos are considerably lower with Crystalens (6.2% and 12.3%, respectively) compared to multifocal IOLs. The incidence of severe and moderate glare are also less with Crystalens (5.4% and 13.8%, respectively) compared to multifocal IOLs.[2-4]

Some patients will develop glare after their YAG capsulotomy. Usually this is due to a small capsulotomy creating a secondary, smaller entrance pupil. Enlarging the capsule opening should take care of this problem.

Michael Colvard, MD, FACS, and developer of the Colvard pupillometer, reports his current experience with glare and halos with the Crystalens Five-O: "In my experience, glare and halos were seldom a problem with the AT-4.5 Crystalens and virtually never a problem with the AT-5.0. My experience, however, is almost entirely with older cataract patients. It seems reasonable to assume that the incidence of glare and halos may be higher in younger patients with more widely dilating pupils. Measurement of the mesopic pupil size should be part of the preoperative evaluation of all presbyopic IOL patients and these measurements should be taken into consideration when counseling our patients."

Injector Loading Techniques

Two injectors have been validated by Eyeonics, Inc., for use with the Crystalens Five-O, the MSI-TF (screw tip) and the MSI-PF (spring loaded) with the MTC-60C cartridge. Of the 7311 Crystalens Five-0's implanted to date, 158 injector-related tears have been reported to the company.[1] Below are some tips for preventing this from occurring.

1. Insert the foam tip plunger into the injector and then place the tip into a beaker of balanced salt solution (BSS). Keep it hydrated until use.

2. After removing the cartridge from the package, inspect it for damage to the tip or sharp edges in the IOL loading zone. If it has damage, set it aside and use another.

3. Lubricate the cartridge with BSS, and then remove excess by suing a gentle shake.

4. Fill the nozzle and coat the bottom and sides of the cartridge loading chamber with Healon.

5. Using the Cummings forceps (Eyeonics, Inc.), remove the lens from the case.

6. Holding the cartridge so that the 2 surfaces of the wings are about 90 degrees to each other, insert the IOL into the cartridge from the back, bringing the IOL into the cartridge loading chamber along the longitudinal axis of the IOL. The leading haptics must be pointed back toward the optic and the trailing haptic pointing backwards away from the topic, with both haptics tucked under the edges of the loading chamber walls (Figure 1).

7. Using the Cummings forceps, move the lens back and forth to insure smooth fluidic motion over the

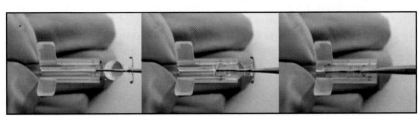

Figure 1. Insert the lens into the injector from the posterior end of the injector toward the forward end.

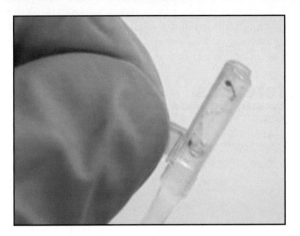

Figure 2. View of Crystalens 5-0 properly loaded in the injector.

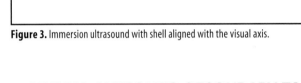

Figure 3. Immersion ultrasound with shell aligned with the visual axis.

cartridge. Center the lens once more verifying placement under the edges of the loading chamber walls.

8. Confirm axial alignment and symmetry of the lens in the nozzle, and that haptic loops are properly located beneath the cartridge wing captures, not between them (Figure 2).

9. Pick up the injector out of the beaker of BSS ensuring the foam tip has been fully hydrated.

10. Slide the cartridge into the front of the injector and snap lock the wing into position in the snap-lock notch.

11. Advance the lens forward until it is visible in the funnel and the lens rests past the collar area. Verify the injector foam tip plunger does not override the lens or capture the haptics. Make sure the lens is not difficult to advance. If it is, get a new cartridge and reload.

12. Gradually move the lens forward by pressing on the injector cap in one motion until the lens is positioned entirely in the cartridge nozzle. After it is positioned, remove pressure from the cap, but do not pull the cap back.

Myopic Outcomes

Myopic outcomes can be suspected when the patient presents with reduced uncorrected distance visual acuity at day 1, and the Crystalens appears anteriorly vaulted. This may be due to a lens implanted upside down (remember "round right" for the leading haptic), a lens poorly positioned in the bag or an episode of early postoperative hypotony. Certainly poor biometric technique can lead to a power miss in either direction.

MYOPIC OUTCOMES SECONDARY TO POOR BIOMETRIC TECHNIQUE

To rule out an error related to biometric technique, check the keratometry, axial length measurement (by IOL Master, ultrasound, or immersion A-Scan), verify K-readings, and the power formula used to select the power of the lens. Axial lengths are an important measurement because inaccuracies can lead to power misses. With Crystalens it is best to measure axial length by either immersion A-scans or optical coherence IOL Master. A-scans are the most important component and are most commonly responsible for power misses. An error of as little as 0.1 mm will result in the following:

* 0.375 D miss in longer eyes (myopes)
* 0.75 D miss in shorter eyes (hyperopes)

METHODS TO MEASURE AXIAL LENGTH

* Contact ultrasound—most common, quick and easy, inexpensive, but least accurate/reproducible due to compression/alignment variable
* Immersion ultrasound—perceived as slow, difficult, and messy, but necessary for reliable measurements; many units dual purpose, simply require shell for immersion (Figure 3)
* Optical coherence (IOL Master)—technology transmits light rather than sound to obtain measurements

Tips to avoid power misses related to biometric technique:

* Have a well-trained, dedicated staff
* Make sure there is a calibrated manual keratometer at all times or an IOL Master for K's
* Do an immersion A-scan or IOL Master for axial length
* Use appropriate formulas and A-constant

- ❖ For Crystalens Five-O, the A-constant is 119.00
- ❖ SRK/T for axial lengths of 22 mm or greater
- ❖ Holladay 2 if eye shorter than 22 mm
- ✳ Always double check versus going on "autopilot"

MYOPIC OUTCOMES SECONDARY TO LENS VAULTS

Myopic outcomes may occur as a result of the lens vaulting forward. Decreased uncorrected distance visual acuity may occur at days 10 to 14 (early onset) or after 14 days (late onset). The myopic shift may be mild (–0.75 to –1.50) with subtle vaulting evident on ultrasound, but not on slit lamp examination. It may be moderate (–1.75 or more), with vaulting that is apparent on slit lamp examination. This may be caused by too large a capsulorrhexis , fibrosis behind the optic, malpositioned loops, or incisional leaks. If this occurs, you should consider cycloplegia for 1 week, reassure the patient, and make sure the patient has functional vision. Have the patient return in 1 to 2 weeks. If the patient is still unhappy, consider reposition or removal and replacement of the lens during the first 3 to 4 postoperative weeks. The Crystalens' polyamide loops bond to the capsular bag by this point in time and become very difficult to dislodge. If there is evidence of fibrosis, consider YAG capsulotomy. If the patient is still unhappy with the visual correction due to power issues, consider a secondary piggyback IOL placed in the sulcus, or a LASIK/ photorefractive keratectomy (PRK) enhancement at 3 months postoperatively when the refraction has stabilized.

References

1. Eyeonics Crystalens Five-O data on file, 2007.
2. Crystalens AT-45 package insert, 2004.
3. AcrySof ReSTOR package insert, 2006.
4. ReZoom package insert, 2005.

CHAPTER 226

YAG CAPSULOTOMY AND CRYSTALENS—CLINICAL PEARLS

Jack A. Singer, MD

Posterior Capsulotomy

It is reasonable to expect the rate of ytrrium-aluminum-garnet (YAG) posterior capsulotomy to be greater for refractive intraocular lenses (IOLs) than for standard IOLs. Refractive IOL patients are more sensitive to small changes in their visual function, and this group includes a greater number of patients who are under 60 years of age.

With the Crystalens (**Eyeonics, Inc. Aliso Viejo, CA**), it is better to treat posterior capsule folds, fibrosis, and cell proliferation at an early stage. Because the Crystalens is designed to flex and move axially in the eye, its function is more sensitive to stiffening and contraction of the lens capsule. Opening the posterior capsule will be more easily performed with greater control before a large degree of capsular tension has developed. That said, the rate of YAG posterior capsulotomy with the Crystalens AT-50SE and AT-52SE is much lower than it was with the AT-45SE.

When performing a YAG laser capsulotomy, use a contact lens and begin with 1.4-mJ energy. Make the initial opening in the center and extend it out towards the plate haptics. Proceed slowly and observe how the capsule reacts after each laser pulse. I aim for an opening that is 0.5 to 1.0 mm smaller than the optic diameter, and reduce the laser energy as I approach the edge of the optic (Figure 1). The posterior capsulotomy will spontaneously enlarge over the course of the early postop period. Anterior vitreous prolapse can occur should the posterior capsulotomy extend beyond the optic, because the anterior capsulorrhexis is also larger than the optic and does not overlap it in many cases.

In the case of reduced posterior vaulting of one or both plate haptics, which is extremely rare with the AT-50SE and AT-52SE, you should open the posterior capsule behind the vaulted plate. When doing this, it is important to leave a bridge of intact posterior capsule behind the hinge, in between the central posterior capsulotomy and the capsulotomy behind the plates, in order to prevent late anterior vitreous prolapse. With the AT-45 and AT-45SE lenses, I will do this at the time of posterior capsulotomy in order to prevent reduced posterior vaulting of one or both plate haptics (Figure 2).

Anterior Capsulotomy

Relaxing cuts in the anterior capsulorrhexis over the plate haptics can enhance accommodation with the Crystalens when the capsular edge is fibrotic and/or overlapping the hinges. When treating the anterior capsule with the YAG, it is important to inactivate any posterior defocus that is otherwise automatically used for posterior capsulotomy.

Another indication for relaxing cuts in the anterior capsulorrhexis is when its diameter is too small and the peripheral capsule bag has not fused. This is characterized by a persistent gap between the anterior and posterior capsules. Four to 6 relaxing cuts in the anterior capsulorrhexis can enhance accommodation and also produce a myopic refractive shift as the unrestrained optic moves slightly forward. This is particularly useful in patients with residual low hyperopia and a greater than average posterior vaulting of the Crystalens. I have seen up to 1.25 diopters (D) of hyperopia eliminated with this easy treatment (Figure 3).

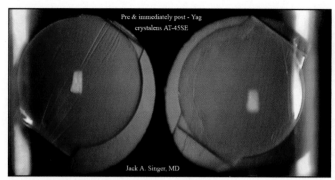

Figure 1. Pre- and immediately post-YAG.

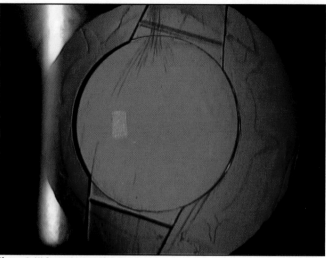

Figure 3. YAG anterior capsulotomy.

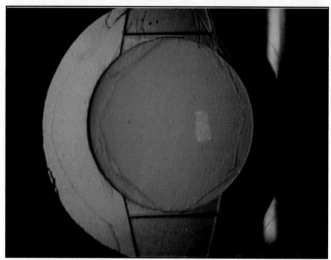

Figure 2. YAG posterior capsulotomy.

CHAPTER 227

CAPSULAR CONTRACTION AFTER CRYSTALENS

Harvey Carter, MD

Capsular contraction has been described with various types and styles of intraocular lenses (IOLs). Although the concept of capsular contraction was previously recognized, it had been of little clinical importance until the development of the first-generation Crystalens (Eyeonics, Aliso Viejo, CA). With previous static monofocal IOLs, the capsular contraction syndrome would occasionally result in anterior capsule phimosis, and slight dislocation, or decentration of the lens implant, typically with very little clinical significance. The first-generation Crystalens was the first dynamic accommodating lens implant that could be moved within the eye by capsular contractile forces. In this context, the potential for capsular contraction syndrome took on new significance.

The most commonly encountered capsular changes previously affecting the outcome of static IOL implant surgery were associated with anterior capsular phimosis and posterior capsular opacification. With the first-generation Crystalens we saw for the first time how capsular contraction could affect the refraction and IOL movement. It should be noted that these refractive changes due to capsular contraction syndrome occurred only with the first-generation Crystalens, the AT-45, and that there have been no cases of "Z" contraction syndrome with the AT-50 third-generation Crystalens.

Embryologically and histologically, the lens capsule epithelium is divided into 3 cell groups. These cell groups are the anterior lens capsule epithelium, the posterior lens capsule epithelium, and the equatorial bow epithelial cells. These three cell types behave in distinctly different ways as they undergo metaplastic changes postoperatively. They exert distinctly different capsular contractile vector forces on a dynamic IOL implant, which cause the IOL implant to move in predictable ways.

Various attempts at mitigating posterior capsular opacification have been tried. Aggressive surgical vacuuming of the anterior and posterior capsules has been advocated by a number of researchers. Unfortunately, it is impossible to vacuum the entirety of the capsule bag with existing technology. There is some controversy as to whether vacuuming the anterior capsule might actually increase the incidence of posterior capsular opacification. A novel approach to controlling changes in the lens capsule epithelial cells was the invention of the Perfect Capsule device by Milvella Limited (Epping, Australia), which provides a sealed system for irrigating epithelial-toxic solutions into the capsular bag without damaging other cells in the eye. Unfortunately, this approach is surgically challenging and can potentially be accompanied by leakage or diffusion of the toxic solution through the capsule or around the seal risking damage to other intraocular structures.

The capsular contraction syndromes can be divided into 3 broad categories corresponding to the distinctly different contractile forces caused by the underlying lens epithelial cell type.

The first category is the anterior capsule contraction syndrome (ACCS). In this syndrome there will be a ground glass to white color change of the anterior capsule that is occasionally associated with anterior capsular striae. Less commonly there will be phimosis of the anterior capsulotomy. The anterior capsule contractile vector forces decrease the equatorial diameter of the capsular bag, resulting in posterior vaulting of the Crystalens with a hyperopic shift.

The second category is the posterior capsule contraction syndrome (PCCS). This syndrome is characterized by whitened striate fibrous capsular changes typically seen in the peripheral posterior capsule between the hinge and the polyimide haptic stakes of the first-generation AT-45 IOL. These posterior capsular striae exhibit contractile changes that radiate from the periphery toward the central optic and sometimes connect with the posterior capsular striae from the opposite haptic. These posterior capsular contractile vector forces cause a decrease in the equatorial diameter of the capsular bag, resulting in asymmetrical vaulting of the AT-45. This asymmetrical vaulting frequently induces a myopic shift with associated astigmatism. The contractile vector forces of the posterior capsule are significantly stronger than those associated with the ACCS. The severity of the

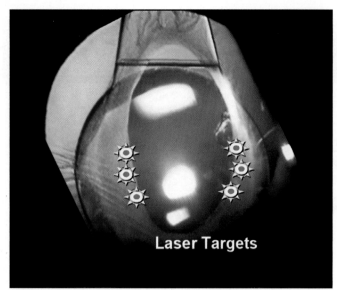

Figure 1. YAG laser targets for opening the phimotic anterior capsule with a vertically oriented AIOL.

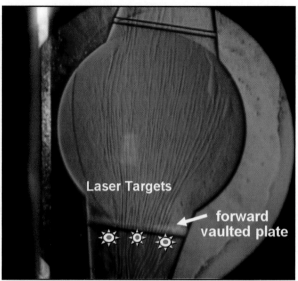

Figure 2. YAG laser targets for selectively opening the posterior capsule in a PCCS "Z" syndrome.

asymmetrical vaulting of the AT-45 can range from very mild (causing only a slight tilt of the optic) to very severe where there is asymmetrical vaulting of the AT-45 haptics in opposite directions, resulting in the "Z" PCCS. It is interesting that the design changes of the third-generation AT-50 Crystalens have eliminated the "Z" syndrome entirely.

The last form of capsule contraction syndrome is extremely rare and is the equatorial capsule contraction syndrome (ECCS). With this syndrome there are little or no anterior or posterior capsule changes seen. The first-generation AT-45 Crystalens would be noted to vault posteriorly, mimicking an ACCS but without any anterior capsule changes. The clinician would notice a decrease in accommodating amplitude, a mild hyperopic change in refraction, and minimal decrease in the equatorial diameter of the capsular bag. The capsular contractile vector forces generated by the equatorial lens capsule epithelium cells are the weakest of the 3 types discussed.

The most severe PCCS caused one haptic to vault anteriorly and the other haptic vaulted posteriorly, giving rise to the "Z" syndrome. As previously mentioned, this syndrome was only seen with the first-generation Crystalens and has not been reported with the current third-generation AT-50 Crystalens. As these capsular contraction syndromes were studied, we found clinical proof that contraction or movement of the lens capsule caused movement of the dynamic lens implant, thereby confirming the proposed mechanism of action of the Crystalens. The ability of the capsular lens epithelial cell to undergo postoperative metaplastic contractile changes will pose a challenge for the development of all future dynamic accommodating IOL platforms.

Multiple strategies were used to treat the capsular contraction syndromes, including surgical manipulations, vitrectomy, and IOL explantation. The most successful and currently accepted treatment modality is the protocol of selective anterior and posterior capsulotomy, which is specifically aimed at controlling the specific capsular contractile vector forces.

These protocols were initially developed to address the changes of ACCS, PCCS, and ECCS seen with the first-generation AT-45 Crystalens, but can likely be applied to milder changes seen with later-generation lens implants as well. The need for pinpoint, and very precise, YAG laser treatments has been aided by newer YAG laser technology. These produce smaller and tighter plasma envelopes that allow us to selectively titrate the size of the capsular opening in order to move the Crystalens haptics within the capsular bag. An incidental finding noted after these selective YAG capsulotomies was that accommodative amplitudes were improved by the treatment.

Treatment Techniques

With the ACCS, which produces an unwanted hyperopic shift, the selective YAG laser anterior capsulotomy is performed along the short axis of the IOL implant. For a 12-to-6 vertically oriented lens implant, as shown in Figure 1, the treatment will begin with one shot at the 3 o'clock position, followed by one shot at the 9 o'clock position. This is followed by one shot at the 2 o'clock position, then another at the 8 o'clock position, followed by shots at the 4 o'clock and 10 o'clock positions in order to gradually expand the anterior capsular diameter in a controlled fashion. A second or third ring of small selectively placed anterior capsule shots can be made to further expand the opening in a controlled, titrated fashion to yield the most predictable refractive change. Using this approach has resulted in reduction of an unwanted hyperopic shift of 1 to 1.5 diopters (D).

With the PCCS, the YAG laser treatment is first directed behind the anteriorly vaulted haptic as shown in Figure 2. It must be carefully aimed at the region of the posterior capsule between the plate haptic hinge and the polyimide haptic stakes. Next, treatment may be directed to the posterior capsule behind the opposite plate haptic. Finally, a small central posterior capsulotomy may also be added. The net effect of these selective posterior capsulotomies is to reduce or eliminate the posterior capsular contractile vector forces, which have resulted in a decrease in the equatorial diameter of the capsular bag. The predictable changes resulting from selective laser capsulotomy allow us to use the YAG laser as a refractive enhancement tool for the Crystalens. It is best if the 2 posterior peripheral capsulotomies do not connect.

CAPSULAR CONTRACTION AFTER MULTIFOCAL IOLs

Richard Tipperman, MD

Compared to monofocal intraocular lenses (IOLs), I have found that multifocal IOL function may be much more sensitive to moderate capsular contraction. The following case illustrates this.

A 67-year-old woman underwent cataract surgery via phacoemulsification with implantation of a ReSTOR IOL (Alcon Laboratories, Fort Worth, TX). Approximately 5 months after her surgery, she was self-referred because of poor vision for distance and near. Her uncorrected distance vision was 20/70 and her near vision was J5.

Slit lamp examination revealed significant anterior capsule contraction, with the edge of the capsulorrhexis actually covering the peripheral portion of the apodized diffractive rings (Figure 1). The patient underwent an anterior Nd:yttrium-aluminum-garnet (YAG) capsulotomy to enlarge their capsulorrhexis opening. The uncorrected distance vision improved to 20/25 and the near vision to J2 (Figure 2).

This case demonstrates the importance of a consistently sized capsulorrhexis. Because the peripheral portion of the ReSTOR IOL contributes 100% to the distance vision, a contracted capsulorrhexis can compromise distance vision. Additionally, by impinging on the apodized diffractive rings, a small capsulorrhexis can limit near vision as well.

We must first strive to avoid a capsulorrhexis whose primary diameter is too small. Postoperatively, consider the effects of moderate capsule contraction as part of the differential diagnosis of visual complaints.

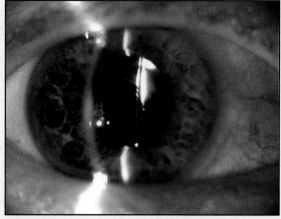

Figure 1. Slit lamp examination revealed significant anterior capsule contraction, with the edge of the capsulorrhexis actually covering the peripheral portion of the apodized diffractive rings.

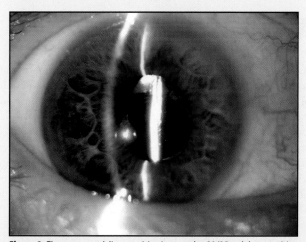

Figure 2. The uncorrected distance vision improved to 20/25 and the near vision to J2.

CHAPTER 228

DECENTRATION OF
MULTIFOCAL IOLs—WHAT NOW?

Renée Solomon, MD and Eric Donnenfeld, MD; William Martin, MD;
and Tom M. Coffman, MD

Renée Solomon, MD and
Eric Donnenfeld, MD

With dramatic improvement in intraocular lens (IOL) technology, multifocal and accommodative IOLs are assuming an increasingly greater role in our refractive surgical armamentarium. Multifocal IOLs and accommodative IOLs have revolutionized the rehabilitation of the cataract patient.[1-5] However, quality of vision issues including reduced contrast sensitivity and symptoms of glare and halos following implantation of multifocal IOLs have been reported.[1] The term "Vaseline vision dysphotopsia" has been coined to describe the reduced quality of vision associated with certain multifocal IOLs.[6] Quality of vision is by definition reduced in all patients receiving a multifocal IOL due to the separation of light and the two images formed on the retina. These issues are compounded with IOL decentration. The optics of multifocal IOLs makes their proper centration very important to the objective and subjective quality of visual function.

Decentration of multifocal contact lenses has been shown to induce significant optical aberrations. All IOLs, whether monofocal or multifocal, exhibit prism and coma when decentered or tilted. Because the center of the capsular bag is along the optical axis of the eye and the pupil is usually nasal by about 3 to 5 degrees (angle Kappa), an IOL perfectly centered in-the-bag is usually temporal to the pupil. The anatomic pupillary axis of the eye, visual axis, and optical axis are not aligned. When the rings of a multifocal IOL are not concentric with the patient's pupil, the pattern becomes asymmetric. Patients may complain of reduced quality of vision of daytime images and asymmetric halos around lights at night.[7] In the case of mild decentration, these visual complaints are worse with diffractive multifocal IOLs than refractive multifocal IOLs.

In evaluating complaints of glare and halos or reduced quality of vision following multifocal IOL implantation, it is important to be sure that all potential causes of these complaints

have been addressed. The five Cs that should be evaluated are: cylinder and residual refractive error, capsular opacities, cornea and ocular surface disease, cystoid macular edema (CME), and centration of the IOL with the pupil. Once the first four potential contributing factors are resolved, then IOL centration should be evaluated.

In a prospective, longitudinal study of eyes in which the multifocal IOL and the pupil were not aligned, laser iridoplasty was used to re-center the pupil over the IOL. The effect of this maneuver on visual acuity outcomes and quality of vision was evaluated. In this study, Argon laser iridoplasty (ALI) was demonstrated to be a safe and effective technique to improve quality of vision following multifocal IOL implantation. There was a statistically significant improvement in photopic and scotopic contrast sensitivity and in patient satisfaction.[8,9] No patient experienced a reduction in quality of vision. Many patients with significant multifocal IOL decentration relative to the pupil will have excellent quality of vision and for these patients there is no reason to perform an ALI. However, we routinely perform ALI on patients with multifocal IOLs and residual refractive error prior to performing excimer laser photoablation. We prefer to center the excimer laser treatment over the center of the IOL rather than over the pupil.

For patients whose IOL is not centered behind the pupil (Figure 1A) the ALI technique is easy to perform. Four laser spots of 500-milliwatt power, 500-μm spot diameter, and 500-millisecond duration are placed in the mid-periphery of iris in the area in which the iris encroaches on the center of the IOL (Figure 1B). The iris in this area will retract, exposing the covered section of the multifocal IOL. The laser energy may need to be increased for blue irises, which absorb less energy and decreased for dark irises. Four laser spots are placed to begin with, but the number is titrated to the amount of pupil movement required to achieve centration of the IOL behind the pupil (Figure 2). The patient is pretreated with one drop of topical ophthalmic anesthetic and no contact lens is used for the laser procedure. No postoperative medications are prescribed. Patients may notice an improvement in the quality of

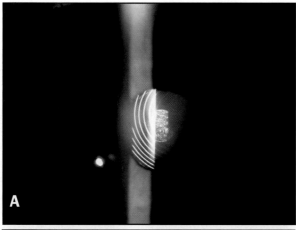

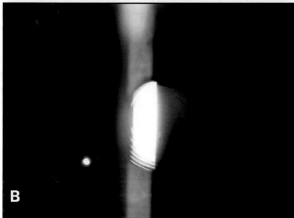

Figure 1. Slit lamp biomicroscopy of a ReSTOR multifocal IOL before (A) and after (B) treatment with argon laser iridoplasty.

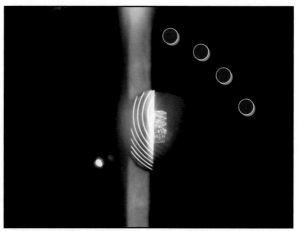

Figure 2. Argon laser iridoplasty spots are placed in iris mid periphery using the following parameters: 500 milliwatt energy, 500 μm diameter, 500 millisecond duration.

References

1. Solomon R, Donnenfeld ED. Refractive intraocular lenses multifocal and phakic IOLs. In: Friedlaender MB, ed. *Int Ophthalmol Clin.* Vol. 46. Philadelphia: Lippincott Williams and Wilkins; 2006:123-143.

2. Rocha KM, Chalita MR, Souza CE, Soriano ES, Freitas LL, Muccioli C, Belfort R Jr. Postoperative wavefront analysis and contrast sensitivity of a multifocal apodized diffractive IOL (ReSTOR) and three monofocal IOLs. *J Refract Surg.* 2005;21:S808-S881.

3. Nijkamp MD, Dolders MG, de Brabander J, van den Borne B, Hendrikse F, Nuijts RM. Effectiveness of multifocal intraocular lenses to correct presbyopia after cataract surgery: a randomized controlled trial. *Ophthalmology.* 2004;111:1832-1839. Erratum in: *Ophthalmology.* 2004;111:2022.

4. Leyland M, Zinicola E. Multifocal versus monofocal intraocular lenses in cataract surgery: a systematic review. *Ophthalmology.* 2003;110:1789-1798.

5. Wang L, Koch DD. Effect of decentration of wavefront-corrected intraocular lenses on the higher-order aberrations of the eye. *Arch Ophthalmol.* 2005;123:1226-1230.

6. Bucci F. Vaseline vision dysphotopsia and explantation of the ReSTOR multifocal implant. Poster presented at: ARVO; May 8, 2007; Fort Lauderdale, FL.

7. Holladay JT. Understanding optics. In: *Quality of Vision.* Thorofare, NJ: SLACK Incorporated; 2005:3-5.

8. Solomon R, Donnenfeld ED, Perry HD, et al. Argon Laser Iridoplasty to Improve Visual Function Following Multifocal IOL Implantation. Presented at the American Academy of Ophthalmology Annual Meeting, New Orleans, Louisiana, November 2007.

9. Donnenfeld ED, Solomon R, Perry HD, et al. Argon Laser Iridoplasty to Improve Visual Function Following Multifocal IOL Implantation. Presented at the Refractive Surgery Subspecialty Day, New Orleans, LA, November 2007. 236/14

vision immediately following the iridoplasty.

One of the surgical techniques that can be performed to avoid IOL decentration is to place the multifocal IOL slightly nasal to the dilated pupil. When the pupil dilates it also moves approximately 0.5 mm nasal as compared to the normal scotopic pupil. By placing the IOL haptics at 12 o'clock and 6 o'clock, the multifocal IOL can be reproducibly placed slightly nasal to the dilated pupil, which will translate to a well-centered IOL under normal illumination and pupil size.

Some cataract surgeons, when they recognize IOL decentration, will perform an intraocular IOL repositioning procedure. ALI avoids the time, expense, and potential complications of additional intraocular surgery and ALI can be titrated and repeated if necessary. ALI is a simple procedure that can be performed in the office to improve the visual function of patients following insertion of multifocal IOL.

William Martin, MD

The importance of intraocular lens (IOL) centration has been discussed in the past as well as different ways to manage poor IOL centration. With the advent of aspheric and multifocal lenses, IOL centration has an even more critical impact on the quality of vision.[1,2] Many authors have emphasized the importance of various factors such as ocular surface abnormalities, early capsular opacification, and residual refractive error, such as astigmatism, on multifocal IOL outcomes.[3] Proper centration, however, is an equally important factor in the quality of vision.

A multifocal IOL that is perfectly centered within the capsular bag may appear misaligned with the patient's pupil, because the latter is frequently slightly nasally decentered.[4]

Surgical rotation and recentering of the lens may not always correct the problem. Misalignment of the IOL and the pupil is usually due to the fact that the center of the capsular bag may not line up with the center of the pupil. The pupil is decentered inferonasally in a significant portion of the population. As a result, the IOL will appear to be decentered superotemporally. The misalignment with the pupil can cause visual symptoms for the patient and surgical recentration of the lens may be unsuccessful due to the fact that the IOL is already properly centered within the capsular bag.

Argon laser pupilloplasty (ALP) can be a valuable tool in the management of these problems.[5-7]

The technique involves placing four spots that straddle the meridian of the direction toward which the pupil should be recentered. A total of 500 mW of energy should be used per spot, and each spot should be 500 µm in size. Exposure time should be 0.15 seconds (Table 1), but may be titrated according to the individual response. The laser beam should be focused on the mid-periphery and two spots should be placed both above and below the meridian in the direction toward which the pupil should be displaced.

Case Description

The patient is a 57-year-old white female with a history of prior radial keratotomy performed in 1993. She developed cataracts within the last several years and underwent bilateral ReSTOR implantation by another physician. The patient was unhappy with her surgical outcome. Her uncorrected vision was 20/50 in the right eye and 20/60 in the left eye. The patient was referred to us by her physician for management of her postoperative complaints. On examination the patient demonstrated significant opacification of the posterior capsule and a refractive error of OD PL −0.50 × 0.89 [20/25], OS +1.75 −0.50 × 122 [20/35]. Corneal topography indicated

well-centered radial keratotomy scars with a relatively regular topographic appearance of the cornea. Schirmer's testing and topography also revealed significant keratoconjunctivitis sicca, for which the patient was started on topical artificial tears and cyclosporine. A yttrium-aluminum-garnet (YAG) posterior capsulotomy was successfully performed and the patient's vision improved to 20/30 in the right eye and 20/60 in the left eye uncorrected. The patient was still unhappy with the visual results. At this point the refraction was OD +075 −075 × 096 20/20, OS +175 −050 × 123 20/20. It was also noted that the ReSTOR lens in the left eye was significantly decentered temporally. At this point it was decided to perform an ALP, which would be centered over the 10-degree axis. Four spots were placed—two just above and two just below the 10-degree meridian. Each spot was 500 µm in diameter and delivered 50 mW of energy with an exposure time of 0.5 seconds.

Immediately upon completion of the treatment, the patient claimed subjective improvement of her vision and reduction of the symptoms that she had described as "doubling of vision and ghost images." Her vision preoperatively was 20/60 uncorrected, and within 5 minutes following the pupilloplasty the vision had improved to 20/30+. At this point the patient still has some refractive error in both eyes for which anterior surface ablation has been scheduled and we expect further improvement of this patient's vision upon this treatment.

This case is very instructive and clearly demonstrates the importance of having a game plan for dealing with postoperative problems in multifocal IOL patients. In addition to assessing and managing ocular surface disease, capsular opacification, and residual refractive error, the alignment of the diffractive IOL optic with the pupil must also be assessed. In the case of pupil misalignment, ALP can displace the pupil in such a way as to improve IOL centration with the pupil.

References

1. Cataract surgical problem consultation - December #6. *J Cataract Refract Surg.* 2004;30(12):2468-2470.
2. Visual performance of patients with bilateral vs. combo Crystalens, ReZoom, ReSTOR. *Am J Ophthalmol.* 2007;144(3):347-352.
3. Effect of OPC on visual function in patients with monofocal and multifocal IOL. *Eye.* December 22, 2006.
4. Visual simulation of retinal images through a decentered monofocal and refractive multifocal IOL. *Jpn J Ophthalmol.* 2005;49(4):586-589.
5. *British J Ophthalmol.* 1998;82:504-507.
6. *Asia Pacific J Ophthalmol.* 1993;5(4):31-33.
7. Pupilloplasty with mobile laser ray. *J French Ophthalmol.* 1996;9(3):249.

Tom M. Coffman, MD

About 1% of all posterior chamber lenses will decenter at some time. This may be due to a zonular dehiscence, uneven capsule contracture, or asymmetric haptic placement. The latter could be one haptic in the bag and one in the sulcus, or one haptic in the bag or sulcus and one in the vitreous.

With a monofocal intraocular lens (IOL), if the patient's optical zone is still within the edge of the decentered IOL, this

often causes no symptoms. However, if the patient has glare or sees a second image beyond the IOL edge, the lens may need to be surgically repositioned.

In the case of a slightly decentered ReZoom IOL, if the patient's visual axis is still within the edge of the central 2.1 mm distance zone, the patient should be asymptomatic. However, once the decentration causes the visual axis to pass through the edge of the central button, the best corrected visual acuity (BCVA) might typically drop to 20/40. Sometimes if the optical center is beyond 1½ mm from the center, the vision is normal and the patient is asymptomatic.

Figure 1. (A) Make two small stab incisions large enough for insertion of Kuglen hooks. (B) Pull haptics out of the capsular tube with a Sinsky or Kuglen hook and into the anterior chamber. These slide out easily even many years later. Sometimes the hook needs to go under the haptic with the hook pointing upward, to tire iron the lens over the anterior capsule. (C) The left Kuglen hook is used to pull the lens superiorly into the angle and held at the haptic lens junction. The right hook is placed over top of it and snags the haptic in the hook so that it may be bent to the right. (D) Slide the right hook along the haptic to bend it back about 90 degrees. Then rotate the lens around and repeat this with the other haptic. Because this requires pulling the lens into the angle, the first haptic is compressed some and one needs to tease it back out again. The end result is an overall length of 15 mm that then fits very well to center in the sulcus. This length has not been found to cause complications in the sulcus. (E) Spin the lens into the sulcus and challenge the fixation by bumping the lens back and forth, perpendicular to the axis of the haptics. If it does not return to center, rotate the lens 30 to 45 degrees and challenge it again until one finds a solid location. Rarely, one will need to spin the lens back into the sulcus and expand the haptics again to make sure the diameter is sufficient to maintain centration.

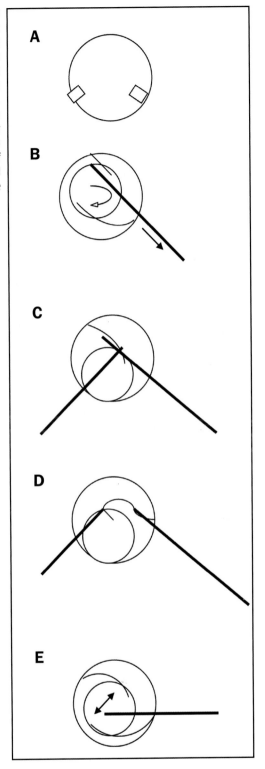

If one recenters the IOL within the capsular bag during the first week, the haptics are still rigid enough to keep it centrally aligned. To recenter the IOL, insert a Kuglen hook through the paracentesis incision and rotate the wayward haptic into the bag. If both haptics are already within the bag try rotating the lens 45 to 90 degrees. Test the lens centration by nudging it back and forth perpendicular to the axes of the haptics. If it does not naturally center itself each time, then try rotating it into a different alignment. Refilling and pressurizing the anterior chamber may also help to center the lens.

If more than 1 week has passed since surgery, the PMMA haptics may already have lost much of their rigidity. If so, the compressed loops may not enable good bag or sulcus centration. One solution is the Coffman Recentration Technique to expand the haptics (Figure 1). First make small paracentesis ports to permit the use of two Kuglan hooks. Place these ports at a comfortable position for both the left and right hands. Irrigate the iris with 1% preservative free xylocaine and then fill the anterior chamber with viscoelastic. The recentration starts by introducing a Sinsky hook and spinning one haptic out of its tunnel into the anterior chamber. Next, continue rotating the IOL until both haptics are in the anterior chamber, and their axis is aligned so that one haptic is pointing away from you and one is pointing toward you. Place the left Kuglen hook just outside of the distal haptic where it is staked into the optic. Place the right hook inside the acute angle of the insertion. Pull each so the right hook bends the haptic back at a right angle from its optic attachment. This usually requires squeezing the lens toward you into the angle to keep it from spinning. Then spin the lens 180 degrees and bend the second haptic backward in the same way. Because the first haptic is now pressed into the angle one should check it and tease it back to a more open position when released. This maneuver will commonly produce a 15-mm overall haptic diameter that seats well in the sulcus and has never caused inflammation in my experience.

Once the haptics have been expanded, the IOL may be rotated back into the capsular bag or the ciliary sulcus. If the bag cannot be reinflated, or alternatively if one desires a 0.5 to 0.75 diopter myopic shift, then the ciliary sulcus is the better location for the lens. For IOL powers less than 6 diopters, moving an IOL from the bag to the sulcus produces a negligible myopic shift. For IOL powers above 26 diopters, moving the lens to the sulcus will produce a myopic shift of at least one diopter.

Once in place nudge the lens as described earlier to make sure it will remain centered. The viscoelastic may be removed by balanced salt solution (BSS) irrigation with a small cannula and depressing the posterior lip. It may also be removed piece meal by re-filling the anterior chamber and then suctioning with a larger cannula and a small syringe. This recentering procedure can be performed with any 3-piece IOL, but will not work with a single-piece lens.

Many surgeons remove and exchange decentered lenses. The Coffman Recentration Technique is easier and much less traumatic to the eye. Only about 2% of IOLs recentered in this way will decenter again due to a capsule or zonular defect. The procedure may be then repeated and the axis of the haptics rotated into a more secure alignment.

CHAPTER 229

REFRACTIVE IOL EXCHANGE— INDICATIONS AND TECHNIQUES

Michael E. Snyder, MD and Robert H. Osher, MD

The goal of this chapter is to outline a written rationale for when a surgeon and the patient should consider explanting a presbyopia-correcting intraocular lens (Pr-C IOL) and to describe techniques that facilitate removing and exchanging the lens. Although each surgeon and patient will need to decide together whether to exchange the IOL in their unique situation, we will outline our general approach. Similarly, we will review several surgical techniques for IOL exchange which we find to be most facile, recognizing that multiple acceptable approaches may exist.

Indications for Presbyopia-Correcting IOL Removal

The reasons that patients may require Pr-C IOL removal typically fall into one of three categories. First, there may be an actual problem with the implanted lens, such as damage to the optic, silicone oil adherence, visually prominent surface scratches, or yttrium-aluminum-garnet (YAG) laser pits. The IOL may be decentered, subluxated, unstable, asymmetrically vaulted,[1] or even backwards. Second, there may be a power error causing unacceptable myopia, hyperopia, or anisometropia.[2] Lastly, patients with Pr-C IOLs may have unwanted optical phenomena intrinsic to the implant design.[3]

When the patient presents with structural optic damage or IOL malposition, the indication for surgical intervention is usually straightforward. We have found that a slightly decentered Pr-C IOL may require repositioning that would not have been necessary if it were a monofocal implant.

The decision to exchange a Pr-C IOL for a power error requires a candid discussion with the patient, reviewing alternatives such as the use of contact lenses or spectacles, laser vision correction, or, occasionally, piggyback IOL implantation. These options may vary depending on surgeon and patient preference and the numerous unique individual circumstances. A patient's desire for a second intervention should not be automatically presumed. In cases of mild ametropia, we

prefer to defer consideration of exchange until the second eye has been implanted, as many patients may tolerate their result in the first eye if the refractive error attained in the fellow eye is "dead on."

The choice for or against IOL exchange in the setting of unwanted optical phenomena becomes far more complex. In these instances many factors, including the amount of time the implant has been in place, the nature and degree of the phenomena, the status of the fellow eye, and the alternative options become critically important. Accordingly, a thorough historical discussion with the patient is crucial in arriving at the optimal solution. One patient who had a ReSTOR lens placed in his first eye elsewhere was so dissatisfied that he and his physician agreed to sever their relationship because of mutual frustration, despite an excellent technical result. This individual sought numerous opinions from a variety of highly qualified ophthalmologists over a period of almost 2 years, most of whom recommended IOL exchange for a monofocal implant. Our careful and lengthy discussion with this patient revealed that the majority of the patient's complaints seemed to stem from his floaters. Therefore, we recommended vitrectomy alone. Following surgery, the patient was delighted with his distance and near vision, and requested ReSTOR IOL placement in his fellow eye. An exchange for a monofocal in this case would have likely compounded this patient's frustrations.

Observations of halos or glare are not uncommon in patients with Pr-C IOLs. These comments must be taken in perspective. Some patients, while they may describe halos, may not actually be bothered by them. Asking "does that bother you?" may end the discussion if the answer is no. Even if the response is positive, the patient may conclude that it is a fair tradeoff for uncorrected near vision. Furthermore, those who notice halos after the surgery on their first eye may not notice halos after they have undergone surgery in the second eye. Some surgeons may be reluctant to implant the fellow eye of the symptomatic patient with a Pr-C IOL, even though ample data supports reduction in halos following second eye implantation and, even elimination of halos in some patients after many months, due possibly to "neuroadaptation." This poorly understood process can continue for a year or more in some individuals. In addition, many patients who notice halos at night can mitigate their symptoms by the judicious use of brimonidine or dilute pilocarpine before night time activities. Negative dysphotopsia, the perception of a dark temporal shadow, may occur with any IOL and an exchange may or may not eliminate that symptom.[4]

Sometimes the multifocal patient may complain about a reduction in the quality of distance vision. Rarely, the complaint may be related to the contrast degradation from multifocality itself. However, a reduced tear film from keratitis sicca or otherwise mild posterior capsule (PC) opacity may tip the contrast sensitivity reduction over the edge and, if compensated, the patient can be satisfied. If dry eye is present, it should be fully treated. Mild PC haze becomes a more challenging issue, because YAG capsulotomy will often alleviate these complaints, but can also make an IOL exchange more difficult. Again, a meticulous history and careful clinical exam are essential. If we observe some PC plaque at the time of cataract surgery, we will have a lower threshold for primary posterior capsulorrhexis if a multifocal IOL is planned. This decision will obviate the issue at a later time, as we believe that IOL exchange is easier and less hazardous in the setting of a primary posterior capsulorrhexis when compared to IOL exchange after YAG capsulotomy.

We caution the surgeon who may consider IOL exchange when the patient's primary complaint is incomplete satisfaction at near without correction (in the absence of other photic aberrations), because it is highly unlikely that such a problem would be improved after IOL exchange. We do not typically advise exchange of one type of Pr-C IOL for another style, except, perhaps, in a very unique case.

Despite the best efforts on the part of both patient and surgeon, some people just cannot tolerate the photic anomalies of a Pr-C IOL and will require IOL exchange. While estimated numbers range around one percent nationwide, it is a small fraction of a percent of patients that require an explantation in our practice.

Presbyopia-Correcting IOL Exchange—Surgical Techniques

The technique chosen for IOL exchange of a Pr-C IOL will depend primarily on several factors, including the type of IOL implanted, the status of the posterior capsule and the status of the capsule-zonular apparatus.

EXCHANGE OF AN ACRYLIC MULTIFOCAL IOL WITH AN INTACT CAPSULAR BAG

Significant ametropia is the most common indication in this group, although rare cases of IOLs causing intolerable photic aberrations will also present with an intact capsular bag. Reopening the capsular bag can usually be achieved without compromise to the capsule structures, regardless of

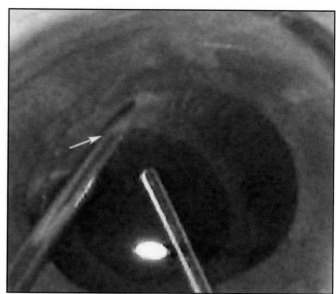

Figure 1. A 25-gauge needle whose tip has been bent toward the bevel is seen on the left side of this surgical photo, with the back side of the needle tip passing under the capsulorrhexis margin (arrow), lifting the CCC margin. An OVD cannula (right instrument) is poised to slide under the CCC edge for viscodissection opening of the capsular bag.

the amount of time since surgery, as originally described by Osher.[5] We will typically fill the anterior chamber with an OVD, and then slip an OVD cannula under the capsulorrhexis margin and viscodissect the capsular bag open. This maneuver should be continued for 360 degrees before trying to liberate the IOL from the bag. Not uncommonly, the anterior capsule will be adherent to the anterior surface of the IOL. One simple maneuver will solve this challenge. After injecting an OVD into the anterior chamber, a 25 gauge 5/8 inch needle is bent about 20 degrees near the tip, toward the bevel. The needle is then inserted through a paracentesis and, with the bevel down toward the IOL surface, the back side of the needle is slipped under the continuous curvilinear capsulorrhexis (CCC) margin. An OVD cannula is placed under that local elevation of the capsular margin, via a separate incision. (Figure 1) As the OVD is injected, viscodissection will reopen the capsular bag.

The IOL can then be gently maneuvered into the anterior chamber where it is folded with a forceps over a spatula that has been introduced through a stab incision opposite the main incision and gently explanted. Alternatively, the IOL can be bisected, trisected, or a quadrant can be excised, removing the implant in pieces. A variety of scissors will cut the ReSTOR IOL, including delicate Vannas scissors. The ReZoom lens material is a bit stiffer in the anterior chamber environment and requires a hardier scissors. We currently prefer the Osher IOL cutting scissors (Duckworth and Kent, Hartfordshire, England; Bausch & Lomb, Rochester, NY). The serrated blades prevent "tiddlywinking" as the cut is made, which is more likely to occur with the silicone lenses. The replacement IOL may be implanted in to the capsular bag or ciliary sulcus, depending on the surgeon's preference.

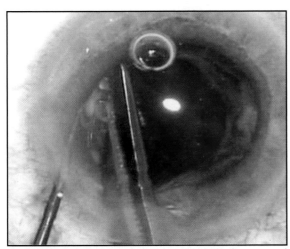

Figure 2. The residual remnant of a Crystalens AT-45 PCIOL silicone-encased polyamide haptic (Eyeonics, Inc., Aliso Viejo, CA) can be seen, firmly anchored into the capsular bag. Viscodissection could not open this dense fibrosis. The stump is trimmed as far peripherally as possible. The iris is retracted by a second instrument for visualization. The serrations in the edge of the IOL cutting scissors prevent the slippery silicone material from sliding out of the jaws of the scissors (Osher IOL scissors, Duckworth and Kent).

EXCHANGE OF AN ACRYLIC MULTIFOCAL IOL WITH AN OPEN POSTERIOR CAPSULE

When the posterior capsule is open, meticulous technique can often prevent vitreous prolapse. However, the surgeon should always be prepared for a possible vitrectomy. While our preference is a pars plana approach, the surgeon should be comfortable with bimanual and "dry" anterior vitrectomy instrumentation and techniques. Although it is possible to open the periphery of the capsular bag when a previous posterior CCC has been performed, it is far more difficult if the capsule has been torn or opened with the YAG laser. A few important maneuvers should be considered in such cases. First, if the patient's medical condition permits, intravenous administration of mannitol 20 to 30 minutes preoperatively will decrease vitreous volume and vitreous cavity pressure, reducing the likelihood of prolapse. Second, the surgeon must attentively maintain an anterior chamber pressure with the OVD that is higher that the vitreous pressure. To prevent vitreous prolapse, the anterior chamber must be adequately pressurized with OVD. An OVD with dispersive properties such as Viscoat or DisCoVisc (Alcon, Fort Worth, TX) can provide excellent tamponade of the opening. Additional OVD should be added any time the viscoelastic agent escapes from the anterior chamber. In complex IOL exchange cases, some amount of OVD may be retained so we often administer intracameral carbachol for IOP control.

With an open capsule, sectioning the IOL for removal in pieces may be more controlled because explantation of a folded IOL from a contained anterior chamber (AC) space may reduce the volume abruptly and create a posterior-to-anterior pressure gradient resulting in vitreous gel prolapse.

EXCHANGE OF A CRYSTALENS IOL

Although many of the aforementioned principles may also apply to an eye harboring a Crystalens, several unique factors must be considered. Opening the capsular bag with viscodissection is more difficult with these implants because the CCC is typically larger than the optic size and, accordingly, the anterior capsule may be fused to the posterior capsule, making it harder to separate the capsulorrhexis from the posterior capsule without breaking one or both.

First, from a timing perspective, after the first 2 weeks the polyamide haptics of this implant become firmly encased within a fibrous cocoon in the periphery of the bag. This can be very difficult and sometimes impossible to open by means of blunt- or viscodissection . Accordingly, in the presence of a significant ametropic surprise, IOL exchange should be considered as soon after surgery as possible, and before such fibrosis develops. When a Crystalens exchange must be performed at a much later time, the surgeon should be prepared to amputate the haptics as far peripherally as possible and leave them behind within the confines of the bag. Cutting a silicone IOL can be challenging as there is a strong tendency for the IOL to slip out of the jaws of most types of IOL scissors. A serrated scissors will limit silicone optic movement during cutting. The optic will typically need to be sectioned because silicone optics in an aqueous environment are too slippery to fold in the anterior chamber. Alternatively, a larger incision could be chosen.

Placing the New IOL

When selecting the "new" IOL to replace the removal Pr-C IOL, the indication for the IOL exchange becomes paramount. For example, if the exchange is for the purpose of an error in power calculation, then one will likely select the same style of IOL with an adjusted power. If the exchange is for the purpose of optical aberrations or photic disturbances, an alternate Pr-C IOL should be considered with caution. The patient must understand that they may be trading one undesirable aberration for another. The Crystalens requires an expanded and intact capsular bag, ideally with minimal if any fibrosis. Because its haptics must be fixated within the fornix of an intact capsular bag and zonular complex in order to achieve accommodative function, the Crystalens is neither suitable for sulcus fixation nor optic capture within a capsulorrhexis.

The replacement IOL may be inserted within the capsular bag if the posterior capsule is capable of providing adequate fixation. Alternatively, capture of a 3-piece Pr-C IOL can be achieved by placing the haptics in the sulcus and prolapsing the optic through an intact and well-centered anterior and/or posterior capsulorrhexis.[6] If the capsulorrhexis diameter is too large to allow optic capture, then passive sulcus fixation is a viable choice as long as the surgeon selects an IOL of sufficient overall diameter with a reduced power reflecting the more anterior position inside the eye. Similarly, for passive sulcus fixation, the zonular apparatus should be sound, especially inferiorly, and an IOL with a rounded anterior edge should be considered to avoid iris chafing.[7] However, when the optic is captured through a CCC and the margin covered by the anterior capsule, there is no vulnerability to iris chafe from the optic, regardless of its anterior edge profile. If capsular and/or zonular stability is not sufficient, fixation of the IOL to the iris or sclera may be performed or an anterior chamber IOL may be implanted. These techniques are beyond the scope of this chapter.

Conclusion

The indications for repositioning exchanging of a Pr-C IOL require a careful history, comprehensive examination, and detailed discussion with the patient. When combined with a meticulously planned surgical approach, the patient may attain an excellent surgical outcome and a satisfying visual result.

References

1. Jardim D, Soloway B, Starr C. Asymmetric vault of an accommodating intraocular lens. *J Cataract Refract Surg.* 2006;32(2):347-350.

2. Jin GJ, Crandall AS, Jones JJ. Changing indications for and improving outcomes of intraocular lens exchange. *Am J Ophthalmol.* 2005;140(4):688-694.

3. Pepose JS, Qazi MA, Davies J, Doane JF, Loden JC, Sivalingham V, Mahmoud AM. Visual performance of patients with bilateral vs combination Crystalens, ReZoom, and ReSTOR intraocular lens implants. *Am J Ophthalmol.* 2007;144(3):347-357.

4. Trattler WB, Whitsett JC, Simone PA. Negative dysphotopsia after intraocular lens implantation irrespective of design and material. *J Cataract Refract Surg.* 2005;31(4):841-845.

5. Osher RH. Late reopening of the capsular bag. *Video J Cataract Refract Surg.* 1993;9(1).

6. Gimbel HV, DeBroff BM. Intraocular lens optic capture. *J Cataract Refract Surg.* 2004;30(1):200-206.

7. Chang WH, Werner L, Fry LL, Johnson JT, Kamae K, Mamalis N. Pigmentary dispersion syndrome with a secondary piggyback 3-piece hydrophobic acrylic lens. Case report with clinicopathological correlation. *J Cataract Refract Surg.* 2007;33(6):1106-1109.

REFRACTIVE IOL EXCHANGE— INDICATIONS AND TECHNIQUES

Harry B. Grabow, MD

Indications for Refractive IOL Removal

Refractive intraocular lenses (IOLs) today, as we have seen discussed in previous chapters, include both phakic IOLs and pseudophakic IOLs. Phakic IOLs can be fixated in the anterior-chamber angle (Figure 1), on the iris (Figure 2), and in the posterior chamber (Figure 3), and can be spherical, toric, and multifocal. Pseudophakic refractive IOLs include those implanted for clear refractive lens exchange or for cataract surgery. Like phakic IOLs, pseudophakic refractive IOLs can be spherical, toric, or multifocal, and also include accommodating IOLs. Indications for removal of an IOL may not be significantly different in the refractive/presbyopic patient compared to the traditional cataract patient. However, refractive/presbyopic IOL patients have higher expectations, and some of the newer IOL designs have new potential complications of their own.

IOL removal is both patient-driven and surgeon-driven. When elected by patients, the indications usually relate to visual symptoms; when elected by surgeons, there may be no patient symptoms, but rather anatomical or pathological indications. In addition, although IOL removal is more common in the postoperative period, there are also indications for removing an IOL intraoperatively immediately after primary implantation.

Intraoperative Indications

An IOL may need to be removed at the time of primary implantation for several possible reasons. It may have been damaged during insertion, or if damage to the capsule during insertion may have rendered the primary IOL unstable in the eye. Finally, it may have been discovered that the incorrect IOL was inadvertently implanted.

Damage to an IOL can occur to its haptic or optic. Haptic damage can include a bent or avulsed haptic, in the case of a

looped 3-piece IOL, or a torn or avulsed portion of a plate-haptic (Figures 4A and 4B), in the case of a single-piece silicone toric IOL or Collamer (STAAR Surgical, Monrovia, CA) plate-haptic IOL. Damage to silicone IOLs is more common due to the more fragile material, particularly when these IOLs are injected through ever diminishing incision sizes. In such cases, the damage must be assessed to determine whether the IOL can be left in or should be removed.[1] Implantation of 3-piece acrylic IOLs can occasionally be accompanied by crimping of a haptic, or by loosening or disinsertion of a trailing haptic. These haptic deformations may be related to improper loading of the IOLs in injectors. If the haptic damage is likely to impair centration, long-term positional stability, or potential visual function, then the damaged IOL must be removed and replaced.[2]

An optic can be damaged in one of several ways: there may be a fracture that involves the visual axis, or there may be a chip or peripheral fracture that does not affect visual performance. In addition, the optic surface may be scuffed by a handling instrument in a way that may or may not affect visual performance.

Although it is extremely rare and uncommon for damage to occur to a polymethylmethacrylate (PMMA) or a foldable acrylic IOL during implantation, it can occur. One-piece or three-piece clear PMMA IOLs are relatively resistant to mechanical stress damage; however, colorization of the PMMA, such as for aniridia IOLs (Figure 5), alters the PMMA's physical characteristics, rendering it brittle and fragile. Implantation of PMMA aniridia IOLs is fraught with the potential hazard of haptic fracture that will necessitate immediate IOL removal and replacement. In these particular cases, it is always wise to have one or two back-up aniridia IOLs in order to be prepared for this contingency.

Damage to the capsule, particularly a large unstable posterior tear, may require primary IOL removal and replacement with an IOL in a different location. If the capsulorrhexis (CCC) is still intact and is smaller than the optic of a looped-haptic IOL, it may be possible to leave the haptics in the

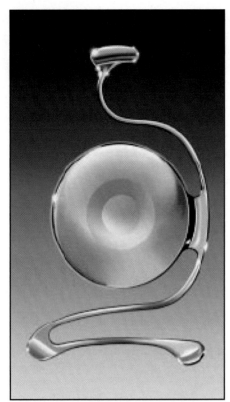

Figure 1. Phakic PMMA anterior-chamber multifocal IOL (Vivarte [Carl Zeiss Meditec, Jena, Germany]).

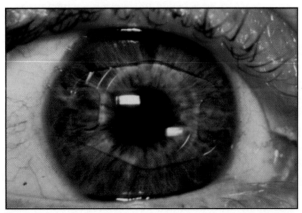

Figure 2. Artisan (Verisyse [Advanced Medical Optics, Santa Ana, CA) PMMA iris-fixated IOL (courtesy of J. Worst).

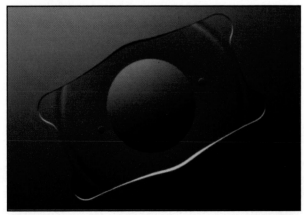

Figure 3. Phakic one-piece plate-haptic collagen posterior-chamber IOL (Visian ICL [STAAR Surgical]).

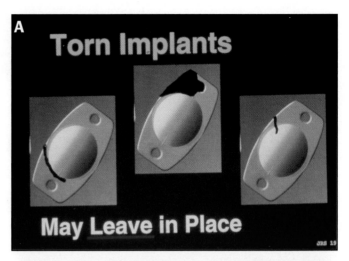

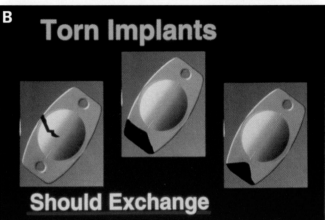

Figure 4. Haptic damage can include a bent or avulsed haptic, in the case of a looped 3-piece IOL, or a torn or avulsed portion of a plate-haptic (courtesy of J. Shepherd).

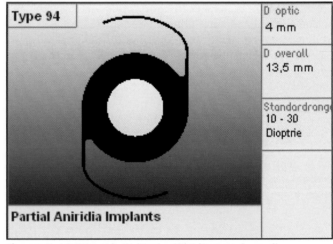

Figure 5. Black PMMA aniridia IOL (Morcher GMbH [Stuttgart, Germany]).

bag and prolapse the optic anteriorly through the A-CCC; however, this may render the eye slightly more minus in refraction. In such a case, the IOL can be elevated with the haptics in the sulcus and the optic captured through and behind the CCC.

Similarly, damage to the zonules may necessitate either relocation or removal of an IOL. If the zonular dialysis is small, and bag implantation is deemed safe, the IOL axis may be

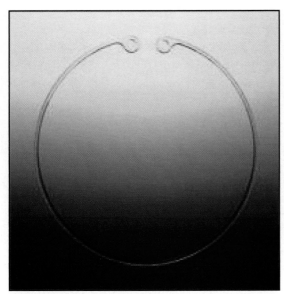

Figure 6. Capsule tension ring (Morcher).

aligned with the meridian of the zonular dialysis. The haptic in that meridian helps to expand the capsule and narrow the peripheral defect where vitreous is exposed. If the zonular dialysis is as wide as 45 degrees to 180 degrees, a capsule tension ring (CTR) (Figure 6) may be added to further expand the equator of the capsule and maintain IOL centration. If it is determined that, despite a standard CTR, the optic may tilt or decenter, then a Cionni modified CTR (M-CTR, Morcher) may need to be inserted. It is important to align the eyelet with the center of the zonular dialysis and to suture the eyelet to the sclera through the ciliary sulcus with 9-0 polypropylene suture. A subtotal zonular dialysis following IOL implantation may necessitate removal of the IOL and a total capsulectomy, along with a possible vitrectomy. The options would then be to suture a posterior-chamber IOL (PC-IOL) to the ciliary sulcus or the posterior surface of the iris, or to implant an anterior-chamber IOL (AC-IOL). If a PMMA AC-IOL is used, a larger incision is required. If the original incision was in clear cornea and is simply extended, sutures will be required. If the original incision was a scleral tunnel, enlargement may not necessitate suturing. In addition, a peripheral iridectomy is required, which can be performed either with microscissors or with an automated vitrector. It is prudent to have all of the potential IOLs needed on hand before surgery begins, with appropriate powers given that the IOL power must decrease as its location moves anterior.

Postoperative Indications

Postoperative indications for explanting refractive IOLs can occur as early as the first postoperative visit or many months or years later. These indications have been reviewed in several large surveys of implant surgeons3 and include these major categories:

* IOL power
* IOL performance
* IOL damage
* IOL malposition

IOL POWER

Incorrect IOL power may be diagnosed by the first postoperative refraction. If, in the setting of a postoperative "refractive surprise," it is determined that the "correct" IOL was implanted as calculated preoperatively, this may indicate an error in IOL power calculation, or, more rarely and unlikely, an error in IOL labeling or packaging by the manufacturer. This complication of incorrect IOL power, or, perhaps more appropriately, undesirable postoperative refraction, is increasingly becoming an indication for secondary surgical intervention following primary lens surgery. The reason for this has less to do with calculation or implantation error, but rather with higher patient expectations of achieving spectacle-free vision. This is particularly true for patients who have had previous keratorefractive surgery, such as radial keratotomy (RK), photorefractive keratectomy (PRK), or laser-assisted in-situ keratomileusis (LASIK). Prior surgical alteration of the corneal curvature affects the accuracy of IOL power calculation, and may often result in up to 3.00 D of refractive error postoperatively. Eyes that have had corneal flattening to treat myopia will attend to have a hyperopic refractive error after IOL surgery, whereas eyes that have had corneal steepening to treat hyperopia will tend to end up more myopic than desired after IOL surgery. When there is an undesired result, it is appropriate to measure the refraction a week after surgery to determine if surgical intervention, such as an IOL exchange, is needed or desired. IOL exchange can usually be safely and easily performed during the first 2 weeks before significant capsular fibrosis occurs.

Late-appearing ametropia, particularly myopia, may be a sign of capsular contraction with anterior movement of an optic that was initially placed in the capsular bag. This is particularly prevalent in cases where the original CCC was made larger than the IOL optic and in cases of round-edged 3-piece silicone IOLs. This may be an indication for IOL exchange. However, if because of excessive capsular fibrosis removing the primary IOL would be too traumatic to the capsular or zonular integrity, then IOL exchange may be contraindicated. Either a secondary sulcus "piggyback" implantation or a keratorefractive procedure may be preferable in this situation.

IOL PERFORMANCE

An IOL may have the correct power and be in the proper location, but may have certain negative optical characteristics that necessitate IOL removal. Certain optical designs, such as truncated 5 × 6 oval-optic PMMA IOLs and square-edged acrylic IOLs (Figure 7), may be associated with significant subjective complaints related to internal edge reflections, and other effects.[4] The undesirable visual symptoms include dark temporal crescent-shaped relative scotomata ("negative dysphotopsias") or bright temporal arcs of light ("positive dysphotopsias")[5,6] Some patients spontaneously report these symptoms as early as the first post-operative day. Multifocal IOLs that have concentric ring designs, whether refractive (such as the ReZoom [Advanced Medical Optics]) or diffractive (such as the ReSTOR [Alcon, Fort Worth, TX]) have required removal due to intolerable nocturnal halos manifest as rings around lights at night[7] that can be disabling to a night driver.

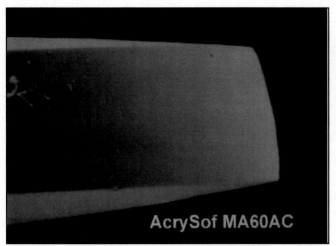

Figure 7. Square-edge acrylic IOL.

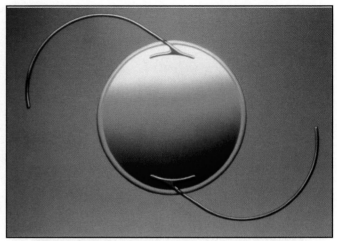

Figure 9. Silicone posterior-chamber IOL.

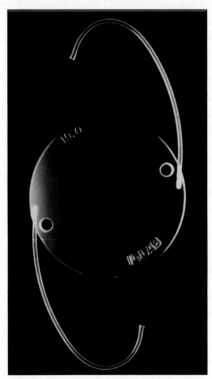

Figure 8 . PMMA posterior-chamber IOL.

IOLs also have varying degrees of biocompatibility. The degree of biologic tolerance depends on IOL design, material, and location within the eye. Although intracapsular sequestration from uveal and corneal tissue is believed to be the most biocompatible location for implantation, different designs and materials perform differently inside the capsular bag. PMMA (Figure 8) and silicone (Figure 9), for example, have been shown to cause more capsular fibrosis than acrylic, hydrogel, and collagen materials. Some investigators believe that silicone IOLs may have higher rates of uveitis and cystoid macular edema (CME) than acrylic and hydrogel IOLs. Persistent anterior chamber cell or flare reaction, keratic precipitates (KP) on the IOL surface[8], posterior synechiae, secondary ocular hypertension, and persistent CME may be indications for removal or replacement of an IOL.

An IOL in the ciliary sulcus may cause ocular tenderness or chronic iridocyclitis (and rarely hyphema). This is especially true for square-edged optics, which may cause pigment dispersion due to iris chafing. Angle-fixated PMMA IOLs, if too long, may fixate posterior to the scleral spur, resulting in progressive ovalization of the pupil in the long axis of the IOL. This may also be associated with ocular pain and tenderness.

Conversely, an angle-fixated PMMA AC-IOL that is too short may move from side-to-side with ocular saccades, exhibiting the so-called windshield wiper form of pseudophakodonesis. Chronic intermittent contact with the corneal endothelium can lead to corneal decompensation. Early recognition of diminishing serial endothelial cell counts may necessitate IOL removal and replacement.

IOL biomaterial incompatibility can occur in special situations, such as when silicone oil in contact with a silicone IOL and silicone oil[9] impairs visibility of the posterior segment for the vitreoretinal surgeon. A posterior segment procedure requiring silicone oil may therefore necessitate removing the silicone IOL. Another biomaterial incompatibility would be the development of interlenticular opacification, when two acrylic-optic IOLs are both piggybacked into one capsular bag, piggyback style, with an anterior capsulorrhexis opening that is smaller than the diameter of the anterior IOL optic.[10] Lens epithelial cells migrate between the acrylic optics forming not only visually symptomatic opacification but also a physico-chemical-biologic bond between the two IOLs that renders them mechanically inseparable.[11] In such cases, simultaneous explantation of both optics or the entire IOL-capsular complex may be necessary.

IOL DAMAGE

The IOL optics may be symptomatically compromised by pitting caused by aggressive Nd:yttrium-aluminum-garnet (YAG) laser posterior capsulotomy.[12] No optic material is immune to this type of laser damage,[13] and silicone and PMMA optics are particularly vulnerable. Rarely, central optic pitting can compromise visual clarity or cause light interference to the point that an IOL exchange becomes necessary.

Additionally, certain IOL materials have been observed to undergo spontaneous discoloration or opacification. Some early generation silicone optics were observed to turn a semiopaque brown color. This was thought to be related to insufficient curing of the liquid silicone during manufacturing.[14]

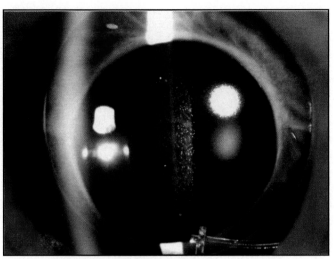

Figure 10. "Glistenings" in hydrophobic acrylic IOL.

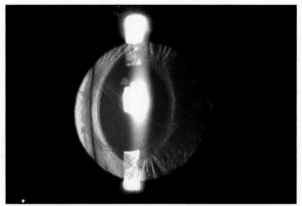

Figure 12. Short-axis decentration of plate-haptic silicone IOL.

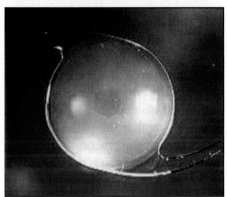

Figure 11 . Calcific surface opacification of hydrophilic acrylic IOL.

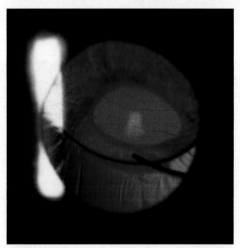

Figure 13 . Superior optic decentration—"sunrise syndrome."

Early-generation hydrophobic acrylic optics developed "glistenings" thought to be actual water vacuoles[15] (Figure 10).

Hydrophilic acrylic IOLs can develop a uniform white opacification of the optic[16-18] (Figure 11) thought to be calcification. Any of these optic opacification syndromes may necessitate an IOL exchange.[20-22]

IOL MALPOSITION

Malpositioned IOLs may be the result of decentration, subluxation, dislocation, and, in the case of toric IOLs, off-axis rotation. An IOL may decenter if it is too short for the space that it occupies. This is particularly true of plate-haptic IOLs,[23] which being only 10.5 or 10.8 mm in diagonal length, may be too short for the capsular bag in large myopic eyes. These IOLs may therefore decenter along their short axis (Figure 12). An IOL may also decenter if displaced by late capsular fibrosis, or if one haptic is in the bag and the other is in the sulcus. If the IOL was placed vertically, with only the inferior loop in the bag, the optic will decenter superiorly with capsular contraction producing a "sunrise syndrome" (Figure 13). An IOL that is too short for the ciliary sulcus may decenter inferiorly, producing a "sunset syndrome" (Figure 14). If an IOL is placed in a capsular bag with insufficient zonular support, capsular fibrosis may cause subluxation, partial anterior dislocation[24], or total posterior dislocation[25] of the lens (Figure 15). In cases of decentration or subluxation, pupil-splitting optic-edge

symptoms, such as glare or monocular diplopia, may be indications for IOL repositioning, removal, or replacement. Likewise, total posterior dislocation into the vitreous may produce annoying symptoms due to excessive IOL motility that would necessitate IOL repositioning[26] or exchange (Figure 16).

Anterior chamber IOLs that are angle-fixated with one or more peripheral iridectomies, may rotate and decenter in such a way that one haptic passes through an iridectomy. This can produce chronic iritis, pigment dispersion, corneal endothelial decompensation, and visual symptoms caused by optic decentration and tilt. Overly long AC-IOLs can result in pupillary ovaling. Anterior chamber IOLs that are iris-fixated, such as the Artisan (Verisyse) style (Figure 17), may become disenclavated producing IOL mobility, corneal endothelial trauma, and visual symptoms. This can usually be corrected by simple re-enclavation.

Phakic PC-IOLs that are too short can move (Figure 18) and can contact the anterior lens capsule causing anterior subcapsular cataract formation. This could necessitate either phakic PC-IOL removal and replacement with either a longer phakic posterior chamber, a phakic AC-IOL, or phakic IOL removal combined with cataract surgery.

Multifocal IOLs, such as the ReSTOR and the ReZoom require perfect centration for proper function. Even slight decentration of 1 mm can cause visual disturbances and undesirable glare symptoms (Figure 19). The Crystalens (Eyeonics, Inc., Aliso Viejo, CA) silicone plate-hap-

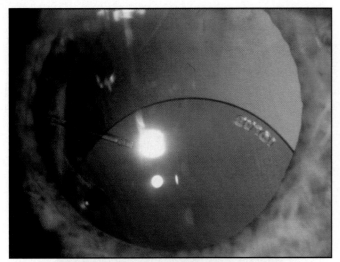

Figure 14 . Inferior decentration—"sunset syndrome."

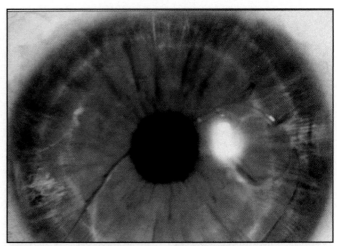

Figure 17. Single dis-enclavation of Artisan (Verisyse) iris-fixated IOL.

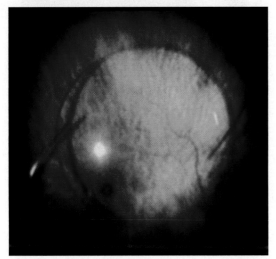

Figure 15 . Total posterior IOL dislocation.

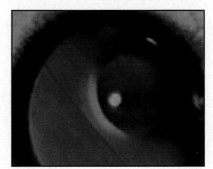

Figure 18. Short phakic PC-IOL (silicone) with decentration.

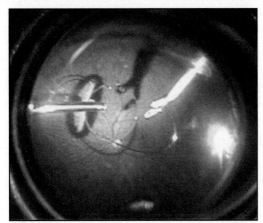

Figure 16. Forceps removal of posteriorly dislocated plate-haptic IOL.

tic accommodating IOL, similar to other single-plane accommodating IOLs, must be positioned posteriorly within the capsular bag to maintain the desired refraction and to have the potential for accommodation.

There are two potential Crystalens malpositions that may require correction. The first is symmetric anterior vaulting of the optic. This induces myopia that may necessitate optic repositioning, an IOL exchange or possibly a corneal refractive enhancement procedure. The second potential Crystalens malposition is the so-called Z-syndrome in which one side of the optic is vaulted anteriorly and the other side remains posterior. Such optic tilting can induce pseudophakic astigmatism of up to 3.00 D. This Z-syndrome may be caused by anterior capsule fibrosis and phimosis (Figure 20) when the capsulorrhexis is made much smaller than the optic. This may be corrected by Nd:YAG-laser anterior and/or posterior capsulotomy. In some cases, an IOL exchange is necessary.

An IOL properly positioned in a capsular bag may become decentered due to late zonular dialysis[27] even in the presence of a capsule tension ring (CTR). This is a potential problem in eyes with pseudoexfoliation (Figure 21), particularly if they are implanted with three piece or plate haptic silicone IOLs. In these eyes, even if a CTR had been implanted, late posterior dislocation of the entire bag–CTR–IOL complex (Figure 22) can occur. Capsular bag–IOL subluxations, can be recentered by sclerally fixating one or both haptics, through the capsular equator (Figure 23), usually under a scleral flap. They can also be recentered, if the capsule can be dissected open with viscoelastic, by secondary implantation of a Cionni-modified capsule tension ring,[28] an Ahmed capsule tension segment (Figures 24 and 25), or an Assiachor Capsular Anchor, that is sutured with 9-0 polypropylene suture to the scleral wall. If these capsular recentering techniques cannot be employed due to extensive zonulodialysis, then the entire capsulo-pseudophakic complex may need to be removed followed by IOL

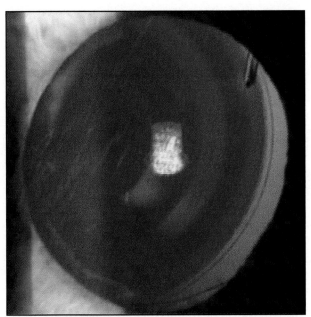

Figure 19. Symptomatic decentration of concentric silicone Array multifocal IOL (Advanced Medical Optics).

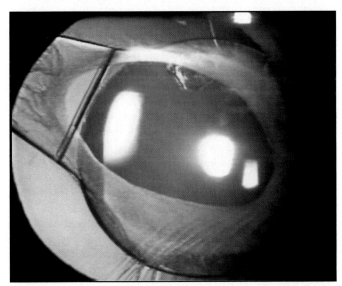

Figure 20. Crystalens with anterior capsular fibrosis and phimosis with 2.00 D of induced pseudophakic astigmatism.

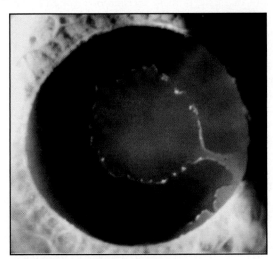

Figure 21. Pseudoexfoliation.

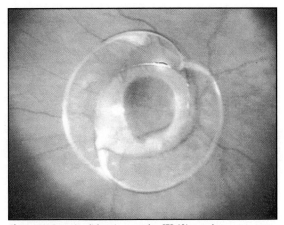

Figure 22. Posterior dislocation capsular-CTR-IOL complex.

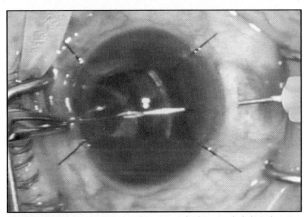

Figure 23. Suturing through capsular equator for late zonulodialysis (courtesy of Ike Ahmed).

replacement. In the absence of a lens capsule, the replacement IOL can be placed in the ciliary sulcus, while suturing the haptics to the sclera or to the posterior surface of the iris.[29,30] Alternatively, and anterior chamber IOL can be implanted.

IOLs can also become malpositioned due to trauma.

Anterior-chamber lenses have been found in the vitreous cavity; posterior-chamber lenses have been found in the anterior chamber; and some times only parts of IOLs are dislocated by the trauma, such as a posterior-chamber IOL optic or haptic entering the anterior chamber through an iridectomy or through the pupil. Some unusual ectopic IOL traumatic dislocations have been reported, such as the almost completely exteriorized case of the posterior-chamber IOL that ended up in the subconjunctival space.[31]

TECHNIQUES OF IOL REMOVAL

The technique of IOL removal and the size of the incision will vary and will depend on the material of the IOL to be removed and the size and design of the replacement IOL. At the present time, removal (or implantation) of a PMMA IOL requires an incision long enough to accommodate the width of the rigid optic, usually in the range of 5.0 to 7.0 mm. This length of incision, if near the cornea, may require suturing and will have astigmatic consequences. Removal of foldable lenses, to the contrary, can be accomplished through smaller incisions, ranging from 3.0 to 4.0 mm. Incisions of this size may be self-sealing without sutures with much less effect on

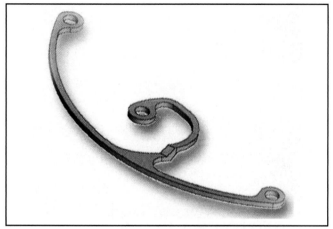

Figure 24. Ahmed capsule tension segment (Morcher).

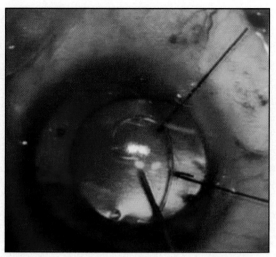

Figure 25. Suturing Ahmed segment (courtesy Ike Ahmed).

corneal curvature. As with all intraocular surgery, the corneal endothelium, iris, capsule, and zonule must be protected and preserved whenever possible. Carefully planned and executed maneuvers, with judicious use of viscoelastics, facilitate these goals. Dispersive viscoelastics usually maintain space better than cohesive viscoelastics, but overinflation of the anterior segment with a dispersive agent can rupture weak zonular fibers and create or extend unstable capsular tears.

Angle-fixated AC-IOLs that have been in place longer than a few months may have developed "fibrotic cocoons" around the haptics, which may be visible on gonioscopy. Attempt at simple linear extraction in such cases may result in avulsion of the iris root and iridodialysis, with attendant hemorrhage (hyphema), and even the possibility of total iridectomy. Testing implant mobility in these cases by gently attempting to rotate the IOL on plane will confirm if the IOL haptics are free or if they can be safely dialed out of their fibrotic tunnels.[32] Significant resistance to rotation may necessitate haptic amputation with scissors, removal of the optic, and then reverse dialing of the amputated haptics out of their fibrotic tunnels. In some cases, it may be advisable to leave the haptics in-situ. The same is true for posterior chamber IOLs with haptics placed in the ciliary sulcus. If these can be rotated and fully mobilized in the plane of the sulcus, they can be easily and safely removed, avoiding uveal hemorrhage.[33]

Bag-fixated PC-IOLs will exhibit different degrees of capsular fixation, depending on their haptic design. Loop-haptic PC-IOLs can usually be rotated clockwise within the capsule after first separating the anterior and posterior capsules and expanding the bag with viscoelastic. If the anterior capsulorrhexis has phimosed and contracted significantly, it may require secondary enlargement or radial relaxing capsulotomies. Two such incisions are usually made 180 degrees apart, to allow safe explanation of the IOL out of the bag without undue zonular trauma. Once a foldable PC-IOL is rotated out of the bag, removal through a 3 to 4 mm is possible by one of two methods: partial or complete optic transection (bisection) or by optic refolding. The former technique can be accomplished by hooking and exteriorizing a haptic through the incision, securing the optic by grasping the optic or the exteriorized haptic with forceps, and then cutting the optic half-way across its diameter along the short axis with scissors (Dodick technique[34]). In this way, a 6-mm optic has been reduced to 3 mm

in the meridian of the hemisection. By pulling one-half of the optic through the incision, the second half will flex and follow the first half out of the eye. With silicone optics, the hemisection may allow complete bisection of the optic by fracturing of the remaining hemi-optic as it is pulled through the incision. The second hemi-optic can then be removed by rotating the optic until its haptic can be hooked and grasped for removal, or by simply grasping the optic with toothed forceps.

Instruments have been designed specifically for foldable IOL sectioning. The Mackool set (Impex Surgical, Staten Island, NY) (Figure 26) facilitates intraocular hemisection or bisection with scissors. Utrata developed a snare (Rhein Medical, Tampa, FL) for bisection of both 3-piece and plate-haptic silicone IOLs (Figure 27). Chu developed heavy-bladed scissors (Rhein) that will bisect both silicone and acrylic optics in one maneuver (Figure 28). Koo developed scissors, one blade of which is a serrated platform, for cutting silicone (and possibly acrylic) IOLs (Figure 29). However, foldable IOLs may also be refolded in the anterior chamber and removed in one piece. This maneuver requires care and adequate viscoelastic, usually with a dispersive or highly retentive cohesive viscoelastic. An instrument to be used as the central folding fulcrum may be introduced parallel to the blades of a folding forceps through the primary incision or through a small paracentesis 180 degrees away. The fulcrum instrument is placed completely across and under the optic and is held firmly while the folding forceps symmetrically depresses each half of the optic posteriorly. The fulcrum instrument is slowly removed before the optic is completely folded and the folded IOL may then be withdrawn from the eye using the folding forceps. This maneuver is more easily performed on acrylic IOLs than on silicone IOLs, which tend to be too slippery and elastic.

Some bag-fixated PC-IOL loop haptics become so fibrosed within the capsular fornix that rotation is not possible without tearing the zonules, despite attempts at separating capsular adhesions with viscoelastic or mechanical means. In these cases, haptic amputation may be the safest way to remove the IOL optic. This may be indicated not only for IOLs with loop haptics, but also for plate-haptic IOLs with large haptic fenestrations through which the anterior and posterior capsules have fused or with the modified plate haptic of the Crystalens (Eyeonics) (Figure 30). Removal of these types of IOLs can

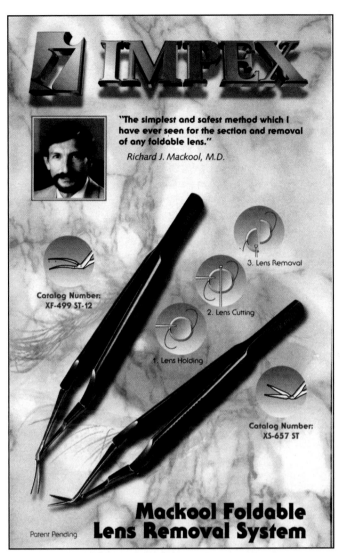

Figure 26. Mackool foldable lens removal system.

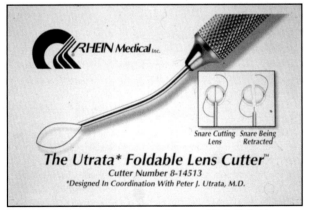

Figure 27. The Utrata foldable lens cutter. (Courtesy of Rhein Medical.)

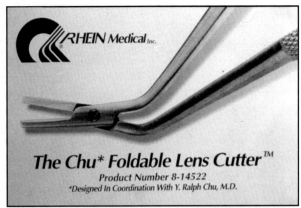

Figure 28. The Chu foldable lens cutter. (Courtesy of Rhein Medical.)

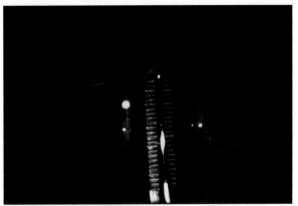

Figure 29. Koo IOL cutter for silicone optic bisection.

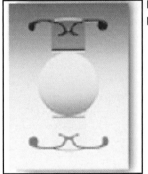

Figure 30. AT-50 Crystalens with combined plate/loop haptics (Eyeonics).

be usually be done in toto within the first 2 to 3 weeks after implantation. After that time, capsular fibrosis may necessitate transecting the plate haptics and removing only the optic.

Posterior-chamber IOLs that dislocate posteriorly, through a posterior capsular defect into the vitreous cavity, usually require a pars plana vitrectomy procedure.[35] If the capsulor-rhexis is still intact, the IOL may be relocated to the ciliary sulcus with or without additional fixation and capture of the optic through the capsular opening. If there is inadequate capsular fixation then scleral or iris suture fixation of the haptics may be necessary[36,37] (Figures 31A and 31B). Relocation of posteriorly dislocated IOLs to the posterior chamber has been done with both loop-haptic and plate-haptic IOLs.[38-40] When sutures are used, 9-0 polypropylene is recommended for its tissue durability. Hoffman et al[41] have developed a technique of suturing haptics to the sclera without making ab externo scleral flaps; and Szurman[42] uses a technique with scleral suture fixation without knots.

References

1. Shepherd, JR. How to avoid complications with plate-haptic-foldable IOLs. *Rev Ophthal.* 1997;Nov:60-65.

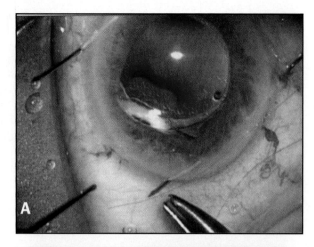

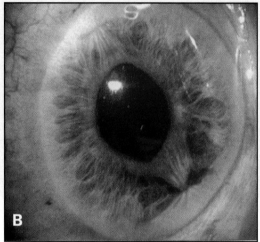

Figure 31. (A) Needle positions for posterior iris haptic fixation. (B) PC-IOL sutured to posterior iris. (Courtesy of G. Condon.)

11. Werner, L, Shugar, JK, Apple, DJ, Pandey, SK, et al. Opacification of piggyback IOLs associated with an amorphous material attached to interlenticular surfaces. *J Cataract Refract Surg.* 2000;26:1612-1619.

12. Bath, PE, Boener, CF, Dang, Y. Pathology and physics of YAG-laser intraocular lens damage. *J Cataract Refract Surg.* 1987;13:47.

13. Auffarth GU, Newland, TJ, Wesendahl, TA, Apple, DJ. Nd:YAG laser damage to silicone intraocular lenses confused with pigment deposits on clinical examination. *Am J Ophthal.* 1994;118(4):526-528.

14. Milauskis, AT. Silicone intraocular lens discoloration in humans. *Arch Ophthal.* 1991;109:913.

15. Dhaliwal DK, Mamalis, N, Olson, RJ, et al. Visual significance of glistenings seen in the AcrySof intraocular lens. *J Cataract Refract Surg.* 1996;22:452-457.

16. Werner L, Apple DJ, Kaskaloglu, M, Pandey, SK. Dense opacification of the optical component of a hydrophilic acrylic intraocular lens: a clinicopathologic analysis of 9 explanted lenses. *J Cataract Refract Surg.* 2001;27:1485-1492.

17. Tehrani, M, Mamalis, N, Wallin T, et al. Late postoperative opacification of MemoryLens hydrophilic acrylic intraocular lenses. *J Cataract Refract Surg.* 2004;30:115-122.

18. Neuhann, IM, Werner, L, Izak, AM, Pandey, SK, et al. Late postoperative opacification of hydrophilic acrylic (Hydrogel) intraocular lens. *Ophthalmol.* 2004;111:2094-2101.

19. Jensen, MK, Crandall, AS, Mamalis, N, Olson, RJ. Crystallization of intraocular lens surfaces associated with the use of HealonGV. *Arch Ophthal.* 1994;112:1037-1042.

20. Olson, RJ, Caldwell, KD, Crandall, AS, Jensen, MK, Huang, S-C. Intraoperative crystallization of the intraocular lens surface. *Am J Ophthal.* 1998;126:177-184.

21. Katai, N, Yokoyama, R, Yoshimura, N. Progressive brown discoloration of silicone intraocular lenses after vitrectomy in a patient on amiodarone. *J Cataract Refract Surg.* 1999;25:451-452.

22. Apple, DJ, Peng Q, Arthur, SN, Werner, L, et al. Snowflake degeneration of polymethylmethacrylate posterior chamber intraocular lens material. *Ophth.* 2002;109:1666-1675.

23. Subramaniam, S, Tuft, SJ. Early decentration of plate-haptic silicone intraocular lenses. *J Cataract Refract Surg.* 2001;27:330-332.

24. Faucher, A, Rootman, DS. Dislocation of plate-haptic silicone intraocular lens into the anterior chamber. *J Cataract Refract Surg.* 2001;27:169-171.

25. Negi, A, Sinha, A. Posterior capsule tear with plate-haptic silicone intraocular lens dislocation. *J Cataract Refract Surg.* 2000;26:1558-1559.

26. Smiddy, WE, Flynn, HW. Management of dislocated posterior chamber intraocular lenses. *Ophth.* 1991;98:889-894.

27. Jehan, FS, Mamalis, N, Crandall AS. Spontaneous late dislocation of intraocular lens within the capsular bag in pseudoexfoliation patients. *Ophthalmology.* 2001;108:1727-1731.

28. Cionni, RJ, Osher, RH. Management of profound zonular dialysis or weakness with a new endocapsular ring designed for scleral fixation. *J Cataract Refract Surg.* 1998;24:1299-1306.

29. Stark, WJ, Bruner, WE, Martin, NF. Management of subluxed posterior-chamber lenses. *Ophthalmic Surg.* 1982;13(2):130-133.

30. Stark, WJ, Michels, RG, Bruner, WE. Management of posteriorly dislocated intraocular lenses. *Ophthalmic Surg.* 1980;11(8):495-497.

31. Sandramouli, S, Kumar, A, et al. Subconjunctival dislocation of posterior chamber intraocular lens. *Ophthalmic Surg.* 1993;24:770-771.

32. Terry, AC, Stark WJ. Removal of closed-loop anterior chamber lens implants. *Ophthal Surg.* 1984;15(7):575-577.

33. Patel, J, Sinskey, RM. The loose posterior chamber lens: diagnosis and management. *J Ocular Ther Surg.* 1983;Jan-Feb;19-21.

34. Batlan, SJ, Dodick, JM. Explantation of a foldable silicone intraocular lens. *Am J Ophthal.* 1996;122(2):270-272.

2. Carlson, AN, Stewart, WC, Tso, PC. Intraocular complications requiring removal or exchange. *Surv Ophthal.* 1998;42:4170440.

3. Mamalis, N. Complications of foldable intraocular lenses requiring explantation or secondary intervention—2001 survey update. *J Cataract Refract Surg.* 2002; 28:2193-2201.

4. Friedberg, HL, Kline, OR, Friedberg, AH. Comparison of the unwanted optical images produced by 6 mm and 7 mm intraocular lenses. *J Cataract Refract Surg.* 1989;15:541-544.

5. Farbowitz, MA, Zabriskie, NA, Crandall, AS, Olson, RJ, Miller, KN. Visual complaints associated with the AcrySof acrylic intraocular lens. *J Cataract Refract Surg.* 2000;26:1339-1345.

6. Davison, JA. Positive and negative dysphotopsia in patients with acrylic intraocular lenses. *J Cataract Refract Surg.* 2000;26:1346-1355.

7. Dick, HB, Krummenauer, F, et al. Objective and subjective evaluation of photic phenomena after monofocal and multifocal lens implantation. *Ophthal.* 1999;106:1878-1886.

8. Wolter, JR, Sugar, A. Reactive membrane on a foldable silicone implant in the posterior chamber of a human eye. *Ophthal Surg.* 1989;20:17-20.

9. Khawly, JA, Lambert, RJ, Jaffe, GJ. Intraocular lens changes after short- and long-term exposure to silicone oil. *Ophthal.* 1998;105:1227-1233.

10. Gayton, JL, Apple, DJ, Peng, Q, et al. Interlenticular opacification: clinicopathological correlation of a complication of posterior chamber piggyback intraocular lenses. *J Cataract Refract Surg.* 2000;26:330-336.

35. Campo, RV, Chung, KD, Oyakawa, RT. Pars plana vitrectomy in the management of dislocated posterior chamber lenses. *Am J Ophthal.* 1989;108:529-534.

36. Panton, RW, Sulewski, ME, Parker, JS, Panton, PJ, Stark, WJ. Surgical management of subluxed posterior-chamber intraocular lenses. *Arch Ophthal.* 1993;111:919-926.

37. Condon, GP, et al. Small-incision iris fixation of foldable intraocular lenses in the absence of capsule support. *Ophthalmology.* 2007;114:1311-1318.

38. Smiddy, WE. Dislocated posterior chamber intraocular lens: a new technique of management. *Arch Ophthal.* 1989;107:1678-1680.

39. Smiddy, WE, Ibanez, GV, Alsonso, E, Flynn, HW. Surgical management of dislocated intraocular lenses. *J Cataract Refract Surg.* 1995;21:64-69.

40. Schneiderman, TE, Johnson, MW, Smiddy, WE, Flynn, HW, et al. Surgical management of posteriorly dislocated silicone plate haptic intraocular lenses. *Am J Ophthal.* 1997;123:629-635.

41. Hoffman, RS, et al. Technique offers scleral fixation without conjunctival dissection. *Ophthal Times,* April 15, 2007:31-36.

42. Szurman, P. Forget the knots—new technique fixates IOLs quickly and efficiently. *EuroTimes,* May 2007:18.

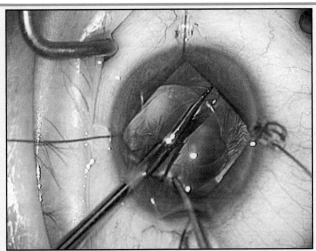

Figure 1. MST Packer Chang IOL Cutter is inserted through a 1.2-mm paracentesis. Toothed forceps fixate the ReSTOR optic within the pupil plane as it is transected.

Figure 2. MST Packer Chang IOL Cutter blades are constructed from a single piece of stainless steel that is bent over itself.

IOL EXPLANTATION

David F. Chang, MD

To remove or exchange an acrylic multifocal intraocular lens (IOL), it is imperative to use a system that minimizes the risk of corneal or capsular trauma. Fortunately, there are several excellent IOL cutting instruments available to cataract surgeons. For a standard scissor design to be used through the phaco incision, my preference is the titanium Osher cutter (Duckworth and Kent). The blades are narrow enough to fit through a phaco incision and have serrations to better grip the silicone or acrylic optic. The scissors are strong enough to cut an acrylic optic, but several repeat cuts are usually necessary to fully penetrate through the optic.

The Packer Chang IOL Cutter (Microsurgical Technologies, Redmond, WA) is an interchangeable attachment that fits onto the universal MST microsurgical handle. Unlike the other MST attachments, which are designed to work through a 0.8-mm paracentesis, the IOL cutting scissors are designed so as to pass through a 1.2- to 1.4-mm incision. This provides the surgeon with the option of grasping and fixating the optic with a toothed forceps through the phaco incision, and using the scissors through a separate side port paracentesis (Figure 1). Secure fixation of the optic is often difficult and yet critical as closure of the blades will tend to push the optic away. Alternatively, the optic can be grasped with MST microforceps through a paracentesis, while the cutting tip is introduced through the IOL incision. Compared to other scissor designs, the narrow profile of the shaft prevents egress of an ophthalmic viscosurgical device (OVD) through the incision.

The other unique characteristic of the Packer Chang IOL Cutter is the strength of the scissor blades. Ordinary paper scissors are constructed from two separate component pieces that are connected by a screw around which the blades pivot. The Packer Chang scissor blades are assembled from a single piece of metal that is folded back upon itself (Figure 2). Similar to the construction of a bolt cutter, this imparts much greater strength to the blades, which can cut through the most rigid of hydrophobic acrylic optics (eg, Advanced Medical Optics Sensar) with little effort and without any tilting or twisting of the lens.

CHAPTER 231

EXPLANTING THE CRYSTALENS— TECHNIQUE

Jeffrey Whitman, MD

It is best to consider removal and replacement of the Crystalens (eyeonics, Aliso Viejo, CA) only after the search for all treatable causes of a patient's dissatisfaction has been exhausted. Potential causes of dissatisfaction may include a power miss, lens vault leading to induced myopia, capsular contraction syndrome which may freeze the lens movement, glare, poor reading ability due to poor lens movement, and unrealistic patient expectations.

When to Remove and Exchange

Repeat biometry should clarify a power miss for which there are several surgical recourses. If the patient is still within the 3 to 4 weeks postoperative period, one may wish to simply perform a removal and exchange with a correctly powered Crystalens. During this period, the polyamide loops should not yet have bonded with the equatorial capsular bag and this will permit easy removal. A temporal 3.2- to 3.5-mm wound is created with a least one side port paracentesis. The anterior chamber is filled with viscoelastic (but not Ocucoat [Bausch & Lomb, Rochester, NY]) as it makes the Crystalens (Eyeonics, Inc., Aliso Viejo, CA) material too slippery), which should also be directed behind the Crystalens haptics, in order to free up the lens from any capsular attachments. The haptic nasal to the wound is then lifted into the anterior chamber (Figure 1) using either the viscoelastic cannula or a lens manipulator (Figure 2). The nasal haptic is then dialed and lifted toward the operative wound. The nearest haptic/loop is then hooked with a lens manipulator and brought through the wound (Figure 3). More viscoelastic is added to maintain adequate clearance between the body of the lens and the corneal endothelium, if needed. The body of the lens is then grasped (foldable lens retriever forceps work well) and pulled through the main incision (Figure 4). The Crystalens will easily mold through the incision, making it unnecessary to bisect the lens while it is still in the eye. Once the Crystalens has been removed, refill the bag with viscoelastic and implant the correctly powered Crystalens as one would have for a primary insertion. A workable formula for

calculating the correct power for the replacement lens is 1.5 times the amount of change desired (eg, a 20-D Crystalens was implanted, ending up in a postoperative refraction of +1.00 D; 1.5 × 1.00 D = 1.5 D, dictating a news lens of 21.5 D).

A lens vault noted in the immediate postoperative period is usually due to a wound leak. If the leak is Seidel positive, consider repositioning of the lens and suturing the wound. If there is no leak, one can still reopen the surgical wound, rotate the lens and push it back with viscoelastic, and then suture the wound. If the lens vaults again, this may not be a true lens vault, but rather an anatomically shallow capsular bag. Consider removal and replacement with a new lens power as above to make up for the more anterior lens position.

When to Remove

Capsular contraction syndrome for the most part was limited to the original Crystalens AT-45 model. The small diameter of the lens coupled with retained cortex could cause contracture of the capsular bag, which would force the lens into unusual positions. This would induce astigmatism along with unpredictable myopia or hyperopia. If recognized early, yttrium aluminum garnet (YAG) laser lysis of contracture bands (well described by Harvey Carter, MD, Dallas, TX) could be used to reposition the lens. However, if laser repositioning fails and the patient is more than 3 weeks postoperative, then the lens must be removed. Again, a 3.2- to 3.5-mm wound is fashioned and the chamber is filled with viscoelastic. If the lens can be loosened from its capsular adhesions with viscoelastic and gentle manipulation, its can be removed as above. More often, the lens loops are adherent to the capsular equator and overly forceful manipulation will only tear or dehisce the bag entirely. Here it is advisable to fill the chamber with viscoelastic as above and then sever the lens haptics as far out to the periphery as possible using Mackool (Impex Surgical, Staten Island, NY) or other intraocular scissors. If the capsular bag is intact, it can then be reopened with additional viscoelastic and a new Crystalens or other monofocal lens can be inserted.

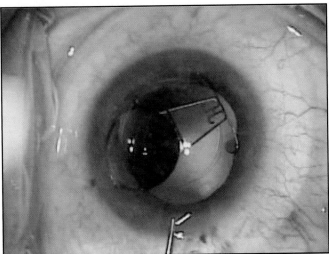

Figure 1. Nasal haptic lifted into the anterior chamber.

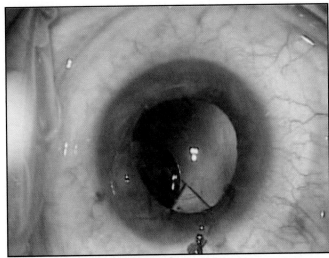

Figure 3. Haptic brought through the wound.

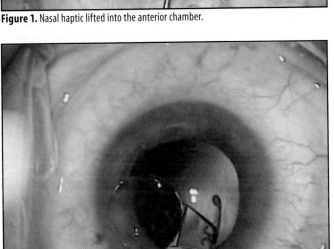

Figure 2. Haptic lifted toward the wound.

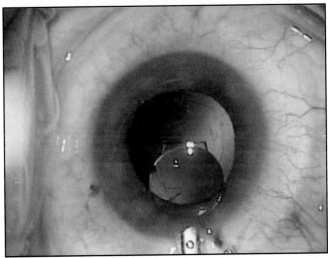

Figure 4. Lens pulled through the wound.

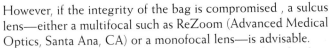

However, if the integrity of the bag is compromised , a sulcus lens—either a multifocal such as ReZoom (Advanced Medical Optics, Santa Ana, CA) or a monofocal lens—is advisable.

Glare is rarely a problem with the Crystalens, but if it does occur, it can be lessened by the use of miotics. If glare is due to clouding of the posterior capsule, a YAG capsulotomy can be performed as long as an intraocular lens (IOL) exchange is not likely to be needed. Certainly if Crystalens removal is necessitated by continued patient complaints or by unrealistic patient expectations, the methods described above can be used depending on how far out postoperatively the patient is.

When to Consider a Piggyback Lens

If the patient has gone through at least 6 months of accommodative training and still lacks satisfactory reading vision, one can either remove the lens as above or replace it with a multifocal or monofocal implant. However, most patients can be made happy by inducing a greater degree of monovision by simply inserting a piggyback lens such as a STAAR AQ5010V (STAAR Surgical, Monrovia, CA) or Advanced Medical

Optics Clariflex into the ciliary sulcus. Always simulate the resulting power change with a contact lens trial prior to initiating a surgical correction. Pick the lens implant power with any suitable formula such as the refractive vergence formula of Warren Hill, MD (http://www.doctor-hill.com). Make a 3.2- to 3.5-mm temporal incision and a temporal paracentesis. Insert a viscoelastic cannula through the paracentesis all the way across the eye just into the sulcus behind the iris and back fill the sulcus/anterior chamber with viscoelastic (Figure 5). Now insert the folded lens through the main incision and gently allow it to unfold into the sulcus (Figure 6). If the capsular bag has been opened with a YAG capsulotomy, add Miostat to bring the pupil down around the edges of the piggyback lens prior to removing the viscoelastic (Figure 7). This lessens the chance of losing vitreous if the capsule has been previously opened. Next, remove the anterior viscoelastic with irrigation and aspiration with the bottle at a very low height (around 50 cm). Refill the anterior chamber with balanced salt solution (BSS) and seal the incisions.

Removal of the Crystalens Five-0 should be very rare; but armed with the correct techniques, patient outcomes can be maximized.

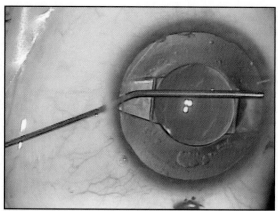

Figure 5. Backfill from the sulcus with viscoelastic.

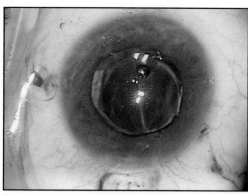

Figure 7. Miostat instilled to constrict the pupil.

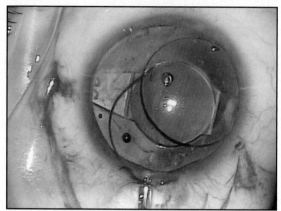

Figure 6. Insert the trailing haptic of the piggyback lens.

CHAPTER 232

PERSONAL EXPERIENCE WITH ENDOPHTHALMITIS IN RLE

Robert Morris, MRCP, FRCS, FRCOphth

Endophthalmitis is a rare and potentially devastating complication of cataract surgery. The incidence reported in the literature is between 1:2000 and 1:4000. There are no published studies reporting the incidence following refractive lens surgery (RLE). I experienced a case of endophthalmitis in a 62-year-old patient 2 years after starting RLE.

Case Report

A 62-year-old man consulted me on the recommendation of a patient who had referred 12 patients in the previous 6 months. He was emmetropic until his early 40s, but now wore varifocals (OD +2.75 / −1.75 × 40 20/20; OS +4.00 / −1.00 × 130 20/20−). He was a jeweller and fly fisherman and desired spectacle independence. After 2 consultations and extensive counselling, I proceeded to perform a refractive lens exchange on the dominant right eye using a ReSTOR (Alcon, Fort Worth, TX) multifocal lens.

Surgery performed in a dedicated ophthalmic operating facility was uneventful. He was pleased with his vision on the fourth postoperative day, but on the fifth postoperative day, he called complaining of reduced vision and pain. I examined him and he had the typical signs of endophthalmitis with mild corneal edema, hypopyon, vitreous cells with a poor retinal view, and vision of counting fingers only. I performed a vitreous tap and injected intravitreal antibiotics (vancomycin 0.2 mg and ceftazidime 2.25 mg). Gram stain was negative and no organisms grew from the culture of a vitreous sample.

The eye remained inflamed and the corneal edema progressed over the next 5 days. The clinical signs finally began to improve and his vision had improved to 20/60 by day 22. The corneal edema had resolved, but he was unable to work or drive. He was back at work part time and driving 2 months post-RLE but complaining of severe floaters as a result of extensive vitreous debris

His vision was 20/20 at 6 months with a reading vision of N10, and he elected to have RLE performed on his left eye with a good outcome. At 9 months, he elected to have a right vitrectomy to clear the vitreous debris.

Subsequently he sought legal advice about compensation for the effect the infection had on his life. After correspondence between lawyers, the case was not pursued because the clinical records documented that the risk and implication of endophthalmitis had been explained, not only preoperatively, but at every stage in the management of the infection. Preoperatively, the clinical information and consent form given to the patient also explained the risks.

Lessons Learned

RLE has a risk of endophthalmitis. The incidence is unknown and may be less than in cataract surgery as patients are generally younger and fitter than the cataract population. All patients undergoing RLE need to be informed that unlike laser in situ keratomileusis (LASIK) the procedure is an intraocular procedure. They should be fully informed not only of the risk of infection and the potential outcome, but also the time taken for recovery in the event of an infection and the potential implications on work and lifestyle.

RLE surgery should, as in this case, be carried out in an accredited ophthalmic operating facility. I do not think this case would have been defensible if surgery had taken place in a nonaccredited office environment.

It is essential that patients are given a fact sheet not only of the benefits of RLE but also the risks. Appropriate informed consent should be obtained by the operating surgeon and a discussion of complications should be documented in the clinical records.

Postoperatively, patients should have 24-hour emergency access to the surgical team who should have access to emergency operating facilities.

Once the diagnosis has been made, the patient should be kept fully informed, given realistic expectations, and receive a thorough explanation of the course of management.

Do not charge self-pay patients for any further consultations or surgery relating to the treatment. What prompted legal action in this case was that the patient, who lived 50 miles away, wished to have his vitrectomy carried out by a local surgeon, and he had to incur the costs for this additional care.

Endophthalmitis Prophylaxis

My current endophthalmitis prophylaxis regime is the application of 0.5% povidone iodine to the ocular surface prior to surgery and intracameral cefuroxime at the end of the surgical procedure.

In the European Society of Cataract and Refractive Surgeons (ESCRS) randomized trial on intracameral antibiotics, 1 mg cefuroxime injected into the anterior chamber at the end of surgery reduced the incidence of endophthalmitis 5 fold.[1] The Swedish national cataract database data showed similar efficacy of intracameral cefuroxime.[2] Both studies question the benefit of topical antibiotics both pre- and postoperatively. The latter study demonstrated a trend for an increased risk of endophthalmitis for corneal and clear temporal wounds.

References

1. Endophthalmitis Study Group, European Society of Cataract and Refractive Surgeons. Prophylaxis of postoperative endophthalmitis following cataract surgery: results of the ESCRS multicenter study and identification of risk factors. *J Cataract Refract Surg.* 2007;33:978-988.
2. Lundstrom M, Wedje G, Stenevi U, et al. A Nationwide Prospective Study Evaluating Incidence in Relation to Incision type and Location. *Ophthalmology.* 2007;114:866-870.

CHAPTER 233

CAPSULAR TEARS, WEAK ZONULES— CAN I STILL IMPLANT A REFRACTIVE IOL?

Uday Devgan, MD, FACS

Capsular Tears and Weak Zonules: Can I Still Implant a Refractive IOL?

Performing premium intraocular lens (IOL) surgery requires premium visual results, and that typically requires a premium anatomic result. Because the capsular bag and zonular apparatus is responsible for fixating and centering the lens implant and for coupling with the ciliary muscle, in the case of accommodating lenses, every effort must be taken to achieve proper positioning and fixation.

Monofocal or multifocal IOLs require good centration, fixation, and placement within the posterior chamber. Accommodating IOLs require the same level of placement but they must also be coupled to the ciliary muscle for optimum function and maximum accommodative amplitude. Capsular weakness, a ruptured posterior capsule, or a large errant capsular tear usually precludes the use of an accommodative IOL but may still allow the use of fixed-position refractive IOLs. For this reason, we will limit our initial discussion to fixed-position refractive IOLs, with a special section devoted to accommodating IOLs at the end of this chapter.

Anterior Capsular Tears/ Radialization

A well-centered, continuous, curvilinear capsulorrhexis of an appropriate size helps to keep the IOL within the capsular bag. However, if the capsulorrhexis is irregular or there is a radial tear, most refractive IOLs can still be implanted. Care should be taken to retrieve the errant tear and complete a continuous capsulorrhexis without having the tear extend to the zonules or beyond. The refractive IOL, both fixed as well as accommodating, can now be placed within the capsular bag with the haptics oriented 90 degrees away from the errant tear.

These patients tend to do well with few postoperative problems related to the errant anterior capsulorrhexis.

Posterior Capsule Rupture

When the posterior capsule ruptures during cataract surgery, the patient is at risk for many sight-threatening complications. Retinal complications such as breaks, detachments, and macular edema are of major concern. Additionally, these patients are more prone to endophthalmitis due to the loss of the barrier function of the posterior capsule.

The surgeon's primary goals when a posterior capsule rupture is detected are to minimize further damage to the capsule, to limit vitreous prolapse, and to prevent posterior displacement of lens fragments. Once the eye has been stabilized and the anterior segment is found to be free of lens material as well as any prolapsed vitreous, options for IOL placement can be evaluated by the surgeon.

If the posterior capsule rupture is limited and a continuous, central, posterior capsulorrhexis can be performed, then the IOL can be placed within the capsular bag (Figure 1).

If the posterior capsule rupture is irregular, then it is better to place the IOL in the ciliary sulcus. Note that only 3-piece fixed-position refractive IOLs should be placed within the sulcus and that any single-piece IOL, particularly acrylic ones, should not be placed in the sulcus. These single-piece acrylic IOLs can cause iris chaffing and pigment dispersion, leading to uveitis, glaucoma, and iris defects, if placed in the ciliary sulcus. The traditional method is to place the entire 3-piece IOL into the sulcus. This will necessitate using a lower IOL power due to the more anterior resting position of the lens (Figure 2).

If there is a well-centered anterior capsulorrhexis, the IOL haptics can be placed within the sulcus and the optic captured behind the capsulorrhexis. This allows for more secure fixation as well as a more accurate postoperative refractive result. This is the preferred technique in cases of a posterior capsule rupture (Figure 3).

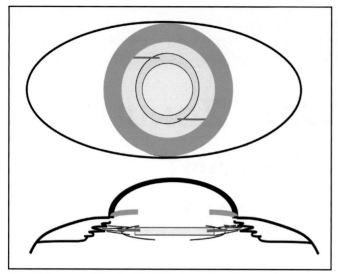

Figure 1. Placement of the entire IOL, both haptics and the optic, within the capsular bag in the presence of a posterior capsular opening.

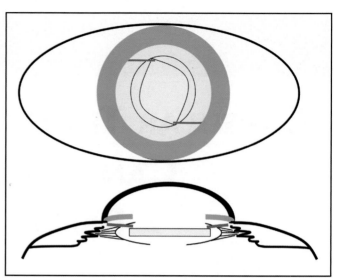

Figure 3. The haptics are in the ciliary sulcus and the optic is captured through the anterior capsulorrhexis into the capsular bag. This allows for very secure fixation of the IOL.

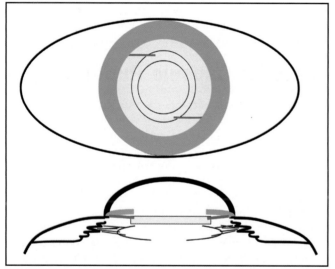

Figure 2. Placement of the entire IOL, both haptics and optic, in the ciliary sulcus in the presence of an open posterior capsule.

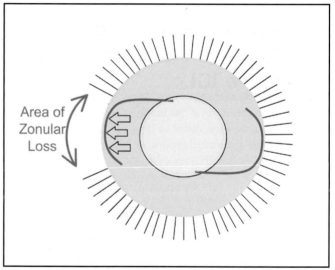

Figure 4. IOL placed in the capsular bag with the haptic at the area of zonular loss to bolster the support at the equator.

Weak and Missing Zonules

Certain ocular conditions, such as pseudoexfoliation or trauma, can result in weak or missing zonules, which can compromise the proper positioning of the refractive IOL. Depending on the degree of zonular instability, there are options for IOL positioning.

If there is a small, focal area of zonular loss, then the IOL can still be placed within the capsular bag, with care taken to ensure that the IOL haptics are positioned at the axis of the zonular loss. This will allow the spring action of the haptic to bolster the capsular equator (Figure 4).

The IOL, if it is of the 3-piece variety, can also be placed in the ciliary sulcus, but with the haptics oriented 90 degrees away from the area of focal zonular loss. The IOL power will need to be adjusted downward due to the more anterior placement of the optic (Figure 5).

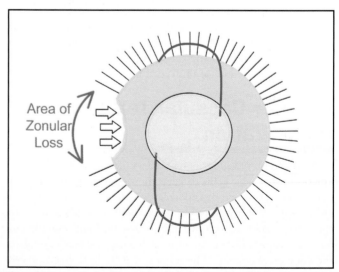

Figure 5. IOL placed in the ciliary sulcus with the haptics oriented 90 degrees away from the area of zonular loss, which tends to move inwards due to lack of support.

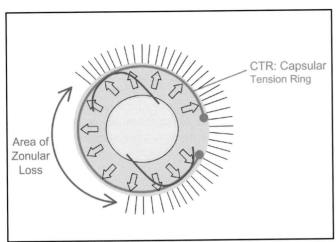

Figure 6. IOL placed in the capsular bag after insertion of a capsular tension ring which distributes force over the entire capsular and addresses the large area of zonular loss.

If the zonular weakness or loss is more extensive, then a capsular tension ring can be placed within the bag to distribute force evenly over the entire capsular equator. The IOL can then be placed within the capsular bag without any adjustment to the calculated IOL power (Figure 6).

For diseases with progressive zonular loss, there exists the possibility that the IOL, even with proper initial positioning or use of a capsular tension ring, will become displaced and decentered. This will result in markedly decreased performance. In these cases, it may be more prudent to implant a monofocal IOL, particularly one with zero spherical aberration, as its optical performance is relatively insensitive to decentration.

Accommodating IOLs

Due to their need to be coupled to the ciliary muscle, accommodating IOLs require more meticulous attention to detail during surgery as they must be placed within the capsular bag for optimum function.

A mild to moderate irregularity in the anterior capsulorrhexis would still allow in-the-bag implantation of an accommodating IOL, but care should be taken to orient the haptics away from this area. A large anterior capsule irregularity will likely cause difficulty with long-term stability of an accommodating IOL.

A posterior capsule rupture usually means that the accommodating IOL cannot be placed. The exception is for a small, central rupture that can be converted into a posterior capsulorrhexis, which is smaller than the optic diameter and is completely covered by the optic. This is rarely achieved and most posterior capsule ruptures will preclude the use of these IOLs.

Similarly, a large defect in the zonular support structures is a contraindication to use of an accommodating IOL because it will not be possible to couple the IOL to the ciliary muscle and the expected accommodative amplitude will be quite low. With a small, focal defect, it may be possible to implant the accommodative IOL in the capsular bag, though this may negatively affect performance.

Although the vast majority of our planned refractive cataract surgeries go as planned, there will be instances where there is an errant capsular tear, a posterior capsular rupture, or significant zonular disruption. In many of these cases, we can still implant a presbyopia-correcting IOL and achieve a good visual outcome. However, in other situations the damage may be so significant that the intended IOL cannot be safely and securely implanted in the eye. For this reason, as part of our routine preoperative discussion, we need to alert the patient to the slim possibility that the intended IOL may not always be the one implanted at the time of surgery.

Can I Put a Multifocal IOL in the Sulcus?

Richard J. Mackool MD

Either a 3-piece ReSTOR (Alcon Laboratories, Fort Worth, TX) or ReZoom (Advanced Medical Optics, Santa Ana, CA) multifocal intraocular lens (IOL) is suitable for sulcus implantation. Placement of either the single-piece ReSTOR or Crystalens (Eyeonics, Aliso Viejo, CA) in the ciliary sulcus is not recommended by their manufacturers.

If there is an intact capsulorrhexis that is smaller than the 6-mm optic of the multipiece ReSTOR or ReZoom lenses, I recommend placement of the IOL in the sulcus, followed by depression of the optic through the capsulorrhexis opening, in order to "capture" the optic within the capsular opening. This provides the same positional stability to the IOL as does standard capsular fixation, and IOL power calculations remain unchanged. In other words, the IOL power remains the same as if calculated for a lens placed entirely within the capsular sac. It has also been my experience that peripheral iris "chafing" does not occur with this type of IOL positioning, most likely because there is neither significant postoperative motion of the atonic peripheral iris nor of the lens haptics.

Can I Put a Multifocal IOL in the Sulcus?

Roger F. Steinert, MD

The truism that "the best way to manage a complication is to avoid it" has never been more true than with presbyopia-correcting intraocular lenses (IOLs).

If the defect is in the integrity of the capsulorrhexis edge, but the posterior capsule is still intact, then secure IOL fixation is usually possible with good centration.

The surgeon should remember to incise the capsulorrhexis edge 180 degrees from the location of the break in order to avoid asymmetric capsule contraction postoperatively that may lead to decentration of the IOL. If the capsulorrhexis is damaged enough to create uncertainty about secure capsular bag fixation, then implantation of an accommodating IOL should not be done. A multifocal IOL with (polymethylmethacrylate) PMMA haptics may be successfully fixated in the ciliary sulcus, as long as the eye is not too large for stable sulcus fixation of the haptics. Use of a smaller diameter IOL intended for capsular bag fixation may lead to decentration or propeller rotation of the IOL, with chronic inflammation in larger eyes. Sulcus fixation of a 1-piece acrylic IOL must be avoided in any eye, as these haptics have a high rate of causing chronic inflammation due to the excessive contact of the thick haptic with the posterior iris and ciliary body. If the IOL is fixated in the sulcus, remember to reduce the IOL power by approximately 0.5 diopter (D), as the optic location will be more anterior than assumed when the IOL power was chosen.

If the posterior capsule has been violated but the capsulorrhexis is intact, then the surgeon has the option of implanting a multifocal lens with the haptics remaining anterior to the anterior capsule and the optic prolapsed posteriorly through and captured by the capsulorrhexis, in the technique originally described by Tobias Nauhann, MD. An accommodating IOL cannot be used in this situation. If this technique is employed for a multifocal IOL, the capsulorrhexis must be well centered on the pupil to avoid postoperative optical problems, so care in performing the capsulorrhexis in every case is especially important. The power of the IOL will be minimally affected, but the surgeon would be wise to check the IOL calculations and, if the power chosen was bordering on being too myopic, then reduce the power by one step (0.5 D). In most cases, no power change will be needed.

If both the posterior capsule and the capsulorrhexis are defective, then the surgeon must determine if there is enough residual capsule to attempt sulcus fixation. A highly experienced surgeon might be successful in performing a McCannel peripheral iris suture fixation of a multifocal IOL. However, the IOL must be nearly perfectly centered to avoid postoperative optical problems, and this can be a challenge with mechanical suture techniques. The safer alternative is to implant a monofocal IOL, either in the anterior or posterior chamber, depending upon the surgeon's preference and experience. The surgeon should have had the discussion with the patient preoperatively about the possibility that operative circumstances might make the use of a monofocal IOL preferable.

CHAPTER 234

Dry Eye After Refractive Surgery

Ahmad M. Fahmy, OD, FAAO and David R. Hardten, MD, FACS

Epidemiology

In order to develop and implement the most appropriate treatment plan for the postsurgical dry eye patient, a good understanding of pathogenesis of chronic dry eye is the key. The perioperative evaluation and treatment of the refractive surgical patient with dry eyes should be approached with a similar strategy used in treating chronically dry eyes. Comparing the physiologic changes postoperatively to eyes without prior surgery can help us understand and anticipate iatrogenic pathology or exacerbation of existing pathology. Patients suffering from ocular irritation caused by tear film instability are very difficult to manage successfully. An estimated 10 million people in the United States comprise this group of patients suffering from dry eye syndrome.1 Chronic dry eye is more prevalent in females than males and more advanced in postmenopausal women using hormone replacement therapy (HRT). Patients developing chronic dry eye after ocular surgery are also more likely to be female, as demonstrated by low Schirmer's scores and corneal punctate epitheliopathy. In our experience, patients suffering from severe dry eye can be considerably functionally impaired due to fluctuation of visual acuity, halos, glare, and discomfort.

Definition and Classification

Dry eye researchers have historically struggled to produce a concise definition and classification of dry eye conditions. In 1995, the National Eye Institute/Industry Dry Eye Workshop defined dry eye, or keratoconjunctivitis sicca, as: "A disorder of the tear film due to tear deficiency or excessive evaporation that causes damage to the intrapalpebral ocular surface and is associated with symptoms of discomfort."[2,3]

This classification of dry eye is further delineated into patients with aqueous tear deficiency and those with increased evaporative loss. Deficient aqueous production is a hallmark finding in patients with Sjögren's syndrome and other autoimmune diseases. Evaporative loss can be exacerbated by meibomian gland disease or other surface abnormalities such as excessive exposure or evaporation due to lid abnormalities. Other terms often used for this constellation of symptoms are dysfunctional tear syndrome or ocular surface disease. In addition to these factors, we have since uncovered additional key components of a dry eye: tear film hyperosmolarity and ocular surface inflammation. As such, the definition of dry eye has been changed after considerable investigation by the International Dry Eye Workshop (DEWS). The definition now reads: "Dry eye is a multifactorial disease of the tears and ocular surface that results in symptoms of discomfort, visual disturbance, and tear film instability with potential damage to the ocular surface. It is accompanied by increased osmolarity of the tear film and inflammation of the ocular surface."[3]

After approximately 3 years of investigation, the DEWS report places focus on damage of the ocular surface caused by hyperosmolarity and inflammation. There is now a growing correlation between these two additional factors and the resultant symptoms in dry eye. Tear film instability and osmolarity are accurate markers of disease, and need to be further investigated in clinical trials targeting the development of new treatments.

Surgical Patient Selection and Education

Patients interested in improving their vision or decreasing their dependence on glasses and contact lenses by undergoing cataract surgery, natural lens replacement (NLR), or refractive surgery but who also report dry eye symptoms should be approached carefully. Patient education regarding postoperative visual acuity fluctuation and irritation should be performed due to the typical increase in dryness, especially during the early phase of recovery. For most patients, increased dryness after surgery is tolerable and not visually significant. Therefore, chronic dry eye is not a definite contraindication to

Table 1

PERTINENT MEDICAL HISTORY

Systemic Pathology	Symptoms	Medications
Systemic lupus erythematosus	Contact lens intolerance	Antidepressants
Stevens-Johnson's syndrome	Foreign body sensation	Antihistamines
Environmental allergies	Fluctuation of vision	Antihypertensives
Neurological pathology	Redness	
Sjögren's syndrome		
Rheumatoid arthritis		
Acne rosacea		
Sarcoidosis		
Menopause		
OCP		

Table 2

PREOPERATIVE CLINICAL EVALUATION

Ocular Surface	Systemic
Punctate epithelial keratopathy	Dental and periodontal disease (Sjögren's)
Meibomian gland inspissation	Rhinophyma
Tear meniscus / Schirmer's	
Eyelid collarette formation	
Conjunctival pleating	
Exposure/ectropion	
Conjunctival tylosis	
Hyperosmolarity	
Palpebral fissure	
Telangiectasia	
Tear break up time	

cataract surgery, NLR or refractive surgery. However, patients with ocular surface disease should be treated aggressively and counseled regarding the likelihood of exacerbation of symptoms postoperatively. Systemic pathology and medications used by the patient can contribute to a dry ocular surface (Table 1).

In our experience, common dry eye symptoms are chronic irritation, fluctuation of visual acuity, and an uncomfortable foreign body sensation. Just as it is important to identify systemic causes of dry eye, there are many clinical findings that can help the careful clinician identify ocular surface pathology (Table 2).

Improving surface lubrication, and if present, controlling a concomitant inflammatory component can considerably improve objective and subjective success postoperatively. Postsurgical patients with a markedly compromised tear film due to a combined mechanism etiology can experience significant fluctuations in visual acuity (Table 3). Most patients report that this fluctuation improves just after a blink or following instillation of artificial tears. It has been reported that the surface regularity index (SRI) does not significantly change immediately after instillation of artificial tears in healthy, nonoperative eyes.[4,5] In the case of treatment with laser in situ keratomileusis (LASIK), it is reasonable to attribute some visual acuity fluctuation to poor tear spread over the newly contoured central depression in myopic cases and the resultant increased dioptric power of the precorneal tear film. Intermittent blur after blinking and irritation are bothersome symptoms that can disappoint cataract or refractive surgery patients whose visual expectations continue to increase with progressive improvements in surgical technology. With improved surgical technique and increased experience of the

Table 3

SIGNIFICANT FACTORS AFFECTING POST- SURGICAL CHRONIC DRY EYE AND REGRESSION

- Moderate to high refractive error / ablation depth
- Subjective reports of dry eye symptoms
- Decreased corneal sensation
- Dry working environment
- Prolonged computer use
- Ocular surface disease
- Size of incision
- Smoking
- Female

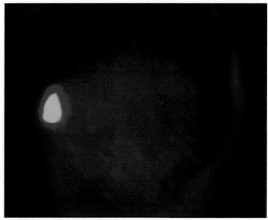

Figures 2. Epitheliopathy in a patient that had normal looking epithelium prior to topical anesthetic and dilating drops.

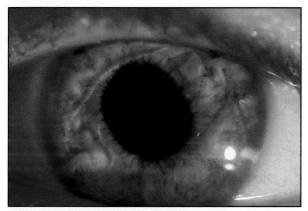

Figure 1. Verisyse phakic anterior chamber lens.

surgeon, LASIK may still be the procedure of choice for mild to moderate levels of myopia in healthy eyes, as well as those with mild to moderate dry eyes, even after cataract surgery.

It is important to carefully look for evaporative as well as inflammatory causes of dry eye, as many patients will present with both a tear production deficiency and an evaporative component.

In a survey conducted in 2001, members of the American Society of Cataract and Refractive Surgeons (ASCRS), listed dry eye as the most common "complication" of LASIK.[6] Once chronic dry eye has been identified and treated aggressively, evidence shows that regression after LASIK is reduced.[7] It is always best to delay any type of refractive surgery until after a smooth, well-lubricated ocular surface has been achieved. In other procedures, such as conductive keratoplasty or implantation of a phakic anterior chamber (Verisyse) lens one should also carefully evaluate the ocular surface (Figure 1).

Optics and the Precorneal Tear Film

The efficiency of light transmission to the inner eye is largely dependent on the refractive relationship between the precorneal tear film and air. A healthy tear film is an essential requirement for superior corneal refraction and transparency,

as well as for protection from disease. Acting in concert, the three components provide a precorneal tear film which is evenly distributed across the ocular surface. This refracting surface must be free of imperfections to avoid disturbing the visual image. A strong lipid layer works to maintain optical integrity by retarding evaporation and maintaining exceptional visual acuity.[4] The precorneal tear film is the ultimate refracting surface of the eye. It is maintained by the total environment provided by the eyelids, conjunctiva, and secretory glands. Malfunction of any of the components of this intricate system can lead to secondary ocular surface disease and compromised vision. When there is advanced tissue compromise secondary to the breakdown of the precorneal tear film, the effect on vision can be so great as to affect Snellen acuity and contrast sensitivity, or to produce glare and halos around a point source of light.[8] Visual symptoms of dry eye may also include considerable photophobia and the induction of higher-order aberrations.[8]

Ocular Surface Stress Test

Environmental induction of dry eye has been carefully studied and provides the careful clinician with more diagnostic tools.[9] As such, investigation of the patient's daily environment is essential. In addition to environmentally induced stress, evaluation of ocular surface changes secondary to topical medications is also helpful in identifying surface disease.

The standard eye examination requires installation of diagnostic eye drops, which may reveal pre-existing disease. Frequent use of preserved topical medications may produce punctate epithelial keratopathy (PEK), which may not have been visible prior to administration of the drops in these patients (Figures 2 and 3).

Ocular surface "stress testing" thus acts much like a stress test that may be performed on any other organ system to help the clinician uncover pathology. If significant PEK is observed after installation of diagnostic drops in clinic, this is a clear indication of the need to consider more aggressive therapy in these patients, especially around the time of surgery.

If a dry eye patient develops an infection, or develops pathology that necessitates short term or prophylactic topical

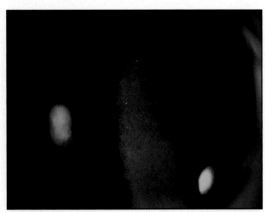

Figure 3. Epitheliopathy in a patient that had normal looking epithelium prior to topical anesthetic and dilating drops.

medications, this becomes a difficult combination to balance. However, there is reliable evidence that non-preserved topical medications, including fortified antibiotics, can retain sterility after opening the vial for 4 weeks if kept in a sterile environment at 4°C.[10]

Tear Production, Clearance, and Sensitivity

The ocular surface and the lacrimal gland work together as a functional unit to stimulate lacrimal tear production. Sensory nerves in the corneal epithelium and stroma trigger the blink mechanism to spread tears uniformly and clear tears from the ocular surface by pumping used tears into the nasolacrimal ducts. Eyelid inflammation, surgical severing of corneal nerves, and laser ablation results in disruption of this important feedback loop, obstructing neural sensory input to the lacrimal gland. As a result, tear production, clearance, and ocular surface sensitivity to touch (including the conjunctiva) decrease. It has been reported that depressed conjunctival sensation after LASIK is caused by placement of the microkeratome suction ring on perilimbal conjunctival nerves.[11] On the question of clearance, it has been suggested that a decreased blink rate caused by corneal denervation and the resultant increased tear film evaporation are important altered tear dynamic factors postoperatively.[11] Decreased tear clearance exacerbates dry eye conditions, as pooling of inflammatory constituents damages the ocular surface. Precorneal tear film dysfunction may be more prominent in eyes that have undergone multiple surgical procedures, including refractive procedures as well as cataract extraction. In such cases, the irregular corneal surface limits sustained and even corneal lubrication.[11]

Neurotrophic Epitheliopathy

A temporarily neurotrophic cornea results from ocular surgery.[12] Nerve bundles course through the corneal tissue to carry neural input through the stroma and the epithelium centrally. This corneal denervation effect is more prominent in higher refractive corrections requiring deeper ablations for myopic, as well as hyperopic cases in laser refractive surgery. Large incision cataract surgery or limbal relaxing incisions can

have a similar effect. Disruption of corneal innervation induces anesthesia and hypoesthesia that result in significant punctate epithelial erosions. Laser ablation results in depression of corneal sensation of surface dryness and results in decreased feedback and stimulation of the lacrimal gland, putting in motion a cycle of events adversely affecting ocular lubrication. The incidence of symptomatic neurotrophic epitheliopathy has been reported to be approximately 4% at 1 to 3 months in LASIK.[12] Postsurgical patients may present early postoperatively without discomfort when the clinical presentation of epithelial erosion is primarily due to early hypoesthesia. Many notice the blur in vision, but not discomfort. It has been demonstrated that the number of stromal nerve fiber bundles decreases by nearly 90% in the early postoperative period after LASIK.[13] The regeneration of these nerve fiber bundles takes place slowly. At 1 year postoperatively, some reports show that the number of nerve fiber bundles remains less than 50% of that just prior to LASIK, although most studies demonstrate corneal sensation returns to normal preoperative levels at approximately the 6 month period.[13] Nasally hinged flaps tend to sever fewer of these nerve fiber bundles and therefore dry eye symptoms postoperatively may be less when creating a nasally hinged flap during LASIK.[13] Enhancement may cause a return of symptoms and clinical evidence of neurotrophic epitheliopathy because lifting the flap once again interrupts reinnervation.

Patients after photorefractive keratectomy (PRK) have been thought not to develop a clinically significant degree of epithelial neuropathy, even though corneal sensation is reduced for approximately 3 months postoperatively. Yet in our experience, PRK can still be associated with relatively long periods of epitheliopathy in some patients.

Patients after cataract surgery also have significant increases in dry eye symptoms and findings.[14] Most patients have some increase in ocular discomfort and exacerbation of ocular discomfort to environmental triggers as measured by the Ocular Surface Disease Index even several months after surgery.

Regression

Sustained dysfunction of the precorneal tear film after LASIK exacerbated by the wound healing response has been reported to contribute significantly to regression of the refractive result. Albietz and colleagues demonstrated an incidence of 27% myopic regression in chronic dry eye patients after LASIK compared to 7% without chronic dry eye in a group of 565 eyes studied retrospectively.[7] There are several proposed mechanisms of regression. One proposed by Albietz and colleagues involves epithelial hyperplasia due to increased release of epidermal growth factor. It is reasonable to consider that repeated mechanical trauma during blinking of the dry ocular surface postoperatively increases the release of epidermal growth factor, leading to epithelial hyperplasia and regression.[7]

A second reasonable mechanism to consider involves keratocyte apoptosis. It has been suggested that dry eye after LASIK is related to apoptosis of stromal keratocytes induced by inflammatory cytokines.[1] Autoimmune disorders direct cytotoxic reactions in which antibodies and lymphocytes damage surrounding tissue. The most common inflammatory disorder encountered is blepharitis, but as discussed earlier, many patients suffer from a variety of autoimmune conditions that cause similar inflammatory cellular damage. When antibodies to specific cells affix to their corresponding antigen and activate complement on their cell surface to accomplish cytolysis, they are referred to as cytotoxic antibodies. When the cells are foreign, cytolysis is protective; when the cells are self, autoimmune disease occurs. Cells containing mediators are activated by stimuli other than an antigen/antibody union on their surface. Neural, chemical, and physical stimuli also induce mediator release, initiating symptoms that resemble allergic reactions, even though no allergen exposure has taken place. Even in the case of the perfectly healthy postoperative eye, during the wound healing inflammatory cascade, infiltration of the ocular surface with T-cells causes tissue damage that leads to apoptosis of stromal keratocytes, underscoring the importance of anti-inflammatory medical treatment.

Dry Eye and Phacoemulsification

Evidence of subjective and objective signs of dry eye is well documented after excimer laser refractive surgery. Clinical trials have also demonstrated lower postoperative Schirmer's I scores in patients undergoing cataract extraction.[15] Extracapsular cataract extraction requires a large limbal incision of approximately 4 to 5 clock hours of limbal tissue, which severs corneal nerve bundles and disrupts the regulation of basal tear secretion in the superior half of the cornea. Resultant loss of corneal sensitivity can often persist for more than 2 years after surgery. Severe dry eye epitheliopathy is more common in patients with associated collagen vascular disorders including rheumatoid arthritis, Sjögren's, and polyarteritis nodosa. Decreased corneal epithelial cell mitosis and delayed wound healing have also been shown to be significantly increased in dry eye patients undergoing cataract extraction.

The healthy tear film is a complex of proteins, glycoproteins, lysozyme, and lipids that work to protect the ocular surface from infection. The large, multifunctional glycoprotein 340 found in tear film isolates demonstrates antimicrobial properties resulting in aggregation and pathogen clearance of *Streptococci, S. Aureus, S. Mutans,* and *H. Influenzae*.[16] Glycoprotein 340 has also been implicated in the regulation of epithelial growth, proliferation, and differentiation.[16] Additionally, SPD, a lipophilic molecule that opsonizes bacteria, is also found in the precorneal tear film, and has been shown to inhibit corneal invasion by *Pseudomonas*.[17] The ability of the healthy tear film to protect the eye underscores the importance of placing a strong emphasis and careful scrutiny of the health of the ocular surface in the cataract patient. Perioperative treatment of the dry eye cataract patient with fourth generation fluoroquinolone is appropriate and very effective. Patients being treated with punctal plugs may also be more likely to become infected due to bacterial colonization within the punctae and punctal plugs.[18] Careful examination of the punctae, replacement of the plugs, and irrigation of the nasolacrimal apparatus is recommended in appropriate cases. In these cases, it may be also more reasonable to consider an alternative treatment for dry eye, and an attempt to stabilize the tear film before moving forward with cataract extraction.

Treatment

TEAR FILM SUPPLEMENTS

There has been a significant increase in our understanding of the pathogenesis of dry eye syndrome and how to successfully treat it. Traditionally, a very common treatment of dry eyes has been supplementing the tear film with artificial tears. Although artificial tear film supplements in solution and ointment form provide immediate lubrication of the ocular surface and patient comfort, it has been shown that use of artificial tear solutions preserved with benzalkonium chloride (BAK) causes significant epithelial toxicity.[19] Nonpreserved formulations provide the added benefit of avoiding increased irritation and are indicated for patients that are increasingly symptomatic shortly after using preserved formulations. Precorneal tear film supplements can alleviate symptoms temporarily and provide an excellent additional treatment, but patients typically achieve long-term relief by addressing the inflammatory component along with decreased tear production. Chronic inflammation of the ocular surface exacerbates early dissipation of the precorneal tear film. In addition to replenishing the tear film, the addition of nutrients and fatty acid-enriched formulations containing eicosapentaenoic acid (EPA) has also been proven to be very helpful in decreasing inflammation, stimulating aqueous tear production, and augmenting the tear film oil layer.[20] Oral administration of essential fatty acids that contain sufficient amounts of gammalinolenic-acid (GLA) stimulate the natural production of anti-inflammatory series one prostaglandins (PGE1).[21] These prostaglandins reduce ocular surface inflammation and reduce the inflammatory process associated with meibomitis. The nutrient cofactors vitamin A, vitamin C, vitamin B6, and magnesium act to facilitate this conversion and are functionally disrupted by alcohol, aging, smoking, elevated cholesterol levels, and other environmental factors.[22] Vitamin E also plays an anti-inflammatory role by stabilizing the essential fatty acids and preventing oxidation. It also works to inhibit cyclooxygenase-2 (CO_2) enzyme activity that promotes the inflammatory response.[22] Vitamin C also enhances the production of immunoglobulin E (IgE) concentrates in tears, which is the first line of basophil and mast cell defense against invading pathogens and allergens that frequently exacerbate dry eye symptoms.[22] These nutrient cofactors also work to modulate goblet cell production.

AUTOLOGOUS SERUM

Another approach aimed at prolonging surface lubrication is the addition of topically applied autologous serum that incorporates growth factors naturally present in the tear film.[23] Autologous serum application has been proven to significantly decrease staining and improve symptoms of ocular surface dysfunction associated with dry eye. This is particularly true in patients with Sjögren's syndrome.[23] Although patients subjectively report autologous serum eye drops are superior to artificial tears in relieving signs and symptoms of dry eye disease, they are not widely used due to limitations, including required special preparation and increased risk of infection.[23]

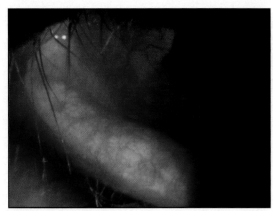

Figure 4. Meibomian Gland Inspissation.

EYELID HYGIENE

In staphylococcal blepharitis (Figure 4), inspissation of the meibomian glands may lead to early evaporation of the tear film and the classic punctate keratopathy that is consistent with symptomatic dry eye. The most effective treatment aimed at improving meibomian gland function and the oily contribution to the tear film is the application of warm compresses to both the upper and lower eyelid, followed by eyelid massage with warm water and a mild soap. During the application of warm compresses, we find it helpful to use heat-absorbing substances rather than repeatedly reheating a clean face towel. We typically advise patients to perform the warm compresses and lid hygiene routine for approximately 5 to 10 minutes twice a day. If the severity of blepharitis is marked, we recommend more sessions (4 times) each day. It is also important to remind the patient to be careful not to use a high concentration of soap that may irritate the eye and break down the tear film further. Meibomitis is significantly improved with diligent application of warm compresses and massage in most patients.

The addition of doxycycline to the treatment regimen may be indicated in many patients with rosacea. Tetracycline (and its derivatives) decreases bacterial lipase activity in vitro.[24] Interestingly, in addition to its bacteriostatic effect, its proposed anti-inflammatory effects plays a significant role in reducing meibomitis. The anti-inflammatory mechanism of action of doxycycline and other antibiotics was proposed by gastrointestinal disease experts who pondered why antibiotics helped many patients with Crohn's disease who had no clinical evidence of infection. Studies suggest that the clinical anti-inflammatory effect of doxycycline is due in part to its antioxidant effects.[24] Free fatty acid concentrations in the meibum from acne rosacea patients have been shown to decrease with oral minocycline treatment. Adding 100 mg of doxycycline orally twice a day or a new form that combines slow release and quick release doxycycline of 40 mg per day reduces meibomitis. This dosage is titrated according to severity and tolerance. Patients using doxycycline should be counseled regarding birth control and possible photosensitivity, nausea, and vaginal candidiasis. Eyelid involvement can also be limited by topically treating the periocular skin and scalp of rosacea patients. Metronidazole (0.75% topical gel) application twice a day and ketoconazole (2.0% shampoo diluted as a lather) once a day are common treatments. With oral and topical skin treatment, 70% to 80% of rosacea patients reported significant improvements in facial redness, papules, pustules, and telangiectasia.[25] In our practice, we typically instruct the patient to avoid applying the metronidazole topical gel close to the eyelid margin, drawing a clear distinction between an eyelid ointment to be applied to the lid margin and a topical gel that is to be applied to the skin around the eye. The brand name version of metronidazole (Noritate, Dermik, Berwyn, PA) is tolerated directly on the lids by many patients who find this helpful in controlling ocular rosacea symptoms. Rosacea patients are also advised to avoid sunlight because it is the single-most common factor triggering exacerbation of rosacea.

CYCLOSPORINE A

In addition to using warm compresses and lid massage, using eyedrops that have an anti-inflammatory effect can improve tear film quality. It has been shown that 0.05% cyclosporine A (CsA) (Restasis, Allergan, Irvine, CA), an immunomodulator, significantly decreases the concentration of the inflammatory cytokine interleukin-6 (IL-6) in the conjunctival epithelium of moderate to severe dry eye patients.[26] This decrease in IL-6 concentration was not different from baseline at the 3-month interval; however, it showed a significant decrease from baseline at 6 months.[26] When adding topical ophthalmic cyclosporine emulsion to the chronic dry eye treatment, the clinician should remind the patient that immediate results are not expected, and consistency in compliance past the 3-month interval is important, although many patients still obtain symptomatic relief with Restasis sooner. We now routinely start patients on topical CsA 1 to 2 months preoperatively when dry eye symptoms or signs are present before cataract or refractive surgery. This regimen is continued for up to 6 months postoperatively. This may help to speed the recovery of vision in the early postoperative period when patients are most symptomatic.

CORTICOSTEROIDS

When a symptomatic patient presents with significant dry eyes, blepharitis, and conjunctival inflammation that is not improved sufficiently with lid hygiene and artificial tear supplements, it may be helpful to use an anti-inflammatory medication such as loteprednol etabonate 0.2% or 0.5% and CsA in combination. Studies demonstrate that dry eye patients treated with loteprednol etabonate showed statistically significant improvement in signs and symptoms, especially those presenting with advanced dry eye and corneal staining. A combined approach could limit further inflammatory damage to the ocular surface by adding a site-specific corticosteroid while CsA begins to deplete cytokine concentrations. As the inflammation and symptoms improve, the regimen can be altered by tapering loteprednol etabonate while continuing to use CsA prophylactically.

NONSTEROIDAL ANTI-INFLAMMATORY DRUGS

Nonsteroidal anti-inflammatory drugs are used to treat mild to moderate pain and relieve inflammation and swelling associated with rheumatoid arthritis. They inhibit prostaglandin synthesis and have been proven to be effective as an added treatment in patients with chronic dry eye symptoms exacerbated by autoimmune inflammation.

ANTI-ALLERGY

If there is an allergic component to the ocular inflammation, targeting the allergic cascade with anti-allergy medications is essential. We typically use olopatadine hydrochloride 0.1% (Patanol [Alcon, Fort Worth, TX]) and epinastine hydrochloride 0.05% (Elestat [Inspire, Durham, NC]) twice a day to limit allergic conjunctival inflammation. Patients suffering from chronic environmental allergies will often already be taking a systemic antiallergy medication such as cetirizine hydrochloride (Zyrtec [Pfizer, New York, NY]). Although its exact mechanism of action has not been identified, an immunomodulator: tacrolimus also was shown to inhibit T-cell activation.[27,28] Pimecrolimus 1% cream and tacrolimus 0.03% or 1.0% ointment (Fujisawa Healthcare, Deerfield, IL) used in the treatment of a common allergic condition affecting the skin have also been shown to be especially effective in treating steroid-induced rosacea.

INVESTIGATIONAL TREATMENTS

Rebamipide 1.0% and 2.0% ophthalmic suspension (Otsuka Maryland Research Institute, Rockville, MD), currently in a phase 3 investigational study, is a quinolinone derivative. The oral form was developed and marketed as a new therapy for gastric ulcers. It causes mucin to cover the internal surface of the stomach, providing a protective coating. It is the increased mucus-producing effect of rebamipide that is spurring the investigation into its use as a promising dry eye treatment.

PUNCTAL OCCLUSION

Conservation of the tear film by punctal occlusion is one of the most useful treatments available for dry eye patients. Having the option of placing punctal plugs in either the lower eyelid or the upper eyelid or both enables the clinician to titrate the amount of tear film conservation needed precisely. While the main therapeutic mechanism of punctal occlusion is simply increasing retention of the tear film, doing so may exacerbate ocular surface dysfunction if inflammatory blepharitis is a factor. Because punctal occlusion also decreases tear clearance by limiting outflow, keeping inflammatory mediators on the ocular surface longer can worsen the condition. In contrast to punctal cautery, reversible occlusion offers needed flexibility as tear production volume fluctuates over time. Cautery is generally a more permanent solution, although we sometimes see cauterized punctae reopen spontaneously. Punctal occlusion has been reported to improve Schirmer's test scores, reduce punctate staining, and, therefore, patient comfort.[29]

Temporary collagen punctal occlusion lasting approximately 4 to 7 days can be used to ascertain if punctal occlusion is effective. If improvement is noted clinically or subjectively, then permanent silicone punctal plugs are implanted. Silicone punctal plugs are permanent in that they do not dissolve; however, they can be removed.

TARSORRHAPHY

Conservation of the tear film can also be accomplished by limiting exposure and evaporation. In severe cases in which other treatments have not been successful, this can be achieved surgically. In the case of the patient who has developed severe epitheliopathy, persistent nonhealing epithelial defects, or sterile corneal ulceration, tarsorrhaphy is indicated. As with punctal occlusion, this can be done permanently or temporarily. Tarsorrhaphy has been proven to be very effective in healing the compromised cornea after chronic corneal tissue damage from dry eye.[1,4]

HORMONE THERAPY

Several studies strongly suggest that the low incidence of Sjögren's syndrome in males is due to the protective effects of androgenic hormones such as testosterone, and that patients suffering from Sjögren's syndrome are significantly androgen deficient.[30,31] Repeatable findings have demonstrated that the meibomian gland is an androgen target organ that becomes dysfunctional with androgen deficiency and that androgens regulate lipid production of sebaceous glands throughout the body. Acinar cells in sebaceous glands respond to these androgens by producing proteins that increase both the synthesis and secretion of lipids that, in turn, contribute to tear film stability. Androgens also act to attenuate autoimmune reactions, whereas estrogens tend to contribute to many autoimmune disorders. The immunosuppressive effects of androgens are due in part to the stimulation of TGF-beta, a potent immunomodulator and anti-inflammatory cytokine.[31]

Conclusion

Dry eye is a very important issue to be considered in patients contemplating ocular surgery of any kind, and during the postoperative management of corneal refractive surgery patients in particular. Postsurgical management is very similar to management in patients without surgery, including careful attention to concomitant lid abnormalities, inflammation, hygiene, artificial tear replacement, and medical therapy such as topical cyclosporine. In most patients, there is a temporary exacerbation of symptoms and signs for 3 to 6 months with eventual return to the preoperative state. By implementing these controlling measures, most patients can actually be more comfortable with their eyes in the long run than they were in their contact lenses.

Key Points

- There is now a paradigm shift in the diagnosis and treatment of dry eye toward the connection of hyperosmolarity and inflammation to tissue damage. The definition submitted by the DEWS report of dry eye now stands as "a multifactorial disease of the tears and ocular surface that results in symptoms of discomfort, visual disturbance, and tear film instability with potential damage to the ocular surface. It is accompanied by increased osmolarity of the tear film and inflammation of the ocular surface."

- For most patients, increased dryness after ocular surgery is tolerable and not visually significant. Therefore, chronic dry eye is not a definite contraindication to refractive surgery or cataract surgery. However, patients with ocular surface disease prior to surgery should be treated aggressively and counseled regarding the likelihood of exacerbation of symptoms postoperatively.

❖ Improving surface lubrication and if present, controlling a concomitant inflammatory component such as blepharitis, will improve objective and subjective success postoperatively.

❖ Postsurgical patients with a markedly compromised tear film due to a combined mechanism etiology can experience significant fluctuations in visual acuity and optical aberration.

❖ Sensory nerves in the corneal epithelium and stroma trigger the blink mechanism to spread tears uniformly, and clear tears from the ocular surface by pumping used tears into the nasolacrimal ducts. Eyelid inflammation, surgical severing of corneal nerves, and laser ablation results in disruption of this important feedback loop, obstructing neural sensory input to the lacrimal gland.

❖ It is well documented that a temporarily neurotrophic cornea results from creation of the flap during LASIK.

❖ Sustained dysfunction of the precorneal tear film after LASIK exacerbated by the wound healing response has been reported to contribute significantly to regression of the refractive result.

References

1. Krachmer J, Mannis MJ, Holland EJ. Dry Eye. *Cornea: Fundamentals, Diagnosis, and Management.* 2nd ed. London, UK: Elsevier Mosby; 2005:521-540.

2. Aim AA, Anderson DR, Berson EL. The lacrimal apparatus. In: Hart WM, ed. *Adler's Physiology of the Eye: Clinical Application.* 9th ed. London, UK: Mosby Yearbook; 1992:18-27.

3. 2007 Report of the International Dry Eye Workshop (DEWS). *Ocular Surf.* 2007;5(2);65-199.

4. Spalton, OJ, Hitchings, RA, Hunter PA. The cornea. *Atlas of Clinical Ophthalmology.* 2nd ed. London, UK: Mosby;1994:6.2-6.30. Dry Eye and Refractive Surgery 371.

5. Nichols KK, Mitchell LG, Zadnik K. Repeatability of clinical measurements of dry eye. *Cornea.* 2004;23:272-285.

6. Solomon KD, Holzer MP, Sandoval HP. Refractive surgery survey 2001. *J Cataract Refract Surg.* 2002;28:346-355.

7. Albietz JM, Lenton LM, McLennan SG. Chronic dry eye and regression after laser in situ keratomileusis for myopia. *J Cataract Refract Surg.* 2004;30:675-684.

8. Puell M, et al. Contrast sensitivity and disability glare in patients with dry eye. *Acta Ophthalmololgica Scandinavica.* 2006;84:527-531.

9. Stefano, B, et al. The controlled-environment chamber: A new mouse model of dry eye. *Invest Ophthalmol Vis Sci.* 2005;46:2766-2771.

10. Pinnita P, et al. Sterility of non-preservative eye drops. *J Med Assoc Thai.* 2005;88 (Suppl 9):S6-10.

11. Battat L, Marci A, Dursun 0, et al. Effects of laser in situ keratomileusis on tear production, clearance, and the ocular surface. *Ophthalmology.* 2001;108:1230-1235.

12. Wilson SE. Laser in situ keratomileusis-induced (Presumed) neurotrophic epitheliopathy. *Ophthalmology.* 2001;108:1082-1087.

13. Toda I, Asano-Kato N, Komai-Hori Y, et al. Laser-assisted in situ keratomileusis for patients with dry eye. *Arch Ophthalmol.* 2002;120:1024-1028.

14. Li X, Hu L, Hu J, Wang W.: Investigation of dry eye disease and analysis of the pathogenic factors in patients after cataract surgery. *Cornea.* 2007;26(Suppl. 1):S16-S20.

15. Jagat R, et al. Outcomes of phacoemulsification in patients with dry eye. *J Cataract Refract Surg.* 2002;28:1386-1389.

16. Jumblatt M, et al. Glycoprotein 340 in normal human ocular surface tissues and tear film. *Infection and Immunity.* 2006;July:4058-4063.

17. Ni, M, Evans DJ, Hawgood S, Anders EM, Sack RA, Fleiszig SM. Surfactant protein D is present in human tear fluid and the cornea and inhibits epithelial cell invasion by *Pseudomonas Aeruginosa. Infect Immun.* 2005;73:2147-2156.

18. Sugita J, et al. The detection of bacteria and bacterial biofilms in punctal plug holes. *Cornea.* 2001;20(4):362-365.

19. Lopez Bernal D, Ubels JL: Quantitative evaluation of the corneal epithelial barrier: effect of artificial tears and preservatives. *Curr Eye Research.* 1991;10(7):645-646.

20. Barham JB, Edens MB, Fonteh AN, et al. Addition of eicosapentaenoic acid to gamma-linolenic acid-supplemented diets prevents serum arachadonic acid accumulation in humans. *I Nut.* 2000;130(8):1925-1931.

21. Barabino S, Ronaldo M, Camicione P. Systemic linoleic and γ-linolenic acid therapy in dry eye syndrome with an inflammatory component. *Cornea.* 2003;22(2):97-101.

22. Fujikawa A, Gong H, Amemiya T, et al. Vitamin E prevents changes in the cornea and conjunctiva due to vitamin A deficiency. *Graefe's Arch Clin Ophthalmol.* 2003;241:287-297.

23. Poon CA, Geerling G, Dart JK. Autologous serum eyedrops for dry eyes and epithelial defects: clinical and in vitro toxicity studies. *Br J Ophthalmol.* 2001;85:1188-1197.

24. Stone DU, Chodosh J. Oral tetracycline for ocular rosacea: an evidence-based review of the literature. *Cornea.* 2004;23:106-109.

25. O'Agostino P, Arocoleo F, Barbera C, et al. Tetracycline inhibits the nitric oxide synthase activity induced by endotoxin in cultured murine macrophages. *Euro J Pharmacal.* 1998;346:283-290.

26. Sail K, Stevenson DO, Mundorf TK, et al. Two multicenter, randomized studies of the efficacy and safety of cyclosporine ophthalmic emulsion in moderate to severe dry eye disease. *Ophthalmology.* 2000;107:631-639.

27. Ashcroft OM, Dimmock P, Garside R, et al. Efficacy and tolerability of topical pimecrolimus and tacrolimus in the treatment of atopic dermatitis: meta-analysis of randomized controlled trials. BMI.doi:10.1136/bmj.38376.439653.D3.

28. Nghiem P, Pearson G, Langley RG. Tacrolimus and pimecrolimus: from clever prokaryotes to inhibiting calcineurin and treating atopic dermatitis. *J Am Acad Dermatol.* 2002;46:228-241.

29. Yen MT, Pflugfelder SC, Feuer Wj. The effect of punctal occlusion on tear production, tear clearance, and ocular surface sensation in normal subjects. *Am J Ophthalmol.* 2001;131:314-323.

30. Schaumberg DA, Buring JE, Sullivan DA, et al. Hormone replacement therapy and dry eye syndrome. *JAMA.* 2001;286:2114-2119.

31. Sullivan DA, Wickam LA, Rocha EM, et al. Androgens and dry eye in Sjögren's syndrome. *Annals New York Academy of Sciences.* 1999;876:312-324.

CHAPTER 235

DO MULTIFOCAL OPTICS COMPROMISE RETINA TREATMENTS?

J. Michael Jumper, MD; Ron P. Gallemore, MD, PhD; and Robert A. Mittra, MD

It is estimated that presbyopia-correcting intraocular lenses (Pr-C IOLs) will account for as many as 20% (≈700,000) of all IOLs placed in the year 2010. These lenses offer presbyopic patients another alternative in surgical refractive correction. At the same time, an aging population and other factors will likely result in higher rates of retinal disease including age-related macular degeneration (AMD) and diabetic retinopathy. It is important to understand what impact, if any, these newer IOLs will have on the diagnosis and management of retinal disease. This chapter discusses the Food and Drug Administration (FDA)-approved and commercially available Pr-C IOLs: Crystalens (Eyeonics, Inc., Aliso Viejo, CA), ReSTOR (Alcon, Fort Worth, TX), and ReZoom (American Medical Optics, Santa Clara, CA) as they relate to retinal examination, laser retinal treatment, and vitreoretinal surgery.

The Ideal IOL for Retinal Evaluation and Treatment

Before discussing Pr-C IOLs, it is important to establish the features of what would be considered an "ideal" intraocular implant lens from a retina specialist perspective (Table 1). First and foremost, this is a lens that would not compromise contrast sensitivity or light transmission in patients with macular disease such as AMD or diabetic macular edema. The "ideal" IOL would also allow excellent viewing of the macula and retinal periphery in both the clinic and operating room; features that are mainly determined by the optic size, material, and design. A large optic is desirable. It allows for a larger anterior capsulorrhexis and improved viewing area. For example, a 6-mm IOL has 44% more optic area than a 5-mm lens, the result being an easier view of the retinal periphery and better stereopsis.[1] The material and design should be such that capsular opacification is minimal. The "ideal" lens would also

be made of a material that would not be affected when in contact with air, gas, perfluorocarbon liquid, silicone oil, or other surgical adjuvants. Silicone oil can adhere irreversibly to IOLs made of silicone.[2] This can lead to vision loss and the need for IOL exchange.

Retinal Examination of Eyes with Presbyopia-Correcting IOLs

In our experience, the refractive optic of the ReZoom lens, the diffractive optic of the ReSTOR lens, and the monofocal Crystalens optic do not compromise examination or diagnostic imaging of the macula including fluorescein angiography and optical coherence tomography. This impression is supported by the experimental work of Negeshi and co-workers who found no significant effect of retinal image quality with a multifocal IOL that was decentered up to 1 mm.[3] As with all IOLs, opacification of the posterior capsule can potentially degrade examination detail. We have not seen opacification rates with these lenses that are out of the ordinary. Laser capsulotomy may have an impact on the movement of the Crystalens. One author (RAM) has performed vitrectomy on a Crystalens patient with vitreous prolapse into the anterior chamber after yttrium-aluminum-garnet (YAG) capsulotomy.

With these IOLs, the peripheral retinal examination is limited only by the extent of peripheral capsular opacification. To date, none of the authors have seen opacification that would limit treatment. Because of the smaller optic of the Crystalens (4.5 to 5.0 mm), capsular opacification may have a greater impact on the peripheral view than with the ReSTOR and ReZoom.

Surgery on Eyes with Presbyopia-Correcting IOLs

There is a greater need for image clarity when performing retinal surgery. In our experience, detailed macular work such as peeling of membranes has not been limited by any of the three optic styles. Our impression is supported by the experimental work by Lim and co-workers who found no significant difference in image quality, stereopsis, and contrast between monofocal and multifocal IOLs.[4]

Capsular opacification remains the main concern with viewing. Because of the smaller optic of the Crystalens, the effective aperture can be 4 mm or less, even with maximal anterior and posterior capsular opening. This can inhibit stereopsis when peeling macular membranes and limit the peripheral view when performing vitrectomy, cryotherapy, or peripheral laser treatment.

An issue unique to vitreous surgery is the effect of image jump, which occurs when, in a well-dilated eye, the view switches from inside the optic to outside the optic. This prism effect can be as great as 1 mm and can lead to disorientation and inadvertent retinal injury. Image jump is more likely to occur in eyes with a smaller diameter IOL optic.

The intraocular lens that a patient has impacts the selection of tamponade when performing vitrectomy. A silicone IOL is a relative contraindication to the use of silicone oil. If the oil makes direct contact with the lens (open posterior capsule or forward migration of oil) it will adhere irreversibly to the lens and may cause optical irregularity. The Crystalens is made of a third-generation silicone material known as biosil. We know of no studies regarding silicone oil adherence to biosil but must assume that it behaves in a similar manner as other silicone IOL material. Both the ReSTOR and ReZoom lenses are made of acrylic and silicone oil should not adhere to them.

Clear Lens Extraction in Presbyopic Myopes

The availability of Pr-C IOLs makes clear lens extraction an attractive refractive option for middle-aged patients with high myopia. We are often asked to evaluate and counsel patients considering such surgery who have peripheral retinal pathology. There is little information regarding the risk of postoperative retinal detachment in this population using modern phacoemulsification techniques, but studies suggest a

detachment risk with an odds ratio proportional to axial length and preoperative refraction (1.21 mm and 0.92 diopter, respectively).[5] In long-term studies of small numbers of patients, the risk of retinal detachment ranges from 2% to 8%. There is no evidence that the retinal detachment risk with Pr-C IOLs differs from that with monofocal IOLs.

There is clear evidence that symptomatic retinal tears and retinal detachment should be treated regardless of whether or not surgery is planned. The evidence is sparse regarding treatment of asymptomatic pathology. For those patients who elect to have surgery, we will often treat asymptomatic retinal tears or round holes with significant subretinal fluid. In general, we do not treat lattice degeneration or round holes with no or minimal associated subretinal fluid. We hope that future studies will better delineate the retinal detachment risks of clear lens extraction.

Conclusion

IOL technology is advancing rapidly. Cataract surgeons, retina specialists, and patients all share the common goal of long-term maximized vision and safety. In general, these lenses do not compromise retinal diagnosis or treatment. Image deterioration is usually from capsular opacification, which is no different than conventional lenses. Based on the differing optic size, design, and material, there are certain circumstances where one Pr-C IOL may be a better selection than another (Table 2):

1. Consider avoiding Pr-C IOLs in patients with known macular disease including high risk dry age-related macular degeneration, wet AMD, active diabetic macular edema, myopic degeneration, and other macular disorders limiting best corrected visual acuity. These are patients who may need the added contrast sensitivity that a monofocal IOL provides and may not have sufficient macular potential to justify the added expense of these lenses.

2. Consider the monofocal Crystalens in patients at risk of macular disease including early AMD, diabetes with no macular edema, and other disorders with the potential to reduce best corrected vision and contrast sensitivity. These patients may benefit from the accommodative properties of this lens but will not experience the decrease in contrast sensitivity and light transmission that can occur with the multifocal IOLs.

3. Consider the larger optic IOLs (6 mm ReZoom and ReSTOR) in patients with peripheral retinal disease. Peripheral capsular opacification can inhibit peripheral retinal treatment to a greater degree if the optic area is smaller (4.5 to 5.0 mm Crystalens).

4. Retinal surgeons should avoid the use of silicone oil in eyes with a Crystalens and an open posterior capsule. The optic material, biosil, is a type of silicone and silicone oil may adhere irreversibly to the optic causing vision compromise.

References

1. McCuen II BW, Klombers L. The choice of posterior chamber intraocular lens style in patients with diabetic retinopathy. *Arch Ophthalmol.* 1991;May;109:615.

2. Khawly JA, Lambert RJ, Jaffe GJ. Intraocular lens changes after short- and long-term exposure to intraocular silicone oil. An in vivo study. *Ophthalmology.* 1998;105:1227-1233.

3. Negishi K, Ohnuma K, Ikeda T, et al. Visual simulation of retinal images through a decentered monofocal and a refractive multifocal intraocular lens. *Jpn J Ophthalmol.* 2005;49:281-286.

4. Lim JI, Kuppermann BD, Gwon A, Gruber L. Vitreoretinal surgery through multifocal intraocular lenses compared with monofocal intraocular lenses in fluid-filled and air-filled rabbit eyes. *Ophthalmology.* 2000;107:1083-1088.

5. Tielsch JM, Legro MW, Cassard SD, et al. Risk factors for retinal detachment after cataract surgery: a population-based case-control study. *Ophthalmology.* 1996;103:1537-1545.

CHAPTER 236

DO MULTIFOCAL OPTICS COMPROMISE RETINAL TREATMENTS?

Abdhish R. Bhavsar, MD

The issue of whether multifocal intraocular lens (IOL) optics compromise retinal treatments is a complex one. A thorough and complete answer would require a systematic examination of the effect of multifocal IOLs on the clinical examination of the retina, on the clinical treatment of the retina with focal and indirect lasers and on retinal surgeries. However, we are unaware of the existence of such a study. In the absence of such a study, the next alternative is to review the experiences of retina surgeons who have had clinical and surgical exposure to multifocal IOL implants.

Multifocal IOLs and Retinal Surgery

Many of the early experiences with multifocal IOLs have taken place in Minnesota. With the clinical trial exposure of and early acceptance of new techniques and technologies by individuals such as Richard L. Lindstrom, David R. Hardten, Thomas Samuelson, MD, and Elizabeth Davis, MD, we had early retinal exposure to patients with multifocal IOLs. We presented our initial surgical experiences performing "Vitrectomy and Membrane Dissection Surgery in Patients with Multifocal Intraocular Lenses" at the annual Vitreous Society Meeting in Alaska on July 6, 1998.[1] We subsequently published our findings in a letter in Ophthalmology in 2001.[2] We reported on the difficulty that we (two different retina surgeons) experienced when performing dissection of epiretinal membranes in two patients with Advanced Medical Optics (Santa Ana, CA) Array multifocal IOLs. These were cases in which the epiretinal membranes were visually symptomatic, but not extremely dense. In addition, the epiretinal membranes did not have any elevated edges. In both of these cases, there was extreme difficulty with fine focusing on the retinal surface and on the macular epiretinal membrane. In both cases, a plano-concave irrigating contact lens was used. In spite of varying the focal distance and magnification of the surgical microscope, there was no improvement in the ability to focus

on the epiretinal membrane or macular surface. It was not simply a loss of depth perception, but an inability to actually focus on the surface of the retina. No matter what magnification was used, there was a blurred view of the macula. This made the epiretinal membrane dissection very difficult (Figure 1).

The other portions of the surgical procedure including the core vitrectomy, peripheral vitrectomy, and air-fluid exchange were performed without difficulty in focusing. The A.V.I. (Advanced Visual Instruments, Inc., New York, NY) wide angle viewing system was utilized for these surgical maneuvers.

Our surgical experience in humans contradicts the findings of an experimental model in rabbits that examined retinal surgical procedures in eyes with multifocal IOLs.[3] While the authors of this animal study concluded that "that multifocal IOLs are compatible with excellent visibility during vitrectomy procedures," we found certain portions of the vitrectomy procedures to be quite difficult. Other retina surgeons have found this to be the case as well.[4-7] One retina surgeon noted that stereo vision is nearly impossible with multifocal IOLs, although a wide angle lens such as the A.V.I. lens can help with visualization.[4]

During the most recent annual meeting of the American Society of Retina Specialists (ASRS) in December 2008, I had asked for a show of hands of the attendees if they had noted difficulty with performing vitrectomy surgery in patients with multifocal IOLs. Approximately one-third of the retina specialists at this meeting raised their hand indicating such difficulty.[5]

I also posted this topic of "multifocal IOLs/accommodative IOLs and retinal disease" for discussion on RetinaTalk, The ASRS Forum for online discussions, on November 18, 2007. There have been a number of cases reported as part of this online forum. One retina surgeon described doing a vitrectomy and membrane dissection in an eye with an "older" multifocal IOL and he was unable to focus on the retina with both eyes open. He had to close one eye to do the case which "worked out okay". In another case in an eye with a retinal detachment and a ReSTOR IOL (Alcon, Fort Worth, TX), the peripheral

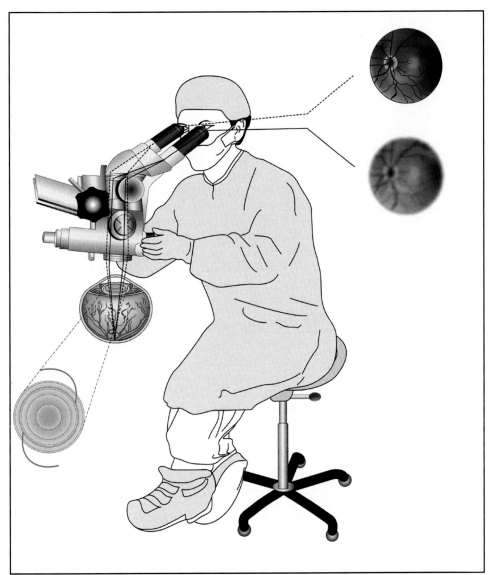

Figure 1. The different optical zones in the multifocal IOL create different images at different focal points. Thus, the surgeon's right eye is viewing one image through one optical zone, which is in focus and clear, and the left eye is viewing a different image through another optical zone, which is out of focus and blurred. This makes good depth perception in the vitreous cavity or on the surface of the retina very difficult or impossible under higher magnification levels.

laser was very difficult due to visualization problems. In a third case involving an eye with proliferative diabetic retinopathy and a ReZoom IOL, the panretinal photocoagulation (PRP) in the office setting was very difficult since a round spot could not be achieved with the laser. Another retina surgeon reported three retinal surgery cases in eyes with multifocal IOLs. He reported difficulty in obtaining "a pristine view with the BIOM". However, a wide field contact lens system helped "a bit in getting a clearer view of the retina, though not as clear as with a biconvex or plano-convex IOL". One case involved vitreomacular traction and the second case involved a macular hole. He found it difficult to perform the membrane dissection and ILM dissection using the contact lens for macular viewing. He had to squint one eye during the surgery "which actually did help somewhat". The third case involved a retinal detachment where he decided to do cryopexy instead of endolaser retinopexy since the view was too difficult through the multifocal IOL to perform endolaser.

It seems that fine focusing under high magnification while performing vitreous surgery and membrane dissection is quite difficult, although performing surgical tasks with a wide-angle lens, such as the A.V.I. lens, is not as difficult. It appears that surgical tasks that do not involve the need for a high degree of depth perception can be performed without issue in eyes that have multifocal IOLs.

With regard to office-based retinal examination with slit-lamp biomicroscopy and indirect ophthalmoscopy, there does not appear to be any notable difficulty. Furthermore, regarding laser procedures with both a contact lens or with an indirect laser, there may be some difficulty but it does not appear that there is any severe difficulty, aside from the difficulty noted above in this section. I have performed a number of retinal exams and laser procedures on patients with multifocal IOLs without incident. However, I would suspect that the application of laser with a contact lens would create aberrations, whereas the application of laser with an indirect lens would be less susceptible to such aberrations.

AMO Array Lens

The Advanced Medical Optics Array lens is made with a zonal progressive multifocal optic with 5 different focus zones on the anterior surface of the lens.[8] The central 2.1 mm of the lens contains the base power. The other peripheral zones contain either the base power or a power that is 3.5 diopters (D) higher than the base power. These zones alternate with the third and the final outer zone having the same base power as the central 2.1-mm zone. Thus, the second and fourth zones contain the higher power, which is 3.5 D greater than the base power. At any time during a retina/vitreous surgical procedure, the surgeon could be viewing images that are as much as 3.5 D disparate in focus between the two eyes. This degree of anisometropia induced by the IOL can significantly alter depth perception. In addition, the multifocal IOL can decrease low-contrast visual acuity in patients by an average of one Snellen line.[8] This loss of contrast may also make surgical maneuvers requiring fine focusing more difficult. Furthermore, other optical aberrations could occur due to retained silicone oil if the Array (Advanced Medical Optics) lens (a silicone lens) is used in an eye that has previously had silicone oil.

It is possible that aside from epiretinal surgery, macular hole, or submacular surgery, the need for high magnification and fine focusing with good depth perception during other retina surgery maneuvers or lasers is not really critical. This may be the case because most other retina procedures and lasers can be performed, albeit to some degree suboptimally, with less-than-perfect depth perception.

ReZoom and ReSTOR IOLs

The ReZoom multifocal IOL is also a refractive IOL with various optical zones and I would expect that the performance during retina surgery would be similar to that of the Array. Although the ReSTOR multifocal IOL is a diffractive IOL with multiple diffractive zones, I would also expect the performance during retina surgery would be similar to that of the Array. With my personal experience in mind, I cannot base this comment in fact, because I have not knowingly performed surgery in a patient with a ReSTOR IOL. However, there have been difficulties reported by other surgeons with these IOLs as described in the previous section entitled, Multifocal IOLs and Retinal Surgery.

Contraindications for Placing Multifocal IOLs

Careful assessment of the retina and of retinal pathology, especially to look for the presence of an epiretinal membrane, should be undertaken prior to considering the placement of a multifocal IOL. If a patient has even a faint epiretinal membrane or other macular pathology, then consideration should be given to foregoing placement of a multifocal IOL. One retina surgeon suggested that all patients who are contemplating having a multifocal IOL should undergo an optical coherence tomography (OCT) examination to rule out the presence of any subclinical epiretinal membrane.[9] If there was any abnormal vitreomacular pathology or epiretinal pathology, then placement of a multifocal IOL would not be recommended.

Accommodating IOLs/ Crystalens

Accommodating IOLs such as the Crystalens (Eyeonics, Inc., Aliso Viejo, CA) can pose some difficulty when viewing or repairing retinal pathology. I have performed many retinal exams with indirect ophthalmoscopy and scleral depression in patients with accommodating IOLs. The small optic size of 4.5 mm does make the view of the peripheral retina more difficult. This permits aberrations from the edge of the optic to more readily interfere with visualization of the peripheral retina. In addition, when there is opacification and/or fibrosis of the anterior capsule and posterior capsule peripheral to the IOL optic, then visualization of the retina is even more difficult. This difficulty of viewing peripheral retinal detail is critical when attempting to rule out a retinal tear or when attempting to treat a peripheral retinal tear or lattice degeneration. Some methods of decreasing the formation of such opacification may include careful removal of any cortical material or even residual lens cells on the posterior capsule and on the posterior surface of the anterior capsule. Special attention should be given to removing lens cells from the peripheral portions of the posterior and anterior capsules. I have repaired a number of retinal detachments in patients with the Crystalens. Viewing the peripheral retina during surgical maneuvers was more difficult due the small optic size. However, the use of the BIOM wide-angle viewing system helped to alleviate some of this difficulty. Other surgical maneuvers such as endolaser and air-fluid exchange were performed with limited difficulty. Although the current model of the Crystalens has a 5.0-mm wide optic, this is still smaller than a standard 6.0-mm IOL and similar principles with respect to edge aberrations and a smaller capsulorrhexis will likely apply.

I am less concerned about accommodating IOLs interfering with retinal management than multifocal IOLs. However, if there is extensive peripheral retinal pathology, that is, lattice degeneration, or a fellow eye history or family history of retinal detachment, then tone must consider the pros and cons of implanting an accommodating IOL with a small optic. At the very least, the anterior segment/refractive surgeon should be aware of these potential difficulties and may opt to discuss these issues with patients who are considering an accommodating IOL.

Small Anterior and Posterior Capsulotomies

Small anterior and posterior capsulotomies are also a concern for the vitreoretinal specialist because they limit and impede visualization of the peripheral retina. Indirect ophthalmoscopy can be affected substantially by an opacified anterior or posterior capsule in the presence of a small capsulotomy. This can make performing laser treatments for peripheral retinal pathology quite difficult. In the case of posterior capsular opacity when an office procedure is performed, the posterior capsule can be readily opened by yttrium-aluminum-garnet

(YAG) capsulotomy. If an intraoperative procedure is performed under such a circumstance, then the vitrectomy cutter can be used to enlarge the posterior capsulotomy. However, in the case of anterior capsular opacity with a small capsular opening, either in the office or in the operating room, the management with either the YAG laser or the vitrectomy cutter requires more effort to clear the axis for better visualization of the peripheral retina.

Modification of Retinal Surgery Techniques in Patients with Multifocal IOLs

Intraocular lens implants have sometimes impeded clear visualization of the vitreous and retina during pars plana vitrectomy surgery. Some modifications of surgical technique have been helpful in these cases. Clear visualization is critical when performing epiretinal surgery. The small central optical zone and the different peripheral optical zones of the multifocal IOL make focusing on the retinal surface difficult. Wide-angle viewing with either the BIOM (Oncothyreon, Bellevue, WA) lens system or 68-degree A.V.I. lens or a green filter on the endoillumination light source may help to improve visualization. Staining epiretinal tissue with Trypan Blue or staining the internal limiting membrane (ILM) with indocyanine green (ICG) may be helpful. Alternatively, Kenalog (Bristol-Myers Squibb Co., Princeton, NJ) can be placed on the retinal surface to help delineate the dissection of epiretinal tissue. Instruments that do not require extremely fine focusing, like the Tano diamond dusted membrane scraper, may be helpful during the epiretinal dissection.

Conclusion

Both anterior segment and vitreoretinal surgeons should be aware of the potential difficulties of performing vitrectomy and membrane dissection surgery in patients who have multifocal IOLs. Pre-existing macular pathology, which may require vitrectomy surgery, may be a relative contraindication for placing a multifocal IOL during cataract extraction. It would be an appropriate practice to discuss these issues with patients who are considering multifocal IOL implants.

In addition, the more that peripheral capsular opacification can be limited in eyes with accommodating IOLs with smaller optics, and the larger that the anterior and posterior capsular openings can be created, the better off your patients will be when retina surgeons have to manage peripheral retinal pathology.

References

1. Vitrectomy and Membrane Dissection Surgery in Patients with Multifocal Intraocular Lenses. Presented at The Vitreous Society Meeting, Alaska, July 6, 1998.

2. Bhavsar AR, Hardten D, Gilbert HD, Lindstrom RL. Vitrectomy and membrane dissection surgery in patients with multifocal intraocular lenses. *Ophthalmology.* 2001;108(9):1513.

3. Lim JI, Kupperman BD, Gwon A, Gruber L. Vitreoretinal surgery through multifocal intraocular lenses compared with monofocal intraocular lenses in fluid-filled and air-filled rabbit eyes. *Ophthalmology.* 2000;107:1083-1088.

4. Personal email communication with Edwin H. Ryan, MD, October 24, 2007.

5. American Society of Retina Specialists Annual Meeting, during the main scientific session, poll of the members present by Abdhish R. Bhavsar, MD, December 4, 2007, Indian Wells, CA.

6. RetinaTalk, The ASRS Forum, posted by Larry Halperin, MD, November 24, 2007 in response to the topic "Multifocal IOLs/Accommodative IOLs and Retinal Disease, authored by Abdhish R. Bhavsar, MD, posted November 18, 2007.

7. RetinaTalk, The ASRS Forum, posted by Narciso Atienza, MD, November 26, 2007, in response to the topic "Multifocal IOLs/Accommodative IOLs and Retinal Disease, authored by Abdhish R. Bhavsar, MD, posted November 18, 2007.

8. Steinert RF, Aker BL, Trentacost DJ, Smith PJ, Tarantino N. A prospective comparative study of the AMO Array zonal-progressive multifocal silicone intraocular lens and a monofocal intraocular lens. *Ophthalmology.* 1999;106:1243-1255.

9. Personal communication with Wendell Danforth, MD, October 2007.

DELL QUESTIONNAIRE

Date_____   Name_____

Cataract and Refractive Lens Exchange Questionnaire

The term "cataract" refers to a cloudy lens within the eye. When a cataract is removed, an artificial lens is placed inside the eye to take the place of the human lens that has become the cataract. Occasionally, clear lenses that have not yet developed cataracts are also removed to reduce or eliminate the need for glasses or contacts. If it is determined that surgery is appropriate for you, this questionnaire will help us provide the best treatment for your visual needs. It is important that you understand that many patients still need to wear glasses for some activities after surgery. Please fill this form out completely and give it to the doctor. If you have questions, please let us know and we will assist you with this form.

1. After surgery, would you be interested in seeing well **without glasses** in the following situations?
     Distance vision (driving, golf, tennis, other sports, watching TV)
     ___Prefer no **Distance** glasses.   ___ I wouldn't mind wearing **Distance** glasses.

     Mid-range vision. (computer, menus, price tags, cooking, board games, items on a shelf)
     ___Prefer no **Mid-range** glasses.   ___ I wouldn't mind wearing **Mid-range** glasses.

     Near vision (reading books, newspapers, magazines, detailed handwork)
     ___Prefer no **Near** glasses.   ___ I wouldn't mind wearing **Near** glasses.

2. Please check the **single** statement that best describes you in terms of **night vision:**
     ___ a. Night vision is extremely important to me, and I require the best possible quality night vision.
     ___ b. I want to be able to drive comfortably at night, but I would tolerate some slight imperfections.
     ___ c. Night vision is not particularly important to me.

3. If you **had** to wear glasses after surgery for one activity, for which activity would you be **most** willing to use glasses?   ____**Distance Vision.**   ____**Mid-range Vision.**   ____**Near Vision.**

4. If you could have good **Distance Vision during the day without glasses**, and good **Near Vision for reading without glasses**, but the compromise was that you might see some **halos or rings** around lights at night, would you like that option?   ____Yes   ____No

5. If you could have good **Distance vision during the day and night** without glasses, and good **Mid-range Vision** without glasses, but the compromise was that you might need glasses for reading the finest print at near, would you like that option?   ____Yes   ____No

6. Surgery to reduce or eliminate your dependence upon glasses for **Distance, Mid-rage and Near Vision** may be partially covered by insurance if you have a cataract that is covered by insurance. Would you be interested in learning more about this option?
    ____Yes   ____No   ____Maybe, it depends on how much is covered by insurance.

7. Please place an "X" on the following scale to describe your personality as best you can:
[--I--]
Easy going   Perfectionist

Please Sign Here_____

DELL QUESTIONNAIRE— COULSON MODIFICATION

Vision Preferences Checklist

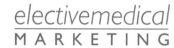

Your Name _____ Date _____

The term "cataract" refers to a cloudy lens within the eye. When a cataract is removed, an artificial lens is placed inside the eye to take the place of the human lens that has become the cataract. Occasionally, clear lenses that have not yet developed cataracts are also removed to reduce or eliminate the need for glasses or contacts. **If it is determined that surgery is appropriate for you,** this questionnaire will help us provide the best treatment for your visual needs. It is important that you understand that many patients still need to wear glasses for some activities after surgery. Please fill this form out completely and return it to us. If you have questions, please let us know and we will assist you with this form.

1. If surgery is recommended for you, would you be interested in seeing well without glasses in the following situations?
   Distance vision (driving, golf, tennis, other sports, watching TV)
   ☐ Prefer no **Distance** glasses.   ☐ I wouldn't mind wearing **Distance** glasses.
   Mid-range vision (computer, menus, price tags, cooking, board games, items on a shelf)
   ☐ Prefer no **Mid-Range** glasses.   ☐ I wouldn't mind wearing **Mid-Range** glasses.
   Near vision (reading books, newspapers, magazines, detailed handwork)
   ☐ Prefer no **Near** glasses.   ☐ I wouldn't mind wearing **Near** glasses.

2. Please check the *single* statement that best describes you in terms of *night vision*:
   ☐ a. Night vision is extremely important to me, and I require the best possible quality night vision.
   ☐ b. I want to be able to drive comfortably at night, but I would tolerate some slight imperfections.
   ☐ c. Night vision is not particularly important to me.

3. If you **had** to wear glasses after surgery for one activity, for which activity would you be **most** willing to use glasses?
   ☐ Distance Vision.   ☐ Mid-range Vision.   ☐ Near Vision.

4. If you could have good **Distance Vision during the day without glasses**, and good **Near Vision for reading without glasses**, but the compromise was that you might see some **halos or rings** around lights at night, would you like that option?
   ☐ Yes   ☐ No

5. If you could have good **Distance Vision during the day and night** without glasses, and good **Mid-Range Vision** without glasses, but the compromise was that you might need glasses for reading the finest print at near, would you like that option?
   ☐ Yes   ☐ No

6. How many hours per day to you spend:
   On the computer _____
   Reading books, newspapers, typed documents or small print _____
   Driving _____

7. Please list up to three favorite hobbies:

   _____   _____   _____

8. Please place an "X" on the following scale to describe your personality as best you can:

   ☐————————————————☐————————————————☐
   Easy going   Perfectionist

Please Sign Here _____

DELL QUESTIONNAIRE— CHANG MODIFICATION

Chang modification of Dell Survey *(for a primarily cataract practice)*

When a cataract is removed, an artificial lens is permanently placed inside the eye to take the place of the human lens that has become the cataract. Occasionally, clear lenses that have not yet developed cataracts are also removed to reduce the need for glasses or contacts. New special lens implants are available that can reduce your dependence upon glasses, compared to standard lens implants. However, the additional "upgrade" cost is not covered by insurance, and most patients still need to wear glasses for some activities after surgery. This questionnaire will assist us in determining which, if any, of these special implants is more appropriate for you (assuming that you do not mind the additional cost and are interested in them).

1. After surgery, would you be interested in seeing well **without glasses** in the following situations?
   Distance vision (driving, golf, tennis, other sports, watching TV)
   ___*Prefer no **Distance** glasses.*   ___*Not important. I wouldn't mind wearing **Distance** glasses.*

   Mid-range vision. (computer, menus, price tags, cooking, board games, items on a shelf)
   ___*Prefer no **Mid-range** glasses.*   ___*Not important. I wouldn't mind wearing **Mid-range** glasses.*

   Near vision (reading books, newspapers, magazines, sewing)
   ___*Prefer no **Near** glasses.*   ___*Not important. I wouldn't mind wearing **Near** glasses.*

2. Please check the **single** statement that best describes you in terms of **night vision:**
   ___ a. Night vision is extremely important to me, and I require the best possible quality night vision.
   ___ b. I want to be able to drive comfortably at night, but I would tolerate some slight imperfections.
   ___ c. Night vision is not particularly important to me.

3. If you **had** to wear glasses after surgery for one activity, for which activity would you be **most** willing to use glasses?   ____**Distance Vision.**   ____**Mid-range Vision.**   ____**Near Vision.**

4. If you could have good **Distance Vision during the day without glasses**, and good **Near Vision for reading without glasses**, but the compromise was that you might see some **halos or rings** around lights at night, would you like that option?   ____Yes   ____No

5. If you could have good **Distance vision during the day and night** without glasses, and good **Mid-range Vision** without glasses, but the compromise was that you might need glasses for reading at near, would you like that option?   ____Yes   ____No

6. Please place an "X" on the following scale to describe your motivation to reduce dependence on glasses:
   [---I---]
   Prefer glasses   somewhat   I hate
   at all times   interested   glasses!

7. Please place an "X" on the following scale to describe your personality as best you can:
   [---I---]
   Easy going   Perfectionist

8. Your occupation or hobbies:

Your Name: _____

PRECONSULTATION HANDOUT

David F. Chang, MD

Prior to their office visit, we mail this introductory handout along with my cataract brochure and the Dell Questionnaire to all new patients with a diagnosis of cataract. This provides the information needed to understand and complete the Dell Questionnaire. See Chapter 93 for details.

Special Lens Implants to Reduce Your Need for Spectacles

Some people mistakenly believe that having cataract surgery will enable them to see perfectly without glasses. Having the eye's natural cataract-clouded lens removed and replaced with a clear artificial lens implant should certainly improve your vision. However, the conventional artificial lens is a single, fixed focus lens. It cannot give distance focus one moment and near focus the next (like the eye's natural lens does in a young person). Thus, even after cataract surgery, eyeglasses are still needed to change and adjust the focus of your eye in order to see things at different distances.

WHY DO WE ALL EVENTUALLY REQUIRE READING GLASSES OR BIFOCALS AS WE AGE?

While we're young, the "focusing" muscles inside our eye change and control the shape of our natural lens. This change in lens shape allows us to shift our focus from far to near, and this natural focusing ability is called accommodation. Like the auto-focus in your camera, accommodation is so fast and automatic that we're not even aware that it's happening. Unfortunately, the eye's natural lens hardens as we age. As it loses flexibility, we progressively lose our accommodation. Presbyopia is the term describing the natural and unavoidable loss of this far-to-near focusing ability over time. By our 40s, the diminishing ability to focus up close must be replaced with reading glasses, bifocals, or trifocals. This is why even laser refractive surgery, such as LASIK, cannot eliminate glasses if you are in your mid-forties or older. Conventional "single-focus" artificial lens implants cannot replace this age-related loss of accommodation or the need for reading glasses either.

When discussing our vision, there are three major "working distances" that most of us regularly use. Driving, watching a movie, or seeing a golf ball require good far distance vision. Seeing the dashboard, a desktop computer, or items on a shelf require good mid-range or intermediate vision. Finally, reading newsprint or sewing require good close-range or near vision. Trifocals literally provide three different lenses in your eyeglass frame so that you can quickly alternate between these three working distances once your natural lens can no longer change focus.

DOES THIS MEAN I WILL ONLY NEED READING GLASSES AFTER CATARACT SURGERY?

Depending on the level of detail you require, you may also need full-time or part-time eyeglasses for far distance vision following cataract surgery. Just as contact lenses come in dozens of different prescription powers, the artificial lenses also come in more than 60 different powers. Absolutely "perfect" distance focus is difficult to achieve with cataract surgery, because there is no opportunity to test or try out several different lens implant powers inside your eye. Another reason that distance eyeglasses may be needed at times is astigmatism. The conventional lens implant does not correct astigmatism, which is a natural blur resulting from the imperfect optical shape of the cornea in many patients. Fortunately, eyeglasses can always be worn to optimize distance focus just as they do for anyone whose eyes are not in perfect focus naturally.

It is important and reassuring to remember that after cataract surgery, you should have the same optical options available to everyone else over age 50 who has never had a cataract. These include bifocals and trifocals, separate reading, computer, or distance glasses, contact lenses (including monovision), and even refractive surgery such as LASIK. However, the goal with standard cataract surgery is to avoid your having to wear strong prescription eyeglasses afterward.

MULTIFOCAL LENS IMPLANTS

There is a special type of lens implant – the multifocal – that provides both near and far focus simultaneously and can significantly reduce your dependence on reading glasses. Conventional single-focus lens implants are called monofocal lenses because they optimize the focus at one location and do not provide the ability to see at both far and near distances without glasses. The term multifocal stands for "multiple focal points" and these lens implants are designed to produce a dual focus - part of the lens is set for distance focus, and part of the lens is set for near. The design is entirely different from bifocal eyeglasses where you look through the top portion for distance and the bottom area for near. With a multifocal lens implant the brain automatically finds the correct focus.

Like the conventional lens implant, the multifocal is a foldable lens that is implanted through an extremely small incision and is equally safe. However, compared to a conventional lens implant selected for distance focus, a multifocal also improves your ability to see up close without glasses. Not everyone with a multifocal lens implant can read equally well without glasses and there are many factors that cause this individual variability. The ability to read without glasses is certainly better if both eyes have a multifocal lens. The younger and healthier the retina is, the better the reading ability will be. Interestingly, the ability to read without glasses improves over time for some patients. It seems that with the multifocal lens system the brain learns to perform better with practice.

Because the lens implant does not correct it, any astigmatism you have will reduce your ability to see both far and near without glasses. Having a very small pupil size can also compromise your near function by limiting the incoming light. While there is no guarantee that you will read as well without glasses as you desire, multifocal lenses give you much better odds of doing so, compared to conventional lens implants.

CAN THESE SPECIAL LENS IMPLANTS ELIMINATE MY EYEGLASSES ALTOGETHER?

This is possible but not very likely. Most people with multifocal lenses still find it easier to read with glasses under certain conditions, such as for prolonged reading, for small print, or when the lighting is poor. While the multifocal lens implant won't totally eliminate reading glasses, it should provide the convenience of "social" reading (e.g. handwritten notes, price tags, receipts, photographs, menus, and a wristwatch or cell phone) without having to put on eyeglasses. With reading glasses on, you should see equally well with a multifocal or a conventional lens implant. Depending upon the amount of detail you need to see, glasses to further sharpen your distance focus may still be worn for some activities. However, compared to standard lens implants, multifocal lenses will provide you with a greater and expanded range of focusing ability without glasses.

WHAT ABOUT THE COST?

Not surprisingly, the multifocal lens implant procedure is more expensive. Health insurance, such as Medicare, covers the costs of cataract surgery with a conventional lens implant. However, the additional premium charge for implanting these special lenses is not covered and must be paid out of pocket by the patient. Remember that the benefit of the multifocal lens implant is the convenience of requiring eyeglasses less frequently. They are not "medically necessary" because they have nothing to do with improving your eye health.

IS THE MULTIFOCAL LENS IMPLANT RIGHT FOR ME?

While the multifocal lens implant should reduce your dependence on eyeglasses, there are some tradeoffs in addition to the added expense. The different focal zones of the lens optic can create the appearance of halos or ghost images around lights at night. While a distant streetlight should be in good focus through the far-focusing portion of the multifocal lens, it appears blurry through the near-focusing portion of the lens. This creates a slight ghost image around the edges of the light. Such halos are not evident during the daytime when your pupils are smaller.

The first multifocal lens implant was introduced in the late 1990s. This first-generation design had one important drawback – the presence of significant glare and halos at night – which limited its popularity. The newer multifocal lens implants have been re-engineered and improved, so that they are less likely to cause bothersome halos compared to the original designs. Fortunately, seeing halos is a distraction that doesn't obscure the focus and the majority of patients describe them as being "minor". The halos will become less noticeable over time as your brain gradually adapts to them. This is similar to the way in which your brain blocks out background noise, such as street traffic sound, over time. Of course, not everyone can adapt as quickly as others. In the rare event that the halos are too bothersome, the multifocal lens can be surgically removed. Because this entails risk, this is more of a last resort.

The multifocal lens implant isn't right for everyone. It doesn't work well if a person has significant astigmatism or other problems involving the cornea, retina, or optic nerve. Patients who have previously had refractive surgery, such as LASIK or radial keratotomy, may not be the best candidates. Finally, your individual lifestyle and activities should be considered. Reducing the need to wear eyeglasses is not a priority for everyone, and since there are some tradeoffs and added costs, the multifocal lens implant would not be important for these individuals. Remember that both multifocal and conventional monofocal artificial lenses will provide excellent vision with glasses following cataract surgery. The difference is in what you can see when you aren't wearing eyeglasses.

ACCOMMODATING LENS IMPLANTS

Accommodating lens implants seek to reduce eyeglass dependence according to a completely different principle. Recall that accommodation is the natural ability of a young eye to focus by changing the lens shape. If the lens implant could also change its shape or position, some focusing ability could be restored. The Crystalens (Eyeonics, Inc., Aliso Viejo, CA) implant is the first accommodating lens to be approved by the FDA. This lens implant has a special hinged design to allow it to flex slightly.

This enables your eye's natural focusing muscles to produce some flexing and movement of the lens. For example, patients who have good distance vision can also see well without glasses at mid-range or intermediate distance with the Crystalens. There is generally not enough lens movement, however, to allow you to see far off in the distance one moment, and to read up close the next. There is also individual variability in the ability of the eye muscles to move the implanted lens. While the Crystalens does increase one's capacity to adjust focus relative to a conventional lens implant, the ability to see at closer distances without eyeglasses is more unpredictable from one patient to the next.

If these special lens implants don't eliminate glasses, what is the advantage?

These special lens implants reduce how often you would need to wear eyeglasses, when compared to the conventional single-focus lens. Someone who dislikes winter would recognize the obvious benefit of warmer weather if they moved to California from Minnesota. Nevertheless, this improvement doesn't mean that they would never wear a coat, but rather that they would need one less often.

WHAT WILL THE FUTURE BRING?

Unfortunately, it is not feasible to replace your lens implant if a newer and improved design comes along in the future. Therefore, if you already have a significant cataract, you should make your choice of lens implant based upon the best technology currently available.

MULTIFOCAL IOL FAQ HANDOUT

David F. Chang, MD

This more detailed discussion provides detailed and written informed consent in the form of an FAQ handout, and is only given to interested candidates, such as those identified by their responses to the Dell Questionnaire. It can be shared with others at home, and reviewed pre and postoperatively. See Chapter 93 for details.

Multifocal Lens Implants—Frequently Asked Questions

Multifocal lens implants are an expensive but exciting technology. They are designed to reduce your dependence upon eyeglasses as compared to if you had a conventional "single focus" lens implant. When you are not wearing glasses, the better you are able to see in the far distance with a conventional lens implant the blurrier it will be up close. You would then wear reading glasses in order to see clearly at near.

HOW DOES THE MULTIFOCAL WORK?

With bifocal eyeglasses, you look through the top part of the lens for distance and through the bottom area of the lens for near. The multifocal lens implant is entirely different because the specially engineered optic provides both a distance focus, and a near focus at all times. Your brain will learn to automatically select the focus that is appropriate for the task at hand. An analogy might be having background music playing in the room during a conversation. Your brain might "tune out" one to listen to the other. There is a brief learning curve for using this unique optical system. For example, you will need to learn the optimal distance to hold reading material—the so-called "sweet spot". For this reason many patients report that their ability to function without glasses continues to improve gradually during the first several months.

WILL THIS EXPENSIVE TECHNOLOGY ELIMINATE THE NEED FOR GLASSES?

Unfortunately, multifocal lens implants usually do not eliminate eyeglasses entirely. There will probably be some situations where the print or the images are simply too small or too far away to see without eyeglasses. The print quality and the amount of available light will make a difference. In addition, your retina must be completely healthy to achieve the optimum results.

Remember that how often an individual requires glasses varies across a broad range of percentages. At one extreme is always (people who must wear their glasses constantly = 100%); at the other end of the continuum is never (some young individuals with perfect vision and a naturally focusing lens never need glasses = 0%). Most of us are somewhere along this continuum in between the two extremes. It is impossible to know in advance how often you will "need" glasses after your multifocal lens implants. This depends upon variables such as your retina, any remaining astigmatism, and how visually demanding your everyday activities are. However, when compared to the conventional single-focus lens implant, the multifocal should put you much closer to the desirable end of the spectrum described above. This is because the multifocal lens provides you with focus at more than one distance ("multifocal" means more than one optimal focal point).

Multifocal lens implants do offer the convenience of less dependence on reading glasses compared to conventional lens implants. People who naturally see well in the distance often go without eyeglasses when outdoors or around the house. However, when they need to see something up close—even for just a moment—they might have to put on reading glasses. Examples of common momentary near tasks would be a looking at a cell phone, a photo, a menu, a boarding pass, an envelope address, a handwritten note, or a price tag or receipt. Having to frequently take their reading glasses on and off is inconvenient for many people. Because of this, they might wear their reading glasses around their neck, scatter multiple pairs around the house, or simply wear bifocals all the time. Although they might still prefer eyeglasses for prolonged reading, most people with multifocal lens implants can enjoy the convenience of performing these simple near tasks without putting on reading glasses.

WILL I SEE HALOS?

Depending upon the size of your pupils you may see halos, which might appear as rings around lights at night. These halos are different from, and less problematic than those typically caused by cataracts. They relate to viewing distant lights through both the near and far focusing zones of the lens. They do not obscure the vision, but rather can create a distracting ghost image.

Fortunately, these halos become less noticeable and distracting over time as the brain learns to selectively ignore them through a process called neuroadaptation. This is the same process that allows us to ignore background noise, such as traffic sounds or an air conditioning fan. Another analogy would be the temporary distraction of having braces or wearing earrings for the first time. As these sensations become more familiar over time, we become less aware of them. How quickly this adjustment occurs varies for different individuals. However, experience has shown that neuroadaptation is a gradual process and that suppression of the nighttime ghost images continues to improve over several months.

Even a conventional lens implant can produce some halos at night, but they are more evident with a multifocal lens implant. Halos are often quite noticeable during the first 24 hours after surgery when your pupil is still dilated. Do not be alarmed or misled by this temporary situation. Compared to their predecessors the newest multifocal lenses have been successfully redesigned so as to significantly reduce the halo effect.

CAN A MULTIFOCAL LENS BE IMPLANTED IN JUST ONE EYE?

Yes, this is possible when the other eye already has a conventional implant, or when there is no cataract in the opposite eye. However, the ability to see both far and near without glasses is better when you have a multifocal lens in both eyes. With a multifocal lens implant in one eye, the brain simply blends together all of the vision that you get with both eyes open. Some individuals may take longer than others to adapt to this situation. For this reason, you shouldn't constantly compare one eye to the other. With a multifocal lens in one eye, you should still have more ability to see things close up, as compared to if you had received a conventional single-focus lens implant.

CAN THE MULTIFOCAL LENS BE REMOVED IF I DON'T LIKE IT?

This is always possible but entails the risks of additional surgery. However, there may be a rare individual for whom the halos continue to be unacceptable and who then elects to have the multifocal replaced with a conventional lens implant. One should not rush into this decision because the ghost images nearly always improve over time. However, removal of any lens implant generally becomes more difficult after 4 months.

DOES INSURANCE COVER THE EXTRA COSTS OF A MULTIFOCAL?

Unfortunately it does not. Health insurance, including PPOs, HMOs, and Medicare, covers a cataract operation with a conventional lens implant when the cataract is bad enough to be considered "medically necessary". The additional fee to upgrade the lens implant to a multifocal is not covered, because the added convenience of reducing your dependence on eyeglasses is not "medically necessary". We ask that you pay this premium out-of-pocket fee in advance. Rarely, unexpected situations might arise during surgery where I determine that a multifocal lens might not be as stable in your particular eye due to the condition of the lens capsule. I would implant a conventional lens implant in this situation and your multifocal lens fee would be refunded.

CAN PATIENTS WITHOUT CATARACTS HAVE MULTIFOCAL LENS IMPLANTS?

The multifocal lens implant is a technology that can allow a 50+ year-old eye to have focus both far and near without glasses. For this reason, people over the age of 50 wearing strong prescription glasses but with no other eye problems may elect to have multifocal lens implants in order to see much better without glasses. Health insurance covers none of the costs, however, if there is no cataract present. Because the natural lens must still be removed before implanting a multifocal lens, the procedure is performed in the same way as for cataract surgery. Thus, patients electing to have lens implant surgery to reduce their need for glasses will never have to worry about developing cataracts later on in life.

WHO MIGHT NEED A LASIK "ENHANCEMENT" AFTER A MULTIFOCAL LENS IMPLANT?

Like contact lenses or eyeglasses, every artificial lens implant model (both conventional and multifocal) is manufactured in more than 60 different "powers". As with prescription eyeglasses or contact lenses, it is important to match the appropriate artificial lens implant power to your eye. To prescribe the correct spectacle or contact lens power, we utilize trial and error to preview different lens powers placed in front of your eye. When you are asked, "which is better, one or two?" you are selecting the lens power that you see best with. However, because the artificial lens implant is inserted inside the eye, and only after your natural lens (cataract) has been removed, it is impossible for you to preview or "try out" different powers before surgery. Furthermore, once it is implanted, we cannot easily exchange the lens implant the way we could with contact lenses or eyeglasses.

Fortunately, an appropriate lens implant power can be estimated using mathematical formulas that utilize preoperative measurements of your eye's dimensions. Although the measurements are very accurate, there are individual variables that prevent this process from being 100% perfect. One variable is the final precise position where the implant will end up inside your eye. Another individual variable is astigmatism, which is a naturally occurring imperfection in the optical shape of your cornea. Astigmatism is therefore not corrected by the lens implant placed inside the eye and is another variable that may reduce your ability to see without glasses. The overall process is accurate enough so that most patients will see quite well without glasses in the distance (assuming that was the target). However, it usually won't be "perfect" and you might choose to wear mild prescription glasses for those occasional tasks that require more precise distance focus.

For a multifocal lens implant to work well, it is very important for the selected lens power to match your individual eye. Despite flawless surgery, some patients with multifocal lens implants are still not able to see as well without glasses as they would like. What can be done if this is because the lens power is "off"? One option is to wear glasses or contact lenses. A theoretical solution might be to exchange the multifocal lens implant for another with a different power. However, because of the risks involved with removing a lens implant, it is usually safer to "enhance" or fine-tune any residual prescription with an external LASIK procedure on the cornea instead. LASIK can also correct any remaining astigmatism coming from your cornea.

All eye operations intending to reduce a person's need for eyeglasses may need to be "enhanced" with a second procedure. For example, nearsighted people choosing to have laser eye surgery (e.g., LASIK) may need a second treatment if the first one does not fully correct their prescription. This unpredictability is understandable because we are working with human tissue and not plastic or metal. Likewise, it is possible that either the conventional or multifocal lens implant that has been selected may not adequately focus your distance vision without glasses. Depending upon how far off we are, laser enhancement may be a good option. The odds that this would need to be done with a multifocal lens are usually less than 5% to 10%, but the chances are greater in patients with a lot of astigmatism or who are wearing very strong prescription glasses to begin with. The need will also depend upon how much better one wants to see without glasses, and I would collaborate with a LASIK specialist, called a refractive surgeon, if this need arose. However, because there would be an additional cost and procedure involved, you should know about this possibility in advance before making your decision to have a multifocal lens implant.

WHAT DO YOU RECOMMEND I DO?

Like cosmetic surgery, taking extra steps to reduce spectacle dependence is a discretionary and personal decision. Because this does not involve health advice or medical needs, the ultimate decision is yours. Start by evaluating how strong your desire is to see as much as possible without glasses. Every individual will value such convenience quite differently. My role, as your eye surgeon, is to explain your options to you.

If you are a patient with cataracts, you are considering surgery because your cataracts prevent you from seeing well with your corrective eyeglasses. After cataract surgery you should be able to see well for both far and near distances with your new eyeglasses (assuming no other eye health problems). The decision about which type of artificial lens implant to have will only affect your ability to see without eyeglasses following cataract surgery. With both conventional and multifocal lens implants, most people will see reasonably well in the distance without any eyeglasses. However, multifocal lens implants will provide the added convenience of being able to read many things up close without glasses.

No current technology can eliminate eyeglasses, and how well you will perform with multifocal lens implants can vary because of individual factors. Nevertheless, they are an excellent option for patients who already need cataract surgery and who want to decrease their reliance upon eyeglasses. While multifocal implants carry no guarantees, they should greatly improve the odds that you will be able to read and see better overall without eyeglasses.

CRYSTALENS **FAQ** HANDOUT

David F. Chang, MD

This more detailed discussion provides detailed and written informed consent in the form of an FAQ handout, and is only given to interested candidates, such as those identified by their responses to the Dell Questionnaire. It can be shared with others at home, and reviewed pre and postoperatively. See Chapter 93 for details.

The Crystalens Implant—Frequently Asked Questions

There are two different types of premium lens implant options—the multifocal and the accommodating lens - that are designed to reduce your dependence on glasses as compared to if you had received a conventional "single-focus" lens implant. When you are not wearing glasses, a conventional lens implant will provide your eye with optimum focus set at one particular distance that does not change. You would then wear glasses in order to change this focus (e.g., moving the focus farther away or closer up).

HOW DO MULTIFOCAL AND ACCOMMODATING LENS IMPLANTS DIFFER?

Conventional single-focus lens implants are called monofocal lenses because they optimize the focus at a single location. Multifocal lens implants are designed to produce a dual focus. Part of the lens is set for distance focus, and part of the lens is set for near, and this technology can significantly reduce your dependence on reading glasses. Accommodating lens implants seek to reduce eyeglass dependence according to a completely different principle. Accommodation is the medical term which describes the natural ability of a young eye to focus by changing the lens shape. If the lens implant could also change its shape or position, some focusing ability could be restored.

The Crystalens (Eyeonics, Inc., Aliso Viejo, CA) implant is the first and only accommodating lens to be approved by the FDA. This lens implant has an ingenious hinged design, to allow it to flex slightly. This enables your eye's natural focusing muscles to cause some flexing and movement of the lens, thereby adjusting the focus. There is generally not enough lens movement, however, to allow you to see far off in the distance one moment, and to read up close the next. As you would imagine, there is also individual variability in the ability of the eye muscles to move the implanted lens. While the Crystalens does increase one's capacity to change focus relative to a conventional lens implant, unfortunately it does not duplicate the focusing ability that we all enjoyed when we were young.

The Crystalens should provide an ability to see without glasses across a greater range of different viewing distances when compared to a single-focus lens implant. For example, if an individual can see well enough to drive with the Crystalens, they should also be able to focus in toward the dashboard. The latter is a good example of our need to see many things at a mid-range or "intermediate" distance—that is neither far off in the distance nor up close. Other examples of tasks performed at an intermediate distance would include working on a desktop computer, playing the piano, cooking, or viewing items on a shelf at arms length. For reading up close, patients with the Crystalens typically wear low power reading glasses.

WILL THIS EXPENSIVE TECHNOLOGY ELIMINATE THE NEED FOR GLASSES?

Unfortunately, neither the Crystalens nor multifocal lens implants are expected to eliminate the need for eyeglasses. There may always be situations where you are trying to see details at some distance that are simply too small to be seen clearly. The print size and the amount of available light will make a difference. In addition, your retina must be completely healthy to achieve the optimum results.

Because a single Crystalens implant does not provide enough focusing range to encompass both the far and near distance extremes, one common strategy is to slightly stagger the separate focusing range of each eye. For example, imagine that after the first eye surgery, you can see well in the distance but cannot read without glasses up close. One option is to implant a Crystalens in your second eye that is focused closer in, rather than far away. Although this particular eye might not see as well far away as the first eye does without glasses, the benefit is that it should see better at near distances when you are not wearing glasses. Unless you were to test each eye separately, this intended slight difference will generally go unnoticed, because the brain "blends" what is seen by the two eyes together. The result would be an expanded ability to see across a greater range of distances (from near to mid-range to far) than would be possible with either eye alone. This concept is similar to the "monovision" strategy that many contact lens wearers over the age of 40 have used, except that it is accomplished without wearing contact lenses.

In a different situation, imagine that your first eye has good vision at the intermediate and near ranges with the Crystalens, but is not very clear in the distance. Your second eye could then be targeted for far distance to complement and supplement what you can already see with the first eye. Again, improved distance focus would come at the cost of decreased near performance in that one eye. Regardless of the strategy, your ability to see without glasses should improve after the second eye receives a Crystalens. Finally, in select circumstances, there is even an option to combine a Crystalens in one eye, with a multifocal lens implant in the second eye.

Remember that how often an individual requires glasses varies across a broad range of percentages. At one extreme is always (people who must wear their glasses constantly = 100%); at the other end of the continuum is never (some young individuals with perfect vision and a naturally focusing lens never need glasses = 0%). Most of us are somewhere along this continuum in between the two extremes. It is impossible to know in advance how often you will "need" glasses after your Crystalens implants. This depends upon variables such as your retina, any remaining astigmatism, and how visually demanding your everyday activities are. However, when compared to a conventional single-focus lens implant, the Crystalens should put you much closer to the desirable end of the spectrum discussed above. This is because the Crystalens provides your eye with some ability to adjust and vary the focus. Therefore, the Crystalens implants do offer the convenience of being less dependent on glasses compared to conventional lens implants.

There is always normal variability in the rate of visual improvement following uncomplicated cataract surgery. Beyond the initial postoperative period, however, many Crystalens patients have observed a gradual improvement in their ability to change focus over time. Since the Crystalens is designed to be flexed and moved by the focusing muscles of the eye, it makes sense that in some eyes, the strength of these focusing muscles improves with greater use.

WILL I SEE HALOS?

The design of the multifocal lens implant will always produce mild ghost images that appear as rings or halos, particularly around lights at night. Although halos are much less apparent with the newest generation of multifocal lens implants, and they always become less distracting over time, there is always some small risk that a given individual may struggle to adapt to them. In general, the quality of vision at night is slightly less with a multifocal lens compared to a conventional single-focus lens implant. Because the Crystalens works according to an entirely different principle, it will not produce the halos that are seen with multifocal lenses. The clarity and quality of vision at night should be equally good as with a conventional lens implant.

DOES INSURANCE COVER THE PREMIUM COST TO UPGRADE TO A CRYSTALENS IMPLANT?

Unfortunately it does not. Health insurance, including PPOs, HMOs, and Medicare, covers a cataract operation with a conventional lens implant when the cataract is bad enough to be considered "medically necessary". The additional fee to upgrade to a Crystalens (accommodating lens implant) or a multifocal lens implant is not covered, because the added convenience of reducing your dependence on eyeglasses is not "medically necessary". We ask that you pay this premium out-of-pocket fee in advance. Rarely, unexpected situations might arise during surgery where I determine that a Crystalens lens might not be as stable in your particular eye due to the condition of the lens capsule. I would implant a conventional lens implant in this situation and your Crystalens fee would be refunded.

CAN PATIENTS WITHOUT CATARACTS HAVE THE CRYSTALENS?

The Crystalens accommodating lens implant is a technology that can allow a 50+ year-old eye to have some focusing ability without glasses. For this reason, people over the age of 50 wearing strong prescription glasses but with no other eye problems may elect to have accommodating lens implants in order to see much better without glasses. Health insurance covers none of the costs, however, if there is no cataract present. Because the natural lens must still be removed before implanting the Crystalens, the procedure is performed in the same way as for cataract surgery. Thus, patients electing to have lens implant surgery to reduce their need for glasses will never have to worry about developing cataracts later on in life.

WHO MIGHT NEED A LASIK "ENHANCEMENT" AFTER A CRYSTALENS IMPLANT?

Like contact lenses or eyeglasses, every artificial lens implant model (conventional, multifocal, or Crystalens) is manufactured in more than 60 different "powers". As with prescription eyeglasses or contact lenses, it is important to match the appropriate artificial lens implant power to your eye. To prescribe the correct spectacle or contact lens power, we utilize trial and error to preview different lens powers placed in front of your eye. When you are asked, "which is better, one or two?" you are selecting the lens power that you see best with. However, because the artificial lens implant is inserted inside the eye, and only after your natural lens (cataract) has been removed, it is impossible for you to preview or "try out" different powers before surgery. Furthermore, once it is implanted, we cannot easily exchange the lens implant the way we could with contact lenses or eyeglasses.

Fortunately, an appropriate lens implant power can be estimated using mathematical formulas that utilize preoperative measurements of your eye's dimensions. Although the measurements are very accurate, there are individual variables that prevent this process from being 100% perfect. One variable is the final precise position where the implant will end up inside your eye. Another individual variable is astigmatism, which is a naturally occurring imperfection in the optical shape of your cornea.

Astigmatism is therefore not corrected by the lens implant placed inside the eye and is another variable that may reduce your ability to see without glasses. The overall process is accurate enough so that most patients will see quite well without glasses in the distance (assuming that was the target). However, it usually won't be "perfect" and you might choose to wear mild prescription glasses for those occasional tasks that require more precise distance focus.

For a Crystalens implant to work well, it is very important for the selected lens power to match your individual eye. Despite flawless surgery, some patients with Crystalens implants are still not able to see as well without glasses as they would like. What can be done if this is because the lens power is "off"? One option is to wear glasses or contact lenses. A theoretical solution might be to exchange the Crystalens implant for another with a different power. However, because of the risks involved with removing a lens implant, it is usually safer to "enhance" or fine-tune any residual prescription with an external LASIK procedure on the cornea instead. LASIK can also correct any remaining astigmatism coming from your cornea.

All eye operations intending to reduce a person's need for eyeglasses may need to be "enhanced" with a second procedure. For example, nearsighted people choosing to have laser eye surgery (e.g., LASIK) may need a second treatment if the first one does not fully correct their prescription. This unpredictability is understandable because we are working with human tissue and not plastic or metal. Likewise, it is possible that either the conventional or Crystalens implant that has been selected may not adequately focus your distance vision without glasses. Depending upon how far off we are, laser enhancement may be a good option. The odds that this would need to be done with a Crystalens are usually less than 5% to 10%, but the chances are greater in patients with a lot of astigmatism or who are wearing very strong prescription glasses to begin with. The need will also depend upon how much better one wants to see without glasses, and I would collaborate with a LASIK specialist, called a refractive surgeon, if this need arose. However, because there would be an additional cost and procedure involved, you should know about this possibility in advance before making your decision to have a Crystalens implant.

WHAT DO YOU RECOMMEND I DO?

Like cosmetic surgery, taking extra steps to reduce spectacle dependence is a discretionary and personal decision. Because this does not involve health advice or medical needs, the ultimate decision is yours. Start by evaluating how strong your desire is to see as much as possible without glasses. Every individual will value such convenience quite differently. My role, as your eye surgeon, is to explain your options to you.

If you are a patient with cataracts, you are considering surgery because your cataracts prevent you from seeing well with your corrective eyeglasses. After cataract surgery you should be able to see well for far, mid-range, and near distances with your new eyeglasses (assuming no other eye health problems). The decision about which type of artificial lens implant to have will only affect your ability to see without eyeglasses following cataract surgery. Compared to a conventional lens implant, the Crystalens should provide the added convenience of being able to adjust your focus across a larger range of different distances without eyeglasses.

No current technology can eliminate eyeglasses, and how well you will perform with Crystalens implants can vary because of individual factors. Nevertheless, they are an excellent option for patients who already need cataract surgery and who want to decrease their reliance upon eyeglasses. While Crystalens implants carry no guarantees, they should greatly improve the odds that you will be able to see better overall without eyeglasses.

Patient Information Sheet for Advanced Elective Options With Cataract Surgery

Barry S. Seibel, MD

All patients undergoing cataract surgery read and sign the following document. It reinforces the fact that a medically indicated (ie, covered by insurance) cataract surgery assumes that a patient has visual symptoms that are interfering with their activities of daily living, that these symptoms are not adequately relieved by spectacle correction, and that cataract surgery has a good prognosis of improving their symptoms by improving their best-corrected visual acuity. In other words, insurance will pay to treat their cataract to allow glasses to work, but will not pay simply to reduce their dependence on glasses; an example that most patients will readily correlate and understand is that most insurances will not cover laser vision correction.

By reiterating the foregoing information in the following document, patients better understand the validity of the need for their out-of-pocket expense for the elective option of reduced dependence on glasses via additional diagnostic and surgical intervention around the time of their medically covered cataract surgery, in addition to extended postoperative care. With this fundamental theme of glasses dependence, a natural corollary is distinguishing between distance and near glasses. They can opt for reduced dependence on distance glasses (option 1) or reduced dependence on both distance and near glasses (option 2). They can of course choose no additional options to avoid additional costs beyond their particular insurance copay and deductible. After considerable collaboration with Alan Reider and Kevin Corcoran, I have placed monovision under option 1.

The theme of postoperative dependence on glasses is related to David Chang's concept of "convenience" with regard to advanced elective options with cataract surgery. Patients need to understand that a standard, no-option surgery still uses a state-of-the-art, Food and Drug Administration (FDA)-approved lens implant, albeit a monofocal model that simply offers less convenience than the more advanced options that decrease glasses dependence. This approach reassures patients who either do not wish or cannot afford the more expensive elective options, and it also explains and validates the concept of additional charges for the elective options that afford greater postoperative convenience.

Following medically indicated routine cataract surgery, most patients will need glasses (or contact lenses). Some patients may wish to reduce or potentially eliminate this need, and several options exist to help achieve this goal. Although most insurance companies will not cover the additional costs associated with these options, many patients may wish to pay themselves in order to achieve the greater convenience of this enhanced lifestyle that is less dependent on glasses.

OPTION 1

Option 1 reduces or eliminates the need for distance vision glasses or contact lenses, increasing the chances of passing a driver's test without glasses. Near-vision glasses (eg, reading, computer) are still usually required, although option 1 often allows the use of nonprescription over-the-counter reading glasses. Monovision (one eye set for distance vision and the other eye set for near vision) may be an option for some patients, especially those who have previously used monovision successfully with contact lenses. Additional evaluation is performed in conjunction with option 1, including advanced mapping of the eye with corneal topography and wavefront aberrometry; these additional tests allow optimization of the choice of lens implant. Corneal limbal relaxing incisions (LRIs) are performed at the time of lens implant surgery, in order to reduce astigmatism, as indicated by the additional testing. An astigmatic lens implant may be used as an addition or alternative to LRIs, depending on your particular eye measurements. The additional cost of option 1 is $XXXX.00 per eye, which is not covered by insurance.

OPTION 2

Option 2 reduces or eliminates the need for glasses or contact lenses for all activities, including distance vision as well as near vision, utilizing advanced presbyopia-correcting lens implants. Seibel Vision Surgery is pleased to offer all three Food and Drug Administration (FDA)-approved presbyopia-correcting lens implants, including the ReSTOR (Alcon, Fort Worth, TX), ReZoom (Advanced Medical Optics, Santa Ana, CA), and Crystalens (Eyeonics, Aliso Viejo, CA). The additional cost is $XXXX.00 per eye, which includes the upgraded lens implant as well as associated professional services, including the option 1 package (see above); this cost is not covered by insurance. A small percentage of the time, laser vision correction (photorefractive keratectomy [PRK] or laser in situ keratomileusis [LASIK]) may be desired to even further enhance glasses independence; Dr. Seibel does not charge any professional fee for this enhancement for his presbyopia-correcting lens patients; they would only pay the laser facility fee of $XXX.00 per eye.

Bear in mind that the additional costs of these options do not guarantee freedom from glasses or contact lenses. Such guarantees are not possible due to the slightly variable healing response in each individual eye that can affect the optical outcome. However, as compared to standard surgery with a standard lens implant, these more advanced options do stack the odds much better in favor of the patient who desires significantly reduced dependence on glasses or contacts for many of life's activities. After a thorough consultation and discussion of your goals, Dr. Seibel will advise you as to which options might be most appropriate for you.

I have read the foregoing and wish to have the following options for my cataract surgery. I understand that the additional costs are not covered by insurance and are my own responsibility.

❑ No options. I realize that I will likely need glasses for most tasks after surgery. No additional charges except usual insurance copay and deductibles.

❑ Option 1. Advanced diagnostic testing, lens implant choice optimization, and astigmatism treatment as needed with limbal relaxing incisions (LRIs) and/or an astigmatism-reducing lens implant for potentially diminished or eliminated need for glasses for distance vision. Reading glasses will still likely be needed. $XXXX.00 per eye.

❑ Option 2. Presbyopia-correcting lens implant for potentially reduced or eliminated need for glasses for both distance and near vision. This option includes the upgrade cost of the lens implant along with associated professional services, including option 1 above. $XXXX.00 per eye.

_____   _____   _____
Patient Name   Patient Signature   Date

OMIC INFORMED CONSENT FOR REFRACTIVE LENSECTOMY

Informed Consent For Refractive Lens Exchange (RLE)
For the Correction of
Hyperopia (Farsightedness) Or Myopia (Nearsightedness)

> NOTE: THIS FORM IS INTENDED AS A SAMPLE ONLY. PLEASE REVIEW IT AND
> MODIFY TO FIT YOUR ACTUAL PRACTICE. IT DOES <u>NOT</u> CONTAIN INFORMATION
> ABOUT LIMBAL RELXING INCSIONS (LRI), SO INCLUDE THAT IF YOU PERFORM
> LRI DURING RLE SURGERY.

INTRODUCTION
This surgery, called a refractive lens exchange or RLE, involves the removal of the clear lens of
your eye, even though there is no cataract. In some cases, the lens may have an early cataract
which does not significantly interfere with corrected vision, and which would normally not
require surgical removal. The eye surgeon, known as an ophthalmologist, surgically removes the
natural lens of the eye and replaces it with an intraocular lens implant (IOL) in order to restore
vision. This is an artificial lens, usually made of plastic, silicone, or acrylic material, surgically
and permanently placed inside the eye.

BENEFITS OF RLE SURGERY
Benefits include improved vision than you presently have without glasses. The farsighted
(hyperopic) eye is out of focus because the length of the eye is too short for the curvature of the
outer lens of the eye (cornea), which causes light rays to focus behind the retina. The
nearsighted (myopic) eye is out of focus because the length of the eye is too long for the
curvature of the outer lens of the eye (cornea), which causes light rays to focus in front of the
retina. The light rays can theoretically be brought to a clearer focus on the retina by substituting
an artificial IOL that has the proper power, thereby improving the natural focus of the eye.
Although this can theoretically improve your natural distance vision if the calculations are
accurate, <u>you will lose the natural focusing power of the eye (accommodation)</u>. As a result, you
will need to have near vision restored. Alternatives for near vision are discussed later in this
document.

NON-SURGICAL ALTERNATIVES TO RLE
Non-surgical alternatives to refractive lens exchange are to continue to wear spectacle lenses or
contact lenses. Contact lenses or glasses are non-surgical, extremely accurate, permit easy
changes in prescription, and also allow the eye to retain its focusing power for near vision.

Although there are essentially no risks to wearing glasses, the quality of vision with strong
farsighted or nearsighted glasses is not normal because of an enlarged image and a slight
decrease in peripheral vision caused by the thickness of the lenses.

Although contact lenses provide higher quality and more normal vision, they have a slight risk of
complications, especially if they are worn overnight. The risks of contact lenses include
infection, which can rarely cause loss of vision if the infection involves the cornea; allergies
(giant papillary conjunctivitis, GPC) which can make wearing the lenses difficult; mild irritation;
and discomfort. There is also evidence that some damage occurs to the important internal layer
of cells that are responsible for keeping the cornea clear. This damage could cause harm if the

I have read and understood this page. Patient's initials _____ Page 1 of 8

contact lenses are worn for many years. Whether this damage will eventually lead to serious long-term complications such as corneal clouding is unknown.

SURGICAL ALTERNATIVES TO RLE, INCLUDING LASER
There are several other procedures for the correction of farsightedness and nearsightedness. The advantage of the procedures described below is that you retain your natural focusing power and do not require an incision into the inside of your eye, which is needed for RLE surgery. You may choose not to have this surgery at all and either continue wearing your glasses or contact lenses, or you may elect to have one of the other procedures discussed in this section.

1. Conductive keratoplasty (CK) is capable of reshaping the cornea, but is only indicated for low degrees of hyperopia.
2. The excimer laser can be used to correct low to moderate amounts of hyperopia (generally +1 to +5 D or diopters) and low to higher amounts of myopia (generally -1 D to –12D) through either PRK (photorefractive keratectomy) or LASIK (laser in situ keratomileusis). LASIK is an operation which combines the creation of a flap with the microkeratome or a laser and the removal of tissue with the excimer laser. PRK involves removing the surface cells on the cornea ("epithelium") and using the excimer laser to remove tissue from the exposed tissue on the corneal surface. Both procedures have been found to be quite successful and relatively safe for the correction of moderate and high myopia up to about –12.00 D. Above 12 diopters, LASIK and PRK are less accurate and cause a high incidence of complications involving the quality of vision, especially at night. Many surgeons have stopped performing either procedure for these extremely nearsighted eyes.
3. In phakic implant surgery, an artificial intraocular lens is surgically placed inside your eye. The lens is made from material similar to the type used for the intraocular lenses currently being implanted in the eye to correct vision after cataract or refractive lens exchange surgery. The difference between phakic implant surgery and other intraocular lens implants is that your natural lens is <u>not</u> removed during phakic implant surgery. The phakic lens is inserted <u>in front of</u> your natural lens.

EXAMINATIONS PRIOR TO SURGERY
If you agree to have the surgery, you will undergo a complete eye examination by your surgeon. This will include an examination to determine your glasses prescription (refraction), measurement of your vision with and without glasses (visual acuity), measurement of the pressures inside your eye (tonometry), measurement of the curvature of your cornea (keratometry), ultrasonic measurement of the length of your eye (axial length), intraocular lens calculation (biometry) to determine the best estimate of the proper power of the implanted lens, microscopic examination of the front part of your eye (slit-lamp examination), and examination of the retina of your eye with your pupils dilated.

NEED TO STOP WEARING CONTACT LENSES PRIOR TO SURGERY
If you wear contact lenses, you will be required to leave them out of the eyes for a period of time prior to having your preoperative eye examination and before your surgery. This is done because the contact lens rests on the cornea, distorting its shape, and this distortion will have an effect on the accuracy of the doctor's measurements of the power of surgical correction needed. Discontinuing contact lens use allows the corneas to return to their natural shape. Soft contact lens wearers should leave lenses out of the eyes for at least one week. Rigid (including gas

I have read and understood this page. Patient's initials _____ Page 2 of 8

permeable and standard hard lenses) contact lens wearers should leave lenses out of the eyes for at least three weeks. Rigid contact lens wearers usually experience fluctuating vision once their lenses have been discontinued due to changes in the shape of the cornea. Although the cornea usually returns to its natural state within three weeks, this process may take longer, and you will need to remain contact lens free until stabilization is complete.

MORE INFORMATION ABOUT INTRAOCULAR LENS BIOMETRY
While biometry, the method used to calculate the power of the IOL, is very accurate in the majority of patients, the final result may be different from what was planned. As the eye heals, the IOL can shift very slightly toward the front or the back of the eye. The amount of this shift is not the same in everyone, and it may cause different vision than predicted. Patients who are highly nearsighted or highly farsighted have the greatest risk of differences between planned and actual outcomes. Patients who have had LASIK or other refractive surgeries are especially difficult to measure precisely. If the eye's visual power after surgery is considerably different than what was planned, surgical replacement of the IOL might be considered. It is usually possible to replace the IOL and improve the situation.

PRESBYOPIA AND ALTERNATIVES FOR NEAR VISION AFTER RLE
Patients who have RLE surgery may have, or will eventually develop, an age-related condition known as presbyopia. Presbyopia is the reason that reading glasses become necessary, typically after age 40, even for people who have excellent distance and near vision without glasses. Presbyopic individuals require bifocals or separate (different prescription) reading glasses in order to see clearly at close range. There are several other options available to you to achieve distance and near vision after RLE surgery.

- GLASSES You can choose to have a monofocal (single focus) IOL implanted for distance vision and wear separate reading glasses, or have an IOL implanted for near vision and wear separate glasses for distance.
- MONOVISION The ophthalmologist could implant IOLs with two different powers, one eye for near vision, and the other eye for distance vision. This combination of a distance eye and a reading eye is called monovision, and enables you to read without glasses. It has been employed quite successfully in many contact lens and refractive surgery patients. Your surgeon will discuss and demonstrate this option.
- MULTIFOCAL IOL The ophthalmologist could implant a "multifocal" IOL. These IOLs, more recently approved by the Food and Drug Administration (FDA), provide distance vision AND restore some or all of the focusing (accommodating) ability of the eye. Depending upon the technological features of the IOLs, they may be described as "accommodating," "apodized diffractive," or "presbyopia-correcting." All of these lenses are "multifocal," meaning they correct for both distance vision and other ranges, such as near or intermediate.
- NEARVISION CK A refractive procedure called NearVision CK uses radiofrequency energy to reshape the cornea in order to improve near vision. This procedure is typically performed in one eye so that the fellow eye remains corrected for distance. This is, therefore, another form of monovision correction.
- **I choose to have near vision after RLE surgery provided by**

_____   Patient initials _____

I have read and understood this page. Patient's initials _____   Page 3 of 8

(**Please write** "glasses," "monovision," "NearVision CK," or "multifocal IOL.")

MORE INFORMATION ABOUT MONOVISION

For most people, depth perception is best when viewing with both eyes optimally corrected and "balanced" for distance. Eye care professionals refer to this as binocular vision. Monovision can impair depth perception to some extent, because the eyes are not focused together at the same distance. Because monovision can reduce optimum depth perception, it is typically recommended that this option be tried with contact lenses (which are removable) prior to contemplating monovision correction involving two IOLs.

Ocular dominance, and choosing the 'distance' eye correctly: Ocular dominance is analogous to right- or left-handedness. Typically, eye care professionals believe that for most individuals, one eye is the dominant or preferred eye for viewing. Several tests can be performed to determine which eye, right or left, is dominant in a particular person. Conventional wisdom holds that if contemplating monovision, the dominant eye should be corrected for distance, and the non-dominant eye corrected for near. While this is a good guideline, it should not be construed as an absolute rule. A very small percentage of persons may be co-dominant (rather analogous to being ambidextrous), and, in rare circumstances, a person may actually prefer using the dominant eye for near viewing.

The methods for testing and determining ocular dominance are not always 100% accurate: there is some subjective component in the measurement process, and different eye doctors may use slightly different methods of testing. It is critical to determine through the use of contact lenses which combination is best for each person (right eye for distance, left for near, or vice versa) prior to undertaking surgical implantation of two different-powered IOLs during RLE. You can imagine how uncomfortable it might be if monovision were to be rendered "the wrong way around." It might be compared to a right-handed person suddenly having to write, shave, apply make-up, etc., with the left hand. Be sure you understand this and have discussed with your surgeon which eye should be corrected for distance, and which for near. If you have any doubts or uncertainty whatsoever, surgery should be delayed until a very solid comfort level is attained through use of monovision contact lenses. **Under no circumstances should you consider undertaking RLE surgery with monovision correction before you are convinced it will be right for you.** Once surgery is performed, it is not always possible to undo what is done, or to reverse the distance and near eye without some loss of visual quality.

FDA STATUS OF IOLs IMPLANTED DURING RLE

When a drug or device is approved for medical use by the Food and Drug Administration (FDA), the manufacturer produces a "label" to explain its use. Once a device/medication is approved by the FDA, physicians may use it "off-label" for other purposes if they are well-informed about the product, base its use on firm scientific method and sound medical evidence, and maintain records of its use and effects. All IOLs were approved for use in patients with cataracts. Their use in patients having refractive lens exchange is considered an "off-label" use of the IOL.

ANESTHESIA, PROCEDURE, AND POSTOPERATIVE CARE

Either the ophthalmologist or the anesthesiologist/nurse anesthetist will make your eye numb with either drops or an injection (local anesthesia). You may also undergo light sedation administered by an anesthesiologist or nurse anesthetist, or elect to have the surgery with only local anesthesia.

An incision, or opening, is then made in the eye. This is at times self-sealing but it may require closure with very fine stitches (sutures) which will gradually dissolve over time. The natural lens in your eye will then be removed by a type of surgery called phacoemulsification, which uses a vibrating probe to break the lens up into small pieces. These pieces are gently suctioned out of your eye through a small, hollow tube inserted through a small incision into your eye. After your natural lens is removed, the IOL is placed inside your eye. In rare cases if complications occur at the time of surgery, it may not be possible to implant the IOL you have chosen, or any IOL at all.

After the surgery, your eye will be examined the next day, and then at intervals determined by your surgeon. During the immediate recovery period, you will place drops in your eyes for about 2 to 4 weeks, depending on your individual rate of healing. If you have chosen monovision or a multifocal IOL to reduce your dependency on glasses or contacts, they may still be required either for further improvement in your distance vision, reading vision, or both. You should be able to resume your normal activities within 2 or 3 days, and your eye will usually be stable within 3 to 6 weeks, at which time glasses or contact lenses could be prescribed.

RISKS OF REFRACTIVE LENS EXCHANGE SURGERY

The goal of RLE surgery is to correct your hyperopia (farsightedness) or myopia (nearsightedness). Depending upon the type of IOL chosen, the goal may also be to restore some or all of the near (and intermediate, depending upon the lens) focusing ability of your eye or to reduce your dependency upon glasses or contact lenses. RLE surgery is usually quite comfortable. Mild discomfort for the first 24 hours is typical, but severe pain would be extremely unusual and should be reported immediately to your surgeon.

Since this surgery is essentially the same as cataract surgery, the same risks apply. As a result of the surgery and local anesthesia injections around the eye, it is possible that your vision could be made worse. In some cases, complications may occur weeks, months or even years later. These and other complications may result in poor vision, total loss of vision, or even loss of the eye in rare situations. Depending upon the type of anesthesia, other risks are possible, including cardiac and respiratory problems, and, in rare cases, death. Although all of these complications can occur, their incidence following RLE surgery is exceptionally low.

These risks of RLE include, but are not limited to:
1. Complications of removing the natural lens may include hemorrhage (bleeding); rupture of the capsule that supports the IOL; perforation of the eye; clouding of the outer lens of the eye (corneal edema), which can be corrected with a corneal transplant; swelling in the central area of the retina (called cystoid macular edema), which usually improves with time; retained pieces of cataract in the eye, which may need to be removed surgically; infection; detachment of the retina, which is definitely an increased risk for highly nearsighted patients, but which can usually be repaired; uncomfortable or painful eye; droopy eyelid; increased astigmatism; glaucoma; and double vision. These and other complications may occur whether or not an IOL is implanted and may result in poor vision, total loss of vision, or even

loss of the eye in rare situations. **Additional surgery may be required to treat these complications.**

2. <u>Complications associated with the IOL</u> may include increased night glare and/or halo, double or ghost images, and dislocation of the lens. Multifocal IOLs may increase the likelihood of these problems. In some instances, corrective lenses or surgical replacement of the IOL may be necessary for adequate visual function following RLE surgery.

3. <u>Complications associated with local anesthesia injections around the eye</u> include perforation of the eye, destruction of the optic nerve, interference with the circulation of the retina, droopy eyelid, respiratory depression, hypotension, cardiac problems, and, in rare situations, brain damage or death.

4. <u>If a monofocal IOL is implanted,</u> either distance or reading glasses or contacts will be needed after RLE for adequate vision.

5. <u>Complications associated with monovision.</u> Monovision may result in problems with impaired depth perception. Choosing the wrong eye for distance correction may result in feeling that things are the "wrong way around." Once surgery is performed, it is not always possible to undo what is done, or to reverse the distance and near eye without some loss of visual quality.

6. <u>Complications associated with multifocal IOLs.</u> While a multifocal IOL can reduce dependency on glasses, it might result in less sharp vision, which may become worse in dim light or fog. It may also cause some visual side effects such as rings or circles around lights at night. It may be difficult to distinguish an object from a dark background, which will be more noticeable in areas with less light. Driving at night may be affected. If you drive a considerable amount at night, or perform delicate, detailed, "up-close" work requiring closer focus than just reading, a monofocal lens in conjunction with eyeglasses may be a better choice for you. If complications occur at the time of surgery, a monofocal IOL may need to be implanted instead of a multifocal IOL.

7. If an IOL is implanted, it is done by a surgical method. It is intended that the small plastic, silicone, or acrylic IOL will be left in the eye permanently.

8. If there are complications at the time of surgery, the doctor may decide not to implant an IOL in your eye even though you may have given prior permission to do so.

9. Other factors may affect the visual outcome of RLE surgery, including eye diseases such as glaucoma, diabetic retinopathy, and age-related macular degeneration; the power of the IOL; your individual healing ability; and, if certain IOLs are implanted, the function of the ciliary (focusing) muscles in your eyes.

10. The selection of the proper IOL, while based upon sophisticated equipment and computer formulas, is not an exact science. After your eye heals, its visual power may be different from what was predicted by preoperative testing. You may need to wear glasses or contact lenses after surgery to obtain your best vision. <u>Additional surgeries such as IOL exchange, placement of an additional IOL, or refractive laser surgery may be needed if you are not satisfied with your vision after RLE.</u>

11. The results of surgery cannot be guaranteed. If you chose a multifocal IOL, it is possible that not all of the near (and intermediate) focusing ability of your eye will be restored. Additional treatment and/or surgery may be necessary. <u>Regardless of the IOL chosen, you may need laser surgery to correct clouding of vision.</u> At some future time, the IOL implanted in your eye may have to be repositioned, removed surgically, or exchanged for another IOL.

12. If your ophthalmologist has informed you that you have a high degree of hyperopia (farsightedness) and/or that the axial length of your eye is short, your risk for a complication known as nanophthalmic choroidal effusion is increased. This complication could result in difficulties completing the surgery and implanting a lens, or even loss of the eye.

13. If your ophthalmologist has informed you that you have a high degree of myopia (nearsightedness) and/or that the axial length of your eye is long, your risk for a complication called a retinal detachment is increased. Retinal detachments can lead to vision loss or blindness.

14. Since only one eye will undergo surgery at a time, you may experience a period of imbalance between the two eyes (anisometropia). This usually cannot be corrected with spectacle glasses because of the marked difference in the prescriptions, so you will either temporarily have to wear a contact lens in the non-operated eye or will function with only one clear eye for distance vision. In the absence of complications, surgery in the second eye can usually be accomplished within 3 to 4 weeks, once the first eye is stabilized.

FINANCIAL IMPLICATIONS OF RLE SURGERY

I understand that I am responsible for the cost of the surgery and the IOL, including the surgeon's fee, the anesthesiologist's fee, if any, and the surgical center's or hospital's fee. This is because health insurance does not pay for removal of the clear lens of the eye for the purposes of correcting natural vision or for removal of an early cataract that is not visually disabling.

I understand that I will be responsible for the costs of any surgery-related injuries. I also understand that no compensation is being offered to me in the event of an injury or complication. In the event of a complication for RLE, it might be possible that other surgery, eye drops, or even hospitalization may be required. Although some or even all of these costs may be covered by my health insurance policy, if they are not, I understand that I will be responsible for these costs as well.

If I need a second surgical procedure, such as replacement or repositioning of my IOL, I understand that although my surgeon will not charge me a surgical fee, there will be additional fees from the surgery center and from the anesthesiologist, if one is required.

Patient initials _____

PATIENT CONSENT

The basic procedures of RLE surgery, the reasons for the type of IOL chosen for me, and the advantages, disadvantages, risks, and possible complications of alternative treatments have been explained to me by my ophthalmologist. Monovision has been discussed with me and my ophthalmologist has either demonstrated it to me with glasses or contact lenses, or offered to do so. Although it is impossible for the doctor to inform me of every possible complication that may occur, the doctor has answered all my questions to my satisfaction.

In signing this informed consent for RLE surgery and implantation of an IOL, I am stating that I have been offered a copy, I fully understand the possible risks, benefits, and complications of RLE surgery and

- I have read this informed consent _____ **(patient initials)**
- The consent form was read to me by _____ **(name).**

CHOOSE ONE OF THESE OPTIONS AND CROSS OUT THE OTHER TWO

Monofocal IOL/Reading Glasses Option
I wish to have a RLE operation with a monofocal IOL on my _____ (state "right" or "left" eye) and wear glasses for _____ (state "near" or "distance") vision.

Monovision with 2 IOLs Option
I wish to have a RLE operation with two different-powered IOLs implanted to achieve monovision.

I wish to have my _____ (state "right" or "left") eye corrected for **distance** vision.

I wish to have my _____ (state "right" or "left") eye corrected for **near** vision.

Multifocal IOL Option
I wish to have a RLE operation with a _____multifocal IOL implant (state name of implant) on my _____ (state "right" or "left") eye.

_____   _____
Patient (or person authorized to sign for patient)   Date

_____   _____
Physician Signature   Date

Version 2/27/06

This is a modified OMIC Informed Consent for Refractive Lens Exchange (RLE) for the Correction of Hyperopia (Farsightedness) or Myopia (Nearsightedness).

I have read and understood this page. Patient's initials _____ Page 8 of 8

LRI Instrumentation

COMPANY	COMPLETE LRI SYSTEM	PRE-SET DIAMOND KNIFE	MICROMETER DIAMOND KNIFE (full range)-	STEPPED DIAMOND KNIFE	BLADE GUIDE RING	MARKERS MARKING SYSTEMS	LRI FIXATION RINGS	WEBSITE
ACCUTOME	NO	YES 500, 550, 600	NO	NO	NO	YES	NO	WWW.ACCUTOME.COM
MASTEL	YES	YES 600	YES	YES	YES	YES	YES	WWW.MASTEL.COM
RHEIN	NO	YES 600	YES	YES	NO	YES	YES	WWW.RHEINMEDICAL.COM
DUCKWORTH & KENT	NO	YES 500, 550, 600	NO	NO	NO	YES	NO	WWW.DANDKUSA.COM
KATENA	NO	YES 600	YES	YES	NO	YES	YES	WWW.KATENA.COM
PELION	NO	YES 500, 600	NO	NO	NO	NO	NO	WWW.PELIONSURGICAL.COM
ASICO	NO	YES 600, 650	YES	YES	NO	YES	YES	WWW.ASICO.COM
STORZ	NO	YES 600	NO	YES	NO	NO	NO	WWW.BAUSCHSURGICAL.COM

FINANCIAL DISCLOSURES

Richard L. Abbott, MD is a board member of Ophthalmic Mutual Insurance Company and a consultant for Santen, Inc.

Natalie A. Afshari, MD has no financial disclosure to report.

Iqbal Ike K. Ahmed, MD is a consultant for Alcon, Advanced Medical Optics, and Carl Zeiss Meditec.

Yachna Ahuja, MD has no financial disclosure to report.

Leonardo Akaishi, MD has no financial disclosure to report.

Alan B. Aker, MD does not have financial interest or affiliation with any of the companies mentioned in his chapters.

Avery Alexander, MD receives no income or royalties from any ophthalmic companies.

José F. Alfonso, MD, PhD has no proprietary interest in any of the materials mentioned in his article.

Jorge L. Alió, MD, PhD has no financial disclosure to report.

David Allen, BSc, FRCS, FRCOphth has no direct financial interest in Alcon Laboratories nor its products. He has received reimbursement of travel and lodging costs from Alcon Laboratories

Noel Alpins, FRANZCO, FRCOphth, FACS states that he has a financial interest in the ASSORT program used for calculation of the treatment parameters and examination of outcomes.

Hussein Amhaz, MD, PhD has no proprietary interest in any of the materials mentioned in this article.

Lisa Brothers Arbisser, MD has research grants and honoraria from Alcon and Advanced Medical Optics.

Pablo Artal, PhD has no financial interest in the research reported.

Kerry K. Assil, MD has the following financial relationships to disclose: AcuFocus, Alcon, Allergan, Advanced Medical Optics, Bausch & Lomb, BioVision AG, EyeSys, EyeTech, Inspire, IntraLase, Ista, Kabi Pharm, KeraVision, KMI Pharm, Neuroptics, Ophtec, ORC, Santen, Tracey Tech, VISK, Vistakon, and VISX.

Jay Bansal, MD has no financial affiliation with any products.

Graham D. Barrett, MBBCh, FRANZCO, FRACS has no financial interest in the subject matter.

George Beiko, BM, BCh, FRCS(C) receives research grant support from Alcon Laboratories Inc, Advanced Medical Optics Inc, and Visiogen Inc.

Roberto Bellucci, MD has no financial disclosure to report.

Joshua Ben-Nun, MD has interest as inventor and founder of NuLens.

Abdhish R. Bhavsar, MD has no financial disclosure to report.

Brian S. Boxer Wachler, MD is a consultant for Alcon Laboratories.

Rosa Braga-Mele, MD, MEd, FRCSC is a consultant for Bausch & Lomb, Alcon, and Advanced Medical Optics, but has no proprietary interest in any products mentioned in her chapter.

Michael B. Brenner, MD, FICS has no financial disclosure to report.

Frank A. Bucci, Jr, MD has no financial disclosure to report.

Carlos Buznego, MD has received funding for research, speaking, and/or consulting from the following: Allergan, Alcon, Glaukos, Inspire, Ista, Lenstec, and Sirion.

Stephen Bylsma, MD is a consultant to STAAR Surgical Company.

Matthew C. Caldwell, MD has no financial disclosure to report.

Fabrizio I. Camesasca, MD has no financial interest in the matter described.

Charles Campbell is a consultant for Advanced Medical Optics and this work was done for the VISX unit of Advanced Medical Optics so that we would know how best to guide the users of the VISX laser refractive systems when used with these eyes. He is self-employed as Consultant, Ophthalmic optics and instruments.

Harvey Carter, MD is a consultant for Advanced Medical Optics, Eyeonics, and Milvella.

Jeffrey J. Caspar, MD has no financial disclosure to report.

David Castillejos, MD is a consultant to Vision Membrane Technologies, Inc.

Timothy B. Cavanaugh, MD has no financial relationship to disclose.

David F. Chang, MD is a consultant for Advanced Medical Optics, Alcon, and Visiogen, and his consultant fees are donated to the Himalayan Cataract Project.

Shiao Chang, PhD is an employee and stockholder of Calhoun Vision, Inc.

William Jerry Chang, MD has no financial disclosure to report.

Geoff Charlton is a shareholder in Allergan, but has no financial relationship to disclose.

Arturo Chayet, MD is a clinical investigator for Calhoun Vision, Inc.

William K. Christian, MD has no financial relationships at this time.

Y. Ralph Chu, MD is a consultant for Advanced Medical Optics, Allergan, Visiogen, and OcuSoft.

John Ciccone has no financial disclosure to report.

Robert J. Cionni, MD has the following financial disclosures: consultant, speaker, and investigator for Alcon and product for Morcher GmbH.

Tom M. Coffman, MD has no financial interest in any product discussed.

D. Michael Colvard, MD, FACS is a consultant with Eyeonics, Advanced Medical Optics, and Oasis Medical.

J. Andy Corley is chairman and CEO of Eyeonics, Inc.

Kay Coulson, MBA serves as a practice-development speaker and consultant for Alcon Laboratories.

Alan S. Crandall, MD is a consultant for Alcon.

William W. Culbertson, MD receives research funding, travel expenses, and honoraria from Advanced Medical Optics; travel expenses and honoraria from Carl Zeiss Meditec; and is a consultant for Optimedica.

James A. Davies, MD, FACS a paid consultant of Eyeonics, Inc.

Dan Davis, OD has no financial disclosures to report.

Elizabeth A. Davis, MD, FACS does consulting for Advanced Medical Optics/Intralase, Allergan, Bausch & Lomb, ISTA Pharmaceuticals, STAAR Surgical.

James A. Davison, MD, FACS is a paid consultant for Alcon Surgical but has no financial interest in any of the items discussed.

James D. Dawes, MHA, CMPE, COE has no financial disclosure to report.

Sheraz M. Daya, MD, FACP, FACS, FRCS(Ed) is a consultant to Bausch & Lomb and Intralase and has a financial interest in Eyeonics.

David J. Deitz, MPhil has no proprietary interest in the material included in his chapters.

Steven J. Dell, MD is a consultant to Advanced Medical Optics, Allergan. and Eyeonics.

Jim Denning, BS is a stockholder in Eyeonics.

Kevin Denny, MD has no financial conflicts.

Uday Devgan, MD, FACS is a consultant to Allergan, Advanced Medical Optics, Bausch & Lomb, Eyeonics, Ista Pharm, and STAAR.

Steven Dewey, MD is a consultant for Advanced Medical Optics and receives royalties from MST.

H. Burkhard Dick has no financial interest in anything mentioned in the paper.

John F. Doane, MD has a financial interest in Eyeonics (research funded).

Eric Donnenfeld, MD is a consultant to Allergan, Advanced Medical Optics, Alcon, and Bausch & Lomb.

Paul Dougherty, MD receives travel support from and owns a small equity interest in Lenstec, Inc.

Paul Ernest, MD has no financial disclosure to report.

Ahmad M. Fahmy, OD, FAAO has no financial disclosure to report.

Luis E. Fernández de Castro, MD has no financial interest.

Luis Fernández-Vega, MD, PhD has no proprietary interest in any of the materials mentioned in this article.

I. Howard Fine, MD is a consultant for Advanced Medical Optics, Inc; Bausch & Lomb, Inc; Carl Zeiss Meditec, Inc.; iScience Surgical Corporation; and Omeros Corporation. He receives honoraria from Alcon Laboratories, Inc; Eyeonics, Inc; Rayner Intraocular Lenses Ltd; and STAAR Surgical Company.

William J. Fishkind, MD, FACS is a paid consultant for Advanced Medical Optics (Advanced Medical Optics) and receives royalty income from Thieme Publishers.

Michael T. Furlong, MD has no financial disclosure to report.

Ron P. Gallemore, MD, PhD has no financial disclosure to report.

Andrea Galvis, MD did not provide a financial disclosure.

William D. Gaskins, MD, FACS has no financial relationship to disclose.

Johnny L. Gayton, MD is on the speaker's bureau at Alcon and Ista. He also receives a grant from Alcon for ReSTOR/ARMD research.

Pietro Giardini, MD has no financial disclosure to report.

James P. Gills, MD has no financial disclosure to report.

Pit Gills, MD has no financial disclosure to report.

Frank Jozef Goes, MD receives travel compensation from Advanced Medical Optics for papers presented at international meetings.

Harry B. Grabow, MD has no financial disclosure to report.
Oscar Gris, MD has no financial or proprietary interest in any material or method mentioned.

Jose L. Güell, MD declares that he does not have any commercial or proprietary interest in the products or companies mentioned in the text. He also certifies that there are no affiliations with any organizations with a direct financial interest in the materials discussed in the chapter.

D. Rex Hamilton, MD, MS, FACS has received honoraria for educational lectures from Alcon, Advanced Medical Optics, Allergan, and Reichert Instruments.

David R. Hardten, MD consults for Allergan, Advanced Medical Optics, and TLCVision and has done research for Alcon, Allergan, Advanced Medical Optics, and STAAR.

R. Lee Harman, MD, FACS has no financial interest in any of the subject materials. (He does not own stock in Advanced Medical Optics or Alcon or any ophthalmic company other than The Harman Eye Clinic and LEGACY Strategic Consultants, LLC.)

David Harmon is president and executive editor or *Market Scope*, a market research, analysis and reporting service for ophthalmic manufacturers, investors, and ophthalmic surgeons

Nicola Hauranieh, MD has no financial disclosure to report.

Weldon W. Haw, MD has no financial disclosure to report.

Bonnie An Henderson, MD is on the speaker's bureau and receives grant support from Alcon and ISTA Pharmaceuticals.

Warren E. Hill, MD, FACS is a consultant for Alcon Laboratories, Carl Zeiss Meditec, Oculus, and Santen.

Jerry Tan Tiang Hin, MBBS, FRCS, FRCOphth has no financial disclosure to report.

Kenneth J. Hoffer, MD, FACS owns EyeLab.com, which sells IOL power calculation software (Hoffer Programs and Holladay IOL Consultant) to ophthalmologists.

Richard S. Hoffman, MD has no financial relationships to disclose.

Jack T. Holladay, MD, MSEE, FACS is author of the Holladay Formula and provides consultation for A-scan companies that use his formulas.

Edward Holland, MD did not provide a financial disclosure.

Jeffrey D. Horn, MD receives research support from Alcon and is a member of Alcon Speakers Bureau.

John A. Hovanesian, MD is a consultant, member of the scientific advisory board, and stockholder of Eyeonics, Inc.

Suber S. Huang, MD, MBA has no financial disclosure to report.

Conall F. Hurley, MB, BCh, BAO, FRCSI has no financial disclosure to report.

Randolph T. Jackson, MD has no financial disclosure to report.

J. Michael Jumper, MD has no financial disclosure to report.

Paul Kaufman, MD has no financial disclosure to report.

Hakan Kaymak, MD has no financial interest in the products mentioned in this article.

Robert Kershner, MD, FACS has no financial disclosure to report.

Guy M. Kezirian, MD, FACS is president of SurgiVision® Consultants, Inc.

Terry Kim, MD is a consultant for Alcon, Allergan, ISTA, Becton Dickinson Ophthalmics, and Hyperbranch Medical Technology

Guy E. Knolle, MD, FACS has no financial disclosure to report.

Michael C. Knorz, MD is a consultant to Advanced Medical Optics Inc.

Olga Konykhov, MD has no financial disclosure to report.

Marie Czenko Kuechel, MA has no financial disclosure relevant to this chapter, but she is a paid consultant/administrator to the Physicians Coalition for Injectable Safety (to which ASOPRS is a member).

George D. Kymionis, MD, PhD has no financial disclosure to report.

Stephen S. Lane MD has no financial disclosure to report.

Michael Lawless, MD has no financial disclosure to report.

Yunhee Lee, MD has no financial disclosure to report.

Robert P. Lehmann, MD, FACS has no financial interest in any products or companies; however, he is a consultant for Alcon.

John Lehr, OD has no financial disclosure to report.

Jess C. Lester, MD, FACS has no financial disclosure to report.

Richard A. Lewis, MD is a consultant for Alcon.

Richard L. Lindstrom, MD has the following disclosures to report: Acufocus, Inc.; Advanced Medical Optics; Advanced Refractive Technologies; Alcon Laboratories, Inc.; AVS; Bausch & Lomb, Inc.; Bio Syntrx; Biovision; Calhoun Vision, Inc.; Citation Ventures; Clarity Ophthalmics; Clear Sight; CoDa Therapeutics; EBV Partners; Egg Factory, Eyemaginations, Inc., Eyeonics, Fziomed; Glaukos Corporation; HEAVEN Fund; High Performance Optics; Improve Your Vision; IntraLase Corporation I-Therapeutix; Lensar; Life Sciences; Midwest Surgical Services; Minnesota Eye Consultants, P.A.; NeuroVision; NuLens; OccuLogix Ocular Surgery News/Slack; Omeros Corporation; Pixel Optics; Quest, Refractec; Revision Optics; RXVP; Santen, Inc.; Schroders; SupplyEye Surgijet/Visijet; 3D Vision Systems; TLC Vision Laser Center; Tracey Technologies; Versant; Viradax; Vision Solutions Technologies; and VISX USA, Inc.

Brian Little, FRCS, FRCOphth, FHEA has no financial disclosure to report.

Dwayne Logan, MD has no financial disclosure to report.

Angel López-Castro, MD has no financial disclosure to report.

Brian D. Lueth, MD has no financial disclosure to report.

Richard J. Mackool, MD is a consultant to Alcon.

Richard J. Mackool, Jr, MD has no financial relationship to disclose.

Scott MacRae, MD is a consultant for Bausch & Lomb.

Shareef Mahdavi, BA is a consultant to the eyecare industry, as well as Advanced Medical Optics and Carecredit. Shareef also serves on the editorial board of *Cataract and Refractive Surgery Today*.

Martin A. Mainster, PhD, MD, FRCOphth serves as a consultant for Advanced Medical Optics, Inc.

Michael W. Malley, BA has no affiliation with any laser manufacturer or product listed in this book.

William F. Maloney, MD has no financial relationship to disclose.

Edward E. Manche, MD is an investor in Calhoun Vision.

Felicidad Manero, MD declares that he does not have any commercial or proprietary interest in the products or companies mentioned in the text. He also certifies that there are no affiliations with any organizations with a direct financial interest in the materials discussed in the chapter.

Paul Mann, MD has received honoraria from Alcon Laboratories, Inc for speaking engagements.

William Martin, MD has the following financial relationships to disclose: Advanced Medical Optics, Alcon, Allergan, VISX, Zeiss, Ista, Otsuka, Pfizer, Xanodyne, Genzyme, Eagle.

Samuel Masket, MD receives grant/research support from Alcon; is a consultant (eg, advisory board) for Alcon, Visiogen, PowerVision, and Othera; and is on the speaker's burea at Alcon, Allergan, and Bausch & Lomb.

W. Andrew Maxwell MD, PhD is a consultant to Alcon Laboratories.

J. E. "Jay" McDonald II, MD is a paid consultant for Bausch & Lomb. However, he has no proprietary interest in the material included in his chapters.

Marguerite B. McDonald, MD, FACS has no financial interest related to the topic of her chapter, and no trade names, companies, or products are mentioned in her chapter.

Javier A. Gaytan Melicoff, MD declares that he does not have any commercial or proprietary interest in the products or companies mentioned in the text. He also certifies that there are no affiliations with any organizations with a direct financial interest in the materials discussed in the chapter.

Ulrich Mester, MD has no financial interest in the products mentioned in this article.

Marc A. Michelson, MD has no financial relationship to disclose.

Kevin M. Miller, MD is a consultant, speaker, and clinical investigator for Alcon Laboratories.

Rick Milne, MD is a consultant for (paid for travel and speaking for) Advanced Medical Optics, Ista, Moria, and Refractec.

Robert A. Mittra, MD has no financial disclosure to report.

Satish Modi, MD, FRCS(C), CPI is on the Speakers' Alliance with Alcon.

Robert Montés-Micó, PhD has no proprietary interest in any of the materials mentioned in this article.

Merce Morral, MD declares that he does not have any commercial or proprietary interest in the products or companies mentioned in the text. He also certifies that there are no affiliations with any organizations with a direct financial interest in the materials discussed in the chapter.

Robert Morris, MRCP, FRCS, FRCOphth has no financial interest in any of the products mentioned in his article.

Con Moshegov, MD, FRANZCO, FRACS receives study grants from Alcon Laboratories and travel subsidies from Alcon Laboratories and Advanced Medical Optics.

Lana J. Nagy, BS has no financial disclosure to report.

Louis D. "Skip" Nichamin, MD is a consultant and stockholder with PowerVision.

Lee T. Nordan, MD is a shareholder and consultant to Vision Membrane Technologies, Inc.

Terrence P. O'Brien, MD has financial interest in Alcon Labs, Allergan, Advanced Medical Optics, an Inspire.

Thomas A. Oetting, MD has no financial disclosure to report.

Roger V. Ohanesian, MD has financial interests in Eyeonics (research funded), Glaukos (research funded), Allergan (shareholder).

Randall J. Olson, MD has no financial disclosure to report.

Robert H. Osher, MD did not provide a financial disclosure.

Ivan L. Ossma, MD, MPH receives research grants from Visiogen Inc and lecture fees from Advanced Medical Optics, Allergan, Alcon, and Novartis Ophthalmics.

Mark Packer, MD, FACS is a consultant for the following companies: Advanced Medical Optics, Inc.; Advanced Vision Science, Inc.; Bausch & Lomb, Inc.; Carl Zeiss Meditec, Inc.; Carl Zeiss Surgical GmbH; Celgene Corporation; Ethicon, Inc.; Gerson Lehman Group, Inc.; iScience Surgical Corporation; i-Therapeutix, Inc.; Johnson & Johnson Vision Care, Inc. (Vistakon Division); Leerink Swann & Company; Visiogen, Inc (he owns stock also); VisionCare, Inc.; WaveTec Vision Systems (he owns stock also). He does travel, research & honoraria for the following companies: Alcon Laboratories, Inc.; Endo Optiks, Inc.; Eyeonics, inc.; and STAAR Surgical, Inc.

Parag D. Parekh, MD, MPA has no financial disclosure to report.

Natalia Pelaez, MD declares that she does not have any commercial or proprietary interest in the products or companies mentioned in the text. She also certifies that there are no affiliations with any organizations with a direct financial interest in the materials discussed in the chapter.

Jay S. Pepose, MD, PhD is a consultant for Bausch & Lomb and Eyeonics.

Matteo Piovella, MD is consultant for Advanced Medical Optics and SLACK Incorporated.

John W. Potter, OD, FAAO is a full-time employee of TLC Vision Corporation.

Thomas C. Prager, PhD, MPH is a consultant for ESI.

Louis Probst, MD is a consultant for Advanced Medical Optics, TLCVision, and Intralase.

Mujtaba A. Qazi, MD has no financial disclosure to report.

Sherman W. Reeves, MD, MPH has no financial disclosure to report.

Paul Rhee, OD is an employee and shareholder in Calhoun Vision.

Allan M. Robbins, MD, FACS has no financial interests in any of the products or techniques discussed.

Kenneth J. Rosenthal, MD, FACS receives travel, honoraria, research funds and is on the speakers bureau for Advanced Medical Optics. He also receives travel and other perquisites from Ophtec.

Sheri L. Rowen, MD, FACS has no financial disclosure to report.

Jonathan B. Rubenstein, MD did not provide a financial disclosure.

James J. Salz, MD is on the board of directors of OMIC.

Thomas W. Samuelson, MD is a consultant for Advanced Medical Optics.

Helga P. Sandoval, MD, MSCR did not provide a financial disclosure.

Christian Sandstedt, PhD is an employee and stockholder of Calhoun Vision, Inc.

John A. Scholl, MS is a PowerVision employee and Vice President of Research & Development.

Daniel M. Schwartz, MD is a stockholder and consultant for Calhoun Vision, Inc.

Jim Schwiegerling, PhD is a consultant to Alcon Laboratories.

Barry S. Seibel, MD receives royalty from both SLACK Incorporated and Rhein Medical.

Mohamed H. Shabayek, MD, PhD has no financial disclosure to report.

Alan Shiller, MD did not provide a financial disclosure.

Joel K. Shugar, MD, MSEE has no financial interest in any of the subject matters discussed in his chapter.

Jack A. Singer, MD is a consultant to Eyeonics.

Maite Sisquella, OPT has no financial disclosure to report.

Stephen G. Slade, MD, FACS is a consultant for Advanced Medical Optics, Alcon, Bausch & Lomb, Eyeonics, STAAR, and Revision Optics

Michael E. Snyder, MD is on the Alcon speaker's bureau and does some research for Alcon.

Kerry D. Solomon, MD is a consultant to Alcon.

Renée Solomon, MD has no financial disclosure to report.

Michael Sopher has no financial relationship to disclose.

Jason E. Stahl, MD has no financial disclosure to report.

George Stamatelatos, BSc Optom is a consultant to ASSORT.

Roger F. Steinert, MD is a consultant for Advanced Medical Optics.

Julian D. Stevens, MRCP, FRCS, FRCOphth did not provide a financial disclosure.

Tracy Swartz, OD, MS, FAAO has no financial disclosures.

Audrey Talley-Rostov, MD is an investigator for Visiogen, speaker and trainer for Addition Technologies, and on the speakers bureau for Allergan and Advanced Medical Optics.

Joshua Teichman, MD has no financial relationship to disclose.

Richard Tipperman, MD is a consultant for Alcon Laboratories and has no other financial disclosure to report.

William Trattler, MD has received funding for research, speaking, and/or consulting from the following: Allergan, Inspire, Ista, Vistakon, Glaukos, Lenstec, and Sirion.

Patricia L. Turner, MD has no financial disclosure to report.

Farrell Tyson, MD, FACS has no financial disclosure to report.

Carlos Vergés, MD, PhD has no financial relationship to disclose.

Paolo Vinciguerra, MD has no financial interest with the matter described.

Vanee Virash, MD did not provide a financial disclosure.

Daniel Vos, MD has no financial interest in the products discussed and is not a paid consultant for any company.

David T. Vroman, MD has no financial disclosure to report.

John A. Vukich, MD is a consultant and has done contract research for STAAR Surgical, Lenstec, Visiogen, Advanced Medical Optics, and Oculus.

R. Bruce Wallace III, MD, FACS is a paid consultant for Allergan, Inc and Advanced Medical Optics, Inc.

Kevin L. Waltz, OD, MD is a consultant to Advanced Medical Optics and Eyeonics and investor in Tracey Technologies.

Ming Wang, MD, PhD is an investor in Tracey Technologies.

Robert D. Watson has financial interest in the IOL Counselor software.

Robert Jay Weinstock, MD is a paid consultant for Eyeonics and Bausch & Lomb.

Darrell E. White, MD is a paid consultant for Allergan.

Jeffrey Whitman, MD is on the speaker's bureau for Eyeonics, Bausch & Lomb, and Advanced Medical Optics. He also has stock warrants in Eyeonics.

Stephen Wiles, MD is a consultant for Eyeonics, Inc.

John R. Wittpenn, MD receives both consulting and speaking fees from Allergan. He receives royalties for an unrelated product from Novartis.

Michael Y. Wong, MD has no financial disclosure to report.

J. Trevor Woodhams, MD did not provide a financial disclosure.

Helen Wu, MD did not provide a financial disclosure.

Sandra Yeh, MD is a consultant with Eyeonics.

Sonia H. Yoo, MD has financial interest in Alcon Labs, Advanced Medical Optics, and Ista.

Geunyoung Yoon, PhD is a consultant for Bausch & Lomb.

Leonard Yuen, MD, MPH has no financial relationship to disclose.

Charles M. Zacks, MD has no financial interest in the subject of his chapter.

Harvey Zalaznick, MD did not provide a financial disclosure.

INDEX

WAIT

...There's More!

SLACK Incorporated's Health Care Books and Journals offers a wide selection of products in the field of Ophthalmology. We are dedicated to providing important works that educate, inform and improve the knowledge of our customers. Don't miss out on our other informative titles that will enhance your collection.

Curbside Consultation in Cataract Surgery: 49 Clinical Questions
David F. Chang, MD
288 pp, Soft Cover, 2007, ISBN 13: 978-1-55642-799-2
Order # 67999, **$79.95**

Curbside Consultation in Cataract Surgery provides quick and direct answers to the thorny questions most commonly posed during a "curbside consultation" between surgical colleagues. This unique reference offers expert advice, preferences, and opinions on tough clinical questions commonly associated with cataract surgery from 49 of the top cataract consultants in North America. Numerous images, diagrams, and references are included to enhance the text and to illustrate surgical pearls.

Phaco Chop: Mastering Techniques, Optimizing Technology, and Avoiding Complications
David F. Chang, MD
288 pp, Hard Cover w/ DVD, 2004,
ISBN 13: 978-1-55642-679-7
Order # 66798, **$184.95**

Phaco Chop covers everything from step by step instruction for the beginner to advanced chopping for complicated cases or bimanual phaco. Additionally, a DVD is included containing 2 hours of instructional video that complement and supplement the text.

Mastering Refractive IOLs: The Art and Science
David F. Chang, MD
960 pp, Hard Cover, 2008, ISBN 13: 978-1-55642-859-3
Order # 68593, **$174.95**

The Little Eye Book: A Pupil's Guide to Understanding Ophthalmology
Janice K. Ledford, COMT; Roberto Pineda II, MD
160 pp, Soft Cover, 2002, ISBN 13: 978-1-55642-560-8
Order# 65600, **$21.95**

Handbook of Ophthalmology
Amar Agarwal, MS, FRCS, FRCOphth
752 pp, Soft Cover, 2006, ISBN 13: 978-1-55642-685-8
Order # 66852, **$67.95**

Phacodynamics: Mastering the Tools and Techniques of Phacoemulsification Surgery, Fourth Edition
Barry S. Seibel, MD
400 pp, Hard Cover, 2005, ISBN 13: 978-1-55642-688-9
Order # 66887, **$169.95**

Wavefront Customized Visual Correction: The Quest for Super Vision II
Ronald Krueger, MD; Raymond Applegate, OD, PhD; Scott MacRae, MD
416 pp, Hard Cover, 2004, ISBN 13: 978-1-55642-625-4
Order # 66259, **$222.95**

Everyday OCT: A Handbook for Clinicians and Technicians
Joel S. Schuman, MD; Carmen A. Puliafito, MD, MBA; James G. Fujimoto, PhD
160 pp, Soft Cover (Spiral Wire), 2007,
ISBN 13: 978-1-55642-781-7
Order # 67816, **$99.95**

Optical Coherence Tomography of Ocular Diseases, Second Edition
Joel S. Schuman, MD; Carmen A. Puliafito, MD, MBA; James G. Fujimoto, PhD
768 pp, Hard Cover, 2004, ISBN 13: 978-1-55642-609-4
Order # 66097, **$299.95**

Please visit
www.slackbooks.com
to order any of these titles!
24 Hours a Day...7 Days a Week!

Attention Industry Partners!
Whether you are interested in buying multiple copies of a book, chapter reprints, or looking for something new and different — we are able to accommodate your needs.

Multiple Copies
At attractive discounts starting for purchases as low as 25 copies for a single title, SLACK Incorporated will be able to meet all of your needs.

Chapter Reprints
SLACK Incorporated is able to offer the chapters you want in a format that will lead to success. Bound with an attractive cover, use the chapters that are a fit specifically for your com-

Please contact the Marketing Communications Director of the Health Care Books and Journals for further details on multiple copy purchases, chapter reprints or custom printing at 1-800-257-8290 or 1-856-848-1000.

*Please note all conditions are subject to change.

CODE: 328

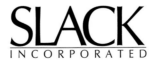

SLACK Incorporated • Health Care Books and Journals
6900 Grove Road • Thorofare, NJ 08086
1-800-257-8290 or 1-856-848-1000
Fax: 1-856-848-6091 • E-mail: orders@slackinc.com • Visit: www.slackbooks.com